HANDBOOK OF HEALTH PSYCHOLOGY

SECOND EDITION

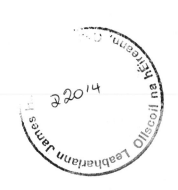

HANDBOOK OF HEALTH PSYCHOLOGY

SECOND EDITION

EDITED BY

ANDREW BAUM
The University of Texas at Arlington

TRACEY A. REVENSON
The Graduate Center – City University of New York

JEROME SINGER
Uniformed Services University of the Health Sciences

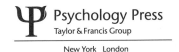

Psychology Press
Taylor & Francis Group

New York   London

Psychology Press
Taylor & Francis Group
711 Third Avenue
New York, NY 10017

Psychology Press
Taylor & Francis Group
27 Church Road
Hove, East Sussex BN3 2FA

© 2012 by Taylor & Francis Group, LLC
Psychology Press is an imprint of Taylor & Francis Group, an Informa business

Printed in the United States of America on acid-free paper
Version Date: 20111031

International Standard Book Number: 978-0-8058-6461-8 (Hardback)

Library of Congress Cataloging-in-Publication Data

Handbook of health psychology / editors, Andrew Baum, Tracey A. Revenson, Jerome Singer. -- 2nd ed.
    p. cm.
    Includes bibliographical references and index.
    ISBN 978-0-8058-6461-8 (hardback)
    1. Clinical health psychology--Handbooks, manuals, etc. 2. Medicine and psychology--Handbooks, manuals, etc. I. Baum, Andrew. II. Revenson, Tracey A. III. Singer, Jerome E.

R726.7.H3645 2012
616.89--dc23
                                    2011044532

Visit the Taylor & Francis Web site at
http://www.taylorandfrancis.com

and the Psychology Press Web site at
http://www.psypress.com

To the memory of Andy Baum (1948–2010) and Jerome E. Singer (1935–2010), who have left their intellectual handprint on the field of health psychology; and to my husband, Ed Seidman, for his unconditional love, to my daughter Molly, my beloved principessa, and to the memory of my father, who believed I could become anything I wanted.

Tracey A. Revenson
New York City
January 2011

Contents

SECTION I   Overarching Frameworks and Paradigms

SECTION II   Cross-Cutting Issues

SECTION III   Risk and Protective Factors

SECTION IV   Macro-Level and Structural Influences on Health

SECTION V   Applications of Health Psychology

Preface

Since the publication of the first edition of the *Handbook of Health Psychology* (Psychology Press, 2001), enormous progress has been made in the connections among biological, psychological, and social components of health, health behavior, and illness. More important, scholars in the field have expanded this tripartite model across even more levels of analysis, including cultural and macrosocial factors at one end and cellular factors at the other. Moreover, a new emphasis has been to translate research evidence in to practice and policy.

The second edition of the handbook reflects these changes and is quite different from the first in terms of both approach and content. The 34 chapters are written by some of the top scholars in health psychology. Each author has taken seriously the task of providing a theoretical foundation, synthesizing and evaluating the empirical evidence, and contemplating how the state of the science can inform future research, clinical practice, and/or policy. The book maintains the first edition's framework of the biopsychosocial model, but the choice of topics reflects the advances that have been made in the field over the past quarter century. Specifically, this new edition adds sections on risk and protective factors for disease and on macro-level factors that affect health. We believe that this structure more closely reflects current scholarship in health psychology.

The first section, "Overarching Frameworks and Paradigms," presents the central theories that inform many areas of research within the field. For example, the concept of allostatic load is a "newer" stress theory that emphasizes the interaction of biological and social systems and may explain the onset of many conditions. The second section, "Cross-Cutting Issues," focuses on the specific mechanisms that help us explain the link between health and behavior across diseases and populations. The third section, "Risk and Protective Factors," new to the revised edition, focuses on specific variables that lead directly or indirectly to the onset and progression of major diseases or are instrumental in promoting health. Most of these risk and protective factors are applicable across many diseases. Some of the risk and protective factors are behavioral (e.g., smoking, exercise), some psychological (e.g., personality, depression), and some a combination of the two (e.g., obesity). The fourth section, "Macro-Level and Structural Influences on Health," also a new addition to the second edition, expands on the previous section. Although many structural factors can be conceptualized as risk or protective factors, this section highlights the larger (extraindividual) social and structural influences on health because this is a direction in which health psychology is moving. The final section, "Application to the Study of Disease," centers on translational research, taking the theories of the earlier sections and applying them to specific disorders.

The primary aim of this handbook is to provide current approaches to many of the critical topics in health psychology at the start of the 21st century. Because the handbook ranges from basic theories to cutting-edge research, to translation of the research to clinical practice and social policy and then cuts across concepts (e.g., behavior change), populations (e.g., women's health), risk and protective factors (e.g., obesity), and diseases, it is appropriate for a wide range of readers from a number of fields—primarily psychology, but also public health, medical sociology, medicine, nursing, and other allied health professions. The chapters are written so that they are accessible to a novice in the area, but they are also deep and detailed enough for a seasoned researcher. We see the handbook being used as a reference volume for those individuals who want to get a broad picture of health psychology as well as those individuals who want only a snapshot in a particular area in which they are working. It can thus also be used in graduate and advanced undergraduate classes, with chapters providing the "frame" for a specific topic.

Acknowledgments

There are many people who have contributed to the development of this volume over the years who deserve our heartfelt thanks. First and foremost is our editor at Taylor & Francis/Psychology Press, Debra Riegert, who remained a stalwart midwife of the second edition during the ups and downs of its birth. We cannot thank her enough for her support, persistence, and friendship. A second person who should be singled out is Phapichaya Chaoprang Herrera, MA, for her stellar work as the editorial assistant for the volume. Pang was always organized and gracious, the ringmaster of a rodeo of nearly 100 contributors and two vocal editors. The book would not have been completed without her, and we can't thank her enough.

We thank the contributors to this volume for their hard work, dedication, and vision, and to their stick-to-it-tive-ness. (You know who you are!) They are the marrow of the field of health psychology, and there would not be a volume without them. We also offer our gracious thanks to Cheryl A. Armstead, Regan A. R. Gurung, and Beverly E. Thorn, who reviewed the proposal for the second edition and made very smart comments.

Most of all, I thank Andy Baum and Jerry Singer for allowing me to be part of this endeavor from the first idea of a handbook in 1993. Though seldom in agreement, we managed to produce a volume that was true to all our visions. Andy, especially, I will miss our "lively" phone conversations the next time around.

Tracey A. Revenson

Editors

Andrew Baum was Jenkins Garrett Professor of Psychology at the University of Texas at Arlington (UTA) and director of the Center for the Study of Health and Illness at the time of his death on November 22, 2010. He earned his BS at the University of Pittsburgh and his PhD at the State University of New York at Stony Brook. Prior to his appointment at UTA, Baum served as professor of psychiatry at the University of Pittsburgh and professor of psychology, psychiatry, and neuroscience at the Uniformed Services University of the Health Sciences. Dr. Baum received multiple awards from such professional organizations as the American Psychological Association (Early Career Award and Senior Investigator Award) and the Society of Behavioral Medicine (Outstanding Service Award) for his contributions to the field of health psychology. Dr. Baum served as editor of two scientific journals, the *Journal of Applied Social Psychology* and the *Journal of Applied Biobehavioral Research*, and was associate editor of *Psychological Bulletin*. He served as president of the Division of Health Psychology from 1988 to 1989. He authored or coauthored more than 250 refereed journal articles, books, book chapters, and abstracts. His early research contributions concerned crowding and the effects of severe and chronic stress on health, best exemplified by his work after the Three Mile Island nuclear accident. More recently, Dr. Baum's work focused on the biobehavioral aspects of cancer and chronic illness, chronic stress and illness, psychoneuroimmunology, and molecular effects of stress and trauma.

Tracey A. Revenson is Professor of Psychology and Deputy Executive Officer at the Graduate Center of the City University of New York, where she is also a member of the Women's Studies Certificate Program. She holds a BA from Yale University and an MA and PhD from New York University; she completed a postdoctoral fellowship in environment, development, and health at the University of California, Irvine. Trained as a one of the first generation of health psychologists, she brings a socioecological perspective to her research on stress and coping processes among individuals, couples, and families facing chronic physical illnesses. She has also examined the influence on interpersonal relationships and gender on adaptation to illness. She is the author or editor of seven volumes, including *Couples Coping With Stress: Emerging Perspectives on Dyadic Coping* (APA Books, 2005), *Ecological Research to Promote Social Change* (Kleuwer Academic, 2000), and *Social Categories in Everyday Life* (APA Books, 2011). She was the founding editor-in-chief of the journal *Women's Health: Research on Gender, Behavior and Policy*. She currently serves as associate editor of the *Annals of Behavioral Medicine* and is on the editorial board of *Health Psychology*. Dr. Revenson was elected president of the Division of Health Psychology of the American Psychological Association in 2004–2005.

Jerome E. Singer was Emeritus Professor, Department of Medical and Clinical Psychology, at the Uniformed Services University until his death on April 21, 2010. As chairman of this department from 1974 to 1999, he founded one of the first health psychology departments and, along with Andrew Baum, one of the first health psychology doctoral programs in the United States. Dr. Singer received his PhD at the University of Minnesota, where he conducted groundbreaking work on emotion with Stanley Schachter, and then held faculty positions at Pennsylvania State University and Stony Brook University. Dr. Singer received numerous honors, including an honorary doctoral degree from the University of Stockholm and the Award for Outstanding Contributions to Health Psychology from the Division of Health Psychology of the American Psychological Association (APA). He served as president of the Division of Health Psychology (38) of the APA in 1981–1982 and of the Academy of Behavioral Medicine Research in 1990–1991. Dr. Singer authored numerous articles and edited numerous books in the areas of stress and health psychology. Along with David C. Glass, he was awarded the Socio-Psychological Prize from the American Association for the Advancement of Science for their monograph *Urban Stress: Experiments With Noise and Social Stressors* (Academic Press, 1972).

Contributors

Leona S. Aiken
Arizona State University
Tempe, Arizona

Michael G. Ainette
Dominican College
Orangeburg, New York

Melissa A. Alderfer
Children's Hospital of Philadelphia
Philadelphia, Pennsylvania
and
Perelman School of Medicine
University of Pennsylvania
Philadelphia, Pennsylvania

Michael H. Antoni
University of Miami
Coral Gables, Florida

Danielle Arigo
Syracuse University
Syracuse, New York

Geniel H. Armstrong
University of Montana
Missoula, Montana

Elizabeth A. Bachen
Mills College
Oakland, California

Andrew Baum
University of Texas at Arlington
Arlington, Texas

Julia D. Betensky
Rutgers, The State University of New Jersey
New Brunswick, New Jersey

Susan Bodnar-Deren
Rutgers, The State University of New Jersey
New Brunswick, New Jersey

Hayden B. Bosworth
Duke University Medical Center
Durham, North Carolina

Glenn S. Brassington
Sonoma State University
Rohnert Park, California
and
Stanford University School of Medicine
Stanford, California

Jessica Y. Breland
Rutgers, The State University of New Jersey
New Brunswick, New Jersey

Addie L. Brewer
San Diego State University
San Deigo, California

Elizabeth Brondolo
St. John's University
Queens, New York

Linda D. Cameron
University of California, Merced
Merced, California

Adam W. Carrico
University of California, San Francisco
San Francisco, California

Charles S. Carver
University of Miami
Coral Gables, Florida

Susan D. Cochran
University of California, Los Angeles
Los Angeles, California

Sheldon Cohen
Carnegie Mellon University
Pittsburgh, Pennsylvania

Zachary Cohen
Stanford University School of Medicine
Stanford, California

Richard J. Contrada
Rutgers, The State University of New Jersey
New Brunswick, New Jersey

Sharon Danoff-Burg
University at Albany, State University of
   New York
Albany, New York

Angela Liegey Dougall
University of Texas at Arlington
Arlington, Texas

Jacqueline Dunbar-Jacob
University of Pittsburgh School of Nursing
Pittsburgh, Pennsylvania

Christine Dunkel Schetter
University of California, Los Angeles
Los Angeles, California

Victoria Egizio
University of Pittsburgh School of Medicine
Pittsburgh, Pennsylvania

Merrill F. Elias
University of Maine
Orono, Maine

Leigh Anne Faul
Georgetown University
Washington, District of Columbia

Adelaide L. Fortmann
San Diego State University
San Diego, California

Theodora Fteropoulli
City University London
London, United Kingdom

Linda C. Gallo
San Diego State University
San Diego, California

Mary A. Gerend
Florida State University
Tallahassee, Florida

Karen Glanz
University of Pennsylvania Schools of
   Medicine and Nursing
Philadelphia, Pennsylvania

David C. Glass
Stony Brook University
Stony Brook, New York

Neil E. Grunberg
Uniformed Services University of the
   Health Sciences
Bethesda, Maryland

Joanne Hash-Converse
Rutgers, The State University of New Jersey
New Brunswick, New Jersey

Eric B. Hekler
Stanford University School of Medicine
Stanford, California

Vicki S. Helgeson
Carnegie Mellon University
Pittsburgh, Pennsylvania

Shashivadan P. Hirani
City University London
London, United Kingdom

Michael A. Hoyt
University of California, Merced
Merced, California

Kristina M. Jackson
Brown University
Providence, Rhode Island

Paul B. Jacobsen
University of South Florida
Tampa, Florida

J. Richard Jennings
University of Pittsburgh School of Medicine
Pittsburgh, Pennsylvania

Michelle C. Kegler
Emory University
Atlanta, Georgia

Abby C. King
Stanford University School of Medicine
Stanford, California

Shonda Lackey
St. John's University
Queens, New York

Stephen J. Lepore
Temple University
Philadelphia, Pennsylvania

Elaine A. Leventhal
University of Medicine and Dentistry of
    New Jersey
New Brunswick, New Jersey

Howard Leventhal
Rutgers, The State University of New Jersey
New Brunswick, New Jersey

Marci Lobel
Stony Brook University
Stony Brook, New York

Erica Love
St. John's University
Queens, New York

Regan M. Maas
University of California, Los Angeles
Los Angeles, California

Anna L. Marsland
University of Pittsburgh
Pittsburgh, Pennsylvania

Lynn M. Martire
Pennsylvania State University
University Park, Pennsylvania

Vickie M. Mays
University of California, Los Angeles
Los Angeles, California

Maura McCall
University of Pittsburgh School of Nursing
Pittsburgh, Pennsylvania

Sara I. McClelland
University of Michigan
Ann Arbor, Michigan

Ilan H. Meyer
The Williams Institute
University of California, Los Angeles
Los Angeles, California

Stanton P. Newman
City University London
London, United Kingdom

Kristina Orth-Gomér
Karolinska Institute
Stockholm, Sweden

Crystal L. Park
University of Connecticut
Storrs, Connecticut

James W. Pennebaker
University of Texas at Austin
Austin, Texas

Suzanne Phelan
California Polytechnic State University
San Luis Obispo, California

Leigh Alison Phillips
Rutgers, The State University of New Jersey
New Brunswick, New Jersey

Courtney C. Prather
University of North Texas
Denton, Texas

Krista W. Ranby
Duke University
Durham, North Carolina

Tracey A. Revenson
Graduate Center, City University of
    New York
New York, New York

Joni Ricks
University of California, Los Angeles
Los Angeles, California

John Ruiz
University of North Texas
Denton, Texas

Michael F. Scheier
Carnegie Mellon University
Pittsburgh, Pennsylvania

Elizabeth Schlenk
University of Pittsburgh School of Nursing
Pittsburgh, Pennsylvania

Neil Schneiderman
University of Miami
Coral Gables, Florida

Richard Schulz
University of Pittsburgh
Pittsburgh, Pennsylvania

Asani H. Seawell
Grinnell College
Grinnell, Iowa

Sarah Shafer Berger
Uniformed Services University of the
    Health Sciences
Bethesda, Maryland

Smriti Shivpuri
San Diego State University
San Diego, California

Ilene C. Siegler
Duke University School of Medicine
Durham, North Carolina

Timothy W. Smith
University of Utah
Salt Lake City, Utah

Joshua M. Smyth
Pennsylvania State University
University Park, Pennsylvania

Caroline M. Stanley
Wilmington College
Wilmington, Ohio

Annette L. Stanton
University of California, Los Angeles
Los Angeles, California

Amy K. Starosciak
Uniformed Services University of the
    Health Sciences
Bethesda, Maryland

Patrick Steffen
Brigham Young University
Provo, Utah

Jan Stygall
City University London
London, United Kingdom

Kimberly S. Swanson
University of Washington
Seattle, Washington

Dennis C. Turk
University of Washington
Seattle, Washington

Thomas A. Wills
University of Hawaii Cancer Center
Honolulu, Hawaii

Hilary D. Wilson
University of Washington
Seattle, Washington

Rena Wing
The Miriam Hospital and the Warren Alpert
    Medical School
Brown University
Providence, Rhode Island

Introduction

Progress, Premises, and Promises of Health Psychology

Tracey A. Revenson

During the past four decades, health psychologists have worked to understand the biological, psychological, and social factors that affect health, health behavior, and illness. Researchers have grappled with probing questions: How do personality and behavior contribute to the pathophysiology of cardiovascular disease? What do women gain from screening mammography if it creates anxiety and avoidance of regular screening? Why do we expect individuals to take responsibility for condom use to prevent HIV transmission when using condoms is an interpersonal negotiation? When are social relationships supportive, and when are they detrimental to health? The chapters in this volume address these and many other questions (for these four questions, see Aiken, Gerend, Jackson, & Ranby, Chapter 6; Antoni & Carrico, Chapter 33; Betensky, Glass, & Contrada, Chapter 27; Smith, Gallo, Shivpuri, & Brewer, Chapter 17; and Wills & Ainette, Chapter 20). The field of health psychology has amassed a body of knowledge that has been—or has the potential to be—translated into clinical and community interventions to improve physical health and emotional well-being.

The discipline of health psychology brought together psychologists from traditional areas of psychology who shared a common interest in problems of health and illness but who brought their own disciplinary paradigms and methodologies to the table. Not surprisingly, this cacophony of models, approaches, methods, and jargon appeared confusing at times, raising the question of whether health psychology has its own paradigms (Friedman & Adler, 2007). That question remains unanswered, although many theories or minitheories exist (see Section I, this volume). At the same time, this cacophony brought a breadth and eclecticism to the study of health–behavior relationships that has been partly responsible for its success as a subdiscipline within U.S. and European psychology.

The original paradigm adopted by health psychology was the *biopsychosocial model* (Engel, 1977; Schwartz, 1982), which posited that physiological, psychological, and social factors are braided together in health and illness processes and cannot be studied in isolation. Contrasting itself with biomedical models, the biopsychosocial model did not give primacy to biological indices, stating that it was impossible to understand disease processes without understanding the psychological mechanisms propelling them or the social context surrounding them. The biopsychosocial model was inclusive enough to be applied to risk estimates for particular diseases as well as health-promoting behaviors and environments, to disease progression as well as psychosocial adaptation to illness, and to individually oriented therapeutic and behavior change interventions as well as broader community-based and media approaches. The biopsychosocial model stimulated theories, research designs, and methods. Most important, it suggested a multicause, multieffect approach to health and illness, rather than the limiting single-cause, single-effect approach. However, there remained a compartmentalization of the components of the biopsychosocial model in the early years of the field in part because most health psychologists had been trained in the traditional areas of psychology (e.g., clinical psychology, social psychology).

The march toward middle age marks a good time to take stock of accomplishments and achievements, to do a little soul searching, and to make midcourse adjustments. Where is the field of health psychology now? What has changed in the past decade, since the original publication of this handbook, and where is the field headed in the next decade? I offer a number of broad insights into the field and invite the reader to look for specific examples within the rich offerings of this handbook.

STABILITY AND CHANGE

Many of the original phenomena of interest in health psychology have remained central to the field over the past 40 years. The topics of stress and coping, health behavior change (including smoking cessation, condom use, and exercise), and cognitive models of why individuals do or do not engage in preventive health behavior (such as screening or treatment adherence) remain important areas for study (see Aiken et al., Chapter 6; Brassington, Hekler, Cohen, & King, Chapter 16; Dunbar-Jacob, Schlenk, & McCall, Chapter 12; Glanz & Kegler, Chapter 5; Grunberg, Berger, & Starosciak, Chapter 14; Hoyt & Stanton, Chapter 10; and Revenson & Lepore, Chapter 9). Because the work in these areas has grown, bringing in new models and methods and broadening the models to include more diverse populations, researchers working in these areas continue to make steady progress with the potential for translation to practice.

At the same time, much has changed in a decade. Some theories, among them the commonsense model of illness (Leventhal et al., Chapter 1, this volume), have undergone substantial revision. Other theories have expanded in new directions and become more complex, particularly those that address behavior change (Glanz & Kegler, Chapter 5, this volume). For example, in the area of stress and illness, we have moved far beyond correlations of the accumulation of self-reported stressful life events with reports of illness or medical visits to demonstrating causal pathways of stress with infectious disease (Marsland, Bachen, & Cohen, Chapter 31, this volume). Similarly, in the understanding of pain, we have models that integrate physiology and psychology (Turk, Wilson, & Swanson, Chapter 7, this volume); but also, with new methods and statistical techniques (e.g., a combination of daily process methods and hierarchical linear modeling), we can examine the causal role of emotions or social support in pain perceptions and coping behavior over time (e.g., Holtzman & DeLongis, 2007).

EXPANDING LEVELS OF ANALYSIS

There are two ways in which new approaches, perhaps better described as paradigmatic world-views, have come into health psychology. Both involve expanding the scope of the work to cross multiple levels of analysis. Anderson (1998) described a framework for health sciences that involve the need to study multiple levels of analysis of any health problem. These levels were the social/environmental, behavioral/psychological, organ systems, cellular, and molecular. More important, he indicated that the great advances would occur not with research that examines the association of variables within levels but with research that focuses on reciprocal and mutually causative processes between levels. At the time, much of health psychology research involved examining how a single variable, or multiple variables within a single level, affected health outcomes in an additive fashion. Anderson urged health psychologists to examine interactions among variables from at least two different levels of analysis to move the field of health psychology forward. Chapter 19 in this volume, by Dunkel Schetter and Lobel, provides an excellent example of research that crosses multiple levels of analysis.

In the past decade, we have seen many examples of such movement. These movements have occurred in two different ways. The first is a centrifugal move inward toward the original "center" of biological and microanalytic processes (Jennings & Egizio, Chapter 2, this volume). An example of this is how stress is implicated in infectious processes (Marsland et al., Chapter 31, this volume). Contemporary research examines the pathways through which stress perceptions affect infection on organ system, cellular, and molecular levels (Dougall & Baum,

Chapter 3, this volume; Miller, Chen, & Cole, 2009). As an exemplar of this research, Epel et al. (2004) demonstrated that among women facing chronic stress as well as women facing "normal" stress, greater perceived stress was associated with the biological indicators of accelerated cellular aging (telomere length, telomerase, and oxidative stress).

The second advance is a centripetal force that moves health psychology outward toward the social/environmental level of analysis. Health psychologists have taken the lead in examining the biological and psychological mechanisms by which socioeconomic status (SES) affects both individual and community health outcomes (Ruiz, Steffen, & Prather, Chapter 23, this volume). For example, Matthews and Gallo (2011) have proposed a "reserve capacity model" to explain how individuals at the lower ends of the socioeconomic ladder may lack the resources to cope with many of the strains and stresses of everyday life, thus making them more vulnerable to illness. Similarly, moving away from simplistic models of race differences, psychologists have examined how perceptions of racism can affect cardiovascular reactivity and heart disease, specifying mediating mechanisms at multiple levels, including everyday racism, coping, and community norms (Brondolo, Lackey, & Love, Chapter 24, this volume).

Another notable change is studying health–behavior processes within the social contexts in which we live: within the context of the family (see this volume, Alderfer & Stanley, Chapter 21; Martire & Schulz, Chapter 13; Revenson & Lepore, Chapter 9); within ascribed social roles (Helgeson, Chapter 22, this volume); and within cultural communities that have received little prior attention by health psychologists (Mays, Maas, Ricks, & Cochran, Chapter 34, this volume; Meyer, Chapter 25, this volume). Health psychology has done a better job of including aspects of the larger sociopolitical context in models, such as social class (Ruiz et al., Chapter 23, this volume), race and racism (Brondolo et al., Chapter 24, this volume) and prejudice (Mays et al., Chapter 34, this volume; Meyer, Chapter 25, this volume). A contextual approach also recognize the fact that health-behavior processes are developmental and that we must understand health and illness processes at different stages of the life cycle (Siegler, Elias, & Bosworth, Chapter 26, this volume). If this handbook is a reflection of the current state of the field, then health psychology research is currently represented at the intersections between all five of Anderson's levels of analysis.

A FOCUS ON HEALTH AND ILLNESS

Despite its name, health psychology tended to focus more on diseases and disease outcomes instead of health. As shown in the chapters in Section III of this volume, this has changed radically over the past decade, with a balancing of risk and resilience factors in the prevention of illness as well as a focus on positive indicators of adjustment to illness. For example, there has been growth in the scientific inquiry into the benefits of spirituality, religion, and meaning making as predictors of overall health and well-being and of adjustment to stress and illness (Masters & Spielmans, 2007; Park, Chapter 18, this volume). Adjustment outcomes involve such positive outcomes as stress-related growth and richer interpersonal relationships as well as such negative outcomes as depression and lowered quality of life (Hoyt & Stanton, Chapter 10, this volume; Park, Lechner, Antoni, & Stanton, 2009; Stanton & Revenson, 2011).

This focus on health as well as illness has occurred in other areas as well. There has been an explosion of research on physical activity and exercise because they maintain health, prevent illness, and speed recovery (Brassington et al., Chapter 16). The field has gone beyond descriptive and correlational research on such stress buffers as social support and dispositional optimism to understanding the mechanisms for these relationships (Scheier, Carver, & Armstong, Chapter 4, this volume; Wills & Ainette, Chapter 20, this volume); prospective studies add causal strength to these explanations.

In addition to understanding the mechanisms by which disease can be prevented, researchers have made great advances in understanding those factors that optimize quality of life for people living with pain and serious illness (see this volume, Danoff-Burg & Seawell, Chapter 32; Hoyt &

Stanton, Chapter 10; Turk et al., Chapter 7; see also Section V, this volume). We now understand in a more sophisticated fashion how others in our social world can help or hinder our coping (see this volume, Alderfer & Stanley, Chapter 21; Martire & Schulz, Chapter 13; Revenson & Lepore, Chapter 9; Wills & Ainette, Chapter 20); whether (and how) disclosing our emotions makes us feel better (Revenson & Lepore, Chapter 9, this volume; Smyth, Pennebaker, & Arigo, Chapter 8, this volume); and in an understudied area within health psychology, how sexual function affects quality of life (McClelland, Chapter 11, this volume).

NEXT STEPS

There are a number of areas where progress has been made, but more needs to come. First is the area of behavioral interventions. The stellar research in many areas of health psychology holds great promise for translation into effective behavioral medicine interventions at both the clinical and community levels. The final section of this volume contains chapters that assess the state of the science in behavioral interventions for people with cardiovascular disease (Newman, Hirani, Stygall, Fteropoulli, Chapter 28, this volume) and cancer (Faul & Jacobsen, Chapter 30, this volume). Although many pilot projects suggest fruitful new directions, the findings from large-scale randomized clinical trials have been more equivocal (Coyne, Lepore, & Palmer, 2006; Schneiderman & Orth-Gomér, Chapter 29, this volume; Wing & Phelan, Chapter 15, this volume).

A second area where growth is needed is what is often referred to as "health disparities." Health disparities are "differences in health that are not only unnecessary and avoidable, but in addition, are considered unfair and unjust" (Whitehead, 1992, p. 433). Health disparities research seeks to measure and reduce or eliminate avoidable differences in health. Most of the research on health disparities within health psychology, as in other disciplines, involves demonstrating between-group differences in some health indicator, most often between groups that differ in race or SES and occasionally in groups that differ in gender or gender orientation. However, between-group studies based on such nominal categories as ethnic-group membership do little to illuminate the mediating pathways that explain these group differences and may suggest loci for intervention (Yali & Revenson, 2004). Moreover, research on racial or gender disparities does not lead us to those answers when it is confounded with poverty or SES on either the individual or neighborhood level. Similarly, poverty does not fully account for race differences in health; these differences occur at every level of the SES gradient (Mays, Cochran, & Barnes, 2007). Our understanding of health disparities, as well as our ability to close the gaps, will increase if we consider the psychological manifestations of such group difference as racism, sexism, heterosexism, and ageism. For example, a number of studies have found that African Americans who attributed interpersonal mistreatment to racial discrimination exhibit greater blood pressure reactivity and recovery to laboratory stressors that bear similarities to an encounter with racial prejudice (Brondolo et al., Chapter 24, this volume); these findings suggest that it is not race per se but perceived racism that may act as a chronic stressor. Similarly, place of birth, years in the United States, and acculturation level are often overlooked when racial health disparities are examined, but they are important moderators along with SES (Adler & Rehkopf, 2008). Including these multiple influences may help explain paradoxical effects in ethnic-minority populations, for example, why Latinas have worse health relative to non-Latino Whites but have lower all-cause mortality rates (e.g., Abraído-Lanza, Chao, & Flóres, 2005).

No individual-level factors (e.g., coping) have emerged as effective for offsetting the impact of racism on health (Brondolo et al., Chapter 24, this volume). It is likely that changes will need to occur at structural, economic, and political levels in order to have the broadest impact on reducing health disparities. In a comprehensive review, Mays et al. (2007) describe several race–discrimination–health pathways that lead to poorer health, including segregation, residential stratification, conditions of violence, lack of social capital, and growing up in poor neighborhoods; Mays' chapter in this volume (Chapter 34) lattices together race, discrimination, geography, and politics to help us understand the HIV epidemic among African American women in the Southern United States. It cannot hurt to reiterate that health psychology will need to include social structural variables more directly into its research to be able to provide answers to these social health problems.

Recognizing the need for structural variables leads to the final point: The next generation of health psychologists needs to be trained to conduct interdisciplinary research and have a tool kit of multiple methods. It may benefit us to bring in the paradigms and methods of such sister fields as medical sociology and medical anthropology, as well as epidemiology and public health, to a greater degree in order to look more broadly and deeply across levels of analysis. Doing so will also move the field forward to be more accepting of multiple methods, including qualitative studies. At the beginning of a program of research or at the end, when research findings seem counterintuitive, qualitative research can not only help frame research questions but can also tell us whether we are asking the right questions. In a study that this author consulted on, the investigator wanted to know why African American women had much lower smoking cessation rates and much higher attrition rates in a behavioral counseling and medication intervention than did White women or Black or White men. Conducting a series of focus groups with women who dropped out of the trial, we learned that the Black women did not understand that the National Institutes of Health protocol stipulated that if they smoked even one cigarette, missed one counseling session, or failed to take the medication even one day, they would be dropped from the trial (Thompson, Revenson, & Covey, 2004). Not surprisingly, the women were outraged about the way they had been treated because this information had not been presented in an understandable fashion. Moreover, more African American than White women experienced physical side effects from the medication, which led to medication nonadherence. These qualitative data provided insight into the quantitative differences found and also suggested culturally sensitive changes for the next trial.

CONCLUSION

The exponential growth in brain and behavioral sciences over the past decade is mirrored in the field of health psychology. But rapid growth also begets growing pains. Health psychologists have taken stock, many times, to assess our progress and our pitfalls (e.g., Folkman & Moskowitz, 2004; Taylor, 1987, 1990). This introduction has served both to document the progress that the field of health psychology has made in the past decade and to suggest directions for greater impact. As Revenson and Baum (2001) quoted in the introduction to the first volume, "There are many miles to go before we sleep" (Frost, 1923). We continue to march forward.

REFERENCES

Abraído-Lanza, A. F., Chao, M. T., & Flóres, K. R. (2005). Do healthy behaviors decline with acculturation? Implications for the Latino mortality paradox. *Social Science & Medicine, 61*, 1243–1255.

Adler, N. E., & Rehkopf, D. H. (2008). U.S. disparities in health: Descriptions, causes, mechanisms. *Annual Review of Public Health, 29*, 235–252.

Anderson, N. B. (1998). Levels of analysis in health science: A framework for integrating sociobehavioral and biomedical research. *Annals of the New York Academy of Sciences, 840*, 563–576.

Coyne, J. C., Lepore, S. J., & Palmer, S. C. (2006). Efficacy of psychosocial interventions in cancer care: Evidence is weaker than it first looks. *Annals of Behavioral Medicine, 32*, 104–110.

Engel, G. L. (1977). The need for a new medical model: A challenge for biomedicine. *Science, 196*, 129–136.

Epel, E. S., Blackburn, E. H., Lin, J., Dhabhar, F. S., Adler, N. E., Morrow, J. D., & Cawthon, R. (2004). Accelerated telomere shortening in response to life stress. *PNAS, 101*(49), 17312–17315.

Folkman, S., & Moskowitz, J. T.(2004). Coping: Pitfalls and promises. *Annual Review of Psychology, 55*, 745–774.

Friedman, H. S., & Adler, N. E. (2007). The history and background of health psychology. In H. S. Friedman & R. C. Silver (Eds.), *Foundations of health psychology* (pp. 3–18). New York, NY: Oxford University Press.

Frost, R. (1923). Stopping by woods on a snowy evening. In *New Hampshire*. New York, NY: Holt.

Holtzman, S., & DeLongis, A. (2007). One day at a time: The impact of daily satisfaction with spouse responses on pain, negative affect and catastrophizing among individuals with rheumatoid arthritis. *Pain, 131,* 202–213.

Masters, K. S., & Spielmans, G. I. (2007). Prayer and health: Review, meta-analysis, and research agenda. *Journal of Behavioral Medicine, 30,* 329–338.

Matthews, K. A., & Gallo, L. C. (2011). Psychological perspectives on pathways linking socioeconomic status and physical health. *Annual Review of Psychology, 62,* 501–530.

Mays, V., Cochran, S. D., & Barnes, N. W. (2007). Race, race-based discrimination, and health outcomes among African Americans. *Annual Review of Psychology, 58,* 201–225.

Miller, G., Chen, E., & Cole, S. W. (2009). Health psychology: Developing biologically plausible models linking the social world and physical health. *Annual Review of Psychology, 60,* 501–524.

Park, C. L., Lechner, S. C., Antoni, M. H., & Stanton, A. L. (Eds.). (2009). *Medical illness and positive life change: Can crisis lead to personal transformation?* Washington, DC: American Psychological Association.

Revenson, T. A., & Baum, A. (2001). Introduction. In A. Baum, T. A. Revenson, & J. E. Singer, (Eds.), *Handbook of health Ppsychology* (pp. xv–xx). Mahwah, NJ: Erlbaum.

Schwartz, G. (1982). Testing the biopsychosocial model: The ultimate challenge facing behavioral medicine? *Journal of Consulting and Clinical Psychology, 50,* 1040–1053.

Stanton, A., & Revenson, T. A. (2011). Adjustment to chronic disease: Progress and promise in research. In H. Friedman (Ed.), *Oxford handbook of health psychology* (pp. 224–272). New York, NY: Oxford University Press.

Taylor, S. E. (1987). The progress and prospects of health psychology: Tasks of a maturing discipline. *Health Psychology, 6,* 73–87.

Taylor, S. E. (1990). Health psychology: The science and the field. *American Psychologist, 45,* 40–50.

Thompson, A. B., Revenson, T. A., & Covey, L. S. (2004, March). *Understanding ethnic disparities in quit rates among women in a smoking cessation study.* Paper presented at the annual meeting of the Society for Behavioral Medicine, Baltimore, MD.

Whitehead, M. (1992). The concepts and principles of equity and health. *International Journal of Health Services, 22,* 429–445.

Yali, A. M., & Revenson, T. A. (2004). How changes in population demographics will impact health psychology: Incorporating a broader notion of cultural competence into the field. *Health Psychology, 23,* 147–155.

Section I

Overarching Frameworks and Paradigms

1 Modeling Health and Illness Behavior

The Approach of the Commonsense Model

Howard Leventhal, Susan Bodnar-Deren, Jessica Y. Breland,
Joanne Hash-Converse, and Leigh Alison Phillips
Rutgers, The State University of New Jersey

Elaine A. Leventhal
University of Medicine and Dentistry of New Jersey

Linda D. Cameron
University of California, Merced

The current chapter updates and reorganizes our earlier handbook contribution, "Representations, Procedures and Affect in Illness Self Regulation" (H. Leventhal, Leventhal, and Cameron, 2001). The changes are a product of our insights into what the common-sense model (CSM) is now telling us and was telling us throughout its history. The CSM has undergone a number of changes in name reflecting the evidence and insights into the mechanisms underlying response to health information. The earliest version, the parallel processing model (H. Leventhal, 1970), emerged from studies of fear communications. The data from these studies showed that cognitive information and affective information were processed as separate, interacting meanings and feelings that affected immediate and delayed response to warnings of threatening health events. The fear studies and the descriptive and experimental studies of preparation for and response to stressful interventions—for example, such medical interventions as endoscopy (Johnson & Leventhal, 1974), such natural but stressful processes as childbirth (E. A. Leventhal, Leventhal, Shacham, & Easterline, 1989), and laboratory tests examining responses to the cold pressor (Ahles, Blanchard, & Leventhal, 1983; H. Leventhal, Brown, Shacham, & Engquist, 1979)—indicated that procedures and action plans, the nondeclarative knowledge involved in self-regulation, were separate from the cognitive representations and emotional reactions to stressful events. These data led us to change the model's name from "parallel processing model" to "self-regulation model" to emphasize the focus on the performance components (perceptions and action plans) of the system. Finally, as we and many other investigators identified the cognitive contents and processes that guided how patients managed chronic conditions in their home environments, we recognized that a patient's cognitive *representations* of a condition and its treatment provided the frameworks guiding everyday management. The cognitive emphasis led to a mix of renaming, including "model of illness cognition" (Croyle & Barger, 1993), "mental representations in health and illness" (Skelton & Croyle, 1991), and "common-sense representation of illness danger" (H. Leventhal, Meyer, & Nerenz, 1980). In sum, the name changes reflect the evolution of the CSM as a framework for understanding how people adapt to health threats in settings ranging from hospitals to clinics and the home.

The CSM identifies variables, constructive processes, and behaviors that reflect how people in these settings perceive, understand, react to, and interact with others in managing threats to health. Although the concepts and processes articulated in the CSM are situated in a particular set of contexts, they are applicable to a wide range of life situations because health, illness, and dying are universal. Thus, the processes underlying how people represent and respond to health and illness in these settings reflect fundamental properties of the human mind and fundamental properties of the processes involved in sharing information when interacting with others. We view the CSM as a work in progress, that is, as a framework for conceptual elaboration and empirical work; it is not a closed system. A basic aim of this chapter is to show how a cognitive approach to health and illness behavior can be elaborated and used as a tool for the development of interventions in clinical settings to improve health outcomes.

The CSM is consistent with a long-standing tradition in social and personality psychology (e.g., Kelly, 1955; Lewin, 1935), as well as in studies of "folk illness" by medical anthropologists (e.g., Kleinman, 1980; Pachter, 1993). As is the case with the CSM, the variation in these names reflects differences in emphasis on various features of perception and action to prevent, treat, cure, and/or adjust to acute or chronic conditions. Three themes are fundamental to all these models:

1. Individuals are conceptualized as active problem solvers trying to make sense of potential or existent changes in their somatic state and to act to avoid or control those changes that are perceived as signs of illness or physical disorder; in effect, individuals are self-regulating systems. In this framework, adaptation is a product of a problem-solving process in which decisions to take one or more specific actions are based on the individual's understanding of the illness threat (*illness representations*), the availability of procedures for management (*representation of procedures and action plans*), and the experienced outcomes contingent on the costs and benefits of specific procedures.

2. The adaptive process is based on beliefs, commonsense perceptions, and available skills. That is, the representation of a disease threat, the representation of the procedures selected for its management, the plans for action, and the appraisal of outcomes are products of the individual's understanding and skills at a given point in time. Thus, neither the representations nor the procedures for management reflect the objective, biomedical nature of the threat or the procedures medically optimal for control.

3. The notion of folk illness, which distinguishes the biomedical concept of disease from the social concept of illness, emphasizes the role of the sociocultural environment in shaping the self-regulation process. Thus, an individual's representation of a threat and selection and evaluation of procedures for management are shaped and moderated by the attitudes and beliefs of his or her social and cultural environment. This environment includes family, friends, biomedical as well as traditional health practitioners, mass media, such socially defined roles as the passive versus active patient, and the linguistic terms used to label and describe specific diseases and treatments. Each of these factors constrains and shapes the substance and behavior of the self-regulation system. Because a wide range of factors shape the content, or *software*, of the self-regulatory behavioral system, assessments across persons within a common sociocultural domain and assessments across cultural domains will reveal both common and unique features of illness representations, coping strategies, and appraisals.

The themes enumerated in the preceding list are visible in each of the sections of this chapter. Section 1, "The Content and Structure of the Commonsense Model," provides an overview of the hierarchical structure of the CSM. It begins by describing the core control unit of the system, comprised of the representation of illness (its five content domains) and the representations of procedures and action plans for the implementation of action. The structure of each component is bilevel, abstract, and perceptually and procedurally concrete. The representations and action plans of the core control unit are engaged in the more or less implicit, or automatic, management of illness and health problems. Section 1 ends with a brief overview of the executive system and the tools it has for monitoring and regulating the behaviors generated by the core control unit.

Section 2, "The Dynamics of Commonsense Self-Regulation," describes the workings of the self-regulatory system, beginning with the detection of deviations from the normal, "healthy" self, and the matching of detected deviations to illness prototypes. The match activates the illness and treatment representations, or *hypotheses*, that control the problem-solving process. The focus here is on the rules governing the interactions among the system's perceptual, cognitive, and affective components as individuals construct representations of threats and procedures for threat control. The self-system is central to our discussion of system dynamics because the meaning of specific illness episodes arises from their impact on the self.

Section 3 briefly examines the ways in which the CSM has been used in interventions and in the construction of clinical trials. It also provides a brief overview of the CSM approach to the cultural and social context, with admittedly limited empirical examples. This section briefly examines ways in which the CSM addresses efforts at intervention and the construction of clinical trials. A possibly unique contribution of the CSM is the identification of specific elements involved in interpersonal exchanges that affect the construction of illness and treatment representations and the criteria patients use for testing the validity of their common-sense models. This approach complements social learning models of interpersonal influence.

Finally, Section 4 offers some final points on the model, the premises underlying the CSM, and the implications of the CSM for reliability of instruments and clinical trials. The reader should be advised that our citations of the literature are selective and cover but a fraction of the diverse empirical literature relevant to the CSM approach to self-regulation. Older, exhaustive reviews are available elsewhere (Petrie & Weinman, 1997; Skelton & Croyle, 1991).

THE CONTENT AND STRUCTURE OF THE COMMONSENSE MODEL

In this section we review the content and structure of the CSM and supporting empirical evidence. The CSM's architecture is hierarchical, with a feedback control system at its base, the executive system at the top, and strategies at intermediate levels. Although all systems are involved in generating behavior, not all are equally salient at a given moment. For example, the base-level control system is dominant for behaviors that are well practiced and relatively automatic, whereas the executive system exerts stronger control when behavior is interrupted and undergoing restructuring. The following four parts of this section cover the content and structure of the system: (1) The Core Control Unit, a feedback loop at the center of problem solving; (2) Illness Representations, Content, and Structure; (3) Procedures, Action Plans, and Appraisals: The Output/Performance Side of the System; and (4) The Self-System: Executive Function and Executive Tools. Any sequence we might choose for describing the system does violence to its operation because the system is not linear; however, because language is linear, we have no choice but to follow a linear sequence.

THE CORE CONTROL UNIT: A FEEDBACK LOOP

The majority of models describing self-regulation to health threats (e.g., Carver & Scheier, 1982; Lazarus & Folkman, 1984; H. Leventhal, 1970; Prochaska, DiClemente, & Norcross, 1992) contain a core feedback control unit that has the following properties: First, it is focused on ongoing self-regulation processes, that is, on *episodic problem solving*. Second, the problem-solving process involves at least three sets of factors: (1) a *representation* of the health problem that is active during the ongoing episode; (2) *procedures and action plans* for controlling the threat; and (3) an *appraisal* of the consequences of the coping efforts. The separation of the representation of the health threat from the procedures and action plans for threat management was a critical feature in the earliest version of the CSM, the parallel processing model (H. Leventhal, 1970). The separation emerged from the repeated finding that messages depicting health threats did not lead to behavior unless they were combined with information suggesting a concrete plan for action. This finding held whether it was the simple act of taking a tetanus shot (H. Leventhal, Jones, & Trembly, 1966; H. Leventhal, Singer, & Jones, 1965) or the more complex act of quitting smoking (H. Leventhal, Watts, & Pagano, 1967). Neither the representation of the health threat (the fear message) alone nor the action plan alone produced action; the combination was essential. These factors—that is, representations, procedures for action, and the appraisals generated by postresponse feedback (a factor not examined in our earlier studies)—are the basic constituents of a TOTE (test-operate-test-exit) unit in control theory (Carver & Scheier, 1982; Miller, Galanter, & Pribram, 1960). The TOTE is, however, a content-free control unit; it can describe such a closed system as a thermostat to regulate heat or the control unit for managing threats to health. The latter is rich in content, open, and accessible to influence by higher order regulatory processes or executive functions. Anticipating our examination of system dynamics, we can expect that representations of threat and the action plans are likely closely interrelated and less independent of one another than is suggested by the stages in the early parallel response model, as shown in Figure 1.1.

Figure 1.1 depicts another important feature of reactions to health threats, namely, the parallel, or independent, processing of information for *controlling danger* and the processing of information for *controlling the emotional responses* elicited by the danger. The separateness of the two processing systems was visible in data showing that such vivid depictions of disease threats as films of surgery for lung cancer and photographs of the contortions of tetanus aroused stronger reports of fear and larger changes in attitudes than such less threatening depictions as risky driving (H. Leventhal & Trembly, 1968). The increase in fear and more favorable attitudes elicited by the strong fear messages were, however, transient and increasing the level of fear did not increase behavior (i.e., getting a chest x-ray or a tetanus shot). By contrast, if the fear messages were combined with an action plan, exposure to either strong or weak fear messages increased reported adherence to efforts to reduce smoking and recorded receipt of tetanus shots over the following weeks and months.

Efforts to understand how fear affects attitudes and behavior have, however, produced varied results. Some studies support the hypothesis that fear facilitates behaviors to prevent disease and inhibits behaviors to detect or approach a disease threat (Millar & Millar, 1996), but more recent work suggests that fear promotes adherence to both types of behavior (Diefenbach, Miller, & Daly, 1999). The findings from the early fear communication studies should not, however, be interpreted

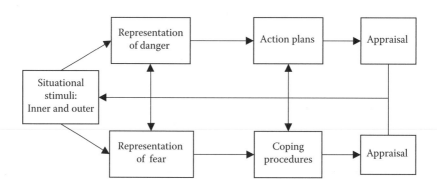

FIGURE 1.1   The parallel processing model. The model posited that two independent, interacting systems processed cues of health threats. The top row represents the cognitive system (i.e., what patients see, feel, and believe), which leads to action plans and action and then to a postaction appraisal. The lower row represents the emotional system (i.e., the experience of emotion), procedures for coping with emotion, and appraisal of coping outcomes. The representations of danger and fear are generated by informational antecedents different than action plans. The diagram is a highly simplified version of the model. (Adapted from Leventhal, H., in *Advances in Experimental Social Psychology*, 5, 176–177, Academic Press, New York, 1970.)

as inconsistent with these more recent data. Given the complexity of the system underlying the CSM, fear can have diverse effects on behavior depending on how it is related to the perceptual/cognitive and procedural/performance factors in the system. Thus, when fear is classically conditioned to perceptual cues to create so-called hot cognitions (Loewenstein, 2005), its consequences will be longer lasting and can drive behavior in different directions depending on the relative strength of procedures and action plans available for directly confronting the threat as opposed to those available for controlling fear (H. Leventhal, 1984; H. Leventhal & Scherer, 1987).

ILLNESS REPRESENTATIONS: STRUCTURE AND CONTENT

It is our contention that a psychological model of the processes involved in coping with specific illness episodes and illness threats must depict the structure and the content of the problem-solving system (the cognitive and emotional material within it). Although such a content-free model as the TOTE and its hierarchical versions (Austin & Vancouver, 1996) provide an approach to modeling dynamic systems, the absence of content is a serious limitation. Sociopsychological and cognitive research often ignores mental contents, seeing the task as secondary and of concern only to applied research. Content is ignored, however, at one's peril, for content affects both structure and process. The content (e.g., ideas about the indicators, duration, causes, and ways of preventing and curing specific diseases) is the software underlying everyday perception, thinking, and action (the commonsense system) and is a product of the individual's declarative and nondeclarative (perceptual and procedural) knowledge (Squire, 2004). The categories in which these common-sense ideas are cast (e.g., the attributes of illness representations, the perceptions and procedures in implicit and explicit awareness and memory, and the rules governing the behavior of the system) are constructions essential for describing and understanding the mechanisms underlying adaptive action (H. Leventhal & Nerenz, 1985). Ignoring structure and content is tantamount to ignoring nucleic acids, genes, proteins, and pathways in cell biology.

The CSM specifies the structure and content of representations of illness that provide the goals or targets for action and the specific procedures and action plans for performance and goal attainment in specific environments. Our approach to the identification of the content of illness representations was influenced by our decision to study illness behavior (Kasl & Cobb, 1966). The typical episode of illness behavior is initiated by somatic stimuli, that is, disease-related sensations (symptoms) and changes in function. Our objective was defined, therefore, as the investigation of the ways in which people understood and/or represented somatic and functional change and how the representations affected behavior (H. Leventhal, Nerenz, & Strauss, 1982; H. Leventhal & Leventhal, 1993). We assumed, incorrectly perhaps, that we would identify the same features of the representation of health threats whether we began our quest by studying how people interpreted somatic symptoms or by studying health-related actions that are undertaken in response to messages in media and/or the observation of illness in others by persons who are asymptomatic and presumed healthy.

The Content of Illness Representations

Open- and closed-ended interviews with patients and studies using multidimensional scaling of illness labels with undergraduates identified five sets of attributes of illness representations (see Figure 1.2): (1) illness *identity*, that is, the symptoms and labels that define the particular illness (Dempsey, Dracup, & Moser, 1995; Lau, Bernard, & Hartman, 1989; Meyer, Leventhal, & Gutmann, 1985); (2) *timelines*, including perceptions and beliefs respecting the onset, duration, and rate of decline with and/or without a home-based or medical intervention, as well as the time from disease onset to death when no treatment is possible (Heidrich, Forsthoff, & Ward, 1994; Meyer, Leventhal, & Gutmann, 1985); (3) *causes* of the threat, which may involve external agents (e.g., bacteria, viruses, job stress, or even bewitchment), internal susceptibilities (e.g., genetic factors), and behaviors (e.g., a lump causing breast cancer; Baumann, Cameron, Zimmerman, & Leventhal, 1989); (4) anticipated and experienced *consequences* of the disease, which may involve physical, emotional, social, and economic outcomes (Cella, Tulsky, Gray, & Sarafian, 1993; Croyle & Jemmott, 1991); and (5) *control*, whether the threat to health is expected and perceived to be responsive to self and/or expert treatments (Lau & Hartman, 1983).

The five content domains of lay representations of illness have been written about from the time of Hippocrates and Galen to the present (Schober & Lacroix, 1991). The variables within these domains guide the selection of procedures for controlling disease and define the targets and time frames for observing outcomes. For example, the sudden onset of chest pain and breathlessness are likely to be experienced immediately as possible symptoms of a heart attack. Once the representation of a heart attack is activated, it will define the cessation of vigorous activities and rapid care-seeking as procedures for management of these symptom targets (Bunde & Martin, 2006; Matthews, Siegel, Kuller, Thompson, & Varat, 1983). Such symptoms as a lump in the breast or difficulty and pain during urination may activate representations of breast cancer and prostate cancer, respectively. The representations of these somatic changes may activate such procedures as "wait and see and test" (e.g., massage, drink fluids) before individuals seek a medical diagnosis (Cameron, Leventhal, & Leventhal, 1993; Facione, 1993; Hackett & Cassem, 1969). Symptoms represented as the "familiar common cold" are likely to become targets for a variety of self-care procedures as getting extra sleep, taking aspirin, taking vitamin C, and drinking fluid.

The Structure of Illness Representations

Representations have structure; they are both abstract and concrete. For example, such words as *cancer* and *heart attack* are labels for the abstract concepts that enrich the meaning of these diseases, and the symptoms and functional changes are their concrete, experienced features. Thus, the identity of a heart attack, cancer, or migraine headache involves an integration of abstract and experienced symptoms, the full or complete meaning of which involves abstract and concrete factors in the domains of timeline, consequences, perceived causes, and response to treatments (Andrews, Vigliocco, & Vinson, 2009). The multilevel nature of disease representations is a salient feature of physician-authors' autobiographies of life-threatening illnesses (Mandell & Spiro, 1987) and is consistent with data showing that concrete experience (symptoms and functional change) are often the main drivers of behavior. For example, concrete, symptomatic experiences are consistent and powerful predictors of utilization of health care (Berkanovic, Hurwicz, & Landsverk, 1988; McKinlay & Dutton, 1974; Pescosolido, 1992). The more interesting examples of the abstract and concrete nature of representations are those in which behavior is a product of interactions among the levels. For example, using data from six large surveys conducted in Africa and Asia, Yoder and Hornik (1996) found that mothers used oral rehydration to treat infant diarrhea if they observed concrete symptoms (e.g., vomiting, fever, reduced play) and judged the child's condition to be serious. Thus, concrete experience had direct effects as well as indirect effects (moderated by severity judgments) on behavior. Concrete experience is clearly critical in acceptance or rejection of injectable antiretroviral therapy for HIV (Horne, Cooper, & Fisher, 2008).

More dramatic evidence appears when abstract and concrete levels of processing generate conflicting goals and different criteria for appraising the efficacy of a procedure for illness management. These conflicts typically focus on differences in time frames. For example, when conditions are represented as acute, perceptual experience and the immediate effects of behavior on symptoms will control action. When a condition is represented as chronic, the time frame is abstract and lifelong and behavior is more likely to be initiated and evaluated by objective cues and indicators. Diabetes, hypertension, asthma, and cardiovascular disease provide examples of the conflicting approaches to management generated by the concrete and abstract levels of representation. Diabetic patients rely on symptoms to vary their insulin and food intake to avoid hypoglycemia even though they are trained to be active users of accurate, objective devices for assessing blood glucose levels; subjective cues often win the competition over objective indicators as guides for action (Gonder-Frederick & Cox, 1991). Hypertensive patients behave similarly. Meyer, Leventhal, and Gutmann

(1985) found that 80% of the patients in their study who were in ongoing treatment agreed with the statement that "people can't tell when their blood pressure is elevated," a response that recognizes hypertension as asymptomatic. However, 90% of these patients believed they could tell whether their blood pressure was elevated and named such somatic cues as heart palpitations, warm face, and headaches as valid indicators. More important, patients were compliant and had better blood pressure control if they believed their medications reduced their symptoms. If the medications were seen as ineffective in controlling symptoms, both adherence and blood pressure control were poor. It is likely that patients agreed with the "people can't tell" statement because doctors told them that elevated blood pressure is asymptomatic or silent. Words can, however, be empty, not anchored in experience or action.

The belief that hypertensive disease is symptomatic is unsurprising on three counts. First, the label *hypertension* suggests that specific somatic experiences accompany elevated blood pressure (Blumhagen, 1980). Second, exertion and psychological stress can produce acute, phasic changes in blood pressure that generate palpable somatic experiences (Pennebaker & Watson, 1988). Third, medical practitioners may inadvertently suggest that hypertension is symptomatic when they conduct the standard, head-to-toe "review of systems" to detect comorbidities and unfavorable sequela of hypertension and its treatment.

That these factors link specific symptoms to the label *hypertension* reflects a fundamental feature of the cognitive system, namely, the need to anchor abstractions in concrete experience (Quinn & Eimas, 1997; Rosch, Mervis, Gray, Johnson, & Boyes-Braem, 1976). We initially conceptualized this linkage as a *symmetry rule*; that is, the experience of symptoms will lead to a search for labels, and the presence of labels will lead to a search for symptoms. The effect of symptoms on the search for labels was demonstrated by Schachter and Singer's (1962) classic study of emotional contagion (1962) and is consistent with early studies showing that concepts with perceptual referents, or concrete concepts, are mastered more easily than abstract concepts (Johnson, 1975). The converse, that labels can stimulate a search for symptoms, was observed in a study where participants told that their blood pressure was elevated actually reported more symptoms, which were identical to those reported by hypertensive patients; symptom reports did not increase among participants given false feedback that their blood pressures were normal (Baumann, Cameron, Zimmerman, & Leventhal, 1989; Croyle, 1990).

A dramatic example of the impact of labeling on blood pressure was uncovered in a recent study of white-coat hypertension, which is the increase in blood pressure that some patients experience when a physician takes their blood pressure at a clinic (Spruill et al., 2007). To determine who was truly hypertensive, the 214 patients in the study were required to wear ambulatory monitoring devices for 36 hours; 119 patients proved to be hypertensive, with base-level blood pressure elevated during that time, whereas 95 were not. In each of these two groups were patients who incorrectly labeled themselves as hyper- or normotensive. The day after monitoring, patients returned to the clinic for evaluation and their blood pressure was taken by the physician. Readings were above ambulatory levels for the patients who believed they were hypertensive regardless of their actual hypertensive status. Thus, the self-characterization was related to the increase in readings and actual, ambulatory classification as hypertensive was not. Patients showing the white-coat effect also reported worry about their blood pressure. Both the elevated worry and the increased blood pressure were reactions specific to the clinic setting; neither worry nor elevated readings were related to the patients' level of trait anxiety.

PROCEDURES, ACTION PLANS, AND APPRAISALS: THE OUTPUT/PERFORMANCE SIDE OF THE SYSTEM

The representation of a health threat creates the framework for action; the response output, or performance, requires the selection of a procedure and the formation of an action plan (Cioffi, 1991; H. Leventhal, 1970). In the CSM, illness representations define the threat and activate motivation for action, identify procedures appropriate for control, define goals or targets for determining efficacy, and sustain performance until the threat is removed (H. Leventhal, Diefenbach, & Leventhal, 1992). For example, an individual suffering from a runny nose and a headache may assume that he has an acute cold (identity and symptoms), one that will last for a week (time frame), is uncomfortable but not life threatening (consequences), and whose symptoms can be managed (control). The representation sets the framework for the selection of such an over-the-counter medication as aspirin or acetaminophen (identity and control) to eliminate or reduce the symptoms in half an hour to an hour, to work for 4 to 6 hours (timelines) with no serious side effects other than stomach irritation, which can be controlled with an antacid (consequences). The representations of procedures for performance are shaped by and reflect the properties of the illness representations. The combination of the procedural representations with an action plan completes the performance, or output, side of the CSM control units.

Representations of Procedures

The variety of procedures available for the management of health threats is enormous. Procedures include such short-term actions as the use of over-the-counter medications, participation in procedures available for the early detection of cardiovascular disease and cancers, annual checkups, and surgery or other one-time repairs. In addition, the individual can engage in such longer term actions as adopting a low-fat diet, quitting smoking and maintaining cessation, adopting any number of lifetime procedures to minimize dysfunction, or living with a chronic condition.

The extraordinary variety of procedures for health maintenance and avoidance and the control of disease reflects the complexities of human biology and the cultural and social systems that have emerged in every known human population. In addition to their enormous variety and specificity, most procedures have multiple objectives; moreover, the very same procedure may have different objectives at varying points in time. Examples of multiple functions can be found for medications, physical activities, and social contacts. Insulin used to control blood glucose levels in diabetics has, for instance, been used to prevent cardiac complications among severely ill hospitalized patients who are not diabetic (Ellaham, 2010). Exercise can enhance endurance and coronary health, reduce depression, and slow and perhaps avoid dementia. Social comparison can assist in determining the cause of symptoms, clarifing expectations, and reducing fear. For example, if two people suffer from stomach pains, vomiting, and diarrhea 12 hours after sharing dessert at lunchtime, it is plausible to assume that both are suffering from food poisoning rather than to conclude they are dealing with an ulcer or stomach cancer (H. Leventhal, Hudson, & Robitaille, 1997). In addition, patients awaiting surgery are comforted if rooming with and able to view healthy survivors of treatment (Kulik & Mahler, 1997). Comparisons provide diagnostic insight and reassurance, depending, of course, on the status of the targets of comparison.

Procedures for appraising the efficacy of procedures for self-management are central to the CSM and to utility and social learning models. The factors most frequently mentioned are *response efficacy*, or the effectiveness of the response in meeting its goal, and *self-efficacy*, or the individual's belief in his or her ability to perform the response (Bandura, 1997). Both social learning theory and the CSM consider a much wider range of factors in the appraisal process than do other models. Here, anticipated and perceived efficacy are related to the magnitude of change achieved in the experience of concrete symptoms and in objective disease indicators, whether alone or in combination, along with unwanted side effects of the treatment (consequences) and timelines for effects.

The contrast between social learning and CSM approaches and models of coping is sharper still. The former focus on specific responses (e.g., taking a medication, endurance versus strength exercises), whereas studies of coping have focused on the identification and assessment of such broad classes of behavior as problem-focused coping and emotion-focused coping and have assessed these factors to predict behavioral and health outcomes (Lazarus & Launier, 1979). In the CSM, illness representations stipulate specific responses or specific classes of response for management in specific settings. For example, if gastric distress is perceived to be caused by food, the representation will encourage the use of a tablet or liquid antacid; whereas if poisoning or recurrence of stomach cancer is the perceived cause, a visit to the emergency department or oncologist would be appropriate. All three responses—taking antacid, visiting the emergency department, and seeing an oncologist—are both problem focused and emotion focused because they resolve the defined problem and minimize associated affect. The CSM can predict response choice, whereas coping theory does not.

Such generic factors as problem-focused and emotion-focused coping, along with such factors as conservation of resources (Hobfoll, 1989)—that is, reduced activity designed to conserve energy (Duke, Brownlee, Leventhal, & Leventhal, 2002)—define the potential focus for behavioral management. Thus, these factors identify strategies that can moderate the selection of a procedure from among the set of procedures consistent with the illness representation. For example, the experience of breathlessness can encourage moderate exercise or block physical activity. The choice of a procedure can be moderated by the patient's strategy; if his or her strategy is to conserve resources and minimize symptom-induced fears, rest would be preferred over exercise. If the individual's strategy is to confront problems and strengthen the system through use (E. A. Leventhal & Crouch, 1997; H. Leventhal, Leventhal, & Schaefer, 1991), moderate exercise would be preferred. Hierarchical models, representations of illness and procedures for management nested under strategies, have been proposed to deal with moderators (Krohne, 1993; E. A. Leventhal, Suls, & Leventhal, 1993). The modest predictive power of coping instruments, the inconsistent outcomes from study to study, and the failure of coping theory–based interventions to improve adherence reflect the absence of solid empirical data on different levels of analysis. Exceptions will be mentioned later (see Stone, Helder, & Schneider, 1988; Stone & Neale, 1984).

Horne and his associates (Horne, 1997; Horne, Wienman, & Hankins, 1999) have examined the range of beliefs and perceptions that people hold respecting medications. These beliefs can focus on medications in general (Figueiras et al., 2009) or on the specific medications taken to manage a particular condition (Horne, 1997, 2003). For example, people may feel medications are necessary and beneficial while simultaneously expressing such concerns about medications as feeling they are overprescribed, are risky because they can be addictive, or have harmful side effects. When evaluating medications prescribed for themselves, patients hold a range of beliefs about what is necessary. Thus, their perceptions of what they need and the benefits they may reap from the medications they take may include beliefs about the best causal route for achieving benefits, a timeline for benefit, and the relief of symptoms as well as improvement in objective indicators, beliefs, and perceptions that underlie simpler notions of efficacy and self-efficacy in use. Beliefs in the need for and concerns about one's prescribed medication affect, for example, how patients managing HIV perceive and adhere to their life-saving medications (Horne, Cooper, Gellaitry, Date, & Fisher, 2007), how individuals adhere to antihypertensive medication (Horne, Clatworthy, Polmear, & Weinman, 2001), and how sufferers adhere to medication for inflammatory bowel disease (Horne, Parham, Driscoll, & Robinson, 2009). The variety, flexibility, and variation in functional utility of specific procedures are central to the CSM. In the CSM, procedures and action plans are the components that combine with illness representations to generate the behaviors that affect health outcomes.

Action Plans

Action plans are the central players for the implementation of procedures. Studies of fear communications indicate that action plans are essential for performance (H. Leventhal, 1970; H. Leventhal, Singer, & Jones, 1965). Action plans play multiple roles in the implementation process. The most obvious role, perhaps, is establishing a cue for behavior; for example, using breakfast as a cue to take a proton pump inhibitor and an antihypertension medication, or using the biggest meal of the day as a cue to take a lipid-lowering agent. Implementation intentions, the mediator between intentions and performance, are also defined by the cueing function (Gollwitzer, 1999; Sheeran & Orbell, 2000). The second and likely most important feature of an action plan involves optimal placement of the cue in the individual's behavioral environment. For example, a patient who always drinks coffee or juice in the morning might place the medication near the coffee pot or juice carton; if liquids or breakfast are a sometime affair but tooth brushing or a mouth rinse is not, the medication should be placed in that context. Action plans must satisfy a third requirement to produce the biological effects desired with adherence: the time for use must consider the half-life of the medication in relation to the environmental context. For example, pantoprazole will be more effective in controlling acid production and lowering the probability of cancer from an esophageal ulcer if it is taken prior to the first meal of the day rather than at night. Creating an action plan to link treatment to an individual's life pattern can be a demanding and complex affair if the individual's work or life patterns are chaotic or if the individual lacks the cognitive competency to assist in designing an appropriate plan.

THE EXECUTIVE SELF: STRATEGIES AND TOOLS FOR FUNCTION

The control system, representations of illness and treatment, and action plans operate in the context of the self and its executive functions. The executive operates in three areas: monitoring the output of automatic subsystems, holding information in working memory, and regulating such behavioral processes as thoughts and overt behavior. Monitoring involves screening and selecting specific cues as targets for action and selecting criteria for evaluating behavioral outcomes. The executive uses a variety of processes to hold information in short-term memory for ongoing problem solving, organizes and rehearses material to ensure later recall when needed, and engages in other transformations of material to increase the availability of material for delayed use. Behavioral regulation involves scanning and selecting procedures or tools for responding to particular settings, modifying routines, and creating action plans.

The Prototype of Self

In addition to monitoring and regulating the monitoring, organizing and storing information, and shaping behaviors for problem solving, the executive plays a central role in evaluating the implications of current function, symptoms and illness, and treatment for future goals (Hooker & Kaus, 1994; Marcus & Nurius, 1986). That each of us possesses an underlying schema or prototype of the self is apparent from the large number of studies showing that self-assessments of health (SAH) are valid predictors of mortality. As global judgments of overall health status on a simple, 5-point scale, answering, "Would you say your health is excellent, very good, good, fair, or poor," health self-assessments predict mortality over time frames of 20 and more years in community samples and perform equally well in patients in clinical settings (Benyamini & Idler, 1999; Idler & Benyamini, 1997; Jylha, 2009). Symptoms and knowledge of existent medical conditions have been shown to be strong predictors of these self-assessments (Idler, Leventhal, McLauglin, & Leventhal, 2004), but the factor most strongly related to SAH is function, that is, the ability to perform everyday tasks, the instrumental activities of daily life. Mora and colleagues (2008) found that reports of functional competence by elderly community-dwelling participants were the strongest predictors of mortality in the 5 following years, and declines in annual reports of functional competence over the 5 years were correlated close to .90 with declines in annual SAH over that same time frame. The combination of baseline SAH and the slope of the change in annual SAH were strong predictors of mortality. (Because of their high correlation, the slope of change in annual judgments of function could be used in place of SAH.) Recent studies found that self-assessments of health and current function predicted mortality among patients with terminal cancers and were, in fact, stronger predictors of mortality than available clinical indicators (Shadbolt, Barresi, & Craft, 2002; Teno, Weitzen, Fennell, & Mor, 2001).

In summary, the more than 200 community studies from different countries and the somewhat smaller but equally impressive number of studies of clinical samples provide incontrovertible support for the assumption that individuals have access to subjective cues that provide valid evidence on the viability of their physical selves. The data stand in stark contrast to the studies on the validity of predictions based on affective states: predictions of future affect are notoriously inaccurate; and projections of future preferences, for example, for thirst (Van Boven & Loewenstein, 2003) or for treatment, are biased by current emotional states. Identification of the specific features of the self that inform SAH is critical for the elucidation of mechanisms underlying prototype checks that lead to the activation of illness representations and affect treatment decisions, including those made when terminally ill (Saraiya, Bodnar-Deren, Leventhal, & Leventhal, 2008). The evidence from the two very different sources, that is, clinical and community studies, converge in suggesting that functional changes are the critical inputs to self-assessments of health. Function, however, is a very broad category; and individuals may differ in the attention and weight they give to one or another functional change. The CSM also suggests that the weight given to a specific functional change may depend on the rate of decline: rapid declines tend to create a sense of urgency, and gradual ones tend to be attributed to general issues in aging. Filling in these details will be critical for understanding the dynamics underlying health and illness decisions. These will be discussed in greater detail in sections 2 and 3.

Tools for Self-Management

Although much, if not most, monitoring of behavioral output, short-term information storage, and response modification occur automatically, these processes are shared and duplicated by executive processes. Executive-level monitoring (screening and target selection), outcome evaluation, and response control differ from monitoring, evaluation, and control at well-practiced, more automatic levels. Executive processes are slower, less detailed, more global, and more resource intensive than well-practiced, implicit processes. These differences are a necessary consequence of the executive position as a general problem solver. Borrowing from other cognitive models, the CSM hypothesizes that the executive requires generic tools and strategies for engaging and managing a broad array of automatic systems and environmental contexts. The cognitive tools or heuristics for managing changing somatic experiences and functional changes—for example, controlling the direction of attention, retrieving information that is "available" and "representative" (Tversky & Kahneman, 1974)—are not necessarily tuned or relevant to the condition at hand. Behavioral tools or heuristics (e.g., stop, step back and take another look, slow down, and monitor while rehearsing) are general strategies or tools and are not designed to fit a specific context; they are similar to the contrast between a variable wrench and one designed to fit a one-quarter-inch-diameter hexagonal bolt. We will discuss these processes in greater detail as we address the dynamics of common-sense regulation in the following section.

THE DYNAMICS OF COMMONSENSE SELF-REGULATION

Studies from the CSM framework have examined some of the processes underlying decisions and actions to control physical illnesses; these studies are an important contribution of the CSM for understanding self-regulation dynamics. We will describe findings in the following areas: (a) the construction of illness representations, a theoretically implicit and largely automatic process; (b) the interaction of executive and automatic processes for the selection of procedures for managing cardiovascular conditions; and (c) the assessment of the prototypes that underlie the constructive process (discussed in section 1).

Examining these dynamic processes provides a view of the interaction between the content and structure of commonsense models; it brings the system to life. Whether the findings are from cross-sectional or longitudinal data, they provide a single picture or a sequence of snapshots of the changing common-sense model at specific time points. We do not have a running, "online" view of the system's operation. Despite this shortcoming, one can see how the system likely operates and can detect issues requiring further empirical study. Our view of the system can be described in the following sequence: (a) the experience of somatic sensations and functions discrepant from the usual, normal self are detected automatically and matched either automatically (nonconscious) or deliberately (conscious) to underlying illness prototypes to form illness representations; (b) once these experiences enter awareness, either because they match a specific prototype to form a representation or because of increases in their intensity, duration, and disruptiveness, the executive functions of the self-system (ES) is engaged in self-examination and treatment; (c) if the condition increases in severity and duration or fails to respond to self-treatment, the ES will discuss the condition with someone close; and (d) medical care will ensue if the close other concurs with the self-expressed concern. The sequence is not linear, however. Individuals strongly predisposed to meditate, exercise, or seek medical care may respond to somatic cues far too subtle and vague to match a prototype of any specific illness and engage in these behaviors preventively, for example, exercising to get rid of a subtle sense of malaise that does not match the prototype of a specific illness.

Our review also highlights issues involved in the processing, selection, appraisal, and formation of action plans—part of the CSM dynamic process—that need further investigation. The first are the details of the "normal" prototype of the physical and functional self. The second is an examination of prototypes of illnesses. An examination of system dynamics makes clear that prototypes are not the same as representations of illnesses and treatments; prototypes underlie the activation of representations. Prototypes also play a critical role in the arousal of emotion; these processes will be discussed briefly. Finally, we will touch upon the need for increased understanding of the processes by which voluntary self-management routines are automated.

DETECTING AND MATCHING DEVIATIONS TO ILLNESS PROTOTYPES

In the absence of distractions, changes in somatic sensations and physical and cognitive functions enter awareness automatically (Pennebaker, 1999). When these sensations deviate from the normal or usual sense of self, they will be compared automatically and matched to one or another underlying prototype or schema (Bishop, 1991). When matched and recognized as an example of such a familiar experience as a stress headache, muscle strain, gastric distress, allergies, or a head cold, the condition will be perceived as acute and self-resolving (Bishop & Converse, 1986). The CSM will engage conscious, executive function to select and perform a procedure that is familiar and expected to be effective: a favorite home remedy, over-the-counter medication, or bed rest, for example. The time frames for the representation of the condition and the self-selected treatment establish a criterion for evaluating efficacy; thus, for example, a headache should go away in half an hour to an hour after taking aspirin or acetaminophen.

Deviations Can Activate Executive Decisions

When symptoms and functional changes exceed the threshold for disruptiveness or do not respond to usually effective self-management, the executive system is "wakened" to further action. An excellent example of this process is seen in Cameron and colleagues' 1993 analysis of the factors leading to the use of medical care in a sample of 111 elderly individuals interviewed immediately prior to their seeing their primary care physician for a self-initiated visit. Not surprisingly, all 111 subjects reported experiencing new or worrisome symptoms. The overpowering role of somatic changes in initiating the visit was clear when these symptomatic care seekers were compared to control participants who had not sought care and were matched to them on age, gender, and family size. These matched control participants were called as soon as possible and asked how they were feeling and if they had any symptoms or functional problems; only 30% had a new or worrisome symptom, a difference of 70% and a clear example of the power of symptoms as initiators of care seeking. Symptoms alone are not, however, sufficient for care seeking; indeed, common sense suggests symptoms have to be painful or disruptive of daily function, fail to respond to self-management, or match to a prototype that activates a representation of a potentially threatening illness. The data supported these assumptions: relative to the representations of symptoms of the 111 care seekers, the symptoms reported by the 33 symptomatic matched controls were rated as less serious and disruptive, of shorter duration, and less likely to be labeled as symptoms of a specific illness. In addition, control participants were less likely to have discussed their symptoms with another person, and those who did were much less likely to be advised to seek care. In sum, the representations of their symptoms were less fleshed out; neither the representations nor their efforts at control had crossed the border from minor deviations to potential threat. Deviations that are sufficiently severe and threatening, that is, deviations that cross a border (the crossing can be fear based and automatic or a deliberate decision), lead to discussion with others and care seeking, all complex processes in the domain of executive function.

Mora and colleagues (2002) replicated and extended Cameron et al.'s findings (1993) by comparing the magnitude of the relationship of personal traits and the attributes of the illness episode in the prediction of care seeking. Personal characteristics, including age, gender, illness burden, trait negative affect, and self-assessments of health, had no relationship to care seeking for either an acute condition or a flare of a chronic condition. By contrast, four characteristics of the unfolding episode were related to care seeking: number of symptoms, severity, duration, and novelty of the symptoms. As with the findings for white-coat hypertension, anxiety specific to the ongoing episode was a strong predictor of care seeking for ongoing chronic conditions, but trait anxiety was not.

Care seeking requires both the elaboration of key features of the representation and evidence of failure to manage or control symptoms. These studies suggest that the initial representation of somatic and functional changes as a familiar, benign event is fragile and readily disrupted if the ongoing changes last and are unresponsive to self-initiated action. The tendency to perceive events as acute is consistent with reality, given that most symptoms and dysfunctions are temporary, and consistent with the need to sustain optimistic expectations (Taylor, 1983, 1991). For example, 40% of the women entering chemotherapy treatment for metastatic breast cancer believed their disease equivalent to an acute, curable illness (H. Leventhal, Easterling, Coons, Luchterhand, & Love, 1986). This statistic is also true of chronic conditions that are less life threatening than cancer, such as asthma. The great majority of patients hospitalized with asthma believe they will have asthma all their lives, but over half also believe they have asthma only when symptomatic (Halm, Mora, & Leventhal, 2006). Patients whose asthma representations are modeled on the episodic nature of flares are less likely to use medication to prevent attacks, to be checked when asymptomatic, or to test pulmonary function and use results to modify medication dosages. Data also suggest that as symptoms decline and function appears to return to normal, the executive self tends to act as though all is well and self-regulation declines. Self-management can stop even when a patient agrees that he or she has such a chronic condition as asthma (Halm et al., 2006), has AIDS (Horne et al., 2004; Reynolds et al., 2009), or experiences myocardial infarction (Sambamoorthi, Moynihan, McSpiritt, & Crystal, 2001).

Matching Experience to Prototypes Activates Illness Representations

If illness and treatment representations are generated from the matching and/or integration of experience with underlying prototypes, how does this matching occur? The CSM is specific about the matching process, identifying the elements involved in matching, suggesting the sequence in which they operate, and distinguishing which portions of the process are automatic and which remain under executive control. Empirical studies within the CSM framework (Bauman, Cameron, Zimerman, & Leventhal, 1989; Bishop, 1991; Bishop & Converse, 1986), related investigations (Godoy-Izquierdo, López-Chicheri, López-Torrecillas, Vélez, & Godoy, 2007), and reviews (Brody & Kleban, 1983; Stoller, 1993, 1997) suggest that representations of illness and treatments, action plans, and overt action are activated by the match of experience to prototypes. Such diagrams as Figure 1.2 are concordant with the suggestion that the process is often linear; that is, somatic and external stimuli generate illness representations that generate procedures implemented by action plans, the outcomes of which are appraised for efficacy. The CSM also includes two sets of reverse arrows, as shown in Figure 1.2. The first identifies a feedback path indicating that postaction feedback can alter any or all of the prior components, beginning with the stimulus inputs (symptom reduction), continuing through changes in dosing and selection of an alternative procedure, and then moving from self-management to expert assistance (solid, leftward pointing arrows). The second, dashed, leftward-pointing arrow defines a feed-forward path by which action plans or the availability of a procedure generates somatic stimuli and creates illness representations. A common example would involve the activation of vague somatic stimuli when thinking about the diagnosis or treatment of a threatening condition, as in the case of white-coat hypertension (Spruill et al., 2007). Pathways such as these are also seen in the "worried well" (Cameron, Leventhal, & Leventhal, 1995) and healthy individuals who seek care for cardiovascular disease (Aikens, Zvolensky, & Eifert, 2001; Bunde & Martin, 2006). These feed-forward pathways exist in many complex systems; however, their influence may be visible only in relatively small percentages of episodes and individuals. Because the traditional linear order is likely most common, we will begin by addressing the processes involved in the conversion of somatic stimuli to symptoms and illness representations.

Specific Elements Convert Sensations to Symptoms: The Matching Process

The ability to distinguish nonself from self, or pathogenic processes from normal and nonthreatening departures from baseline, is typically the initial step in the activation of illness representations. Lazarus (1966) has labeled the interpretive step of translating somatic sensations into symptoms "primary appraisal." The word *appraisal* implies that decoding is a conscious process; this is unfortunate because much of the decoding process takes place automatically and implicitly, that is, outside awareness (Henderson, Hagger, & Orbell, 2007; Shiloh, Peretz, & Iss, 2007).

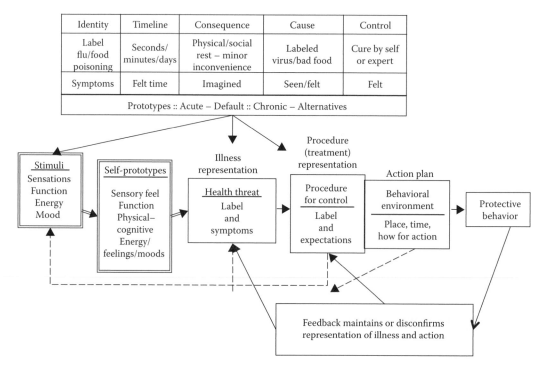

Identity	Timeline	Consequence	Cause	Control
Label flu/food poisoning	Seconds/ minutes/days	Physical/social rest – minor inconvenience	Labeled virus/bad food	Cure by self or expert
Symptoms	Felt time	Imagined	Seen/felt	Felt
Prototypes :: Acute – Default :: Chronic – Alternatives				

FIGURE 1.2　An early view of the CSM. Solid arrows identify pathways for rapid, relatively automatic processing from detection of deviations, through activation of a representation to feedback. The five domains of the representations affect the interpretation of cues, set targets and time frames for action and anticipated outcomes, and efforts to control perceived causes. Dashed arrows represent the effects of action readiness (procedures and plans) to searching for, detecting, and representing cues for action; this is a feed-forward pathway.

The data we have reviewed suggest three processes common to this early step. First, a somatic sensation or change in function will become a source of uncertainty and concern if it deviates significantly from the normal or healthy self, fails to match an existent prototype of an acute but benign condition, and interferes with daily functioning. Expert-care seeking is likely if the deviations are severe, long-lasting, unresponsive to self or family management, and distracting from everyday activities. These factors may also be accompanied by concern that the observed changes may match a chronic or life-threatening condition. Second, if the somatic sensations and functional changes match an illness schemata or prototype of a familiar, acute condition, the match is more rapid, even automatic, if all symptoms match the underlying prototype (Bishop & Converse, 1986). These rapidly formed representations activate treatment procedures embedded in well-learned action plans, making care seeking unlikely if home-based treatments alleviate the initiating discrepancy. Third, the deviations may quickly be matched to a serious, chronic illness (e.g., cancer, diabetes) or a life-threatening acute or episodic condition (e.g., heart attack or asthma).

Perceptual recognition is the initial process in each of the foregoing pathways: a deviation is perceived and represented automatically; or it is perceived, not definitively matched, and remains ambiguous. The prototype-check process does not require the use of abstract symbols or words. The word *headache* is not necessary to feel and recognize headaches any more than the word *table* is needed to see and recognize tables; recognition is automatic and further supplemented by self-involvement; for example, if resting one's arm on the table causes it to wobble, one may be reminded of earlier situations where a wobbly table created an embarrassing spill.

An array of expectations respecting causes, consequences, and the like, will come into play once the deviation is lodged in a prototype because prototypes are amalgams of declarative (semantic and episodic) and nondeclarative (perceptual and procedural) memories (Squire, 2004). Cognitive scientists have described this matching process in general terms, undefined elements linking experience to schemata from the bottom up and linking schemata to experiences from the top down. This bidirectional process is sensitive to context (Kahneman & Miller, 1986). Early versions of the CSM were equally vague, describing matching as a process of finding symmetry between symptoms and labels, that is, as a built-in need to search for and find abstractions to fit concrete experiences and to find concrete experiences to make sense of abstractions (H. Leventhal, Meyer, & Nerenz, 1980), an approach consistent with the English empiricist view espoused by John Locke (Andrews, Vigliocco, & Vinson, 2009).

Data do, however, support the hypothesis that an identifiable set of elements is involved in the linking process. As Bishop (1991) suggested, the elements fall into the five domains of illness representations: identity, timelines, cause, consequences, and control. The linking elements in the identity domain are common sense and based on sensory patterns (e.g., is the sensation sharp, dull, or throbbing?) and location (e.g., chest, leg, or arm)—the real estate of the mind. Linking elements in the timelines domain are equally common sense and complex; they include rates of onset, duration (acute versus chronic), and rates of decline (which overlap with linking elements in the control domain). Control linking elements are highly varied and range from home remedies (e.g., aspirin, chicken soup) and prescribed medications (Horne et al., 2004; Horne & Weinman, 2002) to more complex, threatening, and sometimes noxious interventions (e.g., surgery, chemotherapy). Causal linking elements include triggers (e.g., falls, ingested substances); long-term, slow-acting, potentially changeable lifestyle elements (e.g., smoking, diet, physical activity, stress); and stable features of self (e.g., genes, phenotypic features). Severe pain and physical dysfunction (e.g., the inability to rise from bed or to walk) are examples of immediate consequences with implications for managing activities of daily life.

These elements are used to link experience (i.e., somatic sensations, functional changes, and alterations in experience following the enactment of a procedure for control) to one or more underlying illness prototypes. The result is activation of an illness representation, a concrete and concept-rich hypothesis as to the nature of the condition. The representation creates the framework for further action, that is, "hypothesis testing" in which the passage of time and results of testing confirm and expand the initial representation or disconfirm it and encourage a search for further information (typically social in nature).

THE INTERACTION OF EXECUTIVE AND AUTOMATIC, IMPLICIT PROCESSES IN CARDIAC DISEASE

Executive functions interact continually with the automatic matching process we have just described. This can be seen in the contrast between patient responses to symptoms of myocardial infarction (MI) and heart failure (HF). The dynamics also provide insights into the executive self's reliance on the abstract features of illness representations when integrating its judgments of illness with procedures and action plans. The data also suggest how different methods for conceptualizing and assessing illness and treatment prototypes will affect the development of interventions for the management of these life-threatening conditions (see Figure 1.3).

Myocardial Infarction

Bunde and Martin (2006) conducted a detailed analysis of the factors affecting swiftness of care seeking following the onset of an MI. They interviewed 433 patients, on average, 8 days following hospitalization for MI. The interviews consisted of a detailed review of the emotional experience at symptom onset, the perception of factors affecting symptoms, actions taken to interpret and manage symptoms until deciding to call for care, and the time of arrival at the hospital.

The factors associated with swifter care seeking included prior history of MI, location of symptoms (i.e., the chest and arm pain), severity of symptoms, and sweating. Location and the number and severity of symptoms most likely led to care seeking because they are consistent with a prototype of MI. Sweating, which is usually associated with physical effort, was an ambiguous and unsettling cue because the patients were not exerting themselves. The ambiguity added motivation to seek care in order to define what was happening (Cameron et al., 1995). Increased delay in care seeking was associated with gastrointestinal distress, an experience that did not match the MI prototype, and depressive symptoms as measured by the Patient Health Questionnaire depression scale (PHQ-9; Kroenke & Spitzer, 2002). Although total scores on the PHQ-9 were related to a longer delay, a post hoc analysis showed that the effect was attributable to two items: feelings of fatigue and sleep disturbance, suggesting that lack of energy rather than a true depressive symptoms was responsible for the increased delay in care seeking. An interesting feature of the data was the independence of the three prototype checks from reports of depression; location, pattern, and fatigue had separate and independent effects on delay. Thus, the decision to seek care, an executive action, involved a self-made and socially reinforced response to a commonsense representation of a heart attack, and it was slowed by an overall state of fatigue.

Heart Failure

Heart failure, cardiac muscle dysfunction leading to the reduction of the heart's pumping ability, typically follows a history of hypertension and myocardial infarctions. Heart failure, however, does not manifest the same location and temporal features as symptoms of MI; that is, it is not accompanied by the abrupt onset of severe pains in the chest and/or arm or sweating. Rather, the symptoms of heart failure include chronic fatigue, swollen legs, and breathlessness—symptoms that lack an abrupt onset of pain, are chronic, and do not occur in the heart. In addition to failing to match the prototype of a heart attack, the location and temporal features of heart failure match alternative prototypes. For example, chronic fatigue and swollen legs may be interpreted as part of the aging process, and breathlessness may be interpreted as a symptom of a pulmonary problem. Because the symptoms of heart failure do not match the prototype of a heart condition, it should be no surprise that these symptoms do not lead patients to perceive themselves as having a heart disease. Furthermore, because these patients do not recognize the presence of a heart problem, they fail to seek care when experiencing symptoms of heart failure. That is, the lack of a clear representation results in the inaction of the executive system.

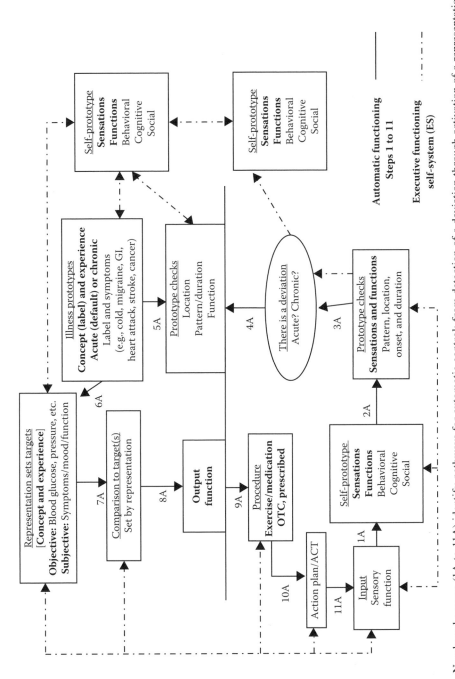

FIGURE 1.3 Numbered arrows (1A to 11A) identify pathways for automatic control: from detection of a deviation through activation of a representation of somatic cues to feedback from action (11A). Dashed arrows represent monitoring and efforts at behavioral control by executive functions of the self-system (ES). The sequence of processing will vary with prior history: automatic preceding EF for familiar illnesses, simultaneously for novel somatic changes that do not immediately match to a prototype. EF is increasingly active in the near term, fading out as self-management is automated. Coherence and long-term maintenance occur when automatic and executive processes have common features.

Qualitative interviews with patients diagnosed with heart failure provide vivid examples of the mismatch between symptoms of heart failure and common-sense models of heart disease (Horowitz, Rein, & Leventhal, 2004). Patients state, for example:

> When you hear about having heart problems you're supposed to feel maybe a pain in your left arm, maybe a pain in your chest, or pressure. I couldn't describe what I felt as pressure but I guess it must have been that, uh because I had to struggle in order to talk … if I had chest pain, and then I would have said, okay, I'll call and say I'm having chest pain but it didn't just seem like anything came together where I could call. (Horowitz et al., 2004, p. 634)

Because heart failure symptoms fail to match a prototype, that is, because the symptoms are not anchored in a conceptual diagnosis, the symptom experience lacks the conceptual component that is critical for connecting different types of symptoms experienced at different time points and integrating these experiences with procedures and action plans for treatment. This is evident in the following exchange:

> Interviewer (I): How do you make that decision that it's time to go to the emergency room?
> Patient (Pt.): These things seem to happen in the middle of the night so I don't call doctors.
> I: You said you weren't feeling that great …
> Pt. I was kind of tired … didn't seem to be anything out of the ordinary.
> I: Were there any warning signs earlier?
> Pt.: Not that I could detect.… I didn't feel that great. Oh, I guess that I could have gone to the doctor after I had that collapse on the hallway floor. (Horowitz et al., 2004, p. 635)

The behavioral response, an executive decision, is symptom driven and time specific when symptoms do not match and activate a conceptual category or prototype (Bishop, Briede, Cavazos, Grotzinger, & McMahon, 1987). Thus, patients know they "have" heart failure, but the concept is an empty label because it is not connected to concrete experience. The symptoms associated with heart failure, for example, fatigue and the collapse on the hallway floor, are related respectively to aging and a chance episode that might be age- but not heart-related. Figure 1.3 depicts the ongoing self-monitoring of discrete experiences as the executive system attempts to make sense of somatic cues that do not automatically fit an illness prototype.

CONCEPTUALIZATION AND ASSESSMENT OF PROTOTYPES

Given the critical role played by prototypes in the generation of illness representations, investigators have used a mix of empirical approaches in attempts to "map" the prototype domain. The differences in methods reflect differences in the conceptualization of these memory structures and how they contribute to the activation of illness representations.

Clustering by Judgments of Similarity and Clustering by Elements

D'Andrade and colleagues (1972) used multidimensional scaling to generate a hierarchical model of people's perceptions of diseases. The picture emerged from an analysis of similarity judgments of pairs of disease labels, every disease paired once with every other one. The multilevel tree structure that emerged showed that diseases branched successively on the basis of their causes, control, symptoms, and impact on function rather than factors involved in diagnosis. The maps of illness labels generated by multidimensional scaling overlapped considerably with the experiences defined in the CSM though they differed somewhat across cultures; that is, the maps generated by multidimensional scaling were more easily interpreted for English-speaking Americans than for Mexican participants. Recent data show that Hispanic Americans are more likely than either whites or African Americans to perceive themselves as having asthma only when they have symptoms (Halm et al., 2006).

Bishop (1991) examined how prototypes affect perception and judgments by investigating how participants would respond to and time their responses to sets of symptoms assembled either randomly or to represent specific prototypes. The symptom sets were based on the assumption that everyone has fairly well defined prototypes for many such everyday acute conditions as head colds, stomachaches, or stress headaches and prototypes for a number of serious and potentially life-threatening conditions, among them diabetes, heart attacks, and cancers. Symptom sets that "fit" specific prototypes were more easily and more quickly identified (labeled) than were randomly selected sets, and they elicited more comprehensive and fully elaborated representations (e.g., perceptions of causes and consequences). Bishop (1991) suggested that illnesses are formed into prototype clusters if they are perceived to be similar to each other with respect to cause, consequences, control, timeline, and the like; he suggests that these shared properties need not correspond to the "biological reality" of these illnesses. For example, people are fearful of and avoid being near and having any physical contact with individuals with HIV/AIDS because they group AIDS with other contagious conditions (Bishop, 1991). The suggestion that the representations of a specific illness can affect behavior because its features (e.g., causal beliefs, symptom experiences) place it in clusters with illnesses with quite different biomedical features testifies to the importance of the conceptual level of illness representations for executive functioning. It also makes clear that categorization or clustering can lead to actions that are biologically invalid. We suspect that the common tendency to respond to chronic, life-threatening conditions as though they are acute and self-limited, namely, treating symptoms and ignoring the underlying condition, occurs far more frequently than not and poses more serious consequences than anticipated for individual health and health care costs.

Clusters, Disease-Specific Prototypes, and Episode-Specific Schemata

Clusters of features forming groups of related-disease prototypes and illness-specific prototypes are two of three suggested ways of conceptualizing the memory structures that capture experience and activate illness representations. The third way suggests that the memory structures are episode specific. Croyle and Barger (1993) have pointed to the contrast between Bishop and Converse's proposal (1986) that the activation of representations involves the matching of symptoms to a generalized prototype and Leventhal and colleagues' description (H. Leventhal, 1982, 1986; H. Leventhal & Diefenbach, 1991) of the process as an integration of current symptoms with an episode-specific prototype. Bishop and Converse's model is supported by data showing that symptom sets constructed to match a prototype are more quickly labeled and better recalled than a randomly constructed symptom set. H. Leventhal and colleagues' initial basis of their formulation, namely, that episode-specific memory schemata underlie the decoding of somatic sensations and the formation of illness representations, was based on clinical reports of phantom pain. Phantom pains are most often reported following limb amputation, and the pain embedded in the phantom limb is typically identical to that experienced in an episode immediately prior to amputation. The somatic sensations of limb and pain appear to be stored in perceptual memory (Melzack, 1992), and the complexity of the memory is highlighted by the manner in which the pain can ebb and flow as the phantom limb changes its apparent position. Croyle and Barger (1993) suggest that "only frequently experienced illness, such as the flu, stimulates the development of prototypes" and that "severe or unusual episodes, however, may serve as a direct basis for comparison" (p. 34). Although Coyle and Barger's position is likely a valid resolution of H. Leventhal and colleagues' and Bishop and Converse's viewpoints, it is basically an issue for future theoretical and empirical analysis. Its significance will become apparent when we discuss the cultural and social contexts of CSM formation in the final section.

SELECTING PROCEDURES AND CONSTRUCTING ACTION PLANS

Early studies on fear communication (summarized in H. Leventhal, 1970), studies on preparing patients for responding to noxious medical examinations and treatments (Johnson, 1975; Johnson &

Leventhal, 1974), and more recent studies of implementation intentions (Gollwitzer, 1999; Orbell & Verplanken, 2010; Sheeran & Orbell, 2000; Sullivan & Rothman, 2008) have all tested the benefits of implementing action plans for behavioral success. Their designs were experimental and involved either providing participants with plans or instructing participants to form intentions to act to specific cues and to reach specific goals. Similarly, H. Leventhal et al. (1965) exposed participants to strong or mild threat messages about the risks of tetanus and randomly assigned some participants to an action plan condition in which they were given a map of their university campus with the health service clearly marked, asked to review their class schedules, and told to find a time when they would pass the health service when changing classes. Action planning involved a review of daily behavior in one's local environment to identify specific cues of place and times that fit ongoing daily behavior patterns and were suitable niches for taking action. The plan was designed to meet an immediate goal (i.e., inoculation) and a longer term goal (i.e., resistance to tetanus). The importance of specifying a goal was clear, for selecting a locus and a cue for action did not lead to inoculation in the absence of a high- or low-fear message that established the goal of avoiding tetanus. The longer term goal justified finding a locus and setting a cue to act on the proximal goal of inoculation. Studies of implementation intentions replicate these conditions by asking subjects to select a cue for action or by specifying a cue for action, specifying the selection of a goal for action, and asking participants to choose the context for cueing action (Orbell & Verplanken, 2010; study 3). Sampling studies in this burgeoning literature reveal, however, that relatively little is known about how people generate action plans in their community and home environments.

Although the CSM has not yet generated studies examining how individuals generate action plans in their local environments, it does point to a number of issues and suggest hypotheses respecting the process of planning. Planning to adopt a new behavior, to stop or reshape an ongoing behavior, requires monitoring the context for action and the action itself, which are executive functions. It also requires selecting and testing cues for initiating and evaluating action, that is, determining whether the cues are available, reliable, and valid indicators for evaluating outcomes. Tools used for focusing attention, monitoring and reviewing the environment, and monitoring and shaping behavior are available and are part of everyday parlance. For example, such comments as "look closely" (focus attention), "stop a minute," "slow down," "take a second look," and "step back" (Hardy, 2006; Landin, 1994; Salomon & Globerson, 1987) identify specific tools that are used for improving performance in sports, playing musical instruments, controlling impulses, and avoiding persuasive scams. They are tools to locate specific places for modifying performance and improving self-regulation in a specific environment.

TRANSLATING THE CSM INTO CLINICAL INTERVENTIONS

Although our understanding of the processes involved in self-management has deepened over the past three decades, few efforts have been made to translate these insights into interventions to improve communication about and management of chronic conditions in clinical settings (see McAndrew et al., 2008, for notable exceptions). The failure to do so is surprising given that five chronic conditions consume approximately 70% of all health care spending (Halverson, 2007) and low-cost treatments are available for effective control of at least four of the five (asthma, two cardiovascular diseases [MI and HF], diabetes, and depression). Furthermore, evidence from randomized trials indicates that some behavioral interventions can control and perhaps prevent disease onset. For example, four randomized trials have shown that behavioral interventions can control, if not stop, the progression from a prediabetic state to diagnosed diabetes, and they do so for a period of 2 to 4 years (Diabetes Prevention Program Research Group, 2002). Behavior change is also more effective than medication in controlling the progression of diabetes (Diabetes Prevention Program Research Group, 2002; Tuomilehto et al., 2001). This evidence is especially important because diabetes is reaching epidemic proportions worldwide. Also, because diabetes is a systemic disorder, it creates the conditions for such comorbidities as cardiovascular disease, kidney failure, and blindness; thus, controlling diabetes can affect multiple conditions (Fleming et al., 2001). Adherence is still a major problem, however; as former U.S. Surgeon General C. Everett Koop stated, "Drugs don't work in patients who don't take them" (quoted in Osterberg & Blaschke, 2005, p. 487).

WHERE DO WE START?

The diabetes prevention trials provide proof of a concept: behavior can be changed, and change can slow or stop disease progression. However, the methods used are unlikely to be translated to practice. Patients in the behavioral arm of the Diabetes Prevention Program trial had face-to-face sessions with a behavior-change therapist, received numerous phone contacts, and were included because they were highly motivated (Diabetes Prevention Program Research Group, 2002). Can we do better given what we know about how patients manage health and illness? Experts in health policy start from the top down, addressing such issues as affordability and access, the integration of care, and what practitioners are paid to do. Psychologists begin at the ground level, moving from how patients understand illness and treatment, through relationships with providers, to barriers to effective self-care in home environments. The diabetes trials support our view that interventions need to start with both top-down and bottom-up approaches. An effective behavioral intervention will be completely useless if it cannot be implemented in real-world settings.

The CSM and Changing the Microsystem

We believe the CSM is particularly well suited as a framework for generating interventions in clinical settings and doing so within the constraints of many health care systems. Although illness representations form an excellent starting point for intervention, it is critical to recognize that illness representations will change with changes in the progression of the underlying disease and in response to treatment and lifestyle behaviors. Because the CSM is based on a control systems approach, it is inherently dynamic. Thus, illness representations create a set of changing goals or targets for behavioral management, some of which are proximal and others of which are remote. In addition, the CSM assumes these targets are both concrete (i.e., experience-based features of representations) and abstract (e.g., such concepts as good health). It is also presumed that concepts differ in connectedness to experience: concrete concepts are more tightly linked to experience, and remote goals are more likely to be abstract. It is also clear that abstract concepts play a critical role in linking temporally separated experiences and targets; for example, patients see some symptoms (e.g., a fall on the floor; breathlessness; swelling feet) as separate events unless they are linked by the data-rich concept of heart failure (Horowitz et al., 2004). Finally, the CSM has generated evidence indicating that one can identify the elements critical for both intrapsychic and interpersonal discourse—the prototype checks that connect ongoing experience with illness prototypes and communicate the details of experience to others. The prototypes underlying the system, that is, the perceptual and procedural content and concepts that define the self and specific diseases, are more stable than representations. The self-system is the most stable and difficult to change.

Representations of procedures for prevention and control and the action plans in which procedures are embedded form the second set of processes involved in the CSM's conceptualization of self-management. These representations are also central in the discourse among patients, practitioners, family, and friends. Behaviors that produce substantial changes in salient, concrete targets of illness representations, and do so more quickly, establishing identity and timeline, will form coherent bonds with the illness model. If these behaviors are not connected to the abstract features of the illness representation, however, the behaviors are very likely to be episodic or present only when symptoms are present; and so they will be stopped when symptoms clear. To initiate and sustain a health-promoting or illness-controlling behavior, the intervention needs to create a plausible link to targets defined by the illness model, specify timelines for effects, and ensure that both the actions and their effects are perceived as action progresses and are anchored in a conceptual framework that links current moments with future goals. These intervention characteristics are complex criteria, and few studies meet these requirements.

Successful Interventions

The studies that preceded the development of the CSM—for example, the examination of the effects of fear communications on attitudes and behavior and the effects of preparation for difficult medical treatments—were intervention based. A main contribution of the fear studies was the validation that action plans played a critical role in translating attitudes (representations of health threats) into active behavior (H. Leventhal, 1970). The fear studies anticipated two important issues validated in later studies: the importance of establishing a cue to elicit behavior and the need to specify a goal or rationale for performing the behavior. Action plans had no effect on performance if not associated with a message that defined the possibility and widespread presence of threat (H. Leventhal, 1970). The fear component of the messages used concrete images to depict the cause and consequences of the disease and embedded the imagery in a conceptual framework that defined the causal agent as universal in the environment; concrete targets were everywhere and unavoidable. Action planning was assisted pictorially with a map of the campus and verbally by instructing participants to locate the recommended action at an optimal point in their daily schedules, thereby defining the cues for action. Timelines were not specified, nor were concrete consequences; participants could think they were safe following inoculation but had no concrete evidence of safety. The college students' prototypes of preventive treatments were sufficient to generate meaningful frameworks for action.

Many of these features have been replicated in studies of implementation intentions that examine how the specification of cues for action bridges the gap between intention and action and how the specification of goals (i.e., making behavioral goals more specific) helps to bridge this gap (Bodemheimer & Handley, 2009; Orbell & Verplanken, 2010). Planning, that is, reviewing ongoing behavioral patterns to locate interstices for performing recommended actions, is ignored or attended to implicitly. By contrast, planning is the most important feature of action plans in the CSM, and it is a key factor in cognitive behavioral therapies (e.g., Wilson & Vitousek, 1999). In addition, studies of implementation intentions tend to ignore the conceptual distinction between the nonverbal (perceptual and procedural processes) and abstract features of plans and goals. We believe that attending to both aspects of plans and targets or goals for action is a necessary component for any successful intervention. The limited attention to perceptual and procedural processes is apparent in an otherwise interesting study contrasting the goals associated with an implementation intention to do something (e.g., exercise), in comparison to the goals associated with a plan to *not* do something (Richetin, Conner, & Perugini, 2010). For example, goals for eating and not eating meat were assessed using attitude questions that measured general feelings about meat eating ("What is your overall attitude toward eating / avoiding eating plenty of meat?") and general beliefs about exercise (e.g., staying fit versus having more time to do other things). The data provide convincing evidence for the hypothesis that the goals for action and for nonaction are different. The attitudes and goals are, however, described in a relatively abstract fashion. For example, it is unclear whether meat avoiders avoid the idea of meat or are repelled by the sight and odor of blood and cooked flesh. Likewise, are meat eaters attracted by the sight and odor of gravy or by the chewing of a tasty piece of beef washed down with a glass of red wine? The CSM would argue that changing these preferences and behaviors requires addressing the concrete experience that will be linked to a new abstract goal structure (e.g., meat eating is conceptualized as providing a source of proteins to build muscle mass). Modifying specific behaviors that create the cognitive and emotional reactions involved in taste preferences would be the likely approach for a cognitive behavioral treatment and the CSM.

The CSM in Clinical Practice

Developing and testing hypotheses in the clinical setting is the major challenge facing the CSM and all situated models. Two different approaches have been taken to implement the CSM in clinical settings. The first and earliest used a structured approach for all patients, whereas recent examples have been more flexible and have incorporated features common to cognitive behavioral therapies. The second approach aims to improve the biomedical validity of patient representations and the efficacy of their action plans by modifying the behavior of the clinician, influencing how the clinician explores information and presents it to the patient.

Using a Structured Approach

Earlier versions of the CSM used the same intervention for all patients to facilitate acceptance of and effective responding to noxious medical interventions. There is also a second, larger set of studies supporting the value of focusing attention on sensory features and providing simple procedures for responding during medical procedures. In the first of these studies, patients scheduled for a morning endoscopy were contacted by a nurse the evening before the examination (Johnson & Leventhal, 1974). Half of the patients were randomly assigned to view photographs and listen to texts that described the basic features of the examination room and its equipment; the other half saw photographs and listened to text that described what someone would feel when undergoing each of the steps depicted (e.g., throat swabbing) and the specific actions to take at each point (e.g., mouth breathing). Focusing attention on somatic sensations normalized patients' interpretations; the sensations were no longer cues of impending threat, and heart rates decelerated during the examination for the patients prepared to respond to the sensory experiences. Numerous studies have replicated these findings (e.g., Johnson, 1996).

Two other sets of investigators have focused on identifying and correcting features of illness representations to affect behavioral responses and outcomes following life-threatening myocardial infarctions. The CSM has been used in a recent approach to the reconceptualizing experience in highly stressful situations (Donovan et al., 2007; Ward et al., 2009). This five-step program is designed to develop shared treatment preferences among patients and proxies (typically a family member) prior to complex cardiac surgery. It begins with a formal assessment of pain representations (the experiences captured by concepts of the five illness domains), followed by the exploration (step 2) of misconceptions uncovered in step 1. Step 3 is a discussion of the deficits created by these misconceptions and is followed by step 4, the provision of information to reshape and replace these misconceptions. The final step involves clarification and a summary discussion. The intervention led to impressive gains in shared treatment preferences in comparison to patients and proxies in the standard care control group (81% versus 19% complete congruence). It also reduced barriers to analgesic use and lowered ratings of usual pain severity; it did not, however, improve coping and well-being. The program focused more on creating valid integrations of experience and concepts than teaching specific responses. This promising approach could be strengthened by constructing action plans with attention to the timing and quantity of changes in pain and the social and psychological context for action.

The second study focuses on the difficult task of reducing the time from first notice of symptoms of myocardial infarction to arrival at hospital emergency rooms for treatment (Dracup et al., 2009). Although promising on several counts, including success in altering an array of such cognitive factors as beliefs respecting heart attacks and need for immediate treatment, the intervention did not reduce total time to care seeking. The failure to achieve this important goal may have been a consequence of insufficient attention to addressing features of illness representations of patients who had prior episodes of MI. Many of these patients may have been told, "You're okay, you can go home now," comments that patients may interpret as meaning they are pain free and cured, an inference that does not distinguish the underlying systemic disease from the manifest episode. Patients also may not realize that future symptoms may differ from past symptoms. A second problem may have been insufficient attention to the formation of action plans, which could have been improved by encouraging patients to call emergency medical services (EMS) when symptomatic and making clear that EMS staff members expect and want patients to call.

Using Cognitive Behavioral Techniques

A second approach involves training clinicians to use psychological models. Many investigators have focused on training to enhance the use of psychological principles and models by medical practitioners. Because this literature is vast, we comment only on selected examples of studies that have examined the use of cognitive behavioral techniques similar to those addressed by the CSM.

A systematic series of studies by Ley (1977, 1982) examined how the organization and sequencing of presentation of information affected patient understanding and adherence. Multiple studies indicated that patients better understood, remembered, and adhered to treatment protocols when information was organized, for example, by presenting all treatment advice and action plans separately from threatening diagnostic information to ensure that patients were not focused on threat when listening to treatment options. Recent efforts demonstrate that physicians and pharmacists can be trained to address illness representations, action plans, and goal setting (De-Ridder, Theunissen, & van Dulmen, 2007; Horne & Weinman, 1998). Both studies highlight the specificity of effects: in the first study, training enhanced communication only in the training's focus area; and in the second, the specification of goals relevant to the biomedical demands of treatment led to better outcomes.

An early study by Inui, Yourtee, and Williamson (1976) trained physicians to use the health belief model when educating patients with hypertension. By focusing on various aspects of management, including the asymptomatic nature of hypertension, patients were found to be more adherent and, most important, their blood pressure control improved over the following months. Although we do not know precisely which components of training affected communication and which aspects of communication affected patient behavior and health outcomes, the description suggests that training focused on both the representation of illness (the asymptomatic nature of hypertension) and plans for implementing treatment. Examination of these studies points to the difficulty in discerning which elements of theory-based interventions are actually used and which of those used are responsible for the intervention's effects.

Using Clinicians as Educators

A third approach conceptualizes the clinician as educator. A central issue raised during our discussion of sharing illness representations is whether a practitioner can infer a patient's illness and treatment representations and action plans during the typical clinical encounter. Given the time constraints and biomedical issues facing practitioners, is it realistic or necessary to take on this burden? A recent study by Phillips, Leventhal, and Leventhal (2011) suggests that it is. They found that patients were more likely to report higher levels of adherence and resolution of their problem at the one-month follow-up interview if they reported during the baseline interview that during the medical visit their physicians (a) discussed the meaning of symptoms, (b) provided a specific response for management, (c) stated treatment outcomes, and (d) discussed possible actions if outcomes were not as expected. In addition, none of the patients who reported that their physicians did all these things had to return for care because their problems had not resolved, whereas the patients who did return for care had not reported these physician behaviors. We do not know why the clinicians informed some patients and not others with these details. It appears, however, that their comments worked and reflected the CSM.

The findings of Phillips, Leventhal, and Leventhal (2011) question the widely held opinion that improving adherence requires improvements in the clinician's psychosocial sensitivity (i.e., the clinician's ability to recognize and accept the patient's cultural background, to display empathy, and, of course, to listen) regardless of how the medically relevant information is integrated with the patient's prior beliefs and experiences. The data from their preliminary study suggest that empathy and liking may be essential contexts for communication, but they are insufficient for adherence and positive health outcomes. Their data found no link between physician psychosocial skills (i.e., bed-side manner) and reported adherence. In fact, satisfaction was negatively related to reported adherence and improvement of the condition at 1-month follow-up. In addition, the patients requiring follow-up treatment were as likely as not to report high levels of practitioner psychosocial skills and satisfaction with the visit. Therefore, addressing illness and treatment representations and action plans appears to be an additional and necessary ingredient for adherence and treatment outcomes.

The results of the Phillips et al. (2011) study, as well as our recordings and observations in clinical practice, suggest the need to specify how to use the CSM to personalize clinical practice at the behavioral and biomedical levels. Specific ingredients of the CSM address personalization, though few have been clearly spelled out. First, it is essential for the clinician to grasp the patient's perspective; even a superficial recognition of the patient's representation can be an effective starting point for communication. Second, the CSM suggests that the patient's experience, symptoms, and function provide tools for communication. A patient's prototype checks link experiences to illness prototypes. Some links, such as recognizing a heart attack, are automatic; others emerge from conscious queries by the executive system. The CSM suggests that effective communication requires that these experiences be made public (i.e., shared with the clinician) and framed appropriately (i.e., attributed to a valid source). The experiences should also be related to management; that is, clinicians should explain how the symptoms should change, identify the time frame for change, discuss the meaning of change, and propose the procedures and plans needed once the cues are gone.

These points are illustrated by an encounter between a patient and his internist after the patient was discharged from the emergency department with negative findings for a heart attack. Prior to discharge, the patient was told that he needed to be checked by his internist in case something had not shown up on his tests. His internist read the history and saw the patient seated with his head down, his hand on his chest, and a worried look on his face. The internist proceeded to address four issues by: (1) acknowledging public recognition of the symptoms suggesting heart attack; (2) discussing the patient's interpretation of his symptoms; (3) locating the actual source of his somatic complaints and reframing their meaning if possible; and (4) suggesting treatments for the current episode as well as long-term treatments for underlying risks. Although the less experienced practitioner might attempt to address these issues with words and test results, the expert clinician attempted to detect the source of the symptoms and by doing so reframed their meaning.

The physical examination provided the tool to explore the chest and was an opportunity to enrich words with experience. Exploring and applying pressure to the patient's chest elicited a complaint from the patient: "That's the pain." A repeat of the pressure reproduced the symptoms again. The symptoms were now public, that is, shared with the physician. By eliciting the symptoms at will, the internist proved that the symptoms were "real." She was now able to understand their causes. She stated, "I can't push your heart, but I can push your sternum, and I suspect that you have an inflammation of the joints between the ribs and sternum, called costochondritis. We can treat it with an over-the-counter anti-inflammatory drug for a short time, three to five days." It is not surprising that the patient no longer appeared terrified; the clinician and his body had provided a persuasive explanation for his symptoms, and the internist had provided a simple treatment.

This encounter meets the conditions for adherence reported by Phillips et al. (2011); the internist prescribed a treatment and discussed the time frame and expectations for outcomes. The clinician did not stop, however. Instead, she used the experience as an opportunity to address the patient's risk factors, for example, his family history of heart attack that led him to suspect he was having a heart attack. This was now the focus of discussion, and the internist provided a set of recommendations to address underlying systemic sources of risk. Clearly, not all presenting complaints permit such a comprehensive approach, but many can be addressed with some of the features of the preceding example. The clinical examples raised at least three interesting issues. The first concerns the similarity between the skilled use of the CSM and the cognitive behavioral approach to treating panic disorder (e.g., Clark, 2004). The second is the problem that arises in creating interventions that address the gaps and misunderstandings in each patient's self-management process. Addressing representations and action plans that are person specific may violate the rules for maintaining the fidelity demanded in the typical behavioral clinical trial. Third, as the complexity of the prescribed behavioral changes increases, there is a need for integrated team care, where the skills of participating specialists address those aspects of treatment relevant to their specialty with knowledge of its fit to other components.

CONCLUSION

PREMISES UNDERLYING THE CSM

It is worth emphasizing the basic premises underlying the overall approach and details elaborated on in this chapter. First, we view the common-sense model as an effort to develop a systems approach to the cognitive and affective processes underlying preferences, decisions, and behaviors for managing illness and improving health. We do not view the CSM as a proprietary framework; it is an approach to analysis from which investigators are encouraged to borrow. Second, the sequence of studies that led to the models that preceded the CSM and the CSM itself parallel findings in the cognitive and biological sciences; investigators should continue to borrow freely from these sources (with attribution, of course, when the borrowing is concept or data specific). The most recent, startling, and amusing parallel is research suggesting that laboratory rats represent objects (e.g., a nest) using features that resemble the domains of underlying illness prototypes (e.g., location; pattern; implied function, cause and consequences; Lin, Chen, Kuang, Wang, & Tsien, 2007).

Our third premise is that CSM differs from other theories of health and illness behavior because its properties parallel those of cognitive and biomedical models. The most fundamental of these properties is the focus on problem-solving processes, that is, how the interaction between information and underlying prototypes activates the representations of specific illnesses, procedures for treatment, and action plans for implementing procedures. The composition of representations (i.e., the variables in the five domains) and their changeability in response to behavioral feedback and social communication is shared with some models of cognitive behavioral therapy. Three key differences in identification of the details involved in information processing illustrate the differences between other models and the CSM model: (1) the specification of prototype checks for the recognition and activation of illness representations and their role in the appraisal of treatment procedures (both intra- and interpersonally); (2) the specification of the cognitive heuristics and behavioral tools available to executive functions; and (3) the search for pathways linking illnesses and treatment representations to psychological distress (anxiety and depression). The CSM also identifies important features of experience and concepts involved in creating action plans to guide behavior. Among the most important of these is the identification of critical treatment time frames (i.e., rate of change and time for benefit) and their relationship to perceived illness-related time frames. From our perspective, if the CSM did not strive for specificity in concepts, it would not merit being called a theory.

IMPLICATIONS OF THE CSM FOR RELIABILITY OF INSTRUMENTS AND CLINICAL TRIALS

This chapter has raised a number of questions respecting hypothesis testing and the development of evidence-based practices; these questions relate to the systems-based framework of the CSM. Both hypothesis testing and clinical application from the CSM framework are centered on the individual. Individuals can be grouped by disease and other broadly defined demographic factors, and these groupings can be used as moderator variables. Individuals differ, however, on the specific properties of their disease (e.g., the genes expressed), their illness and treatment representations, and their action plans. If these individual differences are common among large numbers of individuals, these groups can be identified as moderators in treatment studies. However, the CSM is primarily focused on the dynamic among the processes specific to an individual, his or her specific qualities, life experiences, and illness and treatment.

The dynamic nature of representations and action plans compromises traditional procedures for assessing the reliability of assessment instruments because adequate test-retest reliability assumes the stability of individual differences. Assessments of validity are further complicated because the predictive and discriminant validity of a measure in the commonsense framework depends on context; that is, validity is a function of the values of other factors in the CSM system. What is needed and generally lacking is calibration, or the ability of an instrument to replicate a reading in a context specified by theory. For example, a thermometer would be useless if it consistently gave the same temperature reading; rather, its utility stems from its ability to give the proper reading in the proper situation (e.g., a reading of 0 degrees Celsius in ice water and a reading of 100 degrees Celsius in boiling water). Similarly, any CSM-based assessment must account for the dynamic nature of illness and treatment beliefs.

The CSM also suggests that problems exist in current approaches to intervention trials. Trials are inherently more complex if a theory suggests pretreatment individualization, that is, if the intervention plans to address gaps in individual participants' illness and treatment representations and action plans. A key question is whether the randomized trial—where the same treatment is applied to all persons, with attention to such moderators as age, education, and treatment representations—is the appropriate mechanism for creating and testing clinical interventions. We suspect these traditional designs and their reliance on significance testing is neither the best conceptually nor the most efficient. Indeed, we suspect it is far less efficient and valuable than a combination of time series designs with a more Bayesian flavor (Gallistel, 2009).

Finally, if the reader is entertaining our beliefs about the essential properties of a theory of health and illness behavior and shares some of our concerns about the methods now adhered to in the development and testing of hypotheses and clinical interventions, we can regard our chapter as modestly successful. These issues have motivated the two senior members of our team for many decades, are now embedded in the thinking of our younger members, and we believe they were forces that motivated Dr. Andrew Baum, to whom we dedicate this and our future efforts.

ACKNOWLEDGMENTS

Junior authors are identified in alphabetical order. Funding from the National Institute for Aging of the National Institutes of Health provided the years of funding on which the preparation of this chapter was based (grant numbers 5R24AG023958 and R37AG003501).

REFERENCES

Ahles, T. A., Blanchard, E. B., & Leventhal, H. (1983). Cognitive control of pain: Attention to the sensory aspects of the cold pressor stimulus. *Cognitive Therapy and Research, 7*, 159–177.

Aikens, J. E., Zvolensky, M. J., & Eifert, G. H. (2001). Differential fear of cardiopulmonary sensations in emergency room noncardiac chest pain patients. *Journal of Behavioral Medicine, 24*, 155–167.

Andrews, M., Vigliocco, G., & Vinson, D. (2009). Integrating experiential and distributional data to learn semantic representations. *Psychological Review, 116*, 463–498.

Austin, J. T., & Vancouver, J. B. (1996). Goal constructs in psychology: Structure, process, and content. *Psychological Bulletin, 120*, 338–375.

Bandura, A. (1997). *Self-efficacy: The exercise of control.* New York, NY: Worth.

Baumann, L. J., Cameron, L. D., Zimmerman, R. S., & Leventhal, H. (1989). Illness representations and matching labels with symptoms. *Health Psychology, 8*, 449–469.

Benyamini, Y., & Idler, E. (1999). Community studies reporting association between self-rated health and mortality: Additional studies, 1995 to 1998. *Research on Aging, 21*, 392–401.

Berkanovic, E., Hurwicz, M., & Landsverk, J. (1988). Psychological distress and the decision to seek medical care. *Social Science and Medicine, 27*, 1215–1221.

Bishop, G. D. (1991). Understanding the understanding of illness: Lay disease representations. In J. A. Skelton & R. T. Croyle (Eds.), *Mental representation in health and illness* (pp. 32–59). New York, NY: Springer-Verlag.

Bishop, G. D., & Converse, S. A. (1986). Illness representations: A prototype approach. *Health Psychology, 5*, 95–114.

Bishop, S. D., Briede, C., Cavazos, L., Grotzinger, R., & McMahon, S. (1987). Processing illness information: The role of disease prototypes. *Basic and Applied Social Psychology, 9*, 21–43.

Blumhagen, D. (1980). Hyper-tension: A folk illness with a medical name. *Culture, Medicine, and Psychiatry, 4*, 197–227.

Bodenheimer, T., & Handley, M. A. (2009). Goal-setting for behavior change in primary care: An exploration and status report. *Patient Education and Counseling, 76*, 174–180.

Brody, E. M., & Kleban, M. H. (1983). Day-to-day mental and physical health symptoms of older people: A report on health logs. *The Gerontologist, 23*, 75–85.

Bunde, J., & Martin, R. (2006). Depression and prehospital delay in the context of myocardial infarction. *Psychosomatic Medicine, 68*, 51–57.

Cameron, L. D., Leventhal, E. A., & Leventhal, H. (1993). Symptom representations and affect as determinants of care seeking in a community dwelling adult sample population. *Health Psychology, 12*, 171–179.

Cameron, L. D., Leventhal, E. A., & Leventhal, H. (1995). Seeking medical care in response to symptoms and life stress. *Psychosomatic Medicine, 57*, 37–47.

Carver, C. S., & Scheier, M. F. (1982). Control theory: A useful conceptual framework for personality-social, clinical, and health psychology. *Psychological Bulletin, 92*, 111–135.

Cella, D. F., Tulsky, D. S., Gray, B., & Sarafian, E. (1993). The Functional Assessment of Cancer Therapy Scale: Development and validation of the general measure. *Journal of Clinical Oncology, 11*, 570–579.

Cioffi, D. (1991). Beyond attentional strategies: A cognitive-perceptual model of somatic interpretation. *Psychological Bulletin, 109*, 25–41.

Clark, D. M. (2004). Developing new treatments: On the interplay between theories, experimental science and clinical innovation. *Behaviour Research and Therapy, 42*, 1089–1104.

Croyle, R. T. (1990). Biased appraisal of high blood pressure. *Preventive Medicine, 19*, 40–44.

Croyle, R. T., & Barger, S. D. (1993). Illness cognition. In S. Maes, H. Leventhal, & M. Johnston (Eds.), *International review of health psychology* (Vol. 2, pp. 29–49). Chichester, England: Wiley.

Croyle, R. T., & Jemmott, J. B., III. (1991). Psychological reactions to risk factor testing. In J. A. Skelton & R. T. Croyle (Eds.), *Mental representation in health and illness* (pp. 85–107). New York, NY: Springer-Verlag.

D'Andrade, R. G., Quinn, N. R., Nerlove, S. B., & Romney, A. K. (1972). Categories of disease in American-English and Mexican-Spanish. In A. K. Romney, R. N. Shepard, & S. B. Nerlove (Vol. Eds.), *Multidimensional scaling: Theory and applications in the behavioral sciences: Vol. 2. Applications* (2nd ed., pp. 11–53). New York, NY: Seminar.

Dempsey, S. J., Dracup, K., & Moser, D. K. (1995). Women's decision to seek care for symptoms of acute myocardial infarction. *Heart and Lung, 24*, 444–456.

De-Ridder, D. T. D., Theunissen, N. C. M., & van Dulmen, S. M. (2007). Does training general practitioners to elicit patients' illness representations and action plans influence their communication as a whole? *Patient Education and Counseling, 66*, 327–336.

Diabetes Prevention Program Research Group. (2002). Reduction in the incidence of type 2 diabetes with lifestyle intervention of metformin. *New England Journal of Medicine, 346*, 393–403.

Diefenbach, M. A., Miller, S. M., & Daly, M. (1999). Specific worry about breast cancer predicts mammography use in women at risk for breast and ovarian cancer. *Health Psychology, 18*, 532–536.

Donovan, H. S., Ward, S. E., Song, M. K., Heidrich, S. M., Gunnarsdottir, S., & Phillips, C. M. (2007). An update on the representational approach to patient education. *Journal of Nursing Scholarship, 39*, 259–265.

Dracup, K., McKinley, S., Riegel, B., Moser, D. K., Meischke, H., Doering, L. V., ... Pelter, M. (2009). A randomized clinical trial to reduce patient prehospital delay to treatment in acute coronary syndrome. *Circulation: Cardiovascular Quality and Outcomes, 2*, 524–532.

Duke, J., Brownlee, S., Leventhal, E. A., & Leventhal, H. (2002). Giving up and replacing activities in response to illness. *Journal of Gerontology: Psychological Sciences, 57B*, 367–376.

Ellaham, S. (2010). Insulin therapy in critically ill patients. *Vascular Health and Risk Management, 6*, 1089–1101.

Facione, N. C. (1993). Delay versus help seeking for breast cancer symptoms: A critical review of the literature on patient and provider delay. *Social Science and Medicine, 376*, 1521–1534.

Figueiras, M. J., Alves, N., Marcelino, D. A., Cortes, M., Weinman, J., & Horne, R. (2009). Assessing lay beliefs about generic medicines: Development of the Generic Medicines Scale. *Medical Care, 14*, 311–321.

Fleming, B. B., Greenfield, S., Engelgau, M. M., Pogach, L. M., Clauser, S. B., & Parrot, M. A., for the DQIP Group. (2001). The Diabetes Quality Improvement Project: Moving science into health policy to gain an edge on the diabetes epidemic. *Diabetes Care, 24*, 1815–1820.

Gallistel, C. R. (2009). The importance of proving the null. *Psychological Review, 116*, 439–453.

Godoy-Izquierdo, D., López-Chicheri, I., López-Torrecillas, F., Vélez, M., & Godoy, J. F. (2007). Contents of lay illness models dimensions for physical and mental diseases and implications for health professionals. *Patient Education and Counseling, 67*, 196–213.

Gollwitzer, P. M. (1999). Implementation intentions: Strong effects of simple plans. *American Psychologist, 54*, 493–503.

Gonder-Frederick, L. A., & Cox, D. J. (1991). Symptom perception, symptom beliefs, and blood glucose discrimination in the self-treatment of insulin-dependent diabetes. In J. A. Skelton & R. T. Croyle (Eds.), *Mental representation in health and illness* (pp. 220–246). New York, NY: Springer-Verlag.

Hackett, T. P., & Cassem, N. H. (1969). Factors contributing to delay in responding to the signs and symptoms of acute myocardial infarction. *American Journal of Cardiology, 24*, 651–658.

Halm, E. A., Mora, P., & Leventhal, H. (2006). No symptoms, no asthma: The acute episodic disease belief is associated with poor self-management among inner city adults with persistent asthma. *Chest, 129*, 573–580.

Halverson, G. (2007). *Health care reform now*. San Francisco, CA: Wiley.

Hardy, J. (2006). Speaking clearly: A critical review of the self-talk literature. *Psychology of Sport and Exercise, 7*, 81–97.

Heidrich, S. M., Forsthoff, C. A., & Ward, S. E. (1994). Psychological adjustment in adults with cancer: The self as mediator. *Health Psychology, 13*, 346–353.

Henderson, C. J., Hagger, M. S., & Orbell, S. (2007). Does priming a specific illness schema result in an additional information-processing bias for specific illnesses? *Health Psychology, 26*, 165–173.

Hobfoll, S. E. (1989). Conservation of resources: A new attempt at conceptualizing stress. *American Psychologist, 44,* 513–524.

Hooker, K., & Kaus, C. R. (1994). Health-related possible selves in young and middle adulthood. *Psychology and Aging, 9*, 126–133.

Horne, R. (1997). Representations of medication and treatment: Advances in theory and measurement. In K. J. Petrie & J. A. Weinman (Eds.), *Perceptions of health and illness: Current research and applications* (pp. 155–188). London, England: Harwood Academic Press.

Horne, R. (2003). Treatment perceptions and self-regulation. In L. D. Cameron & H. Leventhal (Eds.), *The self-regulation of health and illness behaviour* (pp. 138–154). London, England: Routledge.

Horne, R., Buick, D., Fisher, M., Leake, H., Cooper, V., & Weinman, J. (2004). Doubts about necessity and concerns about adverse effects: Identifying the types of beliefs that are associated with non-adherence to HAART. *International Journal of STD and AIDS, 15*, 38–39.

Horne, R., Clatworthy, J., Polmear, A., & Weinman, J. (2001). Do hypertensive patients' beliefs about their illness and treatment influence medication adherence and quality of life? *Journal of Human Hypertension, 15*(Suppl. 1), 65–68.

Horne, R., Cooper, V., & Fisher, M. (2008). Initiation of therapy with a subcutaneously administered antiretroviral in treatment-experienced HIV-infected patients: Understanding physician and patient perspectives. *AIDS Care, 20*, 1029–1039.

Horne, R., Cooper, V., Gellaitry, G., Date, H., & Fisher, M. (2007). Patients' perceptions of highly active antiretroviral therapy in relation to treatment uptake and adherence. *JAIDS, 45*, 334–341.

Horne, R., Parham, R., Driscoll, R., & Robinson, A. (2009). Patients' attitudes to medicines and adherence to maintenance treatment in inflammatory bowel disease (IBD). *Inflammatory Bowel Diseases, 15*, 837–844.

Horne, R., & Weinman, J. (1998). Predicting treatment adherence: An overview of theoretical models. In L. Myers & K. Midence (Eds.), *Adherence to treatment in medical conditions* (pp. 24–50). London, England: Informa Healthcare.

Horne, R., & Weinman, J. (2002). Self-regulation and self-management in asthma: Exploring the role of illness perceptions and treatment beliefs in explaining non-adherence to preventer medication. *Psychology and Health, 17*, 1–16.

Horne, R., Weinman, J., & Hankins, M. (1999). The Beliefs About Medicines questionnaire: The development and evaluation of a new method for assessing the cognitive representation of medication. *Psychology and Health, 14*, 1–24.

Horowitz, C. R., Rein, S. B., & Leventhal, H. (2004). A story of maladies, misconceptions and mishaps: Effective management of heart failure. *Social Science and Medicine, 58*, 631–643.

Idler, E. L., & Benyamini, Y. (1997). Self-rated health and mortality: A review of twenty-seven community studies. *Journal of Health and Social Behavior, 38*, 21–37.

Idler, E., Leventhal, H., McLaughlin, J., & Leventhal, E. A. (2004). In sickness but not in health: Self-ratings, identity and mortality. *Journal of Health and Social Behavior, 45*, 336–356.

Inui, T. S., Yourtee, E. L., & Williamson, J. W. (1976). Improved outcomes in hypertension after physician tutorials, a controlled trial. *Annals of Internal Medicine, 84*, 646–651.

Johnson, J. E. (1975). Stress reduction through sensation information. In I. C. Sarason & C. O. Spielberger (Eds.), *Stress and anxiety* (Vol. 2, pp. 361–373). Washington, DC: Hemisphere.

Johnson, J. E. (1996). Coping with radiation therapy: Optimism and the effect of preparatory interventions. *Research in Nursing Health, 19*, 3–12.

Johnson, J. E., & Leventhal, H. (1974). The effects of accurate expectations and behavioral instructions on reactions during a noxious medical examination. *Journal of Personality and Social Psychology, 29*, 710–718.

Jylha, M. (2009). What is self-rated health and why does it predict mortality? Towards a unified conceptual model. *Social Science Medicine, 69*, 307–316.

Kahneman, D., & Miller, D. T. (1986). Norm theory: Comparing reality to its alternatives. *Psychological Review, 93*, 136–153.

Kasl, S. V., & Cobb, J. (1966). Health behavior, illness behavior and sick-role behavior. *Archives of Environmental Health, 12*, 531–541.

Kelly, G. (1955). *The psychology of personal constructs: Vol. 1. A theory of personality.* New York, NY: W. W. Norton.

Kleinman, A. (1980). *Patients and healers in the context of culture: An exploration of the borderland between anthropology, medicine, and psychiatry.* Los Angeles, CA: University of California Press.

Kroenke, K., & Spitzer, R. (2002). The PHQ-9: A new depression diagnostic and severity measure. *Depression in Primary Care.* Retrieved from http://www.lphi.org/LPHIadmin/uploads/.PHQ-9-Review-Kroenke-63754.PDF

Krohne, H. W. (1993). Vigilance and cognitive avoidance as concepts in coping research. In H. W. Krohne (Ed.), *Attention and avoidance* (pp. 19–46). Seattle, WA: Hogrefe and Huber.

Kulik, J. A., & Mahler, H. I. M. (1997). Social comparison, affiliation, and coping with acute medical threats. In B. P. Buunk & F. X. Gibbons (Eds.), *Health, coping, and well-being: Perspectives from social comparison theory* (pp. 227–261). Mahwah, NJ: Erlbaum.

Landin, D. (1994). The role of verbal cues in skill learning. *Quest, 46*, 299–313.

Lau, R. R., Bernard, T. M., & Hartman, K. A. (1989). Further explorations of common sense representations of common illnesses. *Health Psychology, 8*, 195–219.

Lau, R. R., & Hartman, K. A. (1983). Common sense representations of common illnesses. *Health Psychology, 2*, 167–185.

Lazarus, R. S. (1966). *Psychological stress and the coping process.* New York, NY: McGraw-Hill.

Lazarus, R. S., & Folkman, S. (1984). *Stress, appraisal, and coping.* New York, NY: Springer.

Lazarus, R. S., & Launier, R. (1979). Stress-related transactions between person and environment. In L. A. Pervin & M. Lewis (Eds.), *Perspectives in interactional psychology* (pp. 287–327). New York, NY: Plenum Press.

Leventhal, E. A., & Crouch, M. (1997). Are there differences in perceptions of illness across the lifespan? In K. J. Petrie & J. Weinman (Eds.), *Perceptions of health and illness: Current research and applications* (pp. 77–102). London, England: Harwood Academic Press.

Leventhal, E. A., Leventhal, H., Shacham, S., & Easterling, D. V. (1989). Active coping reduces reports of pain from childbirth. *Journal of Consulting and Clinical Psychology, 57*, 365–371.

Leventhal, E. A., Suls, J., & Leventhal, H. (1993). Hierarchical analysis of coping: Evidence from life-span studies. In H. W. Krohne (Ed.), *Attention and avoidance: Strategies in coping with aversiveness* (pp. 71–99). Seattle, WA: Hogrefe and Huber.

Leventhal, H. (1970). Findings and theory in the study of fear communications. In L. Berkowitz (Ed.), *Advances in experimental social psychology* (Vol. 5, pp. 119–186). New York, NY: Academic Press.

Leventhal, H. (1984). A perceptual-motor theory of emotion. In L. Berkowitz (Ed.), *Advances in experimental social psychology* (Vol. 17, pp. 117–182). Orlando, FL: Academic Press.

Leventhal, H. (1986). Symptom reporting: A focus on process. In S. McHugh & T. M. Vallis (Eds.), *Illness behavior: A multi-disciplinary model* (pp. 219–237). New York, NY: Plenum Press.

Leventhal, H., Brown, D., Shacham, S., & Engquist, G. (1979). Effects of preparatory information about sensations, threat of pain, and attention on cold pressor distress. *Journal of Personality and Social Psychology*, *37*, 688–714.

Leventhal, H., & Diefenbach, M. (1991). The active side of illness cognition. In J. A. Skelton & R. T. Croyle (Eds.), *Mental representation in health and illness* (pp. 247–272). New York, NY: Springer-Verlag.

Leventhal, H., Diefenbach, M., & Leventhal, E. A. (1992). Illness cognition: Using common sense to understand treatment adherence and affect cognition interactions. *Cognitive Therapy and Research*, *16*, 143–163.

Leventhal, H., Easterling, D. V., Coons, H., Luchterhand, C., & Love, R. R. (1986). Adaptation to chemotherapy treatments. In B. Andersen (Ed.), *Women with cancer* (pp. 172–203). New York, NY: Springer-Verlag.

Leventhal, H., Hudson, S., & Robitaille, C. (1997). Social comparison and health: A process model. In B. P. Buunk & F. X. Gibbons (Eds.), *Health, coping and well being: Perspectives from social comparison theory* (pp. 411–432). Hillsdale, NJ: Erlbaum.

Leventhal, H., Idler, E., & Leventhal, E. A. (1999). The impact of chronic illness on the self system. In R. Ashmore, L. Jussim, & R. Contrada (Eds.), *Self, social identity, and physical health: Interdisciplinary explorations* (Vol. 2, pp. 185–208). New York, NY: Oxford University Press.

Leventhal, H., Jones, S., & Trembly, G. (1966). Sex differences in attitude and behavior change under conditions of fear and specific instructions. *Journal of Experimental Social Psychology*, *2*, 387–399.

Leventhal, H., & Leventhal, E. A. (1993). Affect, cognition and symptom reporting. In C. R. Chapman & K. M. Foley (Eds.), *Current and emerging issues in cancer pain: Research and practice* (pp. 153–173). New York, NY: Raven Press.

Leventhal, H., Leventhal, E. A., & Cameron, L. (2001). Representations, procedures and affect in illness self regulation: A perceptual-cognitive model. In A. Baum, T. Revenson, & J. Weinman (Eds.), *Handbook of health psychology* (pp. 19–47). New York, NY: Erlbaum.

Leventhal, H., Leventhal, E. A., & Schaefer, P. (1991). Vigilant coping and health behavior: A life span problem. In M. Ory & R. Abeles (Eds.), *Aging, health, and behavior* (pp. 109–140). Baltimore, MD: Johns Hopkins.

Leventhal, H., Meyer, D., & Nerenz, D. (1980). The common sense representation of illness danger. In S. Rachman (Ed.), *Medical psychology* (pp. 7–30). New York, NY: Pergamon Press.

Leventhal, H., & Nerenz, D. (1985). The assessment of illness cognition. In P. Karoly (Ed.), *Measurement strategies in health* (pp. 517–554). New York, NY: Wiley.

Leventhal, H., Nerenz, D., & Strauss, A. (1982). Self-regulation and the mechanisms for symptom appraisal. In D. Mechanic (Ed.), *Monograph Series in Psychosocial Epidemiology 3: Symptoms, illness behavior, and help-seeking* (pp. 55–86). New York, NY: Neale Watson.

Leventhal, H., & Scherer, K. R. (1987). The relationship of emotion to cognition: A functional approach to semantic controversy. *Cognition and Emotion*, *1*, 3–28.

Leventhal, H., Singer, R., & Jones, S. (1965). Effects of fear and specificity of recommendations upon attitudes and behavior. *Journal of Personality and Social Psychology*, *2*, 20–29.

Leventhal, H., & Trembly, G. (1968). Negative emotions and persuasion. *Journal of Personality*, *36*, 154–168.

Leventhal, H., Watts, J. C., & Pagano, F. (1967). Effects of fear and instructions on how to cope with danger. *Journal of Personality and Social Psychology*, *6*, 313–321.

Lewin, K. (1935). *A dynamic theory of personality*. New York, NY: McGraw-Hill.

Ley, P. (1977). Psychological studies of doctor-patient communication. In S. Rachman (Ed.), *Contributions to medical psychology* (pp. 9–42). Oxford, UK: Pergamon Press.

Ley, P. (1982). Satisfaction, compliance and communication. *British Journal of Clinical Psychology*, *21*, 241–254.

Lin, L., Chen, G., Kuang, H., Wang, D., & Tsien, J. Z. (2007). Neural encoding of the concept of nest in the mouse brain. *PNAS*, *104*, 6066–6071.

Loewenstein, G. (2005). Hot-cold empathy gaps and medical decision-making. *Health Psychology*, *24*(Suppl. 4), S49–S56.

Mandell, H., & Spiro H. (1987). *When doctors get sick*. New York, NY: Plenum Medical Book Co.

Marcus, H., & Nurius, P. (1986). Possible selves. *American Psychologist*, *41*, 954–969.

Matthews, K. A., Siegel, J. M., Kuller, L. H., Thompson, M., & Varat, M. (1983). Determinants of decision to seek medical treatment by patients with acute myocardial infarction symptoms. *Journal of Personality and Social Psychology*, *44*, 1144–1156.

McAndrew, L. M., Musumeci-Szabó, T. J., Mora, P. A., Vileikyte, L., Burns, E., Halm, E. A., ... Leventhal, H. (2008). Using the common sense model to design interventions for the prevention and management of chronic illness threats: From description to process. *British Journal of Health Psychology*, *13*, 195–204.

McKinlay, J. B., & Dutton, D. B. (1974). Social-psychological factors affecting health service utilization. In S. J. Mushkin (Ed.), *Consumer incentives for health care* (pp. 251–303). New York, NY: Prodist.

Melzack, R. (1992). Phantom limbs. *Scientific American, 226*, 120–126.

Meyer, D., Leventhal, H., & Gutmann, M. (1985). Common-sense models of illness: The example of hypertension. *Health Psychology, 4*, 115–135.

Millar, M. G., & Millar, K. (1996). The effects of anxiety on response times to disease detection and health promotion behaviors. *Journal of Behavioral Medicine, 19*, 401–413.

Miller, G. A., Galanter, E., & Pribram, K. H. (1960). *Plans and the structure of behavior*. New York, NY: Holt.

Mora, P. A., DiBonaventura, M. D., Idler, E., Leventhal, E. A., & Leventhal, H. (2008). Psychological factors influencing self-assessments of health: Towards an understanding of the mechanisms underlying how people rate their own health. *Annals of Behavioral Medicine, 36*, 292–303.

Mora, P. A., Robitaille, C., Leventhal, H., Swigar, M., & Leventhal, E. A. (2002). Trait negative affect relates to prior-week symptoms, but not to reports of illness episodes, illness symptoms, and care seeking among older persons. *Psychosomatic Medicine, 64*, 436–449.

Orbell, S., & Verplanken, B. (2010). The automatic component of habit in health behavior: Habit as cue-contingent automaticity. *Health Psychology, 29*, 374–383.

Osterberg, L., & Blaschke, T. (2005). Adherence to medication. *New England Journal of Medicine, 353*, 487–497.

Pachter, L. M. (1993). Latino folk illnesses: Methodological considerations. *Medical Anthropology, 15*, 103–108.

Pennebaker, J. W. (1999). Psychological factors influencing the reporting of physical symptoms. In A. A. Stone, J. S. Turkkan, C. A. Bachrach, J. B. Jobe, H. S. Kurtzman, & V. S. Cain (Eds.), *The science of self-report: Implications for research and practice* (pp. 299–316). Mahwah, NJ: Erlbaum.

Pennebaker, J. W., & Watson, D. (1988). Blood pressure estimation and beliefs among normotensives and hypertensives. *Health Psychology, 7*, 309–328.

Pescosolido, B. A. (1992). Beyond rational choice: The social dynamics of how people seek help. *American Journal of Sociology, 97*, 1096–1138.

Petrie, K. J., & Weinman, J. A. (1997). *Perception of health and illness: Current research and applications*. London, England: Harwood Academic.

Prochaska, J. O., DiClemente, C. C., & Norcross, J. C. (1992). In search of how people change: Applications to addictive behaviors. *American Psychologist, 47*, 156–163.

Phillips, L. A., Leventhal, H., & Leventhal, E. (2011). Physicians' communication of the common-sense self-regulation model results in greater reported adherence than physicians' use of interpersonal skills. *British Journal of Health Psychology*. DOI:10.1111/j.2044-8287.2011.02035.x

Quinn, P. C., & Eimas, P. D. (1997). A reexamination of the perceptual-to-conceptual shift in mental representations. *Review of General Psychology, 1*, 271–287.

Reynolds, N. R., Sanzero Eller, L., Nicholas, K., Corless, B., Kirksey, K., Hamilton, M. J., … Holzemer, W. L. (2009). HIV illness representation as a predictor of self-care management and health outcomes: A multi-site, cross-cultural study. *AIDS and Behavior, 13*, 258–267.

Richetin, J., Conner, M., & Perugini, M. (2011). Not doing is not the opposite of doing: Implications for attitudinal models of behavioral prediction. *Personality and Social Psychology Bulletin, 37*, 40–54.

Rosch, E., Mervis, C. B., Gray, W. D., Johnson, D. M., & Boyes-Braem, P. (1976). Basic objective in natural categories. *Cognitive Psychology, 8*, 382–439.

Salomon, G., & Globerson, T. (1987). Skill may not be enough: The role of mindfulness in learning and transfer. *International Journal of Educational Research, 11*, 623–637.

Sambamoorthi, U., Moynihan, P. J., McSpiritt, E., & Crystal, S. (2001). Use of protease inhibitors and non-nucleoside reverse transcriptase inhibitors among Medicaid beneficiaries with AIDS. *American Journal of Public Health, 91*, 1474–1481.

Saraiya, B., Bodnar-Deren, S., Leventhal, E., & Leventhal, H. (2008). End-of-life planning and its relevance for patients' and oncologists' decisions in choosing cancer therapy. *Cancer, 113*, 3540–3547.

Schachter, S., & Singer, J. E. (1962). Cognitive, social, and physiological determinants of emotional state. *Psychological Review, 69*, 379–399.

Schober, R., & Lacroix, J. M. (1991). Lay illness models in the enlightenment and the 20th century: Some historical lessons. In J. A. Skelton & R. T. Croyle (Eds.), *Mental representation in health and illness* (pp. 10–31). New York, NY: Springer-Verlag.

Shadbolt, B., Barresi, J., & Craft, P. (2002) Self-rated health as a predictor of survival among patients with advanced cancer. *Journal of Clinical Oncology, 20*, 2514–2519.

Sheeran, P., & Orbell, S. (2000). Using implementation intentions to increase attendance for cervical cancer screening. *Health Psychology*, *18*, 283–289.

Shiloh, S., Peretz, G., & Iss, R. (2007). Recovery attributions: Explicit endorsement of biomedical factors and implicit dominance of psycho-social factors. *Journal of Behavioral Medicine*, *30*, 243–251.

Skelton, J. A., & Croyle, R. T. (1991). *Mental representation in health and illness*. New York, NY: Springer-Verlag.

Spruill, T. M., Pickering, T. G., Schwartz, J. E., Mostofsky, E., Ogedegbe, G., Clemow, L., & Gerin, W. (2007). The impact of perceived hypertension status on anxiety and the white coat effect. *Annals of Behavioral Medicine*, *34*, 1–9.

Squire L. R. (2004). Memory systems of the brain: A brief history and current perspective. *Neurobiology of Learning and Memory*, *82*, 171–177.

Stoller, E. P. (1993). Interpretations of symptoms by older people: A health diary study of illness behavior. *Journal of Aging and Health*, *5*, 58–81.

Stoller, E. P. (1997). Medical self care: Lay management of symptoms by elderly people. In M. G. Ory & G. DeFries (Eds.), *Self-care in later life: Research, program, and policy issues* (pp. 24–61). New York, NY: Springer.

Stone, A. A., Helder, L., & Schneider, M. S. (1988). Coping with stressful life events. In L. H. Cohen (Ed.), *Research on stressful life events: Theoretical and methodological issues* (pp. 182–210). Beverly Hills, CA: Sage.

Stone, A. A., & Neale, J. M. (1984). New measure of daily coping: Development and preliminary results. *Journal of Personality and Social Psychology*, *46*, 892–906.

Sullivan, H. W., & Rothman, A. J. (2008). When planning is needed: Implementation intentions and attainment of approach versus avoidance health goals. *Health Psychology*, *27*, 438–444.

Taylor, S. (1983). Adjustment to threatening events: A theory of cognitive adaptation. *American Psychologist*, *November*, 1161–1173.

Taylor, S. (1991). Asymmetrical effects of positive and negative events: The mobilization-minimization hypothesis. *Psychological Bulletin*, *110*, 67–85.

Teno, J. M., Weitzen, S., Fennell, M. L., & Mor, V. (2001). Dying trajectory in the last year of life: Does cancer trajectory fit other diseases? *Journal of Palliative Medicine*, *4*, 457–464.

Tuomilehto, J., Lindström, J., Johan, M. S., Eriksson, G., Valle, T. T, Hämäläinen, H., ... Uusitupa, M., for the Finnish Diabetes Prevention Study Group. (2001). Prevention of type 2 diabetes mellitus by changes in lifestyle among subjects with impaired glucose tolerance. *New England Journal of Medicine*, *344*, 1343–1350.

Tversky, A., & Kahneman, D. (1974). Judgment under uncertainty: Heuristics and biases. *Science*, *185*, 1124–1131.

Van Boven, L., & Loewenstein, G. (2003). Social projection of transient visceral feelings. *Personality and Social Psychology Bulletin*, *29*, 1159–1168.

Ward, S. E., Serlin, R. C., Donovan, H. S., Ameringer, S. W., Hughes, S., Pe-Romashko, K., & Wang, K. (2009). A randomized trial of a representational intervention for cancer pain: Does targeting the dyad make a difference? *Health Psychology*, *28*, 588–597.

Wilson, G. T., & Vitousek, K. M. (1999). Self-monitoring in the assessment of eating disorders. *Psychological Assessment*, *11*, 480–489.

Yoder, P. S., & Hornik, R. C. (1996). Symptoms and perceived severity of illness as predictive of treatment for diarrhea in six Asian and African sites. *Social Science and Medicine*, *43*, 429–439.

2 How Psychophysiology Contributes to Health Psychology

J. Richard Jennings and Victoria Egizio
University of Pittsburgh School of Medicine

Psychophysiologists are interested in the physiological states that accompany psychological processes in humans. The area becomes central to health psychology when the question is asked, "How do psychological processes translate into physiological changes that enhance or endanger health?" Do these physiological changes then further impact both psychological processes and health? Neither the accurate assessment of physiological states nor the inference of physiological mechanisms is simple, however. This chapter reviews issues raised in the psychophysiology of health and develops both the promise and the limitations of psychophysiological measures.

There is a long history of attempting to infer mental state from physiological measures, particularly mental states unavailable to awareness (see Stern, Ray, & Davis, 1980). For example, the early psychoanalyst Carl Jung applied skin resistance measurements in conjunction with administration of free association tests. However, psychophysiology only emerged as an integral part of the young field of health psychology in the 1970s. As excitement waned over the possibility that autonomic measures of a general activation system would be central to psychology (Coles, Jennings, & Stern, 1984), many young investigators instead focused on specific physiological changes that might be antecedents to disease states. In particular, Paul Obrist and a group of active students at the University of North Carolina began gathering evidence designed to show that blood pressure reactions to stress might be part of the pathophysiology of hypertension (Obrist, 1976, 1981; Obrist, Light, James, & Strogatz, 1987). Concurrently, epidemiological data supported the possibility that coronary heart disease might be the consequence of a behavior pattern (Type A behavior) consisting of competitiveness, time urgency, impatience, and hostility (Matthews, 1982; Rosenman et al., 1970). It occurred to many researchers that these behaviors were likely to induce habitual increases in heart rate and blood pressure, possibly mediating this epidemiological link. Krantz and Manuck (1984), in particular, in an influential review suggested how different patterns of cardiovascular reactivity to stress might be related more generally to cardiovascular disease. Although reactivity to stress remains a key component of psychophysiological research relevant to health psychology, the applications to disease and health and the types of physiological reactions studied have expanded greatly. To this end, enhanced knowledge of the endocrine and immune systems and the ability to image brain function and structure noninvasively have been particularly notable.

DEFINING PSYCHOPHYSIOLOGY

Psychophysiology is largely a correlative science. Changes in psychological state are related, typically with concurrent measurement, to the presence of or changes in a physiological state. The correlation is rendered more precise when there is a close temporal relationship between psychological and physiological measurements. It remains difficult, however, to show that the psychological state caused the physiological state. Suggestive evidence for causation can be offered by changing the psychological state with different methods, timing, and stimulus materials and showing that the predicted physiological change routinely occurs. Similarly limiting is the less common case in which a physiological change is induced and causation of a psychological state is inferred. With either direction of causation, however, a basic physiologist would typically not be satisfied that a causative mechanism had been isolated. There simply remain too many complex and poorly understood steps in the translation between mind and body. For example, we could consistently observe that inducing attention was accompanied by a slowing of heart rate, but this remains a correlation because it is difficult to prove even that attention preceded the initiation of the heart rate response. Moreover, we are not able to trace each link in the chain of causation through the brain's instantiation of attention, electrophysiologically and neurochemically, to the changes in the cardiac sinus node triggering the slowing of heart rate. Thus, psychophysiology differs from much of physiology and neuroscience in the level of concepts used and the accuracy of inferring causation.

In comparison to epidemiologists, psychophysiologists do strive to study causative mechanisms, distinguishing themselves from the strictly correlative approach typical of epidemiology. Most psychophysiological work focuses on the co-occurrence of psychological and physiological states, typically changing psychological state and observing physiological response. Both physiological and psychological states are measured in some detail. This focus limits the number of participants that can be studied. Thus, the psychophysiologist is oriented more toward mechanism, studies smaller samples, and may be less focused on a disease state than is the typical epidemiologist.

General physiological arousal, a concept nearly synonymous with stress, is a primary construct of interest to psychophysiologists. Psychologists generally associate the physiological measures typical of psychophysiological experiments—palmar sweating, heart rate, and blood pressure—with an individual's level of physiological arousal. The concept of general physiological arousal is intuitively appealing and became popular in the mid-20th century among physiologists. This popularity was fueled by the observation that the brain stem appeared to contain a structure that regulated a single energetic system, which, in turn, modulated general physiological activity, personal motivation, and emotion (Lindsley, 1951). This energetic system was thought to generate an arousal level that could be assessed with measures of the autonomic nervous system, providing a convenient measure of motivation, emotion, and energy for the psychologist. Support for the physiological concept of general arousal has, however, proven limited; indeed, a closer look at the concepts of stress and arousal, independently and jointly, reveals a multitude of issues. Virtually any of the physiological systems that we measure cannot be conceptualized as solely a response mechanism for psychological stress. A list of likely factors to consider when interpreting a physiological change can readily be developed: support for behavior (e.g., exercise, orienting to a novel event, directed thought); metabolism (e.g., ingestion, digestion, water and salt balance); regulation (e.g., adjusting to change of posture, normalizing blood pressure, adjusting to decrease in blood flow); and/or emotion (e.g., fear, anger, happiness). This list is not exhaustive; such other factors as a response to infection can be noted. Historically, the bodily communication systems—autonomic, endocrine, and immune systems—were considered as peripheral response systems with minimal coupling to central nervous system control. All the communication systems are, however, now known to be significantly influenced by the central nervous system and by the multitude of afferent information that such communication systems supply about the state of the rest of the body. Thus, physiological responses of interest to health psychologists must not be considered in isolation and are not as simple as considered in early conceptualizations of physiological arousal. Modern psychophysiologists are charged with the complex task of determining how normal autonomic, endocrine, and immune system responses susceptible to psychological influences relate to etiological disease processes or to health enhancement.

In the context of this chapter, we will focus primarily on electrophysiological measures from which autonomic nervous activity can be inferred. As just noted, the brain and our behavior can influence our bodily function equally as strongly through actions of the endocrine and immune system, but the technical knowledge required to assess all these systems is formidable. The result is the unfortunate tendency, which this chapter will perpetuate, of focusing on one of these communication systems between brain and body. We will focus on the cardiovascular system but will use these findings to illustrate how psychophysiology is used and its results conceptualized differently depending on the focus of the investigator, though some investigators may understand and use multiple perspectives in their work. The remainder of the chapter will be organized in sections with the perspectives of (a) cardiovascular measures as autonomic nervous system indices, (b) cardiovascular measures as health-related psychological concepts, (c) cardiovascular measures as risk factors, and (d) cardiovascular measures as indices of disease or preclinical disease. Interested readers are referred to Steptoe (2007) for another perspective on psychophysiological evidence as well as the related chapter by Uchino Smith, Holt-Lunstad, Campo, and Reblin (2007) in the generally useful *Handbook of Psychophysiology* (Cacioppo, Tassinary, & Berntson, 2007). A brief book-length overview is provided by Lovallo (2005b). A focus on methods is provided by Jennings and Gianaros (2007), and Curtin, Lozano, and Allen (2007) provide advice on establishing a psychophysiological laboratory.

CARDIOVASCULAR MEASURES AS AUTONOMIC NERVOUS SYSTEM INDICES

The basic psychophysiological perspective remains physiological, attempting to infer physiological processes from the observed data. Dysregulation of these processes is then typically seen as relevant to disease mechanisms. Physiological concepts invoked might be general arousal, sympathetic nervous system activation—alpha or beta sympathetic, or parasympathetic activation. Patterns of activation might similarly be inferred as more narrowly related to changes in specific end organs, for example, cardiac activation versus vascular activation.

As noted earlier, psychophysiologists became interested in health psychology at the time when earlier concepts of general physiological arousal and the nature of the autonomic nervous system were being challenged. Autonomic nervous system activation had been seen as primarily a function of changes in the reticular activation system of the brainstem. Changes in the reticular activation system were thought to adjust sympathetic and parasympathetic activation in a reciprocal fashion in tune with the level of alertness or affect, which was also determined by reticular activation level (Lindsley, 1951). Advances in physiology and psychophysiology led to revised concepts that (a) emphasized the independence of sympathetic and parasympathetic activation; that is, an arousal level that controlled both did not exist; (b) found relatively specific effects on organ systems; that is, sympathetic activation influencing the heart might not be concurrently influencing the digestive system; (c) stated the importance of afferent information traveling in the autonomic, primarily parasympathetic, nervous system that informed the brain about the body; and (d) noted the integrated, often central, control of endocrine, autonomic, and immune systems (Berntson & Cacioppo, 2007; Berntson, Norman, Hawkley, & Cacioppo, 2008; Jennings et al., 2002; Llewellyn-Smith & Verberne, 2011; Swanson, 2003).

Given this background and the knowledge that physiological variables are often complex and interrelated, investigators are now interested in demonstrating (a) the presence of a normal regulatory set of processes, or processes potentially contributing to disease, and (b) patterns of activation associated with that regulation. A clear example of emphasis on physiological regulation and dysregulation is disruption of the circadian rhythm of blood pressure. Blood pressure typically falls during the night and increases with activity during waking hours. Through the use of ambulatory measures of blood pressure, individuals were identified that showed none or minimal fall or dip during sleep (Henskens et al., 2008). As might be expected given the chronicity of exposure to higher blood pressure, cerebrovascular disease and all cause mortality has been related to nondipping (Brotman, Davidson, Boumitri, & Vidt, 2008). Nondipping, in turn, has been related to psychosocial factors, among them socioeconomic status (Campbell, Key, Ireland, Bacon, & Ditto, 2008).

Other investigations focus more on patterns of integrated physiological activity that are reactive to stress and possibly lead to dysregulation. For example, observation of sympathetic nervous system activation might indicate the further activation of the adrenal medulla, producing circulating adrenalin activating the beta adrenergic receptors in the heart, increasing cardiac contractility (i.e., activation of a pattern of neural and endocrine response, sometimes termed SAM, sympathetic adrenomedullary activation). Concurrent cardiovascular and endocrine assessment would then identify responses to stress in which transient autonomic activity induced the relatively more sustained endocrine response; evidence is available supporting the reliability of this response pattern (Hawkley et al., 2001). Another hypothesis is that the joint presence of sympathetic activation and activation of the adrenal cortex indicates a distress response that might be distinguished from a normal, and potentially adaptive, response to a stressful challenge, that is, a rapid reaction and prompt recovery. Research from this perspective combines assessment of cortisol, an adrenocortical hormone responsive to stress, with the cardiovascular measures used to infer sympathetic activation (Lovallo, 2005b). A generalization from this hypothesis suggests that the joint activation of systems seeking to overcome biological and psychological stress, that is, to maintain homeostasis, creates load on the system the magnitude of which relates to disease—a concept coined "allostatic load" (McEwen & Lasley, 2007; Schulkin, Gold, & McEwen, 1998).

An attractive psychophysiological speculation is that particular cardiovascular diseases could be linked to specific response patterns observed during particular types of stress challenges. Early concepts of cardiovascular reactivity distinguished between reactivity to physical challenges (e.g., exercise, hand grip) and psychological challenges (e.g., frustration with a task). This developed into the concept that physical challenges would show cardiovascular responses appropriate to current oxygen consumption, but psychological challenges would show vascular perfusion in excess of that related to oxygen consumption (Langer et al., 1985; Langer, Obrist, & McCubbin, 1979). This proposition was supported by both animal and human work. Obrist (Obrist, 1981; Obrist et al., 1987) developed this into the hypothesis that an initiating condition for hypertension was repeated overperfusion of the tissue as a result of stress (cf. Folkow, 2001).

A related concept was that selective effects of stress on the heart and vasculature might show different relationships to cardiovascular disease. To this end, different challenge tasks appear to elicit relatively greater responses in heart rate and stroke volume (e.g., mental arithmetic) than do other tasks that appear to increase blood pressure and peripheral resistance (e.g., cold pressor). These cardiac and vascular reaction patterns seemed to map onto individual differences in reactivity patterns and to the relative distribution of beta-sympathetic receptors on the heart and alpha-sympathetic receptors on the vasculature. Despite success in demonstrating these interrelationships (Allen, Obrist, Sherwood, & Crowell, 1987; Kasprowicz, Manuck, Malkoff, & Krantz, 1990), a task battery embodying this distinction did not show any differential predictivity to preclinical heart disease for cardiac and vascular reactivity (Jennings et al., 1997; Jennings et al., 2004; Kamarck, Jennings, Pogue-Geile, & Manuck, 1994). A recent report, however, found that mental arithmetic, a "cardiac" and "psychological" stressor, induced changes in blood pressure and noradrenalin that predicted blood pressure over an 18-year follow-up period better than did similar changes induced by a cold pressor test, a "vascular" and "physical" stressor (Flaa, Eide, Kjeldsen, & Rostrup, 2008).

Finally, heightened cardiovascular indices may be hypothesized to be more injurious if they are sustained rather than transient. What governs this recovery from a response? Interest in reactivity of the vasculature has continued in part because vascular changes do not adapt rapidly to repetitive stress and persist following a stress challenge after cardiac changes have subsided (Gerin & Pickering, 1995; Kelsey, Soderlund, & Arthur, 2004; Linden, Earle, Gerin, & Christenfeld, 1997). This may indicate an extended vulnerability to vascular damage despite appropriate cardiac recovery. Another perspective on recovery is that an active process, most likely vagal activation, governs the time course of recovery. Conceptually, risk attributable to stress exposure might be reduced if cardiovascular reactivity either occurred in the presence of concurrent vagal activation or was terminated by an increase in vagal activation. Empirically, vagal engagement has been indexed by transient heart rate changes and, most particularly, respiratory-related modulations in heart rate, or respiratory sinus arrhythmia (Allen, Chambers, & Towers, 2007; Katona & Jih, 1975; Kollai & Mizsei, 1990; McCabe, Yongue, Ackles, & Porges, 1985; Porges, 1995; Spyer & Gilbey, 1988).

Using these indices, protection from cardiac arrhythmia resulting from the presence of significant vagal activation has been demonstrated in animals, and enhanced heart rate variability is associated with lower risk of cardiac events in people (Camm et al., 2004; Carney, Freedland, & Veith, 2005; Lombardi, Malliani, Pagani, & Cerutti, 1996; Stauss, 2003; Stein, Domitrovich, Huikuri, Kleiger, & Cast, 2005; Vanoli, Adamson, Foreman, & Schwartz, 2008). Although transient vagal activation has been shown to reduce expression of ischemia (Jennings & Follansbee, 1985), large-scale prospective evidence supporting a specific protective action of rapid recovery from stress reactions is, to our knowledge, lacking. There is, however, promising evidence of longitudinal prediction of blood pressure increases from slowed recovery from a stress challenge (Steptoe & Marmot, 2005).

CARDIOVASCULAR MEASURES AS HEALTH-RELATED PSYCHOLOGICAL CONCEPTS

Psychophysiological measures may be used to index a psychological state rather than a physiological state. Used in this way, psychological states relevant to health, most notably stress or emotion, may be detected and measured. Such experiences may be assessed as they occur, as opposed to self-report measures collected after the experience. The agreement between physiological and other measures is typically far from perfect, as we shall see. It has tempted some to suggest that the discrepancy between self-report and physiological indices is itself an index of dysregulation, but this has not garnered substantial empirical support (Levin & Linden, 2008). Note that this perspective does not demand a robust relationship between physiological change and the health-damaging or -maintaining endpoint. The physiological change indexes the psychological concept, which may in turn relate to a health outcome through pathways other than the physiological change. For example, negative affect is related to a modulation of the startle blink reflex (Vrana, 1994), but blink changes have not been directly related to disease processes.

The modal theory of health psychology may be that stress creates negative affect and that affect drives the physiological changes that are health damaging. We shall see in the next section that this does not seem to be the case for cardiovascular reactivity—a relationship to preclinical disease is present, but it does appear mediated by an affective disposition. Conversely, relationships between a trait, such as hostility, and disease have been shown; but yet again these cannot be shown to be uniformly mediated through cardiovascular reactivity. Further analysis of stress, affect, and physiological reactivity seems required.

Such stress theorists as Richard Lazarus (1966, 2007), for example, have noted that stress likely involves such factors as vigilance toward threat, threat evaluation, selection of a coping response, coping per se, anxiety related to threat, and affect appropriate to the coping response. Do all these processes induce the same psychophysiological stress response? It seems equally as likely that a different response may be generated by each of these states. Most strikingly, attentive vigilance induces a slowing of heart rate even in psychologically arousing situations (Lacey & Lacey, 1974). Different forms of attentive and cognitive processing, largely in the absence of clear stress or affect, have been shown to induce cardiovascular reactions (see the exhaustive review by Jennings & Coles, 1991). Emotional responses themselves have also been posited to develop over time, that is, emotion is not defined as the momentary reaction of experienced affect but, rather, as dynamic, time-varying interaction with the environment. For example, Bradley and Lang (2007) suggest an emotional cascade with initial reactions of vigilance and environmental evaluation inducing cardiovascular responses clearly different than the later reactions to the arousing and valence qualities of a stimulus. Different emotions, defined as the immediate affective experience, also appear to elicit different cardiovascular responses (Gross & Levenson, 1993; Mauss, Levenson, McCarter, Wilhelm, & Gross, 2005), although arguments continue about whether we can determine specific emotions solely from the pattern of change across autonomically controlled response systems. For example, can the intensity of the blood pressure response reliably separate the experience of anger in a stressful situation from the experience of fear? If so, some researchers might argue that only an anger response is health threatening. From the perspective of either a cascade of response or changing responses as affect changes, a number of different physiological responses might be expected within one encounter with a stressful situation. Recognizing and interpreting each is important for a full interpretation of the stress response. Indeed, depending on the stressor, the timing of data collection, and the measures derived, a response may be observed, for example, slowing of heart rate, seemingly inconsistent with the concept of stress.

This complication actually implies a greater utility for psychophysiological measures if an investigator conceptualizes particular processes within the complex of stress reactions that may be toxic to health. For example, if an investigator believes that the anger engendered after threat and coping evaluation is toxic, then measures taken during prior anticipation and evaluation of threat as well as measures taken during subsequent motor reactions are irrelevant to a degree (though they might be evaluated to control for the engagement of participants and strength of their reactions). This strategy may be promising because anger has a somewhat specific physiological pattern associated with it (Scarpa & Raine, 1997; Stemmler, Aue, & Wacker, 2007; Vrana, 2007). Scoring of the psychophysiological response keyed to anger would provide the clearest and most convincing test of the investigator's hypothesis. We hasten to note, though, that the psychophysiological response may not capture the entire meaning of anger. It is rare to see a high correlation between verbal reports of experienced anger (or any other emotion) and a physiological index (Averill, 1974; Lang, Davis, & Ohman, 2002; Ohman, 1986). Emotion, akin to stress, may best be conceptualized as composed intersecting but not overlapping aspects—for example, expressive communication, felt affect, physiological change, activation, and valence. An overlapping, multiple measures approach seems necessary to capture the various aspects of anger. The empirical question of whether some integrated index of the various aspects of anger, or another emotion, will better relate to health and disease than a single facet of the emotion remains.

From the perspective of a multifaceted view of stress and emotion, psychophysiological measures can be useful for separating the facets of stress or emotion that may be relevant to health. For example, such conditions as crowding or noise may elicit individual differences in whether people perceive the situation as exciting or stressful—individual differences that may differ when evaluated through self-report or physiological response to these conditions (Evans & English, 2002; Evans, Kim, Ting, Tesher, & Shannis, 2007; Gomez & Danuser, 2004). Social factors may also modify cardiovascular responses to stress. Cardiovascular reactivity has been shown to be moderated by the presence of another person, although the social relationship between the stressed and the supportive individual has proven to be important in this literature (Uchino, 2006; Uchino, Cacioppo, & Kiecolt-Glaser, 1996).

Processes promoting health and well-being have also been assessed with psychophysiological measures. As with the literature in general, positive affect has been studied less than negative affect, though some studies have compared responses to positive and negative affect (Gehricke & Fridlund, 2002; Lefcourt, Davidson, Prkachin, & Mills, 1997). Current interest in emotion regulation has spurred an interest in whether rapid cardiovascular recovery from stress or challenge may indicate resilience, whereas slow recovery may indicate rumination or worry (Brosschot, Gerin, & Thayer, 2006; Gerin, Davidson, Christenfeld, Goyal, & Schwartz, 2006; Gerin & Pickering, 1995). Thus, cardiovascular measures have been studied as indicators of various psychological concepts. New directions within this area might focus on well-being and positive affect, because the majority of research in this area has examined negative affect.

CARDIOVASCULAR MEASURES AS RISK FACTORS

Assessment of cardiovascular measures as risk factors for cardiovascular disease, typically as physiological responses to laboratory stressors, is the modal application of psychophysiology within health psychology. Heart rate, blood pressure, and potentially other resting, noninvasive measures of cardiovascular function may index disease risk (Palatini & Julius, 2004), but the response of these measures to stress is of greater relevance to health psychology. As noted, the success of the Type A behavior pattern in predicting cardiovascular disease incidence combined with the common perception that stress influences heart disease formed a background for the formulation of the reactivity hypothesis. Everyone seems aware that the heart pounds and blood pressure increases during stress. Most also believe that stress is related to heart disease. It is a small conceptual leap to suggest that the cardiac and vascular changes during stress might be the path that leads from stress to heart disease. This, then, is the generic form of the cardiovascular reactivity hypothesis of psychological influence on heart disease.

As outlined by Krantz and Manuck (1984), individuals prone to robust cardiovascular responses and/or experiencing psychological stress throughout their daily life would experience sustained or multiple bouts of increased cardiovascular activation. This activation through wear and tear on the vascular system and/or activation of injurious endocrine or immune substances would create a vascular injury and risk for later clinical cardiovascular disease (Lovallo, 2005a).

Testing this hypothesis requires analyzing it into testable units; a first, successfully tested unit was the relation between individual differences in the robustness of cardiovascular reactions and subsequent disease indices. Laboratory stress challenges yielded reliable individual differences in the amplitude of heart rate and blood pressure responses (Kamarck & Lovallo, 2003). As reviewed by Treiber and colleagues (2003) blood pressure reactions to laboratory stress are associated with both cardiac and vascular disease indices cross-sectionally and longitudinally. Longitudinal results do not establish causation, but they are more strongly suggestive of this than are cross-sectional relationships. For example, our study of Finnish men showed that blood pressure reactions to a battery of laboratory challenges predicted the change in intima-media thickness of the carotid artery over a 7-year period (Jennings et al., 2004). This study is characteristic of the literature in that a preclinical index of heart disease is the dependent variable. Thickening of the arterial wall is indicative of atherosclerosis, and the carotid artery thickening is related to coronary artery thickening, but carotid intima-media thickness remains an indirect, preclinical index of heart disease. The literature relies on such indices as endpoints and, as Treiber and colleagues (2003) note, prediction from cardiovascular reactivity to the hard endpoint of cardiovascular death has not been established and remains an important area for future research.

Other aspects of the cardiovascular reactivity hypothesis have not been as fully resolved as the relationship between individual differences in laboratory reactivity and preclinical indices of cardiovascular disease. The hypothesis would anticipate that individuals with greater reactivity might also be those with an excess of hostility, which is currently viewed as the potent factor within the original complex of Type A traits (Everson-Rose & Lewis, 2005; Smith & MacKenzie, 2006), or sparse social networks, which is another cardiovascular risk factor (Everson-Rose & Lewis, 2005; Knox & Uvnas-Moberg, 1998; Rozanski, Blumenthal, & Kaplan, 1999). This has not typically been the case; that is, cardiovascular reactivity has not proven to be the mediator explaining risk related to trait hostility or impoverished social network. This issue has not been settled, however; work continues on the how hostility relates to physiological function (Chen, Gilligan, Coups, & Contrada, 2005; Fredrickson et al., 2000; Suls & Wan, 1993) and how social integration and social networks relate to cardiovascular reactivity (Christenfeld & Gerin, 2000).

Similarly, the reactivity hypothesis suggests that individuals experiencing greater everyday stress might show greater cardiovascular reactivity. One approach to testing this hyphothesis is to survey stress experiences using such inventories such as the Perceived Stress Scale (Cohen, Kamarck, & Mermelstein, 1983) and then examine cardiovascular reactivity to laboratory stress in individuals varying in their report of daily stress. Results from such studies have been quite variable; both positive and negative correlations have been reported between stress reports and increased and decreased reactivity to laboratory task (Matthews, Gump, Block, & Allen, 1997; Matthews, Gump, & Owens, 2001). Another approach is to assess cardiovascular variables using ambulatory monitoring in conjunction with behavioral reports of stress throughout the day

(Chobanian et al., 2003; Kamarck, Schwartz, Janicki, Shiffman, & Raynor, 2003; Kamarck et al., 1998). This approach has also met with variable success. Within a day or two of recording, few stressful events might be identified with clear timing and sufficient intensity to relate clearly to physiological change. Other evidence suggests that particular situations or individual characteristics may elicit cardiovascular responses reliably only when that characteristic is activated by the environment; for example, individuals invested in control may be reliably reactive only when the situations appear to challenge such control (Kamarck et al., 2005). In addition, some individuals seem to show discrepant physiological changes in ambulatory and laboratory settings (Matthews, Owens, Allen, & Stoney, 1992). Tivedi et al. (2008) provide a current review of the relationships of ambulatory blood pressure and both blood pressure reactivity and recovery from psychological challenge. As they point out, the prediction of ambulatory blood pressure values from either laboratory blood pressure reactivity or recovery requires care. Blood pressure reactivity to challenge in the laboratory has not been found to readily relate to variable, presumably reactive, blood pressure throughout the day. Highly reactive individuals are not routinely found to show higher daytime or nighttime ambulatory pressures. By aggregating across challenge tasks, though, and separating day and nighttime ambulatory pressure, they were able to show that both blood pressure reactivity and recovery predicted daytime ambulatory pressure (Stewart et al., 2006). Nighttime pressure was related more strongly to recovery only. This finding has potential significance because the degree to which blood pressure falls during sleep has correlated with cardiovascular morbidity and mortality (Staessen et al., 1999).

In sum, the cardiovascular reactivity hypothesis has found support in that cardiovascular reactions to laboratory challenges are predictive of later cardiovascular disease indices. These individual differences in cardiovascular reactivity have not, however, readily explained the relationships between cardiovascular risk and such psychological risk factors as hostility and sparse social networks. Similarly, complex rather than simple relationships seem to be emerging for the association between daily stress and personality characteristics relative to both cardiovascular reactivity and disease. Ambulatory monitoring holds the promise of understanding how stress and cardiovascular reactivity in daily life may relate to disease, but such issues as the sampling of events and the complexity of the stress response challenge this approach. Promising new approaches may, however, clarify how cardiovascular reactivity fits into the overall picture of psychosocial risks for heart disease. Specifically, genetic variation may be used to identify different pathways of risk involving cardiovascular reactivity (McCaffery, Bleil, Pogue-Geile, Ferrell, & Manuck, 2003). Also, conceptualizing stress reactivity in terms of integrated autonomic, immune, and endocrine responsivity seems necessary and may provide a better platform from which to understand daily stress, acute stress reactivity, and translation into disease risk (Manuck, Marsland, Kaplan, & Williams, 1995; Marsland, Bachen, Cohen, Rabin, & Manuck, 2002). A related strategy is to examine the central nervous system control of these response systems with the hypothesis that disease risk may be more clearly identified by variation between individuals in the structure and function of central regulatory areas (or influences upon these areas). Such work is already promising (Gianaros et al., 2007; Gianaros, May, Siegle, & Jennings, 2005; Gianaros et al., 2008).

As an aside, it is important to note that when we consider cardiovascular measures as risk factors for the development of cardiovascular disease, it is equally relevant to consider how cardiovascular measures may function as protective factors against its development. For example, the success of such health-promoting activities as exercise and meditation can also be assessed. Regular exercise induces an overall decrease in heart rate throughout the day, called a training effect (de Geus & Van Doornen, 1993; George, Gates, & Tolfrey, 2005); meditation decreases heart rate and blood pressure transiently (Cuthbert, Kristeller, Simons, Hodes, & Lang, 1981; Holmes, 1984; Sawada & Steptoe, 1988). It is not clear that either acts to reduce cardiovascular stress reactivity (de Geus & Van Doornen, 1993; Holmes, 1984; Sawada & Steptoe, 1988), although both exercise and meditation have been associated with enhanced health maintenance (e.g., Mourad et al., 2008; Walton et al., 2002). Research on health-maintaining processes, most particularly those associated with vagal function, is in its infancy or, at least, early childhood with a number of reasonable speculations suggesting the value of further research in the area (e.g., Thayer & Lane, 2007; Thayer & Sternberg, 2006).

CARDIOVASCULAR MEASURES OF DISEASE

Health psychologists by definition study health and illness. This interest means that psychophysiological measures may be employed not as indices of psychological processes but as indices of disease. What is a psychophysiological measure of cardiovascular disease? Prior to surgery, virtually any medical measure done to diagnose a disease could be considered a psychophysiological measure. Most researchers would emphasize the "physiological" part of the measure, ignoring the "psycho"; but the pervasive influence of the central nervous system could somewhat counter this claim. Focusing on standard cardiovascular measures taken in the psychophysiology laboratory, however, leaves blood pressure, the electrocardiogram, and impedance cardiography as candidate measures of disease or preclinical disease (i.e., an index directly associated with the later, treated expression of the disease).

Blood pressure assessment is both a typical psychophysiological measure and a direct measure of a major chronic disease, essential hypertension (Chobanian et al., 2003). A behavioral intervention designed to reduce hypertension would clearly use this measure pre- and postintervention as a primary outcome variable. Care should be taken, however, to exclude secondary causes of high blood pressure and to collect blood pressure in a diagnostically valid manner (Chobanian et al., 2003). Although superficially a simple measure, blood pressure is often badly measured. The care to be taken with participant posture, cuff management, and other factors are described well in Shapiro et al. (1996). Clinical diagnosis requires repeated readings in a seated posture with rest intervening. Interestingly though, these reading are not uniformly valid. Some people have elevated blood pressure in the doctor's office, but not elsewhere, reflecting a so-called white-coat hypertension (Pickering et al., 1990). Ambulatory assessment of blood pressure over a 24-hour or longer period provides an extensive assessment of blood pressure that is more representative of the person's blood pressure than is the clinic assessment. Ambulatory assessment can also reveal failure to decrease blood pressure during sleep—a factor shown to place someone at greater risk for later disease (Henskens et al., 2008). Thus, factors that are potentially psychological in nature are important to consider even when using blood pressure solely as a measurement of disease state.

The electrocardiogram and impedance cardiography provide further examples. The psychophysiologist typically derives heart rate from the electrocardiogram, but the electrocardiogram also is a direct measure of cardiac arrhythmia. Important early work in biofeedback showed some success in modulating the occurrence of cardiac arrhythmia (Weiss & Engel, 1971). Furthermore, the electrocardiogram can be scored to show the depression of the ST segment that is associated with cardiac ischemia. We used both arrhythmia and ST segment depression as outcome variables in a study of vagal function (Jennings & Follansbee, 1985). Impedance cardiography is sensitive to changes in stroke volume that may be diagnostic of ischemic disease of the heart. These applications are primarily to patients with known heart disease, and appropriate clinical oversight is clearly necessary for such studies.

PROSPECTIVE

From any perspective, psychophysiology is integral to health psychology, and ideally investigators will use all the perspectives reviewed in designing their research. For example, a single project can conceive of blood pressure as a disease index, a measure of sympathetic nervous system activation, and a concomitant of anger elicitation. Although using multiple perspective is not possible with every measure or project, it is always possible to consider all the ways a psychophysiological measure could be conceptualized within a research project. Our brief review has suggested that psychophysiological measures have been effectively used from each of our perspectives. The perspectives illustrate the diversity of our field: The psychologist should be interested in physiological measures of psychological processes, the physiologist in physiological measures of control systems, and the medical scientist in the physiological indices of disease and health. Our role is to integrate these perspectives and develop the utility of each.

The future of psychophysiological measures is tied to technical and conceptual development. The technical advances with brain imaging, for example, provide us with new psychophysiological tools to examine central regulation of bodily function and the translation from psychological events to physiological output. Lane et al. (Lane & Wager, 2009; Lane, Waldstein, Chesney et al., 2009; Lane, Waldstein, Critchley et al., 2009) review the promise of these techniques for health psychology. Over the last 20 years, concepts of disease pathogenesis as well as basic physiology have advanced. Cardiovascular disease, for instance, is no longer thought of as a simple buildup of plaque but is viewed as a complex interaction of predisposing factors, among them wall injury possibly related to autonomic and endocrine activation, the immune system response to that injury, and the interaction of all these factors to yield stable or unstable plaque (Bairey-Merz et al., 2002; Steptoe & Marmot, 2006). This revised concept of disease now requires a consideration of concurrent measures of autonomic, endocrine, and immune function. Advances in physiology make it clear that psychological and central nervous system processes are integral to the moment-to-moment control of each of these systems. Technical advances may be required to have truly comparable measures of these systems in real time. In addition, the great strides in genetics require some attention to these predisposing factors, which may alter pathways to disease between different individuals.

CONCLUSION

Behavioral medicine is necessarily related to psychophysiology, and the examination of physiological indices related to psychological processes in intact organisms. Peripheral psychophysiological measures are important indices of the activation of the two branches of the autonomic nervous system, sympathetic and parasympathetic; whereas, central measures of brain function probe regulatory circuitry of relevant to autonomic activation. Such measures can be employed to examine such psychological concepts as reactions to stress, but the specificity of both physiological and psychological reactions must be considered. As measures of risk factors, psychophysiological indices have been particularly prominent in showing that reactions to laboratory stress relate to later cardiovascular disease. Finally, psychophysiological measures can directly assess presence of disease, for example, white-coat and stable hypertension, cardiac arrhythmia. Thus, a number of different psychophysiological approaches are directly relevant to behavioral medicine.

REFERENCES

Allen, J. J. B., Chambers, A. S., & Towers, D. N. (2007). The many metrics of cardiac chronotropy: A pragmatic primer and a brief comparison of metrics. *Biological Psychology, 74*(2), 243–262.

Allen, M. T., Obrist, P. A., Sherwood, A., & Crowell, M. D. (1987). Evaluation of myocardial and peripheral vascular responses during reaction time, mental arithmetic, and cold pressor tasks. *Psychophysiology, 24*(6), 648–656.

Averill, J. R. (1974). An analysis of psychophysiological symbolism and its influence on theories of emotion. *Journal for the Theory of Social Behaviour, 4*(2), 147–190.

Bairey-Merz, C. N., Dwyer, J., Nordstrom, C. K., Walton, K. G., Salerno, J. W., & Schneider, R. H. (2002). Psychosocial stress and cardiovascular disease: Pathophysiological links. *Behavioral Medicine, 27*(4), 141–147.

Berntson, G. G., & Cacioppo, J. T. (2007). Integrative physiology: Homeostasis, allostasis, and the orchestration of systemic physiology. In J. T. Cacioppo, L. G. Tassinary, & G. G. Berntson (Eds.), *Handbook of psychophysiology* (3rd ed., pp. 433–452). New York, NY: Cambridge University Press.

Berntson G. G., Norman G. J., Hawkley, L. C., & Cacioppo, J. T. (2008). Cardiac autonomic balance versus cardiac regulatory capacity. *Psychophysiology, 45*(4), 643–652.

Bradley, M. M., & Lang, P. J. (Eds.). (2007). *Emotion and motivation*: New York, NY: Cambridge University Press.

Brosschot J. F., Gerin W., & Thayer, J. F. (2006). The perseverative cognition hypothesis: A review of worry, prolonged stress-related physiological activation, and health. *Journal of Psychosomatic Research, 60*(2), 113–124.

Brotman, D. J., Davidson, M. B., Boumitri, M., & Vidt, D. G. (2008). Impaired diurnal blood pressure variation and all-cause mortality. *American Journal of Hypertension, 21*(1), 92–97.

Cacioppo, J. T., Tassinary, L. G., & Berntson, G. G. (Eds.). (2007). *Psychophysiological science: Interdisciplinary approaches to classic questions about the mind*. New York, NY: Cambridge University Press.

Camm, A. J., Pratt, C. M., Schwartz, P. J., Al-Khalidi, H. R., Spyt, M. J., Holroyde, M. J., ... Brum, J. M. G. (2004). Mortality in patients after a recent myocardial infarction: A randomized, placebo-controlled trial of azimilide using heart rate variability for risk stratification. *Circulation, 109*(8), 990–996.

Campbell, T. S., Key, B. L., Ireland, A. D., Bacon, S. L., & Ditto, B. (2008). Early socioeconomic status is associated with adult nighttime blood pressure dipping. *Psychosomatic Medicine, 70*(3), 276–281.

Carney, R. M., Freedland, K. E., & Veith, R. C. (2005). Depression, the autonomic nervous system, and coronary heart disease. *Psychosomatic Medicine, 67*(Suppl. 1), S29–S33.

Chen, Y. Y., Gilligan, S., Coups, E. J., & Contrada, R. J. (2005). Hostility and perceived social support: Interactive effects on cardiovascular reactivity to laboratory stressors. *Annals of Behavioral Medicine, 29*(1), 37–43.

Chobanian, A. V., Bakris, G. L., Black, H. R., Cushman, W. C., Green, L. A., Izzo, J. L., Jr., ... Roccella, E. J. (2003). Seventh report of the Joint National Committee on Prevention, Detection, Evaluation, and Treatment of High Blood Pressure. *Hypertension, 42*(6), 1206–1252.

Christenfeld, N., & Gerin, W. (2000). Social support and cardiovascular reactivity. *Biomedicine & Pharmacotherapy, 54*(5), 251–257.

Cohen, S., Kamarck, T., & Mermelstein, R. (1983). A global measure of perceived stress. *Journal of Health & Social Behavior, 24*(4), 385–396.

Coles, M. G. H., Jennings, J. R., & Stern, J. A. (1984). *Psychophysiological perspectives: Festschrift for Beatrice and John Lacey*. New York, NY: Van Nostrand Reinhold.

Curtin, J. J., Lozano, D. L., & Allen, J. J. B. (2007). The psychophysiology laboratory. In J. A. Coan & J. J. B. Allen (Eds.), *The handbook of emotion elicitation and assessment* (pp. 398–425). New York, NY: Oxford University Press.

Cuthbert, B., Kristeller, J., Simons, R., Hodes, R., & Lang, P. J. (1981). Strategies of arousal control: Biofeedback, meditation, and motivation. *Journal of Experimental Psychology: General, 110*(4), 518–546.

de Geus, E. J., & Van Doornen, L. J. (1993). The effects of fitness training on the physiological stress response. *Work & Stress, 7*(2), 141–159.

Evans, G. W., & English, K. (2002). The environment of poverty: Multiple stressor exposure, psychophysiological stress, and socioemotional adjustment. *Child Development, 73*(4), 1238–1248.

Evans, G. W., Kim, P., Ting, A. H., Tesher, H. B., & Shannis, D. (2007). Cumulative risk, maternal responsiveness, and allostatic load among young adolescents. *Developmental Psychology, 43*(2), 341–351.

Everson-Rose, S. A., & Lewis, T. T. (2005). Psychosocial factors and cardiovascular diseases. *Annual Review of Public Health, 26*, 469–500.

Flaa, A., Eide, I. K., Kjeldsen, S. E., & Rostrup, M. (2008). Sympathoadrenal stress reactivity is a predictor of future blood pressure: An 18-year follow-up study. *Hypertension, 52*(2), 336–341.

Folkow, B. (2001). Mental stress and its importance for cardiovascular disorders: Physiological aspects, "from-mice-to-man." *Scandinavian Cardiovascular Journal, 35*(3), 163–172.

Fredrickson, B. L., Maynard, K. E., Helms, M. J., Haney, T. L., Siegler, I. C., & Barefoot, J. C. (2000). Hostility predicts magnitude and duration of blood pressure response to anger. *Journal of Behavioral Medicine, 23*(3), 229–243.

Gehricke, J.-G., & Fridlund, A. J. (2002). Smiling, frowning, and autonomic activity in mildly depressed and nondepressed men in response to emotional imagery of social contexts. *Perceptual and Motor Skills, 94*(1), 141–151.

George, K. P., Gates, P. E., & Tolfrey, K. (2005). The impact of aerobic training upon left ventricular morphology and function in pre-pubescent children. *Ergonomics, 48*(11–14), 1378–1389.

Gerin, W., Davidson, K. W., Christenfeld, N. J., Goyal, T., & Schwartz, J. E. (2006). The role of angry rumination and distraction in blood pressure recovery from emotional arousal. *Psychosomatic Medicine, 68*(1), 64–72.

Gerin, W., & Pickering, T. G. (1995). Association between delayed recovery of blood pressure after acute mental stress and parental history of hypertension. *Journal of Hypertension, 13*(6), 603–610.

Gianaros, P. J., Jennings, J. R., Sheu, L. K., Greer, P. J., Kuller, L. H., & Matthews, K. A. (2007). Prospective reports of chronic life stress predict decreased grey matter volume in the hippocampus. *Neuroimage, 35*(2), 795–803.

Gianaros, P. J., May, J. C., Siegle, G. J., & Jennings, J. R. (2005). Is there a functional neural correlate of individual differences in cardiovascular reactivity? *Psychosomatic Medicine, 67*(1), 31–39.

Gianaros, P. J., Sheu, L. K., Matthews, K. A., Jennings, J. R., Manuck, S. B., & Hariri, A. R. (2008). Individual differences in stressor-evoked blood pressure reactivity vary with activation, volume, and functional connectivity of the amygdala. *Journal of Neuroscience, 28*(4), 990–999.

Gomez, P., & Danuser, B. (2004). Affective and physiological responses to environmental noises and music. *International Journal of Psychophysiology, 53*(2), 91–103.

Gross, J. J., & Levenson, R. W. (1993). Emotional suppression: Physiology, self-report, and expressive behavior. *Journal of Personality and Social Psychology, 64*(6), 970–986.

Hawkley, L. C., Burleson, M. H., Poehlmann, K. M., Berntson, G. G., Malarkey, W. B., & Cacioppo, J. T. (2001). Cardiovascular and endocrine reactivity in older females: Intertask consistency. *Psychophysiology, 38*(6), 863–872.

Henskens, L. H., Kroon, A. A., van Oostenbrugge, R. J., Haest, R. J., Lodder, J., & de Leeuw, P. W. (2008). Different classifications of nocturnal blood pressure dipping affect the prevalence of dippers and nondippers and the relation with target-organ damage. *Journal of Hypertension, 26*(4), 691–698.

Holmes, D. S. (1984). Meditation and somatic arousal reduction: A review of the experimental evidence. *American Psychologist, 39*(1), 1–10.

Jennings, J. R., & Coles, M. G. H (Eds.). (1991). *Handbook of cognitive psychophysiology: Central and autonomic nervous system approaches.* Oxford, England: John Wiley & Sons.

Jennings, J. R., & Follansbee, W. P. (1985). Task-induced ST segment depression, ectopic beats, and autonomic responses in coronary heart disease patients. *Psychosomatic Medicine, 47*(5), 415–430.

Jennings, J. R., & Gianaros, P. J. (2007). Methodology. In J. T. Cacioppo, L. G. Tassinary, & G. G. Berntson (Eds.), *Handbook of psychophysiology* (3rd ed., pp. 812–833). New York, NY: Cambridge University Press.

Jennings, J. R., Kamarck, T. W., Everson-Rose, S. A., Kaplan, G. A., Manuck, S. B., & Salonen, J. T. (2004). Exaggerated blood pressure responses during mental stress are prospectively related to enhanced carotid atherosclerosis in middle-aged Finnish men. *Circulation, 110*(15), 2198–2203.

Jennings, J. R., Kamarck, T. W., Manuck, S., Everson, S. A., Kaplan, G., & Salonen, J. T. (1997). Aging or disease? Cardiovascular reactivity in Finnish men over the middle years. *Psychology and Aging, 12*(2), 225–238.

Jennings, J. R., van der Molen, M. W., Somsen, R. J. M., Graham, R., & Gianaros, P. J. (2002). Vagal function in health and disease: Studies in Pittsburgh. *Physiology & Behavior, 77*(4-5), 693–698.

Kamarck, T. W., Jennings, J. R., Pogue-Geile, M., & Manuck, S. B. (1994). A multidimensional measurement model for cardiovascular reactivity: Stability and cross-validation in two adult samples. *Health Psychology, 13*(6), 471–478.

Kamarck, T. W., & Lovallo, W. R. (2003). Cardiovascular reactivity to psychological challenge: Conceptual and measurement considerations. *Psychosomatic Medicine, 65*(1), 9–21.

Kamarck, T. W., Schwartz, J. E., Janicki, D. L., Shiffman, S., & Raynor, D. A. (2003). Correspondence between laboratory and ambulatory measures of cardiovascular reactivity: A multilevel modeling approach. *Psychophysiology, 40*(5), 675–683.

Kamarck, T. W., Schwartz, J. E., Shiffman, S., Muldoon, M. F., Sutton-Tyrrell, K., & Janicki, D. L. (2005). Psychosocial stress and cardiovascular risk: What is the role of daily experience? *Journal of Personality, 73*(6), 1749–1774.

Kamarck, T. W., Shiffman, S. M., Smithline, L., Goodie, J. L., Thompson, H. S., Ituarte, P. H. G, … Perz, W. (Eds.). (1998). *The diary of ambulatory behavioral states: A new approach to the assessment of psychosocial influences on ambulatory cardiovascular activity.* Mahwah, NJ: Erlbaum.

Kasprowicz, A. L., Manuck, S. B., Malkoff, S. B., & Krantz, D. S. (1990). Individual differences in behaviorally evoked cardiovascular response: Temporal stability and hemodynamic patterning. *Psychophysiology, 27*(6), 605–619.

Katona, P. G., & Jih, F. (1975). Respiratory sinus arrhythmia: noninvasive measure of parasympathetic cardiac control. *Journal of Applied Physiology, 39*(5), 801–805.

Kelsey, R. M., Soderlund, K., & Arthur C. M. (2004). Cardiovascular reactivity and adaptation to recurrent psychological stress: Replication and extension. *Psychophysiology, 41*(6), 924–934.

Knox, S. S., & Uvnas-Moberg, K. (1998). Social isolation and cardiovascular disease: An atherosclerotic pathway? *Psychoneuroendocrinology, 23*(8), 877–890.

Kollai, M., & Mizsei, G. (1990). Respiratory sinus arrhythmia is a limited measure of cardiac parasympathetic control in man. *Journal of Physiology, 424*, 329–342.

Krantz, D. S., & Manuck, S. B. (1984). Acute psychophysiologic reactivity and risk of cardiovascular disease: A review and methodologic critique. *Psychological Bulletin, 96*(3), 435–464.

Lacey, B. C., & Lacey, J. I. (1974). Studies of heart rate and other bodily processes in sensorimotor behavior. In P. Obrist, A. H. Black, J. Brener, & L. V. DiCara (Eds.), *Cardiovascular psychophysiology* (pp. 538–564). Chicago, IL: Aldine.

Lane, R. D., & Wager, T. D. (2009). The new field of brain-body medicine: What have we learned and where are we headed? *Neuroimage, 47*(3), 1135–1140.

Lane, R. D., Waldstein, S. R., Chesney, M. A., Jennings, J. R., Lovallo, W. R., Kozel, P. J., … Cameron, O. G. (2009). The rebirth of neuroscience in psychosomatic medicine: Part I. Historical context, methods, and relevant basic science. *Psychosom Med, 71*(2), 117–134.

Lane, R. D., Waldstein, S. R., Critchley, H. D., Derbyshire, S. W., Drossman, D. A., Wager, T. D., … Cameron, O. G. (2009). The rebirth of neuroscience in psychosomatic medicine: Part II. Clinical applications and implications for research. *Psychosom Med, 71*(2), 135–151.

Lang, P. J., Davis, M., & Ohman, A. (Eds.). (2002). *Fear and anxiety: Animal models and human cognitive psychophysiology*. Hove, England: Psychology Press.

Langer, A. W., McCubbin, J. A., Stoney, C. M., Hutcheson, J. S., Charlton, J. D., & Obrist, P. A. (1985). Cardiopulmonary adjustments during exercise and an aversive reaction time task: Effects of beta-adrenoceptor blockade. *Psychophysiology, 22*(1), 59–68.

Langer, A. W., Obrist, P. A., & McCubbin, J. A. (1979). Hemodynamic and metabolic adjustments during exercise and shock avoidance in dogs. *American Journal of Physiology, 236*(2), H225–H230.

Lefcourt, H. M., Davidson, K., Prkachin, K. M., & Mills, D. E. (1997). Humor as a stress moderator in the prediction of blood pressure obtained during five stressful tasks. *Journal of Research in Personality, 31*(4), 523–542.

Levin, A. Y., & Linden, W. (2008). Does dissociation of emotional and physiological reactivity predict blood pressure change at 3- and 10-year follow-up? *Biological Psychology, 77*(2), 183–190.

Linden W., Earle, T. L., Gerin, W., & Christenfeld, N. (1997). Physiological stress reactivity and recovery: Conceptual siblings separated at birth? *Journal of Psychosomatic Research, 42*(2), 117–135.

Lindsley, D. B. (1951). Emotion. In *Handbook of experimental psychology* (pp. 473–516). Oxford, England: Wiley.

Llewellyn-Smith, I. J., & Verberne, A. J. M. (2011). *Central regulation of autonomic function,* 2nd ed. New York, NY: Oxford University Press.

Lombardi, F., Malliani, A., Pagani, M., & Cerutti, S. (1996). Heart rate variability and its sympatho-vagal modulation. *Cardiovascular Research, 32*(2), 208–216.

Lovallo, W. R. (2005a). Cardiovascular reactivity: mechanisms and pathways to cardiovascular disease. *International Journal of Psychophysiology, 58*(2–3), 119–132.

Lovallo, W. R. (2005b). *Stress & health: Biological and psychological interactions* (2nd ed.). Thousand Oaks, CA: Sage.

Manuck, S. B., Marsland, A. L., Kaplan, J. R., & Williams, J. K. (1995). The pathogenicity of behavior and its neuroendocrine mediation: An example from coronary artery disease. *Psychosomatic Medicine, 57*(3), 275–283.

Marsland, A. L., Bachen, E. A., Cohen, S., Rabin, B., & Manuck, S. B. (2002). Stress, immune reactivity and susceptibility to infectious disease. *Physiology & Behavior, 77*(4–5), 711–716.

Matthews, K. A. (1982). Psychological perspectives on the type A behavior pattern. *Psychological Bulletin, 91*(2), 293–323.

Matthews, K. A., Gump, B. B., Block, D. R., & Allen, M. T. (1997). Does background stress heighten or dampen children's cardiovascular responses to acute stress? *Psychosomatic Medicine, 59*(5), 488–496.

Matthews, K. A., Gump, B. B., & Owens, J. F. (2001). Chronic stress influences cardiovascular and neuroendocrine responses during acute stress and recovery, especially in men. *Health Psychology, 20*(6), 403–410.

Matthews, K. A., Owens, J. F., Allen, M. T., & Stoney, C. M. (1992). Do cardiovascular responses to laboratory stress relate to ambulatory blood pressure levels? Yes, in some of the people, some of the time. *Psychosomatic Medicine, 54*(6), 686–697.

Mauss, I. B., Levenson, R. W., McCarter, L., Wilhelm, F. H., & Gross, J. J. (2005). The tie that binds? Coherence among emotion experience, behavior, and physiology. *Emotion, 5*(2), 175–190.

McCabe, P. M., Yongue, B. G., Ackles, P. K., & Porges, S. W. (1985). Changes in heart period, heart-period variability, and a spectral analysis estimate of respiratory sinus arrhythmia in response to pharmacological manipulations of the baroreceptor reflex in cats. *Psychophysiology, 22*(2), 195–203.

McCaffery, J. M., Bleil, M., Pogue-Geile, M. F., Ferrell, R. E., & Manuck, S. B. (2003). Allelic variation in the serotonin transporter gene-linked polymorphic region (5-HTTLPR) and cardiovascular reactivity in young adult male and female twins of European-American descent. *Psychosomatic Medicine, 65*(5), 721–728.

McEwen, B., & Lasley, E. N. (2007). Allostatic load: When protection gives way to damage. In A. Monat, R. S. Lazarus, & G. Reevy (Eds.), *The Praeger handbook on stress and coping* (Vol.1, pp. 99–109). Westport, CT: Praeger Publishers/Greenwood Publishing Group.

Mourad, J.-J., Danchin, N., Puel, J., Gallois, H., Msihid, J., Safar, M. E., & Tanaka, H. (2008). Cardiovascular impact of exercise and drug therapy in older hypertensives with coronary heart disease: PREHACOR study. *Heart & Vessels, 23*(1), 20–25.

Obrist, P. A. (1976). The cardiovascular-behavioral interaction: As it appears today. *Psychophysiology, 13*(2), 95–107.

Obrist, P. A. (1981). *Cardiovascular psychophysiology:* A perspective. New York, NY: Plenum Press.

Obrist, P. A., Light, K. C., James, S. A., & Strogatz, D. S. (1987). Cardiovascular responses to stress: I. Measures of myocardial response and relationship to high resting systolic pressure and parental hypertension. *Psychophysiology, 24*(1), 65–78.

Ohman, A. (1986). Face the beast and fear the face: Animal and social fears as prototypes for evolutionary analyses of emotion. *Psychophysiology, 23*(2), 123–145.

Palatini, P., & Julius, S. (2004). Elevated heart rate: A major risk factor for cardiovascular disease. *Clinical & Experimental Hypertension, 26*(7–8), 637–644.

Pickering, T. G., Devereux, R. B., Gerin, W., James, G. D., Pieper, C., Schlussel, Y. R., & Schnall, P. L. (1990). The role of behavioral factors in white coat and sustained hypertension. *Journal of Hypertension, 8* (Suppl. 7), S141–S147.

Porges, S. W. (1995). Orienting in a defensive world: mammalian modifications of our evolutionary heritage: A polyvagal theory. *Psychophysiology, 32*(4), 301–318.

Rosenman, R. H., Friedman, M., Straus, R., Jenkins, C. D., Zyzanski, S. J., & Wurm, M. (1970). Coronary heart disease in the Western Collaborative Group Study. A follow-up experience of 4 and one-half years. *Journal of Chronic Diseases, 23*(3), 173–190.

Rozanski, A., Blumenthal, J. A., & Kaplan, J. (1999). Impact of psychological factors on the pathogenesis of cardiovascular disease and implications for therapy. *Circulation, 99*(16), 2192–2217.

Sawada, Y., & Steptoe, A. (1988). The effects of brief meditation training on cardiovascular stress responses. *Journal of Psychophysiology, 2*(4), 249–257.

Scarpa, A., & Raine, A. (1997). Psychophysiology of anger and violent behavior. *Psychiatric Clinics of North America, 20*(2), 375–394.

Schulkin, J., Gold, P. W., & McEwen, B. S. (1998). Induction of corticotropin-releasing hormone gene expression by glucocorticoids: Implication for understanding the states of fear and anxiety and allostatic load. *Psychoneuroendocrinology, 23*(3), 219–243.

Shapiro, D., Jamner, L. D., Lane, J. D., Light, K. C., Myrtek, M., Sawada, Y., & Steptoe, A. (1996). Blood pressure publication guidelines. Society for Psychophysical Research. *Psychophysiology, 33*(1), 1–12.

Smith, T. W., & MacKenzie, J. (2006). Personality and risk of physical illness. *Annual Review of Clinical Psychology, 2*, 435–467.

Spyer, K. M., & Gilbey, M. P. (1988). Cardiorespiratory interactions in heart-rate control. *Annals of the New York Academy of Sciences, 533*, 350–357.

Staessen, J. A., Beilin, L., Parati, G., Waeber, B., & White, W. (1999). Task force IV: Clinical use of ambulatory blood pressure monitoring. Participants of the 1999 Consensus Conference on Ambulatory Blood Pressure Monitoring. *Blood Pressure Monitoring, 4*(6), 319–331.

Stauss, H. M. (2003). Heart rate variability. *American Journal of Physiology—Regulatory Integrative & Comparative Physiology, 285*(5), R927–R931.

Stein, P. K., Domitrovich, P. P., Huikuri, H. V., Kleiger, R. E., & Cast, I. (2005). Traditional and nonlinear heart rate variability are each independently associated with mortality after myocardial infarction. *Journal of Cardiovascular Electrophysiology, 16*(1), 13–20.

Stemmler, G., Aue, T., & Wacker, J. (2007). Anger and fear: Separable effects of emotion and motivational direction on somatovisceral responses. *International Journal of Psychophysiology, 66*(2), 141–153.

Steptoe A., & Marmot M. (2005). Impaired cardiovascular recovery following stress predicts 3-year increases in blood pressure. *Journal of Hypertension, 23*(3), 529–536.

Steptoe, A., & Marmot, M. (2006). Psychosocial, hemostatic, and inflammatory correlates of delayed poststress blood pressure recovery. *Psychosomatic Medicine, 68*(4), 531–537.

Stern, R. M., Ray, W. J., & Davis, C. M. (1980). *Psychophysiological recording*. New York, NY: Oxford University Press.

Stewart, J. C., Janicki, D. L., Kamarck, T. W., Stewart, J. C., Janicki, D. L., & Kamarck, T. W. (2006). Cardiovascular reactivity to and recovery from psychological challenge as predictors of 3-year change in blood pressure. *Health Psychology, 25*(1), 111–118.

Suls, J., & Wan, C. K. (1993). The relationship between trait hostility and cardiovascular reactivity: A quantitative review and analysis. *Psychophysiology, 30*(6), 615–626.

Swanson, L. W. (2003). *Brain architecture: Understanding the basic plan*. New York, NY: Oxford University Press.

Thayer, J. F., & Lane, R. D. (2007). The role of vagal function in the risk for cardiovascular disease and mortality. *Biological Psychology, 74*(2), 224–242.

Thayer, J. F., & Sternberg, E. (2006). Beyond heart rate variability: Vagal regulation of allostatic systems. *Annals of the New York Academy of Sciences, 1088*, 361–372.

Tivedi, R., Sherwood, A., Strauman, T. J., & Blumenthal, J. A. (2008). Laboratory-based blood pressure recovery is a predictor of ambulatory blood pressure. *Biological Psychology, 77*, 317–323.

Treiber, F. A., Kamarck, T., Schneiderman, N., Sheffield, D., Kapuku, G., & Taylor, T. (2003). Cardiovascular reactivity and development of preclinical and clinical disease states. *Psychosomatic Medicine, 65*(1), 46–62.

Uchino, B. N. (2006). Social support and health: A review of physiological processes potentially underlying links to disease outcomes. *Journal of Behavioral Medicine, 29*(4), 377–387.

Uchino, B. N., Cacioppo, J. T., & Kiecolt-Glaser, J. K. (1996). The relationship between social support and physiological processes: A review with emphasis on underlying mechanisms and implications for health. *Psychological Bulletin, 119*(3), 488–531.

Uchino, B. N., Smith, T. W., Holt-Lunstad, J., Campo, R., & Reblin, M. (2007). Stress and illness. In J. T. Cacioppo, L. G. Tassinary, & G. G. Berntson (Eds.), *Handbook of psychophysiology* (3rd ed., pp. 608–632). New York, NY: Cambridge University Press.

Vanoli, E., Adamson, P. B., Foreman, R. D., & Schwartz, P. J. (2008). Prediction of unexpected sudden death among healthy dogs by a novel marker of autonomic neural activity. *Heart Rhythm, 5*(2), 300–305.

Vrana, S. R. (1994). Startle reflex response during sensory modality specific disgust, anger, and neutral imagery. *Journal of Psychophysiology, 8*(3), 211–218.

Vrana, S. R. (2007). Psychophysiology of anger: Introduction to the special issue. *International Journal of Psychophysiology, 66*(2), 93–94.

Walton, K. G., Schneider, R. H., Nidich, S. I., Salerno, J. W., Nordstrom, C. K., & Merz, C. (2002). Psychosocial stress and cardiovascular disease: Part 2. Effectiveness of the transcendental meditation program in treatment and prevention. *Behavioral Medicine, 28*(3), 106–123.

Weiss, T., & Engel, B. T. (1971). Operant conditioning of heart rate in patients with premature ventricular contractions. *Psychosomatic Medicine, 33*(4), 301–321.

3 Stress, Health, and Illness

Angela Liegey Dougall and Andrew Baum
The University of Texas at Arlington

The customary introduction to stress suggests that it is still a matter of scientific debate, despite the fact that it is a common and influential state. It shares aspects of mind and body, representing a good instance of more holistic integration of these constructs. It is also a crosscutting process, influencing a wide array of illnesses, health behaviors, and aspects of health and well-being. Despite the general lack of a consensus on a precise definition of stress or the best approach to measuring it, there is considerable evidence to suggest that stress has important effects on physical and mental states, pathophysiology of disease, and performance (for reviews, see Baba, Jamal, & Tourigny, 1998; Juster, McEwen, & Lupien, 2010; Norris et al., 2002; Steptoe & Ayers, 2004). Major advances have been made during the last decade, particularly in our understanding of disease processes and the pathophysiological mechanisms that underlie the relationship between stress and health. This chapter considers conceptual models of stress, the broad array of behaviors and bodily systems involved in the stress response, and the impact of stress on chronic disease processes. Differences in the consequences of acute and chronic stress, as well as the implications of observed differences between them, are also explored.

THE STRESS CONSTRUCT

Perhaps the most difficult aspect of studying stress is deriving a widely accepted definition of it. Most theorists agree that stress is (or can be) adaptive, that it is associated with threatening or harmful events, and that it is typically characterized by aversive or unpleasant feelings and mood. Beyond this, there are few areas of universal agreement. Some theorists have argued that stress can be positive, but others have insisted that it is a fundamentally aversive state (e.g., Baum, 1990; Selye, 1956/1984). Some have pointed out apparently simultaneous biological and psychological activation, suggesting that stress is an emotion; and some have described stress as a general state of arousal associated with taking strong action or dealing with a strong stimulus (e.g., Baum, 1990; Mason, 1971). Stress has been variously defined as a stimulus, as a response, and as a process involving both. It has been described as both specific and nonspecific responses to danger with little evidence to support one or another contention. However, it appears to be a fundamental component of adjustment and adaptation to environmental change, and as such it has assumed a critical role in theories of human evolution. From these many notions have come a few major theories of stress that reflect integration and synthesis of prior theories and that describe a pattern of responses to threat, harm, or loss.

BIOLOGICAL THEORIES OF STRESS

A history of the stress concept could begin with early philosophers, but modern stress theory really began with Cannon's work early in the 20th century. Cannon (1914) was interested in the effects of stress on the sympathetic nervous system (SNS) and with application of the concept of homeostasis to interaction with the environment. Stressful events elicited negative emotions associated with SNS activation and disequilibrium in bodily systems. This activation was associated with the release of sympathetic adrenal hormones (i.e., epinephrine, norepinephrine), which prepared the organism to respond to the danger posed, characteristically by fighting or fleeing. This early description of stress did not consider the measures of activation or persistence, focusing solely on SNS arousal and release of sympathetic hormones.

Selye (1956/1984) focused his attention solely on the activation of the hypothalamic-pituitary-adrenal cortical (HPA) axis. Initially interested in the effects of hormonal extracts, Selye (1956/1984) discovered a "universal" response to stressful events that included adrenal hypertrophy, lymphoid involution, and ulceration of the digestive tract. He characterized stress as a nonspecific physiological response to a variety of noxious events and argued that regardless of the stressor presented, the same response was seen, driven by activation of the HPA axis.

In contrast to these more focused approaches, Mason (1971) argued that stress affected many biological systems and that responses were based on the type of stressor presented. He concluded that stress was a unified catabolic response with the primary purpose of maintaining high levels of circulating blood glucose and providing the organism with energy to sustain resistance. Although he viewed emotional reactions as nonspecific, he maintained that responses in endocrine pathways followed response patterns that were specific to the stressor.

Whereas these early biological models of stress were typically narrow in focus and ignored or only hinted at important psychological aspects of stress, their importance can be illustrated in several ways. The systems that received most attention in these early theories were the SNS and the HPA axis. Both are arguably principal drivers of stress responding and persist today as focal points in studies of physiological responses during and after stress. Work by Cannon and Selye accurately identified these systems as integral parts of the stress response and focused attention on consequences of prolonged or excessive activation of these systems as primary consequences of stress. Mason recognized the integrated nature of these responses as well as the broad panoply of responses characterizing stress. Sympathetic arousal and activation of the HPA axis are hallmarks of the stress response and have been used as manipulation checks for stressors and explored as mechanisms underlying stress effects on the body.

These theories of biological activity offered some insights into psychological aspects of stress. Cannon's (1914) notion of critical stress levels suggested that organisms had thresholds, or limits, on normal or nonpathogenic responses to threat, and his discussion of emotional stress suggested that emotional stimuli and responses were important in stress as well. In addition, stressors were stimuli that had to be recognized as a threat in order to elicit a response. Selye (1956/1984) argued that adaptive energy or the capacity to adapt to stressors is limited and depletion of adaptive reserves can have consequences, an idea consistent with notions of life change, stressful life events, and aftereffects of stress (e.g., Cohen, 1980; Holmes & Rahe, 1967; Rahe, 1987).

As critical as they are for understanding bodily responses to threat or challenge, these theories were also important because they introduced the notion that the nervous and endocrine systems jointly produced the arousal state characteristic of stress. Cannon incorporated emotional activation in his physiological model of stress, but Selye did not consider more psychologically relevant events or dynamics directly. Despite this, Selye was responsible for popularizing the construct and made stress theory more accessible and readily integrated into independent and parallel theories in the psychological literature on stress.

PSYCHOLOGICAL THEORIES OF STRESS

Psychological theories of stress that developed largely independent of work on its biological bases, focused on variability of response to stressors. Lazarus (1966) emphasized the contribution of the individual to the interaction with an environmental stressor. Like Mason, Lazarus argued that people actively perceived and reacted to stressors and there was considerable individual variation in this experience. The occurrence of an event alone was not sufficient to induce stress. Instead, the notion of appraisal, or cognitive interpretation of the stressor, was introduced and integrated into a transactional model. For stress to be experienced, it was necessary for an individual to appraise the event as threatening or harmful. Stress appraisals then elicited negative emotions; but unlike other models, it was the appraisal of the event, and not the emotional reaction, that determined subsequent physiological and behavioral responses. Additional appraisal processes were used by the individual to determine what available coping strategies could be used to deal with the situation and whether the problem should be attacked or accommodated.

The primary appraisals and perceived stress in this theory were important because they suggested that psychological variables or central nervous system (CNS) activity mediate the relation between stressful events and bodily reactions. Rather than envisioning a unidirectional process originating from the occurrence of a stressor, Lazarus conceptualized stress as a dynamic process in which an individual was constantly reappraising the situation as new information was obtained. Lazarus and Folkman (1984) later expanded on this model and defined stress as the "particular relationship between the person and the environment that is appraised by the person as taxing or exceeding his or her resources and endangering his or her well-being" (p. 19). Central to this model were the processes of cognitive appraisals and coping, both of which mediated this relationship and determined stress-related outcomes. Sustained behavioral and physiological responding to stress that was not reduced or eliminated with directed coping efforts could lead to illness symptoms and disease.

More recently, McEwen and colleagues (McEwen, 1998; Juster, McEwen, & Lupien, 2010) have proposed a model of allostasis and allostatic load that encompasses most of the preceding theories and literature. Like Lazarus and Folkman (1984), they propose that psychosocial, demographic, background, and environmental characteristics contribute to the perception of an event as a stressor and threaten an individual's homeostasis. Allostatic physiological responses include activation of the sympathetic-adrenal-medullary axis and release of catecholamines and activation of the HPA axis and release of glucocorticoids. Whereas this physiological arousal can be adaptive in the immediate context of dealing with a stressor, long-term activation can have negative effects on many other physiological response systems (e.g., immune, metabolic, and neurological alterations) and lead to such outcomes as behavioral changes, cognitive deficits, and vulnerability to disease. This concept of allostatic load, or chronic wear and tear on the body, has provided a useful framework for organizing research on stress-related diseases. Although it can be challenging to design projects to measure allostatic load adequately, recent research has successfully used allostatic load algorithms to identify risk and protective factors that can be identified across the lifespan (Juster et al., 2010).

DEFINING STRESS

A unifying theme in many of these theories is adaptation and adjustment to changes in a person's environment. Selye (1956/1984) argued that life involves constant change and adaptation. Much of this is minor and hardly noticed, not unlike the continual adjustments a person makes to the steering wheel of a car while driving it. The grooves and bumps in the road represent an uneven environment that requires small changes in steering to maintain a straight path, not unlike minor or routine stressors that one encounters every day. Major stressors present dangers more similar to oncoming cars; they may require dramatic and memorable efforts to avoid collision or driving off the road. Each adjustment involves a specific response (e.g., the minor adjustment of the wheel or more effortful maneuvering to avoid other cars). Each also appears to have a nonspecific component, composed largely of SNS and HPA arousal and bodily "support" for cognitive or behavioral adjustments. When these adjustments are more substantial or sudden, they may also affect mood and behavior. Regardless, this nonspecific arousal both motivates and supports coping, making it faster, "stronger," and more effective in accomplishing the adjustments needed to adapt. Collectively, the specific coping directed at threatening, harmful, or otherwise upsetting situations and the nonspecific activation supporting these responses may be considered "stress."

There remains considerable variability in the way stress is defined or conceptualized. Consistent with the previous emphasis on adjustment and adaptation, stress can be described as "a negative emotional experience accompanied by predictable biochemical, physiological, and behavioral changes that are directed toward adaptation either by manipulating the situation to alter the stressor or by accommodating its effects" (Baum, 1990, p. 653). When challenged or threatened, both specific adjustments and supportive nonspecific activation are likely and both continue until the source of stress is eliminated or the individual has successfully accommodated its effects. In this context, stress is an adaptive process with the goal of either altering a stressful situation or adjusting to and minimizing its negative effects. When confronted with a stressor, the body responds in ways consistent with a catabolic fight-or-flight reaction. Negative health effects occur when these emergency responses are extreme or prolonged. In addition, variability in the stress process occurs through the influence of factors that affect appraisal of stressors and coping efforts.

METHODOLOGICAL APPROACHES

Although these general and more specific models of stress have guided many studies, individual researchers' operational definitions of stress have varied. Historically, there has been an emphasis on the stimulus or stressor end of the model, often either measuring outcomes after an organism confronts a particular stressor or counting the number of accumulating life events. Other researchers focus on the emotional, physiological, or behavioral responses to stressors and use these responses to predict physical and mental health. More researchers are beginning to integrate these two elements and incorporate measures of such personal characteristics as appraisal and coping to more accurately predict who is more resilient or more vulnerable to stress.

Stimulus-based approaches often compare groups of organisms either exposed or not exposed to a particular stressor. Acute stress is often manipulated in the laboratory using such administered stimuli as noise, immobilization, and electric shock (in animals) and challenging mental tasks or threatening situations (in humans). Naturally occurring events are also examined, among them residential crowding, ambient noise, natural disasters, or life-threatening accidents. Differences across levels of exposure allow researchers to determine the impact of the stressor on physical and mental health outcomes. Another common approach is to ask participants to indicate which of a list of events occurred within a given time frame (e.g., 6–12 months). Participants can also rate each event on the amount of adjustment required to adapt to the stressor. The relations observed between life event measures and outcomes were consistent but usually modest, with life events generally accounting for less than 9% of the variance in outcome measures (for reviews, see Rahe, 1972; Sarason, de Monchaux, & Hunt, 1975; Zimmerman, 1983).

Substantial improvements have been made in the prediction of outcomes through the use of such personal interviews as those conducted through the Life Events and Difficulties Schedule (LEDS; G. W. Brown & Harris, 1989). Through the use of interview techniques, specific information regarding the actual event and its context can be gathered and rated by objective reviewers. Therefore, many of the response errors and sources of bias inherent in self-report measures can be minimized. Unfortunately, the extensive training of interviewers and raters, as well as the costs associated with lengthy individual visits with study participants, limits the feasibility of this approach. However, the incorporation of the contextual meaning of the events rather than just the occurrence of the event has increased the magnitude of the relationships found between life stress and outcomes. Using this method, researchers have demonstrated that life events and chronic difficulties contribute to the risk of developing many such mental and physical conditions as depression, schizophrenia, anxiety, myocardial infarction, multiple sclerosis, abdominal hip pain, and menstrual disorders (for a review, see G. W. Brown & Harris, 1989). More recently, chronic stress measured in this way has been linked to susceptibility to viral infection (Cohen, 2005). Clearly, identification of objective predictors of mental and physical health outcomes is valuable for the prediction of stress consequences. However, such an approach reveals little about the way stress works or why it has these effects.

Other theories and measures of stress focus more intently on responses, arguing that it is the response that is most closely linked to outcomes or consequences and that the extent to which the event is experienced as stressful is a better metric than is the event itself. In controlled laboratory settings or in naturalistic environments, researchers can measure cognitive, behavioral, and physiological changes before, during, and/or after a stressor. Changes in these response systems can then be correlated with physical and mental health outcomes. Individual difference variables or other factors affecting how stressful events are experienced are also important predictors of both responses and outcomes. Situational factors affecting appraisals of stressors and a person's ability to resist them, as well as individual differences in appraisal or response, are critical determinants of outcomes.

There are many important intervening variables that affect interactions of the perceiver and the situation and affect appraisals of severity or the likelihood of successful adaptation. Among the more frequently studied stress mediators are perceptions of control, predictability, coping, and the availability of social support (Cohen, Gottlieb, & Underwood, 2000; Lazarus & Folkman, 1984; Revenson & Lepore, Chapter 9, this volume; Thompson, 2009; Wills & Ainette, Chapter 20, this volume). Individuals with greater perceptions of control and more social support, as well as situations characterized by appraisals of greater predictability, typically produce less stress and better outcomes. One reason for these differential effects may be the availability of and the types of coping strategies used to deal with the event. When individuals perceive that they can control the event, their perception may promote their use of more problem-focused techniques or greater acceptance, thereby alleviating much of the distress experienced. In addition, greater predictability of the event allows individuals to prepare in the time before the event to deal effectively with the situation. Similarly, perceptions of available social support may serve to enhance the coping resources of individuals through offers of tangible aid or advice (Wills & Ainette, Chapter 20, this volume).

ACUTE AND CHRONIC STRESS

Not all exposures to stressors are equal, and it can probably be assumed that more or worse exposures have more impact than fewer or less severe exposures. Stressor intensity and duration likely interact to produce a range of potential effects. The most common distinction between acute and chronic stress is based on the duration of the stressor. However, as already noted, there is inter- and intraindividual variability in stress responding even to the same stressor. Therefore, acute and chronic stress may best be conceptualized by examining the interactions among the duration of the event itself (acute or chronic), the duration of threat perception (acute or chronic), and the duration of psychological, physiological, or behavioral responses (acute or chronic; Baum, O'Keeffe, & Davidson, 1990).

A "perfect acute" stress situation would refer to a situation characterized by an acute stressor duration, short-lived threat perception, and an acute response, typical of most laboratory stress situations. A subject in a laboratory study of stress is normally exposed to a brief (5–30-minute) stressor (or combination of stressors), views it as stressful for as long as it is present, and recovers rapidly after termination of the stressor. Chronic stress, however, is more complex. A "perfect chronic" situation would refer to a chronic event, chronic threat, and chronic responding. In reality, most stressful experiences consist of combinations of acute and chronic durations of the event, threat, and response, and this characterization may not be stable. For example, following a hurricane (an acute event), an individual may continue to experience perceived threat or harm and may exhibit such chronic responding as elevations in norepinephrine (NE), epinephrine (EPI), cortisol, heart rate (HR), and blood pressure (BP) and reductions in immune system functions. Over time, however, the individual may start to habituate to the chronic threat and show decreased stress responding (i.e., chronic threat with short-lived responding). The goal for stress reduction is for the individual to adapt to the stress situation and no longer perceive the chronic threat or respond to it. Unfortunately, not all individuals habituate or adapt to a stressor, and chronic stress persists or can even sensitize people to new stressors.

The alterations seen in the physiological, cognitive, and behavioral response systems are generally the same in both acute and chronic stress situations; but where acute stress occurs continuously, chronic stress does not appear to be a steady-state phenomenon. Rather, responding appears to be episodic, occurring repeatedly throughout the day as reminders or unwanted intrusions accost an individual. This appears to be the case whether the stressor is still present or long past. It is unlikely that an individual is conscious of a stressor 24 hours a day, 7 days a week, 365 days a year. Instead, it seems more likely that people experience good and bad days and good and bad moments within each day. Episodes of stress may be triggered by exposures to the event, reminders of the event, or anticipation of the event. Most models of stress fail to consider the impact of this repetitive activation of stress response systems or the possibility that the experience of chronic stress may be best characterized as acute episodes of stress related to an overarching stressor.

The episodic nature of chronic stress is supported by evidence that although certain populations report higher levels of distress than comparison groups, there is considerable day-to-day and within-day variations among individuals within the group (Dougall, Baum, & Jenkins, 1998; Stone, Reed, & Neale, 1987). These variations average to consistent high levels over longer time frames. In addition to experiencing these daily fluctuations, the response systems themselves do not always covary. Each system has it own circadian or activity-based pattern of ups and downs, as well as different reactivity and recovery times (e.g., Mason, 1968; Nesse et al., 1985). For example, EPI and NE show immediate increases in response to an acute stressor, whereas cortisol responses are delayed and last much longer. Therefore, single assessments limit an individual's view of the stress process.

It is not difficult to understand why an individual faced with daily stressors (e.g., hectic commutes to work or longtime care giving to a sick relative) experiences stress or excessive demand when dealing with them. Persistence of chronic stress responding after an event is long over is more difficult to explain and is an important question for stress researchers to tackle. It has been suggested that one important element in understanding chronic stress is the occurrence of stressor-related intrusive thoughts, especially in the absence of an ongoing stressor (Baum, Cohen, & Hall, 1993; Baum, Schooler, & Dougall, 1998; Craig, Heisler, & Baum, 1996). Plenty of evidence suggests that stressor-related intrusive thoughts are a common symptom following threatening events (e.g., Holmes & Bourne, 2008; Kangas, Henry, & Bryant, 2005). Intrusive thoughts are thought to be part of ongoing cognitive processing of the event (Creamer, Burgess, & Pattison, 1992; Greenberg, 1995; Horowitz, 1986). They help an individual work through the situation. Indeed, as individuals recover, they report fewer stressor-related intrusions (e.g., Delahanty, Dougall, Craig, Jenkins, & Baum, 1997). However, intrusive thoughts tend to be unwanted, unbidden, and uncontrollable, which are characteristics common to many other types of stressors. In at least some cases, these characteristics of intrusive thoughts may make them more stressful and are related to greater chronic stress (e.g., Dougall, Craig, & Baum, 1999). Rather than being exclusively adaptive, these thoughts may serve as stressors in their own right, possibly sensitizing individuals to other reminiscent stimuli. Intrusions combined with other environmental event-related stimuli may serve to perpetuate chronic stress by eliciting the acute episodes described earlier.

TRAUMA AND CHRONIC STRESS

Intrusive thoughts are most prevalent following extreme stressors. However, they do occur following less severe events and even after benign and positive events that occur in everyday life (Berntsen, 1996). Although positive and neutral intrusions also occur, intrusive thoughts with negative valences are implicated in chronic stress and are probably one of the most salient hall-mark symptoms of posttraumatic stress disorder (PTSD; American Psychiatric Association, 2000). Posttraumatic stress disorder is a special case of extreme stress responding following life threat-ening or extreme stressors. It has broad-base effects across all domains of functioning, impairing an individual's ability to function normally. Victims experience the persistent recurrence of three categories of symptoms: reexperiencing or reliving the event, emotional numbing and avoidance of trauma-related stimuli, and heightened physiological arousal (APA, 2000). In addition to intrusive thoughts, victims experience such other common symptoms as recurrent and disruptive dreams, sleep disturbances, emotional withdrawal, anxiety, dissociation, aggressiveness, hyperarousal, and an exaggerated startle response (APA, 2000).

Posttraumatic stress disorder is also characterized by unusual physiological response pro-files. When victims are reminded of the trauma, cardiovascular, respiratory, and negative emo-tional responses are typically more exaggerated compared with reactivity to unrelated stimuli. As in chronic stress situations, circulating levels of EPI, NE, and their metabolites are elevated (Southwick et al., 2007). This chronic sympathetic-adrenal-medullary (SAM) activation is accom-panied by down regulation of adrenergic receptors, thereby helping to sustain the increased out-put. Dysregulation of serotonin is also evident with PTSD, and use of selective serotonin reuptake inhibitors has proven effective in treating all three of the key symptom criteria (Friedman & Davidson, 2007; Southwick et al., 2007). In contrast, abnormalities in the functioning of the HPA axis are also associated with PTSD, but the nature of these findings is mixed. One body of research has found consistent suppression of cortisol related to an enhanced negative feedback and reduced adrenal capacity (e.g., Yehuda, 2002). However, these findings appear to be limited to male combat veterans and male and postmenopausal female Holocaust survivors (Southwick et al., 2007). Research with other populations, including premenopausal women and children who have comorbid symptoms of depression, has found increased cortisol levels that are associated with an increased pituitary adrenocorticotropic hormone (ACTH) response to corticotrophin-releasing factor (CRF) from the hypothalamus (Rasmusson et al., 2004; Southwick et al., 2007). ACTH travels to the adrenal cortex, where it stimulates release of cortisol; the adrenal cortex then increases its capacity to release cortisol to meet these demands. Taken together, these complex neuroendocrine alterations associated with PTSD have important implications for physical health outcomes. Research indicates that PTSD not only is a mechanism through which exposure to trau-matic events may impact physical health but also serves as an independent risk factor (Schnurr, Green, & Kaltman, 2007).

The experience of trauma is not limited by the physical presence of the precipitating event. Despite the often acute nature of traumatic events, responding may last for months or years. In addi-tion, time of onset is not limited to the time of exposure, and episodes of acute and chronic PTSD have been defined based on whether or not symptoms last less than or more than 3 months (APA, 2000). Although individual symptoms of PTSD predict subsequent diagnosis, not all the symptoms need to be present for a diagnosis to occur. Also, many of these same symptoms are exaggerations of normal stress reactions to an overwhelming event and may, in fact, serve to promote adaptation to such a situation. This observation is consistent with the pervasive finding that a majority of trauma victims do not develop PTSD, but there are still a significant number of victims (approximately 10%–25%) who are affected (Breslau, 2009; Green, 1994).

These considerations suggest that it is important to identify factors in the environment or in the individual that affect whether or not an individual experiences symptoms of posttraumatic stress or ultimately develops PTSD. Several vulnerability factors have been identified, among them a history of psychopathology and gene by environment interactions (e.g., Kilpatrick et al., 2007; Parslow, Jorm, & Christensen, 2006; Segman et al., 2005), as well as such factors that influence normal stress responses as gender, social class, social support, perceived control, and coping (e.g., Norris et al., 2002; Breslau, 2009; Kilpatrick et al., 2007; Olff, Langeland, & Gersons, 2005; Thompson, 2009).

STRESS RESPONSES AND CONSEQUENCES

Emerging models of stress consider a range of responses and consequences of stress that bear on productivity, health, and well-being. Stress affects mood, behavior, and problem solving, changes individuals' motivation to achieve goals or engage in self-protective behavior, and appears to lessen restraints against harmful behaviors. Stress affects the whole body. The effects of stress on the SAM and the HPA axis were documented in the seminal work of Selye (1956/1984) and Cannon (1914). These systems contribute to stimulation of others and exert direct and indirect effects on metabolism and arousal. Changes in these response systems are thought to account for some of the effects of stress on health but are consistent with a mobilization of energy and as such are inherently adaptive. Increases in heart rate and blood pressure, as well as increases in the release of such neuroendocrine factors as EPI, NE, ACTH, glucocorticoids, and prolactin prepare an individual to face a stressor and fight or flee from the scene. In addition, stress-related decreases in several markers of immune system functioning have been observed (for reviews, see Segerstrom, 2010; Segerstrom & Miller, 2004). These changes could be adaptive in that when an organism is injured in battle, the swelling, fever, and other characteristics of an immune response are delayed and therefore do not interfere with the actions of the organism. However, prolonged suppression of a variety of functions could open windows of heightened vulnerability to infection or progression of neoplastic disease.

In addition to bringing about physiological changes, stress can increase such negative emotions as depression, anxiety, anger, fear, and overall symptom reporting. Unwanted or uncontrollable thoughts and memories about a stressor may also be experienced (Holmes & Bourne, 2008; Kangas et al., 2005). These stressor-related intrusions are both a symptom of stress and a stressor in their own right. Painful event–related images and thoughts may elicit their own stress response and may help to perpetuate chronic stress responding by repeatedly exposing an individual to the stressor.

Stress also affects performance. Because attention is typically focused on dealing with stressors when they are present, people may have problems attending to such more mundane tasks as balancing a checking account, monitoring computer screens, or assembling a product (e.g., Baba et al., 1998; Gilboa, Shirom, Fried, & Cooper, 2008; Kompier & DiMartino, 1995; Krueger, 1989). Unfortunately, many of these tasks may be work or safety related (e.g., writing a report or driving an automobile) and could have severe consequences if done improperly. Further, exposure to even a brief laboratory stressor has been shown to induce transient performance deficits in tasks given during the stressor or after it (Glass & Singer, 1972). These negative aftereffects occur even though physiological and emotional responding has decreased and the individual appears to have adapted to the acute stressor. Other consequences of stress include deterioration of sleep quality and quantity, increases in aggressive behaviors, and changes in such appetitive behaviors as eating, drinking, and smoking (e.g., Brunello et al., 2001; Field, Claassen, & O'Keefe, 2001; Mellman, 1997; Smith, Christiansen, Vincent, & Hann, 1999). These wide-reaching effects of stress illustrate the importance of examining the effects of stress on the whole organism rather than focusing on one system such as the SNS, reports of depression, or alcohol use. Responses across all systems work in concert to help the individual adapt by either altering the situation or accommodating its effects. Whereas these biological, cognitive, and behavioral alterations may be adaptive in the short term, chronic activation of these response systems results in wear and tear on the organism and may make the organism more susceptible to negative mental and physical health outcomes.

STRESS AND HEALTH

Stress can affect health as well as intervene at any point in the disease process—in disease etiology, progression, treatment, recovery, or recurrence. Stress exerts these effects in three basic ways: as direct physiological changes resulting from stress-related arousal (e.g., immunosuppression, damage to blood vessels), as cognitive and behavioral changes that convey physiological changes (e.g., intrusive thoughts, smoking, drug use), and as physiological, cognitive, and behavioral changes associated with an individual's illness that affect exposure or treatment (e.g., viral exposure, drug metabolism, treatment adherence, seeking medical help). As discussed later, stress has important implications for the onset, progression, and treatment of almost every known major disease.

Although often difficult to measure, stress appears to affect pathogenic processes that contribute to the onset of disease. One of the most salient mechanisms through which stress can promote disease is through chronic, sustained, and/or exaggerated responses, making them pathological. Prolonged feelings of depression or anxiety can interrupt normal functioning and result in the development of clinical disorders, whereas transient alterations in mood are considerably less harmful (e.g., Kendler et al., 1995; Terrazas, Gutierrez, & Lopez, 1987). Continued self-medication or use of licit or illicit drugs may lead to addiction, and eating disorders may develop from extreme alterations in eating behaviors (e.g., Meyer, 1997; Sharpe, Ryst, Hinshaw, & Steiner, 1997; Vlahov et al., 2004). Prolonged or often-repeated elevations in blood pressure may result in permanent changes contributing to hypertension, and elevated circulating levels of stress hormones may contribute to atherosclerosis and heart disease (Markovitz & Matthews, 1991). Chronic immune system suppression appears to interfere with the ability to ward off pathogens, making individuals more susceptible to such infectious diseases as colds, flu, and HIV disease (Segerstrom, 2010; Segerstrom & Miller, 2004). Stress also appears to affect tumor suppression and progression of cancer (Baum, Trevino, & Dougall, 2011; Kemeny & Schedlowski, 2007). Although exhaustive evaluations of the direct role of stress in disease etiology are difficult to conduct, recent evidence from studies of controlled viral challenges (Cohen, 2005) and wound healing (Christian, Graham, Padgett, Glaser, & Kiecolt-Glaser, 2006; Marucha & Engeland, 2007) confirm the clinically relevant impact of stress on health and disease.

Behavioral and cognitive deficits seen during stress can also affect disease by increasing an individual's chance of exposure to pathogenic agents. Individuals under stress are more likely to engage in high-risk behaviors like unprotected sex and intravenous drug use (Chiasson et al., 2005; Evans-Campbell, Lindhorst, Huang, & Walters, 2006; Wagner et al., 2009). These activities increase the likelihood that an individual will be exposed to an infectious disease or experience such unplanned consequences as pregnancy. As already discussed, decrements in performance can result in dismissal from work or injury and death as a result of inattention and lack of concentration while engaging in such important activities as driving a car or operating machinery (Baba et al., 1998; Gilboa et al., 2008; Kompier & DiMartino, 1995; Krueger, 1989). Such stress-related behaviors as smoking, alcohol use, and sedentary lifestyles may also contribute to etiology of serious health problems (Kiviniemi & Rothman, 2010).

Disease progression and treatment are also affected by stress. New feelings of depression or anxiety may interfere with treatment of preexisting disorders and can increase the likelihood of such acute disease events as heart attacks (e.g., Frasure-Smith, Lesperance, & Talajic, 1995; Mizrahi, 2010; Steptoe & Brydon, 2009; Zautra et al., 1997). Individuals in treatment for psychiatric disorders (e.g., schizophrenia, depression, substance use, or eating disorders) may relapse and experience a return of their symptoms or return to their abusive behaviors (e.g., Grilo, Pagano, & Stout, 2009; Mizrahi, 2010; Monroe & Harkness, 2005; Park et al., 2009; Sinha, 2007). Physiological changes may also interfere with the metabolism of prescription drugs (Grunberg, Berger, & Hamilton, 2011), and behavioral and cognitive stress effects may impair treatment, reducing the likelihood that patients comply with instructions, prescriptions, and recommendations given by their medical teams (e.g., Brickman & Yount, 1996; Perez, Cruess, & Kalichman, 2011). In addition, transient stressors, especially those producing such strong emotions as depression, anxiety, or outward expressions of anger, can promote platelet aggregation, contributing to the underlying cardiovascular disease state, or can trigger such acute cardiac events as myocardial infarction and sudden cardiac death (Steptoe & Brydon, 2009).

Stress can also retard the speed of recovery, make adjustment to diseases and injuries more difficult, and increase the rates of disease recurrence. Patients who report more stress have a more difficult time recovering from and adjusting to illnesses or injuries than do individuals who report less stress (e.g., Grassi & Rosti, 1996; Kiecolt-Glaser, Stephens, Lipetz, Speicher, & Glaser, 1995; Marucha, Kiecolt-Glaser, & Favagehi, 1998; Mullins, Chaney, Pace, & Hartman, 1997). Stress management interventions given prior to surgery or other medical procedures have improved subsequent healing and rehabilitation, however, and stress management interventions have been incorporated into multidisciplinary cardiac rehabilitation programs to improve cardiovascular risk factors and promote recovery (e.g., Blumenthal et al., 2005; Enqvist & Fischer, 1997; Ross & Berger, 1996; Schneiderman & Orth-Gomér, Chapter 29, this volume). Stress may also make patients in remission more vulnerable to recurrence of their disease; among people with latent viruses (e.g., HSV, EBV, HIV), stress has been linked to reactivation of the viruses and disease symptoms (Aiello, Simanek, & Galea, 2010; Glaser, 2005). Stress has also been linked with recurrence of cancer, which is possibly a result of stress's immunosuppressive effects (Baltrusch, Stangel, & Titze, 1991).

Most of these health effects are linked with episodes of long-term or chronic stress. However, acute stressors may also affect health by making an individual more vulnerable during a time of exposure to an infectious agent or by triggering such acute events as heart attacks, as discussed earlier. The difference between acute and chronic stress is not always clearly defined, and most of the models already discussed fail to make a distinction between the two. Closer examination of the meaning and implications of short- and long-term stress needs to be addressed before examining the relationship between stress and disease more closely.

STRESS AND DISEASE

Although stress affects everyday functioning and well-being, its more profound consequences are manifest as influences on disease processes. Whereas the effects of stress on the immune system are one putative mechanism for explaining the relationship between stress and disease, other stress response systems affect disease processes as well. Further, these effects are apparent at several levels and stages of ill health. By examining the effects of stress on some major diseases, the importance of stress in the disease process as well as the integration of whole body responses are highlighted.

In addition to the effects of stress on the onset, management, and recovery from disease, there is evidence to suggest that people with chronic diseases experience more stress, that is, that these illnesses (or aspects of their management) can cause stress. Patients tend to report more social problems and psychological symptoms than do people in the general population, and more psychiatric morbidity has been associated with poorer disease management (e.g., R. F. Brown, Tennant, Dunn, & Pollard, 2005; Dougall et al., 1998; Irvine, Brown, Crooks, Roberts, & Browne, 1991; Mayou, Peveler, Davies, Mann, & Fairburn, 1991; Mullins et al., 1997). This bidirectional relationship between stress and disease has lead researchers to propose that in some cases a vicious cycle develops, in which chronic diseases predispose individuals to psychiatric symptoms and social problems that then impair self-care and result in poor disease management. Disease flare-ups, recurrence, or increases in symptoms then further exacerbate psychiatric symptoms and social problems (e.g., Mayou et al., 1991). In the next sections of this chapter we review the evidence for the association of stress with several disease conditions.

STRESS AND IMMUNE-MEDIATED DISEASE

One of the most salient mechanisms through which stress can make an individual more vulnerable to disease is the link between stress and immune functioning. Both acute and chronic stress have been linked to alterations in immune system activity (Segerstrom, 2010; Segerstrom & Miller, 2004). In response to acute stressors, there is a redistribution of immune cells, especially increases in numbers of circulating natural killer cells and large granular lymphocytes that are important components of the immune system's first line of defense against pathogens (natural immunity; e.g., Dhabhar & McEwen, 1997). However, there is a concomitant down regulation of such specific immune responses as the ability of B and T lymphocytes to proliferate, which is also evidenced during chronic stress exposure.(e.g., Bachen et al., 1992; Delahanty et al., 1996; Zakowski, Cohen, Hall, Wollman, & Baum, 1994). Further evidence of immunosuppression during chronic stress is seen in decreased activity of natural killer cells that are important for destroying viral and cancer cells (e.g., Esterling, Kiecolt-Glaser, Bodnar, & Glaser, 1994; Ironson et al., 1997). Furthermore, stress can interfere with seroconversion following vaccination, decreasing the amount of protection normally afforded (e.g., Pedersen, Zachariae, & Bovbjerg, 2009; Phillips, 2008). Therefore, stress-induced immunosuppression could render the body less able to fight off pathogens or recover from injuries.

Immune system alterations are related to SAM and HPA activation (i.e., increases in catecholamines and glucocorticoids). Lymphatic tissue and immune cells express adrenergic and noradrenergic receptors and stress-related elevations in catecholamines trigger redistribution of immune cells and alter immune cell function, including production of cytokines and development of inflammation (Glaser & Kiecolt-Glaser, 2005; Kemeny & Schedlowski, 2007). Activation of the HPA axis and release of glucocorticoids work in conjunction with SAM activation to produce suppression of specific immune system activity and further elevate inflammatory markers (Glaser & Kiecolt-Glaser, 2005; Kemeny & Schedlowski, 2007). Chronic inflammation has been implicated in such chronic disease processes as the development and progression of cardiovascular disease, metabolic syndrome, diabetes, and such inflammatory conditions as arthritis. Even acute bouts of stress have been associated with increases in inflammation, suggesting important implications for health outcomes (Steptoe, Hamer, & Chida, 2007). Such psychological variables as control, predictability, social support, and availability of a behavioral response have also been shown to mediate immune system alterations associated with stress. In general, uncontrollable or unpredictable stressors or situations affording little social support produce greater immunosuppression (e.g., Sieber, Rodin, Larson, Ortega, & Cummings, 1992; Uchino, Cacioppo, & Kiecolt-Glaser, 1996; Zakowski, 1995).

INFECTIOUS ILLNESS

Infectious illness refers to diseases caused by pathogens (e.g., viruses, bacteria) that is communicable between two or more individuals. Primary defenses against these illnesses are immune system activity that seeks to control and destroy infectious agents. Because stress is associated with periods of lowered immune activity, it should also be associated with less resistance to infectious illnesses. Research in both controlled and natural settings provides support for the contention that stress is associated with vulnerability to infectious illness (Glaser & Kiecolt-Glaser, 2005; Kemeny & Schedlowski, 2007). In natural environments, increases in stress often precede the onset of illnesses (Kasl, Evans, & Niederman, 1979; Rahe, 1972; Stone et al., 1987). In addition, physiological reactivity moderates the effects of stress on illness, with high reactors developing more respiratory infections than low reactors (Boyce et al., 1995).

Clinical markers of immune system functioning have also been examined as indicators of the effects of stress on immunity. Chronic stress can interfere with the body's ability to heal following an injury. In addition to indicating delays in wound healing, there is evidence for stress-induced alterations in the wound milieu, including changes in proinflammatory cytokines and enzymes (Christian, Graham, Padgett, Glaser, & Kiecolt-Glaser, 2006; Marucha & Engeland, 2007). Reactivations of such latent viral infections as herpes simplex virus (HSV) and Epstein-Barr virus (EBV) also appear more likely when individuals are experiencing ongoing stress (Aiello et al., 2010; Glaser, 2005).

In addition to these, correlational studies are studies in controlled environments. Recent advances in measurement procedures have made it possible to conduct studies in controlled environments, confirming that individuals with high levels of life stress are more likely to become infected and display symptoms, for example, when exposed to cold viruses (Cohen, 2005). In these studies, healthy participants are typically exposed to known amounts of a cold virus and then quarantined in a hotel room for 5 or more days. Two major disease outcomes are examined. One outcome is the rate of viral infection, typically ranging from 69% to 100% of the sample exposed to the virus; and the other is the actual incidence of cold symptoms, ranging from 19% to 71% of the sample (Cohen et al., 1998; Cohen, Tyrrell, & Smith, 1991; Stone et al., 1992). Although individuals cannot have cold symptoms without being infected, they can be infected without showing signs of a cold. Rates of both viral infection and cold symptoms increase in a dose-response fashion with the amount of life stress the participants report (Cohen et al., 1991, 1998; Stone et al., 1992). More severe and chronic stressors tend to have a greater impact on disease development than do less severe or acute stressors (Cohen et al., 1998).

HIV Disease

A chronic illness that affects more than one million Americans (CDC, 2008a), HIV is a retrovirus that preferentially attacks the CD4+ T lymphocytes, ultimately causing depletion of these cells (Westergaard & Gupta, 2009). After an acute infection phase, the virus can remain latent for years in the form of a provirus. Reactivation of the virus leads to viral replication, destruction of the CD4+ T-cells, and progression of the disease to AIDS, the acquired immunodeficiency syndrome, which is characterized by a compromised immune system and development of such symptoms as opportunistic infections and cancers.

Perhaps the most salient effects of stress on vulnerability to HIV infection are the behavioral changes associated with high-risk status, especially greater use of such substances as IV drugs and increases in high-risk sexual encounters (Chiasson et al., 2005; Evans-Campbell et al., 2006; Wagner et al., 2009). HIV disease is an infectious illness. Therefore, reductions in immunocompetence associated with stress, as described earlier, also place an individual at greater risk for contracting HIV if exposed (Solomon, Kemeny, & Temoshok, 1991). In addition, reactivation of latent herpes viruses that can be triggered by chronic stress (e.g., herpes simplex virus Type 2 and Epstein-Barr virus) has been identified as a risk factor for HIV acquisition (Aiello et al., 2010).

Considerable more research has examined the effects of stress on HIV disease progression. Living with HIV disease can be stressful for numerous reasons. For example, the disease can have an unpredictable time course, and patients may experience distrust in the medical system and stigma related to their disease (Whetten, Reif, Whetten, & Murphy-McMillan, 2008). Chronic stress either from living with HIV or from experiencing other stressful events has been associated with greater progression of HIV disease as evidenced by decreases in CD4+ cell numbers and increases in viral load, disability, and mortality (Chida & Vedhara, 2009; Leserman, 2008). Also, patients who are experiencing stress are less likely to adhere to the rigorous highly active antiretroviral therapy (HAART), for which strict adherence is necessary to keep HIV replication suppressed (Whetten et al., 2008). In contrast, there is emerging evidence that such positive psychosocial factors as optimism, spirituality, and active coping are associated with slower disease progression (Ironson & Hayward, 2008). Not surprisingly, interventions designed to reduce stress among patients with HIV disease have substantial effects on decreasing symptoms of stress and depression and improving quality of life (J. L. Brown & Vanable, 2008; Crepaz et al., 2008; Scott-Sheldon, Kalichman, Carey, & Fielder, 2008). A few cognitive behavioral interventions have also demonstrated improvements in such disease-related outcomes as CD4+ cell counts and viral load, especially if combined with a medication adherence intervention (Antoni, Carrico, et al., 2006; Antoni et al., 2005; Crepaz et al., 2008). Therefore, stress management interventions have become a common component of tertiary interventions for patients with HIV disease and AIDS.

Cancer

The relationships among stress, immunity, and cancer appear to be more complex than those underlying the pathophysiology of infectious diseases. In part, this is a consequence of the chronic nature of cancer and the more acute time frames of most infections. In addition, immune activity has an unknown role in controlling initial mutations in the process from benign to malignant neoplastic growth and a suspected, but underexplored, role in resistance to tumor growth and metastatic spread. There is better general evidence that stress is associated with cancer progression and may be linked to survival and quality of life. Again, problems related to the chronic nature of cancer development and treatment have made studies of stress and cancer incidence difficult; and research on disease course, recurrence, and survival share similar problems.

These problems have often left the literature linking stress and cancer weak and open to alternative explanations. Inconsistent findings are also an issue, with few studies finding relationships between major stressors or depression and the development of cancer (Chida Hamer, Wardle, & Steptoe, 2008; Kemeny & Schedlowski, 2007; Lutgendorf, Costanzo, & Siegel, 2007; Reiche, Nunes, & Morimoto, 2004). A recent meta-analysis (Chida et al., 2008) demonstrated that higher levels of distress were associated with higher cancer incidence rates, especially among studies that had large sample sizes and long time frames. However, findings varied based on the quality of the study design, the psychosocial risk factor, and the type of cancer examined. Again, problems of timing and tracking of disease-related events makes this research difficult and uncontrolled. Tumors develop over years or decades and grow irregularly. Furthermore, several different mutagenic events are needed to produce malignancy, suggesting several points at which stress could affect initial development. Such mechanisms as cellular DNA repair have been proposed, and some studies have linked stress and its neuroendocrine changes to poorer DNA-repair capabilities (e.g., Flint, Baum, Chambers, & Jenkins, 2007; Gidron, Russ, Tissarchondou, & Warner, 2006). In addition, chronic stress has been associated with shortening of the telomere length and alterations in telomerase activity that may promote accelerated cell aging and make the cell more vulnerable to DNA damage (Epel et al., 2004; Epel et al., 2006).

There is some evidence of stress-related modulation of cancer course and of immune system involvement. Studies of life stress and cancer have suggested that higher levels of stress are associated with poorer quality of life, cancer recurrence, and shorter survival (e.g., Chida et al., 2008; Golden-Kreutz et al., 2005; Palesh et al., 2007). However, some investigators have not found evidence of life-stress associations with cancer course (Ell, Nishimoto, Mediansky, Mantell, & Hamovitch, 1992; Jamison, Burish, & Wallston, 1987). Nevertheless, stress has been associated with alterations in biological and behavioral responses that have also been implicated in cancer progression: inflammation, hormone levels, immune markers, lack of physical activity, and nonadherence to treatment regimens (Antoni, Lutgendorf, et al., 2006). For example, there is some evidence that coping, social support, and other stress mediators are associated with cancer recurrence and length of survival (Chida, Hamer, Wardle, & Steptoe, 2008; Helgeson & Cohen, 1996; Petticrew, Bell, & Hunter, 2002). The presence of conflicting findings may be because studies have not consistently examined the impact of cancer-related stress on disease course; nor has systematic consideration of stressor timing issues, coping, or social assets been characteristic of this work.

Cancer diagnosis and treatment can be a stressful event in its own right, further complicating the stress and cancer-course relationship. Many patients with cancer do not report psychosocial problems, but a significant group can report symptoms of stress, depression, and even posttraumatic stress disorder (Kangas et al., 2005; Snyderman & Wynn, 2009; Spiegel & Giese-Davis, 2003). These symptoms appear to be more pronounced among patients diagnosed with cancers that have poorer prognoses (Kadan-Lottick, Vanderwerker, Block, Zhang, & Prigerson, 2005).

A multitude of interventions have been developed and disseminated to cancer patients aimed at decreasing stress, improving quality of life, and altering disease outcomes. Many of these interventions are targeted for a particular type of cancer, focusing on the needs and obstacles specific to that disease. For example, interventions with breast cancer patients may have components on body image and sexual functioning, whereas smoking cessation may be a major component of interventions that target patients with head and neck cancers. These interventions appear to improve quality of life, but whether or not they affect disease outcomes and survival are equivocal (Coyne, 2009; Coyne, Stefanek, & Palmer, 2007; McGregor & Antoni, 2009). Therefore, the evidence that stress affects cancer course is suggestive and encouraging but far from definitive or complete.

RHEUMATOID ARTHRITIS

Rheumatoid arthritis (RA) is a debilitating chronic disease that afflicted approximately 1.5 million adults in the United States during 2007 (Myasoedova, Crowson, Kremers, Therneau, & Gabriel, 2010). It is characterized by abnormal autoimmune responses that result in joint inflammation and destruction (Firestein et al., 2008). Some cases also involve the production of autoantibodies called rheumatoid factor. As with other chronic diseases, people with RA experience many limitations and disease-related stressors. The most frequent stressors patients report are taking care of their disease, their lack of control over the disease, and the resultant fatigue, pain, and functional impairment (Katz, 1998; Melanson & Down-Wamboldt, 1995).

In addition to the inherent stressfulness of RA is that disease activity and symptoms are exacerbated by the occurrence of daily stressors (Herrmann, Scholmerich, & Straub, 2000). Similar to the stress and disease relationship observed in diabetes and other chronic diseases, a cyclic pattern can develop in which RA leads to increases in stress, which in turn exacerbates RA symptoms. However, the relationship between stress and disease activity is not clear-cut. The type of stressful event as well as such important psychosocial factors as spousal support, optimism, and coping can alter the relationship between stress and RA (Treharne, Lyons, Booth, & Kitas, 2007; Zautra et al., 1998). For example, pain flares and increases in disease activity in rheumatoid disease tend to be preceded by interpersonal stress (Zautra & Smith, 2001). In addition, symptoms of pain and fatigue may be moderated by such psychosocial factors as depressive symptoms or the interaction of positive and negative interpersonal events (Finan et al., 2010; Smith & Zautra, 2008; Zautra et al., 2007). Minor types of stressors appear to affect RA disease activity and symptoms differently than do such major life events as the death of a loved one. Although daily stress has been linked to exacerbation of RA, major life events have actually been associated with decreases in disease activity (Potter & Zautra, 1997).

This finding is supported by differences in immunological responses in RA patients to minor and major stressors. Some researchers have suggested that acute, minor stressors are generally associated with increases in immune system activity, whereas major stressors are generally associated with decreases in the same immune parameters (Huyser & Parker, 1998; Zautra et al., 1989). Several components of the immune system are responsible for the joint inflammation and destruction seen in RA, especially T-cells, autoantibodies from B-cells, and release of inflammatory cytokines. Therefore, increases in the activity of these cells in response to minor stress should be associated with increases in disease activity. Likewise, the decreases in immune system activity following major stressors should be associated with less disease activity (Herrmann et al., 2000; Huyser & Parker, 1998; Potter & Zautra, 1997).

These differential effects appear to be mediated by the release of catecholamines and cortisol (Herrmann et al., 2000; Huyser & Parker, 1998). Rheumatoid arthritis is typically characterized by decreases in HPA axis activity (i.e., cortisol) and increases in SAM activity (i.e., epinephrine and norepinephrine). Each of these systems has opposing effects on RA management and symptoms. Cortisol has important anti-inflammatory actions that decrease RA activity by reducing the chemical activators of the inflammation process and by suppressing the immune system. Consequently, corticosteroids are often prescribed to RA patients to help manage their symptoms (O'Dell, 2007). In contrast, SAM activation has been associated with changes in immune activity and RA symptoms (Huyser & Parker, 1998). Also, RA patients have heightened SAM reactivity to minor stressors (Zautra et al., 1998). Although both catecholamine and cortisol levels increase in response to stress, it has been proposed that the heightened SAM reactivity to minor stressors counteracts any anti-inflammatory effects of HPA axis activation and cortisol release and results in exacerbations of

RA activity and symptoms (Huyser & Parker, 1998). In contrast, RA patients who report major life events may experience dramatic increases in HPA axis activation and cortisol release, which may in turn result in decreases in disease activity (Huyser & Parker, 1998; McFarlane & Brooks, 1990).

Although stress can have a profound impact on the etiology and course of RA, there is a subset of RA patients who appear to be immune to its effects. In these patients, genetic and etiological influences appear to be more influential in determining RA symptoms (Rimon & Laakso, 1985). Two subgroups of RA patients have been identified based on whether or not RA patients are seropositive for the autoantibody rheumatoid factor. In patients who are seronegative, the occurrence of negative life events is associated not only with increases in disease activity but also with the onset of the disease. In contrast, in people who are seropositive no such relations exist (Stewart, Knight, Palmer, & Highton, 1994), suggesting that vulnerability to stress is linked to the physiology of the disease process.

METABOLIC DISEASE

Stress has been implicated in the development of metabolic disorders, especially the onset and progression of metabolic syndrome, cardiovascular disease, and diabetes. Metabolic syndrome is a constellation of metabolic symptoms that when present confer high risk of development or progression of such disorders as cardiovascular disease, hypertension, and diabetes. The key component of the syndrome is visceral obesity or the accumulation of fat around the middle. To be classified as meeting criteria for metabolic syndrome, a patient must also present with at least two of the four remaining features: high levels of fasting plasma glucose (or diabetes), elevated blood pressure, raised levels of triglycerides, and reduced levels of high-density lipoproteins (Alberti, Zimmet, Shaw, & IDF Epidemiology Task Force Consensus Group, 2005). Physiological arousal associated with stress, especially of the HPA axis, has been identified as a key pathway linking stress to the onset and progression of metabolic syndrome (Kyrou, Chrousos, & Tsigos, 2006; Rosmond, 2005). Chronic increases in cortisol, such as those exhibited during stress, can inhibit insulin excretion from the pancreas, promote insulin resistance, alter lipid metabolism, and change the distribution of adipose tissue to produce visceral obesity. Activation of both the HPA axis and the SAM axis promotes such cardiovascular disease processes as hypertension and atherosclerosis. Metabolic syndrome is also characterized by chronic inflammation in part attributable to increased release of proinflammatory cytokines from the visceral adipose tissue (Kyrou et al., 2006). Increases in inflammation feed back to the HPA axis, signaling further release of cortisol and thereby creating a harmful cycle. Fortunately, there is a greater awareness now of metabolic syndrome, and efforts are being made to develop interventions that will disrupt these physiological pathways through alterations in lifestyle: for example, better nutrition, increased physical activity, or decreased stress (e.g., Diabetes Prevention Program Research Group, 2002; Tuomilehto et al., 2001).

CARDIOVASCULAR DISEASE

Stress can be implicated throughout the natural history of cardiovascular disease (CVD), in its formation, its progression, and its triggering of a cardiac event. Stress affects CVD mainly through its influences on behavioral factors and activation of the SAM and HPA axes. In particular, elevations in epinephrine and norepinephrine lead to increased beta and alpha receptor activity (Kamarck & Jennings, 1991; Markovitz & Matthews, 1991). Briefly, beta activation increases heart rate and heart contractility, therefore increasing cardiac output and blood pressure (Guyton & Hall, 2006). Alpha activation causes vasoconstriction of the arteries and veins and causes increases in total peripheral resistance and venous return, both of which increase blood pressure (Guyton & Hall, 2006). Dysregulation of the HPA axis contributes to elevated lipids and chronic inflammation that promote development and progression of cardiovascular disease processes, among them atherosclerotic plaque development (Kyrou et al., 2006). All these physiological events may contribute to

CVD. For example, with an increase in blood flow, shear stress on the arteries is increased, causing endothelium damage, inflammation, and plaque formation and/or rupture (Traub & Berk, 1998). This, along with sharp increases in epinephrine, stimulates platelet activation and the sequelae that follow (Markovitz & Matthews, 1991; Wenneberg et al., 1997). Activation of the parasympathetic nervous system (PNS) can have opposite effects on the heart and blood vessels, and extensive PNS activation can also lead to cardiac events (Lane, Adcock, & Burnett, 1992; Podrid, 1984).

Stress can contribute to atherosclerosis and other underlying CVD processes by increasing heart rate and decreasing diastolic and washout periods in recirculation zones, leading to increased contact of the blood constituents and vessel walls (Markovitz & Matthews, 1991; Traub & Berk, 1998). Platelet aggregation, along with coronary vasoconstriction and plaque rupture, can lead to such other priming processes as thrombosis, ischemia, and acute myocardial infarction. As discussed earlier, stress and its related emotional indices (e.g., hostility) increase platelet aggregation through induction of the autonomic nervous system (ANS) (Kamarck & Jennings, 1991; Markovitz & Matthews, 1991; Wenneberg et al., 1997).

Psychological stress is also associated with transient changes in coronary circulation and metabolism, along with the other coronary changes discussed earlier. Stress elicits such physiological changes as autonomic activation and inflammation that can trigger arrhythmias, myocardial ischemia, and plaque formation or eruption that can, in turn, ultimately lead to such clinical events as angina, ventricular tachycardia, myocardial infarction, or even sudden cardiac death (Steptoe & Brydon, 2009). For example, stress may reduce oxygen delivery to the heart and thereby lower the threshold for myocardial ischemia or may trigger acute arrhythmic events through activation of the ANS, making myocardial infarction more likely. Recent evidence has also suggested that mental stress–induced ischemic episodes are good indicators of 5-year rates of cardiac events (Jiang et al., 1996). In addition, stress-induced silent ischemia (ischemia without angina) occurs much more frequently than is detectable by some clinical measures (Deanfield et al., 1984; Modena, Corghi, Fantini, & Mattioli, 1989). There is also evidence that such acute stress events as public speaking and anger-provoking situations can disrupt cardiac electrical potential and lead to arrhythmias and other acute cardiac events, including myocardial infarction (Steptoe & Brydon, 2009). Cardiac events may also be linked to an individual's prevailing psychological state. For example, markers of CVD are associated with anxiety and depressive disorders, anger, and coping styles (Dedert, Calhoun, Watkins, Sherwood, & Beckham, 2010; Grippo & Johnson, 2009; Hamer & Malan, 2010; Steptoe & Brydon, 2009). Therefore, intervention efforts are aimed at preventing cardiac events by targeting multiple lifestyle risk factors, among them physical activity, nutrition, and stress management. These multifactorial lifestyle interventions have demonstrated some success at decreasing the incidence of cardiac events and death and may offer promise for CVD patients (Angermayr, Melchart, & Linde, 2010).

Diabetes

Just about every neuroendocrine system responds to stress. Hormonal control is essential for individuals with endocrine disorders; if this control is upset by stress, the hormonal balance is lost and disease symptoms worsen. In addition to having direct effects on hormonal levels, stress affects many of the risk factors associated with disease onset and flare-ups, among them diet, licit and illicit drug intake, and compliance with treatment regimens.

One of the most common neuroendocrine disorders is diabetes mellitus, affecting approximately 8% of the U.S. population (Centers for Disease Control and Prevention, 2008b). There are two primary types of diabetes mellitus, insulin-dependent or Type 1 and insulin independent or Type 2 (Amorosa & Swee, 2007). Both disorders are the result of high blood glucose levels and are characterized by such symptoms as blurred vision, unexplained fatigue, and increases in thirst and urination. A primary fuel for all body cells, circulating glucose enters cells to be used through the action of another hormone called insulin. In Type 1 diabetes, the immune system attacks the insulin-producing cells in the pancreas, slowing insulin production and decreasing the amount of glucose that can be used by cells. The onset of Type 1 diabetes usually occurs during childhood, with 15,000 youths diagnosed a year, and is more common among whites than among other racial groups (CDC, 2008b).

In contrast, Type 2 diabetes typically occurs later in life, but there are still 5.3 new diagnoses per 100,000 youths each year, increasing concerns over such behavioral factors as poor diet and lack of physical activity that contribute to diabetes onset (CDC, 2008b). In addition, Type 2 diabetes is more commonly diagnosed among such minority ethnic groups as American Indian, Hispanic American, and African American populations. Type 2 diabetes develops gradually over time as the cells in the body become resistant to the effects of insulin, thereby decreasing the amount of glucose that can enter the cells to be used. Although both Type 1 and Type 2 diabetes are more prevalent when there is a family history of the disease and appear to have genetic links (Amorosa & Swee, 2007), Type 2 diabetes is also associated with several other behavioral and physiological risk factors. The most common Type 2 risk factors are older age, ethnicity, being overweight, being a smoker, having high blood pressure, having high levels of fat in the blood, and being a woman who has had gestational diabetes (Amorosa & Swee, 2007).

Stress does not directly cause diabetes but may be a risk factor for the onset and progression of both types of the disease (Boyer, 2007; Fisher, Thorpe, DeVellis, & DeVellis, 2007; Ionescu-Tirgoviste, Simion, Mariana, Dan, & Iulian, 1987). For example, part of the stress response is oriented toward liberation of large quantities of glucose for cells to use for energy. In Type 1 diabetes, stress may overwhelm the pancreas's ability to produce insulin and, as a result, unmask the diabetes sooner than the onset would normally occur. Similarly, in Type 2 diabetes, stress hormones interfere with insulin use in an already compromised system, resulting in earlier detection of diabetic symptoms. Furthermore, stress plays a role in the risk factors associated with diabetes onset (e.g., obesity and high blood pressure) and can impact treatment by interfering with glycemic control (Boyer, 2007). Stress-related behaviors (e.g., smoking, drinking, poor nutrition, sleep disruptions, and forgetting to take medications) can impair self-care and result in abnormal glucose levels (Boyer, 2007; Clum, Nishith, & Resick, 2001; McNutt, Carlson, Persaud, & Postmus, 2002; Schnurr & Spiro, 1999).

Stress can also have direct effects on symptoms and disease management. As mentioned earlier, stress increases blood glucose levels. In Type 1 diabetes, the body does not produce enough insulin to handle the high blood glucose levels; and in Type 2 diabetes, the body cells are resistant to insulin, so blood glucose levels remain high. Therefore, high blood glucose levels associated with stress cannot be properly handled by the body (Surwit & Williams, 1996). Untreated high glucose levels are dangerous and can lead to ketoacidosis and diabetic coma (Amorosa & Swee, 2007). As with other chronic diseases, patients benefit from stress management interventions that help to decrease the stress associated with diabetes and its symptoms, improve quality of life and functioning, and improve glycaemic control in patients with either Type 1 or Type 2 diabetes (Ismail, Winkley, & Rabe-Hesketh, 2004; Plack, Herpertz, & Petrak, 2010; Winkley, Landau, Eisler, & Ismail, 2006).

CONCLUSION

Stress is a critical crosscutting process that is basic to research, theory, and application in health psychology. It represents modifiable variance in the etiology of disease, affects nearly every behavior that contributes to good or bad health outcomes, and has direct effects on all or most bodily systems and can thereby contribute to developing health problems as well. Stress is basic to the commerce between organisms and their environments, motivating them to take action against stressors or to insulate themselves from stress effects. It also produces nonspecific catabolic arousal, driven primarily by neural-endocrine regulatory loops that support such adaptive capabilities as fight or flight. More specific aspect of stress responding, tied more closely to the stressful situation and its interaction with the organism's resources and abilities, are reflected in emotional responding and coping as well as in cognitive appraisal processes and memory.

Most people are able to adapt to stressful situations; even in the most extreme cases, it would be expected that most people would be able to cope effectively and move on to new challenges. The multiple changes that occur during stress facilitate adaptation. However, there are negative effects of stress that have been observed, including aspects of the pathophysiology of metabolic syndrome, cardiovascular disorders, infectious illnesses (including HIV disease and hepatitis), cancer, diabetes, and such autoimmune diseases as rheumatoid arthritis. These effects appear most often when stress responses are extremely intense or abnormally prolonged. They can also become manifest when resources and coping are not immediately able to overcome or displace stressful conditions. Uncontrollable stress appears to be more difficult to resist than controllable and predictable periods of threat or demand.

Quantification of contributions of stress to disease etiology and personal susceptibility to major health problems has been a slow project but has been increasingly successful in measuring harmful and beneficial effects of stress. Similarly, the ability to intervene and modify lifestyle, coping, social resources, and appraisals of major chronic illnesses, stressors, and associated conditions has continued to improve. Research during the next 10 years should continue characterizing the relationship between stress and health, with a focus on identifying long-term trajectories of stress on disease and by determining how risk and resilience factors alter this relationship. Future research should also emphasize interdisciplinary collaborations among investigators in order to examine changes among multiple stress pathways within the same sample. Such collaborations would enable researchers to apply multilevel approaches to assessing stress that will allow for more complex covariations and interactions among cognitive, behavioral, social, and physiological pathways. Researchers should also incorporate newer approaches that examine gene by environment interactions, further allowing examination of the system in its entirety rather than focusing on one specific response pathway or disease mechanism.

REFERENCES

Aiello, A. E., Simanek, A. M., & Galea, S. (2010). Population levels of psychological stress, herpesvirus reactivation and HIV. *AIDS and Behavior, 14*, 308–317.

Alberti, K. G., Zimmet, P., Shaw, J., & IDF Epidemiology Task Force Consensus Group. (2005). The metabolic syndrome—A new worldwide definition. *Lancet, 366*, 1059–1062.

American Psychiatric Association. (2000). *Diagnostic and statistical manual of mental disorders* (4th ed., rev.). Washington, DC: American Psychiatric Press.

Amorosa, L. F., & Swee, D. E. (2007). In D. Rakel (Ed.), *Textbook of family medicine* (7th ed.). Philadelphia, PA: Elsevier.

Angermayr, L., Melchart, D., & Linde, K. (2010). Multifactorial lifestyle interventions in the primary and secondary prevention of cardiovascular disease and type 2 diabetes mellitus: A systematic review of randomized controlled trials. *Annals of Behavioral Medicine, 40*, 49–64.

Antoni, M. H., Carrico, A. W., Duran, R. E., Spitzer, S., Penedo, F., Ironson, G., ... Schneiderman, N. (2006). Randomized clinical trial of cognitive behavioral stress management on human immunodeficiency virus viral load in gay men treated with highly active antiretroviral therapy. *Psychosomatic Medicine, 68*, 143–151.

Antoni, M. H., Cruess, D. G., Klimas, N., Carrico, A. W., Maher, K., Cruess, S., ... Schneiderman, N. (2005). Increases in a marker of immune system reconstitution are predated by decreases in 24-h urinary cortisol output and depressed mood during a 10-week stress management intervention in symptomatic gay men. *Journal of Psychosomatic Research, 58*, 3–13.

Antoni, M. H., Lutgendorf, S. K., Cole, S. W., Dhabbar, F. S., Sephton, S. E., McDonald, P. G., ... Sood, A. K. (2006). The influence of bio-behavioural factors on tumor biology: Pathways and mechanisms. *Nature Reviews Cancer, 6*, 240–248.

Baba, V. V., Jamal, M., & Tourigny, L. (1998). Work and mental health: A decade in Canadian research. *Canadian Psychology, 39*, 94–107.

Bachen, E. A., Manuck, S. B., Marsland, A. L., Cohen, S., Malkoff, S. B., Muldoon, M. F., & Rabin, B. S. (1992). Lymphocyte subset and cellular immune response to a brief experimental stressor. *Psychosomatic Medicine, 54*, 673–679.

Baltrusch, H. J., Stangel, W., & Titze, I. (1991). Stress, cancer, and immunity. New developments in biopsycho-social and psychoneuroimmunologic research. *Acta Neurologica*, *13*, 315–327.

Baum, A. (1990). Stress, intrusive imagery, and chronic distress. *Health Psychology*, *9*(6), 653–675.

Baum, A., Cohen, L., & Hall, M. (1993). Control and intrusive memories as possible determinants of chronic stress. *Psychosomatic Medicine*, *55*, 274–286.

Baum, A., O'Keeffe, M. K., & Davidson, L. M. (1990). Acute stressors and chronic response: The case of traumatic stress. *Journal of Applied Social Psychology*, *20*, 1643–1654.

Baum, A., Schooler, T. Y., & Dougall, A. L. (1998). The role of experience in acute and chronic stress. Manuscript submitted for publication.

Baum, A., Trevino, L. A., & Dougall, A. J. L. (2011). Stress and cancers. In R. J. Contrada & A. Baum (Eds.), *The handbook of stress science: Biology, psychology, and health* (pp. 411–424). New York, NY: Springer.

Berntsen, D. (1996). Involuntary autobiographical memories. *Applied Cognitive Psychology*, *10*, 435–454.

Blumenthal, J. A., Sherwood, A., Babyak, M. A., Watkins, L. L., Waugh, R., Georgiades, A., … Hinderliter, A. (2005). Effects of exercise and stress management training on markers of cardiovascular risk in patients with ischemic heart disease: A randomized controlled trial. *JAMA*, *293*, 1626–1634.

Boyce, W. T., Chesney, M., Alkon, A., Tschann, J. M., Adams, S., Chesterman, B., … Wara, D. (1995). Psychobiologic reactivity to stress and childhood respiratory illnesses: Results of two prospective studies. *Psychosomatic Medicine*, *57*, 411–422.

Boyer, B. A. (2007). Diabetes. In B. A. Boyer & M. I. Paharia (Eds.), *Comprehensive handbook of clinical health psychology* (pp. 179–200). Hoboken, NJ: Wiley.

Breslau, N. (2009). The epidemiology of trauma, PTSD, and other posttrauma disorders. *Trauma Violence Abuse*, *10*, 198–210.

Brickman, A. L., & Yount, S. E. (1996). Noncompliance in end-stage renal disease: A threat to quality of care and cost containment. *Journal of Clinical Psychology in Medical Settings*, *3*, 399–412.

Brown, G. W., & Harris, T. O. (Eds.). (1989). *Life events and illness.* New York, NY: Guilford Press.

Brown, R. F., Tennant, C. C., Dunn, S. M., & Pollard, J. D. (2005). A review of stress-relapse interactions in multiple sclerosis: Important features and stress-mediating and -moderating variables. *Multiple Sclerosis*, *11*, 477–484.

Brown, J. L., & Vanable, P. A. (2008). Cognitive–behavioral stress management interventions for persons living with HIV: A review and critique of the literature. *Behavioral Medicine*, *35*, 26–40.

Brunello, N., Davidson, J. R., Deahl, M., Kessler, R. C., Mendlewicz, J., Racagni, G., … Zohar, J. (2001). Posttraumatic stress disorder: Diagnosis and epidemiology, comorbidity and social consequences, biology and treatment. *Neuropsychobiology*, *43*(3), 150–162.

Cannon, W. B. (1914). The interrelations of emotions as suggested by recent physiological researches. *American Journal of Physiology*, *25*, 256–282.

Centers for Disease Control and Prevention. (2008a). HIV prevalence estimates—United States, 2006. *Morbidity and Mortality Weekly Report*, *57*(39), 1073–1076.

Centers for Disease Control and Prevention. (2008b). *National diabetes fact sheet: General information and national estimates on diabetes in the United States, 2007.* Atlanta, GA: U.S. Department of Health and Human Services, Centers for Disease Control and Prevention.

Chiasson, M., Hirshfield, S., Humberstone, M., DiFilippi, J., Koblin, B., & Remien, R. (2005). Increased high risk sexual behavior after September 11 in men who have sex with men: An internet survey. *Archives of Sexual Behavior*, *34*(5), 527–535.

Chida, Y., Hamer, M., Wardle, J., & Steptoe, A. Do stress-related psychosocial factors contribute to cancer incidence and survival? *Nature Clinical Practice Oncology*, *5*, 466–475.

Chida, Y., & Vedhara, K. (2009). Adverse psychosocial factors predict poorer prognosis in HIV disease: A meta-analytic review of prospective investigations. *Brain, Behavior, and Immunity*, *23*, 434–445.

Christian, L. M., Graham, J. E., Padgett, D. A., Glaser, R., & Kiecolt-Glaser, J. K. (2006). Stress and wound healing. *Neuroimmunomodulation*, *13*, 337–346.

Clum, G. A., Nishith, P., & Resick, P. A. (2001). Trauma-related sleep disturbance and self-reported physical health symptoms in treatment-seeking female rape victims. *Journal of Nervous and Mental Disease*, *189*(9), 618–622.

Cohen, S. (1980). Aftereffects of stress on human performance and social behavior: A review of research and theory. *Psychological Bulletin*, *88*, 82–108.

Cohen, S. (2005). Keynote presentation at the Eighth International Congress of Behavioral Medicine. The Pittsburgh common cold studies: Psychosocial predictors of susceptibility to respiratory infectious illness. *International Journal of Behavioral Medicine*, *12*, 123–131.

Cohen, S., Frank, E., Doyle, W. J., Skoner, D. P., Rabin, B. S., & Gawltney, J. M., Jr. (1998). Types of stressors that increase susceptibility to the common cold in healthy adults. *Health Psychology, 17*, 214–223.

Cohen, S., Gottlieb, B., & Underwood, L. (2000). Social relationships and health. In S. Cohen, L. Underwood, & B. Gottlieb (Eds.), *Measuring and intervening in social support* (pp. 3–25). New York, NY: Oxford University Press.

Cohen, S., Tyrrell, D. A. J., & Smith, A. P. (1991). Psychological stress and susceptibility to the common cold. *New England Journal of Medicine, 325*, 606–612.

Coyne, J. C. (2009). Are most positive findings in health psychology false… or at least somewhat exaggerated? *European Health Psychologist, 11*, 49–51.

Coyne, J., Stefanek, M., & Palmer, S. (2007). Psychotherapy and survival in cancer: The conflict between hope and evidence. *Psychological Bulletin, 133*, 367–394.

Craig, K. J., Heisler, J. A., & Baum, A. (1996). Intrusive thoughts and the maintenance of chronic stress. In I. G. Sarason, G. R. Pierce, & B. R. Sarason (Eds.), *Cognitive interference: Theories, methods, and findings. The LEA series in personality and clinical psychology* (pp. 397–413). Mahwah, NJ: Erlbaum.

Creamer, M., Burgess, P., & Pattison, P. (1992). Reaction to trauma: A cognitive processing model. *Journal of Abnormal Psychology, 101*, 452–459.

Crepaz, N., Passin, W. F., Herbst, J. H., Rama, S. M., Malow, R. M., Purcell, D. W., Wolitski, R. J., & the HIV/AIDS Prevention Research Synthesis (PRS) Team. (2008). Meta-analysis of cognitive-behavioral interventions on HIV-positive persons' mental health and immune functioning. *Health Psychology, 27*, 4–14.

Deanfield, J., Shea, M., Kensett, M., Horlock, P., Wilson, R., de Landsheere, C., & Selwyn, A. (1984). Silent myocardial infarction due to mental stress. *Lancet, 11*, 1001–1004.

Dedert, E. A., Calhoun, P. S., Watkins, L. L., Sherwood, A., & Beckham, J. C. (2010). Posttraumatic stress disorder, cardiovascular, and metabolic disease: A review of the evidence. *Annals of Behavioral Medicine, 39*, 61–78.

Delahanty, D. L., Dougall, A. L., Craig, K. J., Jenkins, F. J., & Baum, A. (1997). Chronic stress and natural killer cell activity following exposure to traumatic death. *Psychosomatic Medicine, 59*, 467–476.

Delahanty, D. L., Dougall, A. L., Hawken, L., Trakowski, J. H., Schmitz, J. B., Jenkins, F. J., & Baum, A. (1996). Time course of natural killer cell activity and lymphocyte proliferation in response to two acute stressors. *Health Psychology, 15*, 48–55.

Dhabhar, F. S., & McEwen, B. S. (1997). Acute stress enhances while chronic stress suppresses cell-mediated immunity in vivo: A potential role for leukocyte trafficking. *Brain, Behavior, and Immunity, 11*, 286–306.

Diabetes Prevention Program Research Group. (2002). Reduction in the incidence of type 2 diabetes with lifestyle intervention or Metformin. *New England Journal of Medicine, 346*, 393–403.

Dougall A. L., Baum, A., & Jenkins, F. J. (1998). Daily fluctuation in chronic fatigue syndrome severity and symptoms. *Journal of Applied Biobehavioral Research, 3*, 12–28.

Dougall, A. L., Craig, K. J., & Baum, A. (1999). Assessment of characteristics of intrusive thoughts and their impact on distress among victims of traumatic events. *Psychosomatic Medicine, 61*, 38–48.

Ell, K., Nishimoto, R., Mediansky, L., Mantell, J., & Hamovitch, M. (1992). Social relations, social support and survival among patients with cancer. *Journal of Psychosomatic Research, 36*, 531–541.

Enqvist, B., & Fischer, K. (1997). Preoperative hypnotic techniques reduce consumption of analgesics after surgical removal of third mandibular molars: A brief communication. *International Journal of Clinical and Experimental Hypnosis, 45*, 102–108.

Epel, E. S., Blackburn, E. H., Lin, J., Dhabhar, F. S., Adler, N. E., Morrow, J. D., & Cawthon, R. M. (2004). Accelerated telomere shortening in response to life stress. *Proceedings of the National Academy of Sciences USA, 101*, 17312–17315.

Epel, E. S., Lin, J., Wilhelm, F. H., Wolkowitz, O. M., Cawthon, R., Adler, N. E., … Blackburn, E. H. (2006). Cell aging in relation to stress arousal and cardiovascular disease risk factors. *Psychoneuroendocrinology, 31*, 277–287.

Esterling, B. A., Kiecolt-Glaser, J. K., Bodnar, J. C., & Glaser, R. (1994). Chronic stress, social support, and persistent alterations in the natural killer cell response to cytokines in older adults. *Health Psychology, 13*, 291–298.

Evans-Campbell, T., Lindhorst, T., Huang, B., & Walters, K. L. (2006). Interpersonal violence in the lives of urban American Indian and Alaska Native women: Implications for health, mental health, and help-seeking. *American Journal of Public Health, 96*(8), 1416–1422.

Field, C. A., Claassen, C. A., & O'Keefe, G. (2001). Association of alcohol use and other high-risk behaviors among trauma patients. *Journal of Trauma, 50*(1), 13–19.

Finan, P. H., Okun, M. A., Kruszewski, D., Davis, M. C., Zautra, A. J., & Tennen, H. (2010). Interplay of concurrent positive and negative interpersonal events in the prediction of daily negative affect and fatigue for rheumatoid arthritis patients. *Health Psychology, 29*, 429–437.

Firestein, G. S., Budd, R. C., Harris, E. D., Jr., McInnes, I. B., Ruddy, S., & Sergent, J. S. (2008). *Kelley's textbook of rheumatology* (8th ed.). Philadelphia, PA: Elsevier.

Fisher, E. B., Thorpe, C. T., DeVellis, B. M., & DeVellis, R. F. (2007). Healthy coping, negative emotions, and diabetes management: A systematic review and appraisal. *Diabetes Educator, 33*, 1080–1103.

Flint, M. S., Baum, A., Chambers, W. H., & Jenkins, F. J. (2007). Induction of DNA damage, alteration of DNA repair and transcriptional activation by stress hormones. *Psychoneuroendocrinology, 32*, 470–479.

Frasure-Smith, N., Lesperance, F., & Talajic, M. (1995). The impact of negative emotions on prognosis following myocardial infarction: Is it more than depression? *Health Psychology, 14*, 388–398.

Friedman, M. J., & Davidson, J. R. T. (2007). Pharmacotherapy for PTSD. In M. J. Friedman, T. M. Keane, & P. A. Resick (Eds.), *Handbook of PTSD: Science and practice* (pp. 376–405). New York, NY: Guilford Press.

Gidron, Y., Russ, K., Tissarchondou, H., & Warner, J. (2006). The relation between psychological factors and DNA damage: A critical review. *Biological Psychology, 72*, 291–304.

Gilboa, S. Shirom, A., Fried, Y., & Cooper, C. (2008). A meta-analysis of work demand stressors and job performance: Examining main and moderating effects. *Personnel Psychology, 61*, 227–271.

Glaser, R. (2005). Stress-associated immune dysregulation and its importance for human health: A personal history of psychoneuroimmunology. *Brain, Behavior, and Immunity, 17*, 321–328.

Glaser, R., & Kiecolt-Glaser, J. K. (2005). Stress-induced immune dysfunction: Implications for health. *Nature Reviews Immunology, 5*, 243–251.

Glass, D. C., & Singer, J. E. (1972). *Urban stress: Experiments on noise and social stressors.* New York, NY: Academic Press.

Golden-Kreutz, D. M., Thornton, L. M., Wells-Di Gregorio, S., Frierson, G. M., Jim, H. S., Carpenter, K. M., … Andersen, B. L. (2005). Traumatic stress, perceived global stress, and life events: Prospectively predicting quality of life in breast cancer patients. *Health Psychology, 24*, 288–296.

Grassi, L., & Rosti, G. (1996). Psychosocial morbidity and adjustment to illness among long-term cancer survivors: A six-year-follow-up study. *Psychosomatics, 37*, 523–532.

Green, B. L. (1994). Psychosocial research in traumatic stress: An update. *Journal of Traumatic Stress, 7*, 341–362.

Greenberg, M. A. (1995). Cognitive processing of traumas: The role of intrusive thoughts and reappraisals. *Journal of Applied Social Psychology, 25*, 1262–1296.

Grilo, C., Pagano, M., & Stout, R. (2009). Do stressful life events predict eating disorder relapse? Six-year outcomes from the collaborative personality disorders study. *European Psychiatry, 24*(Suppl. 1), S746.

Grippo, A., & Johnson, A. K. (2009). Stress, depression and cardiovascular dysregulation: A review of neurobiological mechanisms and the integration of research from preclinical disease models. *Stress, 12*, 1–21.

Grunberg, N. E., Berger, S. S., & Hamilton, K. R. (2011). Stress and drug use. In R. J. Contrada & A. Baum (Eds.), *The handbook of stress science: Biology, psychology, and health* (pp. 287–300). New York, NY: Springer.

Guyton, A. C., & Hall, J. E. (2006). *Textbook of medical physiology* (11th ed.). Philadelphia, PA: Elsevier.

Hamer, M., & Malan, L. (2010). Psychophysiological risk markers of cardiovascular disease. *Neuroscience and Biobehavioral Reviews, 35*, 76–83.

Helgeson, V. S., & Cohen, S. (1996). Social support and adjustment to cancer: Reconciling descriptive, correlational, and intervention research. *Health Psychology, 15*, 135–148.

Herrmann, M., Scholmerich, J., & Straub, R. H. (2000). Stress and rheumatic diseases. *Rheumatic Disease Clinics of North America, 26*, 737–763.

Holmes, E. A., & Bourne, C. (2008). Inducing and modulating intrusive emotional memories: A review of the trauma film paradigm. *Acta Psychologica, 127*, 553–566.

Holmes, T. H., & Rahe, R. H. (1967). The Social Readjustment Rating Scale. *Journal of Psychosomatic Research, 11*, 213–218.

Horowitz, M. J. (1986). *Stress response syndromes* (2nd ed.). New York, NY: Jason Aronson.

Huyser, B., & Parker, J. C. (1998). Stress and rheumatoid arthritis: An integrative review. *Arthritis Care and Research, 11*, 135–145.

Ionescu-Tirgoviste, C., Simion, P., Mariana, C., Dan, C. M., & Iulian, M. (1987). The signification of stress in the aetiopathogenesis of type-sub-2 diabetes mellitus. *Stress Medicine, 3*, 277–284.

Ironson, G., & Hayward, H. (2008). Do positive psychosocial factors predict disease progression in HIV-1? A review of the evidence. *Psychosomatic Medicine, 70*, 546–554.

Ironson, G., Wynings, C., Schneiderman, N., Baum, A., Rodriguez, M., Greenwood, D., … Fletcher, M. A. (1997). Post traumatic stress symptoms, intrusive thoughts, loss and immune function after Hurricane Andrew. *Psychosomatic Medicine, 59*, 128–141.

Irvine, D., Brown, B., Crooks, D., Roberts, J., & Browne, G. (1991). Psychosocial adjustment in women with breast cancer. *Cancer, 67*, 1097–1117.

Ismail, K., Winkley, K., & Rabe-Hesketh, S. (2004). Systematic review and meta-analysis of randomised controlled trials of psychological interventions to improve glycaemic control in patients with type 2 diabetes. *Lancet, 363*, 1589–1597.

Jamison, R. B., Burish, T. G., & Wallston, K. A. (1987). Psychogenic factors in predicting survival of breast cancer patients. *Journal of Clinical Oncology, 5*, 768–772.

Jiang, W., Babyak, M., Krantz, D. S., Waugh, R. A., Coleman, R. E., Hanson, M. M., … Blumenthal, J. A. (1996). Mental stress-induced myocardial ischemia and cardiac events. *Journal of the American Medical Association, 275*, 1651–1656.

Juster, R., McEwen, B. S., & Lupien, S. J. (2010). Allostatic load biomarkers of chronic stress and impact on health and cognition. *Neuroscience and Biobehavioral Reviews, 35*, 2–16.

Kadan-Lottick, N., Vanderwerker, L., Block, S., Zhang, B., & Prigerson, H. (2005). Psychiatric disorders and mental health service use in patients with advanced cancer. *Cancer, 104*(12), 872–2881.

Kamarck, T., & Jennings, J. R. (1991). Biobehavioral factors in sudden cardiac death. *Psychological Bulletin, 109*, 42–75.

Kangas, M., Henry, J., & Bryant, R. (2005). The relationship between acute stress disorder and posttraumatic stress disorder following cancer. *Journal of Consulting and Clinical Psychology, 73*(2), 360–364.

Kasl, S. V., Evans, A. S., & Niederman, J. C. (1979). Psychosocial risk factors in the development of infectious mononucleosis. *Psychosomatic Medicine, 41*, 445–466.

Katz, P. P. (1998). The stresses of rheumatoid arthritis: Appraisals of perceived impact and coping efficacy. *Arthritis Care and Research, 11*, 9–22.

Kemeny, M. E., & Schedlowski, M. (2007). Understanding the interaction between psychosocial stressand immune-related diseases: A stepwise progression. *Brain, Behavior, and Immunity, 21*, 1009–1018.

Kendler, K. S., Kessler, R. C., Walters, E. E., MacLean, C., Neale, M. C., Heath, A. C., & Eaves, L. J. (1995). Stressful life events, genetic liability, and onset of an episode of major depression in women. *American Journal of Psychiatry, 152*, 833–842.

Kiecolt-Glaser, J. K., Stephens, R. E., Lipetz, P. D., Speicher, C. E., & Glaser, R. (1985). Distress and DNA repair in human lymphocytes. *Journal of Behavioral Medicine, 8*, 311–320.

Kilpatrick, D. G., Koenen, K. C., Ruggiero, K. J., Acierno, R. Galea, S., Resnick, H. S., … Gelernter, J. (2007). The serotonin transporter genotype and social support and moderation of posttraumatic stress disorder and depression in hurricane-exposed adults. *American Journal of Psychiatry, 164*, 1693–1699.

Kiviniemi, M. T., & Rothman, A. J. (2010). Specifying the determinants of people's health beliefs and health behavior: How a social psychological perspective can inform initiatives to promote health. In J. M. Suls, K. W. Davidson, & R. M. Kaplan (Eds.), *Handbook of health psychology and behavioral medicine* (pp. 64–83). New York, NY: Guilford Press.

Kompier, M. A., & DiMartino, V. (1995). Review of bus drivers' occupational stress and stress prevention. *Stress Medicine, 11*, 253–262.

Krueger, G. P. (1989). Sustained work, fatigue, sleep loss and performance: A review of the issues. *Work and Stress, 3*, 129–141.

Kyrou, I., Chrousos, G. P., & Tsigos, C. (2006). Stress, visceral obesity, and metabolic complications. *Annals of the New York Academy of Sciences, 1083*, 77–110.

Lane, J. D., Adcock, R. A., & Burnett, R. E. (1992). Respiratory sinus arrhythmia and cardiovascular responses to stress. *Psychophysiology, 29*, 461–470.

Lazarus, R. S. (1966). *Psychological stress and the coping process.* New York, NY: McGraw-Hill.

Lazarus, R. S., & Folkman, S. (1984). *Stress, appraisal, and coping.* New York, NY: Springer.

Leserman, J. (2008). Role of depression, stress, and trauma in HIV disease progression. *Psychosomatic Medicine, 70*, 539–545.

Lutgendorf, S. K., Costanzo, E. S., & Siegel, S. D. (2007). Psychosocial influences on oncology: An expanded model of biobehavioral mechanisms. In R. Ader (Ed.), *Psychoneuroimmunology* (pp. 869–895). San Diego, CA: Academic Press.

Markovitz, J. H., & Matthews, K. A. (1991). Platelets and coronary heart disease: Potential psychophysiologic mechanisms. *Psychosomatic Medicine, 53*, 643–668.

Marucha, P. T., & Engeland, C. G. (2007). Stress neuroendocrine hormones and wound healing: Human models. In R. Ader (Ed.), *Psychoneuroimmunology* (4th ed., Vol. 1, pp. 825–836). Burlington, MA: Elsevier.

Marucha, P. T., Kiecolt-Glaser, J. K., & Favagehi, M. (1998). Mucosal wound healing is impaired by examination stress. *Psychosomatic Medicine, 60*, 362–365.

Mason, J. W. (1968). Organization of psychoendocrine mechanisms. *Psychosomatic Medicine, 30*, 565–808.

Mason, J. W. (1971). A re-evaluation of the concept of <@147>non-specificity<@148> in stress theory. *Journal of Psychiatric Research, 8*, 323–333.

Mayou, R., Peveler, R., Davies, B., Mann, J., & Fairburn, C. (1991). Psychiatric morbidity in young adults with insulin-dependent diabetes mellitus. *Psychological Medicine, 21*, 639–645.

McEwen, B. S. (1998). Protective and damaging effects of stress mediators. *New England Journal of Medicine, 338*, 171–179.

McFarlane, A. C., & Brooks, P. M. (1990). Psychoimmunology and rheumatoid arthritis: Concepts and methodologies. *International Journal of Psychiatry in Medicine, 20*, 307–322.

McGregor, B. A., & Antoni, M. H. (2009). Psychological intervention and health outcomes among women treated for breast cancer: A review of stress pathways and biological mediators. *Brain, Behavior, and Immunity, 23*, 159–166.

McNutt, L. A., Carlson, B. E., Persaud, M., & Postmus, J. (2002). Cumulative abuse experiences, physical health and health behaviors. *Annals of Epidemiology, 12*(2), 123–130.

Melanson, P. M., & Downe-Wamboldt, B. (1995). The stress of life with rheumatoid arthritis as perceived by older adults. *Activities, Adaptation, and Aging, 19*, 33–47.

Mellman, T. A. (1997). Psychobiology of sleep disturbances in posttraumatic stress disorder. In R. Yehuda & A. C. McFarlane (Eds.), *Psychobiology of posttraumatic stress disorder. Annals of the New York Academy of Sciences* (Vol. 821, pp. 142–149). New York, NY: New York Academy of Sciences.

Meyer, D. F. (1997). Codependency as a mediator between stressful events and eating disorders. *Journal of Clinical Psychology, 53*, 107–116.

Mizrahi, R. (2010). Advances in PET analyses of stress and dopamine. *Neuropsychopharmacology, 35*, 348–349.

Modena, M., Corghi, F., Fantini, G., & Mattioli, G. (1989). Echocardiographic monitoring of mental stress test in ischemic heart disease. *Clinical Cardiology, 12*, 21–24.

Monroe, S. M., & Harkness, K. L. (2005). Life stress, the "Kindling" hypothesis, and the recurrence of depression: Considerations from a life stress perspective. *Psychological Review, 112*, 417–445.

Mullins, L. L., Chaney, J. M., Pace, T. M., & Hartman, V. L. (1997). Illness uncertainty, attributional style, and psychological adjustment in older adolescents and young adults with asthma. *Journal of Pediatric Psychology, 22*, 871–880.

Myasoedova, E., Crowson, C. S., Kremers, H. M., Therneau, T. M., & Gabriel, S. E. (2010). Is the incidence of rheumatoid arthritis rising? Results from Olmsted County, Minnesota, 1955–2007. *Arthritis and Rheumatism, 62*, 1576–1582.

Nesse, R. M., Curtis, G. C., Thyer, B. A., McCann, D. S., Huber-Smith, M. J., & Knopf, R. F. (1985). Endocrine and cardiovascular responses during phobic anxiety. *Psychosomatic Medicine, 47*, 320–332.

Norris, F. H., Friedman, M. J., Watson, P. J., Byrne, C. M., Diaz, E., & Kaniasty, K. (2002). 60,000 disaster victims speak: Part I. An empirical review of the empirical literature, 1981–2001. *Psychiatry, 65*, 207–239.

O'Dell, J. R. (2007). Rheumatoid arthritis. In L. Goldman & D. A. Ausiello (Eds.), *Cecil medicine* (23rd ed.). Philadelphia, PA: Elsevier.

Olff, M., Langeland, W., & Gersons, B. P. R. (2005). The psychobiology of PTSD: Coping with trauma. *Psychoneuroendocrinology, 30*, 974–982.

Palesh, O., Butler, L. D., Koopman, C., Giese-Davis, J., Carlson, R., & Spiegel, D. (2007). Stress history and breast cancer recurrence. *Journal of Psychosomatic Research, 63*, 233–239.

Park, E. R., Chang, Y., Quinn, V., Regan, S., Cohen, L., Viguera, A., … Rigotti, N. (2009). The association of depressive, anxiety, and stress symptoms and postpartum relapse to smoking: A longitudinal study. *Nicotine and Tobacco Research, 11*, 707–714.

Parslow, R. A., Jorm, A. F., & Christensen, H. (2006). Associations of pre-trauma attributes and trauma exposure with screening positive for PTSD: Analysis of a community-based study of 2,085 young adults. *Psychological Medicine, 36*, 387–395.

Pedersen, A. F., Zachariae, R., & Bovbjerg, D. H. (2009). Psychological stress and antibody response to influenza vaccination: A meta-analysis. *Brain, Behavior, and Immunity, 23*, 427–433.

Perez, G. K., Cruess, D. G., & Kalichman, S. C. (2011). Stress and cancers. In R. J. Contrada & A. Baum (Eds.), *The handbook of stress science: Biology, psychology, and health* (pp. 447–460). New York, NY: Springer.

Petticrew, M., Bell, R., & Hunter, D. (2002). Influence of psychological coping on survival and recurrence in people with cancer: Systematic review. *British Medical Journal, 325*. doi:10.1136/bmj.325.7372.1066

Phillips, A. C. (2008). The influence of psychosocial factors on vaccination response: A review. In A. B. Turley & G. C. Hofmann (Eds.), *Life style and health research progress* (pp. 139–153). Hauppauge, NY: Nova Biomedical.

Plack, K., Herpertz, S., & Petrak, F. (2010). Behavioral medicine interventions in diabetes. *Current Opinion in Psychiatry, 23*, 131–138.

Podrid, P. J. (1984). Role of higher nervous activity in ventricular arrhythmia and sudden cardiac death: Implications for alternative antiarrhythmic therapy. *Annals of the New York Academy of Sciences, 432*, 296–313.

Potter, P. T., & Zautra, A. J. (1997). Stressful life events<@146> effects on rheumatoid arthritis disease activity. *Journal of Consulting and Clinical Psychology, 65*, 319–323.

Rahe, R. H. (1972). Subjects<@146> recent life changes and their near future illness reports. *Annals of Clinical Research, 4*, 250–265.

Rahe, R. H. (1987). Recent life changes, emotions, and behaviors in coronary heart disease. In A. Baum & J. E. Singer (Eds.), *Handbook of psychology and health: Stress* (Vol. 5, pp. 229–254). Hillsdale, NJ: Erlbaum.

Rasmusson, A. M., Vasek, J., Lipschitz, D., Mustone, M. E., Vojvoda, D., Shi, Q., … Charney, D. S. (2004). An increased capacity for adrenal DHEA release is associated negatively with avoidance symptoms and negative mood in women with PTSD. *Neuropsychopharmacology, 29*, 1546–1557.

Reiche, E. M. V., Nunes, S. O. V., & Morimoto, H. K. (2004). Stress, depression, the immune system, and cancer. *Lancet Oncology, 5*, 617–625.

Rimon, R., & Laakso, R. (1985). Life stress and rheumatoid arthritis: A 15-year follow-up study. *Psychotherapy and Psychosomatics, 43*, 38–43.

Rosmond, R. (2005). Role of stress in the pathogenesis of the metabolic syndrome. *Psychoneuroendocrinology, 30*, 1–10.

Ross, M. J., & Berger, R. S. (1996). Effects of stress inoculation training on athletes<@146> postsurgical pain and rehabilitation after orthopedic injury. *Journal of Consulting & Clinical Psychology, 64*, 406–410.

Sarason, I. G., de Monchaux, C., & Hunt, T. (1975). Methodological issues in the assessment of life stress. In L. Levi (Ed.), *Emotions: Their parameters and measurement* (pp. 499–509). New York, NY: Raven.

Schnurr, P. P., Green, B. L., & Kaltman, S. (2007). Trauma exposure and physical health. In M. J. Friedman, T. M. Keane, & P. A. Resick (Eds.), *Handbook of PTSD: Science and practice* (pp. 406–424). New York, NY: Guilford Press.

Schnurr, P. P., & Spiro, A., III (1999). Combat exposure, posttraumatic stress disorder symptoms, and health behaviors as predictors of self-reported physical health in older veterans. *Journal of Nervous and Mental Disease, 187*(6), 353–359.

Scott-Sheldon, L. A. J., Kalichman, S. C., Carey, M. P., & Fielder, R. L. (2008). Stress management interventions for HIV adults: A meta-analysis of randomized controlled trials, 1989 to 2006. *Health Psychology, 27*, 129–139.

Segerstrom, S. C. (2010). Resources, stress, and immunity: An ecological perspective on human psychoneuroimmunology. *Annals of Behavioral Medicine, 40*, 114–125.

Segerstrom, S. C., & Miller, G. E. (2004). Psychological stress and the human immune system: A meta-analytic study of 30 years of inquiry. *Psychological Bulletin, 130*, 601–630.

Segman, R. H., Shefi, N., Goltser-Dubner, T., Friedman, N., Kaminski, N., & Shalev, A. Y. (2005). Peripheral blood mononuclear cell gene expression profiles identify emergent post-traumatic stress disorder among trauma survivors. *Molecular Psychiatry, 10*, 500–513.

Selye, H. (1984). *The stress of life* (rev. ed.). New York, NY: McGraw-Hill. (Original work published in 1956.)

Sharpe, T. M., Ryst, E., Hinshaw, S. P., & Steiner, H. (1997). Reports of stress: A comparison between eating disordered and non-eating disordered adolescents. *Child Psychiatry and Human Development, 28*, 117–132.

Sieber, W. J., Rodin, J., Larson, L., Ortega, S., & Cummings, N. (1992). Modulation of human natural killer cell activity by exposure to uncontrollable stress. *Brain, Behavior, and Immunity, 6*, 141–156.

Sinha, R. (2007). The role of stress in addiction relapse. *Current Psychiatry Reports, 9*, 388–395.

Smith, B. W., & Zautra, A. J. (2008). The effects of anxiety and depression on weekly pain in women with arthritis. *Pain, 138*, 354–361.

Smith, D. W., Christiansen, E. H., Vincent, R., & Hann, N. E. (1999). Population effects of the bombing of Oklahoma City. *Journal—Oklahoma State Medical Association, 92*(4), 193–198.

Snyderman, D., & Wynn, D. (2009). Depression in cancer patients. *Primary Care Clinics Office Practice, 36*, 703–719.

Solomon, G. F., Kemeny, M. E., & Temoshok, L. (1991). Psychoneuroimmunological aspects of HIV. In R. Ader, D. L. Felton, & N. Cohen (Eds.), *Psychoneuroimmunology* (pp. 1081–1113). New York, NY: Simon & Schuster.

Southwick, S. M., Davis, L. L., Aikins, D. E., Rasmusson, A., Barron, J., & Morgan III, C. A. (2007). Neurobiological alterations associated with PTSD. In M. J. Friedman, T. M. Keane, & P. A. Resick (Eds.), *Handbook of PTSD: Science and practice* (pp. 166–189). New York, NY: Guilford Press.

Spiegel, D., & Giese-Davis, J. (2003). Depression and cancer: Mechanisms and disease progression. *Biological Psychiatry, 54*, 269–282.

Steptoe, A., & Ayers, S. (2004). Stress and health. In S. Sutton, A. Baum, & M. Johnston (Eds.), *The Sage handbook of health psychology*. London, England: Sage.

Steptoe, A., & Brydon, L. (2009). Emotional triggering of cardiac events. *Neuroscience and Biobehavioral Reviews, 33*, 63–70.

Steptoe, A., Hamer, M., & Chida, Y. (2007). The effects of acute psychological stress on circulating inflammatory factors in humans: A review and meta-analysis. *Brain, Behavior, and Immunity, 21*, 901–912.

Stewart, M. W., Knight, R. G., Palmer, D. G., & Highton, J. (1994). Differential relationships between stress and disease activity for immunologically distinct subgroups of people with rheumatoid arthritis. *Journal of Abnormal Psychology, 103*, 251–258.

Stone, A. A., Bovbjerg, D. H., Neale, J. M., Napoli, A., Valdimarsdottir, H., Cox, D., ... Gawltney, J. M. (1992). Development of common cold symptoms following experimental rhinovirus infection is related to prior stressful life events. *Behavioral Medicine, 18*, 115–120.

Stone, A. A., Reed, B. R., & Neale, J. M. (1987). Changes in daily event frequency precede episodes of physical symptoms. *Journal of Human Stress, 13*, 70–74.

Surwit, R. S., & Williams, P. G. (1996). Animal models provide insight into psychosomatic factors in diabetes. *Psychosomatic Medicine, 58*, 582–589.

Terrazas, E. E., Gutierrez, J. L. A., & Lopez, A. G. (1987). Psychosocial factors and episode number in depression. *Journal of Affective Disorders, 12*, 135–138.

Thompson, S. C. (2009). The role of personal control in adaptive functioning. In Shane J. Lopez and C. R. Snyder (Eds.), *Oxford handbook of positive psychology* (pp. 271–278). New York, NY: Oxford University Press.

Traub, O., & Berk, B. C. (1998). Laminar shear stress: Mechanisms by which endothelial cells transduce an atheroprotective force. *Arteriosclerosis, Thrombosis, and Vascular Biology, 18*, 677–685.

Treharne, G. J., Lyons, A. C., Booth, D. A., & Kitas, G. D. (2007). Psychological well-being across 1 year with rheumatoid arthritis: Coping resources as buffers of perceived stress. *British Journal of Health Psychology, 12*, 323–345.

Tuomilehto, J., Lindstrom, J., Eriksson, J. G., Valle, T. T., Hamalainen, H., Ilanne-Parikka, P., ... Uusitupa, M. (2001). Prevention of type 2 diabetes mellitus by changes in lifestyle among subjects with impaired glucose tolerance. *New England Journal of Medicine, 344*, 1343–1350.

Uchino, B. N., Cacioppo, J. T., & Kiecolt-Glaser, J. K. (1996). The relationship between social support and physiological processes: A review with emphasis on underlying mechanisms and implications for health. *Psychological Bulletin, 119*, 488–531.

Vlahov, D., Galea, S., Ahern, J., Resnick, H., Boscarino, J. A., Gold, J., ... Kilpatrick, D. (2004). Consumption of cigarettes, alcohol, and marijuana among New York City residents six months after the September 11 terrorist attacks. *American Journal of Drug and Alcohol Abuse, 30*(2), 385–407.

Wagner, K. D., Brief, D. J., Vielhauer, M. J., Sussman, S., Keane, T. M., & Malow, R. (2009). The potential for PTSD, substance use, and HIV risk behavior among adolescents exposed to Hurricane Katrina. *Substance Use & Misuse, 44*(12), 1749–1767.

Wenneberg, S. R., Schneider, R. H., Walton, K. G., MacLean, C. R. K., Levitsky, D. K., Mandarino, J. V., ... Wallace, R. K. (1997). Anger expression correlates with platelet aggregation. *Behavioral Medicine, 22*, 174–177.

Westergaard, R., & Gupta, A. (2009). The infectious diseases: The patient with HIV disease. In E. T. Bope, R. E. Rakel, & R. D. Kellerman (Eds.), *Conn's current therapy, 2010* (1st ed.). Philadelphia, PA: Elsevier.

Whetten, K., Reif, S., Whetten, R., & Murphy-McMillan, L. K. (2008). Trauma, mental health, distrust, and stigma among HIV-positive persons: Implications for effective care. *Psychosomatic Medicine, 70*, 531–538.

Winkley, K., Landau, S., Eisler, I., & Ismail, K. (2006). Psychological interventions to improve glycaemic control in patients with type 1 diabetes: Systematic review and meta-analysis of randomised controlled trials. *British Medical Journal, 333*, 65. doi:10.1136/bmj.38874.652569.55 (published 27 June 2006).

Yehuda, R. (2002). Current status of cortisol findings in post-traumatic stress disorder. *Psychiatric Clinics of North America, 25,* 341–368.

Zakowski, S. G. (1995). The effects of stressor predictability on lymphocyte proliferation in humans. *Psychology and Health, 10,* 409–425.

Zakowski, S. G., Cohen, L., Hall, M. H., Wollman, K., & Baum, A. (1994). Differential effects of active and passive laboratory stressors on immune function in healthy men. *International Journal of Behavioral Medicine, 1*(2), 163–184.

Zautra, A. J., Hoffman, J. M., Matt, K. S., Yocum, D., Potter, P. T., Castro, W. L., & Roth, S. (1998). An examination of individual differences in the relationship between interpersonal stress and disease activity among women with rheumatoid arthritis. *Arthritis Care and Research, 11,* 271–279.

Zautra, A. J., Hoffman, J., Potter, P., Matt, K. S., Yocum, D., & Castro, L. (1997). Examination of changes in interpersonal stress as a factor in disease exacerbations among women with rheumatoid arthritis. *Annals of Behavioral Medicine, 19,* 279–286.

Zautra, A. J., Okun, M. A., Robinson, S. E., Lee, D., Roth, S. H., & Emmanual, J. (1989). Life stress and lymphocyte alterations among patients with rheumatoid arthritis. *Health Psychology, 8,* 1–14.

Zautra, A. J., Parrish, B. P., Van Puymbroeck, C. M., Tennen, H., Davis, M. C., Reich, J. W., & Irwin, M. (2007). Depression history, stress, and pain in rheumatoid arthritis patients. *Journal of Behavioral Medicine, 30,* 187–197.

Zautra, A. J., & Smith, B. W. (2001). Depression and reactivity to stress in older women with rheumatoid arthritis and osteoarthritis. *Psychosomatic Medicine, 63,* 687–696.

Zimmerman, M. (1983). Methodological issues in the assessment of life events: A review of issues and research. *Clinical Psychology Review, 3,* 339–370.

4 Behavioral Self-Regulation, Health, and Illness

Michael F. Scheier
Carnegie Mellon University

Charles S. Carver
University of Miami

Geniel H. Armstrong
University of Montana

Models of behavioral self-regulation are designed to capture the nature of purposive action. These models are not domain specific; rather, they are thought to characterize the general set of processes that underlie all self-guided action. As such, the self-regulatory framework is broadly applicable. The purpose of this chapter is to discuss some of the ways in which self-regulatory models of behavior promote a better understanding of health and illness.

Behavioral self-regulatory models are perhaps most familiar to social and personality psychologists, who have been using them for many years. The self-regulatory framework is less familiar to health psychologists. As a result, it may be less apparent how models of behavioral self-regulation can help understand the phenomena that are at the intersection of health and behavior. We hope that this chapter will help illustrate the utility of this approach.

To provide background, we begin this chapter by describing a set of orienting assumptions and principles embedded in models of self-regulation, placing the heaviest emphasis on our own approach. We then turn to issues that self-regulatory models raise with respect to health and illness behaviors. One set of issues has to do with what is needed for self-regulation to occur, with a specific focus on the importance of feedback. A second set of issues has to do with the impact of illness on goal pursuit and with the implications of goal disruption for well-being. A third set of issues has to do with the importance of maintaining confidence when illness episodes and health threats are encountered. A final set of issues has to do with why it might at times be better to abandon some goals and identify alternative goals to pursue.

A MODEL OF BEHAVIORAL SELF-REGULATION

For the past several decades, our research has been guided by a particular model of behavioral self-regulation (Carver & Scheier, 1981, 1990, 1998). What does the term *behavioral self-regulation* mean? We use this term to refer to the processes by which behavior occurs. For us, human behavior is a continual process of moving toward and away from different kinds of mentally represented goals, either explicitly or implicitly. The idea that human behavior is organized around goals is common among personality theorists (e.g., Austin & Vancouver, 1996; Cantor & Kihlstrom, 1987; Carver & Scheier, 1998; Elliott & Dweck, 1988; Emmons, 1986; Klinger, 1975; Little, 1989; Markus & Nurius, 1986; Pervin, 1982). Although there are variations in how goals and goal-related activities are construed, there are also similarities. All share the view that goals energize and direct activities. All also convey the sense that goals give meaning to people's lives and that understanding a person's goals helps us to understand the person (Scheier & Carver, 2001). As a result, goal-related theories often presume that the self consists partly of the person's goals and values and the organization among them.

GOALS AND FEEDBACK PROCESSES

Goals are important to models of behavioral self-regulation, but the real value of self-regulatory models is in the specification of how goals and behavior are linked. What exactly are the mechanisms by which behavior occurs? For us, goals serve as reference values for feedback processes. A feedback loop is comprised of four elements in a particular organization (cf. Miller, Galanter, & Pribram, 1960; Powers, 1973). The elements are an input function, a reference value, a comparator, and an output function (see Figure 4.1).

An input function is a sensor that brings in information about the current state of affairs. It can be thought of as perception. The reference value provides information about what is intended or desired, thereby providing the target around which the system regulates. In the kinds of feedback loops we will be discussing, reference values are roughly equivalent to goals or intentions. The comparator is a mechanism making comparisons between input and reference value, yielding one of two outcomes: Either the values being compared are detectably different from one another or they are not. Following the comparison is an output function. For present purposes, output is behavior, though sometimes the behavior is internal.

There are two types of feedback loops, and the output differs depending on the type of loop. In a discrepancy-*reducing* feedback loop, the output is aimed at diminishing differences between input and reference value. In human behavior, discrepancy reduction (matching of input to reference value) is reflected in attempts to approach desired goals. For example, a high school student who wrestles might want to maintain a particular body weight and will take appropriate actions (e.g., exercising, counting calories, eating only certain kinds of food, spending time in the steam room) to ensure that the desired weight is maintained.

In a discrepancy-*enlarging* feedback loop, the output increases differences between input and reference value. Thus, the reference value is one to avoid rather than one to approach. It may be simplest to think of such values as "anti-goals." An example from the health domain would be the case of a person who wants not to be heavy. The goal here is not to regulate around a desired weight, or to be light because that is desirable, but to move as far from being heavy as possible. It is easy to see

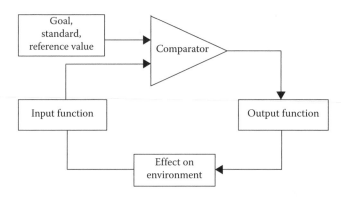

FIGURE 4.1 Schematic depiction of a feedback loop. In such a loop, a sensed value is compared to a reference value or standard, and adjustments are made in an output function (as necessary) to shift the sensed value either in the direction of the standard or away from it, depending on whether the feedback loop is discrepancy reducing or discrepancy enlarging, respectively.

how an avoidance goal can lead a person to engage in maladaptive behavior—from eating less than a healthy amount of food, for example, to purging after food is consumed, all performed to distance the person from his or her conception of what it means to be overweight.

Sullivan and Rothman (2008) addressed the effectiveness of discrepancy-enlarging and discrepancy-reducing goals in reducing fat and caloric intake. In addition to goal types, their study addressed the effects of implementation intentions (contextualized if-then statements about how the goal will be achieved). They found that avoidance goals were generally not as effective as approach goals in reducing caloric and fat intake. However, if participants using avoidance goals also used an implementation plan, they had significantly better results than those using avoidance goals with no implementation plan. This finding suggests that avoidance goals can also promote positive health outcomes, more so under some circumstances than others.

HIERARCHICAL ORGANIZATION AMONG GOALS

One difference between goals is whether they engender approach or avoidance. Another is in level of abstraction (for broader treatment of this issue, see Carver & Scheier, 1998). For example, a man might have the goal, at a very high level of abstraction, of being healthy. He may also have the goal, at a lower level of abstraction, of exercising. The first goal is to be a particular kind of *person,* whereas the second concerns completing particular kinds of *action.* Exercising suggests yet even more concrete goals, for example, walking to the exercise room and stepping on the treadmill machine. Such goals are closer to specifications of individual acts than is the goal of exercising, which is more of a summary statement about the overriding intent that provides the organizational focus for a set of action patterns. However, even these individual acts have lower-level goals. For example, stepping on the treadmill requires the activation of specific muscle groups in the legs in a particular order.

In this example, the concrete goals identified link directly to the more abstract goal guiding behavior. This linkage illustrates the idea that goals can be connected hierarchically. In 1973, William Powers argued that behavior occurs by means of a hierarchical organization of discrepancy-reducing feedback loops. Inasmuch as such loops imply goals, his argument assumed a hierarchical model of goals (see also Vallacher & Wegner's [1985, 1987] theory of action identification). Powers reasoned that the output of a high-level system consists of resetting reference values at the next lower level. To put it differently, higher-order systems "behave" by providing goals to the systems just below them. In this manner, there is a "cascade" of control from higher-order, more abstract loops to lower-order, more concrete loops, as the intent or theme of the higher-order goal is embodied in more and more specific components of action.

Figure 4.2 shows a simple portrayal of Powers's hierarchy. This diagram omits the loops of feedback processes, using lines to indicate only the links among goal values. The lines imply that moving toward a particular lower goal contributes to the attainment of a higher goal (or even several at once). Multiple lines to a given goal indicate that several lower-level action qualities can contribute to its attainment. As indicated previously, there are goals to "be" a particular way and goals to "do" certain things (and at lower levels, goals to create physical movement).

Hierarchical models are not new to the domain of health psychology. For several decades, Leventhal and his colleagues have been studying the commonsense models of illness that people hold (Leventhal & Carr, 2001; Leventhal, Leventhal, & Cameron, 2001; Leventhal, Meyer, & Nerenz, 1980; see also Leventhal's contribution to this handbook). Commonsense models of illness refer to the ways in which people think about and understand illness.

Important for present purposes is the idea that commonsense models of illness are represented in two ways (Leventhal & Carr, 2001). That is, illness attributes are represented both at an abstract, cognitive level and at a more concrete, perceptual level (Meyer, Leventhal, & Gutmann, 1985). Consider illness identity. Concretely, illnesses are identified by a collection of discrete symptoms and bodily cues. More abstractly, these constellations of symptoms give rise to an illness label.

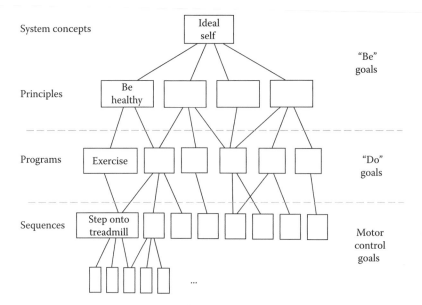

FIGURE 4.2 A hierarchy of goals (or of feedback loops). Terms on the left side of the figure provide the labels that Powers (1973) used to identify the top levels of control in the specific hierarchy that he proposed. Lines indicate the contribution of lower-level goals to specific higher-level goals. They can also be read in the opposite direction, indicating that a given higher-order goal specifies more concrete goals at the next lower level. The hierarchy depicted involves goals of "being" particular ways, which are attained by "doing" particular actions. (Adapted from Carver, C.S. and Scheier, M.F., *On the Self-Regulation of Behavior*, Cambridge University Press, New York, 1998.)

The collection of scratchy throat, cough, and stuffy nose is identified as a cold. Add a fever and achy joints and the combination of symptoms becomes the flu. It is possible to construe these two levels of illness representation as existing within a simple hierarchy of feedback control (Leventhal & Carr, 2001). At the higher level, people regulate their activities so as to avoid the perception that they have a particular illness. They do this by managing and regulating their lower-level symptoms on which the illness label depends.

Interestingly, de Ridder, Theunissen, and van Dulmen (2007) recently found that patients are more likely to express their concerns to their physicians when those physicians take illness representations into account. In addition, adoption of an illness representation framework also causes physicians to be more affectively expressive during their patient consults and leads patients to participate more in the discussion. Research groups have begun to use the commonsense model of illness representations to help inform interventions designed to prevent and help manage chronic illness threats (see e.g., McAndrew et al., 2008).

Affect

People's actions are often accompanied by affective states, varying in both intensity and quality. Where does the affect come from? In our view, feelings arise through the operation of a second feedback process (for details, see Carver & Scheier, 1990, 1998, 1999). The function of this second feedback system is to check on and regulate how well the behavior system is doing at carrying out its job. For discrepancy-reducing behavioral loops, the perceptual input for the affect-creating loop is a representation of the *rate of discrepancy reduction in the action system over time* (we consider discrepancy-enlarging loops shortly).

Rate of discrepancy reduction does not create affect by itself because a given rate of progress has different affective consequences under different circumstances. As in any feedback system, this input is compared against a reference value (cf. Frijda, 1986, 1988): the rate of behavioral discrepancy reduction that is desirable. We believe that the result of the comparison process at the heart of this loop (the error signal from the comparator) is manifest subjectively in two ways. The first way is as a vague and nonverbal sense of confidence or doubt. The second way is as an affective valence—a sense of positivity or negativity.

For example, take the case of a person recovering from a surgical procedure. The person may have a clear idea of how long the recovery should take. If recovery goes faster than expected, positive affect is experienced. If the recovery lags behind schedule, negative affect arises. Several studies have yielded evidence that tends to support this view of the source of affect (e.g., Brunstein, 1993; Guy & Lord, 1998; Hsee & Abelson, 1991; Lawrence, Carver, & Scheier, 2002; for a more thorough discussion, see Carver & Scheier, 1998).

According to the view just advanced, positive feelings arise when an action system is performing well at *what it is organized to do*. We see no reason to presume that approach and avoidance systems are any different in that respect. That is, approach systems promote discrepancy reduction. When approach systems are making good progress toward desired goals, positive affect is experienced. When satisfactory progress is not being made, affect turns more negative. Avoidance systems promote discrepancy enlargement. When avoidance systems are doing well at what they are organized to do—distancing the person from antigoals—positive affect should result (Carver, 2009). If the avoidance systems are doing poorly at what they are organized to do, the affective experience should be negatively valenced.

Confidence and Doubt

This model of affect suggests that one mechanism yields two subjective outputs: affect and a hazy sense of confidence versus doubt. We believe that the affect and expectancies that are generated "online" as behavior unfolds are intertwined. As affect becomes more negative, doubt tends to increase; as affect becomes more positive, hopefulness and confidence also rise. Thus, what we have said about affect also applies to the sense of confidence versus doubt that arises in parallel with affect as rate of progress falls above or below a desired level.

The online sense of confidence and doubt can be blended with, colored by, or over-ridden by other information obtained in a more deliberate way. That is, people often rely on multiple sources of information to generate expectancies for the future, for example, memories of prior outcomes in similar situations, thoughts about alternative approaches to the problem, or thoughts about other resources they might bring to bear (Lazarus, 1966). People also may use social comparison information (Wills, 1981) and attributional analyses of prior events (Abramson, Seligman, & Teasdale, 1978). This additional processing can affect the expectancies that ultimately arise, as well as the nature of the affect that is experienced.

Effort and Giving Up

Expectancies, however derived, have an important influence on behavior. If expectations are favorable enough, the person continues to strive for the goal. If doubts are strong enough, there is an urge to disengage from effort, and even from the goal itself. We have argued that these two classes of reactions form a "watershed" or bifurcation (Carver & Scheier, 1981, 1998, 1999). That is, whereas one set involves continued efforts at movement forward, the other consists of disengagement and quitting (see also Klinger, 1975; Kukla, 1972; Wortman & Brehm, 1975).

Just as goals vary in their specificity, from very concrete to very abstract, so too do expectancies vary in their level of specificity (Armor & Taylor, 1998; Carver & Scheier, 1998). For example, at a concrete level, a person may expect to gain movement in his foot after an auto accident. At a higher level, this person may expect to be able to walk again. At a higher level yet, the person may expect to perform again as a professional athlete, with all the actions, movements, motivations, and demands that being a professional athlete implies.

These various expectancies are associated with goals that are more or less abstract. Expectancies also differ in their level of generality. Generalized expectancies are expectancies that pertain to very diverse outcomes. They operate across the levels of the goal hierarchy described earlier. They pertain not just to one goal with a particular content, but to many goals with many different types of content, across wide domains of behavior. Thus, people who are generally optimistic are those who believe that they are likely to attain not just one higher-order goal, but all of the higher-order goals that their goal hierarchies contain, along with all of the subgoals to which those higher-order goals are linked.

ISSUES IN THE SELF-REGULATION OF HEALTH AND ILLNESS BEHAVIORS

The model of self-regulation presented in the preceding pages was meant to capture the structure and processes underlying "behavior in general." That is, it was meant to provide a generic model of action. The model was not designed specifically with health behaviors and illness episodes in mind. On the other hand, we have shown that the model can readily be applied to phenomena of interest in the health domain (see also Scheier and Carver, 2003a, 2003b).

By providing a theoretical structure, self-regulatory models help to identify variables and processes for study. At the same time, the models raise important issues about the nature of self-regulatory activities and what it is about those activities that may predispose a person to favorable or unfavorable health-related outcomes. In the sections that follow, we explore some of the issues raised by the self-regulatory model as it applies to health and illness behaviors.

ILLNESS-INDUCED GOAL DISRUPTION

The occurrence of illness and the onset of disease can disrupt a person's goal-directed actions, and this disruption can be harmful for emotional, psychological, physical, and functional well-being. Two different case-control studies, for example, have shown that patients report higher levels of goal disturbance than healthy controls (Echteld, van Elderen, & van der Kamp, 2001; Pinquart, Nixdorf-Hanchen, & Silbereisen, 2005). Not surprisingly, goal disruption increases as illness-related physical symptomatology increases. This finding emerges both from cross-sectional and retrospective studies (e.g., Abraido-Lanza & Revenson, 2006; Boerner & Cimarolli, 2005; Katz, Morris, & Yelin, 2006) and from prospective studies (e.g., Affleck, Tennen, Urrows et al., 1998; Affleck, Tennen, Zautra et al., 2001).

Other research has demonstrated that illness-induced goal disruption is directly related to differences in well-being. Much of this research assessed goal disruption indirectly by measuring the extent to which valued activities are obstructed or threatened. For example, Katz and Yelin (2001) assessed activity loss annually across a 4-year time span. The more valued activities that were lost across time, the more likely the participants were to develop depressive symptoms. Nor is this the only study linking goal disruption to lower well-being. A host of studies reinforce the idea that goal disruption is harmful to the person and can produce greater depression, reduced quality of life, and lower levels of psychological well-being (Abraido-Lanza & Revenson, 2006; Affleck et al., 1998; Boerner & Cimarolli, 2005; Boersma, Maes, & Joekes, 2005; Boersma, Maes, & van Elderen, 2005; Echteld et al., 2001; Echteld, van Elderen, & van der Kamp, 2003; Katz & Yelin, 2001; Kuijer & de Ridder, 2003). Goal disruption is also associated with lower levels of life satisfaction and happiness (Boerner & Cimarolli, 2005; Devins, Stam, & Kopmans, 1994), although not all research is consistent on this point (see, e.g., Echteld et al., 2001).

More recently, Joekes, Maes, and Warrens (2007) conducted a longitudinal study looking at the impact of myocardial infarction (MI) on quality of life and self-management. They found that disruption of midlevel goals—for example, engaging in regular physical activities—was related to reduced emotional, physical, social, and global quality of life. Interestingly, disruption of midlevel goals did not seem to promote disruption of such higher-order goals as the desire for better health. This latter finding suggests several possibilities. First, it is feasible that midlevel goals simply do not impact higher-order goals in this context. Given the hierarchical model described earlier, however, we do not think that this is the case. A second possibility is that higher-order goals may be associated with a longer time frame for completion than midlevel goals (Carver & Scheier, 1981). If so, perhaps disruption of higher-order goals would have been detected had follow-up occurred over a sufficiently long period of time. A final possibility is that the measures used in the study do not accurately assess all levels of goals within the goal hierarchy. This possibility is underscored by a recent review of self-regulation assessments and interventions by Maes and Karoly (2005), who noted that a lack of effective assessment tools for the study of self-regulation has clearly been a problem for current research.

The studies just reviewed suggest that goal disruption can have negative effects on well-being. Also relevant are complementary studies showing that unimpeded goal pursuit can result in enhanced well-being. Participants in one study (Hoppmann, Gerstorf, Smith, & Klumb, 2007), recruited from the Berlin Aging Study (Baltes & Mayer, 1999), were asked to provide data regarding their daily activities at five randomly chosen times during the day using paper diaries. This information was then used to investigate links between performance of everyday activities and "possible selves" in three domains (health, everyday cognitions, and social relations). The term *possible selves* refers to an individual's ideas of what he or she might become, as well as hopes, fears, and most important, goals regarding these representations (Markus & Nurius, 1986). For two of the domains (health and social relations), hoped-for selves were associated with an enhanced likelihood of performing activities in those domains during the time period monitored. More important, performance of goal-relevant activities was associated with higher concurrent positive affect and a higher probability of surviving a 10-year follow-up period.

A second study (Hoppmann & Klumb, 2006) examined how performing goal-relevant daily activities (pertaining to self-set goals for work and family) related to affective and neuroendocrine reactions to stress. Participants reported on their self-defined work and family goals at baseline. They later reported on the goal relevance of their daily activities, as well as their concurrent mood, at randomly selected times during the day. In addition, they provided samples of salivary cortisol. The performance of goal-relevant activities was linked to more positive mood and lower salivary cortisol. Further, the relationship between performing goal-related activities and cortisol was partially mediated by differences in mood.

Taken together, these various studies make two points. First, disruption of one's goal-directed activities, whether through the intrusion of illness or other life challenges, undermines positive affect, resulting in lower levels of well-being. Second, engaging in activities that are relevant to the pursuit of valued goals promotes better psychological and physical well-being (as indexed by longer survival time and decreased production of salivary cortisol, which is often taken as a biological marker of stress).

THE IMPORTANCE OF FEEDBACK

Regardless of whether a feedback loop is discrepancy enlarging or discrepancy reducing, feedback is essential to the system's functioning. Without feedback, comparisons cannot be made, and evaluation of the effects of one's self-regulatory actions would not be possible. Research from health psychology suggests that informational feedback matters so much that people will seek it out and rely on it *even when it does not tell them anything,* and even when relying on it creates *problems* for their health. Under such circumstances, the feedback loop governing behavior continues to operate, continues to sense, compare, and guide behavior, but it does so in a manner that is counterproductive.

Several studies of hypertension help illustrate this point (Baumann & Leventhal, 1985; Meyer et al., 1985). Unlike most illnesses, hypertension is an asymptomatic disorder. There are no reliable symptoms that a person can use to monitor whether blood pressure is raised or not. Yet most people who enter treatment for hypertension quickly come to believe that they *can* isolate a symptom of it. Indeed, the longer they are in treatment, the more likely they are to think they can tell when their blood pressure is up (Meyer et al., 1985). Patients then use the symptoms to make medical decisions. Furthermore, they use the symptom to tell them whether to take their medication, or even whether to remain in treatment.

These studies on hypertension underscore the critical nature of feedback. People desire it so much that they will adopt symptoms to enable them to track their illness, even though those symptoms bear no relation to reality, and more often than not they are told so by their physicians. If feedback is so important, then providing accurate feedback should enhance self-regulatory activities and do so in all contexts, including those that are health relevant. Such seems to be the case.

Consider, for example, the case of physicians providing care for their patients. The intention on the part of the physician is to adhere as closely as possible to the standard of care that has evolved for the particular illness being treated or for the particular preventative action being taken. Several studies have shown that when health care providers are given feedback relevant to the care that they are providing, their level of patient care improves so that it more closely approximates the recommended standard of treatment. For example, Sabris, Pomeranz, and Amateau (2003) found that when health care providers were given feedback about times they had missed an opportunity to vaccinate a patient, the rate of missed opportunities declined from 49% preintervention to 13% postintervention (see also McClellan, Millman, Presley, Couzins, & Flanders, 2003).

Providing feedback to health care providers has become a widely used and successful method of intervention to enhance patient care. A recent meta-analysis of health interventions identified 32 studies that used feedback to health care providers (Weingarten et al., 2002). Results of the meta-analysis confirmed that providing feedback significantly improved adherence to recommended treatment guidelines. Collectively, these studies demonstrate the important role that feedback plays in enhancing provider compliance with standard treatment protocols. More generally, the studies underlie the significance of feedback in behavioral self-regulation.

THE IMPORTANCE OF POSITIVE EXPECTATIONS: THE CASE OF DISPOSITIONAL OPTIMISM

Another important theme in our discussion of self-regulatory activities was that expectations play a pivotal role in responses to adversity. Recall that when people encounter adversity during the course of their goal-directed actions, negative affect and doubt begin to arise. The affect and doubt generated online as behavior unfolds can then be modified by more deliberate consideration of one's situation and the likelihood that a good outcome will be obtained. When people expect positive outcomes, even when things are difficult, they should experience less negative emotion and more positive emotion. When people are more pessimistic, they should experience a stronger bias toward negative feelings (Carver & Scheier, 1998; Scheier & Carver, 1992). These differences play themselves out in the various ways in which people respond to illness threats.

The expectancies we have been most interested in are the general sense of optimism and pessimism (Scheier & Carver, 1985; Scheier, Carver, & Bridges, 1994). Dispositional optimism refers to general positive outcome expectancies. In other words, optimists generally believe that things will go their way and that good things, rather than bad things, will happen to them. Pessimists believe the opposite. Other things being equal, these stable individual differences in optimism and pessimism should impact the nature of the outcome expectancies that people generate and thereby the affect experienced when people encounter challenging situations.

Optimism and Psychological Well-Being

There is now ample evidence that optimists experience less distress and more positive affect, and they maintain a higher quality of life in response to adversity than do pessimists. This is true of adversity in general (see, e.g., Scheier, Carver, & Bridges, 2001), and it is true for the challenges and difficulties brought on by illness and other threats to physical well-being (see, e.g., Scheier & Carver, 2003a, 2003b).

Consider, for example, the following set of illustrative studies, all involving medical contexts. The first study focuses on women being treated for breast cancer (Carver et al., 1993). Women were interviewed at diagnosis, the day before surgery, a few days after surgery, and 3, 6, and 12 months later. Optimism (at initial assessment) predicted less distress over time, controlling for effects of medical variables and earlier distress. Thus, optimism predicted resilience against distress during the full year. Allison, Guichard, and Gilain (2000) have reported conceptually similar findings in a study that examined adjustment among a sample of head and neck cancer patients. Patients were assessed before treatment and 3 months afterward. Optimists reported a higher quality of life before treatment and also after treatment, controlling for initial ratings.

Another medical context in which optimism has been studied is in vitro fertilization. The study focused on people who were unsuccessful (Litt, Tennen, Affleck, & Klock, 1992). Eight weeks beforehand, participants reported their optimism, distress, expectancies for fertilization success, and the impact of infertility on their lives. Two weeks after notification of a negative pregnancy test, distress was measured again. Of the initial variables, only optimism predicted follow-up distress (controlling for Time 1 distress). Optimistic participants were the least distressed after the failed fertilization attempt.

Optimism, Coping, and Psychological Well-Being

If optimists experience less distress than do pessimists when under adversity, is it just because they are cheerful people? This apparently is not the full story because the differences often remain when controls are included for prior distress. It now appears that optimists and pessimists differ in their affective responses because of the differences between them in how they cope with the adversity they encounter. The ways in which optimists and pessimists differ in coping resemble the differences in broad behavioral tendencies discussed earlier in the chapter. That is, people who are confident about eventual success continue trying, even when the going is hard. People who are doubtful try to escape the adversity by wishful thinking; they are drawn into temporary distractions that do not help solve the problem, and they sometimes even stop trying.

Differences in coping that correspond to this picture have been found in a number of studies. Early studies examined student reports of situational coping responses and general coping styles (e.g., Scheier, Carver, & Bridges, 2001), finding that optimists appear generally to cope by approaching a problem, whereas pessimists appear to be avoidant of problems.

Other projects have studied coping strategies in specific difficult contexts. Indeed, several of the studies described earlier, in the context of well-being, also looked at coping. For example, Litt et al. (1992) also examined coping in their study of failed in vitro fertilization. They found that pessimism related to escape as a coping response. Escape, in turn, led to more distress after the fertilization failure. Optimists were also more likely than pessimists to report feeling they had benefited from the experience—for example, by becoming closer to their spouse.

Similarly, Carver et al. (1993) also included measures of coping in their study of adjustment during the first year after diagnosis for breast cancer. Both before and after surgery, optimism related to coping that involved accepting the reality of the situation as one that must be dealt with, placing as positive a light on it as possible, and trying to relieve the situation with humor. Pessimism related to overt denial (reports of trying to push the reality of the situation away) and to giving-up tendencies at each time point. The coping responses related to optimism and pessimism were also related to distress. Further analyses revealed that the effect of optimism on distress was largely indirect through coping, particularly at postsurgery.

Another study of coping among women under treatment for breast cancer (Schou, Ekeberg, & Ruland, 2005) focused on two coping responses: fighting spirit (confronting the cancer and trying to beat it) and hopelessness or helplessness (feeling a sense of giving up). These responses mediated the relationship between optimism and quality of life a year after diagnosis. The greater fighting spirit of optimists (assessed before diagnosis) predicted better quality of life at the one-year follow-up. Hopelessness or helplessness (reported by pessimists) predicted poorer quality of life.

Solberg Nes and Segerstrom (2006) recently conducted a meta-analysis of optimism and coping. To do this, they tried to categorize studies into one of four categories that resulted from crossing two major distinctions in coping responses. Perhaps the best known distinction, made very early in the analysis of coping, is between problem-focused coping—aimed at doing something about the stressor itself to blunt its impact—and emotion-focused coping—aimed at soothing distress (Lazarus & Folkman, 1984). Another particularly important distinction is between engagement or approach coping, aimed at dealing with the stressor or emotions stemming from it, and disengagement or avoidance coping, aimed at escaping the stressor or emotions stemming from it (e.g., Roth & Cohen, 1986; Skinner, Edge, Altman, & Sherwood, 2003).

Solberg Nes and Segerstrom (2006) concluded that optimism was positively associated with broad measures of engagement coping, as well as with problem-focused coping. Optimism was also positively, and about equivalently, associated with the two subsets of engagement coping responses: those that are problem focused (e.g., planning, seeking instrumental support) and those that are emotion focused (e.g., cognitive restructuring, acceptance). Furthermore, optimists were responsive to the type of stressor being confronted. Optimism predicted more problem-focused coping with controllable stressors (e.g., academic demands) and more emotion-focused coping with uncontrollable stressors (e.g., trauma). Thus, optimism predicted active attempts to both change and accommodate to stressful circumstances in ways that reflect flexible engagement.

The pattern for disengagement coping was generally opposite that of engagement coping. Optimism related negatively to disengagement coping, as well as to both specific subsets of problem-focused disengagement (e.g., behavioral disengagement) and emotion-focused disengagement (e.g., denial, wishful thinking).

In sum, optimists appear to differ from pessimists in stable coping tendencies and in coping responses that emerge when confronting stressful situations. These coping differences explain, at least in part, the differences in psychological well-being that optimists and pessimists experience (for a more detailed account of optimism, psychological well-being, and coping, see Scheier & Carver, 2003a).

Optimism and Physical Well-Being

We now know that such psychological factors as depression, stress, and purpose in life are linked to physical health outcomes (e.g., Cohen, Alper, Doyle, Treanor, & Turner, 2006; Frasure-Smith, Lespérance, Juneau, Talajic, & Bourassa, 1999; Matthews, Owens, Edmundowicz, Lee, & Kuller, 2006). Given that optimism is a predictor of such outcomes, it should not be surprising that optimism has also been linked to physical well-being.

Research on optimism and health has been diverse in nature, ranging from the prevalence of disabilities and health problems among the elderly (Paúl, Ayis, & Ebrahim, 2007), to recovery from coronary artery bypass graft surgery (Scheier et al., 1989), to mortality (Allison, Guichard, Fung, & Gilain, 2003). Rasmussen, Scheier, and Greenhouse (2009) have recently conducted a meta-analysis of the literature on optimism and health, showing that optimism is a significant predictor of physical well-being. Perhaps not surprisingly, the effect of optimism on health is greater in studies that use more subjective outcomes (e.g., reports of symptoms or pain, or clinical ratings by physicians) than in studies that use more objective, "harder" disease endpoints (e.g., mortality, pregnancy outcomes, or immune responses). Follow-up subgroup analyses examined associations between optimism and health or biological markers of health in a variety of different domains, including studies focusing on mortality, cardiovascular outcomes, pregnancy outcomes, physiological markers, physical symptoms, and pain. In each case, a significant effect size for optimism emerged. In the following sections, we review some specific studies that link optimism to physical well-being. Our purpose is not to be exhaustive, but to provide a flavor of the kind of findings that have emerged.

Outcomes Related to Cardiovascular Disease

Several studies have examined the effects of optimism on outcomes related to heart disease and its treatment. One such study examined the effects of optimism on recovery in men undergoing coronary artery bypass surgery (Scheier et al., 1989). In this study, dispositional optimism, assessed presurgically, predicted the rate and extent of the normalization of the patient's lifestyle 6 months postsurgery. Specifically, optimism was associated with a faster rate of recovery and a more complete recovery.

Also relevant are findings from another study on bypass patients that examined the need for rehospitalization postsurgically (Scheier et al., 1999). This study found that optimists were significantly less likely to be rehospitalized 6 months postsurgery than were pessimists, controlling for medical variables and other factors such as depression and neuroticism.

Optimism has also been related to ambulatory blood pressure in two separate studies. Räikkönen, Matthews, Flory, Owens, and Gump (1999) collected ambulatory blood pressure measures in a sample of 30- to 45-year-old adults. They also had participants report on mood throughout the day. Pessimists had higher blood pressure levels and felt more negative and less positive throughout the period of monitoring. Optimists also exhibited high levels of blood pressure, equaling the blood pressure of the pessimists in the sample, but only when they reported negative mood. Conceptually similar results have recently been obtained in a sample of healthy black and white adolescents (Räikkönen & Matthews, 2008).

Matthews, Räikkönen, Sutton-Tyrell, and Kuller (2004) explored the effects of optimism on progression of carotid atherosclerosis. Healthy middle-aged women underwent two carotid ultrasound scans 3 years apart to measure intima media thickness (IMT). IMT is generally considered to be an early indicator of atherosclerosis. Over the period between scans, optimists were less likely than pessimists to have an increase in carotid IMT, even when statistically controlling for possible biological, lifestyle, and medication covariates. Indeed, those women who were optimistic exhibited virtually no increase in IMT over the time period.

Another study (Tindle et al., 2009) is also relevant here. The study is impressive because of the size of the sample involved, more than 95,000 women from the Women's Health Initiative. Tindle et al. tracked participants, all free of cancer and cardiovascular disease at study entry, across an 8-year period. The results were clear and striking: Optimists were less likely than pessimists to develop new cases of coronary heart disease (CHD) and were less likely to die from CHD-related causes across the 8 years of study (they also had lower total mortality due to all causes). The advantage due to optimism ranged from 9% for incident CHD to 30% for CHD-related mortality. These associations were independent of a host of demographic characteristics, risk factor variables, and comorbidities, as well as hostility, depressive symptoms, and a number of health-related behaviors.

Disease Progression

The relationship between physical well-being and optimism has been further explored in studies addressing the effect of positive expectations on HIV disease progression. A study by Ironson et al. (2005) examined the effect of optimism in the progression of HIV. They followed subjects for 2 years and assessed changes in CD4 levels. They found that participants who were higher in optimism lost significantly fewer CD4 cells over time than those lower in optimism.

Another study followed a group of females diagnosed with HIV for a period of 5 years (Ickovics et al., 2006). They found that women with more psychological resources, including positive affect, positive expectancies regarding their HIV status, and the ability to find meaning in their diagnosis, showed slower rates of CD4 loss. In addition, this group had a much lower mortality rate (16%) than did women with none of these psychological resources (50%). Such findings indicate that positive expectations not only can affect disease progression but also may decrease the likelihood of death in people infected with HIV, underscoring further the importance of positive expectations in health maintenance.

A final study (Roy et al., 2010) is also relevant here. Although it did not directly focus on disease progression, it did focus on a mechanism thought to underlie the progression of a host of different diseases, namely, inflammation. Roy et al. (2010) sampled more than 6,000 participants from the Multi-Ethnic Study of Atherosclerosis. The results showed that pessimism was significantly associated (in the manner expected) with a number of inflammatory markers, including IL-6, C-reactive protein, and fibrinogen, after adjusting for demographics, depressive symptoms, cynical hostility, and health behaviors. The effect of pessimism on fibrinogen remained significant in a fully adjusted model that added body mass index, hypertension, and diabetes to the equation.

Positive Health Behaviors

Positive expectations can also improve health through their effect on behavior change. For example, a study of individuals with diabetes found that higher optimism was related to better self-care behaviors and higher self-efficacy (Yi, Vitaliano, Smith, Yi, & Weigner, 2008). Similarly, Harper et al. (2007) studied a group of cancer patients and found that individuals with higher dispositional optimism were more likely to engage in positive changes in diet and exercise following their cancer diagnosis. In addition, those individuals higher in optimism were more likely to engage in a variety of such prosocial behaviors as spending more time with loved ones and being more active in charity work.

King, Rothman, and Jeffery (2002) have published several articles on their Challenge study, which assessed the effects of positive expectancies on smoking cessation and weight loss (although the expectancies examined were specific to the target behaviors being studied rather than generalized optimism). The smoking cessation portion of the study revealed that initial cessation was higher for groups whose intervention focused on positive expectations (Hertel et al., 2008). Similarly, Finch et al. (2005) found that weight loss was greater over time for those participants whose intervention focused on holding and maintaining positive expectations.

Health behaviors are important throughout one's lifetime, perhaps especially so as people age and health problems become more prominent. Giltay, Geleijnse, Zitman, Buijsse, and Kromhout (2007) addressed the effects of positive expectations on health behaviors in elderly men. The researchers followed a group of men for 15 years and found several health behavior trends. For example, over the 15-year period, dispositional optimism was related to more physical activity and higher intake of fruit, vegetables, and whole-grained bread in comparison to less optimistic individuals. Thus, optimists engaged in more health-promoting behavior.

An important health behavior for individuals diagnosed with a chronic illness is adherence to medical treatment. Milam, Richardson, Marks, Kemper, and McCutchan (2004) followed HIV-infected participants for an average of 18 months. They found that optimism was positively correlated with greater medication adherence, and negatively correlated with levels of cigarette and illicit drug use.

Other research has explored the effects of positive expectations on experiences surrounding heart transplant surgery (Leedham, Meyerowitz, Muirhead, & Frist, 1995). Patient confidence predicted better adherence to the postoperative medical regimen (reflecting engagement) and strongly predicted nurses' ratings of patients' physical health at 6 months after surgery. There was also a tendency for positive expectations to predict longer delays before development of infection, a near-universal side effect of heart transplantation. Such results indicate that optimism may be important in adherence to medical treatments.

WHEN TO PERSIST, WHEN TO GIVE UP

As we have described, positive expectations play an important role in the self-regulation of action. Confidence fosters persistence and perseverance, which often lead to positive outcomes. Positive expectations can help a joint replacement patient endure the hardships associated with physical rehabilitation, and they can help a person continue with chemotherapy in spite of the extreme fatigue and side effects that the treatment causes.

Perseverance is clearly important in a great many activities of life. However, this is only part of the story. An equally important role is played by the exact *opposite* set of processes. A critical role in life is also played by doubt, disengagement, and giving up (Carver & Scheier, 1998, 2003; Wrosch, Scheier, Carver, & Schulz, 2003).

Everyone has to quit sometimes. No one goes through a lifetime without confronting an insoluble problem, and eventually everyone has to die, whether from the progression of a disease, the gradual failure of critical organ systems associated with normal aging, or from something else. People also have accidents, compromising aspects of their physical functioning, which render certain future activities impossible. On a more mundane level, sometimes people have to order a different entrée at a restaurant because their preferred choice is sold out. Yes, disengagement is a necessity—a natural and indispensable aspect of effective self-regulation (Klinger, 1975).

When is disengagement and giving up an adaptive response? In our view, disengagement is adaptive *when it leads to the taking up of other goals,* whether these represent scaled-back versions of the original goal, substitutes for the lost one, or simply new goals in a different domain. By providing for the pursuit of alternative goals, giving up creates an opportunity to reengage and move ahead again (Carver & Scheier, 1998; Scheier & Carver, 2001). In such cases, giving up occurs in service to the broader function of keeping the person engaged with life. Thus, disengagement and reengagement function as complementary processes. Both seem important for adaptive self-regulation (e.g., Rasmussen, Wrosch, Scheier, & Carver, 2006; Wrosch, Scheier, Miller, Schulz, & Carver, 2003).

We have recently collected data that speak directly to the psychological benefits of disengagement and reengagement. In a first study, we examined relations between goal disengagement, goal reengagement, and subjective well-being in college students (Wrosch et al., 2003, Study 1). We found that the capacity to disengage from untenable goals was related to low levels of perceived stress and intrusive thoughts and high levels of self-mastery. In addition, the capacity to reengage and pursue alternative goals was significantly related to high levels of self-mastery and purpose in life and to low levels of perceived stress and intrusive thoughts.

In a second study, we examined whether goal disengagement and reengagement becomes even more important when people face extremely challenging life circumstances. To study this hypothesis, we assessed goal disengagement and goal reengagement, using the Goal Adjustment Scale (GAS; Wrosch et al., 2003), as well as symptoms of depression (using the CES-D) in 20 parents of children with cancer and 25 parents of healthy children (Wrosch et al., 2003, Study 2). As expected, high levels of both goal disengagement and goal reengagement predicted low levels of symptoms of depression, particularly among parents whose children had cancer.

Disengagement and reengagement have also been studied in the context of physical well-being. In one community sample (Wrosch, Miller, Scheier, & Brun de Pontet, 2007, Study 2), participants completed the measure of disengagement and reengagement and provided salivary cortisol at four prescribed times of the day across 4 separate days. When the cortisol was aggregated across the 4 days, a significant difference in the slopes of the diurnal rhythms was found. Participants who had a more difficult time disengaging from unattainable goals had a flatter slope, consistent with the idea that they were under greater stress. Reengagement tendencies did not impact cortisol production in this study.

Miller and Wrosch (2007) examined the associations between disengagement and reengagement and C-reactive protein in 15- to 19-year-old adolescents. This is an interesting sample in that the age of the participants reflects a time of life during which new roles are tried out and discarded as the attempt is made to form a more stable sense of self. As such, it is a time of life at which disengagement and reengagement processes might be quite important. Disengagement and reengagement were assessed at baseline. Blood was also drawn at baseline and again 6 and 12 months later to determine how levels of C-reactive protein changed over the course of one year. C-reactive protein provides a marker for systemic inflammation, and higher levels have been linked to a variety of medical conditions, including diabetes and heart disease (Willerson & Ridker, 2004). Participants with a lower capacity for disengagement showed significant increases in C-reactive protein over time, whereas C-reactive protein levels for participants with a higher capacity for disengagement remained constant over time. Also noteworthy was the fact that reengagement tendencies had no impact on production of C-reactive protein in this study.

Taken together, these various studies on disengagement and reengagement make a strong case that such processes are related to well-being. Interestingly, it also seems clear that a somewhat different pattern emerges depending on whether the outcomes employed are psychological in nature or more biological or disease-related in nature. That is, with respect to psychological well-being, both disengagement and reengagement tendencies seem to contribute to positive outcomes. Both predict psychological well-being. However, a very different picture emerges from the studies done on biomarkers of stress and health. In these studies, it is disengagement, and only disengagement, that is linked to positive results. The reasons for these differences remain unclear. The pattern of results does appear reliable enough, however, that the issue should certainly be pursued in future research.

Two additional studies come at disengagement and reengagement processes from a somewhat different angle. We assume that disengagement and reengagement processes are important and are linked to well-being in part because they help to keep a person engaged in life pursuits; that is, as people abandon unattainable goals and adopt other goals, they are kept engaged in life and are provided with a purpose for living. If so, results conceptually similar to those obtained for disengagement and reengagement should emerge if purpose in life was assessed instead.

Matthews et al. (2006) have recently conducted such a study. They assessed purpose in life using the Life Engagement Test (LET; Scheier et al., 2006) in community-dwelling women who were participating in a larger project on cardiovascular disease. The women had also undergone coronary and aortic electron-beam-tomography scans from which calcification scores were derived. Calcification of the coronary, aortic, and carotid arteries is often taken as a marker of subclinical atherosclerosis. Consistent conceptually with the results described earlier, the Matthews et al. study found that purpose in life was protective. Women with a higher sense of purpose had about half the risk for aortic calcification as those whose purpose in life was lower.

A more recent study explored the association between incidence of Mild Cognitive Impairment (MCI) and incidence of Alzheimer Disease (AD) in a community-dwelling sample of close to 1,000 older persons (Boyle, Buchman, Barnes, & Bennett, 2010). They found that purpose in life, assessed at study entry, predict lower rates of new cases of MCI and AD. The effect for purpose in life remained significant even after adjusting for demographic factors, depressive symptoms, neuroticism, network size, and comorbidities.

CONCLUSION

We began this chapter by describing some of the principles and processes of self-regulatory models and then used those principles and processes to identify a set of issues that might be important to consider when thinking about disease outcomes and health and illness behaviors. In so doing, we demonstrated the importance of feedback in the self-regulatory process. We also described how illness can disrupt a person's ongoing goal-directed efforts and how this disruption can have a negative effect on well-being. We also made a case that positive expectations play a central role in determining one's psychological and physical response to disease and that disengagement processes may at times be as likely as persistence to lead to better well-being. We have long held that self-regulatory models provide a useful heuristic enabling one to better understand the nature of goal-directed activities regardless of the particular domain of behavior in which those goal-directed activities are taking place. We hope the comments offered here will help convince others of the value of self-regulatory principles in understanding the kinds of behaviors involved in maintaining health and dealing with illness.

ACKNOWLEDGMENTS

Preparation of this chapter was supported by funds awarded to the Pittsburgh Mind-Body Center at the University of Pittsburgh and Carnegie Mellon University (NIH HL076852 and HL076858) and by funds awarded to the University of Miami (CA64710 and BCS0544617).

REFERENCES

Abraido-Lanza, A. F., & Revenson, T. A. (2006). Illness intrusion and psychological adjustment to rheumatic diseases: A social identity framework. *Arthritis and Rheumatism, 55*(2), 224–232.

Abramson, L. Y., Seligman, M. E. P., & Teasdale, J. D. (1978). Learned helplessness in humans: Critique and reformulation. *Journal of Abnormal Psychology, 87*, 49–74.

Affleck, G., Tennen, H., Urrows, S., Higgins, P., Abeles, M., Hall, C., … Newton, C. (1998). Fibromyalgia and women's pursuit of personal goals: A daily process analysis. *Health Psychology, 17*(1), 40–47.

Affleck, G., Tennen, H., Zautra, A., Urrows, S., Abeles, M., & Karoly, P. (2001). Women's pursuit of personal goals in daily life with fibromyalgia: A value-expectancy analysis. *Journal of Consulting and Clinical Psychology, 69*(4), 587–596.

Allison, P. J., Guichard, C., Fung, K., Gilain, L. (2003). Dispositional optimism predicts survival status 1 year after diagnosis in head and neck cancer patients. *Journal of Clinical Oncology, 21*(3), 543–548.

Allison, P. J., Guichard, C., & Gilain, L. (2000). A prospective investigation of dispositional optimism as a predictor of health-related quality of life in head and neck cancer patients. *Quality of Life Research, 9*, 951–960.

Armor, D. A., & Taylor, S. E. (1998). Situated optimism: Specific outcome expectancies and self-regulation. In M. Zanna (Ed.), *Advances in experimental social psychology* (Vol. 29, pp. 309–379). San Diego, CA: Academic Press.

Austin, J. T., & Vancouver, J. B. (1996). Goal constructs in psychology: Structure, process, and content. *Psychological Bulletin, 120*, 338–375.

Baltes, P. B., & Mayer, K. U. (1999). *The Berlin Aging Study: Aging from 70 to 100*. New York, NY: Cambridge University Press.

Baumann, L. J., & Leventhal, H. (1985). "I can tell when my blood pressure is up, can't I?" *Health Psychologist, 4*, 203–218.

Boerner, K., & Cimarolli, V. R. (2005). Optimizing rehabilitation for adults with visual impairment: Attention to life goals and their links to well-being. *Clinical Rehabilitation, 19*(7), 790–798.

Boersma, S., Maes, S., & Joekes, K. (2005). Goal disturbance in relation to anxiety, depression, and health-related quality of life after myocardial infarction. *Quality of Life Research, 14*(10), 2265–2275.

Boersma, S., Maes, S., & van Elderen, T. (2005). Goal disturbance predicts health-related quality of life and depression 4 months after myocardial infarction. *British Journal of Health Psychology, 10*, 615–630.

Boyle, P. A., Buchman, A. S., Barnes, L. L., & Bennett, D. A. (2010). Effect of a purpose in life on risk of incident Alzheimer disease and mild cognitive impairment in community-dwelling older persons. *Archives of General Psychiatry, 67*, 304–310.

Brunstein, J. C. (1993). Personal goals and subjective well-being: A longitudinal study. *Journal of Personality and Social Psychology, 65*, 1061–1070.

Cantor, N., & Kihlstrom, J. F. (1987). *Personality and social intelligence*. Englewood Cliffs, NJ: Prentice-Hall.

Carver, C. S. (2009). Threat sensitivity, incentive sensitivity, and the experience of relief. *Journal of Personality, 77*, 125–138.

Carver, C. S., Pozo, C., Harris, S. D., Noriega, V., Scheier M. F., Robinson, D. S., … Clark, K. C. (1993). How coping mediates the effect of optimism on distress: A study of women in early stage breast cancer. *Journal of Personality and Social Psychology, 65*(2), 375–390.

Carver, C. S., & Scheier, M. F. (1981*). Attention and self-regulation: A control-theory approach to human behavior*. New York, NY: Springer Verlag.

Carver, C. S., & Scheier, M. F. (1990). Origins and functions of positive and negative affect: A control-process view. *Psychological Review, 97*, 19–35.

Carver, C. S., & Scheier, M. F. (1998). *On the self-regulation of behavior*. New York, NY: Cambridge University Press.

Carver, C. S., & Scheier, M. F. (1999). Themes and issues in the self-regulation of behavior. In R. S. Wyer, Jr., (Ed.), *Advances in social cognition* (Vol. 12, pp. 1–105). Mahwah, NJ: Erlbaum.

Carver, C. S., & Scheier, M. F. (2003). Three human strengths. In L. G. Aspinwall & U. M. Staudinger (Eds.), *A psychology of human strengths: Fundamental questions and future directions for a positive psychology* (pp. 87–102). Washington, DC: American Psychological Association.

Cohen, S., Alper, C. M., Doyle, W. J., Treanor, J. J., & Turner, R. B. (2006). Positive emotional style predicts resistance to illness after experimental exposure to rhinovirus or influenza A virus. *Psychosomatic Medicine, 68,* 809–815.

de Ridder, D. T. D., Theunissen, N. C. M., & van Dulmen, S. M. (2007). Does training general practitioners to elicit patients' illness representations and action plans influence their communication as a whole? *Patient Education and Counseling, 66*(3), 327–336.

Devins, G. M., Stam, H. J., & Kopmans, J. P. (1994). Psychosocial impact of laryngectomy mediated by perceived stigma and illness intrusiveness. *Canadian Journal of Psychiatry–Rev Canadienne de Psychiatrie, 39*(10), 608–616.

Echteld, M. A., van Elderen, T. M. T., & van der Kamp, L. J. T. (2001). How goal disturbance, coping and chest pain relate to quality of life: A study among patients waiting for PTCA. *Quality of Life Research, 10*(6), 487–501.

Echteld, M. A., van Elderen, T., & van der Kamp, L. J. (2003). Modeling predictors of quality of life after coronary angioplasty. *Annals of Behavioral Medicine, 26*(1), 49–60.

Elliott, E. S., & Dweck, C. S. (1988). Goals: An approach to motivation and achievement. *Journal of Personality and Social Psychology, 54,* 5–12.

Emmons, R. A. (1986). Personal strivings: An approach to personality and subjective well being. *Journal of Personality and Social Psychology, 51,* 1058–1068.

Finch, E. A., Linde, J. A., Rona, L. L., Jeffery, R. W., Rothman A. J., King, C. M., & Levy, R. A. (2005). The effects of outcome expectancies and satisfaction on weight loss and maintenance: Correlational and experimental analysis—A randomized trial. *Health Psychology, 24*(6), 608–616.

Frasure-Smith, N., Lespérance, F., Juneau, M., Talajic, M., & Bourassa, M. G. (1999). Gender, depression, and one-year prognosis after myocardial infarction. *Psychosomatic Medicine, 61*(1), 26–37.

Frijda, N. H. (1986). *The emotions*. Cambridge, England: Cambridge University Press.

Frijda, N. H. (1988). The laws of emotion. *American Psychologist, 43,* 349–358.

Giltay, E. J., Geleijnse, J. M., Zitman, F. G., Buijsse, B., & Kromhout, D. (2007). Lifestyle and dietary correlates of dispositional optimism in men: The Zutphen Elderly Study. *Journal of Psychosomatic Research, 63,* 483–490.

Guy, J. L., & Lord, R. G. (May, 1998). *The effects of perceived velocity on job satisfaction: An expansion of current theory*. Paper presented at the 10th Annual Conference of the American Psychological Society, Washington, DC.

Harper, F. W. K., Schmidt, J. E., Beacham, A. O., Salsman, J. M., Averill, A. J., Graves, K. D., & Andrykowski, M. A. (2007). The role of social cognitive processing theory and optimism in positive psychosocial and physical behavior change after cancer diagnosis and treatment. *Psycho-Oncology, 16,* 79–91.

Hertel, A. W., Finch, E. A., Kelly, K. M., King, C., Lando, H., Linde, J. A., … Rothman, A. J. (2008). The impact of expectations and satisfaction on the initiation and maintenance of smoking cessation: An experimental test. *Health Psychology, 27*(Suppl. 3), S197–S206.

Hoppmann, C. A., Gerstorf, D., Smith, J., & Klumb, P. L. (2007). Linking possible selves and behavior: Do domain-specific hopes and fears translate into daily activities in very old age? *Journal of Gerontology, 62B*(2), 104–111.

Hoppmann, C. A., & Klumb, P. L. (2006). Daily goal pursuits predict cortisol secretion and mode states in employed parents with preschool children. *Psychosomatic Medicine 68,* 887–894.

Hsee, C. K., & Abelson, R. P. (1991). Velocity relation: Satisfaction as a function of the first derivative of outcome over time. *Journal of Personality and Social Psychology, 60,* 341–347.

Ickovics, J. R., Milan, S., Boland, R., Schoenbaum, E., Schuman, P., & Vlahov, D. (2006). Psychological resources protect health: 5-year survival and immune function among HIV-infected women from four US cities. *AIDS, 20,* 1851–1860.

Ironson, G., Balbin, E., Stuetzle, R., Fletcher, M. A., O'Cleirigh, C., Laurenceau, J. P., … Solomon, G. (2005). Dispositional optimism and the mechanisms by which it predicts slower disease progression in HIV: Proactive behavior, avoidant coping, and depression. *International Journal of Behavioral Medicine, 12*(2), 86–97.

Joekes, K., Maes, S., & Warrens, M. (2007). Predicting quality of life and self-management from dyadic support and overprotection after myocardial infarction. *British Journal of Health Psychology*, *12*, 473–489.

Katz, P. P., Morris, A., & Yelin, E. H. (2006). Prevalence and predictors of disability in valued life activities among individuals with rheumatoid arthritis. *Annals of the Rheumatic Diseases*, *65*(6), 763–769.

Katz, P. P., & Yelin, E. H. (2001). Activity loss and the onset of depressive symptoms—Do some activities matter more than others? *Arthritis and Rheumatism*, *44*(5), 1194–1202.

King, C. M., Rothman, A. J., & Jeffery, R. W. (2002). The Challenge study: Theory-based interventions for smoking and weight loss. *Health Education Research*, *17*(5), 522–530.

Klinger, E. (1975). Consequences of commitment to and disengagement from incentives. *Psychological Review*, *82*, 1–25.

Kuijer, R. G., & de Ridder, D. T. D. (2003). Discrepancy in illness-related goals and quality of life in chronically ill patients: The role of self-efficacy. *Psychology & Health*, *18*(3), 313–330.

Kukla, A. (1972). Foundations of an attributional theory of performance. *Psychological Review*, *79*, 454–470.

Lawrence, J. W., Carver, C. S., & Scheier, M. F. (2002). Velocity toward goal attainment in immediate experience as a determinant of affect. *Journal of Applied Social Psychology*, *32*, 788–802.

Lazarus, R. S. (1966). *Psychological stress and the coping process*. New York, NY: McGraw-Hill.

Lazarus, R. S., & Folkman, S. (1984). *Stress: appraisal and coping*. New York, NY: Springer.

Leedham, B., Meyerowitz, B. E., Muirhead, J., & Frist, W. H. (1995). Positive expectations predict health after heart transplantation. *Health Psychology*, *14*, 74–79.

Leventhal, H., & Carr, S. (2001). Speculations on the relationship of behavioral theory to psychosocial research on cancer. In A. Baum & B. L. Andersen (Eds.), *Psychosocial interventions for cancer* (pp. 375–400). Washington, DC: American Psychological Association.

Leventhal, H., Leventhal, E. A., & Cameron, L. (2001). Representations, procedures and affect in illness self-regulation: A perceptual-cognitive model. In A. Baum, T. Revenson, & J. Weinman (Eds.), *Handbook of health psychology* (pp. 19–47). Hillsdale, NJ: Erlbaum.

Leventhal, H., Meyer, D., & Nerenz, D. (1980). The common sense representation of illness danger. In S. Rachman (Ed.), *Medical psychology* (Vol. 2, pp. 7–30). New York, NY: Pergamon Press.

Litt, M. D., Tennen, H., Affleck, G., & Klock, S. (1992). Coping and cognitive factors in adaptation to in vitro fertilization failure. *Journal of Behavioral Medicine*, *15*, 171–187.

Little, B. R. (1989). Personal projects analysis: Trivial pursuits, magnificent obsessions, and the search for coherence. In D. M. Buss & N. Cantor (Eds.), *Personality psychology: Recent trends and emerging directions* (pp. 15–31). New York, NY: Springer-Verlag.

Maes, S., & Karoly, P. (2005). Self-regulation assessment and intervention in physical health and illness: A review. *Applied Psychology: An International Review*, *54*(2), 267–299.

Markus, H., & Nurius, P. (1986). Possible selves. *American Psychologist*, *41*, 954–969.

Matthews, K. A., Owens, J. F., Edmundowicz, D., Lee, L., & Kuller, L. H. (2006). Positive and negative attributes and risk for coronary and aortic calcification in healthy women. *Psychosomatic Medicine*, *68*(3), 355–361.

Matthews, K. A., Räikkönen, K., Sutton-Tyrell, K., & Kuller, L. H. (2004). Optimistic attitudes protect against progression of carotid atherosclerosis in healthy middle-aged women. *Psychosomatic Medicine*, *66*(5), 640–644.

McAndrew, L. M., Musumeci-Szabó, T. J., Mora, P. A., Vileikyte, L., Edith, B., Halm, E. A., … Leventhal, H. (2008). Using the common sense model to design interventions for the prevention and management of chronic illness threats: From description to process. *British Journal of Health Psychology*, *13*(2), 195–204.

McClellan, W. M., Millman, L., Presley, R., Couzins, J., & Flanders, W. D. (2003). Improved diabetes care by primary care physicians: Results of a group-randomized evaluation of the Medicare Health Care Quality Improvement Program (HCQIP). *Journal of Clinical Epidemiology*, *56*, 1210–1217.

Meyer, D., Leventhal, H., & Gutmann, M. (1985). Common-sense models of illness: The example of hypertension. *Health Psychology*, *4*, 115–135.

Milam, J. E., Richardson, J. L., Marks, G., Kemper, C. A., & McCutchan, A. J. (2004). The roles of dispositional optimism and pessimism in HIV disease progression. *Psychology and Health*, *19*(2), 167–181.

Miller, G. A., Galanter, E., & Pribram, K. H. (1960). *Plans and the structure of behavior*. New York, NY: Holt, Rinehart, & Winston.

Miller, G. E., & Wrosch, C. (2007). You've gotta know when to fold 'em: Goal disengagement and systemic inflammation in adolescence. *Psychological Science*, *18*(9), 773–777.

Paúl, C., Ayis, S., & Ebrahim, S. (2007). Disability and psychosocial outcomes in old age. *Journal of Aging and Health*, *19*(5), 723–741.

Pervin, L. A. (1982). The stasis and flow of behavior: Toward a theory of goals. In M. M. Page & R. Dienstbier (Eds.), *Nebraska symposium on motivation* (Vol. 30, pp. 1–53). Lincoln, NE: University of Nebraska Press.

Pinquart, M., Nixdorf-Hanchen, J. C., & Silbereisen, R. K. (2005). Associations of age and cancer with individual commitment. *Applied Developmental Science, 9*(2), 54–66.

Powers, W. T. (1973). *Behavior: The control of perception.* Chicago, IL: Aldine.

Räikkönen, K., & Matthews, K. A. (2008). Do dispositional pessimism and optimism predict ambulatory blood pressure during schooldays and nights in adolescents? *Journal of Personality, 76*(3), 605–629.

Räikkönen, K., Matthews, K. A., Flory, J. D., Owens, J. F., & Gump, B. B. (1999). Effects of optimism, pessimism, and trait anxiety on ambulatory blood pressure and mood during everyday life. *Journal of Personality and Social Psychology, 76*(1), 104–113.

Rasmussen, H. N., Scheier, M. F., & Greenhouse, J. B. (2009). Optimism and physical health: A meta-analytic review. *Annals of Behavioral Medicine, 37,* 239–256..

Rasmussen, H. N., Wrosch, C., Scheier, M. F., & Carver, C. S. (2006). Self-regulation processes and health: The importance of optimism and goal adjustment. *Journal of Personality, 74,* 1721–1747.

Roth, S., & Cohen, L. J. (1986). Approach, avoidance, and coping with stress. *American Psychologist, 41,* 813–819.

Roy, B., Diez-Roux, A. V., Seeman, T., Ranjit, N., Shea, S., & Cushman, M. (2010). Association of optimism and pessimism with inflammation and hemostasis in the Multi-Ethnic Study of Atherosclerosis (MESA). *Psychosomatic Medicine, 72,* 134–140.

Sabris, S. S., Pomeranz, A. J., & Amateau, M. M. (2003). The effect of education, feedback, and provider prompts on the rate of missed vaccine opportunities in a community health center. *Clinical Pediatrics, 42,* 147–11.

Scheier, M. F., & Carver, C. S. (1985). Optimism, coping and health: Assessment and implications of generalized outcome expectancies. *Health Psychology, 4,* 219–247.

Scheier, M. F., & Carver, C. S. (1992). Effects of optimism on psychological and physical well-being: Theoretical overview and empirical update. *Cognitive Therapy and Research, 16,* 201–228.

Scheier, M. F., & Carver, C. S. (2001). Adapting to cancer: The importance of hope and purpose. In A. Baum & B. L. Andersen (Eds.), *Psychosocial interventions for cancer* (pp. 15–36). Washington, DC: American Psychological Association.

Scheier, M. F. & Carver, C. S. (2003a). Self-regulatory processes and responses to health threats: Effects of optimism on well-being. In J. Suls & K. Wallston (Eds.), *Social psychological foundations of health* (pp. 395–428). Oxford, England: Blackwell.

Scheier, M. F., & Carver, C. S. (2003b). Goals and confidence as self-regulatory elements underlying health and illness behavior. In L. D. Cameron & H. Leventhal (Eds.), *The self-regulation of health and illness behaviour* (pp. 17–41). London, England: Routledge.

Scheier, M. F., Carver, C. S., & Bridges, M. W. (1994). Distinguishing optimism from neuroticism (and trait anxiety, self-mastery, and self-esteem): A re-evaluation of the Life Orientation Test. *Journal of Personality and Social Psychology, 67,* 1063–1078.

Scheier, M. F., Carver, C. S. & Bridges, M. W. (2001). Optimism, pessimism, and psychological well-being. In E. C. Chang (Ed.), *Optimism and pessimism: Implications for theory, research, and practice* (pp. 189–216). Washington, DC: American Psychological Association.

Scheier, M. F., Matthews, K. A., Owens, J. F., Magovern, G. J., Lefebvre, R. C., Abbott, R. A., & Carver, C. S. (1989). Dispositional optimism and recovery from coronary artery bypass surgery: The beneficial effects on physical and psychological well-being. *Journal of Personality and Social Psychology, 57,* 1024–1040.

Scheier, M. F., Matthews, K. A., Owens, J. F., Schulz, R., Bridges, M. W., Magovern, G. J., Sr., & Carver, C. S. (1999). Optimism and rehospitalization following coronary artery bypass graft surgery. *Archives of Internal Medicine, 159,* 829–835.

Scheier, M. F., Wrosch, C., Baum, A., Cohen, S., Martire, L. M., Matthews, K. A., … Zdaniuk, B. (2006). The Life Engagement Test: Assessing purpose in life. *Journal of Behavioral Medicine, 29*(3), 291–298.

Schou, I., Ekeberg, O., & Ruland, C. M. (2005). The mediating role of appraisal and coping in the relationship between optimism-pessimism and quality of life. *Psycho-Oncology, 14,* 718–727.

Skinner, E. A., Edge, K., Altman, J., & Sherwood, H. (2003). Searching for the structure of coping: A review and critique of category systems for classifying ways of coping. *Psychological Bulletin, 129,* 216–269.

Solberg Nes, L., & Segerstrom, S. C. (2006). Dispositional optimism and coping: A meta-analytic review. *Personality and Social Psychology Review, 10,* 235–251.

Sullivan, H. W., & Rothman, A. J. (2008). When planning is needed: Implementation intentions and attainment of approach versus avoidance health goals. *Health Psychology*, *27*(4), 438–444.

Tindle, H. A., Chang, Y., Kuller, L. H., Manson, J. E., Robinson, J. G., Rosal, M. C., … Matthews, K. A. (2009). Optimism, cynical hostility, and incident coronary heart disease and mortality in the Women's Health Initiative. *Circulation*. 2009, *120*, 656–662.

Vallacher, R. R., & Wegner, D. M. (1985). *A theory of action identification*. Hillsdale, NJ: Erlbaum.

Vallacher, R. R., & Wegner, D. M. (1987). What do people think they're doing? Action identification and human behavior. *Psychological Review*, *94*, 3–15.

Weingarten, S. R., Henning, J. M., Badamgarav, E., Knight, K., Hasselblad, V., Gano, A., Jr., & Ofman, J. J. (2002). Interventions used in disease management programmes for patients with chronic illness—which ones work? Meta-analysis of published reports. *British Medical Journal*, *325*(7370), 925–939.

Willerson, J. T., & Ridker, P. M. (2004). Inflammation as a cardiovascular risk factor. *Circulation*, *109*, 2–10.

Wills, T. A. (1981). Downward comparison principles in social psychology. *Psychological Bulletin*, *90*, 245–271.

Wortman, C. B., & Brehm, J. W. (1975). Responses to uncontrollable outcomes: An integration of reactance theory and the learned helplessness model. In L. Berkowitz (Ed.), *Advances in experimental social psychology* (Vol. 8, pp. 277–336). New York, NY: Academic Press.

Wrosch, C., Miller, G. E., Scheier, M. F., & Brun de Pontet, S. (2007). Giving up on unattainable goals: Benefits for health? *Personality and Social Psychology Bulletin*, *33*, 251–265.

Wrosch, C., Scheier, M. F., Carver, C. S., & Schulz, R. (2003). The importance of goal disengagement in adaptive self-regulation: When giving up is beneficial. *Self and Identity*, *2*, 1–20.

Wrosch, C., Scheier, M. F., Miller, G. E., Schulz, R., & Carver, C. S. (2003). Adaptive self-regulation of unattainable goals: Goal disengagement, goal re-engagement, and subjective well-being. *Personality and Social Psychology Bulletin*, *29*, 1494–1508.

Yi, J. P., Vitaliano, P. P., Smith, R. E., Yi, J. C., & Weigner, K. (2008). The role of resilience on psychological adjustment and physical health in patients with diabetes. *British Journal of Health Psychology*, *13*, 311–325.

5 Processes of Health Behavior Change

Karen Glanz
University of Pennsylvania Schools of Medicine and Nursing

Michelle C. Kegler
Emory University

When successful interventions to promote positive health behavior change are based on a solid understanding of the individuals, their social milieu and environmental contexts, and the influences on their health behaviors, the chances are good that programs will be effective (Glanz & Rimer, 2008). This understanding is often most efficiently acquired by applying health behavior theories and planning models. This chapter introduces contemporary theoretical bases for health behavior change programs and their applications in practice. Other chapters in this book provide more extensive examinations of health behavior change related to specific health issues. This chapter (a) introduces key concepts related to processes of health behavior change; (b) describes applications of several current theoretical models to health behavior change interventions at the individual, interpersonal, organizational, and community levels; and (c) highlights important overarching issues and constructs that cut across theories.

DETERMINANTS OF HEALTH BEHAVIOR AND HEALTH BEHAVIOR CHANGE

MULTIPLE DETERMINANTS OF HEALTH BEHAVIOR

Many social, cultural, and economic factors contribute to the development, maintenance, and change of health behavior patterns. No single factor or set of factors has been found to adequately account for why people act as they do, either for a specific type of behavior (e.g., smoking) or across multiple behaviors (e.g., obtaining preventive medical exams and exercising regularly). Physiologic and psychological factors, acquired habits, and knowledge about self-care are important individual determinants of healthy behaviors. Families, social relationships, socioeconomic status, culture, and geography are also important influences on health-related behavioral actions. A broad understanding of some of the key factors and models for understanding health behavior can provide a foundation for well-informed behavior change interventions, help identify the most influential factors for a particular patient or population, and focus change processes on the most salient issues for individuals.

MULTIPLE LEVELS OF INFLUENCE

Classic definitions of health behavior emphasize the actions of individuals (Glanz, Rimer, & Viswanath, 2008). Traditionally, health psychologists have focused on such intraindividual factors as a person's beliefs, knowledge, and skills. This focus contrasts with a public health perspective, which is concerned with individuals as part of a larger community. Increasingly, as seen in this handbook, health psychologists are addressing public health concerns and highly prevalent diseases, as well as health risks, including HIV/AIDS, diabetes, and cardiovascular disease. The field of health psychology also focuses on social conditions, among them socio-economic status and racial disparities. Thus, it is important to bear in mind that individuals' actions (i.e., their behaviors) are what determine many of the social conditions that affect people's health. For example, people act collectively to make laws and policies and to implement and enforce them.

Increasingly, experts believe that health behavior change strategies are most likely to be effective if they embrace an ecological perspective of health psychology and health promotion (McLeroy, Bibeau, Steckler, & Glanz, 1988; Sallis, Owen, & Fisher, 2008). That is, they should not only be targeted at individuals but should also affect interpersonal, organizational, and environmental factors influencing behavior. This view can clearly be illustrated when one thinks of the context of selecting and purchasing food and making food choices (Glanz, 2008). Consumers learn about foods through advertising and promotion in the media, by labels on food packages, and through product information in grocery stores and restaurants. Their purchases are influenced by personal preferences, family habits, medical advice, availability, cost, packaging, placement, and intentional meal planning. The process is complex and clearly determined not only by multiple factors but by factors at multiple levels. Still, much food choice—and other health behaviors—can be represented by routines and simple, internalized rules.

Contemporary thinking suggests that strategies that reach beyond the individual to the social milieu and environment can enhance the chance of successful health-enhancing behavior change (Glanz & Rimer, 2008). Understanding the various levels of influence that affect the public or patient's behavior and health status maximizes the chances of positive change. This will be discussed and illustrated with examples later in this chapter.

EXPLANATORY AND CHANGE THEORIES

Theories can guide the search to understand why people do or do not follow medical advice, help identify what information is needed to design an effective intervention strategy, and provide insight into how to design an educational program so it is successful (Glanz et al., 2008). Thus, theories and models help to explain behavior, as well as suggest how to develop more effective ways to influence and change behavior. *Explanatory or predictive theories* help to identify factors that may influence a health behavior; if properly specified, explanatory theories should be able to predict reasonably well who will be more or less likely to perform a given behavior. In contrast, *theories and models of behavior change* focus on the change process; these theories tend to detail stages through which individuals progress before achieving lasting health behavior change. These two types of theory often have different emphases but are quite complementary. For example, understanding why someone chooses the foods he or she eats is one step toward successful nutrition management, but even the best explanations will not by themselves be enough to fully guide change to improve health. Some type of change model will also be needed. Similarly, knowing the reasons why someone smokes is important for the development of effective smoking cessation materials. However, equally important is an understanding of how someone who has made several unsuccessful quit attempts in the past can progress to becoming a nonsmoker. In this chapter, we describe how commonly used theories and models can be particularly useful in guiding change processes, thus zeroing in on the leverage points that health psychologists can consider in developing behavior change programs for individuals and populations.

TYPES OF HEALTH BEHAVIORS AND IMPLICATIONS FOR CHANGE

There are several ways that health behaviors can be characterized that have important implications for the process of behavior change. The ways include whether a behavior is one-time, episodic, or habitual; whether the focus is on single or multiple behaviors; whether the recommended changes are restrictive or additive; and whether the attempted change is in a gradual or strict manner. This section briefly touches on these features of health behaviors.

EPISODIC VERSUS LIFESTYLE BEHAVIORS

A useful distinction can be made between episodic behaviors and lifestyle behaviors, or habits. Health behavior can be engaged in once or periodically, as in getting immunizations or a flu shot. Other health behaviors are actions that are performed over a long period of time, as in eating a healthful (or, conversely, unhealthy) diet, getting regular physical activity, and avoiding tobacco use. It is these latter types of behaviors, presenting as a sustained pattern of behavior, that are usually considered "lifestyle behaviors" or health habits. The process of changing habitual behavior is often more complex and always requires more points of contact over time than does changing a one-time or episodic behavior.

SINGLE VERSUS MULTIPLE BEHAVIORS

Much research and practice focuses on change processes for single behaviors, for example, eating patterns, smoking, or sexual risk taking. In the ideal, the person who practices a variety of behaviors in a health-enhancing manner can be described as having a healthy lifestyle. More realistically, many people practice some, but not all, lifestyle behaviors in a healthy manner. Moreover, most people do not practice all healthful or risky behaviors consistently; for instance, someone might get regular, health-promoting exercise several times a week but be a cigarette smoker who seldom brushes his or her teeth. Or someone might quit smoking, only to begin overeating as a substitute. The complex interplay between health behaviors presents important challenges, whether a given intervention addresses a single behavior or multiple behaviors. More conceptual and empirical development around multiple behavior change is needed (Noar, Chabot, & Zimmerman, 2008).

RESTRICTIVE VERSUS ADDITIVE BEHAVIORS

Many behavior change recommendations focus on advice to restrict, limit, or stop certain behaviors such as overeating, smoking, or drinking in excess. For example, the emphasis of nutrition counseling is often to restrict intake of certain foods or nutrients by, for example, reducing fat and saturated fat intake, limiting calorie intake, and limiting sodium intake. Yet the most often-mentioned obstacle to achieving a healthful diet is not wanting to give up the foods we like (Morreale & Schwartz, 1995). Basic psychological principles hold that when people are faced with a restriction, or loss of a choice, that choice or commodity becomes more attractive. In contrast, emphasizing such additive recommendations as increasing intake of fruits and vegetables and being more active often appeals to people because it sanctions their doing more of something. However, research suggests that it is not necessarily easy to get people to take up a new habit, and some health risk behaviors (e.g., drinking and driving) need first to be limited or stopped before new positive behaviors or substitute behaviors can take their place.

GRADUAL OR STRICT CHANGE

A generally held view is that the chances of long-term health behavior change are greater when efforts to change occur in a gradual, stepwise manner. This might involve reducing cues to a maladaptive behavior (e.g., smoking) or making small dietary changes each week until the total diet comes close to recommendations. A basic principle involved is that small successes (i.e., recognition of each successful behavioral change) increase confidence and motivation for each successive change. Although this approach is effective for many people, others become impatient or even lose their enthusiasm for minimally recognizable changes. An alternative is to begin with a highly restrictive change such as quitting smoking "cold turkey" or following a very low-calorie diet for the first two weeks of a weight loss effort. These types of programs may be useful for people who are highly motivated, newly diagnosed diabetics, or survivors of a coronary incident or for those who have not been successful in making gradual changes. In some cases, a strict change for an initial short time period will help someone get over withdrawal symptoms or will yield highly motivating visible or clinical changes. Such behavior changes often require careful supervision and may not work for everyone.

CROSS-CUTTING ISSUES AND CONSTRUCTS

It is important to note that various theories of health-related behavior often overlap. Not surprisingly, these explanations for behavior and models for change share several constructs and common issues. This section highlights a few of the most important of these.

BEHAVIOR CHANGE AS A PROCESS

One central idea that has gained wide acceptance in recent years is the simple notion that behavior change is a process, not an event. Rather, it is important to think of the change process as one that occurs in stages. Few people can decide one day to stop smoking and the next day become non-smokers for life. The idea that behavior change occurs gradually is not new, but it has gained wider acceptance in the past few years. Indeed, some multistage theories of behavior change date back more than 50 years (Lewin, 1935; Weinstein, 1993). Multiple theories, including the transtheoretical model of behavior change and the precaution adoption process model, propose that people are at different stages of readiness to adopt healthful behaviors (Prochaska, DiClemente, & Norcross, 1992; Prochaska, Redding, & Evers, 2008; Weinstein, Sandman, & Blalock, 2008). People do not always move through the stages of change in a linear manner but often recycle and repeat certain stages; for example, individuals may relapse and go back to an earlier stage depending on their level of motivation and self-efficacy. Stages identified in the transtheoretical model of behavior change include precontemplation (no recognition of a need for or interest in change), contemplation (thinking about changing), preparation (planning for change), action (adopting new habits), and maintenance (ongoing practice of new, healthier behavior; Prochaska et al., 2008). Stages in the precaution adoption process model include being unaware of the issue, unengaged by the issue, or undecided about acting, as well as having decided to act or decided not to act, acting, and maintaining the action (Weinstein et al., 2008). Factors that move people from one stage to another differ between stages. For example, personal experience with a hazard may move people from unengaged to undecided, whereas detailed how-to information may move people from the decided to the acting stage.

CHANGING BEHAVIORS VERSUS MAINTAINING BEHAVIOR CHANGE

Even where there is good initial compliance to health-related behavior change advice or attempts, such as using sunscreen or changing one's diet, relapse is very common. Thus, it has become clear that undertaking initial behavior changes and maintaining behavior change are very different and require different types of programs and/or self-management strategies. People who quit smoking by going cold turkey will probably be tempted again, perhaps at a party where their friends are smoking. To maintain cessation behavior requires developing self-management and coping strategies, as well as establishing new behavior patterns that emphasize perceived control, environmental management, and improved confidence in one's ability to avoid temptation.

Barriers to Actions, Pros and Cons, and Decisional Balance

The concept of barriers to action, or perceived obstacles, is often mentioned in theories of health behavior and is important to understanding health behavior change. An extension of the concept of barriers to action involves the *net benefits* of action, also referred to as the "benefits minus barriers" in the health belief model (Champion & Skinner, 2008). The health belief model is based on an assumption that people fear diseases and that health actions are motivated in relation to the perceived threat and expected threat-reduction potential of actions, as long as that potential outweighs practical and psychological obstacles to taking action, thus resulting in net benefits (Champion & Skinner, 2008). Key constructs of the health belief model are identified as perceived susceptibility and perceived severity (two dimensions of threat) and perceived benefits and perceived barriers (the components of net benefits). More recent adaptations include "cue to action," a stimulus to undertake behavior; and self-efficacy, or confidence in one's ability to perform an action (Champion & Skinner, 2008).

In the stages-of-change model, there are parallel constructs labeled as the pros, which are the benefits of change, and cons, which are the costs of change (Prochaska et al., 1992). Taken together, these are known as "decisional balance," or the pros minus cons, similar to the net benefits of action in the health belief model. The idea that individuals engage in relative weighing of the pros and cons has its origins in models of decision making and has been considered important for many years (Janis & Mann, 1977; Lewin, 1935). Indeed, this notion is basic to models of rational decision making, in which people intellectually think about the advantages and disadvantages, obstacles and facilitators, barriers and benefits, or pros and cons of engaging in a particular action.

INTERVENTIONS TO CHANGE HEALTH BEHAVIOR

As discussed earlier in this chapter, health behaviors are shaped through a complex interplay of determinants at different levels of influence. For example, physical activity is influenced by self-efficacy at the individual level, social support from family and friends at the interpersonal level, and perceptions of crime and safety at the community level (Eyler et al., 2003; Humpel, Owen, & Leslie, 2002; Wilcox, Castro, King, Housemann, & Brownson, 2000). A core principle of ecological models suggests that these multiple levels of influence interact across levels (Sallis et al., 2008; Stokols, 1996). For example, social support for exercise from coworkers may interact with the availability of exercise equipment at the worksite to facilitate increased physical activity.

Traditionally, and especially in clinical settings, strategies to change health behaviors have focused on such individual-level factors as knowledge, beliefs, and skills. As ecological thinking has gained currency, intervention strategies have broadened to target factors at such other levels of influence as organizational policies and the built environment. This recognition of the complex range of factors that shape health behaviors can make the selection of intervention strategies daunting. Deciding on the best intervention approach starts with understanding the population of interest, combined with identifying the most important and changeable determinants of the selected behavior (Gielen, McDonald, Gary, & Bone, 2008).

Fortunately, there are several broadly applicable and widely used theories and models for targeting behavioral determinants at various levels, so a firm grasp of available options makes it unnecessary to "reinvent the wheel" (Glanz & Rimer, 2008). Health psychologists and program planners can select from such individual-level theories as the health belief model, which emphasizes beliefs of susceptibility and severity of a health problem, as well as perceived benefits and barriers of taking action (Champion & Skinner, 2008). Alternatively, an intervention planner might use organizational development theories to create policy or environmental change within an organization such as a clinic or school.

Some widely used health behavior change strategies and related theoretical models are listed in Table 5.1.

TABLE 5.1
Theory-Based Intervention Strategies for Positive Health Behavior Change

Level of Change	Intervention Strategy	Related Theories
Individual	Goal-setting and behavior modification	Social cognitive theory
	Tailoring	Stages of change
Interpersonal	Lay health advisors	Social support
		Social networks
	Support groups and	Social support
	buddy systems	Social networks
Organizational	Provider reminders and feedback	Social cognitive theory (at the organizational level)
Community	Coalition building	Community coalition action theory

Intervention strategies targeting the individual level include goal setting, behavioral contracting, and tailored health communication. These strategies most typically draw on Bandura's (1986) social cognitive theory (SCT) and the stages-of-change construct from the transtheoretical model (Prochaska et al., 2008). Social cognitive theory explains human behavior in terms of a three-way, dynamic, reciprocal model in which personal factors, environmental influences, and behavior continually interact (Bandura, 1986). The theory synthesizes concepts and processes from cognitive, behavioristic, and emotional models of behavior change. A basic premise of SCT is that people learn not only through their own experiences but also by observing the actions of others and the results of those actions (McAlister, Perry, & Parcel, 2008). Key SCT constructs relevant to behavior change interventions include observational learning, reinforcement, self-control, and self-efficacy (Bandura, 1986). *Self-efficacy*, or a person's confidence in his or her ability to take action and to persist in that action despite obstacles or challenges, seems to be especially important for influencing health behavior change efforts (Bandura, 1997). Health psychologists can make deliberate efforts to increase clients' self-efficacy using three types of strategies: (1) setting small, incremental and achievable goals; (2) formalized behavioral contracting to establish goals and specify rewards; and (3) engaging in monitoring and reinforcement, including client self-monitoring by keeping records (McAlister et al., 2008).

Commonly used strategies at the interpersonal level involve lay health advisors and social support programs. Underlying theoretical constructs include social support, social norms, and social networks. Intervention strategies at the organizational level include provider reminders and feedback, as well as other systems changes. The process of creating organizational change is often informed by organizational development theory. At the community level, coalition building is a particularly common intervention strategy. The following sections describe each of these intervention strategies and how they are informed by theory. Brief examples of each strategy are also provided.

INDIVIDUAL-LEVEL INTERVENTIONS

Individual-level interventions target such psychological constructs as attitudes, beliefs, and self-efficacy, as well as such personal attributes as skills. The premise underlying these interventions is that the mechanisms for changing behavior lie within an individual (McLeroy et al., 1988). A large number of the theories used to inform health behavior change—including the health belief model, the theory of planned behavior, and stages-of-change model—were developed for this level of intervention (Rimer, 2008). Constructs from social cognitive theory also have direct implications for individual-level interventions.

Goal Setting and Behavioral Contracting

Goal setting and behavioral contracting involves setting achievable and incremental goals, committing to achieving the goals through a behavioral contract, monitoring and documenting progress, and reinforcing goal achievement through rewards. This approach has been used to help people quit smoking, manage asthma, eat more healthfully, and exercise more (Cullen, Baranowski, & Smith, 2001; McAlister et al., 2008; Shilts, Horowitz, & Townsend, 2004). Goal-setting and behavioral contracting interventions are informed by two major constructs from SCT: reinforcement and self-regulation (McAlister et al., 2008). According to SCT, self-regulation is achieved through (a) goal setting or identifying achievable incremental and long-term goals, (b) systematic observation of one's own behavior or self-monitoring, (c) feedback about the performance of the behavior and suggestions for improvement, (d) self-instruction or active cognitive engagement with oneself during the planning and performance of the behavior, (e) reinforcement with tangible or intangible self-rewards, and (f) obtaining social support from persons to encourage self-control efforts.

Goal-setting interventions must consider such goal properties as difficulty of the goal (e.g., run a marathon versus jog for 20 minutes three times per week), proximity or time frame (e.g., lose one pound per week or lose 40 pounds in a year), and type of goal setting (Shilts et al., 2004). Types of goal setting include self-set, assigned, prescribed, participatory or collaborative, guided, and group-set. Interestingly, self-set goals are not necessarily more effective than assigned goals (Shilts et al., 2004; Strecher et al., 1995), perhaps because self-set goals can be poorly defined or overly ambitious. Additional tenets of goal setting as an intervention strategy are that specific goals linked with performance feedback are more effective than vague goals and that more challenging goals can lead to higher performance. Goal setting is believed to work by motivating effort, persistence, and concentration. Feedback is central to goal-setting interventions, as are rewards.

One example of an intervention that used goal setting is Squire's Quest, a 10-session multimedia game designed to get children to increase their fruit and vegetable intake (Baranowski et al., 2003). The sessions included goal setting, self-regulation, and self-reward, along with fast-food selection, food preparation, and other topics (Cullen et al., 2004). Children were assigned goals related to eating more fruits and vegetables at specific meals or locations (e.g., breakfast or a fast-food restaurant). Parents verified that goals were met by signing a form. The software was designed to give positive rewards for goals attained and to help children problem-solve when goals were not achieved. Evaluation results showed that fruit and vegetable intake increased among intervention participants by 1.0 serving per day relative to the control group (Baranowski et al., 2003).

Tailoring

Tailoring refers to a process of individualizing health messages to a particular person's unique needs with respect to a specific health outcome based on an individualized assessment (Rimer & Kreuter, 2006). Tailoring begins with an individualized assessment that typically measures such theory-based determinants as stage of change from the transtheoretical model and perceived barriers from the health belief model. Health messages are then customized to address a person's unique combination of beliefs and circumstances. For example, a woman may be thinking about getting a mammogram but be worried about the cost. A tailored message might reinforce her interest in getting a mammogram and provide her a list of low-cost mammography services in her community. Tailoring has the potential to increase the relevance and salience of information and thereby increase motivation to process health information (Rimer & Kreuter, 2006). Tailoring is believed to motivate greater information processing by matching content to an individual's unique needs and interests, by contextualizing information in a meaningful way, and by packaging information to appeal to an individual's design and delivery preferences, as well as to their preferences for quantity and type of information (Rimer & Kreuter, 2006).

Many tailoring interventions rely on the stages-of-change construct from the transtheoretical model (Rimer & Kreuter, 2006). The transtheoretical model suggests that people are at different stages of readiness to adopt a behavior. Stages include precontemplation or no intention to take action in the next 6 months, contemplation or the intention to take action in the next 6 months, preparation or an interest to take action in the next 30 days, and action characterized by active behavior change for less than 6 months (Prochaska et al., 2008). Additional stages include maintenance and termination. Maintenance pertains to behavior change that persists more than 6 months, and termination is characterized by the total absence of temptation to relapse.

For tailoring purposes, individuals are classified by stage with a few questions to assess whether they are interested in changing a specific behavior, thinking about a change, or preparing to change, or whether they are already changed or are trying to maintain a change. Following classification by stage, motivational messages can be tailored to move an individual from one stage to another. Using flu shots as the health behavior of interest, if a woman is unaware of the need for a flu shot, she would be classified in the precontemplation stage. Communication strategies tailored for this stage would attempt to capture her attention through an interesting narrative or a compelling image (Rimer & Kreuter, 2006). If the person is vaguely aware of flu shots but does not feel they apply to her, a tailored message may present data about her risk and how a serious case of the flu would affect her and her family. If she is already thinking about getting a flu shot but has not yet decided, a list of the pros and cons of getting a shot may help her to move toward action. A list of nearby locations of flu shots may also facilitate action. Movement to the maintenance stage may be facilitated through annual reminders.

Alternatively, communication strategies beyond health messages can be employed at each stage. According to Prochaska, Redding, and Evers (2008), consciousness raising in the form of messages about the causes and consequences of a behavior would be appropriate at the precontemplation change, whereas self-reevaluation through values clarification would help move people from the contemplation to the preparation stage. Encouraging individuals to seek social support, in contrast, would be appropriate at the maintenance stage.

Early tailoring efforts often focused on such tailored written materials as newsletters (Rimer & Kreuter, 2006). There is now an extensive scientific literature on the impact of health behavior change interventions made through tailored print, and there are many examples of features contributing to their greater or lesser rates of success (Noar, Benac, & Harris, 2007). Tailoring has also been used in such print materials as calendars, in telephone counseling and face-to-face counseling, and more recently through interactive Web-based programs. Puff City was a Web-based program that focused on asthma management among urban African American adolescents (Joseph et al., 2007). The tailoring, delivered through four consecutive computer sessions, was based on constructs from the transtheoretical model and the health belief model. Participation in the intervention had a positive impact on both behavioral and health outcomes. A tailored colon-cancer-risk-counseling intervention for relatives of colorectal cancer patients combined face-to-face meetings with print materials and follow-up phone calls. That tailored strategy, which drew on the precaution adoption process model and the health belief model, was effective at increasing screening adherence among those individuals who received the intervention (Glanz, Steffen, & Taglialatela, 2007).

INTERPERSONAL-LEVEL INTERVENTIONS

Interpersonal interventions attempt to alter the social influences that support and/or undermine health behavior. Rather than focus on the use of social influences to change an individual's beliefs or attitudes directly, interpersonal-level interventions attempt to change the nature of existing social relationships by targeting social support, social networks, and social norms as the proximal leverage points to change behavior (McLeroy et al., 1988).

Lay Health Advisor Interventions

Lay health advisors are a fairly common interpersonal-level behavior change strategy. Lay health advisor interventions involve identifying natural helpers within a community; these are individuals within social networks to whom others turn for advice or assistance of some kind (Eng & Parker, 2002). These "natural helpers" are then taught about a particular health topic such as breast cancer detection and the importance of regular mammograms. The lay health advisors, in turn, educate members of their social networks about the health topic and provide various types of social support to facilitate the desired behavior among network members. Lay health advisor interventions can also strengthen social networks by linking previously disconnected networks, by expanding network size, or by creating new networks (Heaney & Israel, 2008).

Four key types of social support have been identified: emotional or the provision of care, trust, and empathy; informational, including the provision of information, advice, and suggestions; tangible aid and services such as transportation or funds and labeled instrumental support; and appraisal support, such as constructive criticism and affirmation that can be used for self-evaluation (Heaney & Israel, 2008). Social support can be provided by members of one's social networks, including family, friends, and coworkers, or from more formal helping systems such as social workers or case managers employed by a health care organization. Types and levels of support often vary by type of network. For example, longer term emotional support may be more likely to come from family and friends, and informational support may be more likely to come from helping professionals (Heaney & Israel, 2008). The use of lay health advisors attempts to tap the best of professional helping systems such as accurate information in conjunction with the unique assets of informal helping networks (e.g., longer term, empathetic, and reciprocal support).

Several studies have documented the effectiveness of engaging indigenous natural helpers to provide social support (e.g., information and transportation) for such health behavior changes as obtaining annual mammograms or obtaining annual blood lead tests for children. For example, a lay health advisor intervention in rural North Carolina recruited more than 150 African American women to promote breast cancer screening in their communities (Earp et al., 2002). After completing training on breast cancer, breast cancer screening, and existing payment programs, the lay health advisors raised awareness of breast cancer screening through conducting an average of two one-on-one conversations per week with women in their social networks, combined with participating in two community activities per month such as presentations at beauty parlors and churches. The intervention was particularly effective in increasing mammography use among low-income women (Earp et al., 2002).

Social Support Interventions

Another type of interpersonal-level intervention attempts to develop new relationships that can serve as mechanisms for provision of social support (Heaney & Israel, 2008). These intervention approaches include buddy systems and support groups. Buddy systems typically involve pairing individuals who are attempting to change the same behavior, such as to quit smoking or to lose weight. The buddy is given the responsibility of providing various kinds of social support to his or her partner to assist the person in making behavior change efforts. Support usually involves checking in with the partner regularly and encouraging him or her in the behavior change attempts (May & West, 2000; May, West, Hajek, McEwen, & McRobbie, 2006). Alternatively, the buddy may be someone who has already successfully navigated the behavior change process through a sponsor in Alcoholics Anonymous or a cancer survivor, for example. Interventions have also been designed in which the buddy is someone, such as a friend or spouse, from an individual's existing social network (Kidorf et al., 2005).

Support groups and self-help groups are another form of interpersonal intervention. These approaches involve the development of a new social network (Heaney & Israel, 2008). Individuals who share the same health problem convene in a group setting to provide social support to one another. Members both provide and receive social support in these interventions, which often have an informational and emotional support component. An HIV antiretroviral medication adherence intervention, for example, involved having medical providers identify "peers" who were socially skilled and had high levels of adherence (Simoni, Pentalone, Plummer, & Huang, 2007). These peers were then trained on barriers to adherence and how to provide appraisal and emotional, spiritual, and informational support in a sensitive manner. The intervention involved six biweekly group meetings of all peers and participants. The meetings focused on barriers to adherence and strategies to overcome these barriers. Relationships, substance abuse, and mental health issues also emerged in the discussions. In addition, peers also called their partners three times a week to provide one-on-one social support. Although the intervention did not result in improved adherence as measured by electronic drug monitors, it was associated with improvements in self-reported adherence, social support, and depression.

In recent years, Internet-based support groups have grown in popularity. These interventions also involve the creation of new social networks that at the same time allow for anonymity. In an intervention to change perceptions of social support among persons with diabetes, Barrera, Glasgow, McKay, and Boles (2002) provided participants with an opportunity to exchange information, emotional support, and coping strategies by means of an Internet-based diabetes support conference where members could post and respond to messages from other people with diabetes. A second component was more topic oriented, with staff introducing for discussion such topics as stress management. Participants then participated in live-chat discussions. Participants showed significant increases in perceived social support relative to a control group that received information only.

ORGANIZATIONAL-LEVEL INTERVENTIONS

Organizations and communities influence health behaviors in a variety of ways. Organizations provide goods and services and act as the primary mechanisms through which people engage with their community. Moreover, people spend a considerable amount of time in such organizational settings as schools and worksites. Consequently, the social environments (e.g., organizational climate), built environments (e.g., ergonomics and safety from occupational hazards), and organizational policies and practices (e.g., healthy foods at meetings) contribute to shaping health behavior. Organization-level change strategies are often informed by organizational development theory (Butterfoss, Kegler, & Francisco, 2008). Other organizational interventions are based on long-held understanding of how organizations are structured. Provider reminders and feedback in health care settings are typical of this type of strategy, which can be considered to use prompts similar to those based on social cognitive theory, but at the organizational level.

Provider Reminders and Feedback

Interventions that focus on changing office systems to support preventive services are increasingly common in health care settings. The use of assessment and feedback, as well as provider reminders of various types, has been found to be particularly successful in promoting cancer prevention through screening and smoking cessation. Based on a review of 20 research findings of provider assessment and feedback to increase delivery of appropriate cancer-screening services, there was a median increase of 9 to 14 percentage points in the proportion of study participants completing fecal occult blood tests (FOBTs) Pap tests, or mammographies (Sabatino, Habarta, & Baron, 2008). Provider reminders have also been found effective for increasing adherence to cancer-screening guidelines, with an 8.8-percentage-point median increase across the same three tests (Sabatino et al., 2008). A systematic review of published studies of the effectiveness of reminders to providers to discuss the importance of quitting smoking with their patients who smoke also found that various types of reminders (stickers, flow sheets, checklists, etc.) were effective in increasing health care providers' advice to patients to quit (Hopkins et al., 2001).

COMMUNITY-LEVEL INTERVENTIONS

Community-level interventions aim to improve population health by creating healthy environments and increasing community capacity for problem solving through systems changes, improved public policies, and more integrated and effective collaboration between community residents and institutions (McLeroy, Norton, Kegler, Burdine, & Sumaya, 2003).

Community Coalitions

Community coalitions are one form of collaborative structure that enable individuals and organizations to combine their human and material resources in working together toward a common goal (Butterfoss & Kegler, 2009). Coalitions facilitate multilevel, social ecologic interventions that acknowledge that health behaviors are deeply rooted in social and cultural contexts. They provide a vehicle for consensus building and involvement of diverse constituencies in solving a problem. By facilitating community participation, coalitions also help to ensure that resulting interventions meet real community needs, are culturally appropriate, and are more likely to be sustained (Butterfoss & Kegler, 2009).

Coalition approaches have been widely embraced by practitioners and funders alike. As a result, coalitions have been formed to address a long list of health issues, ranging from tobacco control to immunizations to violence prevention (Butterfoss & Kegler, 2009). Until recently, coalition building was loosely based on theoretical work from the fields of political science, community development, interorganizational relations, and group process (Butterfoss & Kegler, 2009). Recent theoretical advances include the construct of partnership synergy developed by Lasker, Weiss, and Miller (2001) and the community coalition action theory (CCAT) by Butterfoss and Kegler (2009). The former posits that such community collaboratives as coalitions gain a collaborative advantage through partnership synergy. Partnership synergy is created through the pooling of diverse perspectives, skills, and resources that lead to more creative, practical, and comprehensive solutions than could be developed by a single organization (Lasker, Weiss, & Miller, 2001).

Community coalition action theory is based on a series of propositions that explain coalition behavior from the formation to institutionalization stage (Butterfoss & Kegler, 2009). Briefly, coalitions typically form because of a threat, opportunity, or mandate, then develop in stages from formation to institutionalization. Coalitions cycle through stages as new issues emerge or member composition changes. In the formation stage, a lead agency organizes a core group that then expands to include diverse community representation. Coalition leadership and staff put processes and structures in place to facilitate successful member engagement. Satisfied and participating members pool resources and create collaborative synergy that leads to comprehensive and appropriate action plans and intervention strategies. Implementation of well-designed intervention strategies leads to community changes in policies, programs, and practices. Community change, in turn, results in changes in the health and social outcomes of interest. Community changes in combination with successful member engagement lead to increases in community capacity.

Coalitions have been particularly effective in tobacco control. Comprehensive state tobacco-control programs, which include community coalitions as described by CDC's *Best Practices* (2007), contributed to a decline in adult smoking prevalence from 29.5% in 1985 to 18.6% in 2003 (Farrelly, Pechacek, Thomas, & Nelson, 2008). Coalitions helped to change social norms, educate the public about tobacco use and the dangers of secondhand smoke, and advocate for policies to create smoke-free environments. Community coalitions have also been successful in improving service delivery systems (Foster-Fishman, Salem, Allen, & Fahrbach, 2001; Rosenthal et al., 2006); advancing the adoption of evidence-based programs that prevent risk behaviors and promote protective behaviors in adolescents (Feinberg, Jones, Greenberg, Osgood, & Bontempo, 2010); improving child vaccination rates (Findley et al., 2008); strengthening alcohol, tobacco, and other drug-related policies and regulations (Hays, Hays, DeVille, & Mulhall, 2000); and increasing community capacity for collaborative problem solving (Kegler, Norton, & Aronson, 2008; Zakocs & Guckenburg, 2007).

CONCLUSION

Successful behavior change strategies take many forms. Theory and research suggest that the most effective behavior change interventions are those that use multiple strategies and aim to achieve multiple goals of awareness, information transmission, skill development, and supportive environments and policies. Goal setting and monitoring are important elements of many successful interventions. The emergence of such information technology tools as the Internet, wireless technology, and personal digital assistants have expanded the range of theory-based strategies available for effective behavior change in health care and community settings. Behavioral interventions should be sensitive to audience and contextual factors, and they should recognize that most behavior change is incremental and that maintenance of change usually requires continued and focused efforts.

REFERENCES

Bandura, A. (1986). *Social foundations of thought and action: Social cognitive theory*. Englewood Cliffs, NJ: Prentice-Hall.

Bandura, A. (1997). *Self-efficacy: The exercise of control*. New York, NY: W. H. Freeman.

Baranowski, T., Baranowski, J, Cullen, K., Marsh, T., Islam, N., Zakeri, I., … deMoor, C. (2003). Squire's Quest! Dietary outcome evaluation of a multimedia game. *American Journal of Preventive Medicine*, *24*(1), 52–61.

Barrera, M., Glasgow, R., McKay, H., & Boles, S. (2002). Do Internet-based support interventions change perceptions of social support? An experimental trial of approaches for supporting diabetes self-management. *American Journal of Community Psychology*, *30*(5), 637–654.

Butterfoss, F., & Kegler, M. (2009). The community coalition action theory. In R. DiClemente, R. Crosby, & M. Kegler (Eds.). *Emerging theories in health promotion practice and research* (2nd ed.). San Francisco, CA: Jossey-Bass.

Butterfoss, F., Kegler, M., & Francisco, V. (2008). Mobilizing organizations for health promotion: Theories of organizational change. In K. Glanz, B. K. Rimer, & K. Viswanath (Eds.), *Health behavior and health education: Theory, research and practice* (4th ed.). San Francisco, CA: Jossey-Bass.

Centers for Disease Control and Prevention. (2007). *Best practices for comprehensive tobacco control programs, 2007*. Atlanta, GA: U.S. Department of Health and Human Services, Centers for Disease Control and Prevention, National Center for Chronic Disease Prevention and Health Promotion, Office on Smoking and Health.

Champion, V. L., & Skinner, C. S. (2008). The health belief model. In: K. Glanz, B. K. Rimer, & K. Viswanath (Eds.), *Health behavior and health education: Theory, research and practice* (4th ed.). San Francisco, CA: Jossey-Bass.

Cullen, K., Baranowski, T., & Smith, S. (2001). Using goal setting as a strategy for dietary behavior change. *Journal of the American Dietetic Association*, *101*, 562–566.

Cullen, K., Zakeri, I., Pryor, E., Barnowski, T., Baronowski, J, & Watson, K. (2004). Goal setting is differentially related to change in fruit, juice and vegetable consumption among fourth-grade children. *Health Education and Behavior*, *31*(2), 258–269.

Earp, J., Eng, E., O'Malley, M. S., Altpeter, M., Rauscher, G., Mayne, L., … Qaqish, B. (2002). Increasing use of mammography among older, rural African American women: Results from a community trial. *American Journal of Public Health*, *92*(4), 646–54.

Eng, E., & Parker, E. (2002). Natural helper models to enhance a community's health and competence. In R. DiClemente, R. Crosby, & M. Kegler (Eds.), *Emerging theories in health promotion practice and research*. San Francisco, CA: Jossey-Bass.

Eyler, A., Matson-Koffman, D., Young, D., Wilcox, S., Wilbur, J., Thompson, J., … Evenson, K. (2003). Quantitative study of correlates of physical activity in women from diverse racial/ethnic groups: The Women's Cardiovascular Health Network Project—Summary and conclusions. *American Journal of Preventive Medicine*, *3*(Suppl. 1), 93–103.

Farrelly, M., Pechacek, T., Thomas, K., & Nelson, D. (2008). The impact of tobacco control programs on adult smoking. *American Journal of Public Health*, *98*(2), 304–309.

Feinberg, M., Jones, D., Greenberg, M., Osgood, D., & Bontempo, D. (2010). Effects of the Communities That Care model in Pennsylvania on change in adolescent risk and problem behaviors. *Prevention Science*, *11*(2), 163–171.

Findley, S., Irigoyen, M., Sanchez, M., Stockwell, M., Mejia, M., Guzman, L., … Ferreira, R., … Andres-Martinez, R. (2008). Effectiveness of a community coalition for improving child vaccination rates in New York City. *American Journal of Public Health*, *98*(11), 1959–1961.

Foster-Fishman, P., Salem, D., Allen, N., & Fahrbach, K. (2001). Facilitating interorganizational collaboration: The contributions of interorganizational alliances. *American Journal of Community Psychology*, *29*(6), 875–905.

Gielen, A. C., McDonald, E. M., Gary, T. L., & Bone, L. R. (2008). Using the PRECEDE-PROCEED model to apply health behavior theories. In K. Glanz, B. K. Rimer, & K. Viswanath (Eds.), *Health behavior and health education: Theory, research and practice* (4th ed.). San Francisco, CA: Jossey-Bass.

Glanz, K. (2008). Current theoretical bases for nutrition intervention and their uses. In A. M. Coulston & C. J. Boushey (Eds.), *Nutrition in the prevention and treatment of disease* (2nd ed.). New York, NY: Elsevier.

Glanz, K., & Rimer, B. K. (2008). Perspectives on using theory. In K. Glanz, B. K. Rimer, & K. Viswanath (Eds.), *Health behavior and health education: Theory, research and practice* (4th ed.). San Francisco, CA: Jossey-Bass.

Glanz, K., Rimer, B. K., & Viswanath, K. (Eds.). (2008). *Health behavior and health education: Theory, research and practice* (4th ed.). San Francisco, CA: Jossey-Bass.

Glanz, K., Steffen, A. D., & Taglialatela, L. A. (2007). Effects of colon cancer risk counseling for first-degree relatives. *Cancer, Epidemiology, Biomarkers and Prevention*, *16*(7), 1485–1491.

Hays, C., Hays, S., DeVille, J., & Mulhall, P. (2000). Capacity for effectiveness: The relationship between coalition structure and community impact. *Evaluation Program Planning*, *23*, 373–379.

Heaney, C., & Israel, B. (2008). Social networks and social support. In K. Glanz, B. K. Rimer, & K. Viswanath (Eds.), *Health behavior and health education: Theory, research and practice* (4th ed.). San Francisco, CA: Jossey-Bass.

Hopkins, D. P., Briss, P. A., Ricard, C. J., Husten, C. G., Carande-Kulis, V. G., Fielding, J. E., … Harris, K. W. (2001). Reviews of evidence regarding interventions to reduce tobacco use and exposure to environmental tobacco smoke. *American Journal of Preventive Medicine*, *20*(2 Suppl.), 16–66.

Humpel, N., Owen, N., & Leslie, E. (2002). Environmental factors associated with adults' participation in physical activity: A review. *American Journal of Preventive Medicine*, *22*(3), 188–199.

Janis, I., & Mann, L. (1977). *Decision making: A psychological analysis of conflict*. New York, NY: Free Press.

Joseph, C., Peterson, E., Havstad, S., Johnson, C., Hoeraut, S., Stringer, S., … Strecher, V. (with Asthma in Adolescents Research Team). (2007). A web-based, tailored asthma management program for urban African American high school students. *American Journal of Respiratory Critical Care Medicine*, *175*(9), 888–895.

Kegler, M., Norton, B., & Aronson, R. (2008). Achieving organizational change: Findings from case studies of 20 California healthy cities and communities coalitions. *Health Promotion International*, *23*, 109–118.

Kidorf, M., King, V., Neufeld, K., Stoller, K., Peirce, J., & Brooner, R. (2005). Involving significant others in the care of opioid-dependent patients receiving methadone. *Journal of Substance Abuse Treatment*, *29*(1), 19–27.

Lasker, R., Weiss, E. & Miller R. (2001). Partnership synergy: a practical framework for studying and strengthening the collaborative advantage. *Milbank Quarterly*, *79*(2), 179–205.

Lewin, K. (1935). *A dynamic theory of personality*. New York, NY: McGraw-Hill.

May, S., & West, R. (2000). Do social support interventions ("buddy systems") aid smoking cessation: A review. *Tobacco Control*, *9*(4), 415–422.

May, S., West, R., Hajek, P., McEwen, A., & McRobbie, H. (2006). Randomized controlled trial of a social support ("buddy") intervention for smoking cessation. *Patient Education and Counseling*, *64*(1–3), 235–241.

McAlister, A., Perry, C., & Parcel, G. (2008). How individuals, environments, and health behaviors interact: Social cognitive theory. In K. Glanz, B. K. Rimer, & K. Viswanath (Eds.), *Health behavior and health education: Theory, research and practice* (4th ed.). San Francisco, CA: Jossey-Bass.

McLeroy, K., Bibeau, D., Steckler, A., & Glanz, K. (1988). An ecological perspective on health promotion programs. *Health Education Quarterly*, *15*(4), 351–377.

McLeroy, K., Norton, B., Kegler, M., Burdine, J., & Sumaya, C. (2003). Editorial. Community-based interventions. *American Journal of Public Health*, *93*(4), 529–533.

Morreale, S. J., & Schwartz, N. E. (1995). Helping Americans eat right: Developing practical and actionable public nutrition education messages based on the ADA Survey of American Dietary Habits. *Journal of the American Dietetic Association*, *95*(3), 305–308.

Noar, S. M., Benac, C. M., & Harris, M. S. (2007). Does tailoring matter? Meta-analytic review of tailored print health behavior change interventions. *Psychological Bulletin*, *133*(4), 673–693.

Noar, S. M., Chabot, M., & Zimmerman, R. S. (2008). Applying health behavior theory to multiple behavior change: Considerations and approaches. *Preventive Medicine, 46*(3), 275–280.

Prochaska, J. O., DiClemente, C. C., & Norcross, J. (1992). In search of how people change: Applications to addictive behaviors. *American Psychologist, 47,* 1102–1114.

Prochaska, J., Redding, C., & Evers, K. (2008). The transtheoretical model and stages of change. In K. Glanz, B. K.. Rimer, & K. Viswanath (Eds.), *Health behavior and health education: Theory, research and practice* (4th ed.). San Francisco, CA: Jossey-Bass.

Rimer, B. (2008). Models of individual health behavior. In K. Glanz, B. K. Rimer, & K. Viswanath (Eds.), *Health behavior and health education: Theory, research and practice* (4th ed.). San Francisco, CA: Jossey-Bass.

Rimer, B., & Kreuter, M. (2006). Advancing tailored health communication: A persuasion and message effects perspective. *Journal of Communication, 56*(Suppl. 1), S184–S201.

Rosenthal, M., Butterfoss, F., Doctor, L., Gilmore, L., Krieger, J., Meurer, J., & Vega, I. (2006). The coalition process at work: Building care coordination models to control chronic disease. *Health Promotion Practice, 7*(2), S117–S126.

Sabatino, S. A., Habarta, N., & Baron, R. C. (2008). Interventions to increase recommendation and delivery of screening for breast, cervical and colorectal cancers by healthcare providers. *American Journal of Preventive Medicine, 35*(1 Suppl.), 67–74.

Sallis, J., Owen, N., & Fisher, E. (2008). Ecological models of health behavior. In K. Glanz, B. K. Rimer, & K. Viswanath (Eds.), *Health behavior and health education: Theory, research and practice* (4th ed.). San Francisco, CA: Jossey-Bass.

Shilts, M., Horowitz, M., & Townsend, M. (2004). Goal setting as a strategy for dietary and physical activity behavior change: A review of the literature. *American Journal of Health Promotion, 19*(2), 81–93.

Simoni, J., Pentalone, D., Plummer, M., & Huang, B. (2007). A randomized controlled trial of a peer support intervention targeting antiretroviral medication adherence and depressive symptomatology in HIV-positive men and women. *Health Psychology, 26*(4), 488–495.

Stokols, D. (1996). Translating social ecological theory into guidelines for community health promotion. *American Journal of Health Promotion, 10*(4), 282–298.

Strecher, V. J., Seijts, G. H., Kok, G. J., Latham, G. P., Glasgow, R., DeVellis, B., … Bulger, D. W. (1995). Goal setting as a strategy for health behavior change. *Health Education Quarterly, 22*(2), 190–200.

Weinstein, N. D. (1993). Testing four competing theories of health-protective behavior. *Health Psychology, 12*(4), 324–333.

Weinstein, N., Sandman, P., & Blalock, S. (2008). The precaution adoption process model. In K. Glanz, B. K. Rimer, & K. Viswanath (Eds.), *Health behavior and health education: Theory, research and practice* (4th ed.). San Francisco, CA: Jossey-Bass.

Wilcox, S., Castro, C., King, A., Housemann, R., & Brownson, R. (2000). Determinants of leisure time physical activity in rural compared with urban older and ethnically diverse women in the United States. *Epidemiology and Community Health, 54,* 667–672.

Zakocs, R., & Guckenburg, S. (2007). What coalition factors foster community capacity: Lessons learned from the Fighting Back initiative. *Health Education and Behavior, 34*(2), 354–375.

6 Subjective Risk and Health-Protective Behavior
Prevention and Early Detection

Leona S. Aiken
Arizona State University

Mary A. Gerend
Florida State University

Kristina M. Jackson
Brown University

Krista W. Ranby
Duke University

This chapter explores the role of perceived risk in health-protective behavior. In models of health behavior, perceived risk for disease occupies the role of distal motivator for health-protective action. We explore the origins of perceived risk, its role in health behavior models, and the linkages between perceived risk and health-related behavior. We intend that the chapter provide a broad picture of the literature on risk perception in health psychology. We have chosen to contextualize the chapter with research on perceived risk for cancer as a putative determinant of cancer prevention and cancer screening. The body of research on the role of perceived risk in cancer detection and prevention is extensive. Moreover, cancer prevention and cancer screening encompass primary and secondary prevention of disease from a public health perspective, that is, primary prevention to both prevent disease onset and promote health, and secondary prevention to detect disease in its earliest state before it becomes symptomatic. Although our empirical research examples are in the main limited to cancer-related behaviors, our presentation is completely general from the perspective of theory and measurement of perceived susceptibility and its empirically supported role in health-protective behavior.

CHAPTER OVERVIEW

We set the stage for the chapter with a brief overview of cancer prevalence and cancer screening in the United States. We then move to the definition of perceived risk and the role of perceived risk in models of health behavior. We follow with the complex issue of the measurement of perceived risk (equivalently perceived susceptibility). We then address how perceived risk comes about, exploring classes of determinants of perceived risk for a range of diseases, including but not limited to cancer. This work leads to an exploration of the relationship between objective and subjective risk. We then provide an extensive examination of the relationship between perceived risk and cancer detection–related behaviors. We follow with the role of perceived risk in interventions to increase screening, with a focus on tailored interventions. Stepping back from the specifics of perceived risk and health behavior, we address the important role of mediation analysis to uncover the mechanisms by which interventions work to bring about behavior change. In a final brief section, we argue for the use of mediation analysis of interventions to understand the constructs, such as perceived susceptibility, that underlie health-protective behavior and health behavior change. Throughout, we integrate considerations of cognitive and emotional aspects of risk perception.

SETTING THE HEALTH CONTEXT FOR PERCEIVED RISK: CANCER PREVALENCE, PREVENTION, AND DETECTION

Prevalence

In the course of their lifetimes, 45% of men and 38% of women will develop invasive cancer (American Cancer Society, 2009), the second leading cause of death in the United States. In all, there were expected to be 1.44 million new cases of cancer and slightly over a half million cancer deaths in the United States in 2008 (Jemal et al., 2009).

Detection and Prevention Recommendations

The American Cancer Society (ACS) recommends cancer screening (American Cancer Society, 2010a) for breast, cervical, and colorectal cancer, as does the U.S. Preventive Services Task Force (2009). New genetic testing for cancer genes has opened a highly complex and difficult area of consideration. As of 2005, the U.S. Preventive Services Task Force (2005) recommended that women at risk for inheritance of the breast cancer susceptibility gene (BRCA1 or BRCA2) be referred for "genetic counseling and evaluation for BRCA testing" (p. 355). Beyond screening are recommendations for cancer prevention through a range of activities, including skin protection, diet, exercise, limitation of alcohol consumption, and, of course, smoking cessation. A new human papillomavirus (HPV) vaccine was approved by the U.S. Food and Drug Administration (FDA) in June 2006; vaccination is recommended for primary prevention of cervical cancer by the Centers for Disease Control (CDC) for all females 11 to 12 years of age (Markowitz et al., 2007). This recommendation opens an avenue of widespread cancer prevention because 70% of cervical cancer cases are associated with viruses targeted by the vaccine (American Cancer Society, 2010b).

Screening Utilization in the United States

The United States is far from achieving universal access to screening and compliance with screening recommendations for major cancers. In 2005, 66% of eligible women received mammography screening, a decline from previous years (Ryerson, Miller, Eheman, Leadbetter, & White, 2008). By 2005, 47% of the population had had some form of colorectal cancer screening, and 43% of men 50 and over had a prostate-specific antigen (PSA) at an appropriate schedule. Race/ethnic disparities are still evident (American Cancer Society, 2008), and socioeconomic differences contribute to race/ethnic disparities (Purc-Stephenson & Gorey, 2008). Screening rates for all tests were substantially higher for those born in the United States than for immigrants. Breen and Meissner (2005) address challenges to cancer screening in the United States from a public health system perspective.

CLASSES OF CANCER-PROTECTIVE BEHAVIORS

For our exploration of perceived risk and behavior, we first divide cancer-protective behaviors into two broad categories: secondary prevention through screening for early detection and primary prevention with protective behaviors. Detection through screening is associated with intermittent access to medical services, whereas most preventive behaviors—among them diet control, exercise, and sun protection—require sustained effort (Gerend, Shepherd, & Monday, 2008). In contrast, new to cancer prevention is the use of HPV vaccine to protect against cervical cancer, which requires simply three vaccine administrations (Markowitz et al., 2007). Our illustrations in the main are taken from literature on screening for early detection; in this regard we note that 16 of the 20 clinical preventive services recommended by the U.S. Preventive Services Task Force (2009) were screening services.

PERCEIVED RISK: DEFINITION AND ROLE IN MODELS OF HEALTH BEHAVIOR

DEFINITION OF PERCEIVED RISK

Health psychology is rich in models of the putative determinants of health-protective behavior (see Glanz and Kegler, Chapter 5, this volume). At the core of essentially all these models is the concept of perceived risk, that is, the extent to which an individual believes that he or she is subject to a health threat (Becker, 1990; Gerrard, Gibbons, & Bushman, 1996; Kowalewski, Henson, & Longshore, 1997; van der Pligt, 1998; Weinstein, 1993). Some but not all authors add to the definition of perceived risk the condition that perceived risk refers to the judgment of risk if no action is taken to protect against the threat (Weinstein, 2000; Weinstein et al., 2007), a characterization termed conditional risk by others (Ronis, 1992). Health psychology draws on a theoretically based literature in risk perception and its determinants (Kahneman & Tversky, 1973; Kasperson et al., 1988; Slovic, 1987; Tversky & Kahneman, 1974). Formal models of risk (Kasperson et al., 1988) postulate that risk is a joint function of the *probability of occurrence* of a negative event and the *magnitude* of its consequences; risk is the product of these factors. Literature applying perceptions of risk to health behavior is less precise. The term *perceived risk*, as well as the terms *perceived susceptibility* and *perceived vulnerability*, are used interchangeably to refer to the subjective likelihood of contracting a disease, absent any consideration of severity. Consistent with typical applications in health, we will use the terms *perceived risk, perceived susceptibility, perceived vulnerability,* and *perceived likelihood* to refer to subjective estimates of the likelihood of personally contracting a disease, not to the combination of likelihood and severity of consequences. Recently, Weinstein et al. (2007) provided a more nuanced characterization in which vulnerability is viewed as a more affective aspect of perceived risk. We will use *perceived severity* to refer to perceptions of seriousness of consequences independent of likelihood (Weinstein, 2000).

Models of health behavior assume that the motivation for health-protective behavior stems from anticipation of some negative health outcome coupled with hope of avoiding the outcome. Anticipation of a negative outcome involves foremost the perception that one is personally susceptible to some disease; for strong health motivation to be achieved, this perception must be coupled with the anticipation that the disease consequences are severe (Weinstein, 1993).

Our particular interest in this chapter is the linkage of perceived susceptibility to health-protective behavior. A theoretical context for this linkage is provided by consideration of how perceived susceptibility is used in models of health-protective behavior. Three widely applicable models of health behavior—the health belief model (HBM; Becker & Maiman, 1975; Rosenstock, 1966, 1974a, 1974b, 1990), protection motivation theory (PMT; Prentice-Dunn & Rogers, 1986; Rogers, 1975, 1983), and the precaution adoption process model (PAPM; Weinstein, 1988; Weinstein & Sandman, 2002)—employ the perceived susceptibility construct as a driving force in health-protective behavior. Perceived risk appears as well in the transtheoretical model of change (TTM; Prochaska, DiClemente, & Norcross, 1992), cognitive-social health information processing (C-SHIP) model (S. M. Miller, Shoda, & Hurley, 1996), and the health action process approach (HAPA; Schwarzer, 2008). Perceived risk is also implicit in the theory of reasoned action (TRA; Ajzen & Fishbein, 1980; Fishbein & Ajzen, 1975) and its extension, the theory of planned behavior (Ajzen, 1991), as well as subjective expected utility theory (Ronis, 1992; Weinstein, 1993), as they are applied to health behavior.

Although perceived susceptibility is consistently cast as the motivating engine for health-protective behavior, the specific role of perceived susceptibility and assumptions about how it combines with other constructs vary in informative ways across models. We provide a brief characterization of the role of the perceived susceptibility construct in several health behavior models. A characterization of the complete health models is beyond the scope of this chapter, however; Conner and Norman (2005), Glanz, Rimer, and Viswanah (2008), Weinstein (1993), and Weinstein, Rothman, and Sutton (1998) provide explications of these and other models. Conner and Norman (2005) also provide extensive reviews of literature employing these models. Curry and Emmons (1994) provide a thorough summary of applications of the HBM, TRA, and the TTM to breast cancer screening.

Perceived Susceptibility as Motivator: Health Belief Model (HBM)

The HBM traces its origins to problems encountered in the U.S. Public Health Service nearly half a century ago—problems of asymptomatic individuals failing to undergo screening tests or to engage in preventive health behaviors (Rosenstock, 1966, 1974a, 1990). According to the HBM, individuals will undertake a health action to the extent that they believe themselves to be susceptible to a health threat (perceived susceptibility), believe that the consequences of the disease are serious (perceived severity or seriousness), believe that the proposed health action will offer protection against the health threat (perceived benefits), and believe that barriers to performing the health action can be overcome (perceived barriers). Finally, individuals must receive some trigger or cue in order to act (cue to action). Both physicians' recommendations for screening (Fox, Siu, & Stein, 1994) and reminder letters (Bastani, Marcus, Maxwell, Das, & Yan, 1994) serve as cues in interventions to increase screening.

Perceived susceptibility is, in a sense, the centerpiece of the HBM. There are two aspects to perceived susceptibility: (1) an individual's belief that contracting a disease is a realistic possibility for him- or herself, and (2) an individual's belief that he or she may have the disease in the complete absence of symptoms (Rosenstock, 1990). Failure to utilize cancer-screening tests may be attributed to a lack of belief that pathology can exist in the absence of symptoms (Rosenstock, 1990). Perceived susceptibility and perceived severity combine to form perceived threat, a determinant of the likelihood of adopting a health action; this combination closely reflects the formal definition of risk (Kasperson et al., 1988), provided earlier. The HBM is silent on the nature of the combinatorial rules for the constructs; in most applications of the health belief model, simple additive effects of the constructs have been explored. The interplay of perceived threat with perceived benefits is important for cancer screening, in that high-risk individuals, though they perceive heightened vulnerability, may avoid seeking screening if they believe that cancer treatment cannot save them (e.g., Lerman & Schwartz, 1993, for breast cancer; M. D. Schwartz, Lerman, Daly, Audrain, Masny, & Griffith, 1995, for ovarian cancer). Ronis (1992) has suggested a combinatorial rule for HBM constructs in which perceived susceptibility and severity are necessary precursors to the perception of benefits of health action, a characterization on which we draw in our discussion of mediational analysis of interventions. The HBM has made sustained contributions as a heuristic for the study of psychosocial correlates of preventive health behavior. (See reviews by Harrison, Mullen, & Green, 1992; Janz & Becker, 1984; Sheeran & Abraham, 1996.) Typically, the perceived barriers construct has been the strongest correlate of nonbehavior, whereas perceived susceptibility has typically exhibited low to moderate positive correlations with protective behavior.

Although perceived susceptibility is expected to combine with perceived severity to motivate health-protective behavior, perceived severity by itself rarely correlates with preventive behavior or screening behavior (Harrison et al., 1992; Janz & Becker, 1984). This finding is certainly true for cancer research: Perceived severity has failed to show predictive utility and has not been amenable to change through intervention because cancer is apparently seen as uniformly serious (Champion, 1994; Curry & Emmons, 1994; Rimer, 1990; but see Ronis & Harel, 1989, for an exception). Researchers often forgo the measurement of perceived severity in characterizing the HBM for cancer-related behavior (e.g., Hyman, Baker, Ephraim, Moadel, & Philip, 1994; Vernon, Myers, &

Tilley, 1997). Thus, perceived susceptibility by itself, rather than the combination of susceptibility and severity, is de facto characterized as the motivating force for cancer protective behavior. In contrast, across a range of diseases Weinstein (2000) found interactions between perceived susceptibility and severity to predict motivation for protection.

FEAR-AROUSING COMMUNICATION, PERCEIVED SUSCEPTIBILITY, AND BEHAVIOR: PROTECTION MOTIVATION THEORY

Perceived susceptibility also plays a central role as a motivator of health-protective behavior in protection motivation theory (PMT), a model that arose from consideration of the impact of fear-arousing communication on the adoption of health-protective behavior (Beck & Frankel, 1981; Rogers, 1975). In PMT, perceptions of susceptibility and severity that result from fear communications are expected to combine with perceptions of the existence of an effective health-protective behavior to arouse protection motivation, which in turn leads to intentions to adopt the health-protective behavior (Rogers, 1975). In its revised form (Rogers, 1983; Prentice-Dunn & Rogers, 1986), PMT provided a special motivational role for perceived susceptibility coupled with perceived severity, that of lowering the probability of a maladaptive response (e.g., delay in seeking treatment for suspected cancer symptoms, persistence in behaviors that put one at increased cancer risk). A number of recent studies have drawn on PMT in studying cancer prevention (e.g., Helms, 2002, for genetic testing for breast cancer; Azzarello, 2006, and Grunfeld, 2004, for skin cancer screening and protection, respectively). De Hoog, Stroebe, and de Wit (2007) provide a comprehensive meta-analysis of the distinct roles of vulnerability to and severity of a health risk on the processing of fear communications.

HOW PERCEPTIONS OF SUSCEPTIBILITY ACCRUE: THE PRECAUTION ADOPTION PROCESS MODEL

Models of health behavior assume that in order for perceived susceptibility to act as a motivational force, perceptions of susceptibility must be personal; that is, individuals must feel that they are themselves vulnerable. Weinstein (1988) proposed the precaution adoption process model (PAPM) as a stage model of the adoption of health behavior. In general, stage models (Weinstein, Rothman, & Sutton, 1998) characterize individuals as falling into a series of ordered categories with regard to adoption of a health behavior. In PAPM, these stages move from lack of awareness of the health issue (Stage 1) through health behavior maintenance (Stage 7). Consistent with this stage structure, beliefs about perceived susceptibility are assumed to develop in a series of cumulative stages. First, an individual is assumed to become aware of a health hazard (awareness), then to believe in the likelihood of the hazard for others (general susceptibility), and finally to acknowledge his or her own personal vulnerability (personal susceptibility). Personal susceptibility is assumed to be critical in the decision to take precautionary action (Weinstein, Rothman, & Sutton, 1998). Assessment of discrepancies between general susceptibility and personal susceptibility has uncovered optimistic biases (Weinstein, 1980). The PAPM has been applied to home testing for radon gas, an environmental cancer threat (Weinstein & Sandman, 1992), and to mammography screening as well (Clemow et al., 2000).

THE GROWTH OF PERCEIVED SUSCEPTIBILITY AND THE PROCESS OF ADOPTING HEALTH BEHAVIORS: TRANSTHEORETICAL MODEL OF CHANGE

The transtheoretical model of change (TTM), like the PAPM, is a stage model of health behavior adoption (Prochaska et al., 1992). It is hypothesized that individuals pass through five stages as they initiate and maintain a health-protective behavior or cease a health-threatening behavior: (1) *precontemplation*, during which the individual has no intention to undertake behavior change and is uninformed of the consequences of the behavior in question; (2) *contemplation*, during which the individual is aware of the benefits (pros) of behavior change but also is strongly aware of the barriers (cons) to behavior change; (3) *preparation*, during which the individual makes definite plans to act in the very near future; (4) *action*, in which a new behavior is in place; and (5) *maintenance*, in which the behavior is carried out over an extended time. Accompanying these stages of change are processes of change; these processes rise and fall in intensity across the stages. The earliest process of change is consciousness raising, through which an individual gains increasing awareness of a health problem and its consequences. According to TTM, consciousness raising as a process begins in the precontemplation stage, peaks during contemplation, and then gives way to other, more action-oriented processes in the remaining three stages. Put another way, progress through the first two stages is hypothesized to be driven by the growth of awareness of perceived risk from a health threat. The TTM has been applied to both cancer screening and cancer prevention. For example, Lipkus, Rimer, and Strigo (1996), Rakowski et al. (1998), and Pruitt et al. (2009) have applied this model to mammography screening; other applications include sun exposure, exercise, dietary change, and alcohol consumption, all related to cancer risk and prevention.

COGNITIVE-SOCIAL HEALTH INFORMATION PROCESSING

The cognitive-social health information processing (C-SHIP) model (S. M. Miller et al., 1996) is a comprehensive model of the genesis and maintenance of health-protective behavior, initially expounded in the context of the complex sustained behavior of breast self-examination (BSE). The model considers five classes of determinants of health behavior that incorporate both cognitions and affect. Among these, two classes address issues of perceived susceptibility: (1) *health-relevant encodings*, including health risks and vulnerabilities, as well as attention strategies for gathering versus avoiding health relevant information; and (2) *health beliefs and expectancies*, including how such vulnerabilities as genetic predisposition affect subjective likelihood of disease development. The model specifies how information about objective risk and resulting perceptions of susceptibility interact with emotions associated with receiving health information, with health goals, and with self-regulation in producing health behaviors. That the model addresses the interplay of emotion with cognitions about one's vulnerability is important for our understanding of cancer screening, especially among individuals at high risk for cancer.

THE HEALTH ACTION PROCESS APPROACH

The health action process approach (HAPA) model (Schwarzer, 2008) is a two-stage model, of which the first stage, or *motivational phase*, characterizes the factors that lead to the intention to adopt a health behavior, and the second stage, or *volitional phase*, characterizes the factors that link these intentions to the initiation of behavior and the maintenance of behavior over time. The model is unique in its elaboration of factors that support the intention–behavior link. In HAPA, as in other models of health behavior, perceived susceptibility is an early motivating factor at the outset of the motivational stage; it is expected to relate to intentions, though less strongly than other predictors of intention, among them outcome expectancies associated with the health behavior. HAPA has been applied to cancer-preventive behaviors, including dietary modification, exercise, cessation of smoking, and sun protection (Lippke, Ziegelmann, Schwarzer, & Velicer, 2009; Scholz, Keller, & Perren, 2009; Schwarzer, Luszczynska, Ziegelmann, Scholz, & Lippke, 2008). An exceptional Web site provides a complete up-to-date bibliography of this research (http://www.hapa-model.de/). Schwarzer (2011) provides a rich summary of the major models of health behavior and their core constructs that complements this brief review.

PERCEIVED SUSCEPTIBILITY AS A PREDISPOSING FACTOR IN COMPLEX MODELS

A number of authors have proposed extensive integrative frameworks of the putative determinants of health-protective behavior, which have been employed in the design of interventions to increase health behavior. Four such frameworks are summarized in Curry and Emmons (1994). Each framework specifies a complex causal chain of variables that ultimately leads to health behavior. Most important for our consideration is the fact that perceived susceptibility is included as a predisposing factor for health behavior adoption early in the causal chain. Perceived susceptibility may facilitate overcoming barriers to the health-protective behavior (McBride, Curry, Taplin, Anderman, & Grothaus, 1993) and lead to receptiveness to health promotion interventions (the PRECEDE-PROCEED model of Green and Kreuter, 1991).

PERCEIVED SUSCEPTIBILITY AS A PREDISPOSING FACTOR FOR HEALTH BEHAVIOR ADOPTION

Not surprisingly, models of health behavior have matured and increased in complexity. Early models have been augmented with new variables, for example, the addition of self-efficacy for health behavior to both the HBM (Rosenstock, Strecher, & Becker, 1988) and PMT (Rogers, 1983). New stage models have viewed health behavior adoption as dynamic, in part driven by perceived susceptibility. The interplay of susceptibility cognitions with emotion has been elucidated. Hybrid models have incorporated a complex network of environmental and medical system variables along with individual cognitions, including perceived susceptibility. The evolution of these models has clarified the role of perceived susceptibility as a potentially powerful predisposing factor at the outset of the process of adoption of health behaviors, a factor that motivates this process of adoption. In sum, health behavior models conceptualize perceived susceptibility to disease as a distal construct in a mediational chain of constructs that eventuate in protective health behavior.

RISK, EMOTION, AND THE PARALLEL RESPONSE MODEL OF SELF-REGULATION

Models of health behavior characterize perceived susceptibility as a cognitive judgment of the likelihood of experiencing a negative health outcome, which judgment influences the decision to act to mitigate the threat. Yet, emotion (or affect) is a powerful factor in decision making (Damasio, 1994), as reflected in the C-SHIP model. Current considerations of how we perceive risk distinguish between *risk as analysis* and *risk as feelings* (Epstein, 1994; Lowenstein, Weber, Hsee, & Welsh, 2001; Slovic, Finucane, Peters, & MacGregor, 2004). Whereas risk as analysis draws on logic and reason, risk as feelings "refers to our fast, instinctive, and intuitive reactions to danger" (Slovic et al., 2004, p. 311). These distinct aspects of risk are argued to arise from two distinct systems of thinking, an analytic system and an experiential system (Slovic et al., 2004), for risk as analysis versus risk as feeling, respectively. Decisions concerning health actions, to obtain cancer screening or genetic screening for cancer heritability, may involve such intense emotions as fear and distress. Emotion or affect may, in fact, mediate the relationship between cognitive risk judgments and behavior (Lowenstein et al., 2001). Leventhal (Cameron & Leventhal, 2003; Leventhal, 1970; Leventhal, Brissette, & Leventhal, 2003; Leventhal, Leventhal, & Cameron, 2001; see also Chapter 1, this volume) proposed a self-regulation theory (or parallel response model) of reaction to health threat. It is characterized by two distinct responses to health threat, reflective of the cognitive and emotional components of risk. The first response, danger control, is problem focused, for mitigating the threat through effective action. The second response, fear control, is emotion focused, for mitigating the strong affective response to the threat. As explained next, which coping mechanism is invoked in response to a health threat depends on an individual's belief as to whether danger control is possible.

MEASUREMENT OF PERCEIVED SUSCEPTIBILITY

Approaches to the measurement of perceived susceptibility are cognitively based. Two broad classes of measures are *absolute measures*, in which personal ratings are made without reference to any outside group, and *comparative measures*, in which personal perceived susceptibility is compared to susceptibility in some normative group (Weinstein & Klein, 1996). There is lack of consensus as to optimal measurement approaches (Vernon, 1999); multiple measures are employed in individual studies (e.g., Gerend, Aiken, West, & Erchull, 2004; McQueen, Swank, Bastian, & Vernon, 2008).

ABSOLUTE MEASURES

Absolute measures vary widely in structure, involving rating scales, frequency scales, and percentage estimates. These scales lead to widely differing estimates of perceived risk. Frequency judgments (e.g., 25 out of 100 people) lead to higher perceived risk than percentage judgments (25%; Peters, McCaul, Stefanek, & Nelson, 2006), perhaps because of the vividness of thinking in terms of individual cases. Anchors on scales (e.g., 1% to 100% versus 1% to 50%) change risk ratings (Peters et al., 2006). Katapodi, Lee, Facione, and Dodd (2004) summarize scale format effects in a meta-analysis of judgments of perceived susceptibility to breast cancer.

Rating Scales

Among absolute measures, typical rating scales ask individuals for Likert-scale judgments of their likelihood of developing cancer, for example, "What do you believe is the chance you will develop breast cancer in your lifetime?" (Gerend, Aiken, West, et al., 2004; see also Bastani, Marcus, & Hollatz-Brown, 1991; McQueen et al., 2008).

Numerical Estimates

Numerical estimates of the chance of contracting cancer are also taken as absolute indicators of perceived susceptibility, for example, "Risk of developing breast cancer in the next 10 years" (< 1%, 1%–5%, 6%–10%, 11%–20% or >20%; Dolan, Lee, & McDermott, 1997; percent risk likelihood, 0% through 100%; McQueen et al., 2008). Perceived risk has also been measured with rate judgments, for example, "the number of women out of 1000 whom you think would develop breast cancer in the next 10 years" (Black, Nease, & Tosteson, 1995; see also L. M. Schwartz, Woloshin, Black, & Welch, 1997).

COMPARATIVE RISK

Direct Comparative Risk

Direct comparative risk is measured with some form of the following question: "What do you believe are your chances of getting (disease) compared to other (men/women) your own age?" with such typical responses as "a lot lower, somewhat lower, about the same, somewhat higher, and a lot higher." This measure has been applied to cancer in general (Kreuter & Strecher, 1995); lung cancer, skin cancer, and cancer in general (Weinstein, 1987); breast cancer (e.g., Aiken, Fenaughty, West, Johnson, & Luckett, 1995; Gerend, Aiken, West, et al., 2004), and colorectal cancer (e.g., Blalock, DeVellis, Afifi, & Sandler, 1990).

Indirect Comparative Risk

Indirect comparative risk is assessed by having an individual rate the likelihood of developing the disease herself and also the likelihood that similar others (e.g., of the same age) will develop the disease. The difference between these two ratings—own absolute minus other absolute—reflects comparative risk (Weinstein & Klein, 1996).

Discrepancies Among Risk Measures

Measures of comparative risk are sometimes used in combination with absolute rating scales in the formation of multi-item susceptibility measures. Some researchers have argued that individuals' perceptions of their own risk appear to drive both own absolute and direct comparative risk judgments (Covey & Davies, 2004; Gerend, Aiken, West, et al., 2004; Klar & Ayal, 2004; Klar & Giladi, 1999); absolute and direct comparative risk form a single factor psychometrically (Gerend, Aiken, West, et al., 2004). Yet, some authors have found that these two measures make independent contributions to prediction; for example, Klein (2003) found differential relationships of comparative and absolute risk information to judgments of safety. Indirect comparative risk does not consistently relate to other perceived susceptibility measures. Moreover, indirect comparative risk may correlate positively, not at all (Covey & Davies, 2004), or even negatively (Price, Pentecost, & Voth, 2002) with risk factors that correlate positively with own absolute and direct comparative risk.

Ranby, Aiken, Gerend, and Erchull (2010) provide an explanation for this discrepancy with indirect comparative risk that draws on recent explications of the cognitive factors underlying social comparative judgments and the algebra of the computation of indirect comparative risk. Following Chambers and Windschitl (2004), we distinguished between the processing of *personal factors* that underlie one's perception of one's own risk (e.g., one's own family history or symptoms experienced, one's perceived similarity to those that contract the disease) versus such *general factors* as base rate, prevalence, or commonness of a disease that underlie perceptions of risk for generalized others' risk. Ranby et al. (2010) provided a straightforward algebraic demonstration that the correlation of a risk factor with indirect comparative risk—computed as own absolute risk minus other absolute risk—is necessarily determined by the correlation of the risk factor with own absolute risk and with other absolute risk. If such a personal risk factor as one's own family history is positively correlated with one's own absolute risk judgment but is not correlated with other absolute risk, then the risk factor must algebraically be correlated with indirect comparative risk. Ranby et al. (2010) found that for perception of risk for breast cancer among a community sample of mature women, women's own Gail epidemiological risk index (an objective risk estimate for breast cancer based on age, menses onset, parity, previous biopsies, and family history; Gail, 1989) positively correlated with their ratings of their own absolute risk ($r = .27$, $p < .001$), was uncorrelated with their ratings of others' absolute risk ($r = -.09$, NS), and was therefore positively correlated with the calculated indirect comparative risk score ($r = .29$, $p < .001$). On the other hand, if such a general risk factor as perceived commonness of a disease exhibits no correlation with own absolute risk but a strong positive correlation with other absolute risk, then the risk factor will correlate negatively with indirect comparative risk; again, an algebraic necessity. Ranby et al. (2010) found that for perception of risk for breast cancer among the same community sample, perceived commonness of breast cancer was uncorrelated with their own absolute risk ($r = .09$, NS), was strongly positively correlated with their ratings of others' absolute risk ($r = .67$, $p < .001$), and therefore was negatively correlated with the calculated indirect comparative risk score ($r = -.41$, $p < .001$). If a risk factor correlates equally with own and other absolute risk, then this risk factor will be uncorrelated with indirect comparative risk. Ranby et al. (2010) recommended against the use of indirect comparative risk measures, having demonstrated that the anomalous patterns of correlations of risk factors with the indirect comparative risk measure were attributable to the algebra of indirect comparative risk.

CONDITIONAL HEALTH THREAT

Perceptions of susceptibility and severity are in part governed by beliefs about personal actions that mitigate or increase cancer risk. Ronis (1992) characterized *conditional health threat* as the perception of threat under some behavior specification, that is, if the individual were to take a specific health-protective action versus taking no health-protective action (see also Rogers, 1983). Ronis (1992) and van der Pligt (1998) argued that the measurement of conditional health threat would provide better understanding of health-protective behavior because such conditional measures untangle the influence of current protective behavior on perceived vulnerability. Weinstein and Nicolich (1993) theorized that the discrepancy in level of perceived risk associated with participation versus nonparticipation in a health-protective behavior reflected perceived effectiveness of the health precaution. Further, Weinstein, Rothman, and Nicolich (1998) argued that the use of conditional health threat clarifies the interpretation of risk. Finally, Cameron (2003) argued that conditional health threat better captures how people think about behavior and health status, as a "dynamic, conditional relationship" (p. 6), rather than in terms of an unconditional level of risk, not tied to specific behavior. We propose that the components of conditional health threat, that is, conditional susceptibility versus conditional severity, will have differential associations with preventive versus screening behavior. For preventive behavior, we expect high perceived susceptibility given inaction coupled with high perceived benefits of the health action to produce preventive behavior, with a subsequent reduction in perceived susceptibility. For screening, the matter is different because susceptibility is not reduced by screening; rather, the argument for screening is that consequences (severity) of cancer will be reduced with early detection, so the appropriate conditional characterizations of perceived severity are "severity if treated early" versus "severity if treated late" (Ronis & Harel, 1989). Ronis and Harel (1989) applied this dual conception of perceived severity to BSE (breast self-examination) performance and showed a link of these severity measures—but not conditional susceptibility—to BSE, yielding new insight into the potential role of perceived severity in screening. Jackson and Aiken (2000) applied conditional perceived susceptibility and severity to skin cancer–preventive behaviors and found the opposite effect—conditional measures of perceived susceptibility but not severity predicted skin protection. Measures of conditional threat may provide help to clarify the links of perceived susceptibility and severity to detection versus preventive behaviors.

PERCEIVED SUSCEPTIBILITY VERSUS CANCER WORRY AND CANCER DISTRESS

Perceived susceptibility has been distinguished from more emotional aspects of vulnerability in studies of cancer-related health behaviors, consistent with theorizing on risk as feelings (Sjoberg, 1998). Measurement of cancer worry has varied widely and has captured a range of levels of emotional effects. The item "During the past month, how often have you thought about your own chances of developing breast cancer" indicates mild worry, whereas "How often have your thoughts about breast cancer affected your mood" indicates moderate worry (M. D. Schwartz, Taylor, & Willard, 2003). More extreme worry is captured by "Thinking about breast cancer makes me feel upset and frightened" (McCaul, Schroeder, & Reid, 1996). Intrusive thoughts about cancer—for example, "I have had dreams about it," from the Impact of Events Scale (Horowitz, Wilner, & Alvarez, 1979)—have served as measures of cancer-related distress (Hay, Buckley, & Ostroff, 2005; M. D. Schwartz et al., 2003). McCaul and Goetz (2003) provide a review of these measures.

The assumption has been made that cancer worry is distinct from perceived susceptibility. Hay et al. (2005) provide a comprehensive analysis of the role of cancer worry in cancer screening, subsuming a variety of terms, including *cancer fear*, *cancer-related distress*, and *cancer anxiety* under the term *cancer worry*. The two variables are moderately related (correlations of .2 to .4; reviewed in Zajac, Klein, & McCaul, 2006; see also McQueen et al., 2008) and form independent factors in the measurement of predictors of colorectal cancer–screening adherence (Ritvo et al., 2008; Vernon et al., 1997). Fear of cancer and cancer treatment (Berman & Wandersman, 1992; Salazar & de Moor, 1995), cancer anxiety (Gram & Slenker, 1992), morbid concern about breast cancer (Irwig et al., 1991), and cancer-related distress (Rees, Fry, Cull, & Sutton, 2004) also have been included in research. A growing literature on breast and ovarian cancer screening among high-risk women (e.g., Audrain et al., 1997; M. D. Schwartz et al., 1999; M. D. Schwartz et al., 2003) has employed such measures of cancer-specific distress.

DETERMINANTS OF PERCEIVED SUSCEPTIBILITY AND THE RELATIONSHIP
OF PERCEIVED SUSCEPTIBILITY TO OBJECTIVE RISK

Two literatures inform the question of the determinants of perceived susceptibility. The first is a broad literature on classes of risk factors that relate to judgments of absolute risk. The second examines individuals' rationales for their comparative ratings of their own risk of cancer relative to some comparison group, typically individuals of the same gender and age (Weinstein, 1984).

THREAT, HEURISTICS, PERSONALITY, EMOTION, AND THE PERCEPTION OF SUSCEPTIBILITY

Gerend, Aiken, and West (2004) identified three traditions in characterizing the determinants of perceived risk. First is a *threat-based approach*, namely, that perceptions of susceptibility are rooted in disease characteristics, for example, the preventability of a disease. Second is a *heuristic-based approach*; rooted in cognitive psychology and decision science, this approach posits that cognitive heuristics shape risk perceptions. Third is an *individual-based approach*, namely, that personality factors color perceptions of risk independent of the particular threat. Gerend, Aiken, and West (2004) integrated these approaches in a mediational model in which threat-based and heuristic-based factors mediated the relationship of individual-based personality factors to perceived susceptibility. Most other research has considered first-order relationships of each class of predictors to perceived susceptibility; Katapodi et al. (2004) and Vernon (1999) provide extensive reviews of this work.

Cognitive Heuristics

Individuals rely on cognitive heuristics in estimating uncertain events (Kahneman & Tversky, 1973; Tversky & Kahneman, 1973, 1974), and these heuristics may underlie inaccurate perceptions of risk in the health domain. Peters, McCaul, Stefanek, and Nelson (2006) provide a comprehensive survey of heuristics that may contribute to the understanding of risk perception. Among these heuristics, the *availability heuristic* (Tversky & Kahneman, 1973) stipulates that we base frequency estimates on the salience of the event in question or the ease with which the event comes to mind. Personal experience with other individuals who have cancer (Wardle, 1995) and the extensive media coverage of cancer may contribute to the observed overestimates of cancer risk (Slovic, Fischhoff, & Lichtenstein, 1979; van der Pligt, 1998). The *representativeness heuristic* (Kahneman & Tversky, 1973) stipulates that we base likelihood estimates for a hypothetical event (e.g., a personal diagnosis of breast cancer) on our similarity to events with comparable characteristics (e.g., our similarity to others diagnosed with breast cancer). Gerend, Aiken, West, et al. (2004) explored the relationship of correlates of perceived risk that reflected both heuristics and disease characteristics; perceived similarity to those who get breast cancer was the strongest correlate of perceived risk. Peters et al. (2006) recommended the use of heuristics to aid the public in understanding risk estimates for cancer and other diseases. Further, they argue that if health providers take into account heuristic thinking about risk, they can improve the information provided to patients, who are increasingly involved in shared medical decision making.

Characteristics of the Health Threat

Bias in perceptions of comparative risk has been hypothesized to depend on disease characteristics (Weinstein, 1984, 1987; Weinstein & Klein, 1996). Harris (1996) and Weinstein (1987) reported a positive relationship between the perceived controllability or preventability of a disease and optimistic bias concerning risk. Both age and heritability play a strong role in risk perception, reflecting an interaction between characteristics of the threat (increasing occurrence with age and genetic risk). Women most often mention heredity as a source of the perceived elevated risk of breast cancer (Aiken et al., 1995; Lipkus et al., 1996). Although cancer incidence increases with age, the "absent/exempt" principle (If I haven't gotten the disease by now, I won't get it; Weinstein, 1987) is associated with lower perceived risk with increasing age (e.g., Aiken, West, Woodward, & Reno, 1994; Gerend, Aiken, West, et al., 2004). Women who may be at genetic risk for breast cancer, because of the possibility of inheriting the BRCA1/2 genetic mutation that greatly increases breast cancer risk, overestimate lifetime risk of developing breast cancer, even following genetic counseling to clarify their risk (Kelly et al., 2005). In a unique study, Fletcher et al. (2006) found that among first-degree relatives (FDRs) of women with newly developed breast cancer, their own perceived risk of developing breast cancer was associated with their perception of their relative's cancer prognosis.

Leventhal (e.g., Leventhal et al., 2003) characterized the lay public's understanding of illness in a *commonsense model* of disease that informs the relationship between disease characteristics and perceived risk. This representation is related to Leventhal's self-regulation theory, with its two coping strategies in the face of health threat: fear control versus danger control. Whether fear control or danger control is the response to a health threat is hypothesized to depend on an individual's preexisting cognitive schema or commonsense (lay) representation of an illness threat, that is, how the individual understands the identity, causes, timeline, consequences, and control of the illness. Rees et al. (2004) found that perceived susceptibility, disease identity, acute timeline, and consequences were all correlated with both cancer worry and general elevated distress among women at increased risk of breast cancer. Three aspects of the lay representation of cancer—the causes of cancer, whether cancer can be controlled or cured, and the timeline for developing cancer—relate to perceptions of lifetime risk of breast cancer (Kelly et al., 2005).

Personality Characteristics and Modes of Information Processing

A variety of personality dimensions have been associated with perceived risk. Among them are monitoring-blunting (M. D. Schwartz, Lerman, Miller, Daly, & Masny, 1995), psychological defense (Dziokonski & Weber, 1977; Paulhus, Fridhandler, & Hayes, 1997), anxiety (MacLeod, Williams, & Berekian, 1991; Robb, Miles, Campbell, Evans, & Wardle, 2006), neuroticism (Darvill & Johnson, 1991; Gerend, Aiken, & West, 2004), emotional distress (Zajac et al., 2006), self-deceptive enhancement, health locus of control, and worry as general aspects of personality (Gerend, Aiken, & West, 2004). This may explain linkages noted between personality factors and breast-screening behavior (Siegler, Feaganes, & Rimer, 1995) reviewed by Siegler and Costa (1994).

Affect and Perceived Susceptibility

Affect contributes strongly to human judgment (Finucane, Alhakami, Slovic, & Johnson, 2000; Lowenstein et al., 2001; Slovic et al., 2004). Finucane has argued that affective reactions to a stimulus may drive perceptions of risk. An affect heuristic for judgments of risk has been characterized (Damasio, 1994) in which the affect associated with mental images of experiences is brought to bear with immediacy when judgments are made (Peters et al., 2006). Decision making depends on the intensity of the affect in a communication. For example, in an experimental study, Slovic, Monahan, and MacGregor (2000) found that the judgment by experienced psychologists and psychiatrists as to whether a mental patient should be released depended on whether or not the communication evoked images of a violent patient.

Considerations of the link between affect and perceived risk have utilized measures of stable affect-related personality traits (e.g., Gerend, Aiken, & West, 2004; McQueen et al., 2008; Zajac et al., 2006) and specific worry about cancer. A substantial literature, summarized in Katapodi et al. (2004), has shown positive relationships between perceived risk of a disease and specific worry, fear, and distress associated with cancer. More recent literature has shown cross-sectional associations among risk perceptions, general emotional distress, and specific worry about cancer (Hay, Coups, & Ford, 2006; Zajac et al., 2006). McQueen et al. (2008) has provided evidence of longitudinal associations of both specific breast cancer worry and general anxiety to perceived susceptibility. Lipkus, Klein, Skinner, and Rimer (2005) showed longitudinal associations in both directions between perceived risk and cancer worry.

Experience of Symptoms

Experience of symptoms is associated with increased perceived risk. For example, breast symptoms, among them having ever found a breast lump (Aiken et al., 1995) and number of previous biopsies and atypical hyperplasia (McQueen et al., 2008), are associated with increased perceived breast cancer risk.

DETERMINANTS OF COMPARATIVE RISK

Weinstein (1984) coded the reasons generated by individuals for their comparative risk judgments into five categories: actions and behavior patterns, heredity, physiology or physical attributes, environment, and psychological attributes. This scheme has been used frequently for studying the determinants of both perceived and absolute risk (Gerend, Erchull, Aiken, & Maner, 2006; Robb, Miles, & Wardle, 2007). For cancer in general, breast cancer (Aiken et al., 1995; Lipkus et al., 1996), and colorectal cancer (Blalock et al., 1990; Hay, Coups, & Ford, 2006; Lipkus, Rimer, Lyna, et al., 1996; Robb et al., 2007), personal lifestyle–related actions were seen as both decreasing risk (e.g., proper diet, exercise) and increasing risk (e.g., red meat consumption, sedentary lifestyle). For lung cancer, personal actions (smoking) were seen as increasing risk (Lek & Bishop, 1995). Across cancers, attributions for heredity were that the absence of disease in the family reduced risk below average. In contrast, women who believed their risk to be above average for breast cancer mentioned heredity most often as the determining factor (Aiken et al., 1995; McCaul & O'Donnell, 1998; Savage & Clarke, 1996). There is lack of understanding of the role of heredity in cancer. Absence of family history is viewed as highly protective, even though most cancers are not associated with family history. Robb et al. (2007) pointed out that experiential and affective influences on judgments of cancer risk appear more salient in judgments of cancer risk than do more cognitive factors, consistent with the conception of risk as analysis and risk as feelings (Slovic et al., 2004).

PROCESSES UNDERLYING OPTIMISTIC BIAS

Optimistic bias for perceived personal risk relative to risk of others has historically been attributed to a motivation to protect oneself from feelings of distress or anxiety about future negative events (see extended discussion in Chambers & Windschitl, 2004). This protection may accrue from downward social comparisons, (i.e., comparisons of one's own risk with the risk of others who are actually more vulnerable; Klein, 1996; Klein & Weinstein, 1997; Perloff & Fetzer, 1986). Chambers and Windschitl (2004) have provided an alternative and comprehensive account that is based on information-processing limitations and biases in judgment processes. A component of their account is the processing of prevalence or base rate information, which people appear to apply more to the judgment of others than to their own risk. Interventions that emphasize only prevalence information may have more impact on one's perception of others' risk than on one's own risk. This finding is of interest for interventions that provide prevalence information to modify perceived risk in service of encouraging cancer prevention and protection.

NUMERACY AND THE RELATIONSHIP BETWEEN OBJECTIVE AND SUBJECTIVE RISK

A fundamental assumption underlying the examination of the relationship of perceived susceptibility to cancer-related behaviors is that perceived susceptibility is a motivator for protective action. Further, there is an implicit assumption that "increasing the match between perceived risk (beliefs) and actual risk (reality) will encourage individuals to initiate and maintain preventive and treatment behaviors at a level that is appropriate to their actual risk and its source" (Leventhal, Kelly, & Leventhal, 1999, p. 81). Here we review literature on the relationship of perceived to objective risk and then discuss fundamental issues in studying these relationships.

OBJECTIVE VERSUS PERCEIVED RISK

Population Estimates

When determined from actual versus estimated population rates, community samples overestimate their probability of developing and dying of cancer (e.g., Helzlsouer, Ford, Hayward, Midzenski, & Perry, 1994, for cancer in general; Ward, Hughes, Hirst, & Winchester, 1997, for prostate cancer).

Epidemiological Estimates and Individual Assessments

Individuals' risk estimates based on epidemiological models have been compared with their own subjective numerical risk estimates (see reviews by Katapodi et al., 2004, and by Vernon, 1999). The Gail model (Gail et al., 1989), a five-factor epidemiological model of breast cancer risk, predicts risk for breast cancer among women who obtain annual mammograms. Using this model, Black et al. (1995), Dolan et al. (1997), Bowen et al. (2003), Katapodi et al. (2004), and Quillin, Fries, McClish, deParedes, and Bodurtha (2004) found on average that women grossly overestimate their chances of developing breast cancer (e.g., 13% by the Gail model versus 51% subjective estimate in Bowen et al., 2003). In more refined analyses, women at heightened risk, including those with a first-degree relative (FDR) or second-degree relative with breast cancer and also women recruited from health care settings greatly overestimated their personal risk (Katapodi et al., 2004). More than 60% of FDRs greatly overestimated their lifetime risk of breast cancer compared to Gail estimates (Lerman et al., 1995). In contrast, optimistic bias, that is, rating one's own risk as lower than that of the average woman, was exhibited in community samples (Aiken et al., 1995; Katapodi et al., 2004). Whereas the average subjective estimate of risk may diverge from actual risk level defined in terms of disease prevalence, subjective and objective estimates do correlate moderately—for example, $r = .46$ (Siegler et al., 1995); $r = .41$ (Gerend, Aiken, West, et al., 2004). Yet, among FDRs, Gail model risk components were found to be unrelated to numerical ratings (0% to 100%) of the chance of getting breast cancer someday (Daly et al., 1996).

COMPARATIVE RISK AND UNREALISTIC OPTIMISM

Although people overestimate their absolute risk of cancer, studies of comparative risk suggest that individuals do exhibit unrealistic optimism, or *optimistic bias* (Weinstein, 1980, 1987; Weinstein & Klein, 1996); that is, they believe they are less likely to contract specific cancers than are others their own age. This bias has been demonstrated for breast cancer (Aiken et al., 1995), skin cancer (A. J. Miller, Ashton, McHoskey, & Gimbel, 1990), and colorectal cancer (Blalock et al., 1990; Lipkus et al., 1996), as well as brain cancer, leukemia, and lung cancer (Lek & Bishop, 1995). When asked to compare their risk to that of women without a family history of breast cancer, FDRs of women with breast cancer accurately estimate their comparative risk as high (Audrain et al., 1997; Lerman, Kash, & Stefanek, 1994). However, when asked to compare their risk to that of others their own age with family history unspecified, a substantial portion of FDRs incorrectly rate their risk as lower than average (Aiken et al., 1995; Blalock et al., 1990). Harris and Smith (2005) found little understanding of communications of either absolute or comparative risk concerning health risks of low probability, and they recommended against providing information about comparative risk to communicate low risk.

NUMERACY AND LAY UNDERSTANDING OF RISK

The level of numeracy in the lay public, defined as "facility with basic probability and numerical concepts" (L. M. Schwartz et al., 1997) is critical in risk-related research (Fischhoff, Bostrom, & Quadrel, 1993), in the comprehension of risk (Reyna, Nelson, Han, & Dieckmann, 2009), and in treatment settings (L. M. Schwartz et al., 1997). Communications to the public about risk are often given in numerical terms; in turn, individuals' numerical estimates of perceived risk are taken as being meaningful assessments of perceived susceptibility. The lay public has difficulty with both comprehending and employing estimates of probability (Weinstein et al., 2007). Gigerenzer, Gaissmaier, Kurz-Milcke, Schwartz, and Woloshin (2008) highlight the pervasiveness of innumeracy among the lay and professional public and how risk communications obscure understanding.

Over four decades ago, a literature developed in applications of Bayesian decision theory in psychology (W. Edwards, Lindman, & Savage, 1963), which examined how individuals estimate the probability of events and revise their probability estimates based on new information. Two principles emerged that may help to explain biases in the lay public's understanding of risk for cancer. First, people overestimate low probabilities and underestimate high probabilities (Mueller & Edmonds, 1967; see also Lichtenstein, Slovic, Fischhoff, Layman, & Combs, 1978). This finding may partially explain the overestimates of rates of specific cancers, which are low percentage on a cancer-by-cancer basis. Second, people are conservative in revising their estimates of probabilities in the face of new information (Phillips & Edwards, 1966), which may partially account for some failures of training to eradicate biases in perceived risk.

Substantial effort has been devoted to improving the communication of risk, including at the federal level by the U.S. National Cancer Institute (1999, 2003). Research has focused on approaches for communication of risk. Ancker, Senathirajah, Kukafka, and Starren (2006) reviewed the design of graphs for communicating health risk. Lipkus (2007) provided a comprehensive review of current practices for communicating health risks verbally, numerically, and visually. He concluded that at the present time there were few overall recommendations for risk communication strategies. In but two examples from a broad literature on risk communication, Galesic, Garcia-Retamero, and Gigerenzer (2009) provided an example of the exploration of effective graphical displays for risk communication; de Wit, Das, and Vet (2008) explored the use of objective statistics versus personal testimonials for increasing perceived personal risk. Lundgren and McMakin (2009) provide a comprehensive handbook on communication of risk.

MODIFYING PERCEIVED SUSCEPTIBILITY AND CANCER DISTRESS THROUGH TRAINING

Interventions have aimed at modifying perceptions of susceptibility, once again, under the assumption that an accurate understanding of one's risk will serve as a motivator to cancer control and prevention–related activities. These interventions may aim either to increase or to decrease perceived susceptibility. Population targets of these interventions include individuals at high risk for cancer, among them FDRs of those with cancer, and also the population at large.

High-Risk Individuals

First-degree relatives of individuals with cancer may exhibit excessive perceived risk and associated high cancer distress associated with failure to follow screening recommendations (M. D. Schwartz et al., 2003). Interventions to reduce perceived susceptibility among FDRs have sometimes been successful (Alexander, Ross, Sumner, Nease, & Littenberg, 1995), though not in all cases (Bloom, Stewart, Chang, & You, 2006). However, women with high cancer distress benefit less from such susceptibility-focused interventions, suggesting that both cancer distress and inaccurate perceptions of risk must be simultaneously addressed (Lerman et al., 1995). Reductions in cancer distress have been achieved through individual counseling (Lerman et al., 1996; M. D. Schwartz et al., 1998). An important issue is whether clarifying that perceived risk is overestimated will lead to underutilization of mammography screening (M. D. Schwartz, Rimer, Daly, Sands, & Lerman, 1999).

General Population

The extent to which estimates of subjective risk can be made more accurate through intervention has also been explored in the general population (Weinstein & Klein, 1995), where perceived risk typically exceeds objective risk. Results have been mixed. Kreuter and Strecher (1995) reported increased accuracy in perceived risk (i.e., decreased perceived risk) for cancer in the general population following an educational intervention. Lipkus, Green, and Markus (2003) were able to increase perceived risk for colorectal cancer in a well-educated sample seen in a laboratory setting. However, providing risk information in the form of mailed pamphlets did not increase cancer worry in an older community sample (Robb et al., 2006), neither did the information on risk have any effect on perceived risk (Robb, Campbell, Evans, Miles, & Wardle, 2008). Both Quillin et al. (2004) and McCaul, Canevello, Mathwig, and Klein (2003) were able to modify perceived risk of developing cancer, but not to the substantially lower level indicated by the Gail epidemiological model. Lipkus et al. (2004) attempted to increase understanding of risk factors for colorectal cancer (CRC) under the assumption that accurate risk attributions might motivate CRC screening in a population with elevated occupational risk for CRC. Greater knowledge of CRC risk factors exhibited small correlations with perceived risk.

Examination of relationships between objective and perceived risk and interventions to improve the accuracy of perceived risk rest on the assumption that levels of objective risk are known. This may be so at a population level or for strata (e.g., ethnic groups) within the population. However, at the individual level, models of cancer risk are becoming increasingly complex, incorporating biologic and genetic data with clinical and epidemiological risk factors. The U.S. National Cancer Institute workshop "Cancer Risk Prediction Models: A Workshop on Development, Evaluation and Application" highlights these complexities (Freedman et al., 2005).

PERCEIVED SUSCEPTIBILITY AND CANCER-RELATED BEHAVIOR

In this section we consider the relationships of perceived susceptibility to both screening for early detection of cancer and cancer-preventive behavior. A critical issue for health psychology is the implication of perceptions of susceptibility for protective behavior. As we have already indicated, models of health behavior conceptualize perceived susceptibility to disease as a distal construct in a mediational chain of constructs that eventuate in health behavior. Relationships of perceived susceptibility to behavior are likely to be complex, to be mediated, moderated, or nullified by other determinants of the particular behavior in question, determinants that we explore in our discussion of perceived susceptibility and protective behavior. Given space limitations, we do not provide a comprehensive review but reference and summarize existing reviews and highlight important themes (see Katapodi et al., 2004, and Vernon, 1999, for comprehensive reviews).

THE MEDICAL CONTEXT OF SCREENING

A vast literature in the public health domain provides documentation of medical system determinants of the use of medically based cancer-screening tests. Health care coverage involves a usual source of care, age, and educational attainment, which are all associated with breast, colorectal, and cervical cancer screening (Meissner et al., 2009). Racial and ethnic disparities persist (Halbert & Wetter, 2008). Beyond financial and health system barriers, these disparities are associated with access, language and acculturation, literacy, and cultural beliefs (Peek & Han, 2004), as well as general mistrust of the health care system, racial profiling, and discrimination (Gerend & Pai, 2008). These variables set limits on the impact of psychosocial variables on screening utilization.

TEMPORAL ISSUES IN THE PERCEIVED RISK–BEHAVIOR RELATIONSHIP

The nature of the relationship of perceived risk to behavior is more complex than a unidirectional conception of perceived risk as a force that motivates behavior. Brewer, Weinstein, Cuite, and Herrington (2004) suggest three hypotheses concerning the manner in which risk and behavior may be related, of which the first two hypotheses propose opposite causal relations between perceived risk and behavior; the third is purely correlational. The behavior *motivation hypothesis*, consonant with models of health behavior, proposes that risk perceptions precede and increase protective action. The reverse is also possible, that taking health-protective action may lower actual risk, leading to a reduction in perceived risk, the *risk reappraisal* hypothesis. The third proposal, the *accuracy hypothesis*, holds that risk perception at any point in time accurately reflects one's level of risk behavior combined with other risk factors operating at that time. Much research linking risk perception to behavior is cross-sectional and correlative in nature and cannot distinguish among these hypotheses (Brewer et al., 2007).

For both prevention and detection, the cross-sectional relationship of perceived risk to behavior changes in complex ways as health innovations diffuse over time (Weinstein & Nicolich, 1993). When a health-protective behavior is first introduced, those who perceive themselves at the highest risk for the health threat may self-select the behavior, occasioning a strong positive correlation between perceived risk and behavior. If the behavior is screening, then perceived vulnerability to the occurrence of the disease should not diminish as the behavior is adopted, because screening is not, of course, preventive. In fact, perceived severity may diminish if people come to believe in the benefits of early detection for cancer survival. However, as a screening innovation is adopted broadly by the medical profession and increasing numbers of individuals are screened, the pool of screened individuals will contain individuals at lower perceived risk, thus diluting the correlation of perceived risk and screening. For preventive behavior, the initial self-selection of high-risk individuals may again result in substantial positive correlations between perceived risk and behavior. However, should the disease risk be mitigated or substantially lessened by the preventive behavior, then a negative correlation may, in time, be observed between perceived risk and behavior; thus those who reliably engage in the behavior may correctly perceive themselves to be at lower risk. (See Aiken et al., 1995, for a consideration of temporal factors in perceived and objective risk as related to mammography screening; see Gerrard et al., 1996, for a critical discussion of these relationships in the HIV/AIDS context.)

PERCEIVED SUSCEPTIBILITY AND CANCER SCREENING

In a review of cervical, breast, and colorectal cancer screening, Vernon (1999) highlighted inconsistent relationships of perceived risk to screening. McCaul, Branstetter, Schroeder, and Glasgow (1996) provided a meta-analysis of the relationship between perceived breast cancer risk and mammography screening, which has been extended by Katapodi et al. (2004). In a combined sample of 52,766 cases across studies, perceived risk exhibited a small significant correlation with mammography-screening adherence (see Katapodi, 2004, Table 9). When considered in the context of Leventhal's characterization of the lay representation of cancer, only perceived risk was associated with intentions to obtain a mammogram or to undergo genetic testing (Bowen et al., 2003). Perceived susceptibility is also associated with colorectal cancer–screening compliance (Brawarsky, Brooks, & Mucci, 2003; Weinberg, Turner, Wang, Myers, & Miller, 2004). Manne et al. (2003) reported a small correlation between perceived susceptibility and intentions for colonoscopy among FDRs with colon cancer. Perceived susceptibility is not a proxy for family history but predicts screening compliance above and beyond family history (Aiken, West, Woodward, & Reno, 1994). Perceived susceptibility also predicts intention to sun protect and to avoid sunbathing more strongly than does objective risk based on skin type (Jackson & Aiken, 2000). As we have argued, the relationship of perceived susceptibility to intentions and behavior has been found to be moderated by other psychosocial variables. Aiken, West, Woodward, and Reno (1994) found that susceptibility related to compliance with mammography screening only when perceived barriers to screening were low; under high perceived barriers, no such relationship was observed.

FEAR, WORRY, CANCER DISTRESS, AND SCREENING BEHAVIOR

In both the general population and in FDRs of individuals with cancer, fear of cancer, worry about cancer, and cancer distress have been associated with both insufficient screening and excessive screening, thus providing a plethora of conflicting results across studies.

General Population

In an extensive literature summary, Hay et al. (2005) reported both positive and negative cross-sectional relationships between worry and cancer screening. They argue that cross-sectional associations may reflect increased screening in response to worry or decreased worry as a result of negative test outcomes. In a meta-analysis of longitudinal studies including both the general population and high-risk individuals, Hay, McCaul, and Magnan (2006) reported an averaged weighted correlation of .12 of cancer worry with subsequent screening. However, in an inner-city population, an inverted U-shaped relationship was observed; moderate worry about breast cancer was associated with greater attendance at a first mammography screening than was either extreme (Sutton, Bickler, Sancho-Aldridge, & Saidi, 1994). The same inverted U-shaped relationship was observed between BSE frequency and breast cancer worries (Lerman et al., 1991).

Ethnic and demographic differences in the association between emotional aspects of cancer and screening have yielded inconsistent results. Among older low-income Mexican American women, fear of and fatalism about cancer were associated with lower Pap smear rates (Suarez, Roche, Nichols, & Simpson, 1997), as was fear of cancer among a wide range of low-acculturated Hispanic women (Coronado, Thompson, Koepsell, Schwartz, & McLerran, 2004). Worry negatively related to mammography screening among African American women (Friedman et al., 1995) but positively in a noteworthy study of the role of emotional characteristics to screening in six urban-residing ethnic groups (Consedine, Magai, & Neugut, 2004). In a sample with a substantial inner-city component, Bastani et al. (1994) reported a strong negative association between fear of finding breast cancer and screening; similar findings were reported for cervical screening among rurally residing women (Coronado et al., 2004).

High-Risk Individuals

There is debate coupled with conflicting results as to whether cancer worry and cancer-specific distress increase or decrease screening among high-risk individuals. Among women who had just received a biopsy for breast cancer diagnosis, a third of the women, those most distressed, did not pursue medical follow-up (Andrykowski et al., 2001). An inverted U-shaped relationship between cancer worry and mammography screening has been observed in a higher risk community sample (Andersen, Smith, Meischke, Bowen, & Urban, 2003). Ovarian cancer worries among FDRs have been positively associated with screening (M. D. Schwartz, Lerman, Daly, et al., 1995). In contrast, high breast cancer distress (i.e., extreme worry, intrusive thoughts about breast cancer) among FDRs is associated with reduced screening (Lerman et al., 1993; see also Kash, Holland, Halper, & Miller, 1992; Lerman et al., 1994), though the opposite has also been found (Stefanek & Wilcox, 1991). Most studies are cross-sectional, posing difficulty in directional interpretation between distress and screening. Among a community sample of FDRs of women with breast cancer, M. D. Schwartz et al. (2003) showed that together cancer worry and general distress both negatively predicted screening at 12-month follow-up. Cancer distress among FDRs of women with breast and ovarian cancer is associated with high perceived risk of cancer and low perceived control over cancer development (Audrain et al., 1997).

Conflicting Findings and the Elusive Inverted U-Shaped Function

In the classic fear communication literature, Janis and Feshbach (1953) argued that fear served as a positive motivator for protective behavior up to some critical level of fear. Above that critical fear level, avoidance of the threat was expected to replace protective behavior, yielding an inverted U-shaped relationship between level of fear and behavior. If this U-shaped relationship exists, then in general community samples with very few highly distressed individuals, the relationship of worry to screening would be positive; it would reverse only in samples with a substantial representation of at-risk highly distressed individuals, as in the findings of M. D. Schwartz et al. (2003). The meta-analyses of susceptibility and worry in relation to screening cited here have included a predominance of individuals who are not at extreme high risk (Hay, McCaul, & Magnan, 2006; Katapodi, 2004; McCaul, Branstetter, et al., 1996); here, positive relationships of perceived risk and cancer worry to screening have been observed. Consedine, Magai, Krivoshekova, Ryzewicz, and Neuget

(2004) provide a critical review of fear, anxiety, and worry in relation to breast cancer screening; they caution that the specificity of fears is critical for the direction of relationship to screening.

INTERVENTIONS TO INCREASE SCREENING

In this section we address interventions to increase cancer screening and, more specifically, attempts to link manipulations of perceived susceptibility to increased screening. There is a vast literature on mammography screening and a newer literature on colorectal screening. Experimental interventions provide the vehicle for untangling the causal impact of such putative determinants as perceived vulnerability on cancer-protective behavior. They potentially speak to the temporal issues in the relationship between perceived susceptibility and screening raised by Brewer et al. (2004). We provide a brief review of screening interventions, particularly those involving tailored messages.

From the perspective of health psychology, theory-based interventions that employ such models as the HBM to design program components are most of interest because they potentially permit us to link changes in constructs in the model (e.g., perceived susceptibility) to changes in screening behaviors. A number of early mammography-screening interventions included components designed to increase perceived susceptibility to breast cancer (e.g., Aiken, West, Woodward, Reno, & Reynolds, 1994; Champion, 1994; Curry, Taplin, Anderman, Barlow, & McBride, 1993; Rimer et al., 1992; Skinner, Strecher, & Hospers, 1994; Zapka et al., 1993). In some studies, the perceived susceptibility component was only one small part of a large complex intervention, and no attempt was made to establish a direct linkage from this component to behavioral outcomes (Champion, 1994; Rimer et al., 1992; Zapka et al., 1993).

TAILORED INTERVENTIONS

With advances in computer technology, a newer generation of tailored intervention has emerged. Tailoring of messages is defined as "any combination of strategies and information intended to reach one specific person, based on characteristics that are unique to that person, related to the outcome of interest, and derived from an individual assessment" (Kreuter, Farrell, Olevitch, & Brennan, 2000, p. 277). From the perspective of perceived susceptibility, the provision of tailored risk information would theoretically modify perceived susceptibility in service of increasing cancer detection and prevention–related behaviors. Early studies of tailored messages (Curry et al., 1993) showed that providing tailored personal objective risk information to FDRs of breast cancer victims increased screening; the same result was reported by Skinner et al. (1994) in a community sample.

Three meta-analyses have addressed the relationship of individualized tailoring of interventions to screening. In a Cochrane review of 13 interventions that communicated individualized risk information, including 10 mammography programs (A. Edwards, Unigwe, Elwyn, & Hood, 2003), individualized risk communication was associated with increased screening (odds ratio = 1.5, 95% CI: 1.11–2.03). However, a reduction in screening was noted in the two interventions that provided the most detailed risk estimate information. This meta-analysis provided no information as to the relationship of perceived susceptibility (rather than objective risk information provided) to screening. In a more recent meta-analysis of 57 behavior change interventions, the 13 interventions for mammography, colorectal, or cervical (PAP) screening yielded a positive effect size ($r = .083$, 95% CI: .069–.097) of tailored messages over generic messages on screening (Noar, Benac, & Harris, 2007). Across all 57 interventions, the presence of perceived susceptibility as a component of the intervention was associated with a smaller effect size than not having this component ($r = .043$, 95% CI: .031–.055; versus $r = .100$, 95% CI: .089–.111, respectively). A third meta-analysis of tailored interventions to promote mammography screening (Sohl & Moyer, 2007) showed a small positive effect of tailoring on screening (odds ratio = 1.42, 95% CI: 1.27–1.60) and also reported that interventions that used the health belief model (which includes perceived susceptibility as a key construct) were associated with higher screening rates (weighted aggregate odds ratio for interventions tailored based on the complete HBM = 3.33).

That Noar et al. (2007) reported a smaller effect size for tailored interventions that included a perceived susceptibility component led us to review in detail the 13 articles from the meta-analysis that targeted mammography, colorectal, or cervical screening. Among these articles, Rimer et al. (2001, 2002) communicated to each participant her own Gail risk score for breast cancer and any specific factor (e.g., nullparity) that led to her particular elevated risk. The intervention substantially reduced the initial great overestimation of breast cancer risk by participants. However, perceived risk following the tailored intervention did not relate to increase in screening. Similarly, Bastani, Maxwell, Bradford, Das, and Yan (1999) found perceived risk to be unrelated to screening. Others of the interventions targeted specific cancer risk in individualized communications but did not provide information that could relate perceived risk to screening. Recent tailored colorectal-screening interventions (Glanz, Steffen, & Taglialatela, 2007; Lipkus, Skinner, et al., 2005) reported increases in perceived risk as a function of intervention but no association between perceived risk and screening. Finally, recent tailored interventions for mammography and colon cancer screening (Champion et al., 2007; Rawl et al., 2008) integrated perceived risk manipulations into tailored messages but did not report the impact on perceived susceptibility or the relationship of perceived susceptibility to screening.

MEDIATION ANALYSIS: UNCOVERING HOW INTERVENTIONS INDUCE CHANGE

It is apparent from the brief review of interventions to increase screening, particularly tailored interventions, that there is a great opportunity to assess not only whether interventions increase screening but also to examine the mechanisms by which interventions have brought about behavior change. Mediation analysis provides a vehicle for uncovering these mechanisms of change (Aiken, in press; MacKinnon, 2008; West & Aiken, 1997). Mediation analysis is a class of statistical procedures employed to establish chains of relationships among a series of constructs. For mediation analysis of interventions, we examine chains from the intervention through one or more constructs (e.g., perceived susceptibility to a disease, perceived benefits of a health action) to some outcome (e.g., mammography screening). We present mediation analyses of three interventions from our own laboratories. These three examples cover the classes of cancer-related behavior we identified at the outset of the chapter: cancer screening, protective behaviors, and new HPV vaccination. Our examples illustrate how mediation analysis characterizes the mechanisms underlying an intervention, with particular emphasis on the role of perceived susceptibility.

We note several other examples of the use of mediation analysis in recent cancer-screening literature. Manne et al. (2003) provide an example of a mediation analysis of a psychosocial study of intention to undergo colonoscopy. Hall, French, and Marteau (2009) provide a mediation analysis of interventions for smoking cessation; Reynolds, Buller, Yaroch, Maloy, and Cutter (2006), for sun protection.

INTERVENTION DESIGN AND MEASUREMENT REQUIREMENTS FOR MEDIATION ANALYSIS

In order to test the theory of an intervention through mediation analysis, the following are required: (a) a specified theoretical model on which the program will be built, (b) a measurement instrument that provides distinct measures of each construct in the model that will serve as a mediator, (c) a translation of each construct of the model into a distinct component of the intervention, (d) assessment of postintervention levels on each of the constructs targeted in the model in an experimental group versus a control group (with adequate statistical control of pretest levels), and (e) measurement of the outcome. West and Aiken (1997) summarize the conditions that must be met in order to demonstrate that a putative mediator is associated with or produced change in the outcome, as specified by Judd and Kenny (1981), Baron and Kenny (1986), and MacKinnon (2008).

MEDIATION ANALYSIS OF A MAMMOGRAPHY-SCREENING INTERVENTION

Aiken, West, Woodward, Reno, et al. (1994) implemented an HBM-based mammography intervention, with individual program components that targeted each of the four HBM constructs: perceived susceptibility, severity, benefits, and barriers. We used mediation analysis to test the linkages from an intervention through intermediate *mediators* (the HBM components) to mammography compliance. We amended the HBM by assessing intentions for screening at immediate posttest, as well as actual compliance 3 months following the intervention. We established paths from perceived susceptibility and perceived benefits to intentions and established a strong link from intentions to subsequent screening. The role of perceived susceptibility in the causal chain from intervention through compliance is of interest here. Our model of the impact of HBM constructs on outcomes is illustrated in Figure 6.1. It differs from typical characterizations of the HBM in that the four HBM constructs are not treated as coequal predictors of the outcome. Rather, following Ronis (1992), we specified a model in which perceived susceptibility and perceived severity were antecedents of perceived benefits, under the assumption that a woman would not perceive the benefits of mammography screening unless she felt threatened (perceived susceptibility plus severity) by breast cancer. Again following Ronis (1992), we specified that the effect of perceived susceptibility on the outcome would be mediated through perceived benefits—that is, that the effect of susceptibility would be an *indirect effect* through benefits—in the following causal sequence: intervention → susceptibility → benefits → intentions → behavioral steps to mammography compliance. This mediational chain was supported. In addition, we observed a *direct path* from susceptibility to intentions: intervention → susceptibility → intentions. The size of the indirect effect of susceptibility, over and above the direct effect, was substantial. The full details of the mediation analysis, including our explorations of possible roles for perceived susceptibility, are provided in West and Aiken (1997). What is criti-

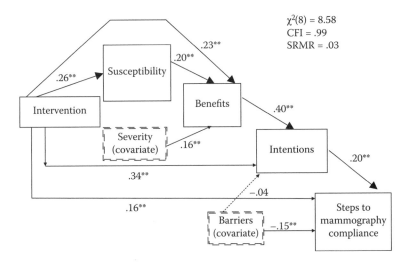

FIGURE 6.1 Mediation analysis of the impact of a health belief model (HBM)–based intervention on compliance with mammography-screening recommendations. The indirect mediational path from intervention to perceived susceptibility through perceived benefits to intentions for screening illustrates how perceived susceptibility serves as an apparent precursor to benefits in the HBM. For paths, ** $p < .01$. (Modified from Aiken, L. S., West, S. G., Woodward, C. K., Reno, R. R., and Reynolds, K. D., *Health Psychology, 13,* 534, 1994. With permission.)

cal here is a conception of perceived susceptibility at the outset of a causal chain that flows through other constructs.

MEDIATION ANALYSIS OF A SUN PROTECTION INTERVENTION

Jackson and Aiken (2006) provided a mediation analysis of a sun protection intervention designed to increase sun protection and decrease sunbathing. Given a youthful female population, the intervention targeted susceptibility to photoaging as a proximal damaging effect of sun exposure. Jackson and Aiken (2006) provided full details of the mediation analysis, which is illustrated in Figure 6.2. The analysis illustrates a powerful role for perceived susceptibility to photoaging. The link from intervention to susceptibility to benefits to intentions was again observed, consistent with Aiken, West, Woodward, Reno, et al. (1994). In addition, there was a link from intervention to susceptibility to both intention to sunbathe and to sun protect and also to hours of sun bathing and of sun protection of the face and body. Mediation analysis offered a characterization of the rich, multifaceted role of perceived susceptibility in effecting behavior change.

PERCEIVED SUSCEPTIBILITY AND HPV VACCINATION

Studies of the new HPV vaccination have examined both the acceptability of the vaccine and the initiation of use as a function of perceived susceptibility to HPV infection. Reiter, Brewer, Gottlieb, McRee, and Smith (2009) found parents' perceived risk for their daughters contracting HPV was associated with initiation of the HPV vaccination among their daughters. Gerend, Shepherd, and Monday (2008) examined the effect of message framing on acceptability of the HPV vaccination. Gain-framed messages highlight the benefits of a health-protective action, whereas loss-framed messages characterize the negative consequences of failure to adopt the action. As explained by Gerend et al. (2008), loss-framed messages are expected to engender increased perceptions of risk and severity of consequences, which should serve as a mediator from the message to action. Gerend

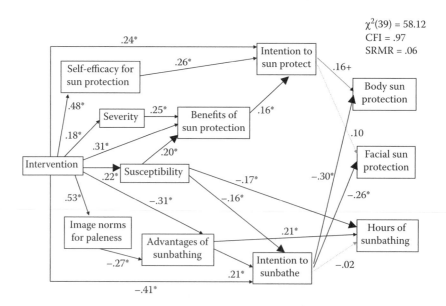

FIGURE 6.2 Mediation analysis of the impact of a hybrid model–based intervention on sun protection and sunbathing. Perceived susceptibility serves as mediator from the intervention to perceived benefits to intentions for sun protection and also through intention to sunbathe to sun protection, and directly to sunbathing. (Modified from Jackson, K. M. and Aiken, L. S., *Health Psychology, 25,* 42, 2006. With permission.)

et al. (2008) found support for a mediational role of perceived susceptibility to HPV in accounting for the acceptability of HPV vaccination among college-aged women. Gerend et al. (2008) provide an extensive discussion of the role of message framing in health behaviors that are effortful over time as opposed to being one-shot behaviors. They expand on an earlier review by Rothman and Salovey (1997). Earlier studies of message framing for cancer-related behavior include Meyerowitz and Chaiken (1987), Rothman, Salovey, Antone, Keough, and Martin (1993), and Banks et al. (1995) for breast self-examination, skin protection, and mammography utilization, respectively.

THE NEED FOR MEDIATION ANALYSIS OF INTERVENTIONS: IDENTIFYING PROCESSES UNDERLYING HEALTH-PROTECTIVE BEHAVIOR

We end with a message to our colleagues about the utility of the examination of interventions to uncover the processes that lead to behavior change. A powerful conception of perceived susceptibility in models of health behavior is that perceived susceptibility stands at the outset of a causal chain that flows through other constructs to health behavior. Clearly, tailored interventions that provide individualized information about risk factors implicitly assume that knowledge of risk factors will lead to modified perceptions of perceived vulnerability that will in turn lead to enhanced health protection through early detection and preventive action. Consideration of mediational chains from intervention to perceived susceptibility to behavior or through other constructs to behavior is critical for advancing our understanding of how health behaviors accrue. Examination of both the direct effect and the indirect effects of susceptibility through other variables on behavior is required to estimate accurately the total effect of perceived susceptibility on health-protective behavior. Examining only the direct effects of susceptibility on intentions or behavior may obscure the role of perceived susceptibility in the behavioral compliance process, potentially leading to underestimates of the total effect of perceived susceptibility on behavior.

What we argue here is not at all limited to perceived risk. Our understanding of whether, how, and to what extent many individual variables operate in determining health-protective behavior is best advanced through the evaluation of model-based interventions, with research structured so that mediation analysis of the effects of putative determinants of behavior can be accomplished (Aiken, in press; West & Aiken, 1997). A distinguishing feature of psychology as a discipline is our strength in theory and experimentation. Thus, health psychologists may provide a special role in health behavior research, providing careful theory testing in controlled settings and placing the refinement of our models of health behavior on a strong empirical base.

CONCLUSION

We conclude where we began, with the theoretical perspective that perceived susceptibility to disease is an important early force in the adoption of health-protective behavior. We caution researchers who seek high correlations of perceived susceptibility with behavior that even when individuals perceive themselves at high risk for a threat to health, other forces mediate and moderate and even nullify the susceptibility–behavior relationship. Critical to the link of perceived susceptibility to behavior is an effective vehicle to mitigate threat. Levanthal's (1970) theorizing over four decades ago rings true—that people who perceive themselves to be at risk will act to protect their health if there is an effective action to be taken, but that they will deny the risk if there is no protective action available. Stated otherwise, the availability of an effective health-protective action moderates the relationship of perceived susceptibility to behavior; the absence of an effective health-protective behavior nullifies the impact of perceived susceptibility. We have seen repeatedly in our own intervention research that perceived benefits of a health action mediate the relationship of perceived susceptibility to health-protective behavior. Even when there is effective protective action, barriers to that action (e.g., access to appropriate medical care, difficulty of carrying out the protective behavior itself) moderate the relationship of perceived susceptibility to health-protective behavior.

There are added complexities in uncovering and understanding the relationship of perceived susceptibility to health-protective behavior. Temporal issues abound—when a health-protective action first becomes available (e.g., mammography screening), the early adopters may be those who perceive themselves at greatest risk. Later, when adoption is widespread, it may be those who have not taken protective action who feel most at risk; thus the correlation between perceived susceptibility and behavior may change from positive to negative over time. The measurement of perceived susceptibility is fraught with challenges—these include the innumeracy of the public and the multiple approaches to measurement. In our own work we have shown that one commonly used measure of perceived susceptibility correlates negatively with behavior if the prevalence of the health risk is high (Ranby et al., 2010); the reason for this anomaly lies in the measurement strategy. Better approaches to communicating and assessing perceived susceptibility are needed. Perceptions of risk are multiply determined, with correlates based in the threat itself (e.g., preventability of the threat), in heuristic thinking (e.g., availability of a positive instance), and individual characteristics (e.g., neuroticism). Other factors, among them worry about a particular disease, often associated with a strong family history, contribute complexity to defining a distinct role for perceived susceptibility.

Despite the challenges to uncovering the role of perceived susceptibility to health-protective behavior, the vast existing literature and our own intervention research program lead us to conclude that perceived susceptibility is, in fact, an important distal force in a chain of constructs leading to health behavior. The strongest tests of hypotheses concerning the role of perceived susceptibility are implemented in the context of randomized trials of interventions that are specifically designed to permit mediation and moderation analyses of the putative mechanisms through which perceived susceptibility may shape health-protective behavior.

REFERENCES

Aiken, L. S. (in press). Advancing health behavior theory: The interplay among theories of health behavior, modeling of health behavior, and behavioral interventions. In H.S. Friedman (Ed.), *Oxford handbook of health psychology*. New York, NY: Oxford University Press.

Aiken, L. S., Fenaughty, A. M., West, S. G., Johnson, J. J., & Luckett, T. L. (1995). Perceived determinants of risk for breast cancer and the relations among objective risk, perceived risk, and screening behavior over time. *Women's Health: Research on Gender, Behavior, and Policy, 1*, 27–50.

Aiken, L. S., West, S. G., Woodward, C. K., & Reno, R. R. (1994). Health beliefs and compliance with mammography-screening recommendations in asymptomatic women. *Health Psychology, 13*, 122–129.

Aiken, L. S., West, S. G., Woodward, C. K., Reno, R. R., & Reynolds, K. D. (1994). Increasing screening mammography in asymptomatic women: Evaluation of a second-generation, theory-based program. *Health Psychology, 13*, 526–538.

Ajzen, I. (1991). The theory of planned behavior. *Organizational behavior and human decision processes, 50*, 179–211.

Ajzen, I., & Fishbein, M. (1980). *Understanding attitudes and predicting social behavior.* Englewood Cliffs, NJ: Prentice-Hall.

Alexander, N. E., Ross, J., Sumner, W., Nease, R. F., & Littenberg, B. (1995). The effect of an educational intervention on the perceived risk of breast cancer. *Journal of General Internal Medicine, 11*, 92–97.

American Cancer Society. (2008). Cancer prevention and early detection facts and figures, 2008. Atlanta, GA: American Cancer Society.

American Cancer Society. (2009). Cancer prevalence: How many people have cancer. Retrieved from http://www.cancer.org/docroot/CRI/content/CRI_2_6x_Lifetime_Probability_of_Developing_or_Dying_From_Cancer.asp?

American Cancer Society. (2010a). American Cancer Society guidelines for the early detection of cancer. Retrieved from http://www.cancer.org/docroot/ped/content/ped_2_3x_acs_cancer_detection_guidelines_36.asp

American Cancer Society. (2010b). Human papilloma virus (HPV), cancer, and HPV vaccines. Retrieved from http://www.cancer.org/docroot/CRI/content/CRI_2_6x_FAQ_HPV_Vaccines.asp

Ancker, J. S., Senathirajah, Y., Kukafka, R., & Starren, J. B. (2006). Design features of graphs in health risk communication: A systematic review. *Journal of the American Medical Information Association, 13*, 608–618.

Andersen, M. R., Smith, R., Meischke, H., Bowen, D., & Urban, N. (2003). Breast cancer worry and mammography use by women with and without a family history in a population-based sample. *Cancer Epidemiology Biomarkers and Prevention, 12*, 314–320.

Andrykowski, M. A., Carpenter, J. S., Studts, L. J., Cordova, M. J., Cunningham, L. L., Mager, … McGrath, P. (2001). Adherence to recommendations for clinical follow-up after benign breast biopsy. *Breast Cancer Research and Treatment, 69*, 165–178.

Audrain, J., Schwartz, M. D., Lerman, C., Hughes, C., Peshkin, B. N, & Biesecker, B. (1997). Psychological distress in women seeking genetic counseling for breast-ovarian cancer risk: The contributions of personality and appraisal. *Annals of Behavioral Medicine, 19*, 370–377.

Azzarello, L. M. (2006). Psychological factors associated with skin cancer detection behaviors. *Dissertation Abstracts International: Section B. The Sciences and Engineering, 66*(7–B), 3937.

Banks, S. M., Salovey, P., Greener, S., Rothman, A. J., Moyer, A., Beauvais, J., & Epel, E. (1995). The effects of message framing on mammography utilization. *Health Psychology, 14*, 178–184.

Baron, R. M., & Kenny, D. A. (1986). The moderator-mediator variable distinction in social psychological research: Conceptual, strategic, and statistical considerations. *Journal of Personality and Social Psychology, 51*, 1173–1182.

Bastani, R., Marcus, A. C., & Hollatz-Brown, A. (1991). Screening mammography rates and barriers to use: A Los Angeles survey. *Preventive Medicine, 20*, 350–363.

Bastani, R., Marcus, A. C., Maxwell, A. E., Das, I. P., & Yan, K. X. (1994). Evaluation of an intervention to increase mammography screening in Los Angeles. *Preventive Medicine, 23*, 83–90.

Bastani, R., Maxwell, A. E., Bradford, C., Das, I. P., & Yan, M. A. (1999). Tailored risk notification for women with a family history of breast cancer. *Preventive Medicine, 29*, 355–364.

Beck, K. H., & Frankel, A. (1981). A conceptualization of threat communications and protective health behavior. *Social Psychology Quarterly, 44*, 204–217.

Becker, M. (1990). Theoretical models of adherence and strategies for improving adherence. In S. A. Shumaker, E. G. Schron, J. K. Ockene, C. T. Parker, J. L. Probstfield, & J. M. Wolle (Eds.), *The handbook of health behavior change* (pp. 5–43). New York, NY: Springer.

Becker, M. H., & Maiman, L. A. (1975). Sociobehavioral determinants of compliance with health and medical care recommendations. *Medical Care, 8*, 10–24.

Berman, S. H., & Wandersman, A. (1992). Measuring fear of cancer: The fear of cancer index. *Psychology and Health, 7*, 187–200.

Black, W. C., Nease, R. F., Jr., & Tosteson, A. N. A. (1995). Perceptions of breast cancer risk and screening effectiveness in women younger than 50 years of age. *Journal of the National Cancer Institute, 87*, 720–731.

Blalock, S. J., DeVellis, B. M., Afifi, R. A., & Sandler, R. S. (1990). Risk perceptions and participation in colorectal cancer screening. *Health Psychology, 9*, 792–806.

Bloom, J. R., Stewart, S. L., Chang, S., & You, M. (2006). Effects of a telephone counseling intervention on sisters of young women with breast cancer. *Preventive Medicine, 2006*, 379–384.

Bowen, D. J., Helmes, A., Powers, D., Anderson, M. A., Burke, W., McTiernan, A., & Drufy, S. (2003). Predicting breast screening intentions and behavior with emotion and cognition. *Journal of Social and Clinical Psychology, 22*, 213–232.

Brawarsky, P., Brooks, D. R., & Mucci, L. A. (2003). Correlates of colorectal cancer screening in Massachusetts men and women. *Preventive Medicine, 36*, 659–668.

Breen, N., & Meissner, H. I. (2005). Toward a system of cancer screening in the United States: Trends and opportunities. *Annual Review of Public Health, 26*, 561–581.

Brewer, N. T., Chapman, G. B., Gibbons, F. X., Gerrard, M., McCaul, K. D., & Weinstein, N .D. (2007). Meta-analysis of the relationship between risk perception and health behavior: The example of vaccination. *Health Psychology, 26*, 136–145.

Brewer, N. T., Weinstein, N. D., Cuite, C. L., & Herrington, J. E. (2004). Risk perceptions and their relation to risk behavior. *Annals of Behavioral Medicine, 27*, 125–130.

Cameron, L. D. (2003). Conceptualizing and assessing risk perceptions: A self-regulatory perspective. Paper presented at the Conceptualizing and Measuring Risk Perceptions Workshop, February 13–14, 2003, Washington, DC. Accessed from http://cancercontrol.cancer.gov/brp/presentations/cameron.pdf

Cameron, L. D., & Leventhal, H. (2003). *The self regulation of health and illness behaviour*. London, England: Routledge.

Chambers, J. R., & Windschitl, P. D. (2004). Biases in social comparative judgments: The role of nonmotivated factors in above-average and comparative-optimism effects. *Psychological Bulletin, 130*, 813–838.

Champion, V. L. (1994). Strategies to increase mammography utilization. *Medical Care, 32*, 118–129.

Champion, V., Skinner, C. S., Hue, S., Monahan, P., Juliar, B., Daggy, J., & Menon, U. (2007). The effect of telephone versus print tailoring for mammography adherence. *Patient Education and Counseling*, *65*, 416–423.

Clemow, L., Stoddard, A. M., Costanza, M. E., Haddad, W. P., Luckmann, R., White, M. J., & Klaus, D. (2000). Underutilizers of mammography screening today: Characteristics of women planning, undecided about, and not planning a mammogram. *Annals of Behavioral Medicine*, *22*, 80–88.

Conner, M., & Norman, P. (Eds.). (2005). *Predicting health behavior: Research and practice with social cognition models* (2nd ed.). Maidenhead, England: Open University Press.

Consedine, N. S., Magai, C., Krivoshekova, Y. S., Ryzewicz, L., & Neuget, A. I. (2004). Fear, anxiety, worry, and breast cancer screening behavior: A critical review. *Cancer Epidemiology Biomarkers and Prevention*, *13*, 501–510.

Consedine, N. S., Magai, C., & Neugut, A. I. (2004). The contribution of emotional characteristics to breast cancer screening among women from six ethnic groups. *Preventive Medicine*, *38*, 64–77.

Coronado, G. D., Thompson, B., Koepsell, T. D., Schwartz, S. M., & McLerran, D. (2004). Use of Pap test among Hispanics and non-Hispanic whites in a rural setting. *Preventive Medicine*, *38*, 713–722.

Covey, J. A., & Davies, A. D. M. (2004). Are people unrealistically optimistic? It depends how you ask them. *British Journal of Health Psychology*, *9*, 39–49.

Curry, S. J., & Emmons, K. M. (1994). Theoretical models for predicting and improving compliance with breast cancer screening. *Annals of Behavioral Medicine*, *16*, 302–316.

Curry, S. J., Taplin, S. H., Anderman, C., Barlow, W. E., & McBride, C. (1993). A randomized trial of the impact of risk assessment and feedback on participation in mammography screening. *Preventive Medicine*, *22*, 350–360.

Daly, M. B, Lerman, C. L., Ross, E., Schwartz, M. D., Sands, C. B., & Masny, A. (1996). Gail model breast cancer risk components are poor predictors of risk perception and screening behavior. *Breast Cancer Research and Treatment*, *41*, 59–70.

Damasio, A. R. (1994). *Descartes' error: Emotion, reason, and the human brain*. New York, NY: Avon.

Darvill, T. J., & Johnson, R. C. (1991). Optimism and perceived control of life events as related to personality. *Personality and Individual Differences*, *12*, 951–954.

De Hoog, N., Stroebe, W., & de Wit, J. B. F. (2007). The impact of vulnerability to and severity of a health risk on processing and acceptance of fear-arousing communications: A meta-analysis. *Review of General Psychology*, *11*, 258–285.

De Wit, J. B. F., Das, E., & Vet, R. (2008). What works best: Objective statistics or a personal testimonial? An assessment of the persuasive effects of different types of message evidence on risk perception. *Health Psychology*, *27*, 110–115.

Dolan, N. C., Lee, A. M., & McDermott, M. M. (1997). Age-related differences in breast carcinoma knowledge, beliefs, and perceived risk among women visiting an academic general medical practice. *Cancer*, *50*, 413–420.

Dziokonski, W., & Weber. S. J. (1977). Repression-sensitization, perceived vulnerability, and the fear appeal communication. *Journal of Social Psychology*, *102*, 105–112.

Edwards, A., Unigwe, S., Elwyn, G., & Hood, K. (2003). Effects of communicating individual risks in screening programs: Cochrane systematic reviews. *British Medical Journal*, *327*, 703–709.

Edwards, W., Lindman, H., & Savage, L. H. (1963). Bayesian statistical inference for psychological research. *Psychological Review*, *70*, 193–242.

Epstein, S. (1994). Integration of the cognitive and psychodynamic unconscious. *American Psychologist*, *49*, 709–724.

Finucane, M. L., Alhakami, A., Slovic, P., & Johnson, S. M. (2000). The affect heuristic in judgments of risks and benefits. *Journal of Behavioral Decision Making*, *13*, 1–17.

Fischhoff, B., Bostrom, A., & Quadrel, M. J. (1993). Risk perception and communication. *Annual Review of Public Health*, *14*, 183–203.

Fishbein, M., & Ajzen, I. (1975). *Belief, attitude, intention, and behavior: An introduction to theory and research*. Reading, MA: Addison-Wesley.

Fletcher, K. E., Clemow, L., Peterson, B. A., Lemon, S. C., Estabrook, B., & Zapka, J. G. (2006). A path analysis of factors associated with distress among first-degree female relatives of women with breast cancer diagnosis. *Health Psychology*, *25*, 413–424.

Fox, S. A., Siu, A. L., & Stein, J. A. (1994). The importance of physician communication on breast cancer screening of older women. *Archives of Internal Medicine*, *154*, 2058–2068.

Freedman, A. N., Seminara, D., Gail, M. H., Hartge, P., Colditz, G. A., Ballard-Barash, R., & Pfeiffer, R. M. (2005). Cancer risk prediction models: A workshop on development, evaluation, and application. *Journal of the National Cancer Institute*, *97*, 715–723.

Friedman, L. C., Webb, J. A., Weinberg, A. D., Lane, M., Cooper, H. P., & Woodruff, A. (1995). Breast cancer screening: Racial/ethnic differences in behaviors and beliefs. *Journal of Cancer Education, 10*, 213–216.

Gail, M. H., Brinton, L. A., Byar, D. P., Corle, D. K., Green, S. B., Schairer, C., & Mulvihill, J. J. (1989). Projecting individualized probabilities of developing breast cancer for white females who are being examined annually. *Journal of the National Cancer Institute, 81*, 1879–1886.

Galesic, M., Garcia-Retamero, R., & Gigerenzer, G. (2009). Using icon arrays to communicate medical risks: Overcoming low numeracy. *Health Psychology, 28*, 210–216.

Gerend, M. A., Aiken, L. S., & West, S. G. (2004). Personality factors in older women's perceived susceptibility to diseases of aging. *Journal of Personality, 72*, 243–270.

Gerend, M. A., Aiken, L. S., West, S. G., & Erchull, M. J. (2004). Beyond medical risk: Investigating the psychological factors underlying women's perceptions of susceptibility to breast cancer, heart disease, and osteoporosis. *Health Psychology, 23*, 247–258.

Gerend, M. A., Erchull, M. J., Aiken, L. S., & Maner, J. K. (2006). Reasons and risk: Factors underlying women's perceptions of susceptibility to osteoporosis. *Maturitas, 55*, 227–237.

Gerend, M. A., & Pai, M. (2008). Social determinants of black–white disparities in breast cancer mortality: A review. *Cancer Epidemiology Biomarkers and Prevention, 17,* 2913–2923.

Gerend, M. A., Shepherd, J. E., & Monday, K. A. (2008). Behavioral frequency moderates the effect of message framing on HBP vaccine acceptability. *Annals of Behavioral Medicine, 35*, 221–229.

Gerrard, M., Gibbons, F. X., & Bushman, B. J. (1996). Relationship between perceived vulnerability to HIV and precautionary sexual behavior. *Psychological Bulletin, 119*, 390–409.

Gigerenzer, G., Gaissmaier, W., Kurz-Milcke, E., Schwartz, L. M., & Woloshin, S. (2008). Helping doctors and patients make sense of health statistics. *Psychological Science in the Public Interest, 8*, 53–96.

Glanz, K., Rimer, B. K., & Viswanah, K. (Eds.). (2008). *Health behavior and health education: Theory, research, and practice* (4th ed.). San Francisco, CA: Jossey-Bass.

Glanz, K., Steffen, A. D., & Taglialatela, L. A. (2007). Effects of colon cancer risk counseling for first-degree relatives. *Cancer Epidemiology Biomarkers and Prevention, 16*, 1485–1491.

Gram, I. T., & Slenker, S. E. (1992). Cancer anxiety and attitudes toward mammography among screening attenders, nonattenders, and women never invited. *American Journal of Public Health, 82*, 249–251.

Green, L. W., & Kreuter, M. W. (1991). *Healthy promotion planning: An educational and environmental approach* (2nd ed.). Mountain View, CA: Mayfield.

Grunfeld, E. A. (2004). What predicts university students' intentions to practice safe sun exposure behaviors. *Journal of Adolescent Health, 35*, 486–492.

Halbert, C. H., & Wetter, D. W. (2008). Introduction to the special section on cancer disparities. *Cancer Epidemiology, Biomarkers, and Prevention, 17*, 2906–2907.

Hall, S., French, D. P., & Marteau, T. M. (2009). Do perceptions of vulnerability and worry mediate the effects of a smoking cessation intervention for women attending for a routine cervical smear test? An experimental study. *Health Psychology, 28*, 258–263.

Harris, P. (1996). Sufficient grounds for optimism: The relationship between perceived controllability and optimistic bias. *Journal of Social and Clinical Psychology, 15*, 9–52.

Harris, P., & Smith, V. (2005). When the risks are low: The impact of absolute and comparative information on disturbance and understanding in US and UK samples. *Psychology and Health, 20*, 319–330.

Harrison, J. A., Mullen, P. D., & Green, L. W. (1992). A meta-analysis of studies of the health belief model with adults. *Health Education Research, 7*, 107–116.

Hay, J., Buckley, T. R., & Ostroff, J. S. (2005). The role of cancer worry in cancer screening: A theoretical and empirical review of the literature. *Psycho-Oncology, 14*, 517–534.

Hay, J., Coups, E., & Ford, J. (2006). Predictors of perceived risk for colon cancer in a national probability sample in the United States. *Journal of Health Communication, 11*, 71–92.

Hay, J., McCaul, R. E., & Magnan, R. E. (2006). Does worry about breast cancer predict screening behavior? A meta-analysis of the prospective evidence. *Preventive Medicine, 42,* 401–408.

Helms, A. W. (2002). Application of the protection motivation theory to genetic testing for breast cancer risk. *Preventive Medicine, 35*, 453–461.

Helzlsouer, K. J., Ford, D. E., Hayward, R. S. A., Midzenski, M., & Perry, H. (1994). Perceived risk of cancer and practice of cancer prevention behaviors among employees in an oncology center. *Preventive Medicine, 23*, 302–308.

Horowitz, M., Wilner, N., & Alvarez, W. (1979). Impact of Events Scale: A measure of subjective stress. *Psychosomatic Medicine, 41*, 209–218.

Hyman, R. B., Baker, S., Ephraim, R., Moadel, A., & Philip, J. (1994). Health belief variables as predictors of screening mammography utilization. *Journal of Behavioral Medicine, 17*, 391–406.

Irwig, L., Cockburn, J., Turnbull, D., Simpson, J. M., Mock, P., & Tattersal, M. (1991). Women's perceptions of screening mammography. *Australian Journal of Public Health*, *15*, 24–32.

Jackson, K. M., & Aiken, L. S. (2000). A psychosocial model of sun-protection and sunbathing in young women: The impact of health beliefs, attitudes, norms, and self-efficacy for sun-protection. *Health Psychology*, *19*, 469–478.

Jackson, K. M., & Aiken, L. S. (2006). Evaluation of a multi-component appearance-based sun-protective intervention for young women: Uncovering the mechanisms of program efficacy. *Health Psychology*, *25*, 34–46.

Janis, I. L., & Feshbach, S. (1953). Effects of fear-arousing communications. *Journal of Abnormal and Social Psychology*, *48*, 78–92.

Janz, N. K., & Becker, M. H. (1984). The health belief model: A decade later. *Health Education Quarterly*, *11*, 1–47.

Jemal, A., Siegel, R., Ward, E., Hao, Y., Xu, J., Murray, T., & Thun, M. J. (2009). Cancer statistics, 2008. *CA: A Cancer Journal for Clinicians*, *58*, 71–96.

Judd, C. M., & Kenny, D. (1981). *Estimating the effects of social interventions*. New York, NY: Cambridge University Press.

Kahneman, D., & Tversky, A. (1973). On the psychology of prediction. *Psychological Review*, *1973*, *80*, 237–251.

Kash, K. M., Holland, J. C., Halper, M. S., & Miller, D. G. (1992). Psychological distress and surveillance behaviors of women with a family history of breast cancer. *Journal of the National Cancer Institute*, *84*, 24–30.

Kasperson, R. E., Renn, O., Slovic, P., Brown, H. S., Emel, J., Goble, R., … Ratick, S. (1988). The social amplification of risk: A conceptual framework. *Risk Analysis*, *8*, 177–187.

Katapodi, M. C., Lee, K. A., Facione, N. C., & Dodd, M. J. (2004). Predictors of perceived breast cancer risk and the relation between perceived risk and breast cancer screening: a meta-analytic review. *Preventive Medicine*, *38*, 388–402.

Kelly, K., Leventhal, H., Andrykowski, M., Toppmeyer, D., Much, J., Dermody, J., … Schwalb, M. (2005). Using the common sense model to understand perceived cancer risk in individuals testing for BRAC1/2 mutations. *Psycho-Oncology*, *14*, 34–48.

Klar, Y., & Ayal, S. (2004). Event frequency and comparative optimism: Another look at the indirect elicitation method of self–others risks. *Journal of Experimental Social Psychology*, *40*, 805–814.

Klar, Y., & Giladi, E. E. (1999). Are most people happier than their peers, or are they just happy? *Personality and Social Psychology Bulletin*, *25*, 585–594.

Klein, W. M. (1996). Maintaining self-serving social comparisons: Attenuating the perceived significance of risk-increasing behaviors. *Journal of Social and Clinical Psychology*, *15*, 120–142.

Klein, W. (2003). Self-prescriptive, perceived, and actual attention to comparative risk information. *Psychology and Health*, *18*, 625–643.

Klein, W. M., & Weinstein, N. D. (1997). Social comparison and unrealistic optimism about personal risk. In B. Buunk & F. X. Gibbons (Eds.), *Health, coping, and social comparison* (pp. 25–61). Hillsdale, NJ: Erlbaum.

Kowalewski, M. R., Henson, K. D., & Longshore, D. (1997). Rethinking perceived risk and health behavior: A critical review of HIV prevention research. *Health Education and Behavior*, *24*, 313–325.

Kreuter, M. W., Farrell, D., Olevitch, L., & Brennan, L. (2000). *Tailoring health messages: Customizing communication with computer technology*. Mahwah, NJ: Erlbaum.

Kreuter, M. W., & Strecher, V. J. (1995). Changing inaccurate perceptions of health risks: Results from a randomized trial. *Health Psychology*, *14*, 56–63.

Lek, Y., & Bishop, G. D. (1995). Perceived vulnerability to illness threats: The role of disease type, risk factor perception and attributions. *Psychology and Health*, *10*, 205–217.

Lerman, C., Daly, M., Sands, C., Balshem, A., Lustbader, E., Heggan, T., … Engstrom, P. (1993). Mammography adherence and psychological distress among women at risk for breast cancer. *Journal of the National Cancer Institute*, *85*, 1074–1080.

Lerman, C., Kash, K., & Stefanek, M. (1994). Younger women at increased risk for breast cancer: Perceived risk, psychological well-being, and surveillance behavior. *Journal of the National Cancer Institute Monographs*, *16*, 171–176.

Lerman, C., Lustbader, E., Rimer, B., Daly, M., Miller, S., Sands, C., & Balshem, A. (1995). Effects of individualized breast cancer risk counseling: A randomized trial. *Journal of the National Cancer Institute*, *87*, 286–292.

Lerman, C., & Schwartz, M. D. (1993). Adherence and psychological adjustment among women at high risk for breast cancer. *Breast Cancer Research and Treatment*, *28*, 145–155.

Lerman, C., Schwartz, M. D., Miller, S. M., Daly, M., Sands, C., & Rimer, B. K. (1996). A randomized trial of breast cancer risk counseling: Interacting effects of counseling, educational level, and coping style. *Health Psychology*, *15*, 75–83.

Lerman, C., Trock, B., Rimer, B. K., Jepson, C., Brody, D., & Boyce, A. (1991). Psychological side effects of breast cancer screening. *Health Psychology*, *10*, 259–267.

Leventhal, H. (1970). Findings and theory in the study of fear communications. In L. Berkowitz (Ed), *Advances In Experimental Social Psychology*, *5,* 119–186.

Leventhal, H., Brissette, I., & Leventhal, E. A. (2003). The common-sense model of self-regulation of health and illness. In L. D. Cameron & H. Leventhal (Eds.), *The self-regulation of health and illness behaviour* (pp. 42–65). London, England: Routledge.

Leventhal, H., Kelly, K., & Leventhal, E. A. (1999). Population risk, actual risk, and cancer control: A discussion. *Journal of the National Cancer Institute Monographs*, *25*, 81–85.

Leventhal, H., Leventhal, E., & Cameron, L. D. (2001). Representations, procedures and affect in illness self-regulation: A perceptual-cognitive approach. In A. Baum, T. Revenson, & J. Singer (Eds.), *Handbook of health psychology* (pp. 19–48). New York, NY: Erlbaum.

Lichtenstein, S., Slovic, P., Fischhoff, B., Layman, M., & Combs, B. (1978). Judged frequency of lethal events. *Journal of Experimental Psychology: Human Learning and Memory*, *4*, 551–578.

Lipkus, I. M. (2007). Numerical, verbal, and visual formats of conveying health risks: Suggested best practices and future recommendations. *Medical Decision Making*, *27*, 696–713.

Lipkus, I. M., Green, L. G., & Marcus, A. (2003). Manipulating perceptions of colorectal cancer threat: Implications for screening intentions and behavior. *Journal of Health Communication*, *8*, 213–228.

Lipkus, I. M., Klein, W. M. P., Skinner, C. S., & Rimer, B. K. (2005). Breast cancer risk perceptions and breast cancer worry: What predicts what? *Journal of Risk Research*, *8*, 439–452.

Lipkus, I. M., Rimer, B. K., Lyna, P. R., Pradhan, A. A., Conaway, M., & Woods-Powell, C. T. (1996). Colorectal screening patterns and perceptions of risk among African-American users of community health center. *Journal of Community Health*, *21*, 409–427.

Lipkus, I. M., Rimer, B. K., & Strigo, T. S. (1996). Relationships among objective and subjective risk for breast cancer and mammography stages of change. *Cancer Epidemiology, Biomarkers and Prevention*, *5*, 1005–1011.

Lipkus, I. M., Skinner C. S., Dement, J., Pompeii, L., Moser, B., Samsa, G. P., & Ransohoff, D. (2005). Increasing colorectal cancer screening among individuals in the carpentry trade: test of risk communication interventions. *Preventive Medicine*, *40*, 489–501.

Lipkus, I. M., Skinner, C. S., Green, L. S. G., Dement, J, Samsa, G. P., & Ransohoff, D. (2004). Modifying attributions of colorectal cancer risk. *Cancer Epidemiology, Biomarkers, and Prevention*, *13*, 560–566.

Lippke, S., Ziegelmann, J. P., Schwarzer, R., & Velicer, W. F. (2009). Validity of stage assessment in the adoption and maintenance of physical activity and fruit and vegetable consumption. *Health Psychology*, *28*, 183–193.

Lowenstein, G. F., Weber, E. U., Hsee, C. K., & Welch, N. (2001). Risk as feelings. *Psychological Bulletin*, *127*, 267–286.

Lundgren, R. E., & McMakin, A. H. (2009). *Risk communication: A handbook for communicating environmental, safety, and health risks* (4th ed.). Hoboken, NJ: Wiley.

MacKinnon, D. P. (2008). *Introduction to statistical mediation analysis*. Mahwah, NJ: Erlbaum.

MacLeod, A. K., Williams, J. M. G., & Berekian, D. A. (1991). Worry is reasonable: The role of explanations in pessimism about future personal events. *Journal of Abnormal Psychology*, *100*, 478–486.

Manne, S., Markowitz, A., Winawer, S., Guillem, J., Meropol, N., Haller, D., … Duncan, T. (2003). Understanding intention to undergo colonoscopy among intermediate-risk siblings of colorectal cancer patients: A test of a mediational model. *Preventive Medicine*, *36*, 71–84.

Markowitz, L. E., Dunne, E. F., Sariaya, M., Lawson, H. W., Chesson, H., & Unger, E. R. (2007). Quadrivalent human papillomavirus vaccine: Recommendations of the Advisory Committee on Immunization Practices. *Morbidity and Mortality Weekly Review*, *56*(RR-2), 1–24.

McBride, C. M., Curry, S. J., Taplin, S., Anderman, C., & Grothaus, L. (1993). Exploring environmental barriers to participation in mammography screening in an HMO. *Cancer Epidemiology, Biomarkers, and Prevention*, *2*, 599–605.

McCaul, K. D., Branstetter, A. D., Schroeder, D. M., & Glasgow, R. E. (1996). What is the relationship between breast cancer risk and mammography screening? A meta-analytic review. *Health Psychology*, *15*, 423–429.

McCaul, K. D., Canevello, A. B., Mathwig, J. L., & Klein, W. M. P. (2003). Risk communication and worry about breast cancer. *Psychology, Health, and Medicine*, *8*, 378–389.

McCaul, K. D., & Goetz, P. W. (2003). Worry. Retrieved from http://dccps.cancer.gov/brp/constructs/worry/worry.pdf

McCaul, K. D., & O'Donnell, S. M. (1998). Naive beliefs about breast cancer risk. *Women's Health: Research in Gender, Behavior, and Policy, 4*, 93–101.

McCaul, K. D., Schroeder, D. M., & Reid, P. A. (1996). Breast cancer worry and screening: Some prospective data. *Health Psychology, 15*, 430–433.

McQueen, A., Swank, P. R., Bastian, L. A., & Vernon, S. W. (2008). Predictors of perceived susceptibility of breast cancer and changes over time: A mixed modeling approach. *Health Psychology, 27*, 68–77.

Meissner, H. I., Yabroff, K. R., Dodd, K. W., Leader, A. E., Ballard,-Barbas, R., & Berrigan, D. (2009). Are patterns of health behavior associated with cancer screening. *American Journal of Health Promotion, 23*, 168–175.

Meyerowitz, B. E., & Chaiken, S. (1987). The effect of message framing on breast self-examination attitudes, intentions, and behavior. *Journal of Personality and Social Psychology, 52*, 500–510.

Miller, A. J., Ashton, W. A., McHoskey, J. W., & Gimbel, J. (1990). What price attractiveness? Stereotype and risk factors in suntanning behavior. *Journal of Applied Social Psychology, 20*, 1272–1300.

Miller, S. M., Shoda, Y., & Hurley, K. (1996). Applying cognitive-social theory to health-protective behavior: Breast self-examination in cancer screening. *Psychological Bulletin, 119*, 70–94.

Mueller, M. R., & Edmonds, E. M. (1967). Effects of information about environmental probability. *Psychonomic Science, 7*, 339–340.

National Cancer Institute (1999). Cancer risk communication: What we know and what we need to learn. *Journal of the National Cancer Institute Monographs*, whole Vol. 25.

National Cancer Institute (2003). Workshop on Conceptualizing (and Measuring) Perceived Risk, February 13–14, 2003, Washington, DC. Retrieved from http://cancercontrol.cancer.gov/brp/conceptual.html

Noar, S. M., Benac, C. N., & Harris, M. S. (2007). Does tailoring matter? Meta-analytic rview of tailored print health behavior change interventions. *Psychological Bulletin, 133*, 673–693.

Paulhus, D. P., Fridhandler, B., & Hayes, S. (1997). Psychological defense: Contemporary theory and research. In R. Hogan, J. Johnson, & S. Briggs (Eds.), *Handbook of personality* (pp. 543–579). San Diego, CA: Academic Press.

Peek, M. E., & Han, J. H. (2004). Disparities in screening mammography. *Journal of General Internal Medicine, 19*, 184–194.

Perloff, L. S., & Fetzer, B. K. (1986). Self-other judgments and perceived vulnerability to victimization. *Journal of Personality and Social Psychology, 50*, 502–510.

Peters, E., McCaul, K. D., Stefanek, M., & Nelson, W. (2006). A heuristics approach to understanding cancer risk perception: Contributions from judgment and decision making. *Annals of Behavioral Medicine, 31*, 45–52.

Phillips, L. D., & Edwards, W. (1966). Conservatism in a simple probability inference task. *Journal of Experimental Psychology, 72*, 346–354.

Prentice-Dunn, S., & Rogers, R. W. (1986). Protection motivation theory and preventive health: Beyond the health belief model. *Health Education Research, 1*, 153–161.

Price, R. C., Pentecost, H. C., & Voth, R. D. (2002). Perceived event frequency and the optimistic bias: Evidence for a two-process model of personal risk judgments. *Journal of Experimental Social Psychology, 38*, 242–252.

Pruitt, S. L., McQueen, A., Tiro, J. A., Rakowski, W., DiClemente, C. C., & Vernon, S. W. (2009). *Journal of Health Psychology, 15*, 64–74.

Prochaska, J. O., DiClemente, C. C., & Norcross, J. C. (1992). In search of how people change: Applications to addictive behaviors. *American Psychologist, 47*, 1102–1114.

Purc-Stephenson, R. J., & Gorey, K. M. (2008). Lower adherence to screening guidelines among ethnic minority women in America: A meta-analytic review. *Preventive Medicine, 46*, 479–488.

Quillin, J. M., Fries, E., McClish, D., deParedes, E. S., & Bodurtha, J. (2004). Gail model risk assessment and risk perceptions. *Journal of Behavioral Medicine, 27*, 205–214.

Rakowski, W., Ehrich, B., Goldstein, M. G., Rimer, B. K., Pearlman, D. N., Clark, M. A., ... Woolverton, H., III (1998). *Preventive Medicine, 27*, 748–756.

Ranby, K. W., Aiken, L. S., Gerend, M. A., & Erchull, M. J. (2010). Perceived susceptibility measures are not Interchangeable: Absolute, direct comparative and indirect comparative risk clarified. *Health Psychology, 29*, 20–28.

Rawl, S. M., Champion, V. L., Scott, L. L., Zhou, H., Monahan, P., Ding, Y., ...Skinner, C. S. (2008). A randomized trial of two print interventions to increase colon cancer screening among first-degree relatives. *Patient Education and Counseling, 71*, 215–227.

Rees, G. Fry, A., Cull, A., & Sutton, S. (2004). Illness perceptions and distress in women at increased risk of breast cancer. *Psychology and Health, 19*, 749–765.

Reiter, P. L., Brewer, N. T., Gottlieb, S. L., McRee, A.-L., & Smith, J. S. (2009). Parents' health beliefs and HPV vaccination of their adolescent daughters. *Social Science & Medicine, 69*, 475–480.

Reyna, V. F., Nelson, W. L., Han, P. K., & Dieckmann, N. F. (2009). How numeracy influences risk comprehension and medical decision making. *Psychological Bulletin, 135*, 943–973.

Reynolds, K. D., Buller, D. B., Yaroch, A. L., Maloy, J. A., & Cutter, G. R. (2006). Mediation of a middle school skin cancer prevention program. *Health Psychology, 25*, 616–625.

Rimer, B. K. (1990). Perspectives on intrapersonal theories in health education and health behavior. In K. Glanz, F. M. Lewis, & B. K. Rimer (Eds), *Health behavior and health education* (pp. 140–157). San Francisco, CA: Jossey-Bass.

Rimer, B. K., Halabi, S., Skinner, C. S., Kaplan, E. B., Crawford, Y., Samsa, G. P., … Lipkus, I. M. (2001). The short-term impact of tailored mammography decision-making interventions. *Patient Education and Counseling, 43*, 269–285.

Rimer, B. K., Halabi, S., Skinner, C. S., Lipkus, I. M., Strigo, T. S., Kaplan, E. B., & Samsa, G. P. (2002). Effects of a mammography decision-making intervention at 12 and 24 months. *American Journal of Preventive Medicine, 22*, 247–257.

Rimer, B. K., Resch, N., King, E., Ross, E., Lerman, C., Boyce, A., … Engstrom, P. (1992). Multistage health education program to increase mammography screening among women ages 65 and older. *Public Health Reports, 107*, 369–380.

Ritvo, P., Myers, R., Del Giudice, M. L., Pazsat, L., Campbell, P. T., Howlett, R. I., … Rabeneck, L. (2008). Factorial validity and invariance of a survey measuring psychosocial correlations of colorectal cancer screening in Ontario, Canada—A replication study. *Cancer Epidemiology, Biomarkers, and Prevention, 17*, 3279–3283.

Robb, K. A., Campbell, J., Evans, P., Miles, A., & Wardle, J. (2008). Impact of risk information on perceived colorectal cancer risk, a randomized trial. *Journal of Health Psychology, 13*, 744–753.

Robb, K. A., Miles, A., Campbell, J., Evans, P., & Wardle, J. (2006). Can cancer risk information raise awareness without increasing anxiety? A randomized trial. *Preventive Medicine, 43*, 187–190.

Robb, K. A., Miles, A., & Wardle, J. (2007). Perceived risk of colorectal cancer: Sources of risk judgments. *Cancer Epidemiology, Biomarkers, and Prevention, 16*, 694–702.

Rogers, R. W. (1975). A protection motivation theory of fear appeals and attitude change. *Journal of Psychology, 91*, 93–114.

Rogers, R. W. (1983). A protection motivation theory of fear appeals and attitude change: A revised theory of protection motivation. In J. R. Cacioppo & R. E. Petty (Eds), *Social psychology: A sourcebook* (pp. 153–176). New York, NY: Guilford Press.

Ronis, D. L. (1992). Conditional health threats: Health beliefs, decisions, and behaviors among adults. *Health Psychology, 11*, 127–134.

Ronis, D. L., & Harel, Y. (1989). Health beliefs and beast examination behaviors: Analysis of linear structural relations. *Psychology and Health, 3*, 259–285.

Rosenstock, I. M. (1966). Why people use health services. *Milbank Memorial Fund Quarterly, 44*, 94–124.

Rosenstock, I. M. (1974a). Historical origins of the health belief model. *Health Education Monographs, 2*, 328–335.

Rosenstock, I. M. (1974b). The health belief model and preventive health behavior. *Health Education Monographs, 2*, 354–386.

Rosenstock, I. M. (1990). Explaining health behavior through expectancies. In K. Glanz, F. M. Lewis, & B. K. Rimer (Eds.), *Health behavior and health education* (pp. 140–157). San Francisco, CA: Jossey-Bass.

Rosenstock, I. M., Strecher, V. J., & Becker, M. J. (1988). Social learning theory and the health belief model. *Health Education Quarterly, 15*, 175–183.

Rothman, A. J., & Salovey, P. (1997). Shaping perceptions to motivate healthy behavior: The role of message framing. *Psychological Bulletin, 121*, 3–19.

Rothman, A. J., Salovey, P., Antone, C., Keough, K., & Martin, C. D. (1993). The influence of message framing on intentions to perform health behaviors. *Journal of Experimental Social Psychology, 29*, 408–423.

Ryerson, A. B., Miller, J. W., Eheman, C. R., Leadbetter, S., & White, M. C. (2008). Recent trends in U.S. mammography use from 2000–2006: A population based analysis. *Preventive Medicine, 47*, 477–482.

Salazar, M. K., & de Moor, C. (1995). An evaluation of mammography beliefs using a decision model. *Health Education Quarterly, 22*, 110–126.

Savage, S. A., & Clarke, V. A. (1996). Factors associated with screening mammography and breast self-examination intentions. *Health Education Research, 11*, 409–421.

Scholz, U., Keller, R., & Perren, S. (2009). Predicting behavioral intentions and physical exercise: A test of the health action process approach at the intrapersonal level. *Health Psychology, 28*, 702–708.

Schwartz, L. M., Woloshin, S., Black, W. C., & Welch, H. G. (1997). The role of numeracy in understanding the benefit of screening mammography. *Annals of Internal Medicine, 127*, 966–972.

Schwartz, M. D., Lerman, C., Audrain, J., Cella, D., Garber, J., Rimer, B., Lin, T. H., Stefanek, M., & Vogel, V. (1998). The impact of a brief problem-solving training intervention for relatives of recently diagnosed breast cancer patients. *Annals of Behavioral Medicine, 20*, 7–12.

Schwartz, M. D., Lerman, C., Daly, M., Audrain, J., Masny, A., & Griffith, K. (1995). Utilization of ovarian cancer screening by women at increased risk. *Cancer Epidemiology, Biomarkers, & Prevention, 4*, 269–373.

Schwartz, M. D., Lerman, C., Miller, S., Daly, M., & Masny, A. (1995). Coping disposition, perceived risk, and psychological distress among women at increased risk for ovarian cancer. *Health Psychology, 14*, 232–235.

Schwartz, M. D., Rimer, B. K., Daly, M., Sands, C., & Lerman, C. (1999). A randomized trial of breast cancer risk counseling: The impact upon self-reported mammography utilization. *American Journal of Public Health, 89*, 924–926.

Schwartz, M. D., Taylor, K. L., & Willard, K. S. (2003). Prospective association between distress and mammography utilization among women with a family history of breast cancer. *Journal of Behavioral Medicine, 26*, 105–117.

Schwartz, M. D., Taylor, K. L., Willard, K., Siegel, J., Lamdan, R., & Moran, K. (1999). Distress, personality, and mammography utilization among women with a family history of breast cancer. *Health Psychology, 18*, 327–332.

Schwarzer, R. (2008). Modeling health behavior change: How to predict and modify the adoption and maintenance of health behaviors. *Applied Psychology: An International Review, 57*, 1–29.

Schwarzer, R. (2011). Health behavior change. In H. S. Friedman (Ed.), *Oxford handbook of health psychology* (pp. 591–611). New York, NY: Oxford University Press.

Schwarzer, R., Luszczynska, A., Ziegelmann, J. P., Scholz, U., & Lippke, S. (2008). Social-cognitive predictors of physical exercise adherence: Three longitudinal studies in rehabilitation. *Health Psychology, 27* (Suppl.), S54–S63.

Sheeran, P., & Abraham, C. (1996). The health belief model. In M. C. Conner & P. Norman (Eds.), *Predicting health behavior* (pp. 23–61). Buckingham, UK: Open University Press.

Siegler, I. C., & Costa, P. T. (1994). Personality and breast cancer screening behaviors. *Annals of Behavioral Medicine, 16*, 347–351.

Siegler, I. C., Feaganes, J. R., & Rimer, B. K. (1995). Predictors of adoption of mammography in women under age 50. *Health Psychology, 14*, 274–278.

Sjoberg, L. (1998). Worry and risk perception. *Risk Analysis, 18*, 85–93.

Skinner, C. S., Strecher, V. J., & Hospers, H. (1994). Physician recommendations for mammography: Do tailored messages make a difference? *American Journal of Public Health, 84*, 43–49.

Slovic, P. (1987). Perception of risk. *Science, 236*, 280–290.

Slovic, P., Finucane, M. L., Peters, E., & MacGregor, D. G. (2004). Risk as analysis and risk as feelings: Some thoughts about affect, reason, risk, and rationality. *Risk Analysis, 24*, 311–322.

Slovic, P., Fischhoff, B., & Lichtenstein, S. (1979). Rating the risks. *Environment, 21*, 17–20; 32–38.

Slovic, P., Monahan, J., & MacGregor, D. J. (2000). Violence risk assessment and risk communication: The effects of using actual cases, providing instructions, and providing probability vs. frequency formats. *Law and Human Behavior, 24*, 271–296.

Sohl, S. J., & Moyer, A. (2007). Tailored interventions to promote mammography screening: A meta-analytic review. *Preventive Medicine, 45*, 252–261.

Stefanek, M. E., & Wilcox, P. (1991). First degree relatives of breast cancer patients: Screening practices and provision of risk information. *Cancer Detection and Prevention, 15*, 379–384.

Suarez, L., Roche, R. A., Nichols, D., & Simpson, D. M. (1997). Knowledge, behavior, and fears concerning breast and cervical cancer among older low-income Mexican-American women. *American Journal of Preventive Medicine, 13*, 137–142.

Sutton, S., Bickler, G., Sancho-Aldridge, J., & Saidi, G. (1994) Prospective study of predictors of attendance for breast screening in inner London. *Journal of Epidemiology and Community Health, 48*, 65–73.

Tversky, A., & Kahneman, D. (1973). Availability: A heuristic for judging frequency and probability. *Cognitive Psychology, 5*, 207–232.

Tversky, A., & Kahneman, D. (1974). Judgment under uncertainly: Heuristics and biases. *Science, 184*, 1124–1131.

U.S. Preventive Services Task Force. (2005). Genetic risk assessment and BRCA mutation testing for breast and ovarian cancer. *Annals of Internal Medicine, 143*, 355–361.

U.S. Preventive Services Task Force. (2009). Guide to clinical preventive services, 2009. U.S. Department of Health and Human Services. Agency for Healthcare Research and Quality. AHRQ Publication No. 09-IP006, August 2009. Retrieved from http://www.ahrq.gov/clinic/pocketgd09

Van der Pligt, J. (1998). Perceived risk and vulnerability as predictors of precautionary behavior. *British Journal of Health Psychology, 3*, 1–14.

Vernon, S. W. (1999). Risk perception and risk communication for cancer screening behaviors: A review. *Journal of the National Cancer Institute Monographs, 25*, 101–119.

Vernon, S. W., Myers, R. E., & Tilley, B. C. (1997). Development and validation of an instrument to measure factors related to colorectal cancer screening adherence. *Cancer Epidemiology, Biomarkers, and Prevention, 6*, 825–832.

Ward, J. E., Hughes, A. M., Hirst, G. H., & Winchester, L. (1997). Men's estimates of prostate cancer risk and self-reported rates of screening. *Medical Journal of Australia, 167*, 240–241.

Wardle, J. (1995). Women at risk for ovarian cancer. *Journal of the National Cancer Institute Monographs, 17*, 81–85.

Weinberg, D. S., Turner, B. J., Wang, H., Myers, R. E., & Miller, S. (2004). A survey of women regarding factors affecting colorectal screening compliance. *Preventive Medicine, 38*, 669–675.

Weinstein, N. D. (1980). Unrealistic optimism about future life events. (1980). *Journal of Personality and Social Psychology, 39*, 806–820.

Weinstein, N. D. (1984). Why it won't happen to me: Perceptions of risk factors and susceptibility. *Health Psychology, 3*, 431–457.

Weinstein, N. D. (1987). Unrealistic optimism about susceptibility to health problems: Conclusions from a community-wide sample. *Journal of Behavioral Medicine, 10*, 481–500.

Weinstein, N. D. (1988). The precaution adoption process. *Health Psychology, 7*, 355–386.

Weinstein, N. D. (1993). Testing four competing theories of health-protective behavior. *Health Psychology, 12*, 324–333.

Weinstein, N. D. (2000). Perceived probability, perceived severity, and health-protective behavior. *Health Psychology, 19*, 65–74.

Weinstein, N. D., & Klein, W. M. (1995). Resistance of personal risk perceptions to debiasing interventions. *Health Psychology, 14*, 132–140.

Weinstein, N. D., & Klein, W. M. (1996). Unrealistic optimism: Present and future. *Journal of Social and Clinical Psychology, 15*, 1–8.

Weinstein, N. D., Kwitel, A., McCaul, K. D., Magnan, R. E., Gerrard, M., & Gibbons, F. X. (2007). Risk perceptions: Assessment and relationship to influenza vaccination. *Health Psychology, 26*, 146–151.

Weinstein, N. D., & Nicolich, M. (1993). Correct and incorrect interpretations of correlations between risk perceptions and risk behaviors. *Health Psychology, 12*, 235–245.

Weinstein, N. D., Rothman, A. J., & Nicolich, M. (1998). Use of correlations data to examine the effects of risk perceptions on precautionary behavior. *Psychology and Health, 13*, 479–501.

Weinstein, N. D., Rothman, A. J., & Sutton, S. R. (1998). Stage theories of health behavior: Conceptual and methodological issues. *Health Psychology, 17*, 290–299.

Weinstein, N. D., & Sandman, P. M. (1992). A model of the precaution adoption process: Evidence from home radon testing. *Health Psychology, 11*, 170–180.

Weinstein, N. D., & Sandman, P. M. (2002). The precaution adoption process model and its application. In R. J. DiClemente, R. A. Crosby, & M. C. Kegler (Eds.), *Emerging theories in health promotion practice and research: Strategies for improving public health*. San Francisco, CA: Jossey-Bass.

West, S. G., & Aiken, L. S. (1997). Toward understanding individual effects in multicomponent prevention programs: Design and analysis strategies. In K. J. Bryant, M. Windle, & S. G. West (Eds.), *The science of prevention: Methodological advances from alcohol and substance abuse research* (pp. 167–209). Washington, DC: American Psychological Association.

Zajac, L. E., Klein, W. M. P., & McCaul, K. D. (2006). Absolute and comparative risk perceptions as predictors of cancer worry: Moderating effects of gender and psychological distress. *Journal of Health Communication, 11*, 37–49.

Zapka, J. G., Costanza, M. E., Harris, D. R., Hosmer, D., Stoddard, A., Barth, R., & Gaw, V. (1993). Impact of a breast cancer screening community intervention. *Preventive Medicine, 22*, 34–53.

Section II

Cross-Cutting Issues

7 Psychological and Physiological Bases of Chronic Pain

Dennis C. Turk, Hilary D. Wilson, and Kimberly S. Swanson
University of Washington

Pain has existed since time in memoriam. Perhaps the first documented mention of pain was in the Ebers papyrus dating back to the fourth century B.C.E. in which the goddess Isis recommends the use of opium to treat the god Ra's headaches. Since that time, pain has been the focus of philosophical speculation and scientific attention, yet it continues to remain a challenging problem for the individual, his or her significant others, health care providers, and society.

Pain is essential for survival because of its alarm function. In acute pain states, nociception—the activation of sensory transduction in nerve fibers that convey information about tissue damage—has a definite purpose: It acts as a warning signal that invokes immediate attention, reflexive withdrawal, and other actions to prevent further damage and to facilitate the healing process. In chronic pain states, this adaptive function plays a significantly smaller role and can often no longer be discerned. In the case of recurrent acute pain diagnoses, such as migraine headaches and sickle cell episodes, the role of pain is even less clear because there is no protective action that can be taken or any tissue damage that can be prevented. Pain associated with neoplastic disease has some features in common with acute pain in that it may be a warning signal, whereas in others it is more like chronic pain because the pain may serve no useful purpose.

Chronic pain affects approximately 20%–30% of the adult population in Western countries (Verhaak, Kerssens, Dekker, Sorbi, & Bensing, 1998). Chronic widespead musculoskeletal pain is reported by approximately 10% of the general population (Gran, 2003). Migraine headache, a recurring acute pain condition, is estimated to affect over 11 milliion Americans (Stewart et al., 1991). Approximately 3.5 million people in the United States have cancer (Raj, 1990), of which, it is estimated, 90% experience at least moderate pain at some point during their illness and over 40% do not experience sufficient relief from their pain treatments (Olivier, Kravits, & Kaplan, 2001).

Given the lengthy history of pain and its prevalence, it might be assumed that pain is well understood and readily treated. Despite advances in the understanding of anatomy and physiological processes, and innovative and technically sophisticated pharmacological, medical, and surgical treatments, pain continues to be a perplexing puzzle for health care providers, as well as a source of significant distress for the individual who is experiencing pain and his or her significant others.

There have been a number of therapeutic advances in the treatment of chronic pain; however, they have several limitations. For example, although therapeutic approaches have resulted in significant improvements, even the most potent drugs reduce pain only by 30%–40% in fewer than 50% of patients (Turk, 2002). Similarly, such sophisticated surgical techniques as implantation of artificial discs in the spine (Deyo, Nachemson, & Mirza, 2004) and implantable drug delivery systems (Taylor, Van Buyten, & Buchser, 2005) provide limited pain reduction and only in a subset of carefully selected patients. Even when medications and invasive procedures effectively reduce pain, they often do not produce concomitant improvements in physical and emotional functioning (Martin et al., 2008). Moreover, many treatments may result in significant adverse effects. For example, over

40% of patients who are implanted with pain-alleviating devices will experience significant adverse events, and premature termination rates from drug clinical trials often exceed 30% (Noble, Tregear, Tradwell, & Schoelles, 2008). Furthermore, opioids, the most potent and frequently prescribed class of drugs to control pain, carry significant risk of misuse and abuse that may exceed 40% (Ives et al., 2006; Michna et al., 2004), and an expanding amount of research has identified important physical problems associated with long-term use (Ballantyne & Shin, 2008). Paradoxically, one of the problems is opioid-induced hyperalgesia whereby patients receiving opioids for the treatment of pain become more sensitive to nociceptive stimuli (Chu, Angst, & Clark, 2008).

The mean duration of pain in patients seeking treatment in chronic pain rehabilitation facilities is approximately 7 years (Flor, Fydrich, & Turk, 1992). Consequently, all domains of their lives have been compromised, and for a significant amount of time. Furthermore, the average age of patients treated at multidisciplinary pain rehabilitation facilities is 44 years old (Flor et al., 1992). Thus, prior to the pain onset, these people had histories spanning 37 years; therefore, their prior experiences are important in understanding how people respond to their symptoms and plight. Moreover, most people live a social context. Significant people in patients' lives likely influence their adaptation and conversely are impacted by living with a person with chronic pain.

People with persistent pain become enmeshed in the medical community as they trek from doctor to doctor and diagnostic test to diagnostic test in a continuing search to have pain diagnosed and successfully treated. For many individuals, the pain becomes the central focus of their lives. As people with pain withdraw from society, they lose their jobs, alienate family and friends, and become isolated. Pain affects their ability to sleep, to function; indeed, it disturbs all facets of their lives. They may develop treatment-related complications and become enmeshed in a legal system that prolongs and compounds their distress. In this ongoing and often elusive quest for relief, it is hardly surprising that they experience feelings of demoralization, helplessness, hopelessness, and outright depression.

In sum, the different forms of persistent pain create a demoralizing situation that confronts the individual not only with pain but with a cascade of ongoing stressors that compromise all aspects of their lives. Living with persistent pain conditions requires considerable emotional resilience and tends to deplete people's emotional reserve, and it taxes not only the individual but also the capacity of family, friends, coworkers, and employers to provide support. It is reasonable to ask a question concerning how a problem as prevalent and costly as pain can be so poorly understood and managed.

This survey begins by reviewing the most common conceptualizations of pain and will then examine the role of psychological factors in the etiology and exacerbation of pain and disability. This is followed by a description of attempts to integrate physiological and psychological variables in comprehensive conceptual models. Finally, the current understanding of the anatomical and neurophysiolgoical bases of pain is reviewed, illustrating the physiological bases of both sensory and psychological components of pain.

CONCEPTUALIZATIONS OF PAIN

Since the middle of the last century, there has been a significant paradigm shift in thinking about pain that was ushered in by the gate control theory (GCT; Melzack, & Wall, 1965) and operant conditioning (Fordyce, 1976), which are described in a following section. First, however, it is helpful to examine the traditional unidimensional conceptualizations that have been dominant since the time of the ancient Greeks (Melzack & Wall, 1982).

UNIDIMENSIONAL SENSORY MODEL

Historically, pain has been understood from the perspective of Cartesian mind-body dualism, in which pain was viewed as a sensory experience dependent on the degrees of noxious sensory stimuli impinging on the individual. From this perspective, similar to a land-line telephone, there are two ends of a pain pathway. Sensory stimulation at one end, at the periphery, has a direct stimulatory effect at the other end, the brain.

The core of sensory-physiological models is that the amount of pain is a direct result of the amount, degree, or nature of sensory input or physical damage and is explained in terms of specific physiological mechanisms. Clinically, it is expected that the report of pain will be directly proportional to the extent of physical pathology (Melzack & Wall, 1982). The production of pain is thus traced back to peripheral pain receptors at the site of the injury. It is assumed that some form of tissue damage will excite receptors that are *specific*, responding exclusively to nociceptive stimuli, initiating pain-specific nerve impulses that are transmitted along specific afferent pain pathways to specific pain centers localized in the brain where the experience of pain will motivate actions to avoid further harm. These views are aptly named specificity theories.

This sensory model has prevailed largely unchanged despite its inability to account for a number of observations. For example, patients with objectively determined, equivalent degrees and types of tissue pathology vary widely in their reports of pain severity. Moreover, the surgical procedures designed to inhibit pain transmission by severing the neurological pathways that are believed to be subserving the reported pain may fail to alleviate it, and patients with equivalent degrees of tissue pathology treated with identical treatments respond in widely different ways (Turk & Burwinkle, 2007).

PSYCHOGENIC VIEW

The psychogenic view is posed as the flip side of the coin from the physical or biomedical model. From this perspective, if the patient's report of pain occurs in the absence of, or is disproportionate to, objective physical pathology, then, ipso facto, the pain reports must have a psychological etiology. Thus, a dichotomy is posed: Pain is either somatagenic or psychogenic. Psychogenic pain is an empty concept. Positive criteria for the identification of psychogenic pain, mechanisms for the production of psychogenic pain, and specific therapies for psychogenic pain are lacking. The diagnosis of psychogenic pain too often only serves to stigmatize further the patient who experiences chronic pain (M. D. Sullivan & Turk, 2001).

MOTIVATIONAL VIEW

A variation of the dichotomous somatic-psychogenic views is a conceptualization that is ascribed to by many third-party payers who suggest that if there is insufficient physical pathology to justify the report of pain, their complaint is invalid, the result of symptom exaggeration, or outright malingering (i.e., the pain "is all in the patient's wallet"). The assumption here is that reports of pain without insufficient objective evidence are motivated primarily by pecuniary interests and other secondary gains. This belief has resulted in a number of attempts to "catch" malingers using surreptitious methods and the use of sophisticated biomechanical machines geared toward uncovering inconsistencies in functional performance. There are, however, no studies that have demonstrated dramatic improvement in pain reports subsequent to receiving disability awards. Yet, Koplow (1990) suggested that it is fear of malingering that drives the entire Social Security disability system.

Although there appears to be little question that psychological factors play an important role in pain perception and response, the aforementioned models view physical and psychological factors as largely independent. Integrated models of pain do not conceptualize physical and psychlogical factors as mutually exclusive but, instead, propose they are interactive. Before examining models that attempt to integrate psychological factors with somatic factors, it is useful to examine in depth the nature of the psychological factors involved.

PSYCHOLOGICAL CONTRIBUTORS TO PAIN

Psychologists have made important contributions to understanding pain by demonstrating the importance of psychosocial and behavioral factors in the etiology, severity, exacerbation, and maintenance of pain. Several effective treatments have been developed based on these factors.

BEHAVIORAL PRINCIPLES

Operant Learning Mechanisms

A new era in thinking about pain began with Fordyce's (1976) description of the role of instrumental reinforcement in chronic pain. The operant conditioning model is not concerned with the initial cause of pain. Rather, it considers pain a subjective experience that may be maintained even after an initial physical basis of pain has resolved. The model focuses on such overt manifestations of pain as limping, moaning, and avoiding activity. The model emphasizes the communicative function of these behaviors and the responses they acquire, rather than being directly involved in the perception of pain per se.

The operant view proposes that acute "pain behaviors" (e.g., limping to protect a wounded limb from producing additional nociceptive input) may come under the control of external contingencies of reinforcement and thus contribute to persistent pain and disability. Pain behaviors may be positively reinforced, for example, by attention from a spouse or health care providers. Pain behaviors may also be maintained by negative reinforcement through escape from noxious stimulation by the use of medications or rest, or avoidance of such undesirable activities as work. In addition, "well behaviors" (e.g., activity, working) may not be sufficiently reinforced; therefore, pain behaviors may be maintained because they are more rewarding. The pain behavior originally elicited by organic factors may be emitted, totally or in part, in response to reinforcing environmental events. Because of the consequences of specific behavioral responses, it is postulated that pain behaviors may persist.

Several studies have provided evidence supporting the underlying assumptions of operant conditioning. For example, Doleys, Crocker, and Patton (1982) showed that pain behaviors (specifically, inactivity) can be decreased and well behaviors (i.e., activity) can be increased by verbal reinforcement with or without feedback and the setting of exercise quotas. Studies (e.g., Thieme, Spies, Sinha, Turk, & Flor, 2005; Turk, Kerns, & Rosenberg, 1992) have found that chronic pain patients reported more intense pain and less activity when they indicated that their spouses were solicitous. These later studies suggest that spouses can serve as discriminative stimuli for the display of pain behaviors by chronic pain patients, including their reports of pain severity.

The operant view has also generated what has proven to be an effective treatment for select samples of chronic pain patients (see Keefe, Dunsmore, & Burnett, 1992; Thieme, Flor, & Turk, 2006). Treatment focuses on extinction of pain behaviors and positive reinforcement of well behaviors.

Although operant factors undoubtedly play a role in the maintenance of disability, exclusive reliance on the operant conditioning model to explain the experience of pain may be inadequate. The model has been criticized for its exclusive focus on motor pain behaviors, failure to consider the emotional and cognitive aspects of pain (e.g., Turk & Flor, 1987), and lack of attention to the subjective experience of pain (Kotarba, 1983).

Respondent Learning Mechanisms

Factors contributing to chronicity that have previously been conceptualized in terms of operant learning may also be initiated and maintained by classical or respondent conditioning (Gentry & Bernal, 1977). In acute pain states it may be useful to reduce movement, and consequently avoid pain, to accelerate the healing process. Over time, however, anticipatory anxiety related to activity may develop and act as a conditioned stimulus (CS) for sympathetic activation (conditioned response, CR) that may be maintained after the original unconditioned stimulus (US, e.g., injury) and unconditioned response (UR, pain and sympathetic activation) have subsided (Lenthem, Slade, Troup, & Bentley, 1983; Philips, 1987).

Lenthem et al. (1983) and Linton, Melin, and Götestam (1984) suggested that once an acute pain problem exists, the expectation that pain will accompany activity results in fear of further injury. This may lead to avoidance of activities. Nonoccurrence of pain is a powerful reinforcer for reduction of activity. Thus the original respondent conditioning may be followed by an operant learning process whereby the nociceptive stimuli and the associated responses no longer need to be present for avoidance behavior to occur.

In addition to the avoidance learning, pain may be exacerbated and maintained through potentially pain-increasing situations due to the anxiety-related sympathetic activation and muscle tension increases that may occur both in anticipation of pain (Flor, Birbaumer, & Turk, 1990). Thus, psychological factors may directly affect nociceptive stimulation and need not be viewed as solely reactions to pain.

Persistant avoidance of specific activities reduces disconfirmations that are followed by corrected predictions (Rachman & Arntz, 1991). The prediction of pain promotes pain avoidance behavior (Schmidt,1985a, 1985b). Insofar as pain avoidance succeeds in preserving the overpredictions from repeated disconfirmation, they will continue unchanged (Rachman & Lopatka, 1988). By contrast, repeatedly engaging in behavior that produces significantly less pain than was predicted is followed by adjustments in subsequent predictions, which also become more accurate. These increasingly accurate predictions are followed by increasingly appropriate behavior, even to elimination of all avoidance if that is appropriate. These observations add support to the importance of physical therapy, with patients progressively increasing their activity levels despite fear of injury and discomfort associated with renewed use of deconditioned muscles.

From a respondent-conditioning perspective, the patient may have learned to associate increases in pain with all kinds of stimuli that were originally associated with nociceptive stimulation (stimulus generalization). Walking, engaging in social interaction, sexual activity, or even thoughts about these activities may increase anticipatory anxiety and concomitant physiological and biochemical changes (Philips, 1987). Subsequently, patients may display maladaptive responses to many stimuli and reduce the frequency of performance of diverse activities other than those that initially induced pain. The physical abnormalities often observed in chronic pain patients (e.g., distorted gait, decreased range of motion, muscular fatigue) may then actually be secondary to changes initiated through learning. In sum, the anticipation of suffering or prevention of suffering may be sufficient for the long-term maintenance of avoidance behaviors in people with persistent pain.

Social Learning Mechanisms

From the perspective of social learning, the acquisition of pain behaviors may occur by means of observational learning and modeling. That is, individuals can acquire responses that were not previously in their repertoires by the observation of others performing these activities. Observational learning plays an important role in many areas of human functioning. Children acquire attitudes about the perception of symptoms and appropriate responses to injury and disease from their parents and social environment, for example, and thus may be more or less likely to ignore or overrespond to symptoms they experience based on observation.

There is a history of both experimental and clinical evidence of the role of social learning in pain experience (Craig, 1986, 1988). For example, Vaughan and Lanzetta (1980, 1981) demonstrated that physiological responses to pain stimuli may be vicariously conditioned during observation of others in pain. Richard (1988) found that children of chronic pain patients chose more pain-related responses to scenarios presented to them and were more external in their health locus-of-control responses than were children with healthy or diabetic parents. Moreover, teachers rated the pain patients' children as displaying more illness behaviors (e.g., whining, visit to school nurse) than children of healthy controls. Fagerhaugh (1975) observed that patients in burn units acquire responses similar to those emitted by other patients on their ward.

Expectancies and actual behavioral responses to nociceptive stimulation are based, at least partially, on prior leaning history. This prior learning may contribute to the marked variability in response to objectively similar degrees of physical pathology noted by health care providers.

PAIN AND AFFECT

As noted, historically, pain has been viewed as a symptom secondary to the presence of tissue pathology and, thus, of secondary importance. However, pain has also been viewed as residing outside the senses and among the emotions— "passions of the soul" (e.g., Aristotle, as cited in Melzack & Wall, 1982).

Pain is ultimately a subjective, private experience, but it is invariably described in terms of sensory and affective properties. Pain, as defined by the International Association for the Study of Pain, "is unquestionably a sensation in a part or parts of the body but it is also always unpleasant and therefore also an *emotional experience*" (Merskey, 1986; emphasis added). The central and interactive roles of sensory information and affective state are supported by an overwhelming amount of evidence (Fernandez, 2002).

The affective component of pain incorporates many different emotions, most commonly the negative emotions of depression, anxiety, and anger. Emotional distress may predispose people to experience pain, be a precipitant of symptoms, be a modulating factor amplifying or inhibiting the severity of pain, be a consequence of persistent pain, or be a perpetuating factor. The literature is replete with studies demonstrating that current mood state modulates reports of pain as well as tolerance for acute pain (e.g., Fernandez & Turk, 1992). Levels of anxiety have been shown to influence not only pain severity but also complications following surgery as well as number of days of hospitalization (e.g., DeGroot et al., 1997; Pavlin, Rapp, & Pollisar, 1998). Level of depression has been observed to play a significant role in premature termination from pain rehabilitation programs (Kerns & Haythornthwaite, 1988). Such individual difference variables as anxiety sensitivity (discussed later) have also been shown to play an important predisposing and augmenting role in the experience of pain (Asmundson, 1999).

Emotional distress is commonly observed in people with chronic pain. People with chronic pain often feel rejected by the medical system, believing that when their pain condition does not respond to treatment they are blamed or labeled as "symptom magnifiers," "whiners," and complainers by their physicians, family members, friends, and employers. As treatments expected to alleviate pain are proven ineffective, people with chronic pain may lose faith and become frustrated and irritated with the medical system. As noted earlier, as their pain persists, they encounter many problems. They may become fearful and have inadequate or maladaptive support systems and other coping resources available to them. They may develop hostility toward the health care system in its inability to eliminate their pain. They may also feel resentment toward their significant others, whom they may perceive as providing inadequate support, and to third-party payers who are skeptical. They are even angry with themselves for allowing their pain to take over their lives. These consequences of chronic pain can result in increasing degrees of self-preoccupation, isolation, depression, anger, and anxiety—an overall sense of demoralization. Because chronic pain persists over long periods of time, affective state will continue to play a role as the impact of pain comes to influence all aspects of life of the person with chronic pain.

ROLE OF COGNITIVE FACTORS IN PAIN

A great deal of research has been directed toward identifying cognitive factors that contribute to pain and disability (e.g., Jensen, Turner, & Romano, 2007; Turk & Rudy, 1992). Studies have consistently demonstrated that patients' beliefs, expectancies about their plight, personal coping repertoires, and personality styles affect reports of pain, activity, disability, and response to treatment (e.g., Jensen, Turner, & Romano, 1994; Tota-Faucette, Gil, Williams, & Goli, 1993).

Beliefs and Appraisals About Pain

Pain appraisal refers to the meaning ascribed to nociception by an individual (Sharp, 2001). If a nociceptive signal is perceived and interpreted as harmful (threat appraisal) and associated with tissue damage, the pain may be interpreted as more intense, more dangerous, and more unpleasant than it otherwise would be and may evoke more escape or avoidance behavior. If no explanation for the symptoms is readily available and the pain is attributed to a trauma, the symptoms will influence the ways to which the individual responds (Robinson, Burwinkle, & Turk, 2007; Turk & Okifuji, 1996). For example, pain associated with cancer has been shown to be more unpleasant than labor pain even when the intensity is equivalent (Price, Harkins, & Baker, 1987). Similarly, Smith, Gracely, and Safer (1998) demonstrate that cancer patients who attributed pain sensations following physical therapy directly to their cancer reported more intense pain than did patients who attributed their pain to other causes.

Perception of danger of an experimental pain stimulus may also lead to avoidance. Arntz and Claassens (2004) experimentally manipulated the appraisal of a mildly painful stimulus (a very cold metal bar) by suggesting that it was either very hot or very cold. It was assumed that heat would be more strongly associated with tissue damage than cold. As expected, participants rated the stimulus as more painful when they were informed that the stimulus was harmful. These studies demonstrate the important role of people's interpretations regarding the meaning of the pain.

Research has also been conducted exploring the effect of positive changes in patients' thoughts and beliefs on treatment efficacy. Newton and Barbaree (1987) used a modified thought-sampling procedure to evaluate the nature of patients' thoughts during and immediately following headache both prior to and following treatment. Results indicated significant changes in certain aspects of headache-related thinking in the treated groups compared to the control group. Reduction in negative appraisal and increase in positive appraisal (e.g., "It's getting worse," "There is nothing I can do") revealed a significant shift in the thoughts of treated as compared to untreated patients, indicating that treated patients were evaluating headaches in a more positive fashion. Treated patients reported experiencing significantly fewer headache per days per week and lower intensity of pain than did untreated patients. Correlational analyses suggested that reports of more intense pain were associated with more negative appraisals of headache episodes. Newton and Barbaree noted that patients who reported the largest positive shift in appraisal also reported the greatest reduction in headache intensity.

Recently, the concept of acceptance of pain has received considerable attention. Acceptance of chronic pain has been defined as "acknowledging that one has pain, giving up unproductive attempts to control pain, acting as if pain does not necessarily imply disability, and being able to commit one's efforts toward living a satisfying life despite pain" (McCracken, 1998; McCracken & Eccleston, 2003). Acceptance has been shown to predict better adjustment on many measures of patient functioning, including depression, disability, daily functioning, and avoidance of activities independent of pain intensity (McCracken, 1998; Viane, Crombez, & Eccleston, 2003). Conversely, a cognitive schema that views disability as a necessary aspect of pain, that activity despite pain is dangerous, and that pain is an acceptable excuse for neglecting responsibilities is associated with decreased function (Jensen, Turner, Romano, & Lawler, 1994; Turk & Okifuji, 1996).

Clearly, it appears essential for patients with chronic pain to develop adaptive beliefs about the relationship among impairment, pain, suffering, and disability and to deemphasize the role of experienced pain in their regulation of functioning. Patients who believe their pain is likely to persist may be quite passive in their coping efforts and fail to make use of cognitive or behavioral strategies to cope with pain. People's cognitions (i.e., beliefs, appraisals, expectancies) regarding the consequences of an event and their ability are hypothesized to impact functioning in two general ways: They may have a direct influence on mood and physiology (e.g., increased muscle tension; Flor, Turk, & Birbaumer, 1985) and an indirect one through their impact on coping efforts.

Coping

Self-regulation of pain and its impact depends on the person's specific ways of dealing with pain, adjusting to pain, and reducing or minimizing pain and distress induced by pain—that is, on their coping strategies. Coping is assumed to be manifested by spontaneously employed purposeful and intentional acts, and it can be assessed in terms of overt and covert behaviors. *Overt* behavioral coping strategies include getting rest and relaxation, using medication, seeking medical attention, and relying on social support. *Covert* coping strategies include various means of distracting oneself from pain, reassuring oneself that the pain will diminish, seeking information, and problem solving. These strategies need not always be adaptive or maladaptive. Coping strategies are thought to act to alter both the perception of intensity of pain and a person's ability to manage or tolerate pain and to continue everyday activities (Turk, Meichenbaum, & Genest, 1983).

Preliminary data based on a large Internet survey of people with fibromyalgia (FM; Robinson, Wilson, Swanson, & Turk, 2008) tend to support the important role of each of these classes of coping resources. In this study, there were few differences in objectively determined medical diseases between respondents who reported high numbers of symptoms compared to those with low numbers of symptoms. However, what did differentiate these two groups were education, perceived availability of social support, and perceived ability to cope with the symptoms. Not surprisingly, those individuals with a larger number of symptoms also reported that they were less able to work and were more likely to apply for disability. These different coping resources are not mutually exclusive and may interact in important ways to contribute to adjustment and adaptation to FM. Essentially, it may be easier to adapt to chronic pain if one has financial resources and adequate social support, as well as an adaptive repertoire of personal coping methods.

Studies have found active coping strategies (i.e., efforts to function in spite of pain or to distract oneself from pain) to be associated with adaptive functioning, and passive coping strategies (i.e., depending on others for help in pain control and restriction of activities) to be related to greater pain and depression (e.g., Lawson, Reesor, Keefe, & Turner, 1990; Tota-Faucette et al., 1993). However, beyond this, there is no evidence supporting the greater effectiveness of one active coping strategy compared to any other (Fernandez & Turk, 1989). It seems more likely that different strategies will be more effective than others for some individuals at some times, but not necessarily for all individuals all of the time.

Catastrophizing

Chronic pain researchers have emphasized the role of a specific set of negative appraisals and beliefs (i.e., catastrophizing). Pain catastrophizing can be defined as an exaggerated negative orientation toward actual or anticipated pain experiences. There has been much debate about the specific nature of catastrophizing as a psychological construct (M. J. L. Sullivan et al., 2001; Turner & Aaron, 2001). Current conceptualizations most often describe it in terms of appraisal or as a set of maladaptive beliefs ("pain is overwhelming, terrible and permanent"; Severeijns, Vlaeyen, & van den Hout, 2004). Catastrophizing appears to be a particularly potent way of thinking that greatly influences pain and disability. People who spontaneously utilize less catastrophizing self-statements reported more pain in both acute and chronic pain studies (Butler, Damarin, Beaulieu, Schwebel, & Thorn, 1989; Martin, Nathan, Milech, & Van Keppel, 1989) and poorer adaptation (Turner, Dworkin, Mancl, Huggins, & Truelove, 2001; Turner, Jensen, & Romano, 2000).

The evidence for the role of pain catastrophizing in chronic pain adjustment has been summarized in review articles (e.g., Keefe, Rumble, Scipio, Giordano, & Perri, 2004; M. J. L. Sullivan et al., 2001). Cross-sectional studies have demonstrated that catastrophizing is associated with increased pain, increased illness behavior, and physical and psychological dysfunction across numerous clinical and nonclinical populations (e.g., Jensen et al., 2002; Turner, Jensen, Warms, & Cardenas, 2002). Prospective studies indicated that catastrophizing might be predictive of the inception of chronic musculoskeletal pain in the general population (Picavet, Vlaeyen, & Schouten, 2002; Severeijns, Vlaeyen, van den Hout, & Picavet, 2005), as well as of more intense pain and slower recovery after surgical intervention (Granot & Ferber, 2005; Pavlin, Sullivan, Freund, & Roesen, 2005). Change in levels of catastrophizing have also been shown to be important mediators of treatment response. For example, Jensen et al. (2007) showed that reductions in catastrophizing following cognitive-behavioral treatment were significantly related to reductions in pain tolerance and physical and psychosocial impairment.

The role of catastrophizing and the belief that pain means harm and therefore activity should be avoided has been incorporated into fear-avoidance models (FAMs) of chronic pain (Asmundson, Norton, & Vlaeyen, 2004; Vlaeyen & Linton, 2000). Although FAMs are multifaceted and include affective (fear) and behavioral (avoidance) components, cognitions are identified as the core determinants of entering into a negative pain cycle (e.g., Asmundson et al., 2004: Philips, 1987). The tenets of contemporary FAMs can be summarized as follows: When pain is perceived following injury, an individual's idiosyncratic beliefs will determine the extent to which pain is catastrophically interpreted. A catastrophic interpretation of pain gives rise to physiological (arousal), behavioral (avoidance), and cognitive fear responses. The cognitive shift that takes place during fear enhances threat perception (e.g., by narrowing of attention) and further feeds the catastrophic appraisal of pain (Asmundson et al., 2004). Appraisals lead to avoidance of activities believed to exacerbate pain or be likely to produce further injury.

Prospective studies have shown that fear avoidance beliefs in patients seeking care for acute pain (e.g., Boersma & Linton, 2005; Buer & Linton, 2002) and chronic pain (Keefe, Brown, Wallston, & Caldwell, 1989) may be predictive of pain persistence, disability, and long-term sick leave. Fear avoidance beliefs are also related to the future inception of (back) pain in the general population (Linton, Buer, Vlaeyen, & Hellsing, 2000; Picavet et al., 2002). Concerns have been raised regarding the amount of variance accounted for by fear avoidance, (Pincus, Vogel, Burton, Santos, & Field, 2006), and in some chronic pain populations (e.g., FM, whiplash-associated disorders) the role of fear avoidance has not been convincingly demonstrated (Vangronsveld, Peters, Goossens, Linton, & Vlaeyen, 2007).

Perceived Control

For chronic pain patients, lack of personal control is typically perceived and likely relates to the ongoing but unsuccessful efforts to control their pain. Perceived control over pain refers to the belief that one can exert influence on the duration, frequency, intensity, or unpleasantness of pain. A large proportion of chronic pain patients tend to believe that they have limited ability to exert control over their pain (Turk & Rudy, 1988). Such negative, maladaptive appraisals of the situation and personal efficacy may reinforce the experience of demoralization, inactivity, and overreaction to nociceptive stimulation commonly observed in chronic pain patients.

Perceived controllability of a pain stimulus may modify the meaning of this stimulus and directly affect threat appraisal. As a consequence, pain may be rated as less intense or less unpleasant, and pain tolerance may increase. However, studies in which the control over pain stimuli was experimentally manipulated have yielded mixed results as to whether perceived controllability affects pain intensity or pain tolerance (e.g., Janssen, Spinhoven, & Arntz, 2004; Salomons, Johnstone, Backonja, & Davidson, 2004). Functional magnetic resonance imaging (fMRI) has shown, however, that manipulation of the controllability of a pain stimulus attenuated the neural response to pain (Salomons et al., 2004). Offering control in an experimental pain situation may interact with such individual characteristics as self-efficacy and feelings of helplessness in determining whether it is effective in reducing pain (Müller & Netter, 2000). Recent advances in brain imaging are permitting opportunities to observe the physical changes occurring in response to psychological variables. The old refrain "it's all in your head" is correct; or as Turk and Salovey (1985) pithily noted, "The reign of pain falls mainly in the brain."

As noted, there may be a downside to trying relentlessly to gain control over pain. The failure of repeated attempts to gain control over pain may lead to frustration and preoccupation with pain and, finally, to exacerbations of distress and disability (Aldrich, Eccleston, & Crombez, 2000; McCracken, Carson, Eccleston, & Keefe, 2004). Instead of futilely trying to gain control over pain itself, one may encounter circumstances when it may be more reasonable and effective to control the effects of pain on one's life rather than the pain per se (Tan et al., 2002). Perhaps a balance needs to be achieved between active attempts to control pain, relinquishing futile attempts, and the resulting distress when pain is not eliminated or substantially reduced. This approach calls to mind Reinhold Niebuhr's "Serenity Prayer": "Give me the serenity to accept the thinks I cannot change, the courage to change the things I can, and the wisdom to know the difference."

Self-Efficacy

Closely related to the sense of control over aversive stimulation is the concept of self-efficacy (SE). An SE expectation is defined as a personal conviction that one can successfully execute a course of action, performing required behaviors, to produce a desired outcome in a given situation. This construct has been demonstrated as a major mediator of therapeutic change.

In chronic pain patients, SE positively affects physical and psychological functioning (Barry, Guo, Kerns, Duong, & Reid, 2003; Woby, Watson, Roach, & Urmston, 2005). Furthermore, improvements in SE after self-management and cognitive-behavioral interventions are associated with improvements in pain, functional status, and psychological adjustment (Keefe et al., 2004; Marks, 2001). Reviews of psychological factors in chronic pain have concluded that the evidence for the role of SE across a broad range of pain populations is impressive (Geisser, Robinson, Miller, & Bade, 2003; Keefe et al., 2004). Moreover, SE also influences the prognosis after such acute physical interventions as surgery. Prospective studies in patients who underwent orthopedic surgery demonstrated that high SE before the start of rehabilitation, as well as larger increases over the course of a rehabilitation, speeds recovery and predicts better long-term outcomes (Dohnke, Knauper, & Muller Fahrnow, 2005; Orbell, Johnston, Rowley, Davey, & Espley, 2001).

Bandura (1977) suggested that given sufficient motivation to engage in a behavior, a person will rely on his or her SE beliefs to determine the choice of activities to initiate, the amount of effort to expend, and how long to persist in the face of obstacles and aversive experiences. Such SE judgments are based on the following four sources of information regarding people's capabilities, in descending order of impact: (1) their own past performance at the task or similar tasks; (2) the performance accomplishments of others who are perceived to be similar to themselves; (3) verbal persuasion by others that they are capable; and (4) perception of their own state of physiological arousal, which is in turn partly determined by prior efficacy estimation. Performance mastery experience can be created by encouraging patients to undertake subtasks that are increasingly difficult or close to the desired behavioral repertoire. From this perspective, the occurrence of coping behaviors is conceptualized as being mediated by the person's beliefs that the demands of the situation do not exceed their coping resources.

Attention

Attention has a selective and amplifying function. The presence of pain may change the way people process pain-related and other information. For example, the presence of chronic pain may focus attention on all types of bodily signals. Chronic pain patients report a multitude of bodily symptoms in addition to pain (e.g., Bennett, Jones, Turk, Russell, & Matallana, 2007). Consistent with the FAM, patients may believe that pain symptoms are indicative of an underlying disease and so they may do everything to avoid pain exacerbations, most often by resorting to inactivity. Patients may use the presence of a disease or symptoms following a trauma to explain common bodily perturbations that might otherwise be ignored (Robinson et al., 2007; Turk, Okifuji, Starz, & Sinclair, 1996).

The processing of internal information may become disturbed in chronic pain patients. It is possible that pain patients become preoccupied with and overemphasize physical symptoms and interpret them as painful stimulation, although they may be less able then healthy controls to differentiate threshold levels (Robinson et al., 2007; Turk et al., 1996). Studies with diverse populations of pain patients (e.g., irritable bowel syndrome: Whitehead, 1980; fibromyalgia: Tunks, Crook, Norman, & Kalasher, 1988; angina pectoris: Droste & Roskamm, 1983; headaches: Borgeat, Hade, Elie, & Larouche, 1984) have supported the presence of what appears to be a hypersensitivity characterized by a lowered threshold for labeling stimuli as noxious.

PERSONALITY STYLE

As discussed earlier, specific pain cognitions (appraisal and beliefs) are largely shaped by an individual's learning history, either through direct experience, result of observation, or information from others. Temperamental or personality factors may predispose some people to make certain kinds of appraisals and to be more susceptible to some beliefs than to others. Temperament is supposed to be at least partly heritable and to show continuity throughout life. Personality in adulthood reflects the molding of underlying temperament by life experiences. Temperament and personality can be vulnerability factors that predispose toward catastrophic misinterpretation of pain sensations and maladaptive pain beliefs, or they can be resilience factors protecting against maladaptive cognitions and promoting SE beliefs.

One personality trait that has received attention in chronic pain is anxiety sensitivity (AS), defined as the fear of anxiety-related sensations. AS is conceived to be a partly heritable personality trait (Reiss, Peterson, Gursky, & McNally, 1986; Stein, Jang, & Livesley, 1999). Individuals with high AS interpret unpleasant physical sensations (e.g., rapid heart beating, feeling dizzy) more often as a sign of danger than do individuals with low AS. There is some evidence that AS may also be a risk factor for the maintenance and exacerbation of chronic pain and disability (Asmundson, Wright, & Hadjistavropoulos, 2000). Furthermore, AS correlates with measures of fear avoidance and is associated with distress, analgesic use, and physical and social functioning in patients across a wide range of different pain-related conditions (Keogh & Asmundson, 2004). Moreover, experimental evidence supports that AS is causally associated with maladaptive pain cognitions and poor behavioral and psychological adjustment to pain; thus AS is not merely a correlate of the chronic pain experience (Keogh & Cochrane, 2002; Keogh & Mansoor, 2001). Trait hope is a personality construct that is closely related to optimism (Snyder, Rand, & Sigmond, 2005), and some research has begun to address its association with adjustment to pain. Using the cold-pressor test to induce experimental pain, Snyder and colleagues found that high-hope people experienced less pain and tolerated the pain stimulus longer than did low-hope people (Snyder, Berg, et al., 2005).

Only a few studies have been looking at the role of dispositional optimism or hope in adaptation to chronic pain. Novy, Nelson, Hetzel, Squitieri, and Kennington (1998) found that optimism was related to less catastrophizing and more use of active coping strategies in chronic pain patients. Affleck and Tennen (1996) reported that dispositional optimism predicts pleasant daily mood in FM but that it is not related to daily pain. Finally, in studying rheumatoid arthritis patients, Treharne, Kitas, Lyons, and Booth (2005) found that optimism was associated with less depression and higher life satisfaction, as well as to less pain for patients in the early and intermediate stages of disease. The main mechanism of the beneficial effect of optimism may be differences in coping behavior between optimistic and pessimistic people (Carver & Scheier, 2005).

INTEGRATIVE MODELS

As evidenced by the extensive discussion of the key role of psychological factors in chronic pain, an integrative model needs to incorporate the mutual interrelations among physical, psychosocial, and behaviorial factors and the changes that occur among these relationships over time (Flor et al., 1990; Turk & Rudy, 1991). Several sets of investigators have proposed integrative models of pain, all with somewhat different emphasis; but each attempts to integrate physiological and psychological variables in the etiology, severity, exacerbation, and maintenance of pain.

GATE CONTROL THEORY

The first attempt to develop an integrative model was the gate control theory (GCT), proposed by Melzack and his colleagues (Melzack & Casey, 1968; Melzack & Wall, 1965), alluded to previously. Perhaps the most important contribution of the GCT is the way it changed thinking about pain perception. Melzack and Casey differentiate three systems related to the processing of nociceptive stimulation—sensory-discriminative, motivational-affective, and cognitive-evaluative—all thought to contribute to the subjective experience of pain. Thus, the GCT specifically includes psychological factors as an integral aspect of the pain experience. It emphasizes the central nervous system (CNS) mechanisms and provides a physiological basis for the role of psychological factors in pain.

The GCT proposes that a mechanism in the dorsal horn substantia gelatinosa of the spinal cord acts as a spinal gating mechanism that inhibits or facilitates transmission of nerve impulses from the body to the brain on the basis of the diameters of the active peripheral fibers as well as the dynamic action of brain processes. The theory postulates that the spinal gating mechanism is influenced by the relative amount of excitatory activity in afferent, large-diameter (myelinated) and small-diameter (unmyelinated nociceptor) fibers converging in the dorsal horns. It further proposes that activity in A-β (large-diameter) fibers tends to inhibit transmission of nociceptive signals (i.e., closes the gate), whereas A-δ and c (small-diameter fibers) primary afferent activity tends to facilitate transmission (i.e., opens the gate). The hypothetical gate is proposed to be located in the dorsal horn, and it is at this point that sensory input is modulated by the balance of activity of A-δ and c and A-β fibers.

In a seminal feature of the GCT, Melzack and Wall (1965) postulated the spinal gating mechanism is influenced not only by peripheral afferent activity but also by efferent neural impulses that descend from the brain. These descending inhibitory pathways were the primary proposed physiological mechanisms to account for the role of psychological factors in pain processing. Although initially proposed as an inhibitory control, according to current research, connections from the brain to the spinal cord are both facilitatory and inhibitory (Millan, 2002).

The GCT maintains that the large-diameter fibers play an important role in pain by inhibiting synaptic transmission in dorsal horn cells. When large-fiber input is decreased, mild stimuli, which are not typically painful, trigger severe pain. Loss of sensory input to this complex neural system, such as occurs in neuropathies, causalgia, and phantom-limb pain, tend to weaken inhibition and lead to persistent pain. Herniated disc material, tumors, and other factors that exert pressure on these neural structures may operate through this mechanism. Emotional stress and medication that affect the reticular formation may also alter the biasing mechanisms and thus the intensity of pain.

From the GCT perspective, the experience of pain is an ongoing sequence of activities, largely reflexive in nature at the outset, but modifiable even in the earliest stages by a variety of excitatory and inhibitory influences, as well as the integration of ascending and descending nervous system activity. The process results in overt expressions communicating pain and strategies by the person to terminate the pain. In addition, considerable potential for shaping of the pain experience is implied because the GCT invokes continuous interaction of multiple systems (sensory-physiological, affect, cognition, and ultimately, behavior).

The GCT describes the integration of peripheral stimuli with such cortical variables as mood and anxiety in the perception of pain. The GCT contradicts the notion that pain is either somatic or psychogenic and instead postulates that both factors have either potentiating or moderating effects on pain. In this model, for example, pain is not understood to be the result of depression or vice versa; rather, the two are seen as evolving simultaneously. Any significant change in mood or pain will necessarily alter the others.

The GCT's emphasis on the modulation of inputs in the dorsal horns and the dynamic role of the brain in pain processes and perception resulted in such psychological variables as past experience, attention, and other cognitive activities being integrated into current research and therapy on pain. Prior to this formulation, psychological processes were largely dismissed as reactions to pain. This new model suggested that cutting nerves and pathways was inadequate because a host of other factors modulated the input. Perhaps the major contribution of the GCT was that it highlighted the central nervous system as an essential component in pain processes and perception.

The physiological details of the GCT have been challenged, and it has been suggested that the model is incomplete (Nathan, 1976; Price, 1987). As additional knowledge has been gathered since the original formulation in 1965, specific points of posited mechanisms have been disputed and have required revision and reformulation (Nathan, 1976; Wall, 1989). Overall, however, the GCT has proved remarkably resilient and flexible in the face of accumulating scientific data and challenges to it, and it still provides a "powerful summary of the phenomena observed in the spinal cord and brain, and has the capacity to explain many of the most mysterious and puzzling problems encountered in the clinic" (Melzack & Wall, 1982, p. 261). The GCT can be credited as a source of inspiration for diverse clinical applications to control or manage pain, including neurophysiologically based procedures (e.g., neural stimulation techniques, from peripheral nerves and collateral processes in the dorsal columns of the spinal cord; North, 1989), pharmacological advances (Abram, 1993), behavioral treatments (Fordyce, Roberts, & Sternbach, 1985), and those interventions targeting modification of attentional and perceptual processes involved in the pain experience (Turk et al., 1983). After the GCT was proposed in 1965, no one could try to explain pain exclusively in terms of peripheral factors.

Although the GCT provided a physical basis for the role of psychological factors in pain, it does not address the nature of the psychological factors in depth. That is, it does not incorporate many of the specific psychological variables reviewed previously. The two models to be described, the diathesis-stress and cognitive-behavioral models, offer more conceptual models of the role of operant, respondent, social learning, and cognitive factors already described.

DIATHESIS-STRESS MODEL

Although everyone experiences acute pain, only a small percentage of people develop chronic pain syndromes. Flor et al. (1990) suggested that neither somatogenic nor psychogenic factors by themselves were sufficient to explain the development of chronic pain. They proposed that preconditions for chronic pain, including predisposing factors, precipitating stimuli, precipitating responses, and maintaining processes, were all required to explain the processes involved. The existence of a physiological predisposition or diathesis involving a specific body system is the first component of this model. This predisposition consists of a reduced threshold for nociceptive activation that may be related to genetic variables, previous trauma, or social learning experiences and results in a physiological response stereotypy of the specific body system. The existence of persistent aversive external and/or internal stimuli (pain-related or other stressors) with negative meaning activate the sympathetic nervous system and muscular processes (e.g., such various aversive emotional stimuli as familial conflicts or pressures related to employment) as unconditioned and conditioned stimuli and motivate avoidance responses. Aversive stimuli may be characterized by "excessive" intensity, duration, or frequency of an external or internal stimulus. An "inadequate" or "maladaptive" behavioral, cognitive, or physiological repertoire of the individual reduces the impact of these aversive environmental or internal stimuli.

Flor et al. (1990) suggested that an important role is played by the cognitive processing of external or internal stimuli related to the experience of stress and pain; for example, increased perception, preoccupation, and overinterpretation of physical symptoms or maladaptive perception of such internal stimuli as muscle tension levels. Moreover, this view suggests that the nature of the coping response (active avoidance, passive tolerance, or depressive withdrawal) may determine the type of problem that develops as well as the course of the illness. The diathesis-stress model (DSM) proposes further that such subsequent maladaptive physiological responding as increased and persistent sympathetic arousal and increased and persistent muscular reactivity may induce or exacerbate pain episodes. The authors suggested that learning processes in the form of respondent conditioning of fear of activity (including social, motor, and cognitive activities), that is, of operant learning of pain behaviors and of pain-related covert and physiological responses as described earlier, make a contribution to chronicity.

Although the DSM focuses more conceptually rather than physiologically on the role of stress and psychological factors on pain processing, physiological responses to chronic stress aid in the understanding of how maladaptive physiological responding may play a role in the development of chronic pain syndromes. Physiologically, during periods of short-term stress and homeostatic imbalance, the hypothalamus activates the pituitary gland to secrete adrenocorticotropic hormone, which acts on the adrenal cortex to secrete cortisol. Secretion of cortisol elevates blood sugar levels and enhances metabolism, an adaptive response that allows the organism to mobilize energy resources to deal with the threat and restore homeostatic balance (i.e., the fight-or-flight response). Prolonged, elevated levels of cortisol associated with chronic stress are, however, related to the exhaustion phase of Selye's general adaptation syndrome (Selye, 1950). The negative effects of this stage of the adaptation syndrome include atrophy of muscle tissue, impairment of growth and tissue repair, and immune system suppression, which together might set up conditions for the development and maintenance of a variety of chronic pain conditions (McBeth et al., 2005; McLean et al., 2005). The degree of these negative effects will vary based on individual differences in psychological processes discussed in depth earlier.

In short, the DSM places greatest emphasis on the role of learning factors in the onset, exacerbation, and maintenance of pain for those people with persistent pain problems. Flor et al. (1990) suggested that a range of factors predispose individuals to develop chronic pain; however, the predisposition is necessary but not sufficient. Conditioning and individual differences are central to this model.

COGNITIVE-BEHAVIORAL MODEL

The DSM tends to give priority to conditioning. The cognitive-behavioral model (CBM) incorporates many of the same constructs as the DSM (viz., anticipation, avoidance, and contingencies of reinforcement) but suggests that cognitive factors, and in particular expectations rather than conditioning factors, are of central importance. It suggests that so-called conditioned reactions are largely self-activated on the basis of learned expectations rather than automatically evoked. The critical factor for the CBM, therefore, is not that events occur together in time, but that people learn to "predict them and to summon appropriate reactions" (Turk et al., 1983). It is the individual patient's processing of information that results in anticipatory anxiety and avoidance behaviors.

From the CBM, people with chronic pain, as is true for all people, are viewed as active processors of information. They have negative expectations about their own ability and responsibility to exert any control over their pain. Moreover, they often view themselves as helpless. Such negative, maladaptive appraisals about their condition, situation, and personal efficacy in controlling their pain and problems associated with pain serve to reinforce the experience of demoralization, inactivity, and overreaction to nociceptive stimulation. These cognitive appraisals are posed as having an effect on behavior, leading to reduced effort, reduced perseverance in the face of difficulty, and increased psychological distress.

The specific thoughts and feelings that people experienced prior to exacerbations of pain, during an exacerbation or intense episode of pain, as well as following a pain episode, can greatly influence the experience of pain and subsequent pain episodes (Newton & Barbaree, 1987). Moreover, the methods people use to control their emotional arousal and symptoms have been shown to be important predictors of both cognitive and behavioral responses (Flor & Turk, 1988; Reesor & Craig, 1988). As described previously, interrelated sets of cognitive variables include thoughts about the controllability of pain, attributions about the person's own ability to use specific pain-coping responses, expectations concerning the possible outcomes of various coping efforts, and common erroneous beliefs about pain and disability. People respond to medical conditions in part based on their subjective representations of illness and symptoms (schema). When confronted with new stimuli, people engage in a "meaning analysis" that is guided by the schema that best match the attributes of the stimulus (Cioffi, 1991). It is on the basis of the person's idiosyncratic schema that incoming stimuli are interpreted, labeled, and acted on.

People build fairly elaborate representations of their physical state, and these representations provide the basis for action plans and coping (Nerenz & Leventhal, 1983; Turk, Rudy, & Salovey, 1986). Beliefs about the meaning of pain and people's ability to function despite discomfort are important aspects of the cognitive schema about pain (Atkinson, Slater, Patterson, Grant, & Garfin, 1991). These representations are used to construct causal, covariational, and consequential information from their symptoms. For example, a cognitive schema that a person has a serious debilitating condition, that disability is a necessary aspect of pain, that activity is dangerous, and that pain is an acceptable excuse for neglecting responsibilities will likely result in maladaptive responses (Jensen et al., 1994; Williams & Thorn, 1989). Similarly, if people believe they have a serious condition that is quite fragile and a high risk for reinjury, they may fear engaging in physical activities (Philips, 1987). Through a process of stimulus generalization, patients may avoid more and more activities, become more physically deconditioned, and consequently become more disabled.

Patients' beliefs, appraisals, and expectations about their pain, their ability to cope, their social supports, their disorder, the medicolegal system, the health care system, and their employers are all important because they may facilitate or disrupt the patient's sense of control and ability to manage pain. These factors also influence people's investment in treatment, acceptance of responsibility, perceptions of disability, adherence to treatment recommendations, support from significant others, expectancies for treatment, and acceptance of treatment rationale (Atkinson et al., 1991; Turk & Rudy, 1991).

Cognitive interpretations also will affect how patients present symptoms to significant others, including health care providers and employers. Overt communication of pain, suffering, and distress (limping and moaning) will enlist responses that may reinforce the pain behaviors and impressions about the seriousness, severity, and uncontrollability of the pain. That is, complaints of pain may lead physicians to prescribe more potent medications, order additional diagnostic tests, and in some cases perform surgery. Family members may express sympathy, excuse the patient from usual responsibilities, and encourage passivity, thereby fostering further physical deconditioning. It should be obvious that the cognitive-behavioral perspective integrates the operant conditioning emphasis on external reinforcement and the respondent view of learned avoidance within the framework of information processing.

The primary focus of the CBM, similar to the DSM, is on the person, rather than on symptoms and pathophysiology. Unlike the DSM, however, the CBM places emphasis on the person's thoughts and feelings because these will influence behavior. Conversely, the CBM acknowledges that environmental factors can also influence behavior and that behavior can affect patients' thoughts and feelings. Bandura (1978) referred to this as a process of reciprocal determinism. From this perspective, assessment of and consequently treatment of the person with persistent pain requires a broader strategy than those based on the previous dichotomous models described, which examined and addressed the entire range of psychosocial, behavioral, and biomedical factors (Turk & Burwinkle, 2007).

In pain management, the CBM focuses on providing patients with techniques to gain a sense of control over the effects of pain on their lives, as well as actually modifying the affective, behavioral, cognitive, and sensory facets of the experience. Behavioral experiences help to show people that they are capable of more than they assumed, increasing their sense of personal competence. Cognitive techniques help to place affective, behavioral, cognitive, and sensory responses under the patient's control. The assumption is that long-term maintenance of behavioral changes will occur only if patients have learned to attribute success to their own efforts. There are suggestions that these treatments can result in changes of beliefs about pain, coping style, and reported pain severity, as well as direct behavior changes (Turner & Clancy, 1986, 1988). Further, treatment that results in increases in perceived control over pain and decreased catastrophizing also are associated with decreases in pain severity ratings and functional disability (Jensen, Turner, Romano, & Karoly, 1991; Turner, 1991).

ANATOMICAL, PHYSIOLOGICAL, AND CHEMICAL BASES OF PAIN

The primitive classical theories of pain processing were based on the idea of a nociceptive stimulus applied at the periphery, connecting by means of a nerve fiber through the spinal cord to the "pain center" in the brain. Our current understanding of the physiological processes involved in pain processing is much more complex but has been built on this primitive tenet. Between the stimulus of tissue injury and the subjective experience of pain is a series of complex electrical and chemical events. In considering pain, it is important to have a conceptual understanding of the physiological processes involved and the anatomical structures that are believed to be important. It is equally important to be aware that the understanding of pain is far from complete, and thus what is described in this section must be viewed as a puzzle with pieces missing and some in the wrong place.

Four distinct physiological processes have been identified in pain: transduction, transmission, modulation, and perception (Fields, 1987). Consideration of these processes will guide our review of anatomical, physiological, and chemical bases subserving the experience of pain.

Transduction

Embedded in the various peripheral tissues are nerve endings that respond best to noxious stimuli (nociceptors). Transduction or receptor activation is the process where one form of energy (chemical, mechanical, or thermal) is converted into another, in this case, the electrochemical nerve impulse in the primary afferents (peripheral fibers that project to the spinal cord). By this process, information about a stimulus is converted to a form that is accessible to the brain. Information is coded by the frequency of impulses in the primary afferents activated by the stimulus. Noxious stimuli lead to electrical activity (action potentials) in the appropriate sensory nerve endings. The transduction process is dependent not only on the mechanical or thermal stimulation of the nerve endings but also on the sensitization related to prolonged stimulation and the release of chemical substances—for example, bradykinin, adenosine triphosphate (ATP), 5-hydroxytryptamine, and potassium—that either stimulate the receptor directly or that sensitize it and lead to such additional phenomena as swelling, vasodilatation, release of histamine from the cells, and hyperalgesia. There are a number of different types of nociceptors, and they vary in the number of neurotransmitters they contain, how fast they conduct electrical messages, how many receptors they express, and how readily they are sensitized during injury. With modern biomedical techniques, significant progress has been made regarding the variation of nociceptors and understanding the specific role each of these subtypes plays in the transduction of nociceptive processing.

Transmission

Transmission refers to the process by which coded information is relayed to those structures of the CNS whose activity produces the sensation of pain. The process of transmission involves the transportation of information from the receptor along the neuron to synapses with other neurons. There are three major neural systems of the pain transmission system: the peripheral sensory nerves (primary afferents), which transmit impulses from the site of transduction to their terminals in the spinal cord; networks of relay neurons that ascend the spinal cord to the brainstem and thalamus; and reciprocal connections between the thalamus and cortical structures. The first stage of transmission is the conduction of impulses in primary afferents to the spinal cord. Nociceptive signals are conducted to the dorsal horns of the spinal cord by means of myelinated (Aδ) and unmyelinated (c) nerve fibers. They differ in the type of pain experience they convey. The Aδ fibers convey a sharp, piercing and "fast" type of pain ("first pain"); the c fibers transmit a secondary and slow pain that tends to be more burning and dull ("second pain"). At the spinal cord, as superficially described in the GCT, primary afferent input is modulated by inhibitory interneurons, descending facilitatory and and inhibitory neurons from the brain, and nonnociceptive primary afferent Aβ fibers. This message will eventually elicit a variety of responses ranging from withdrawal reflexes to the subjective perceptual events ("It hurts!").

The second stage of transmission is conduction of impulses from spinal projection neurons to the thalamus, followed by the third stage, which involves reciprocal connections among the thalamus and various cortical structures. Although a number of pain pathways are described, there are two key pathways in transmitting nociceptive information from the spinal cord to the brain: the lateral and medial pain pathways. The lateral pain system ascends by means of the spinal cord to the lateral thalamus, and from the lateral thalamus to the somatosensory cortex, and has been implicated in the sensory-discriminative component of pain (Hsu & Shyu, 1997; Vogt & Sikes, 2000). Stimulation of neurons in the lateral system evokes perception of a localized (i.e., hand or foot), specific (i.e., burn or prick) type of pain. The medial system ascends by means of the spinal cord, terminates in various nuclei within the medial thalamus, and further projects to cortical structures within the limbic system (e.g., Shyu, Lin, Sun, Chen, & Chang, 2004; Wang & Shyu, 2004) and is thought to play a specific role in the motivational-affective component of pain (Price & Dubner, 1977; Vogt & Gabriel, 1993). Neurons in the medial system have primarily wide receptive fields, and electrial activation evokes perception of diffuse, widespread and nonspecific pain, consistent with a role in affective pain processing.

The neurons are activated by noxious stimuli, and their pattern of activity is thus a complex function of the primary afferent barrage that arrives at the spinal cord and the inhibitory and excitatory influences that are active at the time. In sum, the process of transmission consists of the primary afferent nociceptors terminating in the dorsal horn of the spinal cord. The axons of spinal neurons are activated by these afferent nociceptors and then cross to the anterolateral quadrant on the side opposite to the activated nociceptors. The message then ascends to the brainstem and by means of the thalamus to the cortex.

A number of transmitters, including glutamate and aspartate and neuropeptides, such as substance P and somatostatin, are involved in the transmission of nociceptive input at the dorsal horn. Excitatory amino acids, for example, C-glutamate, are the most important transmitters in nociceptive signaling. They are released by afferent fibers, spinal cord neurons, and alsosupraspinal structures. Most nociceptive neurons have ionotropic N-methyl-D-aspartate (NMDA) and non-NMDA receptors as well as metabotropic glutamate receptors. The NMDA receptors also seem to play an important role in the hyperreactivity of neurons subsequent to tissue damage. Although glutamate has historically been known as the primary excitatory neurotransmitter in pain processing, tachykinins, most notably Substance P, have been receiving increased attention for their role in both central and peripheral facilitatory pain processing. They are also released both peripherally and centrally and are known for their active role in the inflammatory process.

MODULATION

Modulation refers to the neural activity leading to control of the pain transmission pathway. Just as there are several nociceptive mechanisms, there are a number of pain-modulating mechanisms in the central nervous system. Inputs from the frontal cortex and hypothalamus activate cells in the midbrain, which control spinal pain-transmission cells by means of cells in the medulla. The activity of this modulatory system is one reason why people with apparently severe injuries may deny significant levels of pain (Beecher, 1959; Wall, 1979).

Although we are far from understanding all the complexities of the human mind, we know that there are specific pathways in the CNS that control pain transmission, and there is evidence that these pathways can be activated by the psychological factors described earlier. The midbrain, periaqueductal gray matter, and adjacent reticular formation that project to the spinal cord through the rostroventral medulla are all involved in the modulation of nociceptive signals (Fields, 1987). This pathway inhibits spinal neurons that respond to noxious stimuli. There is also a pain-modulating pathway from the dorsolateral pons to the cord. The pathway from the rostral medulla to the cord is partly serotonergic, whereas that from the dorsolateral pons is at least noradrenergic.

In addition to the biogenic amine-containing neurons are endogenous opioid peptides, which are present in all the regions implicated in pain modulation. The opioid-mediated analgesia system can be activated by electrical stimulation or by such opiate drugs as morphine. It can also be activated by pain, stress, and suggestion. Opioids produce analgesia by direct action on the CNS and activate the nociceptive-modulating system. Opioid receptors have two distinct functions: chemical recognition and biological action. Researchers reasoned that the brain itself ought to synthesize molecules that would act at these highly specific receptor sites. Endogenous opioid peptides, namely, leucine-enkephalin, methionine-enkephalin, beta-endorphin, dynorphin, alpha-neoendorphin—pharmacologically similar to morphine reversed by opioid antagonists (e.g., naloxone)—have all been identified.

The important endogenous pain inhibitory system involves descending analgesic pathways from the periaqueductal grey areas of midbrain to spinal dorsal horn by means of the raphe magnus nucleus of the pons; local enkephalinergic interneurons in the spinal cord; and peripheral A-β sensory fibers that presynaptically inhibit A-δ and c fibers at the dorsal horn. The inhibitory system utilizes several neurotransmitters, including serotonin, enkephalin, norepinephrine gamma aminobutyric acid (GABA), and somatostatin. The periaqueductal grey receives neuronal fibers from the cortex, the hypothalamus, and the limbic system, probably explaining the interaction of cognitive and emotional elements with pain perception and inhibition. Given the same noxious stimuli, the pain perception between two people may vary according to the phenomenon of attention or inhibition, both of which are probably modulated by various descending neurons. Emotion, attention, and motivation may all influence pain perception, probably through a complex network of reticular, limbic, and cortical fibers.

Modulation of peripheral pain sensation may occur at any stage in the perception process, either before pain stimuli are perceived or following perception, and may be either facilitatory or inhibitory. For example, if a person is in a traumatic environment or in a traumatizing incident such as a car accident, he or she may be unaware of any painful injury immediately following the incident, suggesting that inhibition occurs at the time of onset or prior to onset of the injury. Conversely, as described, in the presence of chronic pain, some patients may have heigtened attention to all types of sensory experience. The cognitive experience of heightened focus on sensory systems may result in descending excitatory connections that facilitate spinal cord signals, resulting in an increased perception of pain (Millan, 2002).

Perception

The final process involved with pain is perception. Somehow, the peripheral neural activity of the pain transmission neurons interacts with a central process to produce a subjective experience. How objectively observable neural events produce subjective experience is obscure. It is not even clear in which brain structures the activity that produces the perceptual event occurs. Because pain is fundamentally a subjective experience, there are inherent limitations to understanding it.

To understand the variability in individual experiences, it is useful to distinguish between pain detection threshold and pain tolerance. Pain threshold is a property of the sensory system that depends on the stimulus. It is highly reproducible in different people and in the same person at different times. In contrast to this reproducibility, pain tolerance is highly variable. There are several reasons for the variability. There may be an injury to the modulatory system that lowers pain intensity. There may be abnormal neural activity that may produce hypersensitivity that can result from self-sustaining processes set in motion by an injury but may persist beyond the time it takes for the original injury to heal. This self-sustaining process may even create a situation where pain is present without the noxious stimulus produced by an active tissue-damaging process (neuropathic pain, causalgia). Genetic factors are surely involved, and these will be described later. Finally, the psychological processes and factors previously described may affect normal pain intensity, creating unpredictable responses.

Pain tolerance is a manifestation of a person's reaction to pain and is highly dependent on psychological variables, described earlier. Not only does pain tolerance vary between different individuals in the same situation, but the same individual may react differently in different situations.

If pain were simply a sensation, these neural pain mechanisms would probably be sufficient to explain most of the clinically observed variability. However, pain is more than a sensation. The close association of the pain sensory system with the function of protecting the body from damage is unique among sensory systems. To understand pain patients, it is essential to consider the desire to escape from or terminate the sensation. If sensation is not unpleasant, then it is not pain.

As noted in the discussions of the DSM and CBM earlier, the meaning of pain is one important factor in determining pain tolerance. Different people have learned different ways of coping with pain; some minimize it, whereas some overreact. Thus, for many people it may be as important to know what they think their pain means as it is to know its cause. Because of the importance of the patient's interpretation, it is imperative, especially for chronic pain, to make some enquiry about this issue for treatment.

GENETICS

It has long been known that there is wide variation in the way individuals respond to noxious stimulation and treatment. Patients with the same disease and physical pathology often respond quite differently both to the experience and to the treatment. For example, studies have demonstrated sex differences in response to select opioids (Gear et al., 1996). Studies with different species of rats have demonstrated similar variability in responses (e.g., Mogil, Yu, & Basbaum, 2000). Both physical and psychological variables have been explored to assist in better understanding the differences. As we noted, conditioning, affective, and cognitive factors based on prior learning history have an influence on patients' responses. With the explication of the human genome, research is currently expanding to identify haplotypes (subtypes) of individuals with different sensitivity of nociception (e.g., Diatchenko, Nackley, Tchivileva, Shabalina, & Maixner, 2007). It is likely that integrated models that incorporate interactions between physiology and psychology will be provide the best understanding and guide treatment. We are only at the infant stage of understanding each of these classes of mechanisms, let alone the interaction among them.

CONCLUSION

From the patient's point of view, the report of pain connotes distress and is a plea for relief. The subjective experience includes an urge to escape from the cause or, if that is not possible, to obtain relief. It is the overwhelming desire to terminate it that gives pain its power. Pain can produce fear, and if it persists, depression; and ultimately, it can take away the will to live.

It has become abundantly clear that no isomorphic relationship exists between tissue damage and pain report. The more recent conceptualizations discussed view pain as a perceptual process resulting from the nociceptive input and modulation on a number of different levels in the CNS and not as directly proportional to nociceptive input.

Pain is a subjective, perceptual experience, and one characteristic differentiating it from pure sensation is its affective quality. Thus, pain appears to have two defining properties: bodily sensation and an aversive affect (Fernandez & Turk, 1992; Melzack & Casey, 1968). Quintessentially, pain is experienced at a physical level and an affective level.

In this chapter, conceptual models were presented to explain the subjective experience of pain. Current state of knowledge suggests that pain must be viewed as a complex phenomenon that incorporates physical, psychosocial, and behavioral factors. Failure to incorporate each of these factors will lead to an incomplete understanding and thereby inadequate treatment. The range of psychological variables that have been identified as being of central importance in pain, along with current understanding of the physiological basis of pain, were reviewed. Several integrative models were described that try to incorporate the available research and clinical information. Pain has become a vigorous research area and the virtual explosion of information will surely lead to refinements in understanding of pain and advances in clinical management.

REFERENCES

Abram, S. E. (1993). Advances in chronic pain management since gate control. *Regional Anesthesia, 18,* 66–81.

Affleck, G., & Tennen, H. (1996). Construing benefits from adversity: Adaptational significance and dispositional underpinnings. *Journal of Personality, 64,* 899–922.

Aldrich, S., Eccleston, C., & Crombez, G. (2000). Worrying about chronic pain: Vigilance to threat and misdirected problem solving. *Behaviour Research and Therapy, 38,* 457–470.

Arntz, A., & Claassens, L. (2004). The meaning of pain influences its experienced intensity. *Pain, 109,* 20–25.

Asmundson, G. J. G. (1999). Anxiety sensitivity and chronic pain: Empirical findings, clinical implications, and future directions. In S. Taylor (Ed.), *Anxiety sensitivity. Theory, research, and treatment of the fear of anxiety* (pp. 269–286). Mahwah, NJ: Erlbaum.

Asmundson, G. J., Norton, P. J., & Vlaeyen, J. W. S. (2004). Fear avoidance models of chronic pain: An overview. In G. J. Asmundson, J. W. S. Vlaeyen, & G. Crombez (Eds.), *Understanding and treating fear of pain* (pp. 3–24). Oxford, England: Oxford University Press.

Asmundson, G. J. G., Wright, K. D., & Hadjistavropoulos, H. D. (2000). Anxiety sensitivity and disabling chronic health conditions: State of the art and future directions. *Scandinavian Journal of Behaviour Therapy, 29,* 100–117.

Atkinson, J. H., Slater, M. A., Patterson, T. L., Gant, I., & Garfin, S. R. (1991). Prevalence, onset, and risk of psychiatric disorders in men with chronic low back pain: A controlled study. *Pain, 45,* 111–121.

Ballantyne, J. C., & Shin, N. S. (2008). Efficacy of opioids for chonic pain: A review of the evidence. *Clinical Journal of Pain, 24,* 469–478.

Bandura, A. (1977). Self-efficacy: Toward a unifying theory of behavior change. *Psychological Review, 84,* 191–215.

Bandura, A. (1978). The self-system in reciprocal determinism. *American Psychologist, 33,* 344–359.

Barry, L. C., Guo, Z., Kerns, R. D., Duong, B. D., & Reid, M. C. (2003). Functional self-efficacy and pain-related disability among older veterans with chronic pain in a primary care setting. *Pain, 104,* 131–137.

Beecher, H. K. (1959). *Measurement of subjective responses: Quantitative effects of drugs.* New York, NY: Oxford University Press.

Bennett, R. M., Jones, J., Turk, D. C., Russell, J., & Matallana, L. (2007). An internet survey of 2,596 people with fibromyalgia. *BMC Musculoskeletal Disorders, 8,* 27.

Boersma, K., & Linton, S. J. (2005). Screening to identify patients at risk: Profiles of psychological risk factors for early intervention. *Clinical Journal of Pain, 21,* 38–43.

Borgeat, F., Hade, B., Elie, R., & Larouche L. M. (1984). Effects of voluntary muscle tension increases in tension headache. *Headache, 24,* 199–202.

Buer, N., & Linton, S. J. (2002). Fear-avoidance beliefs and catastrophizing: Occurrence and risk factors in back pain and ADL in the general population. *Pain, 99,* 485–491.

Butler, R., Damarin, F., Beaulieu, C., Schwebel, A., & Thorn, B. E. (1989). Assessing cognitive coping strategies for acute post-surgical pain. *Psychological Assessment: A Journal of Consulting and Clinical Psychology, 1,* 41–45.

Carver, C. S., & Scheier, M. F. (2005). Optimism. In C. R. Snyder & S. J. Lopez (Eds.), *Handbook of positive psychology* (pp. 231–243). Oxford, England: Oxford University Press.

Chu, L. F., Angst, M. S., & Clark, D. (2008). Opioid-induced hyperalgesia in humans: Molecular mechanisms and clinical considerations. *Clinical Journal of Pain, 24,* 479–496.

Cioffi, D. (1991). Beyond attentional strategies: A cognitive-perceptual model of somatic interpretation. *Psychological Bulletin, 109,* 25–41.

Craig, K. D. (1986). Social modeling influences: Pain in context. In R. A. Sternbach (Ed.), *The psychology of pain* (2nd ed., pp. 67–95). New York, NY: Raven.

Craig, K. D. (1988). Consequences of caring: Pain in human context. *Canadian Psychologist, 28*, 311–321.

DeGroot, K. I., Boeke, S., van den Berge, H. J., Duivenvoorden, H. J., Bonke, B., & Passchier, J. (1997). Assessing short- and long-term recovery from lumbar surgery with pre-operative biographical, medical and psychological variables. *British Journal of Health Psychology, 2*, 229–243.

Deyo, R. A., Nachemson, A., & Mirza, S. K. (2004). Spinal-fusion surgery—The case for restraint. *New England Journal of Medicine, 350*, 722–726.

Diatchenko, L., Nackley, A. G., Tchivileva, I. E., Shabalina, S. A., & Maixner, W. (2007). Genetic architecture of human pain perception. *Trends in Genetics, 23*, 605–613.

Dohnke, B., Knauper, B., & Muller Fahrnow, W. (2005). Perceived self-efficacy gained from, and health effects of a rehabilitation program after hip joint replacement. *Arthritis and Rheumatism, 53*, 585–592.

Doleys, D. M., Crocker, M., & Patton, D. (1982). Response of patients with chronic pain to exercise quotas. *Physical Therapy, 62*, 1112–1115.

Droste, C., & Roskamm, H. (1983). Experimental pain measurement inpatients with asymptomatic myocardial ischemia. *Journal of the American College of Cardiology, 1*, 940–945.

Fagerhaugh, S. (1975). Pain expression and control on a burn care unit. *Nursing Outlook, 22*, 645–650.

Fernandez, E. (2002). *Anxiety, depression, and anger in pain: Research implications.* Dallas, TX: Advanced Psychology Resources.

Fernandez, E., & Turk, D. C. (1989). The utility of cognitive coping strategies for altering perception of pain: A meta-analysis. *Pain, 38*, 123–135.

Fernandez, E., & Turk, D. C. (1992). Sensory and affective components of pain: Separation and synthesis. *Psychological Bulletin, 112*, 205–217.

Fields, H. L. (1987). *Pain.* New York, NY: McGraw-Hill.

Flor, H., Birbaumer, N., & Turk, D. C. (1990). The psychobiology of chronic pain. *Advances in Behaviour Research and Therapy, 12*, 47–84.

Flor, H., Fydrich, T., & Turk, D. C. (1992). Efficacy of multidisciplinary pain treatment centers: A meta-analytic review. *Pain, 49*, 221–230.

Flor, H., & Turk, D. C. (1988). Chronic back pain and rheumatoid arthritis: Predicting pain and disability from cognitive variables. *Journal of Behavioral Medicine, 11*, 251–265.

Flor, H., Turk, D. C., & Birbaumer, N. (1985). Assessment of stress-related psychophysiological responses in chronic back pain patients. *Journal of Consulting and Clinical Psychology, 53*, 354–364.

Fordyce, W. E. (1976). *Behavioral methods for chronic pain and illness.* St. Louis, MO: C.V. Mosby.

Fordyce, W. E., Roberts, A. H., & Sternbach, R. A. (1985). The behavioral management of chronic pain: A response to critics. *Pain, 22*, 113–125.

Gear, R. W., Gordon, N. C., Heller, P. H., Paul, S., Miaskowski, C., & Levine, J. D. (1996). Gender difference in analgesic response to the kappa-opioid pentazocine. *Neuroscience Letters, 205*, 207–209.

Geisser, M. E., Robinson, M. E., Miller, Q. L., & Bade, S. M. (2003). Psychosocial factors and functional capacity evaluation among persons with chronic pain. *Journal of Occupational Rehabilitation, 13*, 259–276.

Gentry, W. D., & Bernal, G. A. A. (1977). Chronic pain. In R. Williams & W. D. Gentry (Eds.), *Behavioral approaches to medical treatment* (pp. 171–182). Cambridge, MA: Ballinger.

Gran, J. T. (2003). The epidemiology of chronic generalized musculoskeletal pain. *Best Practice and Research Clinical Rheumatology, 17*, 547–561.

Granot, M., & Ferber, S. G. (2005). The roles of pain catastrophizing and anxiety in the prediction of postoperative pain intensity: A prospective study. *Clinical Journal of Pain, 21*, 439–445.

Hsu, M. M., & Shyu, B. C. (1997). Electrophysiological study of the connection between medial thalamus and anterior cingulate cortex in the rat. *Neuroreport, 18*, 2701–2707.

Ives, T. J., Chelminski, P. R., Hammett-Stabler, C. A., Malone, R. M., Perhac, J. S., Potislek, N. M., … Pignoue, M. P. (2006). Predictors of opioid misuse in patients with chronic pain: A prospective cohort study. *BMC Health Services Research, 6*, 46.

Janssen, S. A., Spinhoven, P., & Arntz, A. (2004). The effects of failing to control pain: An experimental investigation. *Pain, 107*, 227–233.

Jensen, M. P., Ehde, D. M., Hoffman A. J., Patterson, D. R., Czerniecki, J. M., & Robinson, L. R. (2002). Cognitions, coping and social environment predict adjustment to phantom limb pain. *Pain, 95*, 133–142.

Jensen, M. P., & Karoly, P. (1991). Control beliefs, coping effort, and adjustment to chronic pain. *Journal of Consulting and Clinical Psychology, 59*, 431–438.

Jensen, M. P., Turner, J. A., & Romano, J. M. (1994). Correlates of improvement in multidisciplinary treatment of chronic pain. *Journal of Consulting and Clinical Psychology, 62*, 172–179.

Jensen, M. P., Turner, J. A., & Romano, J. M. (2007). Changes after multidisciplinary pain treatment in patient pain beliefs and coping are associated with concurrent changes in patient functioning. *Pain*, *131*, 38–47.

Jensen, M. P., Turner, J. A., Romano, J. M., & Karoly, P. (1991). Coping with chronic pain: A critical review of the literature. *Pain*, *47*, 249–283.

Jensen, M. P., Turner, J. A., Romano, J. M., & Lawler, B. K. (1994). Relationship of pain-specific beliefs to chronic pain adjustment. *Pain*, *57*, 301–309.

Keefe, F. J., Brown, G. K., Wallston, K. S., & Caldwell, D. S. (1989). Coping with rheumatoid arthritis pain. Catastrophizing as a maladaptive strategy. *Pain*, *37*, 51–56.

Keefe, F. J., Dunsmore, J., & Burnett, R. (1992). Behavioral and cognitive-behavioral approaches to chronic pain: Recent advances and future directions. *Journal of Consulting and Clinical Psychology*, *60*, 528–536.

Keefe, F. J., Rumble, M. E., Scipio, C. D., Giordano, L. A., & Perri, L. M. (2004). Psychological aspects of persistent pain: Current state of the science. *Journal of Pain*, *5*, 195–211.

Keogh, E., & Asmundson, G. J. (2004). Negative affectivity, catsatrophizing and anxiety sensitivity. In G. J. Asmundson, J. W. S. Vlaeyen, & G. Crombez (Eds.), *Understanding and treating fear of pain* (pp. 91–115). Oxford, England: Oxford University Press.

Keogh, E., & Cochrane, M. (2002). Anxiety sensitivity, cognitive biases, and the experience of pain. *Journal of Pain*, *3*, 320–329.

Keogh, E., & Mansoor, L. (2001). Investigating the effects of anxiety sensitivity and coping on the perception of cold pressor pain in healthy women. *European Journal of Pain*, *5*, 11–22.

Kerns, R. D., & Haythornthwaite, J. A. (1988). Depression among chronic pain patients: Cognitive-behavioral analysis and effect on rehabilitation outcome. *Journal of Consulting and Clinical Psychology*, *56*, 870–876.

Koplow, D. A. (1990, November). *Legal issues.* Paper presented at the annual scientific session of the American Academy of Disability Evaluating Physicians, Las Vegas, Nevada.

Kotarba, J. A. (1983). *Chronic pain: Its social dimensions.* Beverly Hills, CA: Sage.

Lawson, K., Reesor, K. A., Keefe, F. J., & Turner, J. A. (1990). Dimensions of pain-related cognitive coping: Cross-validation of the factor structure of the Coping Strategies Questionnaire. *Pain*, *43*, 195–204.

Lenthem, J., Slade, P. O., Troup, J. P. G., & Bentley, G. (1983). Outline of a fear-avoidance model of exaggerated pain perception. *Behaviour Research and Therapy*, *21*, 401–408.

Linton, S. J., Buer, N., Vlaeyen, J., & Hellsing, A. L. (2000). Are fear-avoidance beliefs related to the inception of an episode of back pain? A prospective study. *Psychology and Health*, *14*, 1051–1059.

Linton, S. J., Melin, L., & Götestam, K. G. (1984). Behavioral analysis of chronic pain and its management. In M. Hersen, R. Eisler, & P. Miller (Eds.), *Progress in behavior modification* (Vol. 18, pp. 1–42). New York, NY: Academic Press.

Marks, R. (2001). Efficacy theory and its utility in arthritis rehabilitation: Review and recommendations. *Disability and Rehabilitation*, *23*, 271–280.

Martin, B. I., Deyo, R. A., Mirza, S. K., Turner, J. A., Comstock, B. A., Hollinworth, W., & Sullivan, S. D. (2008). Expenditures and health status among adults with back and neck problems. *Journal of the American Medical Association*, *299*, 656–664.

Martin, P. R., Nathan, P., Milech, D., & Van Keppel, M. (1989). Cognitive therapy vs. self-management training in the treatment of chronic headaches. *British Journal of Clinical Psychology*, *28*, 347–361.

McBeth, J., Chiu, Y. H., Silman, A. J., Ray, D., Morriss, R., Dickens, C., … Macfarlane, G. J. (2005). Hypothalamic-pituitary-adrenal stress axis function and the relationship with chronic widespread pain and its antecedents. *Arthritis Research & Therapy*, *7*, R992–R1000.

McCracken, L. M. (1998). Learning to live with the pain: Acceptance of pain predicts adjustment in persons with chronic pain. *Pain*, *74*, 21–27.

McCracken, L. M., Carson, J. W., Eccleston, C., & Keefe, F. J. (2004). Acceptance and change in the context of chronic pain. *Pain*, *109*, 4–7.

McCracken, L. M., & Eccleston, C. (2003). Coping or acceptance: What to do about chronic pain? *Pain*, *105*, 197–204.

McLean, S. A., Williams, D. A., Harris, R. E., Kop, W. J., Groner, K. H., Ambrose, K., … Clauw, D. J. (2005). Momentary relationship between cortisol secretion and symptoms in patients with fibromyalgia. *Arthritis & Rheumatism*, *52*, 3660–3669.

Melzack, R., & Casey, K. L. (1968). Sensory, motivational and central control determinants of pain: A new conceptual model. In D. Kenshalo (Ed.), *The skin senses* (pp. 423–443). Springfield, IL: Thomas.

Melzack, R., & Wall, P. D. (1965). Pain mechanisms: A new theory. *Science*, *50*, 971–979.

Melzack, R., & Wall, P. D. (1982). *The challenge of pain.* New York, NY: Basic Books.

Merskey, H. (1986). Classification of chronic pain: Descriptions of chronic pain syndromes and definitions of pain terms. *Pain* (Suppl. 3), S1–S225.

Michna, E., Ross, E. L., Hynes, W. L., Nedeljkovic, S. S., Soumekh, S., Janfaza, D., … Jamison, R. N. (2004). Predicting aberrant drug behavior in patients treated for chronic pain: Importance of abuse history. *Journal of Pain and Symptom Management*, *28*, 250–258.

Millan, M. J. (2002). Descending control of pain. *Progress in Neurobiology*, *66*, 355–474.

Mogil, J. S., Yu, L., & Basbaum, A. I. (2000). Pain genes? Natural variation and transgenic mutants. *Annual Review of Neuroscience*, *23*, 777–811.

Muller, M., & Netter, P. (2000). Relationship of subjective helplessness and pain perception after electric skin stimuli. *Stress Medicine*, *16*, 109–115.

Nathan, P. W. (1976). The gate control theory of pain: A critical review. *Brain*, *99*, 123–158.

Nerenz, D. R., & Leventhal, H. (1983). Self-regulation theory in chronic illness. In T. Burish & L. A. Bradley (Eds.), *Coping with chronic illness* (pp. 13–37). Orlando, FL: Academic Press.

Newton, C. R., & Barbaree, H. E. (1987). Cognitive changes accompanying headache treatment: The use of a thought-sampling procedure. *Cognitive Therapy and Research*, *11*, 635–652.

Noble, M., Tregear, S. J., Treadwell, J. R., & Schoelles, K. (2008). Long-term opioid therapy for chronic non-cancer pain: A systematic review and meta-analysis of efficacy and safety. *Journal of Pain and Symptom Management*, *35*, 214–228.

North, R. B. (1989). Neural stimulation techniques. In C. D. Tollison (Ed.), *Handbook of chronic pain management* (pp. 136–146). Baltimore, MD: Williams & Wilkins.

Novy, D. M., Nelson, D. V., Hetzel, R. D., Squitieri, P., & Kennington, M. (1998). Coping with chronic pain: Sources of intrinsic and contextual variability. *Journal of Behavioral Medicine*, *31*, 19–34.

Olivier, J. W., Kravitz, R. L., & Kaplan, S. H. (2001). Individualized patient education and coaching to improve pain control among cancer outpatients. *Journal of Clinical Oncology*, *19*, 2206–2212.

Orbell, S., Johnston, M., Rowley, D., Davey, P., & Espley, A. (2001). Self-efficacy and goal importance in the prediction of physical disability in people following hospitalization: A prospective study. *British Journal of Health Psychology*, *6*, 25–40.

Pavin, D. J., Rapp, S. E., & Pollisar, N. (1998). Factors affecting discharge time in adult outpatients. *Anesthesia and Analgesia*, *87*, 816–826.

Pavlin, D. J., Sullivan, M. J., Freund, P. R., & Roesen, K. (2005). Catastrophizing: A risk factor for postsurgical pain. *Clinical Journal of Pain*, *21*, 83–90.

Philips, H. C. (1987). Avoidance behaviour and its role in sustaining chronic pain. *Behaviour Research and Therapy*, *25*, 273–279.

Picavet, H. S., Vlaeyen, J. W., & Schouten, J. S. (2002). Pain catastrophizing and kinesiophobia: Predictors of chronic low back pain. *American Journal of Epidemiology*, *156*, 1028–1034.

Pincus, T., Vogel, S., Burton, A. K., Santos, R., & Field, A. P. (2006). Fear avoidance and prognosis in back pain: A systematic review and synthesis of current evidence. *Arthritis & Rheumatism*, *54*, 399–410.

Price, D. D. (1987). *Psychological and neural mechanisms of pain*. New York, NY: Raven.

Price, D. D., & Dubner, R. (1977). Neurons that subserve the sensory-discriminative aspects of pain. *Pain*, *3*, 307–338.

Price, D. D., Harkins, S. W., & Baker, C. (1987). Sensory-affective relationships among different types of clinical and experimental pain. *Pain*, *28*, 297–307.

Rachman, S., & Arntz, A. (1991). The overprediction and underprediction of pain. *Clinical Psychology Review*, *11*, 339–356.

Rachman, S., & Lopatka, C. (1988). Accurate and inaccurate predictions of pain. *Behaviour Research and Therapy*, *26*, 291–296.

Raj, P. P. (1990). Pain relief: Fact or fancy? *Regional Anesthesia*, *15*, 157–169.

Reesor, K. A., & Craig, K. (1988). Medically incongruent chronic pain: Physical limitations, suffering and ineffective coping. *Pain*, *32*, 35–45.

Reiss, S., Peterson, R. A., Gursky, D. M., & McNally, R. J. (1986). Anxiety sensitivity, anxiety frequency and the predictions of fearfulness. *Behaviour Research and Therapy*, *24*, 1–8.

Richard, K. (1988). The occurrence of maladaptive health-related behaviors and teacher-related conduct problems in children of chronic low back pain patients. *Journal of Behavioral Medicine*, *11*, 107–116.

Robinson, J. P., Burwinkle, T., & Turk, D. C. (2007). Perceived and actual memory, concentration, and attention problems following whiplash associated disorders (grades I & II): Prevalence and predictors. *Archives of Physical Medicine Rehabilitation*, *88*, 774–779.

Robinson, J. P., Wilson, H., Swanson, K. S., & Turk, D. C. (2008). Symptom reporting in people with fibromyalgia—High and low endorsers. *Journal of Pain, 9*(suppl 2), 17.

Salomons, T. V., Johnstone, T., Backonja, M. M., & Davidson, R. J. (2004). Perceived controllability modulates the neural response to pain. *Journal of Neuroscience, 24*, 7199–7203.

Schmidt, A. J. M. (1985a). Cognitive factors in the performance of chronic low back pain patients. *Journal of Psychosomatic Research, 29*, 183–189.

Schmidt, A. J. M. (1985b). Performance level of chronic low back pain patients in different treadmill test conditions. *Journal of Psychosomatic Research, 29*, 639–646.

Selye, H. (1950). *Stress*. Montreal, Canada: Acta Medical Publisher.

Severeijns, R., Vlaeyen, J. W., & van den Hout, M. A. (2004). Do we need a communal coping model of pain catastrophizing? An alternative explanation. *Pain, 111*, 226–229.

Severeijns, R., Vlaeyen, J. W., van den Hout, M. A., & Picavet, H. S. (2005). Pain catastrophizing and consequences of musculoskeletal pain: A prospective study in the Dutch community. *Journal of Pain, 6*, 125–132.

Sharp, T. J. (2001). Chronic pain: A reformulation of the cognitive-behavioural model. *Behaviour Research and Therapy, 39*, 787–800.

Shyu, B. C., Lin, C. Y., Sun, J. J., Chen, S. L., & Chang, C., (2004). BOLD response to direct thalamic stimulation reveals a functional connection between the medial thalamus and the anterior cingulate cortex in the rat. *Magnetic Resonance Medicine, 52*, 47–55.

Smith, W. B., Gracely, R. H., & Safer, M. A. (1998). The meaning of pain: Cancer patients' rating and recall of pain intensity and affect. *Pain, 78*, 123–129.

Snyder, C. R., Berg, C., Woodward, J. T., Gum, A., Rand, K. L., & Wrobleski, K. K. (2005). Hope against the cold: Individual differences in trait hope and acute pain tolerance on the cold pressor task. *Journal of Personality, 73*, 287–312.

Snyder, C. R., Rand, K. L., & Sigmond, D. R. (2005). Hope theory: A member of the positive psychology family. In C. R. Snyder & S. J. Lopez (Eds.), *Handbook of positive psychology* (pp. 257–276). Oxford, England: Oxford University Press.

Stein, M. B., Jang, K. L., & Livesley, W. J. (1999). Heritability of anxiety sensitivity: A twin study. *American Journal of Psychiatry, 156*, 246–251.

Stewart, W. F., Lipton, R. B., Celentano, D. D., Verhagen, A. P., Bekkering, G. E., van der Windt, D. A., … Reed, M. L. (1991). Prevalence of migraine headache in the United States: Relation to age, income, race, and other sociodemographic factors. *Journal of the American Medical Association, 267*, 64–69.

Sullivan, M. D., & Turk D. C. (2001). Psychiatric disorders and psychogenic pain. In J. D. Loeser, S. H. Butler, C. R. Chapman, & D. C. Turk (Eds.), *Bonica's management of pain* (3rd ed., pp. 483–500). Philadelphia, PA: Williams and Wilkins.

Sullivan, M. J. L., Thorn, B., Haythornthwaite, J. A., Keefe, F., Martin, M., Bradley, L. A., & Lefebvre, J. C. (2001). Theoretical perspectives on the relation between catastrophizing and pain. *Clinical Journal of Pain, 17*, 52–64.

Tan, G., Jensen, M. P., Robinson Whelen, S., Thornby, J. I., & Monga, T. (2002). Measuring control appraisals in chronic pain. *Journal of Pain, 3*, 385–393.

Taylor, R. S., Van Buyten, J. P., & Buchser, E. (2005). Spinal cord stimulation for chronic back and leg pain and failed back surgery syndrome: A systematic review and analysis of prognostic factors. *Spine, 30*, 152–160.

Thieme, K., Flor, H., & Turk, D. C. (2006). Psychological treatment in fibromyalgia syndrome efficacy of operant behavioural and cognitive behavioural treatments. *Arthritis Research: Therapy, 8*, R121. http://arthritis-reseach-com/content/8/4/R121.

Thieme, K., Spies, C., Sinha, P., Turk, D. C., & Flor, H. (2005). Predictors of pain behaviors in fibromyalgia syndrome patients. *Arthritis Care & Research, 53,* 343–350.

Tota-Faucette, M. E., Gil, K. M., Williams, F. J., & Goli, V. (1993). Predictors of response to pain management treatment: The role of family environment and changes in cognitive processes. *Clinical Journal of Pain, 9*, 115–123.

Treharne, G. J., Kitas, G. D., Lyons, A. C., & Booth, D. A. (2005). Well-being in rheumatoid arthritis: The effects of disease duration and psychosocial factors. *Journal of Health Psychology, 10*, 457–474.

Tunks, E., Crook, J., Norman, G., & Kalasher, S. (1988). Tender points in fibromyalgia. *Pain, 34*, 11–19.

Turk, D. C. (2002). Clinical effectiveness and cost-effectiveness of treatments for patients with chronic pain. *Clinical Journal of Pain, 18*, 355–365.

Turk, D. C., & Burwinkle, T. (2007). Pain: A multidimensional perspective. In S. Ayers, A. Baum, C. McManus, S. Newman, K. Wallston, J. Weinman, & West, R. (Eds.), *Cambridge handbook of psychology, health, & medicine* (2nd ed., pp. 141–147). New York, NY: Cambridge University Press.

Turk, D. C., & Flor, H. (1987). Pain > pain behaviors: The utility and limitations of the pain behavior construct. *Pain, 31*, 277–295.

Turk, D. C., Kerns, R. D., & Rosenberg, R. (1992). Effects of marital interaction on chronic pain and disability: Examining the down-side of social support. *Rehabilitation Psychology, 37*, 259–274.

Turk, D. C., Meichenbaum, D., & Genest, M. (1983). *Pain and behavioral medicine: A cognitive-behavioral perspective.* New York, NY: Guilford Press.

Turk, D. C., & Okifuji, A. (1996). Perception of traumatic onset, compensation status, and physical findings: Impact on pain severity, emotional distress, and disability in chronic pain patients. *Journal of Behavioral Medicine, 19*, 435–453.

Turk, D. C., Okifuji, A., Starz, T. W., & Sinclair, J. D. (1996). Effects of type of symptom onset on psychological distress and disability in fibromyalgia syndrome patients. *Pain, 68,* 423–430.

Turk, D. C., & Rudy, T. E. (1988). Toward an empirically derived taxonomy of chronic pain patients: Integration of psychological assessment data. *Journal of Consulting and Clinical Psychology, 56*, 233–238.

Turk, D. C., & Rudy, T. E. (1991). Persistent pain and the injured worker: Integrating biomedical, psychosocial, and behavioral factors. *Journal of Occupational Rehabilitation, 1*, 159–179.

Turk, D. C., & Rudy, T. E. (1992). Cognitive factors and persistent pain: A glimpse into Pandora's box. *Cognitive Therapy and Research, 16*, 99–112.

Turk, D. C., Rudy, T. E., & Salovey, P. (1986). Implicit models of illness: Description and validation. *Journal of Behavioral Medicine, 9*, 453–474.

Turk, D. C., & Salovey, P. (1985). The reign of pain falls mainly in the brain. *Behavior and Brain Science, 8*, 71–72.

Turner, J. A. (1991). Coping and chronic pain. In M. R. Bond, J. E. Charlton, & C. J. Woolf (Eds.), *Proceedings of the 6th World Congress on Pain* (pp. 219–227). Amsterdam, Netherlands: Elsevier.

Turner, J. A., & Aaron, L. A. (2001). Pain-related catastrophizing: What is it? *Clinical Journal of Pain, 17*, 65–71.

Turner, J. A., & Clancy, S. (1986). Strategies for coping with chronic low back pain: Relationship to pain and disability. *Pain, 24*, 355–363.

Turner, J. A., & Clancy, S. (1988). Comparison of operant behavioral and cognitive-behavioral group treatment for chronic low back pain. *Journal of Consulting and Clinical Psychology, 56*, 261–266.

Turner, J. A., Dworkin, S. F., Mancl, L., Huggins, K. H., & Truelove, E. L. (2001). The role of beliefs, catastrophizing, and copign in the functioning of patients with temporomandibular disorders. *Pain, 92*, 41–51.

Turner, J. A., Jensen, M. P., & Romano, J. M. (2000). Do beliefs, coping, and catastrophizing independently predict functioning in patients with chronic pain? *Pain, 85*, 115–125.

Turner, J. A., Jensen, M. P., Warms, C. A., & Cardenas, D. D. (2002). Catastrophizing is associated with pain intensity, psychological distress, and pain-related disability among individuals with chronic pain after spinal cord injury. *Pain, 98*, 127–134.

Vangronsveld, K., Peters, M., Goossens, M., Linton, S., & Vlaeyen, J. (2007). Applying the fear-avoidance model to the chronic whiplash syndrome. *Pain, 130*, 258–261.

Vaughan, K. B., & Lanzetta, J. T. (1980). Vicarious instigation and conditioning of facial expressive and autonomic responses to a model's expressive display of pain. *Journal of Personality and Social Psychology, 38*, 909–923.

Vaughan, K. B., & Lanzetta, J. T. (1981). The effect of modification of expressive displays on vicarious emotional arousal. *Journal of Experimental Social Psychology, 17*, 1630.

Verhaak, P. F., Kerssens, J. J., Dekker, J., Sorbi, M., & Bensing, M. (1998). Prevalence of chronic benign pain disorder among adults: A review of the literature. *Pain, 77*, 231–239.

Viane, I., Crombez, G., & Eccleston, C. (2003). Acceptance of pain is an independent predictors of mental well-being in patients with chronic pain: Empirical evidence and reappraisal. *Pain, 106*, 65–72.

Vlaeyen, J. W. S., & Linton, S. J. (2000). Fear-avoidance and its consequences in chronic musculoskeletal pain: A state of the art. *Pain, 85*, 317–332.

Vogt, B. A., & Gabriel M. (1993). Anterior cingulate cortex and the medial pain system. In Neurobiology of cingulate cortex and limbic thalamus: A comprehensive handbook (pp. 313–344), Boston, MA: Birkhauser.

Vogt, B. A., & Sikes, R. W. (2000). The medial pain system, cingulate cortex, and parallel processing of nociceptive information. *Progress in Brain Research, 122*, 223–235.

Wall, P. D. (1979). On the relationship of injury to pain. *Pain, 6*, 63–264.

Wall, P. D. (1989). The dorsal horn. In P. D. Wall & R. Melzack (Eds.), *Textbook of pain* (2nd ed., pp. 102–111). New York, NY: Churchill-Livingstone.

Wang, C. C., & Shyu, B. C. (2004). Differential projections from the mediodorsal and centrolateral thalamic nuclei to the frontal cortex in rats. *Brain Research, 995*, 226–235.

Whitehead, W. E. (1980). Interoception. In R. Hölzl & W. E. Whitehead (Eds.), *Psychophysiology of the gastrointestinal tract* (pp. 145–161). New York, NY: Plenum.

Williams, D. A., & Thorn, B. E. (1989). An empirical assessment of pain beliefs. *Pain, 36*, 251–258.

Woby, S. R., Watson, P. J., Roach, N. K., & Urmston, M. (2005). Coping strategy use: Does it predict adjustment to chronic back pain after controlling for catastrophic thinking and self-efficacy for pain control? *Journal of Rehabilitation Medicine, 37*, 100–107.

8 What Are the Health Effects of Disclosure?

Joshua M. Smyth
Pennsylvania State University

James W. Pennebaker
University of Texas at Austin

Danielle Arigo
Syracuse University

Humans are social beings; we rely on others for safety and support, particularly in times of high stress or crisis. Sharing one's experiences is central to creating social bonds but also allows individuals to soothe the negative emotions arising from stressful life events. As a result, individuals have forged connections in various ways throughout history. Although face-to-face contact is the oldest mode of social expression, technological advances have allowed people to communicate over increasingly greater distances. Shouting, drum beating, and signal fires were early ways to convey information. With the advent of written language, it became possible to share our experiences with others through such written means as letters, notes, or even books. In the last 150 years, we have adapted electronic technologies to allow us to communicate over great distances by telegraph, telephone, and radio, culminating in the current array of Internet interactions. Through blogging, social networking sites, and tweets we can now share our current "status" (behavioral, emotional, or otherwise) with the entire world nearly instantaneously. People appear to want others to know what they are experiencing, including their locations, their actions, and—perhaps most important—their emotions.

What is it about sharing, or disclosing, one's personal information that is so appealing? Research has shown that disclosure can create or strengthen bonds between individuals, allow for successful management of a past stressor (Smyth, Hockemeyer, Heron, et al., 2008), and reduce guilt or shame associated with certain experiences (Murray-Swank, McConnell, & Pargament, 2007). Yet colloquial language suggests that there may be additional benefits to "letting out" one's feelings, given that "bottling them up" is generally considered problematic. Over the past two decades, there has been growing interest in the possibility that disclosing one's stressful experiences can lead to good health. Whereas positive experiences have been connected to improved health outcomes (Salovey, Rothman, Detweiler, & Steward, 2000), stressful experiences have been associated with symptoms and illness (Cohen, Doyle, & Baum, 2006; Cohen, Tyrrell, & Smith, 1991, 1993; Wilkerson, Bailey, Bieniasz, Murray, & Ruffin, 2009). Reluctance to disclose one's stressors has recently been associated with increased psychological distress (Barry & Mizrahi, 2005) and depressive affect (Iinying & Huichang, 2003; Zech, de Ree, Berenschot, & Stroebe, 2006). There is also considerable evidence that the failure to recognize or acknowledge emotions is associated with the development of many different disorders (see Singer, 1990). Some prospective studies have linked Type D personality (i.e., having high negative emotional reactivity and coupled with nonexpression and social inhibition) with poor health outcomes, including early mortality (Schiffer et al., 2006).

Despite the potential negative consequences of keeping important feelings to oneself, however, many people choose not to disclose their experiences because of various social constraints. Social constraints exist in the forms of lacking of supportive others in a social network, fear of rejection from others because of social stigma, the perception that others do not understand one's feelings, or role expectations that do not include emotional expression (Lepore & Revenson, 2007; Lepore, Silver, Wortman, & Wayment, 1996). In consideration of such constraints, researchers have sought disclosure methods that can circumvent the occurrence of social punishment (e.g., writing or speaking into a tape recorder). Many studies have now shown that disclosing stressful or traumatic events in these ways promotes physical health, psychological functioning, and subjective well-being (Antoni, 1999; Berry & Pennebaker, 1993; Frattaroli, 2006). This chapter describes existing research on emotional disclosure about personally important topics and how this process may improve health, with a specific focus on disclosure through writing.

ARE DISCLOSURE AND HEALTH OUTCOMES CONNECTED?

Pennebaker and colleagues initially conducted a series of surveys to examine the link between disclosure and general health. These surveys included hundreds of respondents and showed that individuals who had experienced trauma (e.g., abuse, death of a parent) reported increased physical health symptoms relative to individuals who had never experienced trauma (Pennebaker, 1985). Furthermore, those who had experienced trauma and who had not disclosed it reported more health care provider visits, diseases, health symptoms, and use of nonprescription medication than did other participants. Disclosing to others details about a specific trauma (e.g., death of a spouse), in contrast, was associated with fewer health symptoms and fewer ruminative thoughts about the death (Pennebaker & O'Heeron, 1984).

Similarly, a growing body of literature shows that concealing such stigmatized conditions as homosexual orientation or illness diagnosis may negatively affect health. For example, nondisclosure of one's homosexual orientation has been related to poor immune functioning (Strachan, Bennett, Russo, & Roy-Byrne, 2007), higher risk for developing such illnesses as cancer and pneumonia (Cole, Kemeny, Taylor, Visscher, & Fahey, 1996), and higher mortality rates (Cole, Kemeny, Taylor, & Vischer, 1996) among HIV-positive men. Likewise, concealment of an illness diagnosis such as HIV is often concurrent with poor physical health outcomes (e.g., immune function; Strachan et al., 2007), whereas disclosure of one's illness is associated with better health (Pennebaker & Susman, 1988).

Although these and other studies show that negative life experiences, nondisclosure, and health symptoms are somehow linked, such studies employ correlational designs that cannot establish causal connections between disclosure of negative experiences and improved health. For the purpose of determining the impact of disclosure on specific outcomes, an early set of studies asked participants to either disclose or not disclose their prior emotional experiences through writing (Pennebaker & Beall, 1986; Pennebaker, Colder, & Sharp, 1990). These studies resulted in positive health effects among college students who wrote about emotionally charged (i.e., disclosure) topics, but no such benefits were observed for students who wrote about emotionally neutral (i.e., nondisclosure) topics. Several subsequent tests incorporated new populations, health outcomes, and writing topics. Disclosure through writing has now been examined in more than 200 separate studies and has been subject to multiple literature syntheses supporting its efficacy across a variety of psychosocial and physical outcomes. The interest in written disclosure, also called structured expressive writing, is partially a result of its brevity, ease of administration, and potential for cost-effectiveness as an intervention (Pennebaker, 2004).

The standard design for laboratory-based written disclosure uses random assignment to one of two conditions: an experimental group that is asked to disclose about personal, emotional topics and a control group that is asked to disclose about emotionally neutral topics (e.g., daily activities). Groups are asked to write about their assigned topics on three to five consecutive days for 15 to

30 minutes each day. Writing is typically done in a private room with no feedback presented, and participants place their written narratives in a sealed box when completed. The standard instructions for participants assigned to the experimental, expressive writing group are as follows:

> For the next [three] days, I would like for you to write about your very deepest thoughts and feelings about an extremely important emotional issue that has affected you and your life. In your writing, I'd like you to really let go and explore your very deepest emotions and thoughts. You might tie your topic to your relationships with others, including parents, lovers, friends, or relatives. You might tie your writing to your past, your present, or your future, or to who you have been, who you would like to be, or who you are now. You may write about the same general issues or experiences on all days of writing, or write about different topics each day. All of your writing is completely confidential. Don't worry about spelling, sentence structure, or grammar. The only rule is that you once you begin writing, you continue until time is up.

These simple instructions have consistently led individuals to engage in substantively emotional disclosure. Participants have written about such experiences as the death of a loved one, divorce and separation, abuse or attack, and concerns about sexuality, intimacy, appearance, and poor academic or work performance. Although some participants report distress as an immediate result of writing about such topics (e.g., crying, feeling tense), a very large proportion characterize written disclosure as a valuable and meaningful experience. Written disclosure studies thus demonstrate that when individuals are given the opportunity to disclose about personally important topics, they willingly do so, and they perceive the experience as positive. Beyond these aspects, however, there is accumulating evidence that written disclosure may positively impact health and functioning as well.

EXPERIMENTAL EFFECTS OF DISCLOSURE ON OUTCOME MEASURES

Researchers have assessed the effects of disclosure on a variety of health-relevant dimensions, including health reports and health care utilization, physiological outcomes, psychological measures (e.g., measures of emotional state and well-being), employment and academic functioning, health behaviors, and short-term effects on mood. The present review includes only those studies that were conducted in adult samples, including college students, community members, and adult patients. This chapter also focuses mainly on written disclosure because much of the research has been done in this area, but includes relevant findings from the broader process of disclosure (i.e., disclosure through other modes). Readers interested in comprehensive reviews may refer to Frattaroli (2006) and Pennebaker and Chung (2007); the following sections provide a selective overview of key research findings in several important outcome domains.

HEALTH REPORTS AND HEALTH CARE UTILIZATION

As noted, initial written disclosure studies were conducted in college student samples and often examined self-reported physical symptoms and utilization of health care services (both proxies for physical illness). Students who disclosed emotional topics generally had fewer visits to college health centers (obtained from health records; Greenberg & Stone, 1992; Harrist, Carlozzi, McGovern, & Harrist, 2007; Pennebaker & Beall, 1986; Pennebaker et al., 1990; Pennebaker & Francis, 1996) and fewer self-reported health symptoms (Mosher & Danoff-Burg, 2006) relative to students who wrote about neutral topics. Students who engaged in written disclosure about relationship breakups were also protected against increases in upper respiratory infection symptoms that were displayed among control writing students (Lepore & Greenberg, 2002).

Similar benefits have generalized to nonstudent samples. For example, Swanbon, Boyce, and Greenberg (2008) found that gay men who wrote about gay-related experiences (e.g., "coming out") did not report increases in physical symptoms or physician visits, whereas men in the emotionally neutral writing group did report such increases. Maximum-security prisoners who wrote about traumatic events also visited the infirmary less frequently than did prisoners in the control condition (Richards, Beall, Seagal, & Pennebaker, 2000). Among individuals with such medical illnesses as prostate cancer (Rosenberg et al., 2002), breast cancer (Stanton et al., 2002), and fibromyalgia (Gillis, Lumley, Mosley-Williams, Leisen, & Roehrs, 2006), written disclosure resulted in fewer instances of health care utilization than did emotionally neutral writing.

In spite of the demonstrated benefits of written disclosure, there are also studies failing to find such effects. In order to examine the consistency of positive outcomes, several attempts have been made to cumulate research findings analytically (e.g., through meta-analysis). Frattaroli's (2006) recent meta-analysis of over 100 disclosure studies—including disclosure through writing and other modes—showed significant positive effect size for various illness-specific health outcomes and for overall self-reported health (Cohen's $d = .144$, which is equivalent to an $r = .072$); general physical symptoms showed a positive, albeit nonsignificant, effect size.

Combining findings across multiple studies shows a complicated pattern of results for health care utilization. The effect of disclosure on Frattaroli's (2006) broad category of "illness behaviors," which included medication use and medical visits, was significantly positive across various samples. Harris's (2006) meta-analysis, which was specifically focused on heath care utilization, found that written disclosure leads to lower utilization in healthy samples only (i.e., effect sizes for medical and psychiatric samples were not significant). In contrast, Frisina and colleagues (Frisina, Borod, & Lepore, 2004; Frisina, Lepore, & Borod, 2005) found small but significant improvements in utilization among medical and psychiatric patients relative to control writing. Overall, existing literature suggests that disclosure has small positive effects on physical symptoms and health care utilization across a range of study samples. Given that a majority of the literature in this area has tested the effect of written disclosure, it appears that this procedure holds promise for improving general and illness-specific health outcomes.

PHYSIOLOGICAL OUTCOMES AND ILLNESS-RELATED MEDICAL IMPROVEMENT

One of the most commonly assessed physiological processes in written disclosure studies is immune function, which has improved among disclosure-writing participants relative to emotionally neutral writing controls. Students in disclosure conditions demonstrated greater or more efficient immune function (Esterling, Antoni, Kumar, & Schneiderman, 1990; Pennebaker, Kiecolt-Glaser, & Glaser, 1988), better immune control over a latent herpes virus (Esterling, Antoni, Fletcher, Margulies, & Schneiderman, 1994), and higher seroconversion of hepatitis B antibodies following a vaccination (Petrie, Booth, Pennebaker, Davison, & Thomas, 1995). Disclosure also led to improved liver enzyme function (Francis & Pennebaker, 1992) and higher overall circulating lymphocyte counts (Booth, Petrie, & Pennebaker, 1997) in community samples. In patients with HIV, immune function improved for those who increased their use of positive emotion words across writing sessions (Rivkin, Gustafson, Weingarten, & Chin, 2006). In addition, Frattaroli's (2006) comprehensive meta-analysis found a significant positive effect size for written disclosure on immune parameters (Cohen's $d = .199$ or $r = .099$). Participating in written disclosure thus consistently shows improvements in immune function for healthy participants, and there is some evidence that individuals with chronic illness may show greater benefit when writing is structured more carefully (e.g., providing additional instructions to patients).

Patients with chronic illnesses have demonstrated illness-specific improvement as a result of written disclosure in comparison to control writing. For instance, Smyth, Stone, Hurewitz, and Kaell (1999) found disclosure to reduce physician-rated joint swelling in patients with rheumatoid arthritis and improve lung capacity in patients with asthma. Patients with HIV also showed decreased viral load (Petrie, Fontanilla, Thomas, Booth, & Pennebaker, 2004), patients with breast cancer made fewer cancer-related medical appointments (Stanton et al., 2002), and community participants showed faster recovery from a skin biopsy wound (Weinman, Ebrecht, Scott, Dyson, & Walburn, 2008) after written disclosure.

Additional physiological outcomes of disclosure have been explored in healthy and clinical samples, with mixed effects. These outcomes have included, but are not limited to, blood lipids, glucose levels, body composition measures (e.g., body mass index), and liver function. Some outcomes, such as HIV viral load, show positive effect sizes (Cohen's $d = .702$ or $r = .331$; Frattaroli, 2006), but these have been measured in only one study to date. Other outcomes (e.g., blood pressure or other measures of cardiovascular function) have been tested in more than one study, but these show nonsignificant positive effects using meta-analytic techniques (Frattaroli, 2006). These findings show limited support for the efficacy of disclosure across modalities and suggest that further work is necessary to determine the extent of disclosure's benefit on specific physiological outcomes.

PSYCHOLOGICAL FUNCTIONING, AFFECT, AND WELL-BEING

Written and other forms of disclosure have been shown to have positive effects on distress, negative moods, life satisfaction, perceived stress, and depressive symptoms (e.g., Greenberg, Wortman, & Stone, 1996; Gortner, Rude, & Pennebaker, 2006; Koopman et al., 2005; Sloan, Marx, Epstein, & Dobbs, 2008; Spera, Buhrfeind, & Pennebaker, 1994). In contrast, some studies have failed to find similar effects on these outcomes (e.g., Kloss & Lisman, 2002; Pennebaker & Beall, 1986; Pennebaker, Kiecolt-Glaser, & Glaser, 1988; Petrie et al., 1995). Despite such equivocal results among existing studies, both Smyth (1998) and Frattaroli (2006) found significant positive effect sizes for psychological health outcomes across multiple samples using meta-analytic techniques. Both authors have also emphasized that heterogeneous findings in this and other health domains may be a consequence of procedural or measurement differences between studies, or moderating variables (e.g., preintervention level of perceived stress) that influence the magnitude of the effect of disclosure. An additional factor that may impact disclosure's effects on psychological outcomes is the timeframe of follow-up assessment. For example, mood immediately postdisclosure is typically worsened but may over time show a return to baseline or even improvements.

A related area of interest has focused on participants' stress levels, given that some researchers frame disclosure as a "stress management" technique. Doing so suggests that stress reduction is a mechanism through which disclosure improves other health outcomes, yet there is surprisingly limited evidence to support this claim. Participants typically report increased, rather than decreased, psychological distress immediately following written disclosure, with distress alleviation not occurring until days or weeks later (Pennebaker, 1997). Further complication of this issue comes from the results of meta-analytic work: Frattaroli (2006) found a significant positive effect of disclosure for distress symptoms (assessed using symptom questionnaires) but found no such effect for general stress levels (assessed using stress-specific measures). The short-term and moderated effects of disclosure, as well as disclosure's proposed mechanisms, each require further empirical examination. These topics are discussed further later.

There is also some evidence that certain psychiatric populations may not receive psychological benefit from disclosure. For example, Frisina, Borod, and Lepore (2004) found a nonsignificant meta-analytic effect size for psychological functioning among medical and psychiatric samples. This finding suggests that written disclosure may be more effective for improving psychological health in otherwise healthy individuals than in individuals who struggle with physical or mental illness. Similarly, Stroebe, Schut, and Stroebe's (2005) review of disclosure among bereaved individuals found no psychological health benefits for those who disclosed relative to those who wrote or talked about neutral topics. An initial test of disclosure (combing written and oral disclosure) in individuals with posttraumatic stress disorder (PTSD) showed that the intervention might actually be harmful for PTSD symptoms (relative to the control condition; Gidron, Peri, Connolly, & Shalev, 1996). Subsequent studies, however, have provided more encouraging preliminary support for the use of written disclosure for patients with PTSD (Sloan & Marx, 2006; Smyth, Hockemeyer, & Tulloch, 2008).

Examinations of disclosure in healthy samples (e.g., Baikie, 2008; Kraft, Lumley, D'Souza, & Dooley, 2008) and in medical samples (e.g., Junghaenel, Schwartz, & Broderick, 2008; Manne, Ostroff, & Winkel, 2007) suggest that one's coping style and level of emotional expressiveness may also impact the efficacy of emotion-focused interventions (e.g., written disclosure). Awareness and effective regulation of emotional responses may be particularly important for individuals who are bereaved or who exhibit PTSD symptoms because these individuals have experienced severe and irrevocable stressors that challenge even adaptive coping strategies. These individuals may therefore benefit from disclosure activities, written or otherwise, that match their preferred coping mechanisms or that specifically focus on identifying and regulating emotions (Smyth & Arigo, 2009). More work in this area is necessary to elucidate the context and mechanism issues that may limit or enhance the use of written disclosure in clinical psychiatric samples.

EMPLOYMENT AND ACADEMIC FUNCTIONING

Outcomes that affect work and academic performance have been examined in a small number of studies, each demonstrating positive effects. University employees in the written disclosure group showed a reduction in absentee rates (Francis & Pennebaker, 1992), and recently unemployed professionals were reemployed more quickly after disclosure (Spera, Buhrfeind, & Pennebaker, 1994) relative to controls. Pennebaker and colleagues (Pennebaker, 1991; Pennebaker, Colder, & Sharp, 1990), Cameron and Nicholls (1998), and Lumley and Provenzano (2003) found that college students who disclosed through writing had better academic performance (i.e., grade point average) than did students who wrote about neutral topics. Written disclosure about stressful events also led to greater working memory capacity (i.e., task switching and recall) among college students (Klein & Boals, 2001), suggesting that students may see increases in their problem-solving and reasoning abilities as a result of disclosing their emotions. Existing evidence in this area thus indicates that occupationally related outcomes may be improved through disclosing one's feelings about an important topic.

HEALTH BEHAVIORS

Research syntheses have, relatively consistently, found written or broad-based disclosure to have no significant effect on health behaviors (e.g., eating habits, exercise; Frattaroli, 2006; Smyth, 1998). Both Smyth (1998) and Frattaroli (2006) suggest that deliberate modification of behavior requires a complex set of changes in attitudes toward a behavior and behavioral intentions, which may require a more powerful intervention to induce meaningful improvement. Some specific health behavior domains, such as sleep quality, show promise for the benefits of disclosure (e.g., de Moor et al., 2002; Harvey & Farrell, 2003; Mosher & Danoff-Burg, 2006) and suggest that further work in this area might be fruitful.

SHORT-TERM EFFECTS OF DISCLOSURE

Participants typically report that disclosing stressful experiences through writing increases their negative affect from pre- to postdisclosure, whereas participants who write about neutral topics do not report meaningful affective changes (Pennebaker, 1997; Smyth, 1998). Accordingly, disclosure participants demonstrate increased physiological arousal, including skin conductance (Hughes, Uhlmann, & Pennebaker, 1994), heart rate (Low, Stanton, & Danoff-Burg, 2006), blood pressure (McGuire, Greenberg, & Gevirtz, 2005), and salivary cortisol (Smyth, Hockemeyer, & Tulloch, 2008) during and immediately after disclosure. Such changes are typically transient, however; assessments of affect weeks or months postdisclosure show that participants who disclose traumatic or stressful experiences typically report more positive affect and less negative affect than neutral-writing controls.

This observed initial increase and subsequent decrease in negative affect indicates that distress is attenuated at some point in the process. The exact processes of change occurring during and after a disclosure intervention are not yet well understood, and the investigation of the potential mechanisms that link disclosure to health benefits remains an important area of disclosure research, both broadly and writing specific.

WHY DOES DISCLOSURE WORK?

Much of the early literature on disclosure was focused on demonstrating its efficacy as a therapeutic technique. More recently, experimental designs have attempted to identify the underlying mechanisms that may explain its salutary effects. The following sections present several general models that have been proposed to account for the benefits of disclosure; these models apply to disclosure across modalities.

(Dis)Inhibition

The original theory that motivated early studies of disclosure was based on the idea that not talking about important, stressful topics was a form of inhibition. Drawn from an array of animal and psychophysiological literatures, this model suggests that active inhibition is a form of physiological work. Such work is reflected in autonomic and central nervous system arousal and could thus be considered a chronic, low-level stressor, potentially increasing the risk of illness and other stress-related problems. As noted, there is evidence that social constraints may contribute to an environment in which individuals feel pressure to restrict their emotional expression. Disclosure (through writing or talking) was therefore often conceptualized as an opportunity to confront upsetting topics, reducing the constraints or inhibitions associated with nondisclosure (Pennebaker, 1989; Zakowski, Ramati, Morton, Johnson, & Flanigan 2004). Although inhibition may certainly contribute to long-term health problems, the notion that disclosure produces health benefits through disinhibition is not well supported. For example, individuals who wrote about previously disclosed traumas showed the same benefits as those who wrote about traumas they had kept secret (Greenberg & Stone, 1992), and writing about imagined traumas was similarly beneficial to writing about actually experienced events (Greenberg, Wortman, & Stone, 1996).

A barrier to testing the inhibition model is concretely defining inhibition. Across multiple studies, participants have a great deal of difficulty identifying the degree to which they are inhibiting their thoughts or feelings (e.g., "To what degree are you inhibiting or in some way holding back your emotions?"), and friends of participants are unable to reliably report on inhibitory processes. In short, without good measures of the presumed process of inhibition, we are limited in the ability to use the construct as an explanatory mechanism. Inhibition and disinhibition, then, may well be relevant psychological processes in accounting for the health benefits of disclosure, but no satisfactory tests of their existence or roles have been devised.

Integration of Traumatic Memories and Emotion

Memory research has suggested that extremely stressful experiences are stored as sensory or affective information. Converting traumatic memories into language through writing or talking encourages individuals to form coherent narratives, which may allow negative experiences to be integrated with other memories. Integration may reduce both unwanted reexperiencing of the event and autonomic arousal associated with the memory, thereby leading to improved health (Klein, 2002). The experiential model, based on the work of Janet (1909), similarly suggests that reexperiencing a stressful event though disclosure helps to organize related negative emotions into a new schema that is less threatening than the original. The creation of a new schema is thought to result in decreased physiological arousal and tension that may facilitate the salutary effects of disclosure.

EXPOSURE

A related model of exposure proposes that through repeated talking or writing about a stressful event, an individual will habituate to the negative emotions aroused by the experience. The exposure theory of experimental disclosure suggests that repeated disclosure about an emotionally distressing event, whether through writing or speaking, may lead to the extinction of negative emotional associations (e.g., Bootzin, 1997). Sloan, Marx, and Epstein (2005), among others, have shown evidence consistent with the model by examining the immediate effects of disclosure across experimental sessions. These investigators concluded that habituation occurred faster for participants who wrote about the same topic at each session as a result of initial physiological arousal during session 1; participants who switched writing topics demonstrated physiological arousal at both sessions 1 and 2, suggesting that habituation took longer to occur (Sloan et al., 2005). Moreover, significant health improvements were found only for the group that did not switch topics. This finding indicates that instructions to repeat writing on the same topic (which led to more rapid habituation) may have facilitated the positive effects of expressive writing (or, alternatively, that forcing people to change writing topics may be contraindicated; Sloan et al., 2005).

SELF-REGULATION

A great deal of research has demonstrated that emotional dysregulation, or ineffective control over emotional responses and behaviors, is detrimental to physical and mental health (Denollet et al., 2008). Writing or talking about an experience allows an individual to become more aware of thoughts and feelings related to an event. Increased awareness may facilitate habituation to specific triggers and negative feelings and may promote reorganization of thoughts associated with the event. By translating emotional experiences into language, disclosure may thereby help to stabilize an individual's responses to emotionally charged situations.

Several studies have suggested that regulatory writing tasks can lead to positive health effects relative to control writing. Such writing instructions have asked participants to focus on achievement of their long-term goals (King, 2001, 2002) and problem-solving (Cameron & Nicholls, 1998). Health benefits were also found as the result of writing about plans to resolve a current stressful issue, rather than simply disclosing feelings about the issue (Lestideau & Lavallee, 2007). In addition, Sloan and Epstein (2005) demonstrated that individuals with high respiratory sinus arrhythmia, thought to be an indicator of emotion regulation ability, benefited more from disclosure than did individuals low in respiratory sinus arrhythmia. Although this evidence is consistent with a regulatory approach to disclosure, it does not rule out a host of other explanations for improvement.

COGNITIVE AND LINGUISTIC CHANGES

As noted, language is thought to be a key component of disclosure's benefits and is implicated in several of disclosure's proposed mechanisms. With respect to written disclosure, a number of researchers have thus examined changes in word use over the course of multiple writing sessions to determine whether there is an optimal language shift that occurs through writing. Although independent raters initially suggested that individuals who benefited from writing were "smarter," "more thoughtful," and "more emotional" than individuals who had not (Pennebaker, 1993), poor interrater reliability resulted in the development of a computerized text analysis program to objectively verify these conclusions.

The Linguistic Inquiry and Word Count (LIWC; Pennebaker, Booth, & Francis, 2007) calculates the frequency of words in such categories as negative emotions (e.g., sad, angry), positive emotions (e.g., happy, laugh), and insight (e.g., understand, realize). Multiple studies have found that better health is associated with a moderate number of negative emotion words and an increase in the use of positive emotion and insight words over several writing sessions (Pennebaker & Francis, 1996;

Pennebaker, Mayne, & Francis, 1997). The increased use of insight words has been linked to the creation of a coherent narrative and suggests that narrative construction is an important aspect of the disclosure process (Kaufman & Sexton, 2006; Smyth, True, & Souto, 2001). An increasing number of studies also indicate that the ways people change perspectives in their writing predicts health improvements. Specifically, those people who change in their use of pronouns (e.g., from *I* to *we* or *you* or third person) across writing sessions are the ones who evidence the greatest gains (Campbell & Pennebaker, 2003).

What still remains unclear is the process by which narrative construction confers health benefits. The myriad effects of disclosure on biological parameters (e.g., immune function, autonomic activity) demonstrate that cognitive and emotional changes can lead to meaningful physiological changes and improved health, but these findings do not reveal the exact sequencing of events. Whether disclosure leads directly to improved health (with better physiological functioning as a result) is still an open question. Alternatively, better physiological functioning may be the intermediary link between disclosure and improved health (Nazarian & Smyth, 2008). It is also important to note that physiological, cognitive, and emotional processes are interactive, and it may be the case that no one mechanism explains all the benefits of disclosure. Multiple mechanisms may be at work and may differ between people (Smyth & Pennebaker, 2008). Research on disclosure mechanisms typically does not pit multiple theories against each other or test how mechanisms may work together (either within or between individuals), leaving an area of opportunity for further insight into the process that results from disclosure (Nazarian & Smyth, 2008).

FOR WHOM AND UNDER WHAT CONDITIONS IS EMOTIONAL DISCLOSURE BENEFICIAL?

A growing area of research examines the "boundary conditions" of disclosure's positive effects (Smyth & Pennebaker, 2008), suggesting for whom and how disclosure might be optimally implemented. Written disclosure has shown health benefits across a variety of conditions and with populations that have experienced a range of trauma types. Although such findings indicate that written disclosure may be broadly efficacious, researchers and theorists do not yet know how best to synthesize results from such distinct groups as cancer patients, the elderly, and college students. In addition, the existence of studies that have produced null findings suggests that disclosure may not be equally helpful for everyone or that certain circumstances may not be optimal for producing positive health outcomes.

Several studies and reviews provide evidence supporting procedural or participant factors that affect the outcome of disclosure studies (Frattaroli, 2006; Nazarian & Smyth, 2010; Smyth, 1998). For example, mode of disclosure (i.e., writing vs. talking, writing vs. typing) has been examined in multiple studies. "Written" disclosure has been tested through e-mail, showing improvements for college students who typed their narratives at home (Sheese, Brown, & Graziano, 2004). Direct comparisons of various modes have shown mixed results: Whereas Pantchenko, Lawson, and Joyce (2003) found that including written disclosure improved outcomes beyond simply talking about a stressful event, Harrist and colleagues (2007) found no added benefit of writing. Likewise, Frattaroli's (2006) meta-analysis did not reveal a significant moderated effect of disclosure mode. Existing evidence is thus inconclusive regarding the advantage of writing, but it is perhaps the case that disclosure in any form is superior to nondisclosure.

Other boundary conditions that have been tested for moderated effects on disclosure outcomes include topic (i.e., switching vs. not switching across sessions) and individual differences in participants prior to the intervention (e.g., gender, depressive symptoms). Of particular interest are the parameters of disclosure sessions, which can suggest optimal, efficient methods for achieving benefits of writing that are comparable to the benefits of the traditional procedure (i.e., three to five writing sessions of 15–30 minutes each). Tests of parameters have shown that health benefits can be garnered from multiple sessions spaced just 10 minutes apart rather than held on consecutive days or separated by a week (Chung & Pennebaker, 2008), and perhaps from writing sessions that are as brief as 2 minutes (Burton & King, 2008). These findings currently require replication, but they show promise for the power of extremely brief disclosure.

In a similar vein, instructions for written disclosure have been manipulated in order to determine whether the focus or valence of disclosure can impact outcomes. Whereas it was originally believed that the benefits of disclosure resulted from expressing negative feelings about a stressful experience, multiple studies have demonstrated the benefits of positively charged disclosure. For example, instructions that are focused on "benefit finding" typically ask participants to write about what good may have resulted from a negative experience (Danoff-Burg, Agee, Romanoff, Strosberg, & Kremer, 2006; King & Miner, 2000; Stanton et al., 2002). Other positively focused writing instructions have targeted "intensely positive experiences" (Burton & King, 2004) and one's "best possible future self" (King, 2001). An ongoing issue in these studies is the degree to which such writing instructions actually promote benefit finding or other growth-related changes. Participants who receive instructions to find benefits do write about such positive experiences as increased closeness in relationships and the shifting of priorities. Yet it is not clear that these changes are seen as personally meaningful to the extent that they can improve health outcomes.

Writing instructions that purport to encourage positive emotions have outperformed emotionally neutral instructions with consistency (e.g., Burton & King, 2004) but may not provide health benefits superior to trauma-focused writing (Danoff-Burg et al., 2006; King, 2001). In fact, certain outcomes have responded more favorably to trauma-focused writing than to positively focused writing (e.g., working memory capacity; Klein & Boals, 2001). Drawing strong conclusions from studies that alter writing instructions is complicated by the fact that presenting conditions may influence reactions to different types of writing, and thus individuals may respond uniquely to different instructional sets. Given that this problem has been demonstrated in multiple studies that have included positively focused instructions (Austenfeld, Paolo, & Stanton, 2006; Austenfeld & Stanton, 2008; Danoff-Burg et al., 2006; Stanton et al., 2002), this line of enquiry must be pursued thoughtfully (Nazarian & Smyth, 2010).

The presumed audience of disclosure is of considerable interest as well. Brody and Park (2004) proposed that an important aspect of disclosure is the implication that one's information is shared with others rather than kept private. A handful of studies have supported the notion that the disclosure audience has an effect on outcomes, with equivocal results. Pennebaker, Hughes, and O'Heeron (1987) initially showed that individuals who disclosed into a tape recorder were more expressive than those who disclosed to an anonymous other person. These results suggest that some form of censoring occurs in the physical presence of another individual, perhaps because of anticipated social consequences, and may be detrimental for certain domains of health. Although written disclosure is completed while alone, participants have the implicit understanding that narratives will be read by researchers. These participants may write differently than do individuals whose narratives are kept private, and they may thus receive different, if any, benefits from disclosure.

In line with this view, recent work has shown audience effects on physical health. For instance, fewer physical symptoms were endorsed by those study participants who submitted their written disclosure narratives to a researcher, whereas comparable benefits were not observed for those who kept their writing private (Radcliffe, Lumley, Kendall, Beltran, & Stevenson, 2007). Meta-analytic evaluation suggests that reported physical health was not affected by the presence of a disclosure audience. Conversely, effect sizes for psychological functioning were marginally higher when narratives were kept private, rather than being shared (Frattaroli, 2006). Although one might conclude from this and similar evidence that writing for an audience may be beneficial for physical health, whereas private writing can have positive effects on psychological health, one must also consider methodological differences between studies and analytic techniques.

In the case of audience effects, Frattaroli's (2006) meta-analysis included studies of both written or typed disclosures and verbal disclosure and tested for between-study differences in the presence versus absence of an audience (i.e., the researcher). Radcliffe and colleagues (2007) tested the merits of *written*-disclosure audience presence versus absence the in same study, allowing for a stronger test of audience effects and thus for stronger conclusions about these effects. This inconsistency provides an example of a potential problem associated with current methods for testing moderators of disclosure benefits.

Also of concern is the confusion between within-person and between-person effects. In many studies and in meta-analyses, within-person conclusions are drawn from between-person designs. Take, for instance, the finding that individuals who report higher perceived stress levels at the outset of a disclosure intervention benefit more from disclosure than those who report less stress at the outset (Frattaroli, 2006). This finding does not imply that disclosure will be more effective when a person is in a state of high perceived stress, relative to when that person experiences low perceived stress, but it is occasionally interpreted as such. Confusion on this point might lead to the incorrect conclusion that disclosure should be most beneficial if completed when a person experiences heightened distress. On the contrary, if increased insight is essential to disclosure's benefits, disclosing when highly distressed might prevent individuals from writing in a way that will produce positive effects. In light of such issues, more work needs to be done carefully in order to determine which individuals benefit most from disclosure and what conditions lead to optimal outcomes.

CONSIDERATIONS FOR THE USE OF DISCLOSURE IN A CLINICAL CONTEXT

Disclosure of one's thoughts and feelings has traditionally been an integral aspect of psychotherapy. In a review of treatment outcome literature for individuals with a history of childhood sexual abuse, Bradley and Follingstad (2001) suggest that disclosure about a traumatic experience with a therapist can provide habituation through repeated exposure, cognitive reframing of the event, and/or insight into one's ability to tolerate emotional distress. Evidence supports each of these pathways as methods for decreasing symptoms of PTSD (e.g., intrusive thoughts), but more tightly controlled research is necessary to confirm the conclusion that any type of disclosure has positive effects. Bradley and Follingstad (2001) also emphasize the need for clinicians to tailor a disclosure-based approach to the client's symptoms in order for disclosure to produce optimal outcomes.

Although written disclosure has most often been tested as a stand-alone intervention, it has long been suggested that expressive writing may serve as a homework assignment or as an adjunct to other forms of more intensive psychotherapy. In order to make these recommendations with confidence, however, researchers must demonstrate the benefits of disclosure in real-world settings (i.e., effectiveness) in addition to showing the positive effects in controlled laboratory trials (i.e., efficacy; see Smyth & Catley, 2002). Effectiveness research has generated mixed results, with some studies supporting the use of stand-alone, at-home writing (e.g., Warner et al., 2006). The positive findings from studies that have tested expressive writing as a homework adjunct to psychotherapy have been more encouraging, showing greater improvement among those participants who engaged in writing along with therapy than among participants who received therapy alone.

The benefits of written disclosure in conjunction with psychotherapy have been demonstrated in both college and community samples. College students in outpatient psychotherapy showed lower anxiety and depressive symptoms with written disclosure as homework, relative to college students in standard psychotherapy (Graf, Gaudiano, & Geller, 2008). Spouses whose partners had engaged in extramarital affairs experienced greater forgiveness, lower PTSD symptoms, and less anger toward their partners when expressive letter-writing was included as part of psychotherapy (Gordon, Baucom, & Snyder, 2008). And compared to young adult smokers who received only a brief smoking cessation intervention, participants who also completed at-home written disclosure about smoking cessation initially stopped smoking at a higher rate (Ames et al., 2007). Such evidence suggests that adding written disclosure as homework for outpatient psychotherapy may bolster the positive effects of treatment.

An advantage of using written disclosure as a psychotherapy adjunct is its versatility, for it can be modified to fit the needs of individual clients. Written disclosure in the context of psychotherapy should be carefully considered, however; the parameters of writing should be outlined prior to the first assignment, including whether written narratives will be discussed with the therapist and whether feedback will be provided. Based on existing findings, Smyth, Nazarian, and Arigo (2008) also recommend that clients write in a private, quiet space that is free from outside interference and that clients write continuously for 30–45 minutes per session without consideration for spelling or grammar. Time set aside for writing should include a few minutes beforehand to orient oneself to writing and a few minutes afterward to manage any distress triggered by writing. Sessions may be spaced over days, weeks, or longer, depending on what is therapeutically indicated. Writing topics should be important to the client and may include associations between prior experiences and the client's current situation.

In all cases, prior to the initiation of homework sessions, clients should be equipped with strategies for coping with any negative emotions that arise from writing. If these concerns are addressed in the context of treatment, written disclosure may provide a brief but useful extension of in-session work that can increase the benefits of psychotherapy. Additional work is necessary to determine whether at-home, written disclosure may complement disclosure-based psychotherapy for PTSD and other disorders.

CONCLUSION

Both narrative and quantitative research syntheses of existing evidence support the conclusion that disclosure about traumatic or stressful events, particularly written disclosure about such events, can produce physical and psychological health benefits. There is also, however, abundant evidence that there are people for whom, and contexts within which, expressive writing is more or less effective. Exploring these boundary conditions and moderating factors is a critical next step in this line of research inquiry. Although several theoretical accounts of disclosure's salutary effects exist, there is no clear and discriminant evidence in support of any one of these mechanisms. Contrary to such a view, it is likely that expressive writing "kick-starts" a range of processes and mechanisms that produce benefits by acting in concert with one another. Overall, however, existing research suggests that when carefully considered and implemented, written disclosure—and perhaps other forms of disclosure as well—is a potentially useful intervention that can be utilized on its own or as supplement to other ongoing treatment. Ongoing research and practice will certainly continue to explore and document the broad and important effects of emotional disclosure in a wide range of contexts and samples.

REFERENCES

Ames, S. C., Patten, C. A., Werch, C. E., Schroeder, D. R., Stevens, S. R., Fredrickson, P. A., ... Hurt, R. D. (2007). Expressive writing as a smoking cessation treatment adjunct for young adult smokers. *Nicotine & Tobacco Research, 9*, 185–194.

Antoni, M. H. (1999). Empirical studies of emotional disclosure in the face of stress: A progress report. *Advances in Mind–Body Medicine, 15*, 163–166.

Austenfeld, J. L., Paolo, A. M., & Stanton, A. L. (2006). Effects of writing about emotions versus goals on psychological and physical health among third-year medical students. *Journal of Personality, 74*, 267–286.

Austenfeld, J. L., & Stanton, A. L. (2008). Writing about emotions versus goals: Effects on hostility and medical care utilization moderated by emotional approach coping processes. *British Journal of Health Psychology, 13*, 35–38.

Baikie, K. A. (2008). Who does expressive writing work for? Examination of alexithymia, splitting, and repressive coping style as moderators of the expressive writing paradigm. *British Journal of Health Psychology, 13*, 61–66.

Barry, D. T., & Mizrahi, T. C. (2005). Guarded self-disclosure predicts psychological distress and willingness to use psychological services among East Asian immigrants in the United States. *Journal of Nervous and Mental Disease, 193*, 535–539.

Berry, D. S., & Pennebaker, J. W. (1993). Nonverbal and verbal emotional expression and health. *Psychotherapy and Psychosomatics, 59*, 11–19.

Booth, R. J., Petrie, K. J., & Pennebaker, J. W. (1997). Changes in circulating lymphocyte numbers following emotional disclosure: Evidence of buffering? *Stress Medicine, 13*, 23–29.

Bootzin, R. (1997). Examining the theory and clinical utility of writing about emotional experiences. *Psychological Science, 8*, 167–169.

Bradley, R. G., & Follingstad, D. R. (2001). Utilizing disclosure in the treatment of the sequelae of childhood sexual abuse: A theoretical and empirical review. *Clinical Psychology Review, 21*, 1–32.

Brody, L. R., & Park, S. H. (2004). Narratives, mindfulness, and the implicit audience. *Clinical Psychology: Science and Practice, 11*, 147–154.

Burton, C. M., & King, L. A. (2004). The health benefits of writing about intensely positive experiences. *Journal of Research in Personality, 38*, 150–163.

Burton, C. M., & King, L. A. (2008). Effects of (very) brief writing on health: The two-minute miracle. *British Journal of Health Psychology, 13*, 9–14.

Cameron, L. D., & Nicholls, G. (1998). Expression of stressful experiences through writing: Effects of a self-regulation manipulation for pessimists and optimists. *Health Psychology, 17*, 84–92.

Campbell, R. S., & Pennebaker, J. W. (2003). The secret life of pronouns: Flexibility in writing style and physical health. *Psychological Science, 14*, 60–65.

Chung, C. K., & Pennebaker, J. W. (2008). Variations in the spacing of expressive writing sessions. *British Journal of Health Psychology, 13*, 15–21.

Cohen, S., Doyle, W. J., & Baum, A. (2006). Socioeconomic status is associated with stress hormones. *Psychosomatic Medicine, 68*, 414–420.

Cohen, S., Tyrrell, D. A., & Smith, A. P. (1991). Psychological stress and susceptibility to the common cold. *New England Journal of Medicine, 325*, 606–612.

Cohen, S., Tyrrell, D. A., & Smith, A. P. (1993). Negative life events, perceived stress, negative affect, and susceptibility to the common cold. *Journal of Personality and Social Psychology, 64*, 131–140.

Cole, S. W., Kemeny, M. E., Taylor, S. E., & Visscher, B. R. (1996). Elevated physical health risk among gay men who conceal their homosexual identity. *Health Psychology, 15*, 243–251.

Cole, S. W., Kemeny, M. E., Taylor, S. E., Visscher, B. R., & Fahey, J. L. (1996). Accelerated course of human immunodeficiency virus infection in gay men who conceal their homosexual identity. *Psychosomatic Medicine, 58*, 219–231.

Danoff-Burg, S., Agee, J. D., Romanoff, N. R., Strosberg, J. M., & Kremer, J. M. (2006). Benefit finding and expressive writing in adults with lupus or rheumatoid arthritis. *Psychology & Health, 21*, 651–665.

De Moor, C., Sterner, J., Hall, M., Warneke, C., Gilani, Z., & Amato, R., & Cohen, L. (2002). A pilot study of the effects of expressive writing on psychological and behavioral adjustment in patients enrolled in a phase II trial of vaccine therapy for metastatic renal cell carcinoma. *Health Psychology, 21*, 615–619.

Denollet, J., Nyklíček, I., Vingerhoets, A. J. J. M., Vingerhoets, A., Nyklíček, I., & Denollet, J. (2008). Introduction: Emotions, emotion regulation, and health. In *Emotion regulation: Conceptual and clinical issues* (pp. 3–11). New York, NY: Springer.

Esterling, B. A., Antoni, M. H., Fletcher, M. A., Margulies, S., & Schneiderman, N. (1994). Emotional disclosure through writing or speaking modulates latent Epstein-Barr virus antibody titers. *Journal of Consulting and Clinical Psychology, 62*, 130–140.

Esterling, B. A., Antoni, M. H., Kumar, M., & Schneiderman, N. (1990). Emotional repression, stress disclosure responses, and Epstein-Barr viral capsid antigen titers. *Psychosomatic Medicine, 52*, 397–410.

Francis, M. E., & Pennebaker, J. W. (1992). Putting stress into words: The impact of writing on physiological, absentee, and self-reported emotional well-being measures. *American Journal of Health Promotion, 6*, 280–287.

Frattaroli, J. (2006). Experimental disclosure and its moderators: A meta-analysis. *Psychological Bulletin, 132*, 823–865.

Frisina, P. G., Borod, J. C., & Lepore, S. J. (2004). A meta-analysis of the effects of written emotional disclosure on the health outcomes of clinical populations. *Journal of Nervous and Mental Disease, 192*, 629–634.

Frisina, P. G., Lepore, S. J., & Borod, J. C. (2005). Written emotional disclosure in clinical populations: Confirming and updating our meta-analytic findings. *Journal of Nervous and Mental Disease, 193*, 425–426.

Gidron, Y., Peri, T., Connolly, J. F., & Shalev, A. Y. (1996). Written disclosure in posttraumatic stress disorder: Is it beneficial for the patient? *Journal of Nervous and Mental Disease, 184*, 505–507.

Gillis, M. E., Lumley, M. A., Mosley-Williams, A., Leisen, J. C. C., & Roehrs, T. (2006). The health effects of at-home written emotional disclosure in fibromyalgia: A randomized trial. *Annals of Behavioral Medicine, 32*, 135–146.

Gordon, K. C., Baucom, D. H., & Snyder, D. K. (2008). Optimal strategies in couple therapy: Treating couples dealing with the trauma of infidelity. *Journal of Contemporary Psychotherapy, 38*, 151–160.

Gortner, E. M., Rude, S. S., & Pennebaker, J. W. (2006). Benefits of expressive writing in lowering rumination and depressive symptoms. *Behavior Therapy, 37*, 292–303.

Graf, M. C., Gaudiano, B. A., & Geller, P. A. (2008). Written emotional disclosure: A controlled study of the benefits of expressive writing homework in outpatient psychotherapy. *Psychotherapy Research, 18*, 389–399.

Greenberg, M. A., & Stone, A. A. (1992). Emotional disclosure about traumas and its relation to health: Effects of previous disclosure and trauma severity. *Journal of Personality and Social Psychology, 63*, 75–84.

Greenberg, M. A., Wortman, C. B., & Stone, A. A. (1996). Emotional expression and physical heath: Revising traumatic memories or fostering self-regulation? *Journal of Personality and Social Psychology, 71*, 588–602.

Harris, A. H. S. (2006). Does expressive writing reduce health care utilization? A meta-analysis of randomized trials. *Journal of Consulting and Clinical Psychology, 74*, 243–252.

Harrist, S., Carlozzi, B. L., McGovern, A. R., & Harrist, A. W. (2007). Benefits of expressive writing and expressive talking about life goals. *Journal of Research in Personality, 41*, 923–930.

Harvey, A. G., & Farrell, C. (2003). The efficacy of a Pennebaker-like writing intervention for poor sleepers. *Behavioral Sleep Medicine, 1*, 115–124.

Hughes, C. F., Uhlmann, C., & Pennebaker, J. W. (1994). The body's response to processing emotional trauma: Linking verbal text with autonomic activity. *Journal of Personality, 62*, 565–585.

Iinying, L., & Huichang, C. (2003). Self-disclosure and its relationships with personality traits, loneliness, and mental health in college students. *Chinese Mental Health Journal, 17*, 666–668.

Janet, P. (1909). *Les nervoses.* Paris: Flammarion.

Junghaenel, D. U., Schwartz, J. E., & Broderick, J. E. (2008). Differential efficacy of written emotional disclosure for subgroups of fibromyalgia patients. *British Journal of Health Psychology, 13*, 57–60.

Kaufman, J. C., & Sexton, J. D. (2006). Why doesn't the writing cure help poets? *Review of General Psychology, 10*, 268–282.

King, L. A. (2001). The health benefits of writing about life goals. *Personality and Social Psychology Bulletin, 27*, 798–807.

King, L. A. (2002). Gain without pain? Expressive writing and self-regulation. In S. J. Lepore & J. M. Smyth (Eds.), *The writing cure: How expressive writing promotes health and emotional well-being* (pp. 119–134). Washington, DC: American Psychological Association.

King, L. A., & Miner, K. N. (2000). Writing about the perceived benefits of traumatic events: Implications for physical health. *Personality and Social Psychology Bulletin, 26*, 220–230.

Klein, K. (2002). Stress, expressive writing, and working memory. In S. J. Lepore & J. M. Smyth (Eds.), *The writing cure: How expressive writing promotes health and emotional well-being* (pp. 119–134). Washington, DC: American Psychological Association.

Klein, K., & Boals, A. (2001). Expressive writing can increase working memory capacity. *Journal of Experimental Psychology: General, 130*, 520–533.

Kloss, J. D., & Lisman, S. A. (2002). An exposure-based examination of the effects of written emotional disclosure. *British Journal of Health Psychology, 7*, 31–46.

Koopman, C., Ismailji, T., Holmes, D., Palesh, O., Wales, T., & Classen, C. C. (2005). The effects of expressive writing on pain, depression and posttraumatic stress disorder symptoms in survivors of intimate partner violence. *Journal of Health Psychology, 10*, 211–221.

Kraft, C. A., Lumley, M. A., D'Souza, P. J., & Dooley, J. A. (2008). Emotional approach coping and self-efficacy moderate the effects of written emotional disclosure and relaxation training for people with migraine headaches. *British Journal of Health Psychology, 13*, 67–71.

Lepore, S. J., & Greenberg, M. A. (2002). Mending broken hearts: Effects of expressive writing on mood, cognitive processing, social adjustment and health following a relationship breakup. *Psychology & Health, 17*, 547–560.

Lepore, S. J., & Revenson, T. A. (2007). Social constraints on disclosure and adjustment to cancer. *Social and Personality Psychology Compass, 1*, 313–333.

Lepore, S. J., Silver, R. C., Wortman, C. B., & Wayment, H. A. (1996). Social constraints, intrusive thoughts, and depressive symptoms among bereaved mothers. *Journal of Personality and Social Psychology, 70*, 271–282.

Lestideau, O. T., & Lavallee, L. F. (2007). Structured writing about current stressors: The benefits of developing plans. *Psychology & Health, 22*, 659–676.

Low, C. A., Stanton, A. L., & Danoff-Burg, S. (2006). Expressive disclosure and benefit finding among breast cancer patients: Mechanisms for positive health effects. *Health Psychology, 25*, 181–189.

Lumley, M. A., & Provenzano, K. M. (2003). Stress management through written emotional disclosure improves academic performance among college students with physical symptoms. *Journal of Educational Psychology, 95*, 641–649.

Manne, S., Ostroff, J. S., & Winkel, G. (2007). Social-cognitive processes as moderators of a couple-focused group intervention for women with early stage breast cancer. *Health Psychology, 26*, 735–744.

McGuire, K. M. B., Greenberg, M. A., & Gevirtz, R. (2005). Autonomic effects of expressive writing in individuals with elevated blood pressure. *Journal of Health Psychology, 10*, 197–209.

Mosher, C. E., & Danoff-Burg, S. (2006). Health effects of expressive letter writing. *Journal of Social & Clinical Psychology, 25*, 1122–1139.

Murray-Swank, A. B., McConnell, K. M., & Pargament, K. I. (2007). Understanding spiritual confession: A review and theoretical synthesis. *Mental Health, Religion & Culture, 10*, 275–291.

Nazarian, D., & Smyth, J. M. (2008). Expressive writing. In W. O'Donohue & N. A. Cummings (Eds.), *Evidence-based adjunctive treatments* (pp. 221–241). New York, NY: Academic Press.

Nazarian, D., & Smyth, J. (2010). Context moderates the effects of an expressive writing intervention: A randomized two-study replication and extension. *Journal of Social and Clinical Psychology, 29*, 903–929.

Pantchenko, T., Lawson, M., & Joyce, M. R. (2003). Verbal and non-verbal disclosure of recalled negative experiences: Relation to well-being. *Psychology and Psychotherapy: Theory, Research and Practice, 76*, 251–265.

Pennebaker, J. W. (1985). Traumatic experience and psychosomatic disease: Exploring the roles of behavioural inhibition, obsession, and confiding. *Canadian Psychology / Psychologie canadienne, 26*, 82–95.

Pennebaker, J. W. (1989). Confession, inhibition, and disease. In L. Berkowitz (Ed.), *Advances in experimental social psychology* (Vol. 22, pp. 211–244). San Diego, CA: Academic Press.

Pennebaker, J. W. (1991). Writing your wrongs. *American Health, 10*, 64–67.

Pennebaker, J. W. (1993). Putting stress into words: Health, linguistic, and therapeutic implications. *Behaviour Research and Therapy, 31*, 539–548.

Pennebaker, J. W. (1997). Writing about emotional experiences as a therapeutic process. *Psychological Science, 8*, 162–166.

Pennebaker, J. W. (2004). Theories, therapies, and taxpayers: On the complexities of the expressive writing paradigm. *Clinical Psychology: Science and Practice, 11*, 138–142.

Pennebaker, J. W., & Beall, S. K. (1986). Confronting a traumatic event: Toward an understanding of inhibition and disease. *Journal of Abnormal Psychology, 95*, 274–281.

Pennebaker, J. W., Booth, R. E., & Francis, M. E. (2007). Linguistic inquiry and word count: LIWC2007 operator's manual. Austin, TX: LIWC.net.

Pennebaker, J. W., & Chung, C. K. (2007). Expressive writing, emotional upheavals, and health. In H. S. Friedman & R. C. Silver (Eds.), *Foundations of health psychology* (pp. 263–284). New York, NY: Oxford University Press.

Pennebaker, J. W., Colder, M., & Sharp, L. K. (1990). Accelerating the coping process. *Journal of Personality and Social Psychology, 58*, 528–537.

Pennebaker, J. W., & Francis, M. E. (1996). Cognitive, emotional, and language processes in disclosure. *Cognition & Emotion, 10*, 601–626.

Pennebaker, J. W., Hughes, C. F., & O'Heeron, R. C. (1987). The psychophysiology of confession: Linking inhibitory and psychosomatic processes. *Journal of Personality and Social Psychology, 52*, 781–793.

Pennebaker, J. W., Kiecolt-Glaser, J. K., & Glaser, R. (1988). Disclosure of traumas and immune function: Health implications for psychotherapy. *Journal of Consulting and Clinical Psychology, 56*, 239–245.

Pennebaker, J. W., Mayne, T. J., & Francis, M. E. (1997). Linguistic predictors of adaptive bereavement. *Journal of Personality and Social Psychology, 72*, 863–871.

Pennebaker, J. W., & O'Heeron, R. C. (1984). Confiding in others and illness rate among spouses of suicide and accidental-death victims. *Journal of Abnormal Psychology, 93*, 473–476.

Pennebaker, J. W., & Susman, J. R. (1988). Disclosure of traumas and psychosomatic processes. *Social Science & Medicine, 26*, 327–332.

Petrie, K. J., Booth, R. J., Pennebaker, J. W., Davison, K. P., & Thomas, M. G. (1995). Disclosure of trauma and immune response to a hepatitis B vaccination program. *Journal of Consulting and Clinical Psychology, 63*, 787–792.

Petrie, K. J., Fontanilla, I., Thomas, M. G., Booth, R. J., & Pennebaker, J. W. (2004). Effect of written emotional expression on immune function in patients with human immunodeficiency virus infection: A randomized trial. *Psychosomatic Medicine, 66*, 272–275.

Radcliffe, A. M., Lumley, M. A., Kendall, J., Beltran, J., & Stevenson, J. K. (2007). Written emotional disclosure: Testing whether social disclosure matters. *Journal of Social & Clinical Psychology, 26*, 362–384.

Richards, J. M., Beal, W. E., Seagal, J. D., & Pennebaker, J. W. (2000). Effects of disclosure of traumatic events on illness behavior among psychiatric prison inmates. *Journal of Abnormal Psychology, 109*, 156–160.

Rivkin, I. D., Gustafson, J., Weingarten, I., & Chin, D. (2006). The effects of expressive writing on adjustment to HIV. *AIDS and Behavior, 10*, 13–26.

Rosenberg, H. J., Rosenberg, S. D., Ernstoff, M. S., Wolford, G. L., Amdur, R. J., Elshamy, M. R., ... Pennebaker, J. M. (2002). Expressive disclosure and health outcomes in a prostate cancer population. *International Journal of Psychiatry in Medicine, 32*, 37–53.

Salovey, P., Rothman, A. J., Detweiler, J. B., & Steward, W. T. (2000). Emotional states and physical health. *American Psychologist, 55,* 110–121.

Schiffer, A. A., Pavan, A., Pedersen, S. S., Gremigni, P., Sommaruga, M., & Denollet, J. (2006). Type D personality and cardiovascular disease: Evidence and clinical implications. *Minerva Psichiatrica, 47*, 79–87.

Sheese, B. E., Brown, E. L., & Graziano, W. G. (2004). Emotional expression in cyberspace: Searching for moderators of the Pennebaker disclosure effect via e-mail. *Health Psychology, 23*, 457–464.

Singer, J. L. (1990). *Repression and dissociation.* Chicago, IL: University of Chicago Press.

Sloan, D. M., & Epstein, E. M. (2005). Respiratory sinus arrhythmia predicts written disclosure outcome. *Psychophysiology, 42*, 611–615.

Sloan, D. M., & Marx, B. P. (2006). Exposure through written emotional disclosure: Two case examples. *Cognitive and Behavioral Practice, 13*, 227–234.

Sloan, D. M., Marx, B. P., & Epstein, E. M. (2005). Further examination of the exposure model underlying the efficacy of written emotional disclosure. *Journal of Consulting and Clinical Psychology, 73*, 549–554.

Sloan, D. M., Marx, B. P., Epstein, E. M., & Dobbs, J. L. (2008). Expressive writing buffers against maladaptive rumination. *Emotion, 8*, 302–306.

Smyth, J. M. (1998). Written emotional expression: Effect sizes, outcome types, and moderating variables. *Journal of Consulting and Clinical Psychology, 66*, 174–184.

Smyth, J. M., & Arigo, D. (2009). Recent evidence supports emotion regulation interventions for improving health in at-risk and clinical populations. *Current Opinion in Psychiatry, 22*, 205–210.

Smyth, J., & Catley, D. (2002). Translating research into practice: Potential of expressive writing in the field. In S. J. Lepore & J. M. Smyth (Eds.), *The writing cure: How expressive writing promotes health and emotional well-being* (pp. 199–214). Washington, DC: American Psychological Association Press.

Smyth, J. M., Hockemeyer, J. R., Heron, K. E., Pennebaker, J. W., & Wonderlich, S. A. (2008). Prevalence, type, disclosure, and severity of adverse life events in college students. *Journal of American College Health, 57*, 69–76.

Smyth, J. M., Hockemeyer, J. R., & Tulloch, H. (2008). Expressive writing and post-traumatic stress disorder: Effects on trauma symptoms, mood states, and cortisol reactivity. *British Journal of Health Psychology, 13*, 85–93.

Smyth, J. M., Nazarian, D., & Arigo, D. (2008). Expressive writing in the clinical context. In A. Vingerhoets, I. Nyklíček, & J. Denollet (Eds.), *Emotion regulation: Conceptual and clinical issues* (pp. 215–233). New York, NY: Springer Science.

Smyth, J. M., & Pennebaker, J. W. (2008). Exploring the boundary conditions of expressive writing: In search of the right recipe. *British Journal of Health Psychology, 13*, 1–7.

Smyth, J. M., Stone, A. A., Hurewitz, A., & Kaell, A. (1999). Effects of writing about stressful experiences on symptom reduction in patients with asthma or rheumatoid arthritis: A randomized trial. *JAMA: Journal of the American Medical Association, 281*, 1304–1309.

Smyth, J. M., True, N., & Souto, J. (2001). Effects of writing about traumatic experiences: The necessity for narrative structuring. *Journal of Social & Clinical Psychology, 20*, 161–172.

Spera, S. P., Buhrfeind, E. D., & Pennebaker, J. W. (1994). Expressive writing and coping with job loss. *Academy of Management Journal, 37*, 722–733.

Stanton, A. L., Danoff-Burg, S., Sworowski, L. A., Collins, C. A., Branstetter, A. D., Rodriguez-Hanley, A., ... Austenfeld, J. L. (2002). Randomized, controlled trial of written emotional expression and benefit finding in breast cancer patients. *Journal of Clinical Oncology, 20*, 4160–4168.

Strachan, E. D., Bennett, W. R. M., Russo, J., & Roy-Byrne, P. P. (2007). Disclosure of HIV status and sexual orientation independently predicts increased absolute CD4 cell counts over time for psychiatric patients. *Psychosomatic Medicine, 69*, 74–80.

Stroebe, W., Schut, H., & Stroebe, M. S. (2005). Grief work, disclosure and counseling: Do they help the bereaved? *Clinical Psychology Review, 25*, 395–414.

Swanbon, T., Boyce, L., & Greenberg, M. A. (2008). Expressive writing reduces avoidance and somatic complaints in a community sample with constraints on expression. *British Journal of Health Psychology*, *13*, 53–56.

Warner, L. J., Lumley, M. A., Casey, R. J., Pierantoni, W., Salazar, R., Zoratti, E. M., … Simon, M. R. (2006). Health effects of written emotional disclosure in adolescents with asthma: A randomized, controlled trial. *Journal of Pediatric Psychology*, *31*, 557–568.

Weinman, J., Ebrecht, M., Scott, S., Dyson, M., & Walburn, J. (2008). Enhanced wound healing after emotional disclosure intervention. *British Journal of Health Psychology*, *13*, 95–102.

Wilkerson, J. E., Bailey, J. M., Bieniasz, M. E., Murray, S. I., & Ruffin, M. T. (2009). Psychosocial factors in risk of cervical intraepithelial lesions. *Journal of Women's Health*, *18*, 513–518.

Zakowski, S. G., Ramati, A., Morton, C., Johnson, P., & Flanigan, R. (2004). Written emotional disclosure buffers the effects of social constraints on distress among cancer patients. *Health Psychology*, *23*, 555–563.

Zech, E., de Ree, F. D. R., Berenschot, F., & Stroebe, M. (2006). Depressive affect among health care seekers: How it is related to attachment style, emotional disclosure, and health complaints. *Psychology, Health & Medicine*, *11*, 7–19.

9 Coping in Social Context

Tracey A. Revenson
Graduate Center, City University of New York

Stephen J. Lepore
Temple University

The topic of coping with stress has occupied a central place in health psychology for almost four decades. A number of volumes have been devoted to defining what coping is, whether it improves health and well-being; and if it does do so, how it works, for whom, at what times, and in what ways (e.g., Aldwin, 1994; Carpenter, 1992; Eckenrode, 1991; Folkman, 2011; Gottlieb, 1997; Lazarus, 1999; Lazarus & Folkman, 1984; Snyder, 1999; Snyder & Ford, 1987; Zeidner & Endler, 1996). Researchers have created checklists of coping strategies to measure coping (e.g., Carver, Scheier, & Weintraub, 1989; Endler & Parker, 1990; Folkman, Lazarus, Dunkel-Schetter, DeLongis, & Gruen, 1986; Moos, 1993) and taxonomies of coping strategies to understand those measures (Skinner, Edge, Altman, & Sherwood, 2003). We have some clues as to which coping strategies are associated with better physical and mental health, although this is tempered by personality, situation, place, and history. We have so much research on coping—a basic search combining the terms *coping* and *stress* led to 1,652 articles—and yet know so little that some researchers have suggested that we do away with the concept of coping altogether (Coyne & Gottlib, 1996).

The lion's share of research on stress and coping processes tends to conceptualize coping as an individual attribute, describing "ways" of coping and their effects on physical and mental health outcomes. However, even if one could be characterized as having a particular style of coping with stressors, perhaps based on responses to a standard coping checklist, coping is a changeable process with indeterminate benefits that may be applied by individuals to some stressors and not others or to a particular stressor at one time and not another. We have argued that examining coping in its social context will result in a deeper and more precise understanding of how and why people cope with stressors in particular ways at particular times (e.g., Lepore, 2001; Lepore & Evans, 1996; Lepore & Revenson 2006, 2007; Revenson, 1990, 2003). Coping does not take place in a social vacuum (Revenson, 1994); rather, it takes place, implicitly or explicitly, in an interpersonal context that can shape and change it.

How can scholars think about coping without thinking about coping in its social context? How, we wondered, can so much of the literature examine individual efforts to cope with stress and their effects without considering that these efforts are influenced, reshaped, and enhanced by feedback from others? We have not been the only ones to raise these questions; see, for example, the papers and commentaries in special sections of the *Journal of Health Psychology* (1997, Vol. 2, No. 2) and the *American Psychologist* (2000, Vol. 55, No. 6). So when we embarked upon writing this chapter, we decided not to write a review chapter about the coping literature over the past 10 years but instead to examine the phenomenon of coping in social context. Other scholars have addressed this issue in the past (e.g., Eckenrode, 1991). As Folkman and Moskowitz (2004) wrote, "Although most models of coping view the individual as embedded in a social context, the literature on coping is dominated by individualistic approaches that generally give short shrift to social aspects" (p. 758). Similarly, the literatures on coping and social support have remained rather separate despite the fact that both are seen as moderators of the relationship between stress and health. Thus, we wanted to examine how the social environment is incorporated in theories of coping and how to reconcile the literatures into more unified theories.

In this chapter we will examine how the inclusion of social contextual variables broadens the investigation of coping and its effects on physical and mental health by providing clues as to why people cope as they do and relating this to the effectiveness of their coping efforts. To make this argument, we go back historically to find evidence of social context in the essential theories of coping, particularly Lazarus's stress and coping paradigm (e.g., Lazarus, 1981, 1999; Lazarus & Folkman, 1984; Lazarus & Launier, 1978), which remains the gold standard in the area. We then highlight two areas of research and measurement that we feel have moved the area forward over the past decade by combining social context and coping: social constraints and dyadic coping. We end with suggestions for future work.

COPING IN SOCIAL CONTEXT: A BRIEF HISTORICAL JOURNEY

Reading the literature on coping from its early days in the 1970s (Coelho, Hamburg, & Adams, 1974), through its heyday in the 1980s and 1990s (Carver et al., 1989; Lazarus & Folkman, 1984), and to its exaggerated demise at the turn of the century (Coyne, 1997), one senses a fairly homogeneous approach: Coping is conceptualized as an individual-level concept, a characteristic of a person. This conceptualization of coping permeates the literature despite the emergence and centrality of Lazarus's transactional stress and coping paradigm in the field during this same time period (Lazarus, 1966, 1981, 1999; Lazarus, Averill, & Opton, 1974; Lazarus & Folkman, 1984; Lazarus & Launier, 1978).

In Lazarus's model, coping is conceptualized as a dynamic process that involves transactions between persons and their environments. People appraise situations as stressful when environmental demands exceed their personal and social resources (Lazarus & Folkman, 1984). Stress appraisals, in turn, determine how individuals choose to cope with the stressors, although other factors are also involved (e.g., experience, stakes, feedback from others). Coping strategies were described originally as serving either a problem-focused or emotion-focused function (Folkman & Lazarus, 1980). In the former, coping efforts are aimed at managing or eliminating the source of stress; in the latter, coping is directed toward managing the emotional distress that arises from stress appraisals. Coping was defined as "constantly changing cognitive and behavioral efforts to manage, [i.e., master, tolerate, reduce, minimize], specific external and/or internal demands, [and conflicts among them], that are appraised as taxing or exceeding the resources of the person" (Lazarus & Folkman, 1984, p. 141). This transactional paradigm of stress and coping has served, and still serves, as the guiding framework by researchers in the United States, Western Europe, and Asia; but in practice, many researchers have tended to study coping as a trait-like variable.

The stress and coping paradigm brought together a number of germinal ideas. Coping is a dynamic process that unfolds over time. Coping is goal directed and effortful. Coping is not the same as adaptation (its outcome). Two tenets guided the stress and coping paradigm. First, individuals' experience of stress is dependent on their cognitive and affective appraisals of an event; second, both intrapersonal resources and interpersonal factors shape coping. Some early empirical studies found that people varied in the type of coping they used across situations, for example, depending on whether the situations were appraised as posing a harm, loss, or threat (McCrae, 1984). Influenced historically by the cognitive revolution in psychology and Mischel's (1968) person-situation interactionist approach, the stress and coping paradigm examined individuals within their life contexts, giving much emphasis to their subjective perceptions of stressful events and the stakes for making particular coping choices.

At the same time that the transactional stress and coping paradigm appeared, sociologists were studying the influence of social structures and roles on stress and coping processes (Pearlin, 1989; Pearlin & Schooler, 1978). In contrast to the predominant psychological focus on cognitive stress appraisals as determinants of coping, in this approach stress was nested within role theory, especially role conflict or role overload. Predominant were such stresses and strains that required a sustained coping effort as parenting or economic strains. This broader view of stress, in turn, required a broader view of coping, one that examined coping within the context of ongoing social stressors and social roles (also see Lepore, 1995, 1997).

This approach can be exemplified by a prospective, longitudinal study of the partners of men with AIDS conducted by Folkman, Moskowitz, Ozer, and Park (1997). The research examined the coping processes of partners of men with HIV during a profoundly stressful experience: caring for an extremely ill partner. (Antiretroviral drugs had not yet turned HIV into a chronic illness.) Although the self-report data represented the caregiver's perspective, the heart of the coping process was conceptualized as interpersonal for three reasons. First, and most obvious, the object of coping was an interpersonal stressor: caring for another person. Second, the psychological constructs of coping, control, and meaning making were couched within the interpersonal relationship, as opposed to being seen as individual-level characteristics. Third, the methodology organically incorporated the social context. Because Folkman and her colleagues assessed caregivers' coping choices using a narrative methodology, they were able to describe the richness and complexity of interpersonal stress and coping processes in a way that coping checklists could not. Folkman and her colleagues parsed the narratives for their relational aspects and by doing this put coping in its social context. For example, one caregiver's narrative describes the horrific night sweats his partner had up to 12 times a night, the instrumental and emotional support he offers to his ill partner by changing the bedclothes, sitting with him quietly between episodes, and comforting him without showing his own exhaustion.

SEEKING SOCIAL SUPPORT

Early attempts to include social factors in coping research did so by examining support-seeking behavior as a type of coping. Seeking social support is a coping strategy in almost every coping measure (Skinner et al., 2003). Based on these measures, it is not clear whether the support being sought is received or simply expected; or if it was received, whether it was helpful or not in meeting individuals' needs. The original binary classification of coping strategies as either problem- or emotion-focused reinforced this omission. Seeking support clearly served both emotion- and problem-focused functions. Information or feedback on coping choices might lead to a more instrumental handling of the problem, but at the same time expressions of being cared for and valued might minimize the emotional distress caused by the stressor.

This led to the question of where social support fit in the schema of coping taxonomies and what its coping functions were. Early on, the problem-focused versus emotion-focused binary distinction was deemed too simple. In an influential empirical paper, *Dynamics of a Stressful Encounter*, Folkman and her colleagues (1986) empirically delineated eight types of coping, including two clearly interpersonal processes: confrontation and seeking emotional support. Moreover, many aspects of social relationships were embedded in the items of the Ways of Coping Scale and other coping inventories. For example, items having to do with one's social environment or interpersonal relationship can be found in four of the subscales of the revised Ways of Coping Scale (Folkman et al., 1986): (1) "Talked to someone who could do something concrete about the problem" (seeking social support); (2) "I expressed anger to the person(s) who caused the problem" (confrontive coping); (3) "Kept others from know how bad things were" (self-controlling); and (4) "Avoided being with people in general" (escape-avoidance). In another frequently used measure, the COPE (Carver et al., 1989), items tapping the social environment reside in at least three strategies: (1) use of instrumental social support, (2) use of emotional social support, and (3) focus on and venting of emotions.

In a tour-de-force attempt to conceptualize the structure of coping, Skinner and her colleagues (2003) examined both rationale and empirical systems of classifying coping. Using empirical criteria that crossed systems, they came up with five core categories of coping. Support seeking is one of the core categories (along with problem-solving, avoidance, distraction, and positive cognitive restructuring). Strategies from numerous coping scales fell in this category, including many different types of cognitions, emotions, behaviors, and evaluations across multiple sources of support (e.g., friends, family, coworkers).

Whereas social factors are evident in many measures of coping, the relation of social factors to coping is not addressed by such measures. Support seeking often takes its place alongside other types of coping that are treated as stable individual attributes rather than a process that varies across stressors, time, and, most importantly, social contexts.

RELATIONSHIP-FOCUSED COPING

A major move toward linking social factors and coping emerged in a reformulation of the stress and coping paradigm by two members of the original Berkeley Stress and Coping Project. Coyne (Coyne & Fiske, 1992; Coyne & Smith, 1991) and DeLongis (DeLongis & O'Brien, 1990; O'Brien & DeLongis, 1997) added a third coping function to the original stress and coping paradigm: *relationship-focused or relational coping.* This conceptualization of relationship-focused coping rests on the assumption that maintaining relatedness with others is a fundamental human need, as fundamental to coping as eliminating or minimizing stressors and regulating emotions. Relationship-focused coping involves cognitive and behavioral efforts to manage and sustain social relationships during stressful episodes. In doing so, partners attend to each other's emotional needs while maintaining the integrity of the relationship. Relationship-focused coping also encompasses efforts to manage one's own stress without creating upset or problems for others. Relationship-focused coping strategies include negotiating or compromising with others, considering the other person's situation, and being empathic and open in communication (Manne & Badr, 2009; DeLongis & O'Brien, 1990; O'Brien, DeLongis, Pomaki, Puterman, & Zwicker, 2009). Coping was now defined within the context of one's social network. Moreover, the construct of relationship-focused coping incorporated the notion that coping could lead to both adaptive and maladaptive outcomes.

Active Engagement and Protective Buffering

Two relationship-focused coping strategies that have dominated the coping literature are *active engagement* and *protective buffering* (Coyne & Smith, 1991). Active engagement strategies involve the partner in discussions and asking how he or she feels; they are characterized by instrumental or problem-focused coping efforts. Protective buffering involves hiding concerns from the partner and not disclosing personal worries and concerns in order to protect the patient from upset and conflict.

For the most part, these strategies have been studied among couples coping with serious illness (heart disease or cancer). Active engagement has been related to the patient's well-being in couples coping with a myocardial infarction (Coyne & Smith, 1991; Suls, Green, Rose, Lounsbury, & Gordon, 1997) and to marital satisfaction among persons with cancer (Hagedoorn et al., 2000; Kuijer et al., 2000) and their partners (Ybema, Kujer, Buunk, DeJong, & Sanderman, 2001). Patients with the greatest physical impairment or psychological distress benefit the most from active engagement (Hagedoorn et al., 2000).

Active engagement may allow patients to regain control over their lives (Hagedoorn et al., 2000). It also may signify that the partner sees the illness as a shared stressor. Active engagement by partners appears to be a response to the patient's coping with the illness; those individuals who were perceived as coping better were provided more active engagement coping (Kuijer et al., 2000). Similarly, in a German study of couples facing cancer, partners provided the most support to patients who used a good deal of instrumental coping and actively mobilized support; they gave the least support to patients who had accepted the illness but were not coping actively (Luszczynska, Gerstorf, Boehmer, Knoll, & Schwarzer, 2007). Ironically, those patients who were most in need of support may not have received the "best," most active type of support from partners (see also the experimental evidence in Silver, Wortman, & Crofton, 1990).

Protective buffering is ostensibly used to avoid disagreements and "protect" the relationship, but across a number of studies of coping with illness it appears to exact psychological costs for the person using it. In studies of couples coping with a husband's myocardial infarction (Coyne & Smith, 1991; Suls et al., 1997), wives' coping efforts to shield husbands from stress in the post-MI period may have contributed to their own distress, as did husbands' efforts to protect their wives. In a study of spouses of rheumatoid arthritis patients, the wives of ill men confided that they had lessened their own requests for emotional support, for fear of increasing their ill husbands' distress (Revenson & Majerovitz, 1990, 1991). The evidence for studies of cancer is mixed: In one study of patients with various cancers, protective buffering had no effect on patients' distress (Kuijer et al., 2000); whereas in a study of women with breast cancer, greater use of protective buffering (by patient or partner) was associated with greater distress experienced by the person doing the buffering (Manne, Dougherty, Veach, & Kless, 1999).

Although protective buffering is most often conceptualized as a coping strategy, it also can be conceptualized as ways that partners attempt to provide support to each other. The idea of "invisible" support suggests that support transactions in which the recipient is unaware that support is provided may lead to lower psychological distress than support transactions in which the recipient is aware that support is provided (Bolger, Zuckerman, & Kessler, 2000; Maisel & Gable, 2009). Visible support can potentially cause distress in support recipients (e.g., Lepore, Glaser, & Roberts, 2008), possibly by threatening recipients' sense of mastery, self-esteem, and self-efficacy (Bolger & Amarel, 2007; Schwarzer & Knoll, 2007). In contrast, invisible support may proactively minimize or eliminates stress before it occurs, without damaging the self-image of the unknowing recipient of support. Research has not yet examined whether invisible support is beneficial to the provider as well as the recipient. It is easy to imagine that providers of invisible support could feel unappreciated by the support recipient and possibly experience distress or relationship dissatisfaction if their support efforts go unnoticed.

Communication and Relationship Maintenance

Maintaining close relationships in the face of stress protects individuals from the negative effects of stressful episodes. Engaging in "relationship talk" is a potentially useful coping strategy (Acitelli & Badr, 2005). Relationship talk involves taking a relationship perspective and talking about one's relationship as an entity. It is difficult to focus on relationship maintenance during times of extreme stress (Badr, Acitelli, & Carmack Taylor, 2007), but the benefits are apparent: In a study of recently diagnosed lung cancer patients and their partners, engaging in relationship maintenance early on was associated with the psychological and marital adjustment of both patients and partners concurrently and over the next six months (Badr, Acitelli, & Carmack Taylor, 2008; Badr & Carmack Taylor, 2008). Similarly, in a study of breast cancer patients and their husbands (Manne et al., 2006), communication styles were related to the partner's psychological distress nine months later, with mutual constructive communication related to lower distress and demand-withdraw and mutual avoidance communication related to higher distress. Moreover, both mutual constructive communication and demand-withdraw communication were associated with relationship satisfaction in the predicted directions.

Couples in higher-quality marriages tend to communicate in a more relationship-maintaining manner during conflict (e.g., less negative affect reciprocity, less cross-complaining, and more expressions of empathy, understanding, and validation). These communication patterns may allow couples with better marital quality to manage conflict more effectively (Fincham & Beach, 1999).

Empathic Responding

One critical determinant of maintaining satisfying relationships during times of stress may be the extent to which persons can respond with an empathic orientation. Empathy has long been considered an essential component of emotional attunement, promoting caring actions between people (Eisenberg, 2000). Though few coping measures directly assess empathy as a mode of coping, the notion that people use empathy as a means of managing stress within the social context is not new; Haan (1977) identified empathy as a mode of coping that involves attempts to formulate an understanding of another person's feelings and thoughts. Whether conceptualized as coping or support, empathic responding serves to manage or prevent conflict; minimize the distress of loved ones, negative cognitions, or blaming orientations toward others; and promote closeness, emotional intimacy, and relationship quality (Davis, 1994; Gottman, 1998; O'Brien & DeLongis, 1997). Research conducted in laboratory settings indicates that marital tension or conflict is diminished when partners convey empathy during interactions (Gottman, 1998).

Empathic responding as a mode of relationship-focused coping differs significantly from the strategy of seeking social support. Support seeking is generally construed as efforts to get support from another person. Empathic responding is construed as efforts to understand another person and efforts to behaviorally respond to the other person in the stressful situation in a supportive, caring manner as a means to defuse interpersonal stress and maintain the relationship. With empathic responding, the person coping with stress engages in empathic processes and provides caring gestures to the other person in the stressful situation. With social support seeking, the person who is actively coping tries to elicit empathy from others. Thus, the difference is in the focus of investigation and the potential source of change.

Using a measure of relationship-focused coping that incorporates empathic responding, Bodenmann and colleagues (Bodenmann & Cina, 2005; Bodenmann, Pihet, & Kayser, 2006) found that relationship-focused coping predicted marital quality and stability among community-residing couples two to five years later. In an intervention study, improving these coping skills resulted in higher marital satisfaction in the intervention group relative to the control group (Bodenmann & Shantinath, 2004). Observational studies also suggest that using empathic responding leads to higher interaction satisfaction in both members of the couple (Cutrona & Suhr, 1992).

In sum, relationship-focused coping research has greatly enhanced our understanding of the diverse and complex set of influences, especially motivations, for coping with stressors in particular ways. This line of research also has revealed that individuals do not always seek to maximize personal gains by engaging others only in ways that will facilitate the removal of a stressor or psychological and physical adaptation to a stressor but instead take into account the needs of significant others and relationship outcomes. This area of research also helps to explain why individuals might engage in coping behaviors that research suggests is maladaptive, such as inhibiting negative emotions and avoiding thinking or talking about stressors. People might engage in such behaviors for social ends, including promoting relationship harmony and protecting others despite personal costs.

THE CONCEPT OF COPING WITHIN THE SOCIAL SUPPORT LITERATURE

Up to this point, we have focused on theories of coping and how the social context plays a role in defining the construct of coping and operates within certain types of coping. We now examine the other side of the coin: how coping has played a part in theories of social support, which is the most frequently studied social factor in the stress literature.

Social support is defined as the perception or experience that one is loved, valued, and cared for by others and part of a social network of mutual assistance (Wills & Ainette, Chapter 20, this volume). Social support plays a key role in the stress and coping process, serving as a resource that shapes cognitive stress appraisals and coping choices (and ultimately outcomes). Research has shown a consistent association between support and such mental health outcomes as lowered depression and better adjustment to a diverse array of stressors (Stanton & Revenson, 2011).

In the most basic sense, greater support leads to better coping, although this result is moderated by the match between support needs and provision (Cutrona & Russell, 1990), the source or provider of support (Revenson, 1993), and the type of stressor (McCrae, 1984). If we have learned anything after four decades, it is that social support is a complex multifaceted construct, almost a family of constructs (Schwarzer, Dunkel-Schetter, & Kemeny, 1994). It has held many health psychologists' interest because of its potential for optimizing health and well-being.

DEFINITIONS OF SOCIAL SUPPORT

Broadly defined, social support refers to the processes by which interpersonal relationships promote psychological well-being and protect people from health declines, particularly when they are facing stressful life circumstances (Wills & Ainette, Chapter 20, this volume). Mapping onto the functions of affiliation, social support is generally classified into several types, or functions. Functional measures are based on the assumption that social relationships provide certain resources. The functions of support include (a) emotional support (expressing positive affect, caring, and love); (b) esteem support (validating beliefs, emotions, and actions); (c) informational support (providing information or advice, giving instrumental or tangible support, and providing material aid or help); and (d) companionship support, also termed belonging (reminding recipients that they are part of a meaningful social group).

Receiving, using, or requesting social support has costs as well as benefits. In describing the costs, it is important to distinguish between negative social interactions never meant to be helpful (e.g., criticism, avoidance, angry outburst) and well-intended social support attempts that go awry. Support may be perceived as problematic when it is not desired, needed, or requested, or when the type of support offered does not match the recipient's needs (Cutrona & Russell, 1990; Hagedoorn et al., 2000; Lanza, Cameron, & Revenson, 1995). Relative to positive aspects of relationships, the negative aspects are more strongly related to symptoms of distress (e.g., Lepore, 1992; Pagel, Erdly, & Becker, 1987; Revenson, Schiaffino, Majerovitz, & Gibofsky, 1991). We will return to the notion of negative support when we discuss new directions in research.

HOW DOES SOCIAL SUPPORT PROMOTE EFFECTIVE COPING?

A major theme running throughout the social support literature has been that social support can help (or hinder) coping efforts. Thoits (1986) defined social support as "coping assistance." Supportive relationships were conceptualized primarily as available resources that could aid individuals' coping in a number of ways—namely, by influencing stress appraisals, providing information about coping options, giving feedback validating or criticizing individuals' coping choices, providing instrumental assistance in carrying out the coping actions, or simply being present to help sustain coping efforts.

A number of studies have provided empirical support for the theory of social support as coping assistance. For example, in a longitudinal study of cancer surgery patients and their support providers, partner-provided support assessed one month postsurgery was positively related to coping (e.g., fighting spirit) and posttraumatic growth six months after surgery, with received support six months postsurgery acting as a mediator (Luszczynska, Mohamed, & Schwarzer, 2005; Schulz & Schwarzer, 2004). Similarly, in a study of women with early-stage breast cancer, unsupportive behavior from both the provider's perspective and the recipient's perspective was related to greater avoidance coping and greater patient distress (Manne, Ostroff, Winkel, Grana, & Fox, 2005).

Other theoretical approaches suggest that the benefit experienced from receiving social support is a consequence of individuals' proactive coping efforts within their social environment (Ouellette & DiPlacido, 2001; Sarason, Sarason, & Pierce, 1990). Early work focused on additive models with coping and social support as independent moderators of the relationship between stress and mental health outcomes. In some studies, such psychological factors as personality, coping, and support were combined into a stress-resistance index, making it impossible to untangle additive effects or explore interactive ones (e.g., Holahan & Moos, 1986; Nuckolls, Cassel, & Kaplan, 1972). In other work, coping and support could be seen working at cross-purposes: Coping that involved damaging ones' social relationships (e.g., expressing anger toward others) was deemed to be ineffective coping because it minimized potential social support in the present and future (e.g., Felton & Revenson, 1984; Lane & Hobfoll, 1992; Lazarus, 1981).

Many other pathways have been hypothesized to explain how support functions to enhance coping efforts and promote better adaptation to stress; they include mechanisms at many different levels, from the cellular to the psychological (e.g., personality) to the cultural (e.g., social norms). A number of excellent articles and chapters review the multiple pathways through which support leads to coping outcomes (Schwarzer & Knoll, 2007; Taylor, Repetti, & Seeman, 1997; Taylor & Stanton, 2007; Wills & Ainette, Chapter 20, this volume). Support may aid coping by encouraging health-promoting behaviors or decreasing risky behaviors and may thereby also modulate stress responses on the biological level, for example, lowering cortisol levels and autonomic responses to challenge.

An underlying assumption of the social support literature is that people need support at times of crisis and that any support is better than no support (Lanza et al., 1995). Yet requesting social support or receiving unwanted support has its costs (e.g., Revenson et al., 1991). The efficacy of social support seems to depend on a number of contextual factors, including the timing of the support, the type of support that is needed, and the source of the support (Cutrona & Russell, 1990). For example, in studies of patients with cancer (Dakof & Taylor, 1990) and rheumatoid arthritis (Lanza et al., 1995), emotional support was rated as most helpful when it was provided by family members, whereas informational support was rated as most helpful when it was provided by medical professionals. Help may be counterproductive if it threatens autonomy or self-worth (Lepore et al., 2008) or if it immobilizes coping efforts (Coyne & Bolger 1990). Similarly, judgments about how well a person is coping can lead to readiness to provide help or not (Silver, Wortman, & Crofton, 1990).

Social Support as a Coping Resource

In most coping theories, social support is conceptualized as a resource that individuals draw on in order to cope effectively with the stressor at hand (Moos & Schaefer, 1993; Pearlin & Schooler, 1978; Taylor & Stanton, 2007). For example, Holahan and Moos (1990) proposed a resources model of coping in which coping functions as one mechanism through which such resources as social support influence adjustment. In a study that included community-residing healthy and depressed individuals, family support, among other resources, was related to greater active-behavioral and active-cognitive coping and lower avoidance coping (Holahan & Moos, 1987). In a prospective study examining coping and support as predictors of depression among heart disease patients a year later, support predicted decreases in depression both directly and through the mediator of adaptive coping (Holahan, Moos, Holahan, & Brennan, 1997).

Another resource model that focuses on the integration of coping and the social context is conservation-of-resources theory (COR; Hobfoll, 1989). Resources are defined as personal characteristics, conditions, or energies that are valued by the individual and that serve as a means for attainment of what one wants in life. Psychological adjustment depends on individuals' abilities to reverse the losses suffered and efficiently use the remaining coping resources. Specifically, when confronted with stress, individuals strive to minimize net loss of resources. This prediction is not inconsistent with Lazarus and Folkman's (1984) coping model, but it goes beyond their conceptualization of coping as an attempt to minimize, master, or manage stress. Thus, COR theory holds that individuals strive to obtain and retain those resources they centrally value and that loss and gain are expected in the future; there is no "resolved coping episode." Social relationships are a central resource and also appear as loss of support, a central loss. In this regard, COR theory overlaps with relationship-focused coping models, which argue that people strive to maintain or "conserve" positive social relationships. According to COR, families are a critical conduit of resource losses and gains, and they are nested within such broader social contexts as neighborhoods, which can both augment and compensate for family resources (Hobfoll, 2011).

In sum, theories of stress and coping and theories of social factors in stress are intertwined and interdependent. The cognitive appraisal of stress depends partly on the availability of social coping resources. The effectiveness of some coping strategies is dependent on the social context in which they occur. Some coping strategies involve seeking or utilizing social support, and some types of social support involve coping efforts.

WIDENING OUR UNDERSTANDING OF THE SOCIAL CONTEXT OF COPING

A number of recent advances in the stress and coping literature continue to bring the notion of social context to the fore; these include the constructs of social constraints and dyadic coping. We will briefly discuss each in turn. These recent approaches embed the notion of social context in their theories of coping; as a result, they provide illumination of how the social world influences coping processes and vice versa.

SOCIAL CONSTRAINTS ON DISCLOSURE

The concept of social constraints was first introduced as a component of the social-cognitive processing (SCP) model of adjustment to bereavement (Lepore, Silver, Wortman, & Wayment, 1996). A basic premise of the SCP model is that when facing major stressors or traumas, people have a strong urge to talk with others to process the experience, particularly in the initial phases of exposure to the stressor or when they are having difficulty accepting or cognitively processing the stressor. Talking with others may facilitate cognitive processing, as well as emotional adaptation, to the stressor. However, the benefits of such emotional disclosure will depend, in part, on the response of others: If social-network members are receptive to a person's disclosure (or are, at least, perceived as receptive), then disclosure would be beneficial. In contrast, if a person is or perceives herself or himself to be constrained in discussing negative thoughts and feelings, then the potential benefits of disclosure might be negated.

Lepore and Revenson (2007) defined social constraints on disclosure as "objective social conditions and individuals' construal of those conditions that lead individuals to refrain from or modify their disclosure of stress- and trauma-related thoughts, feelings, or concerns" (p. 3). Social constraints involve verbal or nonverbal interpersonal interactions that lead individuals to feel unsupported, misunderstood, or otherwise alienated from their social network at a time when they are attempting to disclose their thoughts, feelings, or concerns or are seeking support. The construct of social constraints is related to such constructs as social conflict (Lepore, 1992), social control (Lewis, Butterfield, Darbes, & Johnston-Brooks, 2004), problematic social support (Revenson, 1993), and miscarried helping (Coyne, Wortman, & Lehman, 1988), but it is not identical to them. Theoretically, the social behaviors of others that are tapped by these various constructs can lead to social constraints on disclosure, but it depends on appraisals made about the intent of the behaviors.

Social constraints can emerge from a history of negative social exchanges with a network member, but they can also emerge in the context of well-intended social exchanges. Furthermore, social constraints are not the absence of social support or reports of unhelpful support. Instead, constraints arise from mismatches between desired and received support, such as when support exchanges that were intended by the provider to be helpful are perceived by the recipient as harmful, unwanted, or inconsequential (Dakof & Taylor, 1990; Reynolds & Perrin, 2004). Thus, many different kinds of social interactions—well-intentioned, positive, neglectful, or critical—have the potential to create social constraints on disclosure to the extent that they lead individuals to restrict or modify their disclosures of stress-related thoughts and feelings.

HOW DO SOCIAL CONSTRAINTS HINDER COPING?

If social network members are receptive to a person's disclosure (or, at least, are perceived as receptive), the SCP model would predict a number of potential benefits of disclosure (Lepore, 2001).

A nonconstraining, supportive social environment could help people to cognitively process the stressor. By cognitively processing the stressor, emotional habituation might be facilitated. Social-network members also could facilitate cognitive processing by suggesting new and positive perspectives, providing information on how to cope or encouraging acceptance. Talking with supportive others could facilitate the creation of a narrative that consolidates disparate thoughts, emotions, and memories shaken by the stressful event, thereby reducing the need for further processing.

Mirroring these processes, social constraints could have an adverse effect on coping by increasing avoidance in thinking and talking about the problem, having the unintended effect of prolonging intrusive thoughts and psychological distress. In addition, avoidance can diminish opportunities for habituation, gaining new perspectives from others, and finding meaning in the stressor (Lepore & Kernan, 2008). Socially constraining behaviors of significant others can also be distressing if they violate individuals' expectations about the nature of their relationship with those significant others, possibly undermining feelings of belonging, trust, and security at a time of heightened vulnerability.

Research with a number of stressful events or traumas supports this perspective. A higher level of social constraints on disclosure has been associated with increased psychological distress in a number of studies covering a wide range of traumas, including bereavement (Lepore et al., 1996), rheumatoid arthritis (Danoff-Burg, Revenson, Trudeau, & Paget, 2004), HIV infection (Ullrich, Lutgendorf, & Stapleton, 2002), cancer risk (Schnur et al., 2004), cancer caregiving (Manne, DuHamel, Redd, 2000), abortion (Major & Gramzow, 1999), traumatic injuries (Cordova, Walser, Neff, & Ruzek, 2005), chronic pain (Herbette & Rime, 2004; Hoffman, Meier, & Council, 2002), and community violence (Kliewer, Lepore, Oskin, & Johnson, 1998; Ozer, Weinstein, Ozer, & Weinstein, 2004).

SOCIAL CONSTRAINTS AND COPING WITH CANCER

Many studies have tested the SCP model's predictions about the role of social constraints in adjustment to cancer (for a review, see Lepore & Revenson, 2007). One fairly robust finding is the direct association between a higher level of social constraints and poorer psychological adjustment in people who have had cancer (Agustsdottir et al., 2010; Cordova, Cunningham, Carlson, & Andrykowski, 2001; Cordova et al., 2007; Eton, Lepore, & Helgeson, 2001; Lepore, 1997, 2001; Lepore & Helgeson, 1998; Lepore & Ituarte, 1999; Manne et al., 2005; Roberts, Lepore, & Helgeson, 2006; Schmidt & Andrykowski, 2004; Widows, Jacobsen, & Fields, 2000; Wingard et al., 2010; Zakowski et al., 2003; Zakowski, Ramati, Morton, Johnson, & Flanigan, 2004).

Coping may partially mediate the association between social constraints and adjustment to such stressors as cancer. A central prediction of the SCP model is that when individuals feel socially constrained, they will use the coping strategy of avoidance. That is, they will avoid thinking about or discussing cancer-related thoughts and feelings and avoid others who are "too close" to the problem. Consistent with these predictions, research with various cancer populations has revealed a positive association between level of social constraints and level of avoidance in thinking and talking about cancer (Cordova et al., 2001; Hughes et al., 2010; Lepore & Helgeson, 1998; Manne et al., 2005; Schmidt & Andrykowski, 2004; Widows et al., 2000; Zakowski et al., 2004). Also consistent with the SCP model, avoidance accounts for some of the association between social constraints and psychological distress. Research has found evidence consistent with mediation among men treated for prostate cancer (Lepore & Helgeson, 1998), women treated for breast cancer (Manne et al., 2005), and women at risk for breast cancer (Schnur et al., 2004). It is not yet clear why social constraints might increase avoidance, but avoidance could be motivated by a patient's desire to minimize strains and conflict with others who send constraint signals.

Another prediction of the SCP model is that social constraints will reduce opportunities for people to cognitively process and make sense of their cancer. One symptom of incomplete cognitive processing might be prolonged intrusive thoughts about cancer (Lepore, 2001). Studies have shown a positive relationship between level of social constraints and level of intrusive thoughts in various cancer populations (Cordova et al., 2001; Manne, 1999; Schmidt & Andrykowski, 2004). The heightened intrusive thoughts can, in turn, be distressing. A high level of uncertainty about illness is another marker of incomplete cognitive processing. Cordova et al. (2001) found a positive association between level of social constraints and expression of uncertainty words (e.g., *perhaps*, *might*) in women's written journals about their breast cancer. In addition to influencing the frequency or duration of intrusive thoughts, to the extent that a high level of social constraints limits cognitive and social processing of cancer-related thoughts and concerns, it can impede habituation processes because of limited exposure to cancer-related stimuli. Thus, cancer patients who have a high level of social constraints should be more distressed by intrusive thoughts than their counterparts with relatively low social constraints. Several studies have shown results consistent with the hypothesis that social constraints moderate the association between intrusive thoughts and distress in people with cancer (Lepore, 2001; Lepore & Helgeson, 1998).

Social constraints may change over time, just as relationships are dynamic and ever changing. Interpersonal exchanges may be perceived as more or less constraining at various times in the coping process, and this perception may change as a result of situational and stress-related changes, relationship changes, or changes in the network members' responses. An excellent example of this dynamic can be found in a study of recently diagnosed lung cancer patients and their spouses (Badr & Carmack Taylor, 2006). Slightly over one third of the patients reported avoiding or having difficulties talking about their cancer, and two thirds of the spouses had difficulties or avoided discussing prognosis, death, or funeral arrangements, ostensibly for fear of upsetting the patient. This resembles the dyadic coping strategy of protective buffering (Coyne & Smith, 1991). Some patients reported that their partner's denial and avoidance was distressing, made them change how they interacted with the partner, and strained the marital relationship.

Current Limitations and Future Directions

Current understanding of the construct of social constraints on disclosure is hampered by the fact that most studies measure it as a perceptual variable, through self-reports. Thus, we do not know much about the characteristics of social transactions that relate to perceptions of social constraints. A next step will be to examine the relative and joint contributions of social support and social constraints to particular coping modes.

Although the literature examining social constraints is beginning to grow with the availability of simple self-report measures and its applicability to a diverse array of stressors (Barnett, Revenson, & Cross, 2011), there are many questions begging to be answered about effects and mechanisms. What are the physical health consequences of social constraints? In one study, Lepore (2001) found that among women who had been treated for localized breast cancer and had relatively high intrusive thoughts about cancer, frequency of engaging in breast self-exams for recurrence was lower if they had high social constraints than if they had relatively low social constraints. Although research has focused on avoidance and intrusive thoughts as important mediating variables, other behavioral, cognitive, and emotional processes could be in play. For example, social constraints might relate to such schemas about the self or others as beliefs about interpersonal trust, self-worth, and self-efficacy, or it might involve such psychological processes relevant to coping, as perceived threat or perceptions of coping efficacy. In an innovative application of SCP theory to diabetes control, researchers found that higher social constraints were associated with lower adherence to certain self-care activities (diet and exercise) among diabetics (Braitman et al., 2008). Further, these associations were mediated by lower self-efficacy to perform diabetes self-care activities and by higher negative mood states.

Broad social and contextual influences (e.g., norms, laws, customs, culture, media), as well as historical factors, can also shape social constraints. For example, when such highly visible and respected members of society as Sheryl Crow can publicly and candidly talk about such medical conditions as breast cancer, the broader population perceives that it has "permission" to discuss these things more freely. Looking at social-level variables that influence social constraints could point to important upstream intervention targets: If modeling open communication with community leaders can reduce social constraints in everyday interpersonal interactions for people with cancer, it could do a lot of good and at a relatively low cost compared to individual- or couple-level interventions.

DYADIC COPING

Within the past decade, a literature has emerged on dyadic coping with stress (Revenson, Kayser, & Bodenmann, 2005). Dyadic coping recognizes mutuality and interdependence in coping responses to a shared stressor. Dyadic coping goes beyond the concept of relationship-focused coping (individual coping efforts within the context of a relationship) and beyond the effects of mutual-influence coping (one person's coping on the other person's coping and adjustment). Each partner's well-being depends upon the couple's ability to draw on each other and their network(s) as social resources.

Drawing on Lazarus's stress and coping paradigm for its ancestry, dyadic coping is a dynamic, transactional process, and stressors are framed as shared (Bodenmann, 2005). The coping process begins with a stress communication: Each member of the dyad communicates his or her own stress to the other in hopes of receiving support and coping feedback. The other partner can respond in either a supportive or unsupportive fashion. Supportive responses include providing advice and practical help with daily tasks, showing empathy and concern, expressing solidarity, and helping one's partner to relax and engage in positive reframing. Unsupportive responses include showing disinterest; providing support that is accompanied by criticism, distancing, or sarcasm; and minimizing the severity of the stressor.

Although the provision of social support is a central component of dyadic coping (Berg & Upchurch, 2007; Bodenmann, 1997, 2005; Manne & Badr, 2008), the construct of dyadic coping goes beyond the exchange of social support. In addition to providing support, couples engage in such shared coping efforts as joint problem solving. These coordinated coping efforts also have both positive and negative forms. Common (with *common* meaning "in common" and not "ordinary") positive dyadic coping involves joint problem solving, coordinating everyday demands, relaxing together, as well as mutual calming, sharing, and expressing solidarity. Common negative dyadic coping involves such strategies as mutual avoidance and withdrawal (Bodenmann, 2005).

In a number of studies of community-living couples, couples in marital therapy, or couples coping with a specific stressor, such as serious illness, common positive dyadic coping was significantly associated with higher marital quality, lower experienced stress, and better psychological and physical well-being (e.g., Badr, 2004; Badr, Carmack, Kashy, Cristofanilli, & Revenson, 2010; Bodenmann, 2000; Bodenmann et al., 2006; Cutrona & Suhr, 1992; Dehle, Larsen, & Landers, 2001; Pasch & Bradbury, 1998; Walen & Lachman, 2000). A study of community-dwelling adults found that couples who reported low levels of common positive dyadic coping at study entry were more likely to divorce or separate five years later (Bodenmann & Cina, 2005).

Dyadic coping has been shown to be positively associated with marital quality through two mechanisms: first, by alleviating the negative impact of stress on marriage; second, by strengthening feelings of mutual trust and intimacy and cognitively representing the relationship as helpful and supportive (Bodenmann, 2005). When spouses report receiving helpful support, they tend to engage in more adaptive ways of coping with chronic stress. For example, in a study of the role of support in coping and pain severity among patients with rheumatoid arthritis, Holtzman, Newth, and DeLongis (2004) found that support indirectly influences pain severity through encouraging the use of such specific coping strategies as positive reappraisal as well as impacting the effectiveness with which these coping strategies were employed. Moreover, support from the spouse attenuated the impact of maladaptive responses to pain, disrupting the vicious cycle of catastrophizing and pain.

This pattern of findings is consistent with research on couples suggesting that the benefits of accommodation (i.e., one's willingness to respond in a constructive manner when a partner has behaved negatively) may depend on the extent to which these responses are met with accommodating responses by one's partner (O'Brien & DeLongis, 1997; Rusbult, Verette, Whitney, Slovik, & Lipkus, 1991). If one spouse engages in efforts to compromise and provide empathy during stressful situations, and his or her spouse does not reciprocate, these coping efforts, though generally expected to have positive effects, may actually result in heightened levels of distress.

Current Limitations and Future Directions

The study of dyadic coping is in its childhood though growing in leaps and bounds, largely benefited by methodologies that can test dependent data from multiple sources (Bolger, Stadler, Paprocki, & DeLongis, 2010; DeLongis, Hemphill, & Lehman, 1992). In a recent chapter on dyadic coping with the stressor of chronic illness, Revenson and DeLongis (2011) made four recommendations for future dyadic research; these suggestions resonate with those we have suggested for the construct of social constraints. First, Revenson and DeLongis suggested that we move toward including the larger social context in the study of dyadic coping. This ranges from gender roles to family environments to cultural mores. To accomplish this, it will be important to move toward interdisciplinary research, specifically, mixing paradigms and methods from different disciplines to create a more integrated picture of dyadic coping processes.

Second, researchers should identify the developmental trajectories of dyadic coping over the life of the stressor and the lifespan of the dyad. For example, among dyads, is there a move toward greater consistency over time? How do attributes of the preexisting relationship affect dyadic coping with a specific stressor? Third was a suggestion to conduct dyadic coping research at multiple levels of analysis. Specifically, it seems important to link individual-level coping processes to dyadic coping; this requires embedding individual goals with dyadic ones and focusing on microanalytic processes without losing the larger relationship context. Finally, Revenson and DeLongis (2011) intimated that it was time to translate the research findings into dyadic coping interventions. Where, when, for whom, and how should we intervene to change dyadic coping processes?

COPING IN THE LARGER MACROLEVEL SOCIAL CONTEXT

To this point, we have focused on intra- and interpersonal aspects of the social context as it affects coping, that is, interpersonal relationships and social support. In an earlier critique Revenson (1997) made the case for a "wider lens" for coping research, stating that "individual behavior can be understood only within its social context, and individuals exist within a number of interdependent or overlapping systems, including family, school and peer domains, as well as broader political, social and cultural contexts" (p. 164; see also Lepore & Revenson, 2006).

Such macrolevel contextual factors as socioeconomic status (SES), culture, ethnicity, and gender affect coping processes through their influence on vulnerability to stress and availability of support, among other phenomena. Although macrolevel factors are major aspects of the social context, we discuss them in a limited fashion here and refer readers to the specific chapters in this volume (Brondolo, Lackey, & Love, Chapter 24; Helgeson, Chapter 22; Mays, Maas, Ricks, & Cochran; Chapter 34; Ruiz, Steffen, & Prather, Chapter 23).

Culture, SES, politics, and social change (e.g., urbanization) affect social-network structure and social capital that, in turn, provide opportunities for such psychosocial mechanisms as coping to influence adjustment. Taylor et al. (1997) proposed a similar conceptualization. In their model, SES and race affect health indirectly through their influence on key environments, including the physical and social environments. Greater social support, access to more social resources, and neighborhoods with greater social capital have been shown to lead to resilience, even among populations facing adversity (Lepore & Revenson, 2006).

Culture

The social context, and the behaviors and interactions that take place within it, is infused with values, belief systems, and worldviews that emanate from cultural phenomena. The concept of culture is applicable across standard social categories, including gender, sexual orientation, race/ethnicity, nationality, religious preference, and disability status. Most conceptualizations of culture include such external referents as customs, artifacts, and social institutions, as well as such internal referents as ideologies, belief systems, attitudes, expectations, and epistemologies.

Coping processes occur within one or more cultural contexts. Cultural schemata provide "lenses" that inform people's worldviews, for example, whether one should trust and follow the advice of medical providers (Dunbar-Jacob, Schlenk, & McCall, Chapter 12, this volume). Culture may also define the acceptability of particular coping responses, among them emotional expression or anger, and place boundaries on coping options (Stanton & Revenson, 2011). Culture might exert some influence on the value of particular coping responses within groups, too, as evident in the value of relationship-focused versus self-focused coping among persons from collectivist versus individualistic cultures. The relations between culture and coping are reciprocal; for example, culture shapes beliefs and cognitions (Landrine & Klonoff, 1992), which are then strengthened by feedback from social ties and socialization practices (Berkman & Glass, 1999).

Socioeconomic Status

In social science research, SES has been conceptualized alternately as financial status (income), occupational status, educational status, or some combination of these, as the position in society into which one is born (which creates hierarchies of majority and minority statuses), or according to subjective perceptions of social status or relative deprivation (Ruiz et al., Chapter 23, this volume). Framing socioeconomic status as a coping resource, Gallo and Matthews (2003; see also Matthews & Gallo, 2011) offered the reserve capacity model as a framework for understanding how SES affects health. Individuals of lower SES experience more stressful life events and events of greater magnitude and have fewer social and psychosocial resources to cope with them, which leads to poorer mental and physical health. There is some empirical evidence for the reserve capacity model (Matthews & Gallo, 2011).

Poverty and its correlates (e.g., low education) can provide a qualitatively different context in which individuals cope (Evans, 2003). The constant struggle for resources to meet basic human needs can severely constrain coping resources. In addition to signaling a lack of fundamental resources, poverty often creates a sense of helplessness and hopelessness.

Race/Ethnicity

Social science researchers typically use demographic markers (e.g., Hispanic, black, nationality, immigrant status) to define ethnic minority cultural groups. However, it is these groups' experiences with racism, discrimination, and social exclusion, on both interpersonal and structural levels, that create stress, attenuate coping resources, and lead to maladaptive coping efforts (see Brondolo et al., Chapter 24, this volume). Research has shown that African American women who attributed interpersonal mistreatment to racial discrimination exhibit greater blood pressure reactivity and recovery to laboratory stressors that bear similarities to an encounter with racial prejudice (e.g., Lepore et al., 2006) than do women who do not make the same attribution. These findings suggest that perceived racism may act as a chronic stressor for which many underresourced individuals cannot cope effectively.

No individual-level coping strategy has emerged as effective for offsetting the impact of racism on health (Brondolo, Brady ver Halen, Pencille, Beatty, & Contrada, 2009). It is likely that changes will need to occur at structural, economic, and political levels in order to have the broadest impact on reducing health disparities. Mays, Cochran, and Barnes (2007) describe several of the race-discrimination-health pathways, including segregation, residential stratification, conditions of violence, lack of social capital, and growing up in poor neighborhoods (see also Mays et al., Chapter 34, this volume).

GENDER

Many of the ways of coping are correlated not only with better adjustment but also sometimes constitute the definition of better adjustment (see Helgeson, Chapter 22, this volume). Two examples may help illustrate how gender socialization translates into differentially effective modes of coping, the first focusing on personality as a determinant of coping and the second on social support.

In the area of personality, the gender-linked personality orientations of *agency* and *communion* (and in their extreme forms, *unmitigated agency* and *unmitigated communion*) are related to adjustment to a number of chronic diseases (Helgeson, 2003a, 2011). Individuals with an agentic orientation focus more on themselves and use more instrumental strategies to cope with stress. Individuals with a more communal orientation focus on others' needs and interpersonal relationships and are more emotionally expressive. Unmitigated agency involves orientation toward oneself without regard for others and difficulty expressing emotions; whereas unmitigated communion refers to an extreme orientation toward others, in which individuals become overinvolved with others to the detriment of their own well-being.

Agency has been linked to better physical and mental health across a number of chronic diseases, including coronary heart disease (Helgeson, 1993), prostate cancer (Helgeson & Lepore, 2004), diabetes (Helgeson, 1994), and rheumatoid arthritis (Trudeau, Danoff-Burg, Revenson, & Paget, 2003). Unmitigated agency has, however, been related to greater difficulty in expressing emotions, which has in turn been associated with negative general and cancer-related adjustment in a group of men with prostate cancer (Helgeson & Lepore, 2004) and to maladjustment in women with breast cancer (Piro, Zeldow, Knight, Mytko, & Gradishar, 2001). Unmitigated communion has been associated with poor health behavior, negative social interactions, and greater depression and cardiac symptoms following a first coronary event (Fritz, 2000); poorer metabolic control and greater psychological distress among adolescents with diabetes (Helgeson, Escobar, Siminerio, & Becker, 2007); and greater functional disability and depressive symptoms among women and men with rheumatoid arthritis (Danoff-Burg et al., 2004; Trudeau et al., 2003) and women with breast cancer (Helgeson, 2003b).

The second example illustrates how gendered enacting of interpersonal relationships creates differential pathways. Interpersonal relationships are essential coping resources for women: Women draw on their support networks more often than men; and these interpersonal contacts serve as a place to express emotions, acquire feedback on coping choices, and obtain assistance with such life tasks as child care. Women are more likely to ask for support, use support, and not feel demeaned by it (Shumaker & Hill, 1991). At the same time, women are more emotionally vulnerable to events that happen to members of their social networks, such that their coping resources may create additional stress (Wethington, McLeod, & Kessler, 1987). A meta-analysis of couples coping with cancer revealed that women report more psychological distress than men whether they are the patient or the caregiver (Hagedoorn, Sanderman, Bolks, Tuinstra, & Coyne, 2008). One prominent explanation is that caring for others is a more central aspect of women's identity (Gilligan, 1982), and the loss of that role is too great a threat to self-esteem and well-being to abandon (Abraído-Lanza & Revenson, 2006).

In sum, it is difficult to isolate the effect of any of these cultural variables because they are tightly intertwined. Moreover, seldom have macrocontextual variables been examined in conjunction with each other for their synergistic influences. However, when one studies coping in social context, this macrosocial context cannot be ignored.

Coping With Shared Community Stressors

Most studies view social support and coping primarily as individual-level or, at best, interpersonal phenomena, failing to take into account community-level structures (Felton & Shinn, 1992). One way to think about social support and coping is in terms of community stressors. Much of the research on community coping has occurred in the aftermath of natural disasters, both naturally produced (e.g., floods, hurricanes) and a result of human behavior (e.g., terrorist attacks, train wrecks). Disasters are interesting social phenomena in that they affect large numbers of persons, so one can see the variation in coping responses and adjustment trajectories (Norris, Tracey, & Galea, 2009). Although much of the work in this area focuses on individual-level coping (e.g., the search for meaning; Park, Aldwin, Fenster, & Snyder, 2008) and individual-level outcomes (e.g., PTSD; Norris et al., 2009), other studies have focused on social relationships as a moderator of the relation between exposure and distress (e.g., MacGeorge, Samter, Feng, Fillihan, & Graves, 2007).

Kaniasty and Norris's work on community disasters (e.g., Kaniasty & Norris, 1995) emphasizes the interdependence of people in their efforts to cope with trauma and make sense of the world. For example, victims of Hurricane Hugo received support from each other and also provided support to each other. However, because large-scale community stressors affect so many people, either because they happen to all family members and neighbors or the effects of one member's adversity affects them all, communitywide disasters can deteriorate social support resources (Kaniasty & Norris, 1993).

NEW DIRECTIONS FOR RESEARCH ON COPING IN SOCIAL CONTEXT

It is customary in such chapters as these to include a final section that evaluates progress and suggests future research directions. Fifteen years ago, in an article titled "Stress, Coping and Social Support Processes: Where Are We? What Next?" Peggy Thoits (1995) reviewed "promising new directions" for each of those three constructs separately. We will look back on a number of those promising new directions as they related to coping in social context and evaluate the progress we have made.

New Methods to Study Changes in Stress and Coping

Along with many others, Thoits questioned whether the methods we were using could really provide answers to questions of causality and change in coping processes as they affected physical and mental health outcomes. Some critics contended that the discrepancies in the coping literature were a result of an overreliance on cross-sectional, between-person, retrospective research designs (e.g., Tennen, Affleck, Armeli, & Carney, 2000). Cross-sectional methods fail to capture the dynamic nature of the coping process (Bolger & Zuckerman, 1995; Coyne & Gottlieb, 1996; Tennen et al., 2000) and as such could not truly test transactional models (Somerfield, 1997). Despite these grim predictions, this new direction has turned from "promising" to "problem partially solved."

Daily process methodology, also referred to as daily diaries, addresses these concerns (Bolger et al., 2010; DeLongis et al., 1992). Because this approach involves multiple assessments over time, daily process methods permit a more accurate assessment of coping. Daily process methods capture such important details as timing, frequency, and emotional reactivity that cannot be assessed using conventional self-report measures of coping. This proximity to events is important in examining changes in such rapidly fluctuating processes as coping. Although daily process studies are labor-intensive research designs, and debate continues regarding ways to improve the methodology (Tennen et al., 2000), they offer a method for testing complex transactional models that examined coping processes across time, people, and situations with longitudinal data.

A second, related development is the statistical procedure of multilevel modeling to analyze daily process data (Bryk & Raudenbush, 1992). From a social-contextual perspective, multilevel modeling takes into account the dependency in data caused by multiple data points and by data from multiple individuals coping with the same stressor (e.g., dyadic data). Multilevel modeling allows for the simultaneous analysis of within-person and between-person variation, within- and between-dyads, and in the case of longitudinal data, same-day and cross-day effects (Bryk & Raudenbush, 1992; Kashy & Kenny, 2000, Kenny, Kashy, & Cook, 2006). For example, in dyadic coping, the coping of each member of the dyad can be examined within the context of one person's coping across time, as well as within the context of the other's coping and the coping of other dyads. Although not able to answer all coping questions, daily process studies are better suited to elucidate dynamic stress and coping processes within their social context.

DOCUMENTATION OF "FLEXIBILITY OR VERSATILITY" IN COPING

Thoits urged us to study coping processes in combination and as they mutually influence each other (1995, p. 3). The isolation of particular coping strategies had been designated as a problem early on in the literature by Vitaliano, Maiuro, Russo, and Becker (1987), who developed the notion of relative coping, that is, determining to what extent a particular strategy is employed, and how effectively, when used in relation to other strategies. Unfortunately, relational coping also relied on self-report measures, quantifying use of a particular coping technique as a proportion versus an absolute score. The ability to gauge how social and nonsocial strategies mutually influence each other is yet to be developed, and whether these strategies work in a synergistic fashion remains an unanswered question in the coping literature.

However, more sophisticated theories of coping go beyond the focus on individual strategies and link coping with the social context. The matching hypothesis (Cutrona & Russell, 1990) suggests that the most effective type of support is that which matches the individual needs; this idea expanded to the timing of support (Revenson, 1993) and the source of support (Dakof & Taylor, 1990; Lanza et al., 1995). Similarly, we have begun to consider the demands of a stressful situation with more precision in order to determine what types of coping efforts might be most effective for particular aspects of stressful situation. We have moved from coping "in general" to coping with specific stressors (your cancer) to coping with particular aspects of stressors (e.g., chemotherapy, hair loss; Somerfield, 1997).

Flexibility in coping has also been demonstrated in the coping literature by findings that different strategies are differentially effective for different groups. That is, we do not unilaterally believe that a particular strategy is adaptive or maladaptive; how a strategy functions depends on the social and cultural context. For example, Stanton's notion of emotional approach coping (Austenfeld & Stanton, 2004; Stanton et al., 2000) addressed the social context implicitly in two ways. First, Stanton differentiated emotional processing from emotional expression—the former an intrapersonal modality and the latter an interpersonal one. Second, in a number of studies she found that emotional approach coping was used more by women than by men and was more effective for them. One could also describe this as an aspect of "matching."

THE COSTS OF SOCIAL RELATIONSHIPS AND THEIR EFFECTS ON COPING

Solid progress has been made here. The idealistic original theory that social support was "good" was quickly invalidated by studies distinguishing structural social network measures from functional ones. Current measures of support asked not only about positive functions but also about such negative interpersonal interactions as criticism, unfulfilled promises, or avoidance. The notion of negative or problematic support—that is, support that was not perceived to be helpful by the recipient or support that led to negative outcomes—begat the new constructs of social constraints and invisible support reviewed earlier in the chapter. This duality has carried over to the study of dyadic coping, where both supportive and unsupportive behaviors, as well as common positive and common negative dyadic coping, are assessed. These constructs and studies testing the mechanisms by which they operated provide new clues as to how support aids coping and vice versa.

CONCLUSION

We would like to be bold enough to say that all coping occurs within a social context and that all coping research and interventions must take that into account. As one critique of the field said over a decade ago:

> We cannot get an adequate evaluation of how people cope in stressful circumstances without taking into account what other persons in their lives are doing. How others are coping; how much our respondents depend on them; and what others leave to these respondents are crucial determinants of what the respondents themselves must do to cope effectively. ... The notion that coping can be relationship-focused as well as problem- and emotion-focused is an acknowledgment of some issues, but hardly sufficient as a solution. (Coyne, 1997, p. 155)

Much has changed since that statement was written. Despite a plethora of critiques, much has been learned about the social context of coping over the past four decades and the past 10 years in particular. Coping is a complex process braiding cognitions, emotions, behaviors, interpersonal relationships, and cultural blueprints. Some strategies work for some people some of the time; perhaps it is time to abandon the pursuit of universal models in favor of contextual stressor-specific ones (see also Folkman & Moskowitz, 2004). We understand that coping appraisals depend on many personal and situations determinants and change rapidly as those determinants change. Although we have not been successful in coming up with measures of coping that address all the theoretical issues, the methods by which coping processes are studied better reflect the transactional, interpersonal nature of coping.

REFERENCES

Abraído-Lanza, A. F., & Revenson, T. A. (2006). Illness intrusion and psychological adjustment to rheumatic diseases: A social identity framework. *Arthritis and Rheumatism: Arthritis Care & Research, 55,* 224–232.

Acitelli, L. K., & Badr, H. J. (2005). My illness or our illness? Attending to the relationship when one partner is ill. In T. A. Revenson, K. Kayser, & G. Bodenmann (Eds.), *Couples coping with stress: Emerging perspectives on dyadic coping* (pp. 121–136). Washington, DC: American Psychological Association.

Agustsdottir, S., Kristinsdottir, A., Jonsdottir, K., Laursdottir, S. O., Smari, J., & Valdimarsdottir, H. B. (2010). The impact of dispositional emotional expressivity and social constraints on distress among prostate cancer patients in Iceland. *British Journal of Health Psychology, 15*(1), 51–61.

Aldwin, C. M. (1994). *Stress, coping, and development: An integrative perspective.* New York, NY: Guildford.

Austenfeld, J. L., & Stanton, A. L. (2004). Coping through emotional approach: A new look at emotion, coping, and health-related outcomes. *Journal of Personality, 7*(6), 1336–1363.

Badr, H. (2004). Coping in marital dyads: A contextual perspective on the role of gender and health. *Personal Relationships, 11,* 197–211.

Badr, H., Acitelli, L. K., & Carmack Taylor, C. L. (2007). Does couple identity mediate the stress experienced by caregiving spouses? *Psychology and Health, 22,* 211–229.

Badr, H., Acitelli, L. K., & Carmack Taylor, C. L. (2008). Does talking about their relationship affect couples' marital and psychological adjustment to lung cancer? *Journal of Cancer Survivorship, 2*(1), 53–64.

Badr, H., & Carmack Taylor, C. L. (2006). Social constraints and spousal communication in lung cancer. *Psycho-Oncology, 15,* 673–683.

Badr, H., & Carmack Taylor, C. L. (2008). Effects of relationship maintenance on psychological distress and dyadic adjustment among couples coping with lung cancer. *Health Psychology, 27*(5) 616–627.

Badr, H., Carmack, C. L., Kashy, D. A., Cristofanilli, M., & Revenson, T. A. (2010). Dyadic coping in metastatic breast cancer. *Health Psychology, 29*(2), 169–180.

Barnett, S., Revenson, T. A., & Cross, W. (2011). The effects of racial identity and social constraints on personal and collective esteem among multiracial individuals. Unpublished manuscript.

Berg, C. A., & Upchurch, R. (2007). A developmental-contextual model of couples coping with chronic illness across the adult life span. *Psychological Bulletin, 133*(6), 920–954.

Berkman, L. F., & Glass, T. (1999). Social integration, social networks, social support, and health. In L. F. Berkman & T. Glass (Eds.), *Social epidemiology* (pp. 137–173). New York, NY: Oxford University Press.

Bodenmann, G. (1997). Dyadic coping: A systemic-transactional view of stress and coping among couples: Theory and empirical findings. *European Review of Applied Psychology, 47*, 137–140.

Bodenmann, G. (2000). *Stress and Coping bei Paaren* [Stress and coping in couples]. Göttingen, Germany: Hogrefe.

Bodenmann, G. (2005). Dyadic coping and its significance for marital functioning. In T. A. Revenson, K. Kayser, & G. Bodenmann (Eds.), *Couples coping with stress: Emerging perspectives on dyadic coping* (pp. 33–50). Washington, DC: American Psychological Association.

Bodenmann, G., & Cina, A. (2005). Stress and coping among stable-satisfied, stable-distressed and separated/ divorced swiss couples: A 5-year prospective longitudinal study. *Journal of Divorce & Remarriage, 44*, 71–89.

Bodenmann, G., Pihet, S., & Kayser, K. (2006). The relationship between dyadic coping and marital quality: A 2-year longitudinal study. *Journal of Family Psychology, 20*(3), 485–493.

Bodenmann, G., & Shantinath, S. D. (2004). The couples coping enhancement training (CCET): A new approach to prevention of marital distress based upon stress and coping. *Family Relations, 53*, 477–484.

Bolger, N., & Amarel, D. (2007). Effects of social support visibility on adjustment to stress: Experimental evidence. *Journal of Personality and Social Psychology, 92*(3), 458–475.

Bolger, N., Stadler, G., Paprocki, C., & Delongis, A. (2010). Grounding social psychology in behavior in daily life: The case of conflict and distress in couples. In C. Agnew, D. E. Carlston, W. G. Graziano, & J. R. Kelly (Eds.), *Then a miracle occurs: Focusing on behavior in social psychological theory and research* (pp. 368–390). New York, NY: Oxford University Press.

Bolger, N., & Zuckerman, A. (1995). A framework for studying personality in the stress process. *Journal of Personality and Social Psychology, 69*(5), 890–902.

Bolger, N., Zuckerman, A., & Kessler, R. C. (2000). Invisible support and adjustment to stress. *Journal of Personality and Social Psychology, 79*(6), 953–961.

Braitman, A. L., Derlega, V. J., Henson, J. M., Robinett, I., Saadeh, G. M., Janda, L. J., … Miranda, J. (2008). *Journal of Social and Clinical Psychology, 27*, 949–969.

Brondolo, E., Brady ver Halen, N., Pencille, M., Beatty, D., & Contrada, R. J. (2009). Coping with racism: A selective review of the literature and a theoretical and methodological critique. *Journal of Behavioral Medicine, 32*, 64–88.

Bryk, A. S., & Raudenbush, S. W. (1992). *Hierarchical linear models: Applications and data analysis methods.* Newbury Park, CA: Sage.

Carpenter, B. N. (1992). *Personal coping: Theory, research and application.* Westport, CT: Greenwood.

Carver, C. S., Scheier, M. F., & Weintraub, J. K. (1989). Assessing coping strategies: A theoretically based approach. *Journal of Personality and Social Psychology, 56*, 267–283.

Coelho, G. V., Hamburg, D. A., & Adams, J. E. (Eds.). (1974). *Coping and adaptation.* Oxford, England: Basic Books.

Cordova, M. J., Cunningham, L. L., Carlson, C. R., & Andrykowski, M. A. (2001). Social constraints, cognitive processing, and adjustment to breast cancer. *Journal of Consulting and Clinical Psychology, 69*(4), 706–711.

Cordova, M. J., Giese-Davis, J., Golant, M., Kronenwetter, C., Chang, V., & Spiegel, D. (2007). Breast cancer as trauma: Posttraumatic stress and posttraumatic growth. *Journal of Clinical Psychology in Medical Settings, 14*(4), 308–319.

Cordova, M. J., Walser, R., Neff, J., & Ruzek, J. I. (2005). Predictors of emotional adjustment following traumatic injury: Personal, social, and material resources. *Prehospital & Disaster Medicine, 20*(1), 7–13.

Coyne, J. C. (1997). Improving coping research: Raze the slum before any more building! *Journal of Health Psychology, 2*(2), 153–172.

Coyne, J. C., & Bolger, N. (1990). Doing without social support as an explanatory concept. *Journal of Social Clinical Psychology, 9,* 148–158.

Coyne, J. C., & Fiske, V. (1992). Couples coping with chronic and catastrophic illness. In M. A. P. Stephens, S. E. Hobfoll, & J. Crowther (Eds.), *Family Health Psychology* (pp. 129–149). Washington, DC: Hemisphere.

Coyne, J. C., & Gottlieb, B. H. (1996). The mismeasure of coping by checklist. *Journal of Personality*, *64*(4), 959–991.

Coyne, J. C., & Smith, D. A. F. (1991). Couples coping with a myocardial infarction: A contextual perspective on wives distress. *Journal of Personality and Social Psychology*, *61*(3), 404–412.

Coyne, J. C., Wortman, C. B., & Lehman, D. R. (1988). The other side of support: Emotional overinvolvement and miscarried helping. In B. Gottlieb (Ed.), *Marshaling social support: Formats, processes, and effects* (pp. 305–330). New York, NY: Sage.

Cutrona, C. E., & Russell, D. W. (1990). Type of social support and specific stress: Toward a theory of optimal matching. In B. R. Sarason, I. G. Sarason, & G. R. Pierce (Eds.), *Social support: An interactional view* (pp. 319–366). New York, NY: Wiley.

Cutrona, C. E., & Suhr, J. A. (1992). Controllability of stressful events and satisfaction with spouse support behaviours. *Communication Research*, *19*(2), 154–174.

Dakof, G. A., & Taylor, S. E. (1990). Victims' perceptions of social support: What is helpful from whom? *Journal of Personality and Social Psychology*, *58*(1), 80–89.

Danoff-Burg, S., Revenson, T. A., Trudeau, K. J., & Paget, S. A. (2004). Unmitigated communion, social constraints, and psychological distress among women with rheumatoid arthritis. *Journal of Personality*, *72*, 29–46.

Davis, M. H. (1994). *Empathy: A social psychological approach*. Madison, WI: Brown & Benchmark.

Dehle, C., Larsen, D., & Landers, J. E. (2001). Social support in marriage. *American Journal of Family Therapy*, *29*(4), 307–324.

DeLongis, A., Hemphill, K. J., & Lehman, D. R. (1992). A structured diary methodology for the study of daily events. In F. B. Bryant, J. Edwards, R. S. Tindale, E. J. Posavac, L. Heath, E. Henderson, & Y. Suarez-Balcazar (Eds.), *Methodological issues in applied social psychology* (pp. 83–109). New York, NY: Plenum Press.

DeLongis, A., & O'Brien, T. B. (1990). An interpersonal framework for stress and coping: An application to the families of Alzheimer's patients. In M. A. P. Stephens, J. H. Crowther, S. E. Hobfoll, & D. L. Tennenbaum (Eds.), *Stress and coping in later-life families* (pp. 221–239). Washington, DC: Hemisphere.

Eckenrode, J. (1991). *The social context of coping*. New York, NY: Plenum Press.

Eisenberg, N. (2000). Emotion, regulation, and moral development. *Annual Review of Psychology*, *51*, 665–697.

Endler, N. S., & Parker, J. D. (1990). Multidimensional assessment of coping: A critical evaluation. *Journal of Personality and Social Psychology*, *58*(5), 844–854.

Eton, D. T., Lepore, S. J., & Helgeson, V. S. (2001). Early quality of life in patients with localized prostate carcinoma—An examination of treatment-related, demographic, and psychosocial factors. *Cancer*, *92*(6), 1451–1459.

Evans, G. W. (2003). A multimethodological analysis of cumulative risk and allostatic load among rural children. *Developmental Psychology*, *39*(5), 924–933.

Felton, B. J., & Revenson, T. A. (1984). Coping with chronic illness: A study of illness controllability and the influence of coping strategies on psychological adjustment. *Journal of Consulting and Clinical Psychology*, *52*(3), 343–353.

Felton, B. J., & Shinn, M. (1992). Social integration and social support: Moving "social support" beyond the individual level. *Journal of Community Psychology*, *20*(2), 103–115.

Fincham, F. D., & Beach, S. R. H. (1999). Conflict in marriage: Implications for working with couples. *Annual Review of Psychology*, *50*, 47–77.

Folkman, S. (2011). *The Oxford handbook of stress, health, and coping*. New York, NY: Oxford University Press.

Folkman, S., & Lazarus, R. S. (1980). An analysis of coping in a middle-aged sample. *Journal of Health and Social Behavior*, *21*, 219–239.

Folkman, S., Lazarus, R. S., Dunkel-Schetter, C., DeLongis, A., & Gruen, R. J. (1986). Dynamics of a stressful encounter: Cognitive appraisal, coping, and encounter outcomes. *Journal of Personality and Social Psychology*, *50*(5), 992–1003.

Folkman, S., & Moskowitz, J. T. (2004). Coping: Pitfalls and promises. *Annual Review of Psychology*, *55*, 745–774.

Folkman, S., Moskowitz, J. T., Ozer, E. M., & Park, C. L. (1997). Positive meaningful events and coping in the context of HIV/AIDS. In B. H. Gottlieb (Ed.), *Coping with chronic stress* (pp. 293–314). New York, NY: Plenum Press.

Fritz, H. L. (2000). Gender-linked personality traits predict mental health and functional status following a first coronary event. *Health Psychology*, *19*, 420–428.

Gallo, L. C., & Matthews, K. A. (2003). Understanding the association between socioeconomic status and physical health: Do negative emotions play a role? *Psychological Bulletin, 129*, 10–51.

Gilligan, C. (1982). *In a different voice: Psychological theory and women's development.* Cambridge, MA: Harvard University Press.

Gottlieb, B. (Ed.). (1997). *Coping with chronic stress.* New York, NY: Plenum Press.

Gottman, J. M. (1998). Psychology and the study of marital processes. *Annual Review of Psychology, 49*, 169–197.

Haan, N. (1977). *Coping and defending: Processes of self-environment organization.* New York, NY: Academic Press.

Hagedoorn, M., Kuijer, R. G., Buunk, B. P., DeJong, G. M., Wobbes, T., & Sanderman, R. (2000). Marital satisfaction in patients with cancer: Does support from intimate partners benefit those who need it most? *Health Psychology, 19*, 274–282.

Hagedoorn, M., Sanderman, R., Bolks, H. N., Tuinstra, J., & Coyne, J. C. (2008). Distress in couples coping with cancer: A meta-analysis and critical review of role and gender effects. *Psychological Bulletin, 134*(1), 1–30.

Helgeson, V. S. (1993). Implications of agency and communion for patient and spouse adjustment to a first coronary event. *Journal of Personality and Social Psychology, 64*, 807–816.

Helgeson V. S. (1994). Relation of agency and communion to well-being: Evidence and potential explanations. *Psychological Bulletin, 116*, 412–428.

Helgeson, V. S. (2003a). Gender-related traits and health. In J. Suls & K. A. Wallston (Eds.), *Social psychological foundations of health and illness* (pp. 367–394). Oxford, England: Blackwell.

Helgeson, V. S. (2003b). Unmitigated communion and adjustment to breast cancer: Associations and explanations. *Journal of Applied Social Psychology, 33*, 1643–1661.

Helgeson, V. S. (2011). Gender, stress, and coping. In S. Folkman (Ed.), *The Oxford handbook of stress, health, and coping* (pp. 63–85). New York, NY: Oxford University Press.

Helgeson, V. S., Escobar, O., Siminerio, L., & Becker, D. (2007). Unmitigated communion and health among adolescents with and without diabetes: The mediating role of eating disturbances. *Personality and Social Psychology Bulletin, 33*, 519–536.

Helgeson, V. S., & Lepore, S. J. (2004). Quality of life following prostate cancer: The role of agency and unmitigated agency. *Journal of Applied Social Psychology, 34*, 2559–2585.

Herbette, G., & Rime, B. (2004). Verbalization of emotion in chronic pain patients and their psychological adjustment. *Journal of Health Psychology, 9*, 661–676.

Hobfoll, S. E. (1989). Conservation of resources: A new attempt at conceptualizing stress. *American Psychologist, 44*(3), 513–524.

Hobfoll, S. E. (2011). Conservation of resources theory: Its implication for stress, health, and resilience. In S. Folkman (Ed.), *The Oxford handbook of stress, health, and coping* (pp. 127–147). New York, NY: Oxford University Press.

Hoffman, P. K., Meier, B. P., & Council, J. R. (2002). A comparison of chronic pain between an urban and rural population. *Journal of Community Health Nursing, 19*, 213–224.

Holahan, C. J., & Moos, R. H. (1986). Personality, coping and family resources in stress resistance: A longitudinal analysis. *Journal of Personality and Social Psychology, 51*(2), 389–395.

Holahan, C. J., & Moos, R. H. (1987). Personal and contextual determinants of coping strategies. *Journal of Personality and Social Psychology, 52*(5), 946–955.

Holahan, C. J., & Moos, R. H. (1990). Life stressors, resistance factors, and improved psychological functioning: An extension of the stress resistance paradigm. *Journal of Personality and Social Psychology, 58*(5), 909–917.

Holahan, C. J., Moos, R. H., Holahan, C. K., & Brennan, P. L. (1997). Social context, coping strategies, and depressive symptoms: An expanded model with cardiac patients. *Journal of Personality and Social Psychology, 72*, 918–928.

Holtzman, S., Newth, S., & DeLongis, A. (2004). The role of social support in coping with daily pain among patients with rheumatoid arthritis. *Journal of Health Psychology, 9*, 677–695.

Hughes Halbert, C., Wrenn, G., Weathers, B., Delmoor, E., Ten Have, T., & Coyne, J. C. (2010). Sociocultural determinants of men's reactions to prostate cancer diagnosis. *Psycho-Oncology, 19*, 553–560.

Kaniasty, K., & Norris, F. H. (1993). A test of the social support deterioration model in the context of natural disaster. *Journal of Personality and Social Psychology, 64*, 395–408.

Kaniasty, K., & Norris, F. H. (1995). In search of altruistic community: Patterns of social support mobilization following Hurricane Hugo. *American Journal of Community Psychology, 23*, 447–477.

Kashy, D. A., & Kenny, D. A. (2000). The analysis of data from dyads and groups. In H. Reis & C. M. Judd (Eds.), *Handbook of research methods in social psychology* (pp. 451–477). New York, NY: Cambridge University Press.

Kenny, D. A., Kashy, D. A., & Cook, W. L. (2006). *Dyadic data analysis.* New York, NY: Guilford.

Kliewer, W., Lepore, S. J., Oskin, D., & Johnson, P. D. (1998). The role of social and cognitive processes in children's adjustment to community violence. *Journal of Consulting and Clinical Psychology, 66*(1), 199–209.

Kuijer, R. G., Ybema, J. F., Buunk, B. P., De Jong, G. M., Thijs-Boer, F., & Sanderman, R. (2000). Active engagement, protective buffering, and overprotection: Three ways of giving support by intimate partners of patients with cancer. *Journal of Social & Clinical Psychology, 19*, 256–275.

Landrine, H., & Klonoff, E. (1992). Culture and health-related schemas: A review and proposal for interdisciplinary integration. *Health Psychology, 11*, 267–276.

Lane, C. & Hobfoll, S. E. (1992). How loss affects anger and alienates potential supporters. *Journal of Consulting and Clinical Psychology, 60*(6), 935–942.

Lanza, A. F., Cameron, A. E., & Revenson, T. A. (1995). Helpful and unhelpful support among individuals with rheumatic diseases. *Psychology & Health, 10(6)*, 449–462.

Lazarus, R. S. (1966). *Psychological stress and the coping process.* New York, NY: McGraw-Hill.

Lazarus, R. S. (1981). The stress and coping paradigm. In C. Edisdorfer, D. Cohen, A. Kleinman, & P. Maxim (Eds.), *Models for clinical psychopathology* (pp. 177–214). New York, NY: Spectrum Medical and Scientific Books.

Lazarus, R. S. (1999). *Stress and emotion: A new synthesis.* New York, NY: Springer.

Lazarus, R. S., Averill, J. R., & Opton, E. M., Jr. (1974). The psychology of coping: Issues of research and assessment. In G. V. Coelho, D. A. Hamburg, & J. E. Adams (Eds.), *Coping and adaptation* (pp. 249–315). New York, NY: Basic Books.

Lazarus, R. S., & Folkman, S. (1984). *Stress, appraisal, and coping.* New York, NY: Springer.

Lazarus, R. S., & Launier, R. (1978). Stress-related transactions between person and environment. In L. A. Pervin & M. Lewis (Eds.), *Perspectives in interactional psychology* (pp. 287–327). New York, NY: Plenum Press.

Lepore, S. J. (1992). Social conflict, social support, and psychological distress: Evidence of cross-domain buffering effects. *Journal of Personality and Social Psychology, 63*, 857–867.

Lepore, S. J. (1995). Measurement of chronic stressors. In S. Cohen, R. Kessler, & L. Gordon (Eds.), *Measuring stress: A guide for health and social scientists* (pp. 102–120). New York, NY: Oxford University Press.

Lepore, S. J. (1997). Social-environmental influences on the chronic stress process. In B. Gottlieb (Ed.), *Coping with chronic stressors* (pp. 133–160). New York, NY: Plenum Press.

Lepore, S. J. (2001). A social-cognitive processing model of emotional adjustment to cancer. In A. Baum & B. L. Andersen (Eds.), *Psychosocial interventions for cancer* (pp. 99–116). Washington, DC: American Psychological Association.

Lepore, S. J., & Evans, G. W. (1996). Coping with multiple stressors in the environment. In M. Zeidner & N. S. Endler (Eds.), *Handbook of coping: Theory, research, and applications* (pp. 350–377). New York, NY: Wiley.

Lepore, S. J., Glaser, D., & Roberts, K. (2008). On the positive relation between received social support and negative affect: A test of the triage and self-esteem threat models in women with breast cancer. *Psycho-Oncology, 17*, 1210–1215.

Lepore, S. J., & Helgeson, V. S. (1998). Social constraints, intrusive thoughts, and mental health after prostate cancer. *Journal of Social and Clinical Psychology, 17*, 89–106.

Lepore, S. J., & Ituarte, P. H. G. (1999). Optimism about cancer enhances mood by reducing negative social interactions. *Cancer Research, Therapy and Control, 8*, 165–174.

Lepore, S. J., & Kernan, W. (2008). Positive outcomes in the context of serious illness: An expanded social-cognitive processing model. In C. Park, S. Lechner, A. Stanton, & M. Antoni (Eds.), *Positive life changes in the context of medical illness* (pp. 139–152). Washington, DC: American Psychological Association.

Lepore, S. J., & Revenson, T. A. (2006). Resilience and posttraumatic growth: Recovery, resistance, & reconfiguration. In L. Calhoun & R. G. Tedeschi (Eds.), *The handbook of posttraumatic growth: Research and practice* (pp. 24–46). Mahwah, NJ: Erlbaum.

Lepore, S. J., & Revenson, T. A. (2007). Social constraints on disclosure and adjustment to cancer. *Social and Personality Psychology Compass, 1*, 313–333.

Lepore, S. J., Revenson, T. A., Weinberger, S., Weston, P., Frisina, P. Robertson, R., ... Cross, W. (2006). Effects of social stressors on cardiovascular reactivity in Black and White women. *Annals of Behavioral Medicine, 31*, 120–127.

Lepore, S. J., Silver, R. C., Wortman, C. B., & Wayment, H. A. (1996). Social constraints, intrusive thoughts, and depressive symptoms among bereaved mothers. *Journal of Personality and Social Psychology, 70*(2), 271–282.

Lewis, M. A., Butterfield, R. M., Darbes, L. A., & Johnston-Brooks, C. (2004). The conceptualization and assessment of health-related social control. *Journal of Social and Personal Relationships, 21*(5), 669–687.

Luszczynska, A., Gerstorf, D., Boehmer, S., Knoll, N., & Schwarzer, R. (2007). Patients' coping profiles and partners' support provision. *Psychology & Health, 22*, 749–764.

Luszczynska, A., Mohamed, N. E., & Schwarzer, R. (2007). Self-efficacy and social support predict benefit finding 12 months after cancer surgery: The mediating role of coping strategies. *Psychology, Health & Medicine, 10*(4), 365–375.

MacGeorge, E. L., Samter, W., Feng, B., Fillihan, S. J., & Graves, A. R. (2007). After 9/11: Goal disruption, emotional support, and psychological health in a lower exposure sample. *Health Communication, 21*, 11–22.

Maisel, N. C., & Gable, S. L. (2009). The paradox of received social support: The importance of responsiveness. *Psychological Science, 20*(8), 928–932.

Major, B., & Gramzow, R. H. (1999). Abortion as stigma: Cognitive and emotional implications of concealment. *Journal of Personality and Social Psychology, 77*(4), 735–745.

Manne, S. L. (1999). Intrusive thoughts and psychological distress among cancer patients: The role of spouse avoidance and criticism. *Journal of Consulting and Clinical Psychology, 67*(4), 539–546.

Manne, S. L., & Badr, H. (2008). Intimacy and relationship processes in couples' psychosocial adaptation to cancer. *Cancer, 112*, 2541–2555.

Manne, S. L., & Badr, H. (2009) Intimacy processes and psychological distress among couples coping with head and neck or lung cancers. *Psycho-Oncology.* doi:10.1002/pon.1645

Manne, S. L., Dougherty, J., Veach, S., & Kless, R. (1999). Hiding worries from one's spouse: Protective buffering among cancer patients and their spouses. *Cancer Research Therapy and Control, 8*, 175–188.

Manne, S. L., DuHamel, K., & Redd, W. H. (2000). Association of psychological vulnerability factors to post-traumatic stress symptomatology in mothers of pediatric cancer survivors. *Psycho-Oncology, 9*, 372–384.

Manne, S., Ostroff, J., Norton, T., Fox, K., Goldstein, L., & Grana, G. (2006). Cancer-related relationship communication in couples coping with early stage breast cancer. *Psycho-Oncology, 15*, 234–247.

Manne, S. L., Ostroff, J., Winkel, G., Grana, G., & Fox, K. (2005). Partner unsupportive responses, avoidant coping, and distress among women with early stage breast cancer: Patient and partner perspectives. *Health Psychology, 24*, 635–641.

Matthews, K. A., & Gallo, L. C. (2011). Psychological perspectives on pathways linking socioeconomic status and physical health. *Annual Review of Psychology, 62*, 501–530.

Mays, V. M., Cochran, S. D., & Barnes, N. W. (2007). Race, race-based discrimination, and health outcomes among African Americans. *Annual Review of Psychology, 58*, 201–225.

McCrae, R. R. (1984). Situational determinants of coping responses: Loss, threat, and challenge. *Journal of Personality and Social Psychology, 46*, 919–928.

Mischel, W. (1968). *Personality and assessment.* New York, NY: Wiley.

Moos, R. H. (1993). *Coping responses inventory.* Odessa, FL: Psychological Assessment Resources.

Moos, R. H., & Schaefer, C. J. A. (1993). Coping resources and processes: Current concepts and measures. In L. Goldberger & S. Breznitz (Eds.), *Handbook of stress: Theoretical and clinical aspects* (2nd ed., pp. 234–257). New York, NY: Free Press.

Norris, F. H., Tracy, M., & Galea, S. (2009). Looking for resilience: Understanding the longitudinal trajectories of responses to stress. *Social Science & Medicine, 68*, 2190–2198.

Nuckolls, K. B., Cassel, J., & Kaplan, B. H. (1972). Psychological assets, life crisis and the prognosis of pregnancy. *American Journal of Epidemiology, 95*, 431–441.

O'Brien, T. B., & DeLongis, A. (1997). Coping with chronic stress: An interpersonal perspective. In B. Gottlieb (Ed.), *Coping with chronic stress* (pp. 161–190). New York, NY: Plenum Press.

O'Brien, T. B., DeLongis, A., Pomaki, G., Puterman, E., & Zwicker, A. (2009). Couples coping with stress: The role of empathic responding. *European Psychologist, 14*, 18–28.

Ouellette, S. C., & DiPlacido, J. (2001). Personality's role in the protection and enhancement of health: Where the research has been, where it is stuck, how it might move. In A. Baum, T. A. Revenson, & J. E. Singer (Eds.), *Handbook of health psychology* (pp. 175–190). Mahwah, NJ: Erlbaum.

Ozer, E. J., Weinstein, R. S., Ozer, E. J., & Weinstein, R. S. (2004). Urban adolescents' exposure to community violence: The role of support, school safety, and social constraints in a school-based sample of boys and girls. *Journal of Clinical Child & Adolescent Psychology, 33*(3), 463–476.

Pagel, M. D., Erdly, W. W., & Becker, J. (1987). Social networks: We get by with (and in spite of) a little help from our friends. *Journal of Personality and Social Psychology, 53*(4), 793–804.

Park, C. L., Aldwin, C. M., Fenster, J. R., & Snyder, L. B. (2008). Pathways to posttraumatic growth versus posttraumatic stress: Coping and emotional reactions following the September 11, 2001 terrorist attacks. *American Journal of Orthopsychiatry, 78*, 300–312.

Pasch, L. A., & Bradbury, T. N. (1998). Social support, conflict, and the development of marital dysfunction. *Journal of Consulting and Clinical Psychology, 66*(2), 219–230.

Pearlin, L. I. (1989). The sociological study of stress. *Journal of Health and Social Behavior, 30*, 241–256.

Pearlin, L. I., & Schooler, C. (1978). The structure of coping. *Journal of Health and Social Behavior, 19*, 2–21.

Piro, M., Zeldow, P. B., Knight, S. J., Mytko, J. J., & Gradishar, W. J. (2001). The relationship between agentic and communal personality traits and psychosocial adjustment to breast cancer. *Journal of Clinical Psychology in Medical Settings, 8*, 263–271.

Revenson, T. A. (1990). All other things are *not* equal: An ecological perspective on the relation between personality and disease. In H. S. Friedman (Ed.), *Personality and disease* (pp. 65–94) New York, NY: Wiley.

Revenson, T. A. (1993). The role of social support with rheumatic disease. *Bailliere's Clinical Rheumatology, 7*(2), 377–396.

Revenson, T. A. (1994). Social support and marital coping with chronic illness. *Annals of Behavioral Medicine, 16*, 122–130.

Revenson, T. A. (1997). Wanted: A wider lens for coping research. *Journal of Health Psychology, 2*(2), 164–165.

Revenson, T. A. (2003). Scenes from a marriage: Examining support, coping, and gender within the context of chronic illness. In J. Suls & K. Wallston (Eds.), *Social psychological foundations of health and illness* (pp. 530–559). Oxford, England: Blackwell Publishing.

Revenson, T. A., & DeLongis, A. (2011). Couples coping with chronic illness. In S. Folkman (Ed.), *The Oxford handbook of stress, health, and coping* (pp. 101–123). New York, NY: Oxford University Press.

Revenson, T. A., Kayser, K., & Bodenmann, G. (Eds.). (2005). *Couples coping with stress: Emerging perspectives on dyadic coping*. Washington, DC: American Psychological Association.

Revenson, T. A., & Majerovitz, D. M. (1991). The effects of chronic illness on the spouse: Social resources as stress buffers. *Arthritis Care and Research, 4*, 63–72.

Revenson, T. A., & Majerovitz, S. D. (1990). Spouses' support provision to chronically ill patients. *Journal of Social and Personal Relationships, 7*, 575–586.

Revenson, T. A., Schiaffino, K. M., Majerovitz, S. D., & Gibofsky, A. (1991). Social support as a double-edged sword: The relation of positive and problematic support to depression among rheumatoid arthritis patients. *Social Science and Medicine, 33*(7), 807–813.

Reynolds, J. S., & Perrin, N. A. (2004). Mismatches in social support and psychosocial adjustment to breast cancer. *Health Psychology, 23*(4), 425–430.

Roberts, K. J., Lepore, S. J., & Helgeson, V. (2006). Social-cognitive correlates of adjustment to prostate cancer. *Psycho-Oncology, 14*, 1–10.

Rusbult, C. E., Verette, J., Whitney, G. A., Slovik, L. F., & Lipkus, I. (1991). Accommodation processes in close relationships: Theory and preliminary empirical evidence. *Journal of Personality and Social Psychology, 60*(1), 53–78.

Sarason, B. R., Sarason, I. G., & Pierce, G. R. (Eds.). (1990). *Social support: An interactional view*. Oxford, England: John Wiley & Sons.

Schmidt, J. E., & Andrykowski, M. A. (2004). The role of social and dispositional variables associated with emotional processing in adjustment to breast cancer: An Internet-based study. *Health Psychology, 23*(3), 259–266.

Schnur, J. B., Valdimarsdottir, H. B., Montgomery, G. H., Nevid, J. S., & Bovbjerg, D. H. (2004). Social constraints and distress among women at familial risk for breast cancer. *Annals of Behavioral Medicine, 28*(2), 142–148.

Schulz, U., & Schwarzer, R. (2004). Long-term effects of spousal support on coping with cancer after surgery. *Journal of Social and Clinical Psychology, 23*(5), 716–732.

Schwarzer, R., Dunkel-Schetter, C., & Kemeny, M. (1994). The multidimensional nature of received social support in gay men at risk of HIV infection and AIDS. *American Journal of Community Psychology, 22*(3), 319–339.

Schwarzer, R., & Knoll, N. (2007). Functional roles of social support within the stress and coping process: A theoretical and empirical overview. *International Journal of Psychology, 42*(4), 243–252.

Shumaker, S., & Hill, D. R. (1991). Gender differences in social support and physical health. *Health Psychology, 10*, 102–111.

Silver, R. C., Wortman, C. B., & Crofton, C. (1990). The role of coping in support provision: The self-presentational dilemma of victims of life crises. In B. R. Sarason, I. G. Sarason, & G. R. Pierce (Eds.), *Social support: An interactional view.* (pp. 397–426). New York, NY: Wiley.

Skinner, E., Edge, K., Altman, J., & Sherwood, H. (2003). Searching for the structure of coping: A review and critique of category systems for classifying ways of coping. *Psychological Bulletin, 129,* 216–269.

Snyder, C. R. (1999). *Coping: The psychology of what works.* New York, NY: Oxford.

Snyder, C. R., & Ford, C. E. (1987). *Coping with negative life events: Clinical and social psychological perspectives.* New York, NY: Plenum Press.

Somerfield, M. R. (1997). The utility of systems models of stress and coping for applied research: The case of cancer adaptation. *Journal of Health Psychology, 2*(2), 133–151.

Stanton, A., Danoff-Burg, S., Cameron, C. L., Bishop, M., Collin, C. A., Kirk, S. B., … Twillman, R. (2000). Emotionally expressive coping predicts psychological and physical adjustment to breast cancer. *Journal of Consulting and Clinical Psychology, 68*(5), 875–882.

Stanton, A., & Revenson, T. A. (2011). Adjustment to chronic disease: Progress and promise in research. In H. Friedman (Ed.), *The Oxford handbook of health psychology* (pp. 244–272). New York, NY: Oxford University Press.

Suls, J., Green, P., Rose, G., Lounsbury, P., & Gordon, E. (1997). Hiding worries from one's spouse: Associations between coping via protective buffering and distress in male post–myocardial infarction patients and their wives. *Journal of Behavioral Medicine, 20,* 333–349.

Taylor, S. E., Repetti, R., & Seeman, T. E. (1997). Health psychology: What is an unhealthy environment and how does it get under the skin? *Annual Review of Psychology, 48,* 411–447.

Taylor, S. E., & Stanton, A. L. (2007). Coping resources, coping processes, and mental health. *Annual Review of Clinical Psychology, 3,* 377–401.

Tennen, H., Affleck, G., Armeli, S., & Carney, M. A. (2000). A daily process approach to coping: Linking theory, research, and practice. *American Psychologist, 55*(6), 626–636.

Thoits, P. A. (1986). Social support as coping assistance. *Journal of Consulting & Clinical Psychology, 54,* 416–423.

Thoits, P. A. (1995). Stress, coping, and support processes: Where are we? What next? *Journal of Health and Social Behavior,* (Extra Issue), 53–79.

Trudeau, K. J., Danoff-Burg, S., Revenson, T. A., & Paget, S. (2003). Gender differences in agency and communion among patients with rheumatoid arthritis. *Sex Roles, 49,* 303–311.

Ullrich, P. M., Lutgendorf, S. K., & Stapleton, J. T. (2002). Social constraints and depression in HIV infection: Effects of sexual orientation and area of residence. *Journal of Social and Clinical Psychology, 21*(1), 46–66.

Vitaliano, P. P., Maiuro, R. D., Russo, J., & Becker, J. (1987). Raw versus relative scores in the assessment of coping strategies. *Journal of Behavioral Medicine, 10,* 1–18.

Walen, H. R., & Lachman, M. E. (2000) Social support and strain from partner, family, and friends: Costs and benefits for men and women in adulthood. *Journal of Social and Personal Relationships, 17*(1), 5–30.

Wethington, E., McLeod, J. D., & Kessler, R. (1987). The importance of life events for explaining sex differences in mental health. In R. C. Barnett, L. Biener, & G. K. Baruch (Eds.), *Gender and stress* (pp. 144–155). New York, NY: Free Press.

Widows, M. R., Jacobsen, P. B., & Fields, K. K. (2000). Relation of psychological vulnerability factors to posttraumatic stress disorder symptomatology in bone marrow transplant recipients. *Psychosomatic Medicine, 62*(6), 873–882.

Wingard, J. R., I-Chan, H., Sobocinski, K. A., Andrykowski, M. A., Cella, D., Rizzo, J. D., … Bishop, M. M. (2010). Factors associated with self-reported physical and mental health after hematopoietic cell transplantation. *Biology of Blood and Marrow Transplantation, 16*(12), 1682–1692.

Ybema, J. F., Kuijer, R. G., Buunk, B. P., DeJong, G. M., & Sanderman, R. (2001). Depression and perceptions of inequity among couples facing cancer. *Personality and Social Psychology Bulletin, 27*(1), 3–13.

Zakowski, S. G., Harris, C., Krueger, N., Laubmeier, K. K., Garrett, S., Flanigan, R., & Johnson, P. (2003). Social barriers to emotional expression and their relations to distress in male and female cancer patients. *British Journal of Health Psychology, 8*(Pt 3), 271–286.

Zakowski, S. G., Ramati, A., Morton, C., Johnson, P., & Flanigan, R., (2004). Written emotional disclosure buffers the effects of social constraints on distress among cancer patients. *Health Psychology, 23*(6), 555–563.

Zeidner, M., & Endler, N. (1996), *Handbook of coping: Theory, research, applications.* New York, NY: Wiley.

10 Adjustment to Chronic Illness

Michael A. Hoyt
University of California, Merced

Annette L. Stanton
University of California, Los Angeles

Most adults are affected by chronic illness, whether directly or through the experience of a loved one. Chronic, noncommunicable diseases account for 70% of all deaths in the United States (Centers for Disease Control and Prevention, 2009) and for 60% of mortality worldwide (Daar et al., 2007). Moreover, prolonged illnesses can disrupt the lives of individuals and those around them in profound ways. Over the past few decades, health psychologists and others have devoted intense empirical and clinical attention to identifying psychosocial and biobehavioral contributors to and consequences of chronic disease, as well as approaches to help individuals and families reduce physical and psychological morbidity. This chapter provides a synthesis of current knowledge regarding psychological adjustment to chronic health conditions.

Hundreds of studies address adaptation to chronic illness. This review focuses on pertinent studies of adults with cancer, cardiovascular disease, diabetes, HIV/AIDS, and rheumatic diseases. These conditions comprise significant causes of morbidity and mortality, and they have received substantial empirical attention by researchers in health psychology and related fields. The aim is not to present an exhaustive review of this voluminous literature. Rather, the focus is on presenting crosscutting issues in the conceptualization of psychological adjustment to these conditions, as well as theoretical frameworks and empirical findings regarding determinants of adjustment to chronic disease. For this revised handbook edition, we focused on recent empirical literature to advance a model of influences on psychological adjustment. The discussion centers on individual adult adjustment, though relevant literatures on adjustment to chronic disease in children (Roberts, 2003) and in families and caregivers (see Martire & Schulz, Chapter 13, this volume; Revenson & Lepore, Chapter 9, this volume) also exist.

CONCEPTUALIZING ADJUSTMENT TO CHRONIC ILLNESS

Sometimes when I wake up in the morning, I forget for a moment that I have cancer. Then it hits me like a ton of bricks and I think, "Will I live to see my little girl graduate from college?" Who wouldn't have these fears?

The doctor brought the psychologist with him when I got my diagnosis. He thought I would fall apart at my third diagnosis of cancer. I figure I'll get rid of it and go on, just like I've done the last two times.

So much positive has come from my experience with cancer. But I've also never been so scared or angry or sad in my life.

To me having a good life after cancer is all about learning how to find balance between what you can control and what you can't.[1]

---

[1] All quotes from individuals with cancer in the chapter are from the authors' research programs.

INDICATORS OF ADJUSTMENT

The foregoing reflections from individuals with cancer, all of whom viewed themselves as adjusting well, are a sampling of the array of reactions that accompany a diagnosis of chronic disease. What constitutes positive adjustment to chronic conditions? Researchers have advanced conceptualizations that incorporate cognitive, emotional, behavioral, social, and physical processes. These interrelated domains include (a) mastery of illness-related adaptive tasks; (b) absence of psychological disorder; (c) experience of relatively low negative affect; increasingly, researchers also are incorporating reports of positive affect and experiences; (d) maintenance of adequate functional status and social roles; and (e) perceptions of high quality of life.

Mastery of tasks associated with meeting the myriad demands of chronic illness signals successful adjustment. S. E. Taylor (1983) offered a model of cognitive adaptation that identifies self-esteem enhancement, maintenance of a sense of mastery, and engagement in a search for meaning. As another example, Low, Beran, and Stanton (2007) outlined illness-related tasks in individuals with advanced cancer, which include managing pain and physical symptoms, locating and interpreting relevant information, communicating with the medical team, and managing financial matters, among others. More general tasks include managing complex emotions, negotiating uncertain circumstances, and sustaining close relationships.

The prevalence of diagnosable psychological disorders is documented in samples of individuals with chronic illness (e.g., Fann et al., 2008; Golden et al., 2008; Miovic & Block, 2007; Müller-Tasch et al., 2008; van 't Land et al., 2010), with a focus on adjustment disorders, depression and related mood disorders, and anxiety disorders (including acute and posttraumatic stress disorders). However, most individuals with chronic disease do not develop symptoms meeting diagnostic threshold for psychopathology. Therefore, subclinical levels of depressive or anxiety-related symptoms are commonly used to indicate adjustment. In a meta-analysis, 19.3% of patients with heart failure experienced clinically significant depression when determined by diagnostic interview versus 33.6% when assessed by self-report questionnaire (Rutledge et al., 2006).

Relatively high negative affect, particularly when sustained over time, is widely used to signal poor adjustment. Assessment has included both general (e.g., state anxiety, global distress) and disease-specific (e.g., fear of disease recurrence) measures. Positive affect and other indicators of positive functioning are garnering increased attention. Daily diary and other momentary assessment methods are increasingly being employed to determine dynamic patterns of affect (e.g., Finan, Zautra, & Davis, 2009).

Functional status and role-related behaviors also indicate adjustment. An example is vocational functioning, including resumption of employment (e.g., Bhattacharyya, Perkins-Porras, Whitehead, & Steptoe, 2007). In a meta-analysis, de Boer, Tashika, Ojajarvi, van Dijk, and Verbeek (2009) found that cancer patients were 1.37 times more likely to be unemployed than the general healthy population. Functional status might also include mobility and ability to complete routine activities. In the social realm, adjustment is indicated by the ability to maintain social roles and relationships. Perceived satisfaction or functioning in various life domains, either overall life satisfaction or perceptions of quality of life within specific domains (e.g., social, sexual, emotional, physical, spiritual), can also denote adjustment. Researchers also often examine the experience of disease- and treatment-related symptoms or related life disruption (e.g., Gore, Kwan, Lee, Reiter, & Litwin, 2009; Jim, Andrykowski, & Munster, 2009).

OBSERVATIONS FROM THE LITERATURE ON ADJUSTMENT TO CHRONIC ILLNESS

Several broad observations emerge from examining the array of conceptualizations of adjustment. First, adjustment to chronic illness is multidimensional, including both intra- and interpersonal dimensions. Second, the dimensions are interrelated. Negative emotional responses (e.g., depressive symptoms) can contribute to functional status (e.g., poor glycemic control) in individuals with diabetes, for example (Lustman & Clouse, 2005).

A third observation is that heterogeneity in adjustment is apparent across individuals and diseases. Although research demonstrates that individuals diagnosed with chronic disease are at heightened risk for distress and dysfunction (e.g., Lazovich, Robien, Cutler, Virnig, & Sweeney, 2009; Polsky et al., 2005; Reeve et al., 2009; Rutledge et al., 2006; Slatkowsky-Christensen, Mowinckel, Loge, & Kvien, 2009), the majority appears to adjust well. Increasingly, researchers are examining trajectories of adjustment indicators over time to identify distinct patterns of adjustment between subgroups of individuals and over the disease course (e.g., Costanzo, Ryff, & Singer, 2009; Donovan, Small, Andrykowski, Munster, & Jacobsen, 2007; Helgeson, Snyder, & Seltman, 2004; Hinnen et al., 2008; Murphy et al., 2008; Rose et al., 2009). In a prospective study demonstrating variability among diseases, Polsky and colleagues (2005) examined five biennial waves of data for more than 8,300 adults and found that individuals with cancer had the highest risk of depressive symptoms within two years after diagnosis (hazard ratio [HR] = 3.55), followed by chronic lung disease (HR = 2.21) and heart disease (HR = 1.45), versus those with no incident of disease. Risk of depressive symptoms did not emerge for those with arthritis (HR = 1.46) until two to four years after diagnosis, and it extended through eight years after diagnosis for those with heart disease. Much of the research reviewed in this chapter centers around specification of factors that explain the heterogeneity in adjustment to chronic diseases.

Another observation is that psychological adjustment involves both positive and negative dimensions. Positive and negative affect are separable constructs with differential determinants and consequences (see Diener, 1984). Even when faced with difficult life circumstances, individuals have the capacity to experience joy and other positive feelings, as well as to discover meaning in their experience. Individuals commonly report constructive life changes resulting from their illness (e.g., Bellizzi, Miller, Arora, & Rowland, 2007). Costanzo, Ryff, and Singer (2009) compared positive (e.g., positive affect, social well-being, self-acceptance) and negative (e.g., depression, anxiety) adjustment indicators before and after cancer diagnosis to those of a matched healthy control group; cancer survivors scored equally as well or better than healthy controls on positive indicators. Using only indication of distress as an outcome will yield only a partial picture of adjustment; it is also limited in that acute distress does not necessarily presage long-term interference with functioning and goal pursuit. Under stressful conditions, positive and negative affect tend to become negatively correlated, suggesting that positive affect might buffer or repair the effects of distress (e.g., B. W. Smith & Zautra, 2008b; Strand et al., 2006). Incorporation of positive adjustment indicators also helps to counter socially constructed notions that unremitting suffering and despair are guaranteed with diagnosis.

Clearly, adjustment to chronic illness is a complex and dynamic phenomenon that unfolds over time. It is recommended that researchers carefully consider their assumptions with regard to what constitutes positive adjustment, tailor their assessments to the theoretical question of interest, recognize that any particular assessment is likely to provide only a snapshot of circumscribed dimensions of functioning, and limit their conclusions regarding adjustment accordingly. Only through research tapping multiple dimensions of adjustment can a comprehensive portrait of adaptation to chronic disease be achieved.

THEORETICAL PERSPECTIVES ON CONTRIBUTORS TO ADJUSTMENT TO CHRONIC ILLNESS

Theories of adjustment to chronic illness often derive from more general conceptual frameworks regarding adjustment to persistent stressful experiences. Among the most prominent is stress and coping theory (e.g., Lazarus & Folkman, 1984), in which central determinants of adaptive outcomes include attributes of the situation, personal resources, cognitive appraisals, and individual coping responses. The theory emphasizes the role of cognitive processes that unfold in response to a stressor, including primary cognitive appraisals of the potential for threat or benefit, and secondary appraisals, or appraisals of one's ability to manage stressor-related demands. The process of appraisal catalyzes the initiation of coping strategies, or "cognitive and behavioral efforts to control or manage specific external and/or internal demands that are appraised as taxing or exceeding the resources of the person" (p. 141). According to Lazarus and Folkman (1984), cognitive appraisals and coping strategies engaged in response to a stressor substantially determine adaptive outcomes in emotional, social, and somatic realms.

Theoretical developments elaborate on appraisal processes pertinent to adjustment to chronic disease. First, appraisals relevant to goal pursuit have received attention. In his cognitive-motivational-relational theory of emotion, Lazarus (1991) expanded the original conceptualization of primary appraisal to include goal-related motivational processes. When one is committed to the pursuit of important goals, appraising satisfactory progress toward their attainment will lead to positive emotional experience, and negative emotions will result from appraisals of goal blockage. The more a disease is perceived as threatening individuals' central goals, the greater the perception of stress, and the more coping processes are engaged. Self-regulation theories also highlight the importance of perceived goal blockage in shaping coping processes and adjustment (Detweiler-Bedell, Friedman, Levanthal, Miller, & Leventhal, 2008; Leventhal, Halm, Horowitz, Leventhal, & Ozakinci, 2005; Rasmussen, Wrosch, Scheier, & Carver, 2006; Scheier & Bridges, 1995; Scheier, Carver, & Armstrong, Chapter 4, this volume). To the extent that an individual expects that goals are obtainable despite chronic illness, or to the extent that he or she is able to identify and engage in alternative goal pursuit, then initiation of approach-oriented coping strategies is likely. However, if a person expects unremitting goal blockage and does not engage in new goals, disengagement might ensue. Likewise, continued pursuit of truly unobtainable goals will likely exert a negative effect on adjustment over time.

Self-regulation theories also address the implications of specific illness perceptions for adjustment. Illness may be perceived as a threat to the self-system with regard to disease cause, identity, timeline, controllability, and consequences (e.g., Leventhal et al., 2005), with associated consequences for adjustment. For example, individuals who view their cancer as chronic (vs. acute or time limited) before chemotherapy evidence greater distress several months after completing treatment, controlling for actual disease stage (Rabin, Leventhal, & Goodin, 2004). Regarding controllability appraisals, chronic disease can destabilize perceptions of control over bodily integrity, ability to engage in day-to-day activities, and fulfillment of social roles. Individuals are likely to discover controllable aspects of their disease, and the adaptive potential of control appraisals might depend on whether the threat is responsive to control attempts (Christensen & Ehlers, 2002; Helgeson, 1992). For example, perceived control over disease consequences (e.g., symptom management) often is associated more strongly with adjustment than is perceived control over disease outcome (e.g., Affleck, Tennen, Pfeiffer, & Fifield, 1987; Thompson, Sobolew-Shubin, Galbraith, Schwankovsky, & Cruzen, 1993).

Extending from examinations of perceptions of personal growth following trauma (e.g., Calhoun & Tedeschi, 2006; Janoff-Bulman & Franz, 1997), theoretical and empirical work is emerging to illuminate the meaning and consequences of perceiving benefit in chronic disease (see Park, Lechner, Antoni, & Stanton, 2009). Individuals commonly construe their illness experience as conferring benefits in a number of realms, including enhanced relationships, greater appreciation of life, enhanced personal strength, sharpened awareness of priorities, and deepened spirituality (e.g., see Affleck et al., 1987, on heart disease; Danoff-Burg & Revenson, 2005, on rheumatoid arthritis [RA]; Milam, 2006, on HIV/AIDS; Stanton, Bower, & Low, 2006, on cancer). Appraisals of benefit or personal growth from illness experiences might allow individuals to reprioritize (Tedeschi & Calhoun, 1995) or maintain (S. E. Taylor & Brown, 1988) goals and self-schemas disrupted by illness-related stressors. Implications of such perceptions of benefit and enhanced sense of meaning for adjustment to chronic disease and for observable behavior change are receiving empirical scrutiny.

Theories of adjustment to chronic illness also specify various contexts that can influence appraisal and coping processes, ultimately shaping adjustment (e.g., Moos & Schaefer, 1993). These include such macrolevel factors as socioeconomic status (SES), gender, and culture (e.g., Gallo & Matthews, 2003; S. E. Taylor et al., 2000; Whitfield, Weidner, Clark, & Anderson, 2002; Yali & Revenson, 2004), as well as the interpersonal, intrapersonal, and disease-related contexts. Integrating theoretical perspectives on adjustment to chronic disease, we offer a conceptual model of influences on adjustment in Figure 10.1. Recursive links and additional moderating and mediating factors are likely. In the following sections, we synthesize empirical support for the various contributors to adjustment to chronic illness and suggest that longitudinal research over the past several decades bolsters support for causal inferences regarding risk and protective factors for adjustment in individuals who experience chronic disease.

EMPIRICAL RESEARCH ON CONTRIBUTORS TO ADJUSTMENT TO CHRONIC ILLNESS

Before cancer I was the man of the house, the "go-to" guy. Now people tiptoe around me. I can't work. I can't be a man anymore.

My wife and I can no longer have sex. Medication for such things must be for the rich. I cannot afford it. I am failing all the way around.

MACROLEVEL CONTEXT

Increasingly, understanding disparities in health related to such macrolevel contextual factors as race, ethnicity, gender, social class, and sexual orientation is a priority for research. Such contexts also shape individual and environmental responses to illness-related experiences, including beliefs about health and health care (e.g., Landrine & Klonoff, 2003; Revenson & Pranikoff, 2005), and they determine the availability and quality of resources. Of course, macrolevel factors do not affect outcomes in isolation. For example, culturally determined behaviors in Latino families (e.g., familial dietary practices) likely interact with socioeconomic factors (e.g., the availability of healthy foods within a low-income neighborhood) to influence individual responses to diabetes (Castro, Shaibi, & Boehm-Smith, 2009). Such interactions prompt the need for analysis of the influence of broader social and historical environments on individuals' coping and adjustment processes. To elucidate the complexities of disparities in adjustment, more critical work will also be needed to understand how intersectionality (see E. R. Cole, 2009) of multiple group membership affects adaptation to chronic illness.

Race/Ethnicity

Substantial evidence demonstrates that incidence and consequences of chronic illness do not occur equally across ethnic and racial groups (Adler & Rehkopf, 2008). Few studies address racial and ethnic influences on psychological adjustment to chronic disease longitudinally. Cross-sectional studies and literature reviews reveal some group differences in quality of life and other indicators of psychological adjustment that suggest less favorable adjustment among ethnic minorities, particularly among Latino and African American groups (e.g., C. K. Holahan, Moerkbak, & Suzuki, 2006; Prowe et al., 2006). For instance, Maly, Stein, Unezawa, Leake, and Anglin (2008) found that Latina women with breast cancer reported poorer quality of life compared to African American and other women. Notably, mistrust in the medical system was a significant mediator of this relationship.

It is essential to investigate mechanisms for any obtained group differences in adjustment. Health care delivery and medical interactions are likely pathways. For example, relative to their White counterparts, ethnic minority patients are reported to receive less health-related information (Cooper-Patrick et al., 1999; Maly, Leake, & Silliman, 2003), perceive less positive affect from their physicians (R. L. Johnson, Roter, Powe, & Cooper, 2004), be less likely to receive particular medical procedures such as breast-conserving surgery in breast cancer patients (Maly et al., 2008), and be less likely to receive antidepressant medication for depressive symptoms (Waldman et al., 2009). Racism and discrimination also may underlie racial disparities in physical health (see Brondolo, Gallo, & Myers, 2009). As Myers (2009) suggests, recipients of ethnic discrimination disproportionately encounter chronic stressors and daily hassles. Disease-related stressors may act synergistically to tax coping resources and negatively influence adjustment. Research that moves

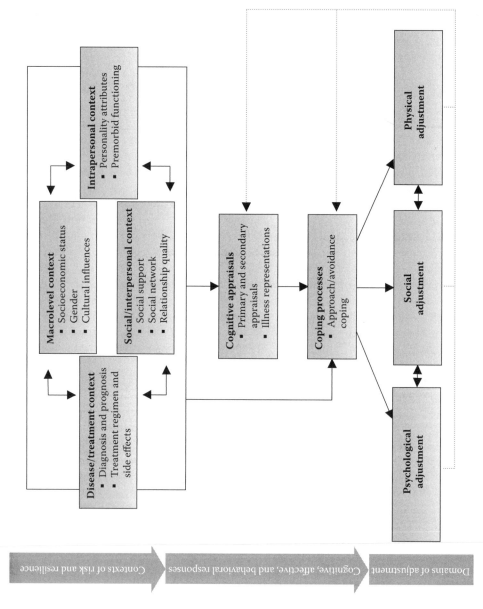

FIGURE 10.1　Contributors to adjustment to chronic illness.

beyond documenting between-group differences to examine culturally relevant processes and to adopt an intersectional approach to understanding how multiple identities affect adjustment promises to make a contribution. Classification of individuals into such broad ethnic categories as Latino might disregard variation in such factors as cultural practices, SES, and acculturation processes. Differences between cultural subgroups (e.g., Mexican Americans vs. Dominican Americans) might be as large as those between ethnic groups, and distinct mechanisms for their relations with adjustment might exist.

Gender-Related Processes

Women consistently report poorer self-rated health than men, though the gender gap shrinks when SES is controlled (Read & Gorman, 2006). Gender differences in illness-related distress mirror evidence on depressive symptoms in the general population (Kessler, 2000; Kessler et al., 2003) in that women report higher distress than do men with chronic illness (Hagedoorn, Buunk, Kuijer, Wobbes, & Sanderman, 2000; Polsky et al., 2005), though exceptions exist. However, indicators of adjustment might be experienced differently across gender groups. For instance, Addis (2008) and others (e.g., Kessler, 2000; Nolen-Hoeksema, 2008; D. J. Smith et al., 2008) suggest that depressive symptoms manifest differently for men and women. For example, men are more likely to mask emotional distress by outward physical symptoms or externalizing behaviors (Brownhill, Wilhelm, Barclay, & Parker, 2002). To elucidate gender differences in adjustment, conceptualizations and assessment of adjustment that are sensitive to gender-related processes and stress appraisals are needed.

The gender-linked personality orientations of agency and communion (and their extreme forms, unmitigated agency and unmitigated communion) have been explored with respect to adjustment to a number of chronic diseases (see Helgeson, 1994; Helgeson & Fritz, 1998, for reviews). Individuals with an agentic orientation focus more on themselves and use more instrumental, problem-solving strategies to cope with stress. Individuals with a more communal orientation focus on others' needs and interpersonal relationships and are more emotionally expressive. Unmitigated agency is characterized by focusing on oneself to the point of exclusion of other people and is marked by difficulty in expressing emotions; unmitigated communion refers to an extreme orientation toward others in which individuals become overly involved with others to the detriment of their own well-being.

Agency is linked to better adjustment across a number of chronic diseases, including coronary heart disease (Helgeson, 1993). However, unmitigated agency is related to poorer mental health, difficulty expressing emotions, and decrements in physical functioning and health-related quality of life in men with prostate cancer (Helgeson & Lepore, 2004) and to maladjustment in women with breast cancer (Piro, Zeldow, Knight, Mytko, & Gradishar, 2001). Unmitigated communion is associated with failure to adhere to behavior change recommendations following hospitalization for a first coronary event (Helgeson, 1990), as well as greater disease-related distress in individuals with RA (Danoff-Burg, Revenson, Trudeau, & Paget, 2004; Trudeau, Danoff-Burg, Revenson, & Paget, 2003), cardiac patients (Fritz, 2000; Helgeson, 1993), and cancer survivors (Piro et al., 2001).

Both unmitigated agency and unmitigated communion are linked to social interaction processes (e.g., Hoyt & Stanton, 2011). Unmitigated agency is related to lower social resources (e.g., supportive social exchanges) over time; thus, unmitigated agency might be at odds with offers of assistance and emotional support that individuals facing a chronic illness often receive and that are typical components of psychosocial interventions. Unmitigated communion is related to high support provision and low support receipt (Helgeson, 1994), as well as intensity of the harmful impact of negative relationship events in women with fibromyalgia (Nagurney, 2008).

In addition to personality traits influenced by gender socialization, other processes may help to explain gender differences. For instance, gender role expectations can shape the acceptability of particular coping responses, such as the use of emotional expression in men (Hoyt, 2009). Moving beyond the documentation of gender differences in adjustment, specification of the ways in which gender shapes emotional, behavioral, and physiological responses to illness-related stressors is needed. S. E. Taylor and colleagues (2000) identified potential gender differences in models of sympathetic-adrenal-medullary system and hypothalamic-pituitary-adrenal (HPA) axis activation in response to stress. They argued that a tend-and-befriend model is more reflective of stress responses in women, versus the traditional fight-or-flight model. In the tend-and-befriend model, adaptive responses to illness-related stressors would involve nurturance of oneself and others and maintenance of social networks. The model purports that oxytocin and endogenous opioids maintain a prominent role in down-regulating stress responses in women. Discussing the treatment of gender in psychoneuroimmunology research, Darnell and Suarez (2009) emphasize the importance of examining gender differences in biobehavioral outcomes and highlight the possibility that in addition to hormonal differences, gender differences in inflammatory or neuroendocrine processes may be mediated by gender-related differences in stress appraisals and emotional responses to stressors.

Socioeconomic Status

The constant struggle for resources to meet basic human needs can severely constrain coping resources and constitutes a significant vulnerability for poor adjustment to a chronic condition. Inequalities in SES are associated with morbidity and mortality (e.g., Mackenbach et al., 2008; Marmot, 2005), as well as receipt and quality of health care (e.g., Asch et al., 2006). Reflected in educational attainment, income, occupational status, geographic location, or some combination of these variables, SES affects health outcomes directly and through environmental and psychosocial mechanisms, including access to and quality of health care, as well as circumstances influencing risky and protective health behaviors (e.g., smoking, substance use, healthy eating, physical activity).

Low-SES environments can inflict a physical and psychological toll, leading to more consistent exposure to stressful life events coupled with fewer social and psychological resources to manage them (Gallo & Matthews, 2003). Low social status and perceptions of illness and its treatment as burdensome or out of one's control signal appraisals of helplessness and hopelessness and therefore predict greater depressive symptoms and poorer functional status among the chronically ill (e.g., Harrison et al., 2005; Havranek, Spertus, Masoudi, Jones, & Rumsfeld, 2004; Stommel, Kurtz, Kurtz, Given, & Given, 2004). Barbareschi, Sanderman, Kempen, and Ranchor (2008) demonstrated that a sense of control mediated the relation between lower SES and quality of life in a prospective study of older coronary heart disease patients. Although we conceptualize SES as a predictor of adjustment, the relation is bidirectional. For example, chronic, disabling diseases have enormous impact on work ability. In a large national sample, Minkler, Fuller-Thomson, and Guralnik (2006) demonstrated a social-class gradient up to the age of 85 years, showing that those individuals with higher incomes have fewer functional limitations. Studies of RA patients show that people often terminate employment early in the disease process (e.g., Reisine, Fifield, Walsh, & Feinn, 2001). Such work-related disability can create a downward drift in SES.

More work is needed to understand how SES is related to various indicators of adjustment for individuals with chronic illness, as well as to the contributors to maladjustment that may be particularly salient in low-SES environments. Research on the influence of other macrolevel factors (e.g., gender, ethnicity) when positioned within a lower SES context is also needed.

Disease and Treatment Context

Disease course (e.g., progressive versus remitting), prognosis, toxicity of treatment, degree of associated pain, and necessity for lifestyle changes all vary in controllability, predictability, and severity across different chronic diseases. Even within disease category, heterogeneity exists. For instance, the daily experience of a newly diagnosed diabetic patient initiating behaviors toward tight insulin control may be very different than adaptive tasks for someone diagnosed years prior with well-established daily practices and controlled insulin.

The impact of the disease and treatment context on adjustment often is examined in samples of patients at similar phases in the disease course or with similar treatment profiles. For example, Jim, Andrykowski, Munster, and Jacobsen (2007) found that physical symptoms experienced during chemotherapy and/or radiotherapy predicted an increase in distress in women with ductal carcinoma in situ at four months after treatment completion. However, individual differences can contribute to across- and within-disease variability. For instance, the individual's degree of uncertainty or acceptance toward the pain of rheumatic disease partially determines the impact of pain on adjustment (L. M. Johnson, Zautra, & Davis, 2006; Kratz, Davis, & Zautra, 2007). Also, disease processes themselves can be influenced by one's internal and external resources and adjustment (e.g., Antoni et al., 2006; B. W. Smith & Zautra, 2008a; Whooley et al., 2008).

It is noteworthy that many studies demonstrate nonsignificant relationships between objective disease-related factors and adjustment. Bardwell et al. (2006) examined the relative contribution of early-stage breast cancer parameters (e.g., treatment type, time since diagnosis, cancer stage), health behaviors, and psychosocial variables (e.g., social support, stress, optimism) to depressive symptoms in a large sample ($n = 2,595$) of women in treatment; disease and treatment factors were not significant predictors. As Bardwell and colleagues suggest, subjective interpretations and appraisals of disease factors, as well as coping responses and social functioning, may be more important to psychological adjustment than objective indicators.

Several research implications exist. Although disease and treatment variables are typically considered within disease category, comparing results across chronic illnesses may present opportunities to discover important mechanisms of adjustment. Further, researchers often control statistically for disease and treatment variables without reporting the magnitude of their relations with adjustment, leaving little to be learned about the impact of disease factors. In addition, investigators seldom report testing for interactions of disease-related variables with other predictors, missing not only a statistical requirement of covariate analysis but also the potential for new insights. Finally, modeling the impact of disease-related factors across time is needed. Different phases of the disease trajectory might be marked by unique psychological vulnerabilities and resilience factors.

SOCIAL/INTERPERSONAL CONTEXT

People don't understand that I don't want their help. I can take care of things myself. I don't need to talk about cancer all the time.

My partner, my daughter, and my friends have been lifesavers for me. I don't know how I could have made it through cancer without them.

A large literature is available on the impact of the social context on health and positive adjustment to chronic illness (see S. E. Taylor, 2007). In general, emotionally supportive relationships set the stage for positive adjustment to chronic disease, whereas criticism, social constraints, and social isolation impart risk. Satisfying interpersonal relationships can provide a forum for emotional expression and processing, practical assistance in managing illness, and reinforcement of one's sense of meaning, joy, and connectedness. Support can encourage positive health behaviors or minimize risky behaviors and can diminish physiological reactivity to stress. Although exceptions exist (e.g., Lepore, Glaser, & Roberts, 2008), compared to those reporting less support, patients receiving more social support exhibit more effective coping, higher self-esteem and life satisfaction, and fewer depressive symptoms. Sound social support partially explains trajectories of psychological adjustment to chronic illness (e.g., Helgeson et al., 2004). It is also important to note that chronic disease itself can change the dynamics within one's interpersonal environment by restricting one's ability to engage in typical social activities or changing the communication climate (e.g., Fryand, Moum, Finset, & Glennas, 2002). Social support affects adjustment through a number of physiological, affective, and cognitive pathways (Lepore, 2001; Uchino, 2006; Wills & Ainette, Chapter 20, this volume), including influencing how one appraises and responds to problems. Conceptualizations of social support include its use as a coping strategy as well as a coping resource. In their review of studies assessing coping and social support in chronic disease, Schreurs and de Ridder (1997) found that prospective studies consistently revealed approach-oriented coping as a mechanism by which social support promotes positive well-being. For example, Holahan, Moos, Holahan, and Brennan (1997) demonstrated that a positive social context at study entry predicted greater relative use of approach-oriented coping by cardiac patients four years later, which in turn contributed to a reduction in depressive symptoms. Likewise, an unsupportive social context can prompt avoidance-oriented coping under stress, which in turn predicts an increase in distress in women with breast cancer (Manne, Ostroff, Winkel, Grana, & Fox, 2005) and poorer adherence and higher viral load in HIV-positive individuals (Weaver et al., 2005).

Both structural aspects of social ties (e.g., marital status, network size) and functional dimensions (e.g., validating emotions, providing information) can yield benefit (e.g., Carpenter, Fowler, Maxwell, & Andersen, 2010; Demange et al., 2004; Ertel, Glymour, & Berkman, 2008; Lett et al., 2007; Molloy, Perkins-Porras, Strike, & Steptoe, 2008). Prospective studies of patients with rheumatic diseases reveal both direct and buffering effects of support on depressive symptoms (Demange et al., 2004), functional status (Fitzgerald et al., 2004), and disease activity (Holtzman & DeLongis, 2007). Although social support is typically assessed as a fairly stable characteristic of an individual's social environment, its effects can change over time. Thus, the dynamic nature of adjustment may reflect the unfolding of interpersonal as well as intrapersonal factors. In an examination of five waves of data over 13 years, Strating, Suurmeijer, and van Schur (2006) found that higher satisfaction with emotional support and social companionship predicted lower distress in RA patients, though this association decreased over time. In fact, social companionship influenced distress only for those earlier in the disease course. Similarly, among couples coping with lung cancer, partners' prorelationship behaviors (e.g., communication of positivity and hopefulness) appear to be more beneficial to patients' long-term adjustment when offered early in the disease course (Badr & Taylor, 2008). More longitudinal studies are needed that model change in social support over time, as well as effects of support dynamics at various stages in the disease course.

Just as relationships can be a powerful positive influence on adjustment to chronic illness, support attempts can be ill timed or a poor match to an individual's needs. Expectations for what constitutes appropriate support and the manner in which one mobilizes and uses available support varies across gender and cultural groups (see S. E. Taylor, 2007, for a discussion). Many well-intended attempts at helping can go awry, particularly when the provided support is not perceived as helpful, desired, or requested (Dunkel-Schetter & Wortman, 1982; Revenson, 1993). For instance, women with advanced osteoarthritis who do not centrally value independence perceive less powerlessness and incompetence in response to instrumental assistance with daily activities than do women who strongly value independence, perhaps because support is matched with their needs (Martire, Druley, Stephens, & Wojno, 2002). It is important to distinguish problematic or unhelpful support from the absence of support. Social isolation prior to a breast cancer diagnosis in the Nurses' Health Study cohort predicted poorer quality of life four years postdiagnosis, explaining greater variance than did treatment- and tumor-related factors (Michael, Berkman, Colditz, Holmes, & Kawachi, 2002). Similarly, breast cancer patients without a confiding intimate relationship are at greater risk for the development of depressive symptoms over time than those who have such a relationship (Burgess et al., 2005).

Social constraint, or the perception that others are unreceptive to one's experiences, is associated with poorer adjustment in persons with cancer (Cordova, Cunningham, Carlson, & Andrykowski, 2001; Hoyt, 2009; Lepore, 2001; Manne et al., 2005), arthritis (Danoff-Burg et al., 2004), diabetes (e.g., Braitman, Derlega, Henson, Robinett, & Saadeh, 2008), and HIV/AIDS (Ullrich, Lutgendorf, & Stapleton, 2002). In a study of gynecological cancer patients, perceived unsupportive behavior by family and friends, involving avoidance and criticism, predicted women's trajectory of depressive symptoms independent of measures of supportive behaviors, which also predicted symptoms (Manne et al., 2008). Low social constraint also buffers the relationship between disease-related intrusive thoughts and subsequent distress among cancer patients (Lepore, 2001). Within couples, perceptions of partner involvement influence adjustment. Dismissal of emotions to avoid disagreements or to protect the patient from difficult feelings (i.e., protective buffering) may work to prevent successful cognitive and emotional processing and increase distress (e.g., Hinnen, Ranchor, Baas, Sanderman, & Hagedoorn, 2009; Langer, Brown, & Syrjala 2009; Manne et al., 2007).

Research examining social support and interpersonal interactions in the context of dyadic relationships, particularly partner and caregiver relationships, has surged (see Berg & Upchurch, 2007, for a review). Dissatisfaction in marital relationships predicts poorer adjustment over time (e.g., Yang & Schuler, 2009). C. L. C. Taylor et al. (2008) found that qualities of the partner relationship (i.e., relationship satisfaction) affect adjustment to lung cancer, such that couples with high relationship satisfaction are better able to engage in supportive dyadic coping and assist each other in regulating distress. Higher marital satisfaction also predicted shorter hospitalization following coronary artery bypass graft (CABG) in women, but not men (Kulik & Mahler, 2006). In a daily interview study with patients with RA (Holtzman & DeLongis, 2007), satisfaction with spousal support attenuated the negative impact of pain catastrophizing on adjustment. Accumulating evidence demonstrates that the traits and coping processes of partners can affect patients' adjustment. In a study of men receiving elective CABG (Ruiz, Matthews, Scheier, & Schulz, 2006), partners' presurgical neuroticism predicted higher depressive symptoms in patients at 18-month follow-up (moderated by relationship satisfaction).

Research has begun to tease out the effects of patterns of appraisal and coping that exist within couples. *Congruence*, or the degree to which partners' responses to illness fit together, can have a salutary effect on adjustment (Revenson, 2003). For instance, married women with RA evidence better psychological adjustment over time when both members of the couple share similar levels of optimism and perceptions of personal control over her illness (Sterba et al., 2008). However, couples need not necessarily share similar responses to chronic illness. A good fit between partners might also be determined by the degree to which partners' coping behaviors complement each other (Badr, 2004). Well-matched differences in coping can increase a couple's overall coping repertoire or fill in gaps. For example, husbands' use of coping through emotional approach compensated for their wives' low use of that strategy in buffering against an increase in depressive symptoms after an unsuccessful infertility treatment attempt (Berghuis & Stanton, 2002). However, similar use of maladaptive coping (e.g., protective buffering) between partners can exert a negative influence on adjustment (see Berg & Upchurch, 2007).

Disentangling the effects of gender differences in adjustment and dyadic role can be difficult. Although some studies show that distress levels of partners are the same or greater than those of patients, a meta-analysis suggests that gender (i.e., being a woman) is more important than dyadic role (partner or patient) in predicting higher cancer-related distress (Hagedoorn, Sanderman, Bolks, & Coyne, 2008).

INTRAPERSONAL CONTEXT

Dispositional or historical factors constitute risk and protective factors for adjustment. For instance, a history of depression or psychosocial dysfunction prior to chronic illness confers vulnerability to poorer adjustment following diagnosis (Burgess et al., 2005; Conner et al., 2006; Tennen, Affleck, & Zautra, 2006). Individual differences in personality attributes also influence responses to stress, as well as behaviors associated with risk and resilience to illness. For instance, neuroticism, or the tendency to experience negative affect, is associated with maladaptive responses to stressful events (see Bolger & Schilling, 1991) and with health outcomes (see Smith, Gallo, Shivpuri, & Brewer, Chapter 17, this volume).

Optimism (i.e., generalized expectancy for positive outcomes) and pessimism are the most frequently examined personality attributes in relation to disease-related adjustment. Higher optimism predicts fewer depressive symptoms among individuals with ischemic heart disease (Shnek, Irvine, Stwart, & Abbey, 2001) and faster in-hospital recovery and return to normal life activities one year after CABG surgery (Scheier et al., 2003). Low pessimism predicts more positive affect and lower pain 6 to 12 months after CABG surgery (Mahler & Kulik, 2000). Optimism's benefits also are documented in people with various cancers and at several phases in the disease trajectory (e.g., Allison, Guichard, & Laurent, 2000; Carver et al., 2005; Petersen et al., 2008; Steginga & Occhipinti, 2006; Trunzo & Pinto, 2003). Optimism's protective effects appear to work by bolstering the use of approach-oriented coping strategies and emotional social support, as well as reducing disease-related threat appraisals and avoidant coping (Brissette, Scheier, & Carver, 2002; Scheier et al., 2003; Schou, Ekeberg, & Ruland, 2005; Trunzo & Pinto, 2003; see also Rasmussen et al., 2006).

Physical health outcomes associated with optimism also are receiving attention. Overall, optimists tend to have better health than pessimists, and they engage in more protective and adherent health practices. Although there are null findings, some evidence suggests that dispositional optimism predicts slower disease progression and decreased risk for subsequent adverse health events (see Rasmussen, Scheier, & Greenhouse, 2009; Tindle et al., 2009). Researchers are just beginning to explore the seemingly complex relationships between optimism and immune processes (see Segerstrom, 2005), though few studies have examined these relations in individuals with chronic illness. In a prospective study of ovarian cancer patients receiving chemotherapy, optimism predicted decreased levels of CA 125, an angiogenic inflammatory marker (de Moor et al., 2006). Further examination of biological and behavioral mechanisms for the effects of optimism is warranted.

Other personality traits have received study. For instance, in a longitudinal study of individuals with HIV, higher conscientiousness was related to lower depressive symptoms and greater use of active coping strategies (O'Cleirigh, Ironson, Weiss, & Costa, 2007). Clusters of personality traits also have been examined. Type D (distressed) personality is a tendency toward negative affectivity across situations coupled with social inhibition. In a five-year prospective study of 319 cardiac patients, Type D personality conferred an increased risk of impaired quality of life (OR = 8.9), independent of depressive symptoms and other behavioral risk factors (Denollet, Vaes, & Brutsaert, 2000). Social transactions may also be involved in distinguishing the effects of personality. For instance, interpersonal sensitivity, the predisposition to perceive or elicit criticism and rejection from others, influences adjustment through social processes. In a cross-sectional study, Siegel and colleagues (2007) found that more interpersonally sensitive men with prostate cancer reported lower efficacy in physician interactions, poorer spousal support, and more symptoms of sexual dysfunction. Dispositional factors can moderate effects of other risk and resilience factors. For example, interpersonal stress predicted increases in negative affect and disease activity in arthritis patients only for those who reported excessive interpersonal sensitivity in a longitudinal study (B. W. Smith & Zautra, 2002). Similarly, emotionally expressive coping predicted decreased distress and fewer medical appointments for cancer-related morbidities in breast cancer patients high in hope, a construct reflecting a sense of goal-directed determination and ability to achieve goals (Stanton et al., 2000).

As the foregoing illustrates, investigation of dispositional factors (e.g., optimism, neuroticism) can illuminate risk and protective factors in adjustment to illness. Such factors can often be assessed easily in the earliest phases of diagnosis and treatment. Because interventions are not readily available to modify stable personal dispositions, the examination of mechanisms (e.g., coping, appraisal) through which enduring attributes carry their effects also is essential.

Cognitive Appraisals

I have taken on prostate cancer—it hasn't taken me. When the doctor told me I might have long-term problems after surgery, I said "That's what you think!"

The most frustrating part is the loss of control, from not being able to work right now to not knowing if the cancer will come back and not being able to do a lot to prevent it. I hate feeling out of control.

Individuals' appraisals and expectancies regarding illness can affect adjustment, and cognitive processes are a potentially productive target of therapeutic intervention. Numerous appraisal processes have been examined in relation to chronic illness; here we focus on appraisal processes as they map onto the stress and coping framework of Lazarus and Folkman (1984).

Primary Appraisals

Primary appraisal, involving the individual's determination of a potentially stressful encounter's significance for well-being through assessments of threat/harm and challenge/benefit, plays a pivotal role in stress and coping theory. Simultaneous appraisals of threat and benefit occur in chronic disease (e.g., Stanton & Snider, 1993), and both predict adjustment. Prospective studies demonstrate that appraisals of illness as a threat to be a strong predictor of increased distress and depressive symptoms (e.g., Park, Fenster, Suresh, & Bliss, 2006; Lynch, Steginga, Hawkes, & Pakenham, 2008; Waltz, Badura, Pfaff, & Schott, 1988).

Chronic illness can disrupt the ability to maintain social and family roles (e.g., Vileikyte et al., 2005); related threat appraisals are associated with worse mental health, particularly when one's role is highly valued within one's cultural context (e.g., Abraido-Lanza, 1997). Such illness-related appraisals can signal a threat to the achievement of distal or higher level (e.g., to be a good parent) and proximal or lower level (e.g., to complete the daily cleaning) goals. In a daily process study with fibromyalgia patients, Affleck et al. (2001) found that goal-oriented processes (e.g., perceived barriers to goals) were related to greater pain and fatigue across time. The study also revealed a buffering role for dispositional optimism, suggesting that threatened goals may be responsive to adaptive self-regulation. Withdrawal of commitment and pursuit of unobtainable goals and reengagement in identification, commitment to, and pursuit of alternative obtainable goals comprise such adaptive processes (e.g., Wrosch, Scheier, Miller, Schulz, & Carver, 2003). Cross-sectional studies have connected goal reengagement with positive affect (but not negative effect) in cancer patients (Shroevers, Kraaij, & Garnefski, 2008), and men with prostate cancer who altered life goals to accommodate their illness were less affected by physical dysfunction than were men who did not (Lepore & Eton, 2000). Continued research on how chronically ill individuals appraise and regulate goal pursuits is needed.

What is the adaptive significance of appraising the experience of chronic illness as conferring benefit? Although perceptions of benefit from this experience have been conceptualized in several ways (e.g., S. E. Taylor, 1983; Tedeschi & Calhoun, 1995), one reasonable conceptualization involves challenge/benefit appraisals. Evidence for a relation between finding benefit and adjustment to chronic illness is mixed (see Algoe & Stanton, 2009, for a review of longitudinal studies). Among the most notable positive findings, perceived positive meaning resulting from the breast cancer experience at one to five years after diagnosis predicted an increase in positive affect five years later (Bower et al., 2005), and finding benefit in the year after breast cancer surgery predicted lower distress and depressive symptoms four to seven years later (Carver & Antoni, 2004). Negative findings and curvilinear relationships with adjustment also are documented (e.g., Lechner, Carver, Antoni, Weaver, & Phillips, 2006).

The links of benefit finding with indicators of physical health appears more consistently positive (see Algoe & Stanton, 2009; Bower, Epel, & Moskowitz, 2009). For example, men reporting benefits from a heart attack had lower cardiac morbidity eight years later (Affleck, Tennen, Croog, & Levine, 1987). Likewise, HIV-positive men with a recent loss of a close other to AIDS who also reported benefit from the loss showed a less rapid decline in CD4 T-cells and a lower rate of AIDS-related mortality over a two- to three-year follow-up (Bower, Kemeny, Taylor, & Fahey, 1998). Significant theoretical and empirical attention is required to address limitations in the conceptualization, operationalization, and conclusions related to the potential adaptive consequences of finding meaning and benefit in chronic illness (e.g., Tennen & Affleck, 2009).

Secondary Appraisals

Maintaining perceptions of control over aspects of chronic disease and having confidence in one's ability to affect a desired outcome (i.e., self-efficacy) have long been considered valuable in adapting to chronic illness (see DeVellis & DeVellis, 2001). Likewise, perceived helplessness related to one's illness predicts maladjustment and poor physical functioning independent of disease severity in RA patients (e.g., Hommel, Wagner, Chaney, White, & Mullins, 2004; C. A. Smith & Wallston, 1992). Few studies have modeled changes in appraisals over time. Bárez, Blasco, Fernández-Castro, and Viladrich (2009) assessed control appraisals at five points in the year following surgery for early-stage breast cancer. Initial appraisals of greater control over breast cancer–related concerns, as well as a faster rate of change in appraisals of control over time, predicted decreases in distress independent of physical symptoms. In another study of breast cancer patients, higher perceived control over the illness was associated with a decline in physical and mental health for women who experienced cancer recurrence, whereas women who remained disease free benefited from high control appraisals (Tomich & Helgeson, 2006). Control appraisals also affect adjustment to cardiac events and surgical interventions. Among CABG patients, individuals who expect more control over their recovery have briefer hospital stays, report less pre- and postoperative distress, and demonstrate an improvement in physical functioning (Barry, Kasl, Lictman, Vaccarino, & Krumholz, 2006; Mahler & Kulik, 1990).

Appraisals of control and self-efficacy are associated with the choice of coping strategies. In general, greater self-efficacy and having a sense of control over one's illness is associated with greater use of approach-oriented coping, which in turn tends to be related to more positive adjustment (see Roesch & Weiner, 2001). Coping self-efficacy refers to expectations about one's ability to carry out various coping strategies. Thus, individuals are more likely to employ coping strategies for which they have higher efficacy expectations. Likewise, disease-related self-efficacy expectancies predict positive adjustment (e.g., Culos-Reed & Brawley, 2003; Engel, Hamilton, Potter, & Zautra, 2004). Increases in self-efficacy predict less anxiety and more vigor among individuals in cardiac rehabilitation (Blanchard, Rodgers, Courneya, Daub, & Black, 2002), and self-efficacy expectancies assessed premorbidly predict subsequent depressive symptoms and physical functioning among older adults with heart disease (van Jaarsveld, Ranchor, Sanderman, Ormel, & Kempen, 2005).

Perceptions of control and other coping appraisals likely set the stage for expectations about one's illness and treatment (see Carver et al., 2000). These might include anticipation of how one will respond to medical treatment or expectations about disease cure or recurrence. Expectations about treatment response may also contribute to aspects of adjustment (e.g., Montgomery & Bovbjerg, 2001, 2004). For instance, expectancies regarding nausea in response to chemotherapy for breast cancer assessed prior to treatment predict severity of posttreatment vomiting, controlling for pre-surgery distress and treatment characteristics (Zachariae et al., 2007). Folkman and Moskowitz (2000) and Tennen and Affleck (2000) offer speculations regarding the contexts in which disease-related control and outcome expectancies might affect well-being. Studies are needed to elucidate the impact of changes in expectations on adjustment over time.

Coping Processes

> I do a bunch of things. I talk to my wife. I get as much information as I can about treatments and the latest research. I rely on my faith. I try to live each day as I want to.

The ways in which individuals respond to the demands of illness influences physical and mental health (e.g., see S. E. Taylor & Stanton, 2007). Broadly, coping efforts are directed toward approaching or avoiding such demands (Suls & Fletcher, 1985). For instance, an individual faced with job-related limitations from arthritic symptoms might disengage from career-related pursuits or might investigate adaptive technologies to overcome obstacles. The approach–avoidance continuum reflects fundamental motivation processes (see Carver, 2007). Approach-oriented coping includes such active strategies as problem solving, seeking information or social support, and expressing and processing stressor-related emotions. In contrast, avoidance-oriented coping involves such cognitive strategies as attempts at denial and suppression and such behavioral strategies as disengagement and using alcohol and drugs as a means of escape. Other coping efforts, such as spiritual coping, can serve either approach or avoidance goals.

Heterogeneity across studies exists in how coping is assessed, relationships obtained between coping strategies and outcomes, and inferences made. However, overarching conclusions can be extracted. A meta-analysis of 63 studies on coping and adjustment to HIV/AIDS (Moskowitz, Hult, Bussolari, & Acree, 2009; note that most studies were cross-sectional) yielded several findings that reflect and inform the broader literature on coping with chronic illness. Avoidant strategies were associated with lower positive affect, higher negative affect, poorer health behaviors, and poorer physical health; whereas approach-oriented coping attempts, particularly direct action and positive reappraisal, evidenced opposite relations (see also Duangdao & Roesch, 2008; Penley, Tomaka, & Wiebe, 2002; Roesch et al., 2005; S. E. Taylor & Stanton, 2007). Daily process research produces similar findings; for example, Carels et al. (2004) found among heart failure patients that a day that included efforts to improve symptoms was followed by a day of fewer illness symptoms, whereas a day that included trying to distract oneself from the illness was followed by a day with more symptoms.

Although both approach strategies and avoidance strategies can be used in an attempt to regulate emotions, efforts to express and process stressor-related emotions promote positive adjustment under particular conditions (see Stanton, 2011). In longitudinal studies, emotional expression and other emotion regulation efforts predict adjustment in breast cancer survivors (e.g., Iwamitsu et al., 2005; Stanton et al., 2000) and arthritis patients (e.g., Hamilton, Zautra, & Reich, 2005). Emotion regulation efforts also predict reports of physical health and disease processes (e.g., Stanton et al., 2000; Temoshock et al., 2008; van Middendorp, Greenen, Sorbi, van Doornen, & Bijlsma, 2005).

Findings regarding the salutary effects of approach-oriented coping have not been as consistent as those for the harmful impact of avoidant coping. One explanation is that specific demands of chronic illness are responsive to approach-oriented coping efforts at particular points during the disease course. This explanation is supported by the Moskowitz et al. (2009) meta-analysis, which revealed that taking direct action to cope with HIV/AIDS is most effective in the early stages of disease. It also is possible that avoidant coping is a more powerful predictor of adjustment when both approach and avoidant coping strategies are examined simultaneously. Researchers might consider theory-driven models in which approach and avoidance strategies are examined separately. Approach-oriented coping also might have unique relationships with positive indicators of adjustment (e.g., positive affect), which are less often measured in longitudinal studies than are negative adjustment indicators. Also, important moderators might condition the utility of approach coping (e.g., emotional expression can be more effective within a supportive interpersonal environment; e.g., Stanton et al., 2000).

It is important to identify the conditions under which specific coping strategies are most effective or detrimental. Yang, Brothers, and Andersen (2008) observed that approach-oriented coping was most helpful for those experiencing relatively high stress. The combination of high avoidance-oriented coping and low social support has been identified as a risk factor for distress in individuals with chronic illness (Devine, Parker, Fouladi, & Cohen, 2003; Jacobsen et al., 2002). Mediational models also warrant study. Avoidance coping can mediate the impact of cancer-related symptom stress on quality of life (Yang et al., 2008) and can serve as a mechanism for the relations between unsupportive behaviors by the partner and cancer patients' distress (Manne et al., 2005). Rather than focusing solely on coping as a predictor of adjustment, research is needed to evaluate mediational and moderational models in longitudinal and experimental designs.

CONCLUSION

This chapter presents a broad synthesis of the literature that supports a biopsychosocial framework for adjustment to chronic illness in which the process of adaptation is multiply determined. Although page limitations precluded addressing the determinants here, related literatures on psychosocial contributors to disease progression, psychoneuroimmunology, and intervention strategies also inform the knowledge base on adjustment to chronic disease.

We recommend several directions for research. First, although enduring psychological distress certainly is an important dependent variable, expansion of outcomes to additional domains, including functional and biobehavioral variables and positive indicators of adjustment, is recommended. Examination of how adjustment indicators influence each other also is warranted. For instance, depressive symptoms predict nonadherence to medication and completion of medical treatment in cardiac patients (e.g., Casey, Hughes, Waechter, Josephson, & Rosneck, 2008; Rieckmann et al., 2006) and other groups (for a review, see DiMatteo, Lepper, & Croghan, 2000).

Continued investigation of distal and proximal contextual factors is an important direction for research. The combined presence of multiple risk factors can potentiate their effects. For instance, a tendency toward negative affectivity is more damaging to adjustment when individuals are socially isolated (e.g., Denollet et al., 2000). Investigations of macrolevel contextual factors are necessary to illuminate the determinants of between- and within-group disparities in adjustment. Prospective and longitudinal studies are needed to identify adjustment trajectories relative to significant events in the disease and treatment course, as well as the contextual circumstances that confer risk and resilience. Sophisticated quantitative and methodological consideration of the temporal context of the disease course will help to identify key periods in the chronic disease trajectory to which specific biopsychosocial processes are most relevant. Modeling the nuanced ways in which changes in contextual factors, cognitive appraisals, and coping processes dynamically affect adjustment over time is increasingly possible.

Researchers are making strides in investigating the relations of biological markers with psychological factors in chronic disease. Biological processes, such as autonomic and inflammatory responses, contribute to the composition of clusters of such adjustment-related symptoms as fatigue, pain, and depression. An innovative direction of empirical work involves characterizing pathophysiological processes that might interfere with positive adjustment. Individual differences in one's perceptions of and responses to disease- and treatment-related events shape variability in sympathetic nervous system activity, HPA axis activity, and related immune responses, affecting both mental and physical adjustment (though reverse causation is also possible). For instance, flatter diurnal cortisol patterns are well replicated among subsets of depressed individuals with chronic disease (e.g., Giese-Davis et al., 2006; Raison & Miller, 2001), and emotional responses to acute and sustained stressors contribute to the modulation of neuroendocrine activity that may provide a link between stress responses, suppressed immunity, and disease-related processes (Brown, Varghese, & McEwen, 2004; Cohen, Janicki-Deverts, & Miller, 2007; Sephton et al., 2009). Further, some evidence indicates that trajectories of psychological and related biological processes covary across time (e.g., Thornton, Andersen, Crespin, & Carson, 2007).

Recent research addresses the role of inflammatory processes, particularly proinflammatory cytokine activity across a number of chronic diseases. Dysregulation of inflammatory processes can induce a constellation of nonspecific symptoms, or *sickness behavior*, including social withdrawal, lethargy and fatigue, and depressionlike symptoms (Brydon et al., 2009; Dantzer, 2001; Wright, Strike, Brydon, & Steptoe, 2005). Such symptoms can compound the burden associated with chronic disease and influence adjustment. Research characterizing fatigue associated with chronic illness provides an illustration. Fatigue is a subjective feeling of low vitality that affects overall daily functioning. Cancer-related fatigue is the most commonly reported symptom associated with cancer and its treatment, with prevalence estimates ranging from 25% to 99% (Bower, 2008; Lawrence, Kupelnick, Miller, Devine, & Lau, 2004). In daily diary studies in patients with rheumatic disorders, day-to-day increases in fatigue co-occur with decreases in positive affect and increases in negative affect, when depressive symptoms and sleep quality are controlled (Zautra, Frasman, Parish, & Davis, 2007). In addition to fatigue's associations with depression and maladaptive coping strategies (e.g., catastrophic thinking), Bower (2008; Bower et al., 2007) and others have determined that biological mechanisms such as anemia, blunted cortisol responses, and proinflammatory cytokine activity are associated with persistent fatigue in cancer survivors. Similar findings link inflammatory markers with fatigue in patients with rheumatic disease (e.g., Davis et al., 2008).

Future research will advance biopsychosocial model of adjustment to chronic illness by characterizing relations among systemic (e.g., inflammation) and disease-specific biological parameters, psychosocial predictors, and adaptive outcomes. A promising direction in biobehavioral research is in identifying genetic and other biological vulnerabilities that might affect risk and resilience, as well as the capacity of the social and intrapersonal contexts to influence gene expression and biological processes (e.g., S. W. Cole, 2009; Miller, Chen, & Cole, 2009). For example, a study with HIV+ men yielded a three-way interaction between ethnicity, disclosure of HIV serostatus, and HIV-related familial support on viral load (Fekete et al., 2009). Non-Hispanic White men who had disclosed their HIV serostatus to their mothers and were receiving high family support demonstrated lower viral load and higher CD4+ cell count, whereas Latino men who also had disclosed to their mothers but were receiving low family support had a higher viral load.

Relatively few studies have tested comprehensive models of adjustment in longitudinal designs. In a study of prostate cancer patients and spouses, Kershaw and colleagues (2008) found support for a stress and coping model in which cognitive appraisals (i.e., uncertainty, hopelessness, negativity) and coping processes (i.e., approach and avoidance) mediated the impact of macrolevel (i.e., SES), interpersonal (i.e., social support and communication), intrapersonal (i.e., self-efficacy, current concerns), and disease-related (i.e., physical symptoms, disease phase) contextual factors on psychological and physical quality of life. Eight months after study entry, variables in the model accounted for 40% and 34% of the variance in psychological and physical quality of life, respectively. Such evaluations of comprehensive models will allow investigators to hone theories of adjustment to chronic disease, learn more about contextual determinants of adjustment trajectories, and sharpen psychosocial interventions that effectively target biopsychosocial processes to improve adaptive outcomes.

Finally, experimental and intervention studies can provide tests of conceptual models of adjustment that translate basic findings into strategies to bolster adjustment and that allow for stronger causal inference. A good example of the translation of the stress and coping framework to an effective intervention strategy is Folkman and colleagues' (1991) coping effectiveness training. Effective in bolstering adjustment in HIV+ men (e.g., Chesney, Chambers, Taylor, Johnson, & Folkman, 2003) and other patient groups, this approach involves group-based skill building focused on disaggregating global appraisals to distinguish immutable and alterable stressors, matching adaptive coping strategies to situational contexts, and selecting and maintaining effective social resources and support. Other effective psychosocial interventions exist for enhancing quality of life, improving medical-regimen adherence, and potentially improving disease endpoints in individuals across several chronic diseases (e.g., Linden, Phillips, & Leclerc, 2007, on cardiovascular disease; Scott-Sheldon, Kalichman, Carey, & Fielder, 2008, on HIV; Dixon, Keefe, Scipio, Perri, & Abernethy, 2007, on arthritis pain; Gonder-Frederick, Cox, & Ritterband, 2002, on diabetes). Such interventions typically involve multiple components including an emotionally supportive context to address disease-specific worries, illness-related education, and training in cognitive and behavioral coping strategies (e.g., Penedo, Antoni, & Schneiderman, 2008). As Stanton, Revenson, and Tennen (2007) suggested, theoretically grounded research on adjustment to chronic illness can refine such interventions by: pointing to effective targets of intervention (e.g., Broadbent, Ellis, Thomas, Gamble, & Petrie, 2009, on illness perceptions); suggesting potential mechanisms by which interventions may gain their utility (e.g., decreasing avoidant coping and increasing approach-oriented strategies; see Andersen, Shelby, & Golden-Kreutz, 2007); identifying at-risk patients for whom interventions might be appropriate (e.g., patients low in optimism, younger cancer patients); and targeting intervention components for maximal effectiveness (e.g., bolstering self-efficacy in relation to specific disease-related tasks). Finally, examining prospective trajectories of adjustment will allow for the implementation of interventions at critical periods in the disease course when they are likely to be most beneficial and help to identify vulnerable groups.

The knowledge base on adjustment to chronic disease is advancing. Along with experimental research, theoretically guided research on contributors to adjustment in longitudinal designs will require relatively large samples, modeling of the dynamic relations among contextual factors, and use of prospective research designs that span long time frames. The next decade of research is likely to produce culturally and socioeconomically-informed models, elaboration of biological and psychosocial mechanisms for adaptive outcomes, and greater translation of theory and research into clinical intervention.

REFERENCES

Abraido-Lanza, A. F. (1997). Latinas with arthritis: Effects of illness, role identity, and competence on psychological well-being. *American Journal of Community Psychology, 25,* 601–627.

Addis, M. E. (2008). Gender and depression in men. *Clinical Psychology, 15,* 154–168.

Adler, N. E., & Rehkopf, D. H. (2008). U.S. disparities in health: Descriptions, causes, and mechanisms. *Annual Review of Public Health, 29,* 235–252.

Affleck, G., Tennen, H., Croog, S., & Levine, S. (1987). Causal attribution, perceived benefits, and morbidity after a heart attack: An 8-year study. *Journal of Consulting and Clinical Psychology, 55,* 29–35.

Affleck, G., Tennen, H., Pfeiffer, C., & Fifield, J. (1987). Appraisals of control and predictability in adapting to chronic disease. *Journal of Personality and Social Psychology, 53,* 273–279.

Affleck, G., Tennen, H., Zautra, A., Urrows, S., Abeles, M., & Karoly, P. (2001). Women's pursuit of personal goals in daily life with fibromyalgia: A value-expectancy analysis. *Journal of Consulting and Clinical Psychology, 69,* 587–596.

Algoe, S. B., & Stanton, A. L. (2009). Is benefit finding good for individuals with chronic disease? In C. L. Park, S. C. Lechner, M. H. Antoni, & A. L. Stanton (Eds.), *Medical illness and positive life change: Can crisis lead to personal transformation?* (pp. 173–193). Washington, DC: American Psychological Association.

Allison, P. J., Guichard, C., & Laurent, G. (2000). A prospective investigation of dispositional optimism as a predictor of health-related quality of life in head and neck cancer patients. *Quality of Life Research, 9,* 951–960.

Andersen, B. L., Shelby, R. A., & Golden-Kreutz, D. M. (2007). RCT of a psychological intervention for patients with cancer: I. Mechanisms of change. *Journal of Consulting and Clinical Psychology, 75,* 927–938.

Antoni, M. H., Lutgendorf, S. K., Cole, S. W., Dhanhar, F. S., Sephton, S. E., McDonald, P. G., … Sood, A. K. (2006). The influence of bio-behavioural factors on tumour biology: Pathways and mechanisms. *Nature Reviews Cancer, 6,* 240–248.

Asch, S. M., Kerr, E. A., Keesey, J., Adams, J. L., Setodji, C. M., Malik, S., & McGlynn, E. A. (2006). Who is at greatest risk for receiving poor-quality health care? *New England Journal of Medicine, 354,* 1147–1156.

Badr, H. (2004). Coping in marital dyads: A contextual perspective on the role of gender and health. *Personal Relationships, 11,* 197–211.

Badr, H., & Taylor, C. L. (2008). Effects of relationship maintenance on psychological distress and dyadic adjustment among couples coping with lung cancer. *Health Psychology, 27,* 616–627.

Barbareschi, G., Sanderman, R., Kempen, G. I., & Ranchor, A. V. (2008). The mediating role of perceived control on the relationship between socioeconomic status and functional changes in older patients with coronary heart disease. *Journal of Gerontology: Psychological Sciences, 63B,* 353–361.

Bardwell, W. A., Natarajan, L., Dimsdale, J. E., Rock, C. L., Mortimer, J. E., Hollenbach, K., & Pierce, J. P. (2006). Objective cancer-related variables are not associated with depressive symptoms in women treated for early-stage breast cancer. *Journal of Clinical Oncology, 24,* 2420–2427.

Bárez, M., Blasco, T., Fernández-Castro, J., & Viladrich C. (2009). Perceived control and psychological distress in women with breast cancer: A longitudinal study. *Journal of Behavioral Medicine, 32,* 187–196.

Barry, L. C., Kasl, S. V., Lictman, J., Vaccarino, V., & Krumholz, H. M. (2006). Perceived control and change in physical functioning after coronary artery bypass grafting: A prospective study. *International Journal of Behavioral Medicine, 13,* 229–236.

Bellizzi, K. M., Miller, M. F., Arora, N. K., & Rowland, J. H. (2007). Positive and negative life changes experienced by survivors of non-Hodgkin's lymphoma. *Annals of Behavioral Medicine, 34,* 188–199.

Berg, C. A., & Upchurch, R. (2007). A developmental-contextual model of couples coping with chronic illness across the adult life span. *Psychological Bulletin*, *133*, 920–954.

Berghuis, J. P., & Stanton, A. L. (2002). Adjustment to a dyadic stressor: A longitudinal study of coping and depressive symptoms in infertile couples over an insemination attempt. *Journal of Consulting and Clinical Psychology*, *70*, 433–438.

Bhattacharyya, M. R., Perkins-Porras, L., Whitehead, D. L., & Steptoe, A. (2007). Psychological and clinical predictors of return to work after acute coronary syndrome. *European Heart Journal*, *28*, 160–165.

Blanchard, C. M., Rodgers, W. M., Courneya, K. S., Daub, B., & Black, B. (2002). Self-efficacy and mood in cardiac rehabilitation: Should gender be considered? *Behavioral Medicine*, *27*, 149–160.

Bolger, N., & Schilling, E. A. (1991). Personality and the problems of everyday life: The role of neuroticism in exposure and reactivity to daily stressors. *Journal of Personality*, *59*, 355–386.

Bower, J. E. (2008). Behavioral symptoms in patients with breast cancer and survivors. *Journal of Clinical Oncology*, *26*, 768–777.

Bower, J. E., Epel, E., & Moskowitz, J. T. (2009). Biological correlates: How psychological components of benefit finding may lead to physiological benefits. In C. L. Park, S. C. Lechner, M. H. Antoni, & A. L. Stanton (Eds.), *Medical illness and positive life change: Can crisis lead to personal transformation?* (pp. 155–172). Washington, DC: American Psychological Association.

Bower, J. E., Ganz, P. A., Aziz, N., Olmstead, R., Irwin, M. R., & Cole, S. W. (2007). Inflammatory responses to psychological stress in fatigued breast cancer survivors: Relationship to glucocorticoids. *Brain Behavior & Immunity*, *21*, 251–258.

Bower, J. E., Kemeny, M. E., Taylor, S. E., & Fahey, J. L. (1998). Cognitive processing, discovery of meaning, CD4 decline, and AIDS-related mortality among bereaved HIV-seropositive men. *Journal of Consulting and Clinical Psychology*, *66*, 979–986.

Bower, J. E., Meyerowitz, B. E., Desmond, K. A., Bernaards, C. A., Rowland, J. H., & Ganz, P. A. (2005). Perceptions of positive meaning and vulnerability following breast cancer: Predictors and outcomes among long-term breast cancer survivors. *Annals of Behavioral Medicine*, *29*, 236–245.

Braitman, A. L., Derlega, V. J., Henson, J. M., Robinett, I., & Saadeh, G. M. (2008). Social constraints in talking about diabetes to significant others and diabetes self-care: A social-cognitive processing perspective. *Journal of Social and Clinical Psychology*, *27*, 949–969.

Brissette, I., Scheier, M. F., & Carver, C. S. (2002). The role of optimism in social network development, coping, and psychological adjustment during a life transition. *Journal of Personality and Social Psychology*, *82*, 102–111.

Broadbent, E., Ellis, C. J., Thomas, J., Gamble, G., & Petrie, K. J. (2009). Further development of an illness perception intervention for myocardial infarction patients: A randomized controlled trial. *Journal of Psychosomatic Research*, *67*, 17–23.

Brondolo E., Gallo, L. C., & Myers, H. F. (2009). Race, racism and health: Disparities, mechanisms, and interventions. *Journal of Behavioral Medicine*, *32*, 1–8.

Brown, E. S., Varghese, F. P., & McEwen, B. S. (2004). Association of depression with medical illness: Does cortisol play a role? *Biological Psychiatry*, *55*, 1–9.

Brownhill, S., Wilhelm, K., Barclay, L., & Parker, G. (2002). Detecting depression in men: A matter of guesswork. *International Journal of Men's Health*, *1*, 259–280.

Brydon, L., Walker, C., Wawrzyniak, A., Whitehead, D., Okamura, H., Yajima, J., … Steptoe, A. (2009). Synergistic effects of psychological and immune stressors on inflammatory cytokine and sickness responses in humans. *Brain, Behavior, & Immunity*, *23*, 217–224.

Burgess, C., Cornelius, V., Love, S., Graham, J., Richards, M., & Ramirez, A. (2005). Depression and anxiety in women with early breast cancer: Five year observational cohort study. *BMJ*, *330*, 702.

Calhoun, L. G., & Tedeschi, R. G. (Eds.). (2006). *Handbook of posttraumatic growth: Research and practice.* Mahwah, NJ: Erlbaum.

Carels, R. A., Musher-Eizenman, D., Cacciapaglia, H., Perez-Benitez, C. I., Christie, S., & O'Brien, W. (2004). Psychosocial functioning and physical symptoms in heart failure patients: A within-individual approach. *Journal of Psychosomatic Research*, *56*, 95–101.

Carpenter, K. M., Fowler, J. M., Maxwell, G. L., & Andersen, B. L. (2010). Direct and buffering effects of social support among gynecologic cancer patients. *Annals of Behavioral Medicine*, *39*, 79–90.

Carver, C. S. (2007). Stress, coping, and health. In H. S. Friedman & R. Cohen Silver (Eds.), *Foundations of health psychology* (pp. 117–144). Oxford, England: Oxford University Press.

Carver, C. S., & Antoni, M. H. (2004). Finding benefit in breast cancer during the year after diagnosis predicts better adjustment 5 to 8 years after cancer. *Health Psychology*, *23*, 595–598.

Carver, C. S., Harris, S. D., Lehman, J. M., Durel, L. A., Antoni, M. H., Spencer, S. M., & Pozo-Kaderman, C. (2000). How important is the perception of personal control? Studies of early stage breast cancer patients. *Personality and Social Psychology Bulletin, 26*, 139–150.

Carver, C. S., Smith, R. G., Antoni, M. H., Petronis, V. M., Weiss, S., & Derhagopian, R. P. (2005). Optimistic personality and psychosocial well-being during treatment predict psychosocial well-being among long-term survivors of breast cancer. *Health Psychology, 24*, 508–516.

Casey, E., Hughes, J. W., Waechter, D., Josephson, R., & Rosneck, J. (2008). Depression predicts failure to complete phase-II cardiac rehabilitation. *Journal of Behavioral Medicine, 31*, 421–431.

Castro, F. G., Shaibi, G. Q., & Boehm-Smith, E. (2009). Ecodevelopmental contexts for preventing type 2 diabetes in Latino and other racial/ethnic minority populations. *Journal of Behavioral Medicine, 32*, 89–105.

Centers for Disease Control and Prevention, U.S. Department of Health and Human Services. (2009). Chronic diseases: The power to prevent, the call to control. Retrieved from http://www.cdc.gov/nccdphp/publications/AAG/chronic.htm (accessed September 20, 2009).

Chesney, M. A., Chambers, D. B., Taylor, J. M., Johnson, L. M., & Folkman, S. (2003). Coping effectiveness training for men living with HIV: Results from randomized clinical trial testing a group-based intervention. *Psychosomatic Medicine, 65*, 1038–1046.

Christensen, A. J., & Ehlers, S. L. (2002). Psychological factors in end-stage renal disease: An emerging context for behavioral medicine research. *Journal of Consulting and Clinical Psychology, 70*, 712–724.

Cohen, S., Janicki-Deverts, D., & Miller, G. E. (2007). Psychological stress and disease. *JAMA, 298*, 1685–1687.

Cole, E. R. (2009). Intersectionality and research in psychology. *American Psychologist, 64*, 170–180.

Cole, S. W. (2009). Social regulation of human gene expression. *Current Directions in Psychological Science, 18*, 132–137.

Conner, T. S., Tennen, H., Zautra, A. J., Affleck, G., Armeli, S., & Fifield, J. (2006). Coping with rheumatoid arthritis pain in daily life: Within-person analyses reveal hidden vulnerability for the formerly depressed. *Pain, 126*, 198–209.

Cooper-Patrick, L., Gallo, J. J., Gonzales, J. J., Vu, H. T., Powe, N. R., Nelson, C., & Ford, D. E. (1999). Race, gender, and partnership in the patient-physician relationship. *JAMA, 282*, 583–589.

Cordova, M. J., Cunningham, L. L., Carlson, C. R., & Andrykowski, M. A. (2001). Posttraumatic growth following breast cancer: A controlled comparison study. *Health Psychology, 20*, 176–185.

Costanzo, E. S., Ryff, C. D., & Singer, B. H. (2009). Psychosocial adjustment among cancer survivors: Findings from a national survey of health and well-being. *Health Psychology, 28*, 147–156.

Culos-Reed, S. N., & Brawley, L. R. (2003). Self-efficacy predicts physical activity in individuals with fibromyalgia. *Journal of Applied Behavioral Research, 8*, 27–41.

Daar, A. S., Singer, P. A., Persad, D. L., Pramming, S. K., Matthews, D. R., Beaglehole, R., & Bell, J. (2007). Grand challenges in chronic non-communicable diseases. *Nature, 450*, 494–496.

Danoff-Burg, S., & Revenson, T. A. (2005). Benefit-finding among patients with rheumatoid arthritis: Positive effects on interpersonal relationships. *Journal of Behavioral Medicine, 28*, 91–103.

Danoff-Burg, S., Revenson, T. A., Trudeau, K. J., & Paget, S. A. (2004). Unmitigated communion, social constraints, and psychological distress among women with rheumatoid arthritis. *Journal of Personality, 72*, 29–46.

Dantzer, R. (2001). Cytokine-induced sickness behavior: Mechanisms and implications. *Annals of the New York Academy of Sciences, 933*, 222–234.

Darnell, B. D., & Suarez, E. C. (2009). Sex and gender in psychoneuroimmunology research: Past, present, and future. *Brain, Behavior, & Immunity, 23*, 595–604.

Davis, M. C., Zautra, A. J., Younger, J., Motivala, S. J., Attrep, J., & Irwin, M. R. (2008). Chronic stress and regulation of cellular markers of inflammation in rheumatoid arthritis: Implications for fatigue. *Brain, Behavior, & Immunity, 22*, 22–23.

De Boer, A. G., Taskila, T., Ojajarvi, A., van Dijk, F. J., & Verbeek, J. H. (2009). Cancer survivors and unemployment: A meta-analysis and meta-regression. *JAMA, 301*, 753–762.

Demange, V., Guillemin, F., Baumann, M., Suurmeiher, B. M., Moum, T., Doelas, D., & Van Den Heuvel, W. J. (2004). Are there more than cross-sectional relationships of social support and social networks with functional limitations and psychological distress in early rheumatoid arthritis? *Arthritis & Rheumatism, 51*, 782–791.

De Moor, J. S., De Moor, C. A., Basen-Engquist, K., Kudelka, A., Bevers, M. W., & Cohen L. (2006). Optimism, distress, health-related quality of life, and change in cancer antigen 125 among patients with ovarian cancer undergoing chemotherapy. *Psychosomatic Medicine, 68*, 555–562.

Denollet, J., Vaes, J., & Brutsaert, D. L. (2000). Inadequate response to treatment in coronary heart disease: Adverse effects of type D personality and younger age on 5-year prognosis and quality of life. *Circulation, 102*, 630–635.

Detweiler-Bedell, J. B., Friedman, M. A., Leventhal, H., Miller, I. W., & Leventhal, E. A. (2008). Integrating co-morbid depression and chronic physical disease management: Identifying and resolving failures in self-regulation. *Clinical Psychology Review, 28*, 1426–1446.

DeVellis, B. M., & DeVellis, R. F. (2001). Self-efficacy and health. In A. Baum and T. Revenson (Eds.), *Handbook of health psychology* (1st ed., pp. 235–247). New York, NY: Lawrence Erlbaum Associates.

Devine, D., Parker, P. A., Fouladi, R. T., & Cohen, L. (2003). The association between social support, intrusive thoughts, avoidance, and adjustment following an experimental cancer treatment. *Psycho-Oncology, 12*, 453–462.

Diener, E. (1984). Subjective well-being. *Psychological Bulletin, 95*, 542–575.

DiMatteo, M. R., Lepper, H. S., & Croghan, T. W. (2000). Depression is a risk factor for noncompliance with medical treatment: A meta-analysis of the effects of anxiety and depression on patient adherence. *Archives of Internal Medicine, 160*, 2101–2107.

Dixon, K. E., Keefe, F. J., Scipio, C. D., Perri, L. M., & Abernethy, A. P. (2007). Psychological interventions for arthritis pain management in adults: A meta-analysis. *Health Psychology, 26*, 241–250.

Donovan, K. A., Small, B. J., Andrykowski, M. A., Munster, P., & Jacobsen, P. B. (2007). Utility of a cognitive-behavioral model to predict fatigue following breast cancer treatment. *Health Psychology, 26*, 464–472.

Duangdao, K. M., & Roesch, S. C. (2008). Coping with diabetes in adulthood: A meta-analysis. *Journal of Behavioral Medicine, 31*, 291–300.

Dunkel-Schetter, C., & Wortman, C. B. (1982). The interpersonal dynamics of cancer: Problems in social relationships and their impact on the patient. In H. S. Friedman & M. R. DiMatteo (Eds.), *Interpersonal issues in health care* (pp. 69–100). New York: Academic Press.

Engel, C., Hamilton, N. A., Potter, P. T., & Zautra, A. J. (2004). Impact of two types of expectancy on recovery from total knee replacement surgery (TKR) in adults with osteoarthritis. *Behavioral Medicine, 30*, 113–123.

Ertel, K. A., Glymour, E. M., & Berkman, L. F. (2008). Social networks and health: A life course perspective integrating observational and experimental evidence. *Journal of Social and Personal Relationships, 26*, 73–92.

Fann, J. R., Thomas-Rich, A. M., Katon, W. J., Cowley, D., Pepping, M., McGregor, B. A., & Gralow, J. (2008). Major depression after breast cancer: A review of epidemiology and treatment. *General Hospital Psychiatry, 30*, 112–126.

Fekete, E. M., Antoni, M. H., Lopez, C. R., Durán, R. E., Penedo, F. J., Bandiera, F. C., … Schneiderman, N. (2009). Men's serostatus disclosure to parents: associations among social support, ethnicity, and disease status in men living with HIV. *Brain, Behavior, & Immunity, 23*, 693–699.

Finan, P. H., Zautra, A. J., & Davis, M. C. (2009). Daily affect relations in fibromyalgia patients reveal positive affective disturbance. *Psychosomatic Medicine, 71*, 474–482.

Fitzgerald, J. D., Orav, E. J., Lee, T. H., Marcantonio, E. R., Poss, R., Goldman, L., & Mangione, C. M. (2004). Patient quality of life during the 12 months following joint replacement surgery. *Arthritis & Rheumatism, 51*, 100–109.

Folkman, S., Chesney, M., McKusick, L., Ironson, G., Johnson, D., & Coates, T. J. (1991). Translating coping theory into intervention. In J. Eckenrode (Ed.), *The social context of coping* (pp. 239–259). New York, NY: Plenum Press.

Folkman, S., & Moskowitz, J. T. (2000). The context matters. *Personality & Social Psychology Bulletin, 26*, 150–151.

Fritz, H. L. (2000). Gender-linked personality traits predict mental health and functional status following a first coronary event. *Health Psychology, 19*, 420–428.

Fryand, L., Moum, T., Finset, A., & Glennas, A. (2002). The impact of disability and disease duration on social support of women with rheumatoid arthritis. *Journal of Behavioral Medicine, 25*, 251–268.

Gallo, L. C., & Matthews, K. A. (2003). Understanding the association between socioeconomic status and physical health: Do negative emotions play a role? *Psychological Bulletin, 129*, 10–51.

Giese-Davis, J., Wilhelm, F. H., Conrad, A., Abercrombie, H. C., Sephton, S., Yutsis, M., … Spiegel, D. (2006). Depression and stress reactivity in metastatic breast cancer. *Psychosomatic Medicine, 68*, 675–683.

Golden, S. H., Lazo, M., Carnethon, M., Bertoni, A. G., Schreiner, P. J., Diez Roux, A. V., … Lyketsos, C. (2008). Examining a bidirectional association between depressive symptoms and diabetes. *JAMA, 299*, 2751–2759.

Gonder-Frederick, L. A., Cox, D. J., & Ritterband, L. M. (2002). Diabetes and behavioral medicine: The second decade. *Journal of Consulting and Clinical Psychology, 70*, 611–625.

Gore, J. L., Kwan, L., Lee, S. P., Reiter, R. R., & Litwin, M. (2009). Survivorship beyond convalescence: 48-month quality-of-life outcomes after treatment for localized prostate cancer. *Journal of the National Cancer Institute, 101*, 888–892.

Hagedoorn, M., Buunk, B. P., Kuijer, R. G., Wobbes, T., & Sanderman, R. (2000). Couples dealing with cancer: Role and gender differences regarding psychological distress and quality of life. *Psycho-Oncology, 9*, 232–242.

Hagedoorn, M., Sanderman, R., Bolks, H. N., & Coyne, J. C. (2008). Distress in couples coping with cancer: A meta-analysis and critical review of role and gender effects. *Psychological Bulletin, 134*, 1–30.

Hamilton, N. A., Zautra, A. J., & Reich, J. W. (2005). Affect and pain in rheumatoid arthritis: Do individual differences in affective regulation and affective intensity predict emotional recovery from pain? *Annals of Behavioral Medicine, 29*, 216–224.

Harrison, M. J., Tricker, K. J., Davies, L., Hassell, A., Dawes, P., Scott, D. L., … Symmons, D. P. (2005). The relationship between social deprivation, disease outcome measures, and response to treatment in patients with stable, long-standing rheumatoid arthritis. *Journal of Rheumatology, 32*, 2330–2336.

Havranek, E. P., Spertus, J. A., Masoudi, F. A., Jones, P. G., & Rumsfeld, J. S. (2004). Predictors of the onset of depressive symptoms in patients with heart failure. *Journal of the American College of Cardiology, 44*, 2333–2338.

Helgeson, V. S. (1990). The role of masculinity in a prognostic predictor of heart attack severity. *Sex Roles, 22*, 755–774.

Helgeson, V. S. (1992). Moderators of the relation between perceived control and adjustment to chronic illness. *Journal of Personality and Social Psychology, 63*, 656–666.

Helgeson, V. S. (1993). Implications of agency and communion for patient and spouse adjustment to a first coronary event. *Journal of Personality and Social Psychology, 64*, 807–816.

Helgeson, V. S. (1994). Relation of agency and communion to well-being: Evidence and potential explanations. *Psychological Bulletin, 116*, 412–428.

Helgeson, V. S., & Fritz, H. L. (1998). A theory of unmitigated communion. *Personality and Social Psychology Review, 2*, 173–183.

Helgeson, V. S., & Lepore, S. J. (2004). Quality of life following prostate cancer: The role of agency and unmitigated agency. *Journal of Applied Social Psychology, 34*, 2559–2585.

Helgeson, V. S., Snyder, P., & Seltman, H. (2004). Psychological and physical adjustment to breast cancer over 4 years: Identifying distinct trajectories of change. *Health Psychology, 23*, 3–15.

Hinnen, C., Ranchor, A. V., Baas, P .C., Sanderman, R., & Hagedoorn, M. (2009). Partner support and distress in women with breast cancer: The role of patients' awareness of support and level of mastery. *Psychology & Health, 24*, 439–455.

Hinnen, C., Ranchor, A. V., Sanderman, R., Snijders, T. A., Hagesoor, M., & Coyne, J. C. (2008). Course of distress in breast cancer patients, their partners, and matched control couples. *Annals of Behavioral Medicine, 36*, 141–148.

Holahan, C. J., Moos, R. H., Holahan, C. K., & Brennan, P. L. (1997). Social context, coping strategies, and depressive symptoms: An expanded model with cardiac patients. *Journal of Personality and Social Psychology, 72*, 918–928.

Holahan, C. K., Moerkbak, M., & Suzuki, R. (2006). Social support, coping, and depressive symptoms in cardiac illness among Hispanic and non-Hispanic White cardiac patients. *Psychology & Health, 21*, 615–631.

Holtzman, S., & DeLongis, A. (2007). One day at a time: The impact of daily satisfaction with spouse responses on pain, negative affect and catastrophizing among individuals with rheumatoid arthritis. *Pain, 131*, 202–213.

Hommel, K. A., Wagner, J. L., Chaney, J. M., White, M. M., & Mullins, L. L. (2004). Perceived importance of activities of daily living in rheumatoid arthritis: A prospective investigation. *Journal of Psychosomatic Research, 57*, 159–164.

Hoyt, M. A. (2009). Gender role conflict and emotional approach coping in men with cancer. *Psychology & Health, 24*, 981–996.

Hoyt, M. A., & Stanton, A. S. (2011). Unmitigated agency, social support, and psychological adjustment in men with cancer. *Journal of Personality, 79*, 259–276.

Iwamitsu, Y., Shimoda, K., Abe, H., Tani, T., Okawa, M., & Buck, R. (2005). Anxiety, emotional, suppressional, and psychological distress before and after breast cancer diagnosis. *Psychosomatics, 46*, 19–24.

Jacobsen, P. B., Sadler, I. J., Booth-Jones, M., Soety, E., Weitzner, M. A., & Fields, K. K. (2002). Predictors of posttraumatic stress disorder symptomatology following bone marrow transplantation for cancer. *Journal of Consulting and Clinical Psychology, 70*, 235–240.

Janoff-Bulman, R., & Frantz, C. M. (1997). The impact of trauma on meaning: From meaningless world to meaningful life. In M. Power & C. Brewin (Eds.), *The transformation of meaning in psychological therapies: Integrating theory and practice* (pp. 91–106). Sussex, England: Wiley.

Jim, H. S., Andrykowski, M. A., Munster, P. N., & Jacobsen, P. B. (2007). Physical symptoms/side effects during breast cancer treatment predict posttreatment distress. *Annals of Behavioral Medicine, 34,* 200–208.

Johnson, L. M., Zautra, A. J., & Davis, M. C. (2006). The role of illness uncertainty on coping with fibromyalgia symptoms. *Health Psychology, 25,* 696–703.

Johnson, R. L., Roter, D., Powe, N. R., & Cooper, L. A. (2004). Patient race/ethnicity and quality of patient–physician communication during medical visits. *American Journal of Public Health, 94,* 2084–2090.

Kershaw, T. S., Mood, D. W., Newth, G., Ronis, D. L., Sanda, M. G., Vaishampayan, U., & Northouse, L. L. (2008). Longitudinal analysis of a model to predict quality of life in prostate cancer patients and their spouses. *Annals of Behavioral Medicine, 36,* 117–128.

Kessler, R. C. (2000). Gender differences in major depression: Epidemiological findings. In E. Frank (Ed.), *Gender and its effects on psychopathology* (pp. 61–84). Arlington, VA: American Psychiatric Publishing.

Kessler, R. C., Berglund, P., Demler, O., Jin, R., Koretz, D., Merikangas, K. R., … Wang, P. S. (2003). The epidemiology of major depressive disorder: Results from the National Comorbidity Survey Replication (NCS-R). *JAMA, 289,* 3095–3105.

Kratz, A. L., Davis, M. C., & Zautra, A. J. (2007). Pain acceptance moderates the relation between pain and negative affect in female osteoarthritis and fibromyalgia patients. *Annals of Behavioral Medicine, 33,* 291–301.

Kulik, J. A., & Mahler, H. I. M. (2006). Marital quality predicts hospital stay following coronary artery bypass surgery for women but not men. *Social Science and Medicine, 63,* 2031–2040.

Landrine, H., & Klonoff, E. A. (2003). Diversifying health psychology: The sociocultural context. In P. Bronstein & K. Quina (Eds.), *Teaching gender and multicultural awareness: Resources for the psychology classroom* (pp. 125–136). Washington, DC: American Psychological Association.

Langer, S. L., Brown, J. D., & Syrjala, K. L. (2009). Intrapersonal and interpersonal consequences of protective buffering among cancer patients and caregivers. *Cancer, 115,* 4311–4325.

Lawrence, D. P., Kupelnick, B., Miller, K., Devine, D., & Lau, J. (2004). Evidence report on the occurrence, assessment, and treatment of fatigue in cancer patients. *Journal of the National Cancer Institute Monographs, 32,* 40–50.

Lazarus, R. S. (1991). *Emotion and adaptation.* New York, NY: Oxford University Press.

Lazarus, R. S., & Folkman, S. (1984). *Stress, appraisal, and coping.* New York, NY: Springer.

Lazovich, D., Robien, K., Cutler, G., Virnig, B., & Sweeney, C. (2009). Quality of life in a prospective cohort of elderly women with and without cancer. *Cancer, 115,* 4283–4297.

Lechner, S. C., Carver, C. S., Antoni, M. H., Weaver, K. E., & Phillips, K. M. (2006). Curvilinear associations between benefit finding and psychosocial adjustment to breast cancer. *Journal of Consulting and Clinical Psychology, 74,* 828–840.

Lepore, S. J. (2001). A social-cognitive processing model of emotional adjustment to cancer. In A. Baum & B. L. Andersen (Eds.), *Psychosocial interventions for cancer* (pp. 99–116). Washington, DC: American Psychological Association.

Lepore, S. J., & Eton, D. T. (2000). Response shifts in prostate cancer patients: An evaluation of suppressor and buffer models. In C. Schwartz & M. Sprangers (Eds.), *Adaptations to changing health: Response shift in quality-of-life research* (pp. 37–51). Washington, DC: American Psychological Association.

Lepore, S. J., Glaser, D. B., & Roberts, K. J. (2008). On the positive relation between received social support and negative affect: A test of the triage and self-esteem threat models in women with breast cancer. *Psycho-Oncology, 17,* 1210–1215.

Lett, H. S., Blumenthal, J. A., Babyak, M. A., Catellier, D. J., Carney, R. M., Berkman, L. F., & Schneiderman, N. (2007). Social support and prognosis in patients at increased psychosocial risk recovering from myocardial infarction. *Health Psychology, 26,* 418–427.

Leventhal, H., Halm, E., Horowitz, C., Leventhal, E. A., & Ozakinci, G. (2005). Living with chronic illness: A contextualized, self-regulation approach. In S. Sutton, A. Baum, & M. Johnston (Eds.), *The Sage handbook of health psychology* (pp.197–240). Thousand Oaks, CA: Sage.

Linden, W., Phillips, M. J., & Leclerc, J. (2007). Psychological treatment of cardiac patients: A meta-analysis. *European Heart Journal, 28,* 2972–2984.

Low, C. A., Beran, T., & Stanton (2007). Adaptation in the face of cancer. In M. Feurstein (Ed.), *Handbook of cancer survivorship* (pp. 211–228). New York, NY: Springer Science & Business Media.

Lustman, P. J., & Clouse, R. E. (2005). Depression in diabetic patients: The relationship between mood and glycemic control. *Journal of Diabetes and Its Complications*, *19*, 113–122.

Lynch, B. M., Steginga, S. K., Hawkes, A. L., & Pakenham, K. I. (2008). Describing and predicting psychological distress after colorectal cancer. *Cancer*, *112*, 1363–1370.

Mackenbach, J. P., Stirbu, I., Roskam, A. J. R., Schaap, M. M., Menvielle, G., Leinsalu, M., & Kunst, A. E. (2008). Socioeconomic inequalities in health in 22 European countries. *New England Journal of Medicine*, *358*, 2468–2481.

Mahler, H. I. M., & Kulik, J. A. (1990). Preferences for health care involvement, perceived control and surgical recovery: A prospective study. *Social Science and Medicine*, *31*, 743–751.

Mahler, H. I. M., & Kulik, J. A. (2000). Optimism, pessimism and recovery from coronary bypass surgery: Prediction of affect, pain and functional status. *Psychology, Health, & Medicine*, *5*, 347–358.

Maly, R. C., Leake, B., & Silliman, R. A. (2003). Health care disparities in older patients with breast carcinoma: Informational support from physicians. *Cancer*, *97*, 1517–1527.

Maly, R. C., Stein, J. A., Umezawa, Y., Leake, B., & Anglin, M. D. (2008). Racial/ethnic differences in breast cancer outcomes among older patients: Effects of physician communication and patient empowerment. *Health Psychology*, *27*, 728–736.

Manne, S. L., Norton, T. R., Ostroff, J. S., Winkel, G., Fox, K., & Grana, G. (2007). Protective buffering and psychological distress among couples coping with breast cancer: The moderating role of relationship satisfaction. *Journal of Family Psychology*, *21*, 380–388.

Manne, S. L., Ostroff, J., Winkel, G., Grana, G., & Fox, K. (2005). Partner unsupportive responses, avoidant coping, and distress among women with early stage breast cancer: Patient and partner perspectives. *Health Psychology*, *24*, 635–641.

Manne, S., Rini, C., Rubin, S., Rosenblum, N., Bergman, C., Edelson, M., & Rocereto, T. (2008). Long-term trajectories of psychological adaptation among women diagnosed with gynecological cancers. *Psychosomatic Medicine*, *70*, 677–687.

Marmot, M. (2005). Social determinants of health inequalities. *Lancet*, *365*, 1099–1104.

Martire, L. M., Druley, J. A., Stephens, M. A. P., & Wojno, W. C. (2002). Negative reactions to received spousal care: Predictors and consequences of miscarried support. *Health Psychology*, *21*, 167–176.

Michael, Y. L., Berkman, L. F., Colditz, G. A., Holmes, M. D., & Kawachi, I. (2002). Social networks and health-related quality of life in breast cancer survivors: A prospective study. *Journal of Psychosomatic Research*, *52*, 285–293.

Milam, J. (2006). Posttraumatic growth and HIV disease progression. *Journal of Consulting and Clinical Psychology*, *74*, 817–827.

Miller, G., Chen, E., & Cole, S. W. (2009). Health psychology: Developing biologically plausible models linking the social world and physical health. *Annual Review of Psychology*, *60*, 501–524.

Minkler, M., Fuller-Thomson, E., & Guralnik, J. M. (2006). Gradient of disability across the socioeconomic spectrum in the United States. *New England Journal of Medicine*, *355*, 695–703.

Miovic, M., & Block, S. (2007). Psychiatric disorders in advanced cancer. *Cancer*, *110*, 1665–1676.

Molloy, G. J., Perkins-Porras, L., Strike, P. C., & Steptoe, A. (2008). Social networks and partner stress as predictors of adherence to medication, rehabilitation attendance, and quality of life following acute coronary syndrome. *Health Psychology*, *27*, 52–58.

Montgomery, G. H., & Bovbjerg, D. H. (2001). Specific response expectancies predict anticipatory nausea during chemotherapy for breast cancer. *Journal of Consulting and Clinical Psychology*, *69*, 831–835.

Montgomery, G. H., & Bovbjerg, D. H. (2004). Presurgery distress and specific response expectancies predict postsurgery outcomes in surgery patients confronting breast cancer. *Health Psychology*, *23*, 381–387.

Moos, R. H., & Schaefer, J. A. (1993). Coping resources and processes: Current concepts and measures. In L. Goldberger & S. Breznitz (Eds.), *Handbook of stress: Theoretical and clinical aspects* (2nd ed., pp. 234–257). New York, NY: Free Press.

Moskowitz, J. T., Hult, J. R., Bussolari, C., & Acree, M. (2009). What works in coping with HIV? A meta-analysis with implications for coping with serious illness. *Psychological Bulletin*, *135*, 121–141.

Müller-Tasch, T., Frankenstein, L., Holzapfel, N., Schellberg, D., Löwe, B., Nelles, M., … Herzog, W. (2008). Panic disorder in patients with chronic heart failure. *Journal of Psychosomatic Research*, *64*, 299–303.

Murphy, B. M., Elliott, P. C., Worcester, M. U. C., Higgins, R. O., Le Grander, M. R., Roberts, S. B., & Goble, A. J. (2008). Trajectories and predictors of anxiety and depression in women during the 12 months following an acute cardiac event. *British Journal of Health Psychology*, *13*, 135–153.

Myers, H. F. (2009). Ethnicity- and socio-economic status–related stresses in context: An integrative review and conceptual model. *Journal of Behavioral Medicine*, *32*, 9–19.

Nagurney, A. J. (2008). The effects of unmitigated communion and life events among women with fibromyalgia syndrome. *Journal of Health Psychology*, *13*, 520–528.

Nolen-Hoeksema, S. (2008). It is not what you have; it is what you do with it: Support for Addis's gendered responding framework. *Clinical Psychology: Science and Practice*, *15*, 178–181.

O'Cleirigh, C., Ironson, G., Weiss, A., & Costa, P. T., Jr. (2007). Conscientiousness predicts disease progression (CD4 number and viral load) in people living with HIV. *Health Psychology, 26,* 473–480.

Park, C. L., Fenster, J. R., Suresh, D. P., & Bliss, D. E. (2006). Social support, appraisals, and coping as predictors of depression in congestive heart failure patients. *Psychology & Health*, *21*, 773–789.

Park, C. L., Lechner, S. C., Antoni, M. H., & Stanton, A. L. (Eds.). (2009). *Medical illness and positive life change: Can crisis lead to personal transformation?* Washington, DC: American Psychological Association.

Penedo, F. J., Antoni, M. H., & Schneiderman, N. (2008). *Cognitive-behavioral stress management for prostate cancer recovery: Facilitator guide. Treatments that work*. New York, NY: Oxford University Press.

Penley, J. A., Tomaka, J., & Wiebe, J. S. (2002). The association of coping to physical and psychological health outcomes: A meta-analytic review. *Journal of Behavioral Medicine*, *25*, 551–603.

Petersen, L. R., Clark, M., Novotny, P., Kung, S., Sloan, J. A., Patten, C. A., … Colligan, R. C. (2008). Relationship of optimism-pessimism and health-relation quality of life in breast cancer survivors. *Journal of Psychosocial Oncology*, *26*, 15–32.

Piro, M., Zeldow, P. B., Knight, S. J., Mytko, J. J., & Gradishar, W. J. (2001). The relationship between agentic and communal personality traits and psychosocial adjustment to breast cancer. *Journal of Clinical Psychology in Medical Settings*, *8*, 263–271.

Polsky, D., Doshi, J. A., Marcus, S., Oslin, D., Rothbard, A., Thomas, N., & Thompson, C. L. (2005). Long-term risk for depressive symptoms after a medical diagnosis. *Archives of Internal Medicine*, *165*, 1260–1266.

Prowe, B. D., Hamiliton, J., Hannock, N., Johnson, N., Finnie, R., Ko, J., & Boggan, M. (2006). Quality of life of African American cancer survivors: A review of the literature. *Cancer*, *109*, 435–445.

Rabin, C., Leventhal, H., & Goodin, S. (2004). Conceptualizations of disease timeline predicts posttreatment distress in breast cancer patients. *Health Psychology*, *23*, 407–412.

Raison, C. L., & Miller, A. H. (2001). The neuroimmunology of stress and depression. *Seminars in Clinical Neuropsychiatry*, *6*, 277–294.

Rasmussen, H. N., Scheier, M. F., & Greenhouse, J. B. (2009). Optimism and physical health: A meta-analytic review. *Annals of Behavioral Medicine*, *37*, 239–256.

Rasmussen, H. N., Wrosch, C., Scheier, M. F., & Carver, C. S. (2006). Self-regulation processes and health: The importance of optimism and goal adjustment. *Journal of Personality*, *74*, 1721–1748.

Read, J. G., & Gorman, B. K. (2006). Gender inequalities in US adult health: The interplay of race and ethnicity. *Social Science & Medicine*, *62*, 1045–1065.

Reeve, B. B., Potosky, A. L., Smith, A. W., Han, P. K., Hays, R. D., Davis, W. W., … Clauser, S. B. (2009). Impact of cancer on health-related quality of life of older Americans. *Journal of the National Cancer Institute*, *101*, 860–868.

Reisine, S., Fifield, J., Walsh, S. J., & Feinn, R. (2001). Factors associated with continued employment among patients with rheumatoid arthritis: A survival model. *Journal of Rheumatology*, *28*, 2400–2408.

Revenson, T. A. (1993). The role of social support with rheumatic disease. In S. Neuman & M. Shipley (Eds.), Psychological aspects of rheumatic disease. *Balliere's Clinical Rheumatology*, *7*(2), 377–396. London, England: Balliere Tindal.

Revenson, T. A. (2003). Scenes from a marriage: Examining support, coping and gender within the context of chronic illness. In J. Suls & K. A. Wallston (Eds.), *Social psychological foundations of health and illness* (pp. 530–559). Malden, MA: Blackwell.

Revenson, T. A., & Pranikoff, J. R. (2005). A contextual approach to treatment decision making among breast cancer survivors. *Health Psychology*, *24*, S93–S98.

Rieckmann, N., Gerin, W., Kronish, I. M., Burg, M. M., Chaplin, W. F., Kong, G., … Davidson, K. W. (2006). Course of depressive symptoms and medication adherence after acute coronary syndromes: An electronic medication monitoring study. *Journal of the American College of Cardiology*, *48*, 2218–2222.

Roberts, M. C. (Ed.). (2003). *Handbook of pediatric psychology* (3rd ed.). New York, NY: Guilford Press.

Roesch, S. C., Adams, L., Hines, A., Palmores, A., Vyas, P., Tran, C., & Vaughn, A. A. (2005). Coping with prostate cancer: A meta-analytic review. *Journal of Behavioral Medicine*, *28*, 281–93.

Roesch, S., & Weiner, B. (2001). A meta-analytic review of coping with illness: Do causal attributions matter? *Journal of Psychosomatic Research*, *41*, 813–819.

Rose, J. H., Kypriotakis, G., Bowman, K. F., Einstadter, D., O'Toole, E. E., Mechekano, R., & Dawson, N. V. (2009). Patterns of adaptation in patients living long term with advanced cancer. *Cancer, 115,* 4298–4310.

Ruiz, J. M., Matthews, K. A., Scheier, M. F., & Schulz, R. (2006). Does who you marry matter for your health? Influence of patients' and spouses' personality on their partners' psychological well-being following coronary artery bypass surgery. *Journal of Personality and Social Psychology, 91,* 255–267.

Rutledge, T., Reis, V. A., Linke, S. E., Greenberg, B. H., & Mills, P. J. (2006). Depression in heart failure: A meta-analytic review of prevalence, intervention effects, and associations with clinical outcomes. *Journal of the American College of Cardiology, 48,* 1527–1537.

Scheier, M. F., & Bridges, M. W. (1995). Person variables and health: Personality predispositions and acute psychological states as shared determinants of disease. *Psychosomatic Medicine, 57,* 255–268.

Scheier, M. F., Matthews, K. A., Owens, J. F., Magovern, G. J., Lefebvre, R. C., Abbott, A. R., & Carver, C. S. (2003). Dispositional optimism and recovery from coronary artery bypass surgery: The beneficial effects on physical and psychological well-being. In P. Salovey & A. J. Rothman (Eds.), *Social psychology of health: Key readings in social psychology* (pp. 342–361). New York, NY: Psychology Press.

Schou, I., Ekeberg, Ø., & Ruland, C. M. (2005). The mediating role of appraisal and coping in the relationship between optimism-pessimism and quality of life. *Psycho-Oncology, 14,* 718–727.

Schreurs, K. M. G., & de Ridder, D. T. D. (1997). Integration of coping and social support perspectives: Implications for the study of adaptation to chronic diseases. *Clinical Psychology Review, 17,* 89–112.

Schroevers, M., Kraaij, V., & Garnefski, N. (2008). How do cancer patients manage unattainable personal goals and regulate their emotions? *British Journal of Health Psychology, 13,* 551–562.

Scott-Sheldon, L. A., Kalichman, S. C., Carey, M. P., & Fielder, R. L. (2008). Stress management interventions for HIV+ adults: A meta-analysis of randomized controlled trials, 1989 to 2006. *Health Psychology, 27,* 129–139.

Segerstrom, S. C. (2005). Optimism and immunity: Do positive thoughts always lead to positive effects? *Brain, Behavior, & Immunity, 19,* 195–200.

Sephton, S. E., Dhabhar, F. S., Keuroghlian, A. S., Giese-Davis, J., McEwen, B. S., Ionan, A. C., & Spiegel, D. (2009). Depression, cortisol, and suppressed cell-mediated immunity in metastatic breast cancer. *Brain, Behavior, & Immunity, 23,* 1148–1155.

Shnek, Z. M., Irvine, J., Stewart, D., & Abbey, S. (2001). Psychological factors and depressive symptoms in ischemic heart disease. *Health Psychology, 20,* 141–45.

Siegel, S. D., Molton, I., Penedo, F. J., Llabre, M. M., Kinsinger, D. P., Traeger, L., . . . Antoni, M. H. (2007). Interpersonal sensitivity, partner support, patient-physician communication, and sexual functioning in men recovering from prostate carcinoma. *Journal of Personality Assessment, 89,* 303–309.

Slatkowsky-Christensen, B., Mowinckel, P., Loge, J. H., & Kvien, T. K. (2009). Health-related quality of life in women with symptomatic hand osteoarthritis: A comparison with rheumatoid arthritis patients, healthy controls, and normative data. *Arthritis and Rheumatism, 57,* 1404–1409.

Smith, B. W., & Zautra, A. J. (2002). The role of personality in exposure and reactivity to interpersonal stress in relation to arthritis disease activity and negative affect in women. *Health Psychology, 21,* 81–88.

Smith, B. W., & Zautra, A. J. (2008a). The effects of anxiety and depression on weekly pain in women with arthritis. *Pain, 138,* 198–209.

Smith, B. W., & Zautra, A. J. (2008b). Vulnerability and resilience in women with arthritis: Test of a two-factor model. *Journal of Consulting and Clinical Psychology, 76,* 799–810.

Smith, C. A., & Wallston, K. A. (1992). Adaptation in patients with chronic rheumatoid arthritis. *Health Psychology, 11,* 151–162.

Smith, D. J., Kyle, S., Forty, L., Cooper, C., Walters, J., Russell, E., ... Craddock, N. (2008). Differences in depressive symptom profile between males and females. *Journal of Affective Disorders, 108,* 279–284.

Stanton, A. L. (2011). Regulating emotions during stressful experiences: The adaptive utility of coping through emotional approach. In S. Folkman (Ed.), *Oxford handbook of stress, health, and coping* (pp. 369–386). New York, NY: Oxford University Press.

Stanton, A. L., Bower, J. E., & Low, C. A. (2006). Posttraumatic growth after cancer. In L. G. Calhoun & R. G. Tedeschi (Eds.), *Handbook of posttraumatic growth: Research and practice* (pp. 138–175). Mahwah, NJ: Erlbaum.

Stanton, A. L., Danoff-Burg, S., Cameron, C. L., Bishop, M. M., Collins, C. A., Kirk, S. B., ... Twillman, R. (2000). Emotionally expressive coping predicts psychological and physical adjustment to breast cancer. *Journal of Consulting and Clinical Psychology, 68,* 875–882.

Stanton, A. L., Revenson, T. A., & Tennen, H. (2007). Health psychology: Psychological adjustment to chronic disease. *Annual Review of Psychology, 58,* 565–592.

Stanton, A. L., & Snider, P. R. (1993). Coping with a breast cancer diagnosis: A prospective study. *Health Psychology, 12*, 16–23.

Steginga, S. K., & Occhipinti, S. (2006). Dispositional optimism as a predictor of men's decision-related distress after localized prostate cancer. *Health Psychology, 25*, 135–143.

Sterba, K. R., DeVellis, R. F., Lewis, M. A., DeVellis, B. M., Jordan, J. M., & Baucom, D. H. (2008). Effect of couple illness perception congruence on psychological adjustment in women with rheumatoid arthritis. *Health Psychology, 27*, 221–229.

Stommel, M., Kurtz, M. E., Kurtz, J. C., Given, C. W., & Given, B. A. (2004). A longitudinal analysis of the course of depressive symptomatology in geriatric patients with cancer of the breast, colon, lung, or prostate. *Health Psychology, 23*, 564–73.

Strand, E. B., Zautra, A., Thoresen, M., Odegard, S., Uhlig, T., & Finset, A. (2006). Positive affect as a factor of resilience in the pain-negative affect relationship in patients with rheumatoid arthritis. *Journal of Psychosomatic Research, 60*, 477–484.

Strating, M. M. H., Suurmeijer, T. P. B., & van Schur, W. H. (2006). Disability, social support, and distress in rheumatoid arthritis: Results from a thirteen-year prospective study. *Arthritis & Rheumatism, 55*, 736–744.

Suls, J., & Fletcher, B. (1985). The relative efficacy of avoidant and nonavoidant coping strategies: A meta-analysis. *Health Psychology, 4*, 249–288.

Taylor, C. L. C., Badr, H., Lee, J. H., Fossella, F., Pisters, K., Gritz, E. R., & Schover, L. (2008). Lung cancer patients and their spouses: Psychological and relationship functioning within 1 month of treatment initiation. *Annals of Behavioral Medicine, 36*, 129–140.

Taylor, S. E. (1983). Adjustment to threatening events: A theory of cognitive adaptation. *American Psychologist, 38*, 1161–1173.

Taylor, S. E. (2007). Social support. In H. S. Friedman & R. C. Silver (Eds.), *The Oxford handbook of health psychology* (pp. 145–171). New York, NY: Oxford University Press.

Taylor, S. E., & Brown, J. D. (1988). Illusion and well-being: A social psychological perspective on mental health. *Psychological Bulletin, 103*, 193–210.

Taylor, S. E., Klein, L. C., Lewis, B. P., Gruenewald, T. L., Gurung, R. A. R., & Updegraff, J. A. (2000). Biobehavioral responses to stress in females: Tend-and-befriend, not flight-or-flight. *Psychological Review, 107*, 411–429.

Taylor, S. E., & Stanton, A. L. (2007). Coping resources, coping processes, and mental health. *Annual Review of Clinical Psychology, 3*, 377–401.

Tedeschi, R. G., & Calhoun, L. G. (1995). *Trauma and transformation: Growing in the aftermath of suffering.* Thousand Oaks, CA: Sage.

Temoshok, L. R., Waldstein, S. R., Wald, R. L., Garzino-Demo, A., Synowski, S. J., Sun, L., & Wiley, J. A. (2008). Type C coping, alexithymia, and heart rate reactivity are associated independently and differentially with specific immune mechanisms linked to HIV progression. *Brain, Behavior, & Immunity, 22*, 781–792.

Tennen, H., & Affleck, G. (2000). The perception of personal control: Sufficiently important to warrant careful scrutiny. *Personality & Social Psychology Bulletin, 26*, 152–156.

Tennen, H., & Affleck, G. (2009). Assessing positive life change: In search of meticulous methods. In C. L. Park, S. C. Lechner, M. H. Antoni, & A. L. Stanton (Eds.), *Medical illness and positive life change: Can crisis lead to personal transformation?* (pp. 31–49). Washington, DC: American Psychological Association.

Tennen, H., Affleck, G., & Zautra, A. (2006). Depression history and coping with chronic pain: A daily process analysis. *Health Psychology, 25*, 370–379.

Thompson, S. C., Sobolew-Shubin, A., Galbraith, M. E., Schwankovsky, L., & Cruzen, D. (1993). Maintaining perceptions of control: Finding perceived control in low-control circumstances. *Journal of Personality and Social Psychology, 64*, 293–304.

Thornton, L. M., Andersen, B. L., Crespin, T. R., & Carson, W. E. (2007). Individual trajectories in stress covary with immunity during recovery from cancer diagnosis and treatments. *Brain, Behavior, & Immunity, 21*, 185–194.

Tindle, H. A., Chang, Y. F., Kuller, L. H., Manson, J. E., Robinson, J. G., Rosal, M. C., … Matthews, K. A. (2009). Optimism, cynical hostility, and incident coronary heart disease and mortality in the Women's Health Initiative. Circulation. doi:10.1161/CIRCULATIONAHA.108.827642

Tomich, P. L., & Helgeson, V. S. (2006). Cognitive adaptation theory and breast cancer recurrence: Are there limits? *Journal of Consulting and Clinical Psychology, 74*, 980–987.

Trudeau, K. J., Danoff-Burg, S., Revenson, T. A., & Paget, S. (2003). Gender differences in agency and communion among patients with rheumatoid arthritis. *Sex Roles, 49*, 303–311.

Trunzo, J. J., & Pinto, B. M. (2003). Social support as a mediator of optimism and distress in breast cancer survivors. *Journal of Consulting and Clinical Psychology, 71,* 805–811.

Uchino, B. (2006). Social support and health: A review of physiological processes potentially underlying links to disease outcomes. *Journal of Behavioral Medicine, 29,* 377–387.

Ullrich, P. M., Lutgendorf, S. K., & Stapleton, J. T. (2002). Social constraints and depression in HIV infection: Effects of sexual orientation and area of residence. *Journal of Social and Clinical Psychology, 21,* 46–66.

Van Jaarsveld, C. H. M., Ranchor, A. V., Sanderman, R., Ormel, J., & Kempen, G. I. J. M. (2005). The role of premorbid psychological attributes in short- and long-term adjustment after cardiac disease: A prospective study in the elderly in the Netherlands. *Social Science and Medicine, 60,* 1035–1045.

Van Middendorp, H., Geenen, R., Sorbi, M. J., van Doornen, L. J. P., & Bijlsma, J. W. J. (2005). Emotion regulation predicts change of perceived health in patients with rheumatoid arthritis. *Annals of Rheumatic Diseases, 64,* 1071–1074.

Van 't Land, H., Verdurmen, J., Ten Have, M., Van Dorsselaer, S., Beekman, A., & De Graaf, R. (2010). The association between arthritis and psychiatric disorders; results from a longitudinal population-based study. *Journal of Psychosomatic Research, 68,* 187–193.

Vileikyte, L., Leventhal, H., Gonzalez, J. S., Peyrot, M., Rubin, R. R., Ulbrecht, J. S., … Boulton, A. J. (2005). Diabetic peripheral neuropathy and depressive symptoms: The association revisited. *Diabetes Care, 28,* 2378–2383.

Waldman, S. V., Blumenthal, J. A., Babyak, M. A., Sherwood, A., Sketch, M., Davidson, J., & Watkins, L. L. (2009). Ethnic differences in the treatment of depression in patients with ischemic heart disease. *American Heart Journal, 157,* 77–83.

Waltz, M., Badura, B., Pfaff, H., & Schott, T. (1988). Marriage and the psychological consequences of a heart attack: A longitudinal study of adaptation to chronic illness after 3 years. *Social Science and Medicine, 27,* 149–158.

Weaver, K. E., Llabre, M. M., Duran, R. E., Antoni, M. M., Penedo, F. J., Ironson, G., & Schneiderman, N. (2005). A stress and coping model of medication adherence and viral load in HIV+ men and women on highly active antiretroviral therapy (HAART). *Health Psychology, 24,* 385–392.

Whitfield, K. E., Weidner, G., Clark, R., & Anderson, N. B. (2002). Sociodemographic diversity and behavioral medicine. *Journal of Consulting and Clinical Psychology, 70,* 463–481.

Whooley, M. A., De Jonge, P., Vittinghoff, E., Otte, C., Moos. R., Carney, R. M., & Browner, W. S. (2008). Depressive symptoms, health behaviors, and risk of cardiovascular events in patients with coronary heart disease. *JAMA, 300,* 2379–2388.

Wright, C. E., Strike, P. C., Brydon, L., & Steptoe, A. (2005). Acute inflammation and negative mood: Mediation by cytokine activation. *Brain, Behavior, & Immunity, 19,* 345–350.

Wrosch, C., Scheier, M. F., Miller, G. E., Schulz, R., & Carver, C. S. (2003). Adaptive self-regulation of unattainable goals: Goal disengagement, goal reengagement, and subjective well-being. *Personality and Social Psychology Bulletin, 29,* 1494–1508.

Yali, A. M., & Revenson, T. A. (2004). How changes in population demographics will impact health psychology: Incorporating a broader notion of cultural competence into the field. *Health Psychology, 23,* 147–155.

Yang, H. C., Brothers, B. M., & Andersen, B. L. (2008). Stress and quality of life in breast cancer recurrence: Moderation or mediation of coping? *Annals of Behavioral Medicine, 35,* 188–197.

Yang, H. C., & Schuler, T. A. (2009). Marital quality and survivorship: Slowed recovery for breast cancer patients in distressed relationships. *Cancer, 115,* 217–228.

Zachariae, R., Paulesen, K., Mehlsen, M., Jensen, A. B., Johansson, A., & Von der Maase, H. (2007). Anticipatory nausea: The role of individual differences related to sensory perception and autonomic reactivity. *Annals of Behavioral Medicine, 33,* 69–79.

Zautra, A. J., Fasman, R., Parish, B. P., & Davis, M. C. (2007). Daily fatigue in women with osteoarthritis, rheumatoid arthritis, and fibromyalgia. *Pain, 128,* 128–135.

11 Measuring Sexual Quality of Life

Ten Recommendations for Health Psychologists

Sara I. McClelland
University of Michigan

Over the past 20 years, sexual quality of life has become of increasing interest to psychologists studying quality of life with ill and/or aging populations. As people are living longer with chronic illnesses, the maintenance of sexual health has become a topic of concern and an essential domain of overall quality of life (QoL; see Arrington, Cofrancesco, & Wu, 2004). This concern has mainly focused on the retention of sexual function after diagnosis and treatment. At the same time, the parameters of the definition of sexual function have been dramatically affected by the rapid development of new treatment techniques and pharmaceutical interventions aimed to treat sexual dysfunction. Together, this interest in maintaining patients' sexual health and testing new sexual function interventions in patient populations has generated a great deal of empirical research in a relatively short period of time. For example, from 1980 to 1989, only 607 articles were published on sexual function, sexual dysfunction, and sexual health. This number grew to 1,428 articles from 1990 to 1999. By the turn of the 21st century, we see this number jump to 5,202 articles published from 2000 to 2009—a nearly ninefold increase over two decades. This emerging body of research has undoubtedly helped to guide clinical interventions and to increase quality of life for patients and their intimate partners. However, questions remain as to whether definitions and operationalizations of sexual function commonly used in research settings are sufficient to describe the range and scope of sexual quality of life (SQoL) experienced by both men and women, especially those who are ill, recovering from illness, or living with a chronic illness.

This chapter offers 10 suggestions to help guide researchers in this burgeoning area of study. The recommendations include measurement as well as research design considerations in order to help enrich researchers' understanding of the psychological qualities of sexual quality of life as experienced across diverse populations who are coping with aging and/or conditions of illness, and perhaps treatment. Although there are a number of resources from a psychometric viewpoint that can help guide researchers as they choose among the various scales that are currently available to measure sexual health and function (Barton, Wilwerding, Carpenter, & Loprinzi, 2004; Berman, Berman, Zierak, & Marley, 2002; Corona, Jannini, & Maggi, 2006; Meston & Derogatis, 2002; Rosen, 2002), this chapter has a more targeted objective: to help researchers capture important and often underexplored aspects of sexual quality of life in their own work, whether they are designing new measurement techniques or using previously validated scales. The aim of this chapter is to raise issues about the conceptualization of sexual quality of life that will inform measurement so that research findings can be increasingly applicable to men and women of all ages, in various types of intimate relationships, and with varying degrees of sexual interactions. Without attention to these definitional issues, researchers run the risk of missing important characteristics of sexual quality of life and ignoring the wide array of sexual expressions that patients experience.

SEXUAL QUALITY OF LIFE AND ILLNESS

For the purposes of this discussion, sexual quality of life is defined as encompassing multiple dimensions that an individual may associate with a healthy and pleasurable sexual life. These include sexual responses, cognitions, and attitudes, as well as dimensions related to intimate relationships and a sense of one's physical body as capable and entitled to experiencing sexual sensations. The physiological dimension of sexual response, and genital response in particular, has often dominated sexual function research. Research on sexuality in illness settings is often characterized by its interest in negative sexual outcomes with a focus on the potential loss of genital response (i.e., erection or lubrication) before or during sexual activity. This extreme focus on the genitals has in large part been a consequence of the changes that have been observed in patients' bodies wrought by illness and its treatments. For example, the research in cancer has consistently found that surgery, radiation, and chemotherapy result in dramatic changes to patients' genitals and, as a result, to their genital and sexual response. For women, these changes may include vaginal stenosis, atrophy and irritation of the mucosa, and inadequate lubrication (Crane & Skibber, 2003; Havenga, Maas, DeRuiter, Welvaart, & Trimbos, 2000; Killackey, 2000; Pocard et al., 2002). For men, these changes may include loss of erectile rigidity, ejaculatory dysfunction, and urinary and bowel dysfunction (Litwin et al., 1998; Schover et al., 2002). Research on these outcomes is essential to help patients and their doctors prepare for the possibility of short- and/or long-term impaired sexual functioning. However, though genital and physiological functioning remain essential components of sexual quality of life, it is important to recognize additional SQoL dimensions, including the psychological, relational, and social contexts in which sexual responsiveness exists. These additional dimensions include addressing sexual activities other than penile-vaginal intercourse, the role of altered body image (not limited to illnesses that affect genital function or appearance), and the effect of gender norms on determinations of what counts as a "successful" sexual activity.

The focus on the physiology of sexual response is in large part a consequence of the model of the human sexual response cycle proposed by Masters and Johnson more than 40 years ago (Masters & Johnson, 1966, 1970). Masters and Johnson's model has remained the most common method to describe the expectation of how a human anticipates and resolves a sexual experience. This model has been the basis for a number of scales used to assess sexual health (Andersen & Cyranowski, 1994; Andersen, Cyranowski, & Espindle, 1999; Rosen et al., 2000; Rosen et al., 1997) and still largely determines the model by which normal sexual responsiveness is assessed. Masters and Johnson's four-phase cycle (excitement, plateau, orgasm, and resolution) has had enormous staying power, in part, because this model guided the development of diagnostic criteria for sexual dysfunction as described in the *Diagnostic and Statistical Manual* (DSM IV; APA, 1994; also DSM IV-TR; APA, 2000), which has been used to guide clinical practice in the United States.

Although this model has come under scrutiny in recent years, particularly in terms of defining female sexual response (Basson, 2000; Kaschak & Tiefer, 2001; Tiefer, 1996, 2004), a detailed discussion of the critiques of the human sexual response is beyond the scope of this chapter. What is important to note is how critiques of "normal sexual response" have in many ways paralleled developments within the research on illness and sexuality. Both of these groups have recently begun to encourage health researchers to look beyond long established models of sexual health and to define "normal" sexuality as more varied than a simple linear progression from desire to activity to orgasm. The challenge remains how best to approach understanding the diverse sexual lives among people facing illness, the changes that illnesses and their treatments bring, and ultimately how sexual well-being is affected by these changes.

For patients and people living with illness, sexual quality of life has been a relatively recent addition to the list of activities that are assumed to be important in research on health-related quality of life (Basson, 2007). For example, in cancer research, sexual health has been shown to play an important role in survivorship trajectories (Gotay & Muroaka, 1998; Hordern, 1999, 2000; NCI, 2004) and is repeatedly cited by patients as an important aspect of their lives they fear will diminish when ill (Yost & Cella, 2003). Research in this area extends to individuals who are coping with sexual outcomes that are a result of office procedures (Inna, Phianmongkhol, & Charoenkwan, 2009), chronic illness (Schmidt, Hofmann, Niederwieser, Kapfhammer, & Bonelli, 2005; Schover & Jensen, 1988), and end-of-life issues (Lemieux, Kaiser, Pereira, & Meadows, 2004; Stausmire, 2004). However, some diseases and some disease sites—for example, breast and prostate cancer—have been more frequently investigated for potential negative sexual outcomes, creating an uneven set of studies in the field of illness and sexuality.

Several factors influence how easily and automatically a disease is associated with potential negative sexual quality of life. Whereas, on the one hand, certain diseases are seen as inherently damaging to sexuality because of the proximity to sexual organs (e.g., gynecological cancers; Gamel, Hengeveld, & Davis, 2000), other diseases are less frequently associated with sexual outcomes and may be more frequently overlooked (e.g., rheumatoid diseases; for exceptions, see Majerovitz & Revenson, 1994; Schmidt et al., 2005; van Berlo et al., 2007). Some treatment regimens are seen as directly damaging sexual function, for example, prostate surgery's effect on erectile function or chemotherapy's impact on vaginal lubrication (e.g., Schover et al. 2002), whereas others may negatively impact sexual relationships through more indirect routes. For example, such physical changes as the presence of a stoma after colorectal cancer surgery may affect a patient's body image, which may also create threats to sexual identity and self-esteem, personal control over bodily functions, and ultimately negatively affect intimacy with a partner (Sprangers, Taal, Aaronson, & te Velde, 1995).

In addition, some disease sites are associated with more subtle aspects of sexuality, including feeling a loss of masculinity or femininity as a result of diagnoses or treatment. This result might include, for example, the incapacity to perform penetrative sex with a partner or the loss of a woman's breasts as a result of mastectomy (Fergus, Gray, & Fitch, 2002; Lund-Nielsen, 2005; Oliffe, 2005). The close association between sexual organs and gender ideals within sexual relationships encourages researchers, patients, and their partners who fall within these disease categories to consider sexual function and adjustment issues as primary issues. At the same time, individuals who have illnesses that do not involve sexual organs may not be counseled to guard against these effects (e.g., kidney or liver disease; Sorrell & Brown, 2006). In sum, whereas concerns of sexual organs, sexual identity, and intimate relationships may inherently be of interest to patients and their families regardless of their disease, disease site, or treatment regimen, the research on these issues has concentrated on a much smaller and specific set of patients.

This uneven attention to sexuality concerns has important outcomes: It can dramatically influence the frequency with which doctors question their patients about their sexual health. For example, in a survey of rheumatologists, only 12% of patients were screened for sexual activity (Britto, Rosenthal, Taylor, & Passo, 2000, cited in Tristano, 2009). Reasons offered by rheumatologists for this low screening pattern rate were time constraints, discomfort with the subject, and ambivalence about whether such screening is in their domain. The degree to which an illness is associated with potential negative SQoL outcomes influences the amount of information available for patients and doctors alike, as well as the quality research on that disease and its treatments.

One small indication of this uneven level of interest in sexual health across disease types can be observed in how frequently major U.S. foundations dedicated to supporting funding, research, and patient education address the issue of sexual health. A quick scan of foundations' Web sites, including the American Cancer Society (http://www.cancer.org), the Multiple Sclerosis Foundation (http://www.msfacts.org), the Arthritis Foundation (http://www.arthritis.org), and the Cardiovascular Disease Foundation (http://www.cvdf.org), demonstrated the enormous variability in the amount of SQoL information provided by these foundations. For example, the American Cancer Society's Web site includes 25 Web pages about sexual health and intimate relationships, for a total of 32,792 words on the subject. In comparison, the Arthritis Foundation's Web site includes two pages, for a total of 691 words on the subject. Neither the American College of Rheumatology Research and Education Foundation Web site nor the Cardiovascular Disease Foundation Web site includes any information pertaining to sexual health. Although this varying amount of Web site information is one, albeit limited, indicator of the varying level of attention that a topic receives, it demonstrates that sexual quality of life is viewed as more salient within certain disease types than others.

Finally, the saliency of the association between sexual health and an illness may influence patient and partner assumptions and expectations about changes in sexual function caused by or attributed to the illness. In research with ill participants, sexual dysfunction can be traced to many possible different sources, including aging, illness effects, and treatment effects, as well as surgery and/or medication and any combination of these. This complex set of etiologies for sexual dysfunction sets sexuality research with ill populations apart from sexuality research with healthy people, where the origin of sexual problems is often treated as emerging from purely psychological causes within the person or relational issues (see Heiman, 2002). This complex set of co-occurring factors means that health psychologists working on sexuality not only can improve quality of life among patients and their partners, but also must define sexual health in a way that addresses an enormous diversity of human experience.

At the same time, the complexity that health psychologists must deal with has the potential to shape the field of sexuality research more broadly. Individuals throughout the life span are contending with multiple influences on their sexuality, changes in their body as a result of illness and/or aging, and an evolving set of concerns relating to their sexual lives. Health psychologists are in the unique position to theorize and empirically observe this complex set of factors in their research and contribute to the emerging body of research on sexual quality of life for all individuals.

DEFINING AND MEASURING SEXUAL QUALITY OF LIFE

Quality-of-life research among people facing serious physical illness has grown tremendously over the last 20 years. The best exemplar is in the area of cancer, where new treatments and longer survivorship trajectories have encouraged the development of scales and interventions aimed to improve aspects of a cancer survivor's life (Bottomley, 2002; Fortune-Greeley et al., 2009; Jeffery et al., 2009; Penson, Wenzel, Vergote, & Cella, 2006). Within this larger body of quality-of-life research lies the domain of sexual quality of life.

A number of self-report instruments to assess quality of life have been developed and validated in diverse populations. In some instruments, sexual function subscales are one domain within the larger construct of quality of life. Other instruments include sexual health items in disease- or site-specific modules (e.g., EORTC QLQ 30 core questionnaire and breast cancer module QLQ-BR23; Aaronson et al., 1993; Sprangers et al., 1996; and the FACT-G and FACT-B; Cella et al., 1993; Sprangers, Cull, Groenvold, Bjordal, Blazeby, & Aaronson, 1998; Brady et al., 1997). In these QoL measures, items tapping sexual desire and satisfaction have provided researchers with ways to track the effects of treatment effects (e.g., Robinson, Saliken, Donnelly, Barnes, & Guyn, 2000), develop psychosocial interventions (see Stanton, 2006, for discussion), and measure change over time (e.g., change from end of treatment to 12 months post-treatment; Jensen et al., 2003). These types of data have been essential in helping guide interventions, increase patient education, and have provided both patients and providers with enormous insight into how sexual quality of life is affected by illness.

These disease- and disease site–specific measures have, however, been limited in how much detail they can include for each dimension of QoL, usually including at most three to five items to measure sexual well-being and often only one item pertaining to sexual quality of life. These targeted QoL sexual function subscales lend themselves to reducing patient burden and increasing clinical efficacy, but they reduce the ability for such psychological concepts as sexual adjustment and adaption to illness to be understood more broadly.

In addition to scales that have been developed to study specific diseases and disease sites, there have also been scales used to study sexual function that, though not developed specifically to study patients with physical illnesses, have been taken up enthusiastically by researchers studying ill populations (e.g., Derogatis, 1997; Taylor, Rosen, Leiblum, 1994). Two scales that are most commonly used by health psychologists are the International Index of Erectile Function (IIEF; Rosen et al., 1997) and the Female Sexual Function Index (FSFI; Rosen et al., 2000). These instruments are used widely in clinical, psychological, and pharmaceutical research and have become the gold standard for research on sexual function in clinical samples of all types. As an indicator of the popularity of these two measures, according to the Web of Science (http://thomsonreuters.com/products_services/science/ science_products/a-z/web_of_science; searched in January 2010), the IIEF has been cited 1,311 times since its publication in 1997 and the FSFI has been cited 481 times since its publication in 2000.

I will not review measures of sexual function here, as a number of others have done this already (see Arrington et al., 2004; Corona et al., 2006; Cull, 1992; Daker-White, 2002; Jeffery et al., 2009; Jones, 2002; Meston & Derogatis, 2002; Rosen, 2002; West, Vinikoor, & Zolnoun, 2004). The available measures of *sexual function* make enormous contributions to the understanding of many aspects of sexual outcomes but are less effective in assessing *sexual quality of life*, a broader construct that requires attention to an individual's psychological, relational, and physical well-being, in addition to characteristics of sexual health that currently fall outside the scope of sexual function definitions (see DSM IV and IV-TR).

As a step toward theorizing this construct more broadly, I will discuss three central issues when designing research on sexual quality of life: measurement and operationalization decisions, definitions of sex in research settings, and issues of research design in studies of medical populations. My hope is that these recommendations will encourage health psychologists to remain attentive to issues of sexuality as they affect adjustment to illness and reveal the psychological mechanisms underlying sexual well-being that are currently understudied and/or not yet well understood. Because the chapter focuses on definitional and measurement issues, I will not review needs assessments or clinical interventions (see Lenahan, 2004, for discussion of sexual health issues across variety of chronic illnesses; see also Andersen, 2002; Andersen, Shelby, & Golden-Kreutz, 2007). Nor do I discuss the etiology of or sexual sequelae of medical disorders (for discussion, see Basson & Schultz, 2007; Bhasin, Enzlin, Coviello, & Basson, 2007; Clayton & Ramamurthy, 2008; Rees, Fowler, & Maas, 2007). I have also limited this discussion to physical illnesses and have therefore not included discussion of mental illness and sexuality (see Zemishlany & Weizman, 2008). Finally, while I am addressing these recommendations to researchers studying sexuality in the medical context, I am not proposing a general theoretical model to address SQoL issues across all chronic illnesses (see Verschuren, Enzlin, Dijkstra, Geertzen, & Dekker, 2010, for discussion of a generic conceptual framework for studying chronic disease and sexuality).

With an eye on the wide spectrum of research issues that health psychologists contend with in designing research, the 10 recommendations are grouped into three broad areas of interest. The first group of recommendations concern *measurement issues* that researchers face when evaluating sexual quality of life. The recommendations included in this group address measurement from a both a broader theoretical perspective (e.g., the role of gender socialization), as well as from a traditional psychometric perspective (e.g., issues of construct equivalency). The second group of recommendations concerns the *definition of terms* in sexuality research. By evaluating the consequences of limiting which activities and behaviors are included within the parameters of research on sexual health, these recommendations encourage investigators to expand the definition of what "counts" as sex. Finally, the third group of recommendations concern *research design decisions* that an investigator makes about how a study will be conducted and what kinds of questions will be answered by these designs (e.g., using a cross-sectional vs. longitudinal design). Although these 10 recommendations do not address every aspect of the research process, each is designed to address important decisions that health psychologists face when designing research to study sexual quality of life in illness contexts.

TEN RECOMMENDATIONS FOR MEASURING SEXUAL QUALITY OF LIFE AMONG PEOPLE FACING MEDICAL ILLNESS

1. Acknowledge the Role of Gender Socialization in Sexual Appraisals

Many research findings regarding sexual outcomes are interpreted as the result of simple sex differences (i.e., men and women rate their level of sexual satisfaction differently). However, an alternative perspective emphasizes the impact of gender role socialization when understanding why men and women do this. In an *American Psychologist* review on men, masculinity, and help seeking, Addis and Mahalik (2003) defined the gender role socialization perspective as follows: "Role socialization paradigms begin with the assumption that men and women learn gendered attitudes and behaviors from cultural values, norms, and ideologies about what it means to be men and women" (p. 7). Expanding on this definition, Range and Jenkins (2010) defined gender socialization as the process by which women and men learn that certain feelings, thoughts, and behaviors are appropriate depending on gender. For example, women are commonly taught, through both verbal and nonverbal cues, that expressions of nurturance and warmth are highly valued, whereas men are commonly instructed that these same expressions are negatively valued. These messages coalesce, and over the life course these gendering practices result in men and women developing varied expectations concerning sexual norms, relationships, and experiences (see McClelland, 2010, for discussion of gendered development of sexual expectations).

Researchers have argued that the sexual domain is one of the most powerful areas in which men and women feel pressure to enact gender roles (Sanchez, Crocker, & Bioke, 2005). Although there is a history of documenting gender differences in sexual outcomes and attitudes (Kinsey, Pomeroy, & Martin 1948; Kinsey, Pomeroy, Martin, & Gebhard, 1953; Oliver & Hyde, 1993; Peterson & Hyde, 2010), research on the mechanisms that link gender socialization with sexual outcomes is much more recent. For example, Kiefer and Sanchez (2007) found that gender norm conformity affected sexual passivity, which was, in turn, associated with women's reduced rates of sexual arousal, sexual function, and sexual satisfaction. In addition, research has demonstrated links between gender conformity and increased rates of consenting to unwanted sex with male partners (Bay-Cheng & Eliseo-Arras, 2008) and lower rates of sexual pleasure (Sanchez et al., 2005). In their research on sexual compliance in heterosexual relationships, Impett and Peplau (2003) articulated how gender norms affected what men and women prioritized when they evaluated their level of sexual satisfaction.

Unfortunately, much of the research on gender socialization has remained outside the scope of the literature on sexual adaptation and medical illness, but this is beginning to change. For example, in a study of women diagnosed with vulvodynia (i.e., vulval pain and vulval vestibulitis), Marriott and Thompson (2008) found that women prioritized their male partner's sexual enjoyment to the extent that they often participated in sexual activities they found extremely painful. As one woman stated, "He used to say, am I hurting you? And I used to say no, and clench my teeth and think, actually I'm in agony here" (p. 251). In a related body of research, investigators have looked extensively at the impact of breast cancer on women's sense of femininity, body image, and intimate relationships with partners (Avis, Crawford, & Manuel, 2004; Pikler & Winterowd, 2003). In interviews with 40 individuals who had been treated with surgery for a variety of chronic illnesses, Manderson (1999) found that women were more self-conscious of their general appearance than the men in the sample and reported feeling less desirable because of changes in body parts beyond just their sexual organs.

Men experience the negative effects of gender norms on their sexual health as well. Schover et al. (2004) developed the Erectile Dysfunction Help-Seeking model in order to measure how traditional masculine attitudes about sex could inhibit help-seeking behavior; men with prostate cancer who held more traditional beliefs about sex and gender roles were less likely to seek medical help for erectile dysfunction. In an interview study of low-income Latino and African American men,

Maliski, Rivera, Connor, Lopez, and Litwin (2008) found participants struggled to maintain a masculine image of themselves during treatment for prostate cancer and its sequelae and in particular, they struggled with the loss of ideal male sexual performance. Participants discussed what it meant to "not being able to be united with my wife," and a fear of losing the partner because of the inability to have an erection (p. 1614). Interestingly, participants also revealed that when they were with other male friends, they talked as if they were still sexually active when, in fact, they were not. The authors conclude, "By doing this, men were able to maintain a public masculine image consistent with the image they perceived others to hold" (p. 1614), a finding that highlights the often powerful and sometimes restrictive role that gender socialization can have in individuals' lives.

Gender norms not only influence individuals' sexual health outcomes but also can inhibit the quality of data that researchers collect by overdetermining what participants report in research settings. In a cognitive debriefing study designed to assess how respondents interpreted the meaning of scale items, McCabe, Tanner, and Heiman (2010) found that participants' responses to questions about sex often conformed to gender norms even though their own personal descriptions of sexual experiences and relationships often contradicted these same gender norms. In other words, there is a strong pull for participants to endorse traditional gender norms for both themselves and their partners when asked about sex and sexuality in research settings.

When asking participants to recall the quality, frequency, or evaluation of their sexual experiences and/or relationships, researchers often forget that these responses are highly influenced by social norms. For example, in an experimental study examining how research conditions affect men's and women's reported rates of sexual experiences and attitudes, investigators examined how responses to sex questions varied over three conditions (Alexander & Fisher, 2003). In one condition, the respondents believed their answers were anonymous; in a second condition, respondents believed their responses might be seen by a peer; in a third condition, respondents answered while they were attached to a nonfunctioning polygraph (known as the bogus pipeline methodology). With each level of exposure, women's responses varied more than did men's. For example, more women reported masturbating and viewing erotica when attached to the polygraph than when responding in the anonymous condition. The authors conclude that "reports of sex differences based on self-reports may reflect conformity to normative expectations for men and women rather than actual differences in behavior" (2003, p. 33). These findings, and studies that have replicated them (e.g., Fisher, 2007, 2009; Lucas & Parkhill, 2009), make clear the challenge involved in designing studies that both prioritize the individuals' experience through the use of self-report measures and at the same time account for the (often unconscious) role that social norms play when participants decide how comfortable they are expressing aspects of their sexual experience and behaviors.

Taking this complex range of factors into account is not a simple or easy task. First, sexual quality of life should be measured independently for men and women. Sexual experiences are unique experiences for men and women both physiologically and socially, unlike fatigue, for example. Ignoring the uniquely gendered conditions of sexuality means that investigators risk obscuring these conditions and missing important elements of patients' lives. This means using measures that are gender specific or tailoring items so they tap the experience of sexual quality of life specifically for men and women in one's population of interest.

Second, SQoL scales should measure gender norms. As Range and Jenkins (2010) argued in their comprehensive analysis of gender theories, "If and when gender differences occur, the causal mechanism may not be biological sex, but instead one or more social or psychological correlates such as gender schema that might mediate or moderate effects otherwise misattributed to biological sex" (p. 152). There are a number of scales that have been developed in other fields for use with other populations that could easily be adapted to suit research with ill populations. These measures include gender ideology scales (Levant & Richmond, 2007; Levant, Richmond, Cook, House, & Aupont, 2007; Thompson & Pleck, 1986; Tolman & Porche, 2000), measures of sexual self-concept (Rostosky, Dekhtyar, Cupp, & Anderman, 2008), and measures of sexual subjectivity (Horne & Zimmer-Gembeck, 2006).

The Female Sexual Subjectivity Inventory is a good example of a scale developed to measure the relationship between gender and sex. Sexual subjectivity is defined as the perception of pleasure from the body and the experience of being sexual (Horne & Zimmer-Gembeck, 2006) and is a concept that is relevant to all ages and genders and across the continuum of health and illness. Sample items include "I think it is important for a sexual partner to consider my sexual pleasure" and "My sexual behavior and experiences are not something I spend time thinking about." Scales that measure gender beliefs would allow investigators to understand how social and sexual norms have been internalized by research participants and how these subsequently affect sexual attitudes and beliefs. These could be used as potential covariates, enabling investigators to understand the role of gender socialization as it interacts with SQoL outcomes.

2. Evaluate Construct Equivalency When Assessing Group Differences

When measuring sexual responsiveness and other qualities of an individual's sexual life, as with any topic, researchers must decide on the best way to operationalize their construct of interest (Cronbach & Meehl, 1955; Machado & Silva, 2007). When health psychologists include SQoL items in a study, there is often an interest in examining group differences in terms of such attributes as gender, age, or experimental condition (as in a clinical trial). Construct equivalency is especially important when making group comparisons to ensure that the same experience (physical sensation, genital response, emotion, etc.) is being evaluated. In this discussion, I will use gender as an exemplar of issues that arise when making group comparisons and the problems that arise when using operationalizations of sexual experiences that may not be equivalent for men and women. However, it is important to keep in mind that construct equivalency is an issue for all types of research that investigate group differences. The choices we make in terms of operationalizing psychological constructs are some of the most important decisions we make as researchers—and some of the most difficult.

In sexual function research, investigators have often operationalized function using observable behaviors that allow participants to report on their genital response. For example, such physical factors as dyspareunia (pain on intercourse) or failure to maintain an erection are examined as similar types of physical sexual experiences that allow researchers to understand important aspects of genital health (Aaronson et al., 1993). However, taking a closer look at issues of construct equivalency, we might ask: Is the experience of erection difficulty the same (or similar enough) to the experience of dyspareunia that ratings on these items can be effectively compared? There are a number of related questions that are pertinent: Are the two physical experiences psychologically similar? What kinds of unstated assumptions are implied in these experiences? For example, the colorectal cancer supplement of the EORTC (CRC-38) includes five items that directly assess sexual quality of life. Three items are designed to be answered by both men and women and concern sexual interest, activity, and satisfaction. In addition, two items are gender specific: Men are asked if they had "difficulty getting or maintain an erection" and if they had a "problem with ejaculation." Women are asked if they had "a dry vagina during intercourse" and if they had "pain during intercourse" (Aaronson et al., 1993). Taking up the question of construct equivalency, one should ask whether men's ability to maintain an erection and women's rate of pain with intercourse are equivalent, particularly when they will be compared with t-tests to document sex differences.

I would argue that the constructs underlying these gender-specific items are, in fact, not equivalent. As a result, this is not an effective way of comparing male and female sexual function. Historical perceptions of male and female sexuality (and the various stigmas attached particularly to female sexuality; see McClelland, 2010, for discussion) can be observed in the assumptions that male sexual response is the norm. This implicit belief can be seen in such statements by researchers, such as, "The simple endpoints equivalent to potency and ejaculation in men are not available [in women]" (Banerjee, 1999, p. 1901). As a result, researchers have often limited their assessment of female sexual function to measures of pain during intercourse (just as they often limit the assessment of male sexual function to erectile function). These implicit associations have resulted in defining female sexual health as the absence of pain and men's sexual health as the presence of pleasure. It is by examining these unstated assumptions inherent in construct equivalency that one is able to see how discrepant these measures have become.

Solving issues of construct equivalency is not simple. Given the recommendation made earlier about the benefits of gender-specific items when assessing sexual quality of life, researchers who want to make group comparisons are faced with a difficult challenge. A first step is to examine how participants interpret and experience items. For example, in a recent study (Flynn et al., 2011), the investigators found that when they asked participants across a variety of group differences (gender, cancer site, and cancer stage) what sexual health meant to them, they found that though genitals were important to participants, they were not the only thing that was important. Some participants had broadened the conceptualization of sexuality to include intimacy in the absence of any sexual activity. For example, one participant with prostate cancer said, "We didn't have intercourse, but we hugged and you go down the street and you hold hands ... this way, you're having sex all the time" (p. 383). Findings such as this should encourage researchers to examine the range of definitions that participants bring to the construct of sexual activity. More important, this type of research question also presents an opportunity for health researchers to inform sexuality research more broadly about the diversity of sexual experiences that individuals imagine as relevant to their sexual quality of life. A second recommendation is to examine the unstated assumptions when making group comparisons, for example, ensuring that items measuring pleasure and pain are compared with like items when comparing the sexual well-being of men and women.

3. Include Body Image as a Dimension of Sexual Quality of Life

How medical illness and/or treatment affect body image is a very popular area of research (Andersen & LeGrand, 1991), particularly for studies of women and research on illnesses that affect what are often considered the "sexual organs" (breasts, uterus, cervix, ovaries; for exception, see Syrjala et al., 1998, for discussion of bone marrow transplant patients). However, body image is often conceptualized and measured as separate from sexual quality of life. In other words, it may be measured, but it is not necessarily analyzed along with those items measuring sexual function. In comparison, research on female sexual function and breast cancer has continuously been interested in the role of body image; researchers not only regularly include body image measures but also analyze the body image data for its associations with sexual function (e.g., Ganz, Rowland, Desmond, Meyerowitz, & Wyatt, 1998).

Studies that have conceptually linked the domains of sex and body image have produced compelling findings that challenge assumptions concerning the parameters of sexual function. For example, Hendren and colleagues (2005) examined sexual function after treatment for rectal cancer and asked a sample of men and women if they had been embarrassed about or ashamed of their body or reluctant to have sex because they felt their body was undesirable. Similar proportions of men (22%) and women (18%) reported this was true. This finding and others like it (Andersen, Woods, & Copeland, 1997; Scott, Halford, & Ward, 2004; Yurek, Farrar, & Andersen, 2000) highlight that body image is not a domain limited to women, nor is it limited to illnesses that affect sexual organs. It also draws attention to the important psychological link between body image and sexual feelings.

In a focus-group study of men and women with different stages of cancer and cancer sites, body image concerns were mentioned in each of the 16 focus groups (Flynn et al., 2011). Moreover, body image concerns negatively affected sexual function and intimacy with partners. Participants named common changes as important to their sexual well-being, including scarring, treatment-related hair loss, and weight gain. Women, more than men, described feeling sexually attractive as important to their sexual motivation. Men described the negative effects of weight gain and such treatment outcomes as colostomy bags as important in how sexually attractive they felt.

Researchers are advised to examine body image and sexuality as related domains. In doings so, they might include such measurement strategies as including body image scores within QoL scales or creating subscale scores. Body image scores should be used as both predictors and outcomes of sexual quality of life. To do this, one should avoid such general items as "Have you felt physically less attractive as a result of your disease or treatment?" or "Have you been dissatisfied with your body?" (Aaronson et al., 1993). Instead, consider using items and methods equipped to collect multiple ways that patients may be psychologically and physiologically imagining their (often altered) body image.

In addition, researchers are advised to avoid items that may unconsciously link body image and femininity because this approach may overly determine what researchers learn about men's experience of body image and sexual well-being. Women are often asked about femininity concerns in breast cancer research, but concerns about how individuals' masculinity and femininity concerns affect sexual quality of life should be extended to all illnesses and to studies with men as well. It is important to examine mechanisms that link body image and sexual quality of life to address important questions: Is sexual quality of life driven by self-perceptions or by partner perceptions of attractiveness? What relational qualities help to support experiences of positive body image? How do men experience changes to their bodies, especially in illness contexts where the physical body is salient in a new way? Qualitative studies of women with breast cancer have identified a wide range of issues related to one's body and bodily integrity. Wilmoth (2001), for example, found that participants described their sexual health in terms of missing parts of their bodies as a result of surgery; loss of menstruation and associations with aging; loss of sexual sensations, including arousal and libido; and an altered sense of womanhood. Thus, it is important to create definitions of sexual quality of life and genital responsiveness that are linked with psychological and physiological constructs.

Items that address the links between body image and sexual quality of life include those that inquire about participants' level of comfort being naked or their interest in physical contact more generally. These items include "I avoid close contact such as hugging," "I am satisfied with the shape of my body," and "I feel that part of me must remain hidden" (Body Image After Breast Cancer Questionnaire, from Baxter et al., 2006, p. 254). In addition, items that assess participants' evaluations of how they feel about their bodies (e.g., "I like the appearance of my body"), measured alongside sexual outcomes, would allow researchers to understand potential mechanisms that link how individuals feel about their bodies and the kinds of sexual thoughts, behaviors, and outcomes that result.

4. Measure the Importance of Sex for Individuals

Although many researchers have argued that sexuality is an essential aspect of quality of life (e.g., Arrington et al., 2004), sexual experiences and/or feelings may not be equally important for everyone. With this idea in mind, researchers should consider including measures that allow for varied levels of importance attached to the sexual domain. Not everyone will be bothered by diminished sexual function; this response may be a result of an individual's history of unsatisfying or perhaps traumatic sexual experiences, as well as a result of physical changes because of aging or illness that make sexual contact uncomfortable or painful. For example, Lindau et al. (2007) noted that "women were more likely than men to rate sex as an unimportant part of life and to report lack of pleasure with sex" (p. 772). The fact that some individuals experience varying levels of investment in the sexual domain suggests that researchers should consider sexual activities, behaviors, and interactions in the context of the importance that individuals place on them. Without attention to overall importance of sexual experiences, researchers are at risk of conflating the lack of sexual activity with sexual dysfunction among participants who report no sexual activity or sexual desire. By including the concept of importance, it is easier to tease apart the motivation behind this reported lack of sexual activity or desire.

This idea of importance has more recently been developed in sex researchers' recommendations to measure levels of distress as a necessary component of a diagnosis of sexual dysfunction (Bancroft, Loftus, & Long, 2003; Derogatis, Rosen, Leiblum, Burnett, & Heiman, 2002). Bancroft et al. (2003) found that a significant portion of women in heterosexual relationships who reported high levels of sexual dysfunction were not distressed by their dysfunction. A similar finding was reported in a study of men treated for prostate cancer who reported that although their sexual function was poor, "they had adjusted to the change and were not terribly bothered, especially if they believed they were cured of the cancer" (Litwin et al., 1998, p. 1008). Given these findings, the role of importance in the sexual domain and its potential associations with related constructs *bother* and *distress* are worth investigating.

Raphael, Rukholm, Brown, Hill-Bailey, & Donato (1996) have developed a quality-of-life measure that blends how important a domain is to the individual with how satisfied he or she is in this domain. This model holds enormous potential for measuring how two dimensions are related. As the investigators explained, "Importance scores serve as a weight for converting satisfaction scores into quality of life (QoL) scores" (Raphael et al., 1996, p. 368). For example, a low satisfaction score weighted by a high importance score results in a low QoL score. This kind of weighting would allow for the separate domains within quality of life to be differentially important and to examine which domains individuals emphasize throughout their lives and at what stages of the illness trajectory.

Similarly, Avis and colleagues (1996) developed a scale that tapped perception of importance as well as satisfaction in their Multidimensional Index of Life Quality. The authors describe how during the scale development phase, they had created QoL scores that were weighted by each participant's importance ratings of each QoL domain. Although Avis and her colleagues found that the importance-weighted measures did not increase the accuracy of satisfaction scores (and were subsequently dropped from analyses), I argue that the practice of measuring importance may hold more promise for research in a domain where variability in importance has already been demonstrated. In a recent national study, Waite, Laumann, Das, and Schumm (2009) found that nearly one quarter of women (24.0%) ages 57–64 responded that sex was "not at all important" when asked how important a part of the participant's life sex was. In this study, the prevalence of reporting the low importance of sex increased with women's age (34.9% in ages 65–74; 52.3% in ages 75–85). For men, this rate was much lower, ranging from 6.2% in ages 57–64, to 14.1% in ages 65–74, and to 25.9% in ages 75–85.

Given that Waite et al. (2009) do not report on the health status of this sample, generalizability to patients living with illness is not immediately possible. Nevertheless, these findings demonstrate that there is enormous variability in how individuals rate the importance of sex. Including items that can measure attitudes toward intercourse, sexual behaviors more broadly, or even thinking about sex, would provide an important frame through which to analyze such other SQoL items as frequency of orgasm and genital function. Taking up the model that Avis and her colleagues presented, researchers are encouraged to create importance-weighted sexual domain scores that account for individuals who report low SQoL and low importance. Analyses with importance-weighted scores may offer insight into individuals and groups that are qualitatively different than those who report, for example, a low SQoL score with high importance.

It is important to note that data reflecting low importance of sex should not be confused with how much men and women like sexual activity or how one gender is inclined toward sex more than the other. Instead, data on importance tell us something about the quality of sexual experiences that men and women imagine when asked to evaluate the relative importance of sex in their lives. Low importance in the sexual domain is not a necessarily dysfunctional, nor is it a "natural" outcome or a gendered one. Because the etiology of sex may be complex for some individuals, researchers are encouraged to investigate not only the range of importance that individuals may attach to sex but also the history and genealogy of these attitudes.

5. DO NOT IGNORE DATA FROM PARTICIPANTS WHO ARE "NOT SEXUALLY ACTIVE"

Many sexual function measures include a skip pattern where participants are asked whether they are partnered and/or whether they have been sexually active during a recent period (e.g., during the past month). The language of "sexual activity" privileges sexual behaviors over sexual intimacy, physical closeness, and nonactivity-based sexuality, including sexual daydreams, masturbation, and fantasies (Wilson, 2010). In just one example of this type of skip pattern, it is possible to see how those participants who have not been sexually active are not asked to provide any further data regarding their sexual well-being: "The first two questions asked if [the participants] were in an intimate relationship and if they were sexually active." If these two questions were answered yes, "participants were asked to complete the seven remaining [sexual function] questions" (Barber, Visco, Wyman, Fantl, & Bump, 2002, p. 292).

Items and skip patterns such as these limit SQoL data to only those participants who are both partnered and recently sexually active. More important, this conditional pattern unnecessarily eliminates data on individuals who fall outside these categories. In some cases, researchers will ask the participant to note such reasons for sexual inactivity as "too tired" or "no current partner" (Barber et al., 2002; Basson et al., 2004). Although these additional data shed light on the relational contexts of the people answering the questions, they do not shed sufficient light on how sexual quality of life is experienced by individuals who are not currently sexually partnered but are still sexually active and/or may be sexual, but without participating in sexual activities. These types of assessments may be particularly limiting for people who still are adjusting to their illness and may be learning to cope with a new form and idea of what "sexual" means in a newly altered body. Asking only about sexual behavior or sexual activities allows fewer opportunities to understand how patients adjust to illness and the effects of illness on their bodies and their intimate relationships (Meyerowitz, Desmond, & Rowland, 1999).

Researchers are encouraged not to confine their samples only to those individuals who are partnered and/or who are currently sexually active. Although this type of skip pattern is often used to ensure that research sample participants share basic characteristics, the cost in terms of lost information is too great. By eliminating responses of participants who are nonpartnered or nonactive, researchers are at risk of missing important issues and ignoring subpopulations who fall outside these parameters. One suggestion is to collect SQoL data that do require participants be sexually active but nevertheless inquires about dimensions of their sexual well-being. This assessment might include items that inquire about sexual thoughts or fantasies (e.g., Changes in Sexual Functioning Questionnaire; Clayton, McGarvey, & Clavet, 1997). A second suggestion is to collect data on the criteria individuals use to decide if they want to be sexual alone or with a partner (i.e., sexual motivations), as well as the psychological, physiological, or relational barriers they believe stand in their way of feeling or enacting sexual expression (e.g., "My partner's health is poor," "I'm too tired"). These types of items expand the potential for research samples to be included in SQoL research and allow researchers to investigate a much larger range of factors when individuals are asked to reflect on their sexual quality of life.

6. Widen the Scope of Inquiry to Examine Nonpartnered Sexual Behaviors

Put simply, individuals outside of relationships still experience SQoL issues. When evaluating sexual quality of life, researchers consistently miss nonpartnered sexual experiences if items ask only about intercourse or ask nonpartnered individuals to skip items concerning sexuality. In addition to retaining those participants who may not be sexually active, researchers should also consider sexual quality outside of relationships. Although many researchers have assumed that sexuality is a dyadic process, individuals are, in fact, born with and develop sexuality regardless of whether they ever experience partnered sex (Pluhar, 2007; Tolman & Szalacha, 1999). Research on sexuality within illness contexts should allow for SQoL appraisals across a wide range of sexual expressions, including when alone, with a regular partner, or across multiple partners (Bockting & Coleman, 2002; Das, 2007).

By linking assessments of sexual function with relational status, researchers may not be accurately capturing nonpartnered sexual behaviors, particularly in the aging populations, who are more likely to have a medical illness (Stanton, Revenson, & Tennen, 2007). For example, in a nationally representative sample of masturbation rates, results for women ranged from 31.6% in the younger group (57–64 years old) to 16.4% in the older group (75–85 years old); and for men, from 63.4% in the younger group (57–64 years old) to 27.9% in the older group (75–85 years old; Lindau et al., 2007). These data illustrate that although the frequency of masturbation decreases with age, it does not disappear and remains quite high into old age.

Nonpartnered sexual behaviors may also be important indicators for patients who are recovering from or coping with medical illness and its treatment. Sexual feelings or behaviors when alone may be an early indicator of the (re)emergence of sexual feelings, for example, after surgery. They may also signal an important point for clinical intervention, one that does not require the patient to contend with such issues as attractiveness to a partner, adequate genital response, and potentially new physical limitations resulting from the illness or its treatment. In sum, researchers should consider not restricting data collection or analysis to only those individuals who report being partnered. To the contrary, researchers may want to widen the definition of sexual activity to include nonpartnered activities.

7. Consider Assessing Nonpenetrative Sex in Addition to Intercourse

In addition to expanding definitions of sex to include masturbation and other sexual behaviors that do not require a sexual partner, it is also imperative to expand definitions to include sexual behaviors that are not limited to vaginal-penile intercourse. Sexual function is only one dimension of sexuality and intimacy (Gamel, Hengeveld, & Davis, 2000), yet sexuality is often equated singularly with and measured as sexual intercourse (Bruner & Boyd, 1999). One of the most common trends in this field has been the use of heterosexual intercourse as the primary benchmark for sexual function. For example, the FSFI (the current gold standard for assessing women's sexual function) includes three items about vaginal penetration and four items that ask about vaginal lubrication, a physiological response that is assessed in order to inquire about the ability to have penetrative sex. The conceptual conflation of sex, vaginal intercourse, and sexual function results in less knowledge about the range of sexual behaviors that participants engage in, as well as limiting the generalizability of research findings for nonheterosexual participants and/or those individuals who are not engaging in heterosexual intercourse (Schneidewind-Skibbe, Hayes, Koochaki, Meyer, & Dennerstein, 2008).

Lindau et al. (2007) found a wide variety of sexual activities reported in their nationally representative study of older adults, 57–85 years old, in the United States. Men and women reported high rates of oral sex and masturbation in the previous year: In the study, 58% of the younger group (57–64 years old) and 31% of the older group (75–85 years old) reported participating in oral sex in the previous year. These rates of sexual activity outside of vaginal-penile intercourse should alert researchers to include measures that are not solely focused on penetrative sex. While not all the participants in this sample were coping with the effects of illness, approximately one quarter of the sample participants rated their health status as poor or fair. Arthritis, diabetes, and hypertension were reported by approximately one half of the respondents, suggesting that the data from this study have important implications for researchers working with ill and aging populations.

Mansfield, Koch, and Voda (1998) found that one fifth of their sample of midlife women reported an increased desire for nongenital sexual expression ("e.g., cuddling, hugging, kissing," p. 297). The authors offered a number of interpretations of this finding. One interpretation offered was that this response did not mean that women wanted to avoid intercourse; instead, it meant that the respondents wanted to increase their responsiveness to intercourse (i.e., through foreplay) or increase their ability to orgasm more readily. This finding also suggests that women may find nonpenetrative sex more enjoyable, a finding that has been replicated in a variety of studies over the years. For example, in a study of African American women over 60, women expressed a great deal of interest and pleasure from various forms of sexual expression, but reported low interest and enjoyment in intercourse (Conway-Turner, 1992). Studies consistently show that vaginal dryness as a result of menopause is a significant factor in sexual (dis)satisfaction (e.g., Tomic et al., 2006). Because dyspareunia and vaginal dryness are frequent outcomes of many medications and surgery, as well as a common menopausal symptom, it is important to consider nonpenetrative sexual expression when measuring sexual quality of life.

Finally, Barsky, Friedman, and Rosen (2006) described the importance of flexibility when coping with long-term sexual dysfunction. The authors argue that individuals with chronic illness best cope by shifting their cognitive and behavioral ideals of what constitutes sexual functioning. This strategy used by the chronically ill might include shifting from intercourse as the only way to be intimate with a partner, for example, to engaging in oral sex as an alternative. This same type of flexibility needs to be reflected in measures that do not solely measure a male patient's ability to penetrate his partner or a female patient's ability to receive penetration. Researchers have argued that our culture's prioritizing of the erect penis above and beyond the experience of sexual pleasure places men (and their partners) in a position of caring more about the function of the penis and less about the pleasure that the penis is capable of (Potts, 2000; Potts, Grace, Gavey, & Vares, 2004). Perhaps even more important, this focus on penetration may obscure aspects of male sexual well-being, including diminished desire and low motivation for sexual activity (Meuleman & van Lankveld, 2005). For all these reasons, researchers should consider the widest possible array of sexual behaviors, including, but not limited to, sexual intercourse. This expanded definition would not only include men and women who do not engage in heterosexual intercourse, but would also better represent the range of sexual behaviors that individuals engage in over the course of their lifetime.

8. Avoid Attribution Errors That Occur When Premorbid Sexual Health Is Not Assessed

Because a diagnosis of a serious medical illness is often sudden and unpredictable, few studies can assess premorbid levels of sexual activity, function, importance, and distress. As a result, researchers often attribute the lack of sexual activity or dysfunction postdiagnosis exclusively to the patient's illness without explicit data on change over time.

Most researchers evaluate premorbid sexual health some time after the diagnosis is made or treatment has begun. Although there are many problems with this approach (see later), even retrospective data may contribute important information. Items asking people to report on their sex life before the illness allow for the evaluation of perceived changes in sexuality following diagnosis. Although these perceptions may be retrospectively flawed, they allow for the patient to evaluate the changes instead of assuming perfect health and function prior to illness (see Bruner et al., 1998, for examples of retrospective items). This approach is essential if researchers are to avoid falsely attributing declining sexual quality of life to illness when sexual activity may have been infrequent or even absent prior to illness. For example, Dennerstein and Lehert (2004) found that when assessing current levels of sexual functioning in middle-aged women, "premorbid functioning [had] a major and essential effect, compared with concomitant cross factors" (p. 180), including change in partner status and feelings for one's partner.

The issue of retrospective data collection, that is, comparing "before surgery" with "after surgery," presents a potential, but not ideal, first step. Hendren and colleagues (2005) assessed sexual dysfunction retrospectively in a sample of men and women who had been treated for rectal cancer. Because the researchers chose not to exclude patients based on preexisting sexual inactivity or dysfunction (exclusions that bias results toward higher rates of sexual function), the researchers were able to make a number of within-group comparisons based on surgery type, recent sexual activity, and pre- and postoperative sexual function. In fact, 35% of men and 47% of women reported they had experienced sexual problems prior to cancer treatment. In terms of investigating the effects of surgery, their decision to measure perceived presurgical sexual dysfunction allowed the authors to exclude participants who reported dysfunction symptoms prior to treatment in order to examine the specific effects of cancer treatment.

Researchers are encouraged to use validated measures of sexual quality of life that include retrospective items that ask participants to reflect specifically on the role of their illness on their own sexual health. This specificity is needed not only to disentangle premorbid sexual dysfunction from illness-related dysfunction, but also to disentangle the potential influence of a partner's illness or the effects of the participant's illness on a partner. One example of a scale that includes an assessment of premorbid sexual quality of life is the Psychosocial Adjustment to Illness Scale (PAIS; Derogatis & Lopez, 1983), which was designed to measure changes an individual experiences as a result of illness. The sexual function subscale has six items that ask the participant to reflect on changes in their sexual interest, satisfaction, and relationship since becoming ill (e.g., "Sometimes when people are ill they report a loss of interest in sexual activities. Have you experienced less sexual interest since your illness?"). A small cross-sectional study of patients with advanced heart failure using the PAIS found that one quarter of the participants reported little or no change in the frequency of sexual activity and one half reported minimal changes in their sexual satisfaction since their illness (Jaarsma, Dracup, Walden, & Stevenson, 1996). In order to tease apart the effects of illness and and/ or treatment from preexisting sexual quality of life, researchers are encouraged to include measures that enable participants to reflect on the changes they perceive in their own sexual well-being.

9. Examine the Reemergence of Sexual Quality of Life Over Time

The role of time and change over time is essential and not yet well understood in studies of sexual quality of life (Talcott et al., 2003). Change over time is even more salient for people living with a medical illness. When does sexual function return? Does sexual quality of life precede sexual function? If so, under what conditions? And what form does it take? Most studies have looked at relatively short periods after diagnosis or treatment. As a result, the reemergence of physical intimacy and characteristics of the psychological adjustment period are not well understood. Research questions addressing change over time require not only longitudinal research designs, but also measures that are sensitive enough to pick up on early SQoL indicators, including the experience of physical intimacy, masturbation, sexual thoughts, and anticipation of sexual activities. For example, Andersen et al. (1997) examined the influence of sexual self-schemas in a sample of women with gynecological cancer and found that a positive self-schema predicted higher rates of sexual responsiveness, including desire, excitement, orgasm, and resolution. Andersen (1999) has suggested that those with positive sexual schemas are better able to adjust to illness and make the necessary changes to their cognitive schemas and sexual behaviors that allow for the experience of pleasure to reemerge.

Researchers are encouraged to measure sexual quality of life over time using longitudinal designs, but perhaps more important, also to assess the emergence of sexual quality of life using measures that assess not only functionality but also the emergence of sexual feelings and fantasy that may or may not be accompanied by sexual behaviors. An example of a measure that assesses these more subtle changes in sexual quality of life over time is the Short Personal Experiences Questionnaire (Dennerstein, Anderson-Hunt, & Dudley, 2002: Dennerstein & Lehert, 2004). Items include, for example, "Give an approximate estimate of how many times you have had sexual thoughts or fantasies (e.g., daydreams) during the last month." This assessment of sexual thoughts may be more accessible to patients at early stages of recovery than assessments of sexual desire or libido, which may be perceived to be too closely related to sexual activities. Patients who are nervously anticipating and/or coping with sexual changes as a result of illness may be relieved to see that resuming normal sexual activities (i.e., intercourse) is not the only threshold to cross in order to be considered healthy, sexually active, or functional. Earlier and more subtle thresholds of sexual characteristics and feelings may offer considerable comfort and information on the way to recovering or adapting to illness.

In addition to including measures that assess early (re)emergence of sexual quality of life, researchers are encouraged to include repeated measures in order to understand the patterns of adjustment over time, including the variation of trajectories that individuals experience (Hegelson,

Snyder, & Seltman, 2004). An important point, which is reflected in the foregoing recommendations, is that in their longitudinal designs, researchers need to consider strongly the definitions
used to determine when individuals "resume sexual activity." As I argued earlier in this discussion,
limiting the definition of successful and functional sex to intercourse results in a tremendous loss of
data on individuals, the diversity of their lives, and the wide variety of sexual experiences, thoughts,
and relationships that individuals—especially those who are adapting or recovering from illness—
might include in their definition of a healthy and vibrant sexual life.

10. EVALUATE THE PSYCHOLOGICAL CONTEXTS OF SEXUAL QUALITY OF LIFE

As discussed in the foregoing recommendations, there is more to sexual quality of life than genital
response. There are many contexts in which sexual quality of life flourishes, but one of the most
important is the psychological health and well-being of an individual. Andersen (1985) was one of
the first health psychologists to find that having a more negative self-view predicted greater sexual
morbidity after cancer than having a positive self-view, a finding that has been replicated in many
studies over the last 25 years (Andersen et al., 1997; Andersen, Woods, & Cyranowski, 1994).
Psychological correlates may impair sexual functioning through perceptual changes in the sexual
self (Cyranowski & Andersen, 2000). A patient's self-esteem can potentially be eroded by physical
changes resulting from treatment, cosmetic issues, and loss of functional ability, as well as numerous other changes after illness. In turn, the loss of self-esteem can adversely affect sexual response.
In addition, stress and depression have been shown to predict decreased sexual response (Brassil &
Keller, 2002; Wilmoth & Spinelli, 2000).

There has been a long history of examining the relationship between anxiety and negative sexual
outcomes (Beck, 1967; Fenichel, 1945; Kaplan, 1974, 1979; Wolpe, 1958). This relationship has
been more recently explored by researchers at the Kinsey Institute who have consistently found a
strong link between negative mood states such as depression and anxiety and subsequent decreased
sexual interest (Bancroft & Janssen, 2000; Lykins, Janssen, & Graham, 2006). For medical populations, negative mood states might be triggered by not only life events and daily stress, but also
thoughts of expected pain and discomfort, anticipation of sexual distress, or anxiety that may be
related to genital function or an altered body image.

Lindau et al. (2007) found that anxiety and avoidance were important factors affecting the sexual health of individuals in three illness groups—arthritis, diabetes, and hypertension—and that
negative psychological responses varied across both gender and illness type. Women in the arthritis
group reported significantly higher rates of anxiety about sexual performance than did men (odds
ratios of 1.26 for women vs. 0.78 for men); whereas the reverse was seen in the diabetes group,
where men were more anxious than women (odds ratios of 1.20 for men vs. 0.86 for women). In the
hypertension group, both men and women reported approximately equal levels of anxiety about
sexual performance. These findings demonstrate the role that psychological conditions can have on
sexual quality of life. Similarly, in their recommendations for studying sexual dysfunction in men,
Lue et al. (2004) emphasized the importance of anxiety, depression, and self-esteem in evaluations
of men's sexual health. They also highlighted the role of expectations and their potential underlying role in sexual disappointment, which may affect sexual satisfaction and an individual's intimate
relationships. More broadly, it is clear that negative psychological experiences, including but not
limited to depression, anxiety, and low self-esteem, play important and often understudied roles
in individuals' experiences of sexual quality of life, particularly for those who are recovering or
adapting to illness.

CONCLUSION

Sexual quality of life is an area that is becoming more important within the literature on adaptation
to medical illness. Thus, it is important to think about measurement issues in terms of construct

validity and appropriate measurement tools (Basson, 2000; Basson et al., 2004; Kaschak & Tiefer, 2001; McClelland, 2010; Moynihan, 2003; Tiefer, 1996, 2004). Definitions of sexual function have become increasingly controversial in the role that for-profit companies have had in the development of clinical and pharmaceutical interventions to treat male and female sexual dysfunction (see Moynihan, 2003). As this controversy around definitions continues to develop, health psychologists will be faced with a set of difficult but important questions: Is sexual health the same as genital functioning? Can I measure men's and women's sexual health using the same items? Is there a short scale I can use in my study that will help me understand the relationship between sexual health and overall well-being? What is the best way for me to evaluate an intervention aimed to help patients' sexual and relational health? The 10 recommendations provided in this chapter offer a starting point for health psychologists to navigate these questions and choose (or adapt) the most appropriate measure to answer these questions. In turn, doing this will help to ensure that the data we collect are not only representative of patients' lives, but are also attentive to diverse sexual experiences.

REFERENCES

Aaronson, N. K., Ahmedzai, S., Bergman, B., Bullinger, M. Cull, A., Duez, N. J., … Takeda, F. (1993). The European organization for research and treatment of cancer QLQ-C30: A quality-of-life instrument for use in international clinical trials in oncology. *Journal of the National Cancer Institute*, *85*(5), 365–476.

Addis, M. E., & Mahalik, J. R. (2003). Men, masculinity, and the contexts of help seeking. *American Psychologist*, *58*, 5–14.

Alexander, M. G., & Fisher, T. D. (2003). Truth and consequences: Using the bogus pipeline to examine sex differences in self-reported sexuality. *Journal of Sex Research*, *40*(1), 27–35.

American Psychiatric Association (APA). (1994). *Diagnostic and statistical manual of mental disorders* (DSM-IV, 4th ed.). Washington, DC: American Psychiatric Press.

American Psychological Association (APA). (2000). *Diagnostic and statistical manual of mental disorders* (DSM-IV-TR, 4th ed.). Washington, DC: American Psychiatric Press.

Andersen, B. L. (1985). Sexual functioning morbidity among cancer survivors: Current status and future research directions. *Cancer*, *55*(8), 1835–1842.

Andersen, B. L. (1999). Surviving cancer: The importance of sexual self-concept. *Medical and Pediatric Oncology*, *33*(1), 15–23.

Andersen, B. L. (2002). Biobehavioral outcomes following psychological interventions for cancer patients. *Journal of Consulting and Clinical Psychology*, *70*(3), 590–610.

Andersen, B. L., & Cyranowski, J. M. (1994). Women's sexual self schema. *Journal of Personality and Social Psychology*, *67*, 1079–1100.

Andersen, B. L., Cyranowski, J. M., & Espindle, D. (1999). Men's sexual self-schema. *Journal of Personality and Social Psychology*, *76*(4), 645–661.

Andersen, B. L., & LeGrand, J. (1991). Body image for women: Conceptualization, assessment, and a test of its importance to sexual dysfunction and medical illness. *Journal of Sex Research*, *28*(3), 457–478.

Andersen, B. L., Shelby, R., & Golden-Kreutz, D. (2007). RCT of a psychological intervention for patients with cancer: I. Mechanisms of change. *Journal of Consulting and Clinical Psychology*, *75*(6), 927–938.

Andersen, B. L., Woods, X. A., & Copeland, L. J. (1997). Sexual self schema and sexual morbidity among gynecologic cancer survivors. *Journal of Consulting and Clinical Psychology*, *65*, 221–229.

Andersen, B. L., Woods, X. A., & Cyranowski, J. M. (1994). Sexual self-schema as a possible predictor of sexual problems following cancer treatment. *Canadian Journal of Human Sexuality*, *3*, 165–170.

Arrington, R. Cofrancesco, J., & Wu, A. W. (2004). Questionnaires to measure sexual quality of life. *Quality of Life Research*, *13*(10), 1643–1658.

Avis, N., Crawford, S., & Manuel, J. (2004). Psychosocial problems among younger women with breast cancer. *Psycho-Oncology*, *13*(5), 295–308.

Avis, N. E., Smith, K. W., Hambleton, R. K., Feldman, H. A, Selwyn, A., & Jacobs, A. (1996). Development of the multi-dimensional index of life quality (MILQ): A quality of life measure for cardiovascular disease. *Medical Care*, *34*, 1102–1120.

Bancroft, J., & Janssen, E. (2000). The dual control model of male sexual response: A theoretical approach to centrally mediated erectile dysfunction. *Neuroscience & Biobehavioral Reviews*, *24*(5), 571–579.

Bancroft, J., Loftus, J., & Long, J. S. (2003). Distress about sex: A national survey of women in heterosexual relationships. *Archives of Sexual Behavior, 32*, 193–208.

Banerjee, A. K. (1999). Sexual dysfunction after surgery for rectal cancer. *Lancet, 353*(9168), 1900–1902.

Barber, M. D., Visco, A. G., Wyman, J. F., Fantl, J. A., & Bump, R. C. (2002). Sexual function in women with urinary incontinence and pelvic organ prolapse. *Obstetrics and Gynecology, 99*(2), 281–289.

Barsky, J. L., Friedman, M. A., & Rosen, R. C. (2006). Sexual dysfunction and chronic illness: The role of flexibility in coping. *Journal of Sex & Marital Therapy, 32*(3), 235–253.

Barton, D., Wilwerding, M., Carpenter, L., & Loprinzi, C. (2004). Libido as part of sexuality in female cancer survivors. *Oncology Nursing Forum, 31*(3), 599–607.

Basson, R. (2000). The female sexual response: A different model. *Journal of Sex and Marital Therapy, 26*, 51–65.

Basson, R. (2007). Sexuality in chronic illness: No longer ignored. *Lancet, 369*(9559), 350–352.

Basson, R., Leiblum, S., Brotto, L., Derogatis, L., Fourcroy, J., Fugl-Meyer, K., ... Weijmar Schultz, W. C. (2004). Revised definitions of women's sexual dysfunction. *Journal of Sex Medicine, 1*, 40–48.

Basson, R., & Schultz, W. W. (2007). Sexual sequelae of general medical disorders *Lancet, 369*(9559), 409–424.

Baxter, N. N., Goodwin, P. J., Mcleod, R. S., Dion, R., Devins, G., & Bombardier, C. (2006). Reliability and validity of the body image after breast cancer questionnaire. *Breast Journal, 12*(3), 221–232.

Bay-Cheng, L. Y., & Eliseo-Arras, R. K. (2008). The making of unwanted sex: Gendered and neoliberal norms in college women's unwanted sexual experiences. *Journal of Sex Research, 45*(4), 386–397.

Beck, A. T. (1967). Depression: Causes and treatment. Philadelphia, PA: University of Pennsylvania Press.

Berman, L., Berman, J., Zierak, M. C., & Marley, C. (2002). Outcome measurement in sexual disorders (pp. 273–287). In W. W. IsHak, T. Burt, & L. I. Sederer (Eds.), *Outcome measurement in psychiatry: A critical review*. Washington, DC: American Psychiatric Publishing.

Bhasin, S., Enzlin, P., Coviello, A., & Basson, R. (2007). Sexual dysfunction in men and women with endocrine disorders. *Lancet, 369*(9561), 597–611.

Bockting, W. O., & Coleman, E. (Eds.). (2002). Masturbation as means of achieving sexual health. New York, NY: Haworth Press.

Bottomley, A. (2002). The cancer patient and quality of life. *Oncologist, 7*(2), 120–125.

Brady, M. J., Cella, D. F., Mo, F., Bonomi, A. E., Tulsky, D. S., Lloyd, S. R., ... Shiomoto, G. (1997). Reliability and validity of the functional assessment of breast cancer therapy quality-of-life instrument. *Journal of Clinical Oncology, 15*, 974–986.

Brassil, D. F., & Keller, M. (2002). Female sexual dysfunction: Definitions, causes, and treatment. *Urologic Nursing, 22*(4), 237–244.

Britto, M. T., Rosenthal, S. L., Taylor, J., & Passo, M. H. (2000). Improving rheumatologists' screening for alcohol use and sexual activity. *Archives of Pediatric and Adolescent Medicine, 154*(5), 478–483.

Bruner, D. W., & Boyd, C. P. (1999). Assessing women's sexuality after cancer therapy: Checking assumptions with the focus group technique. *Cancer Nursing, 22*, 438–447.

Bruner, D. W., Scott, C. B., McGowan, D., Lawton, C., Hanks, G., Prestidge, B., ... Asbell, S. (1998). The RTOG modified sexual adjustment questionnaire: Psychometric testing in the prostate cancer population. *International Journal of Radiation Oncology, Biology, Physics, 42*(1), 202.

Cella, D. F., Tulsky, D. S., & Gray, G., Sarafian, B., Linn, E., Bonomi, A., ... Brannon, J. (1993). The functional assessment of cancer therapy scale: development and validation of the general measure. *Journal of Clinical Oncology, 11*, 570–579.

Clayton, A. H., McGarvey, E. L., & Clavet, G. J. (1997). The changes in sexual functioning questionnaire (CSFQ): Development, reliability, and validity, *Psychopharmacology Bulletin, 33*(4), 731–745.

Clayton, A. H., & Ramamurthy, S. (2008). The impact of physical illness on sexual dysfunction. *Advances in Psychosomatic Medicine, 29*, 70–88.

Conway-Turner, K. (1992). Sex, intimacy and self esteem: The case of the African American older. *Women & Aging, 4*, 91–104.

Corona, G., Jannini, E. A., & Maggi, M. (2006). Inventories for male and female sexual dysfunctions. *International Journal of Impotence Research, 18*, 236–250.

Crane, C. H., & Skibber, J. (2003). Preoperative chemoradiation for locally advanced rectal cancer: Rationale, technique, and results of treatment. *Seminars in Surgical Oncology, 21*(4), 265–70.

Cronbach, L. J., & Meehl, P. E. (1955). Construct validity in psychological tests. *Psychological Bulletin, 52*, 281–302.

Cull, A. (1992). The assessment of sexual function in cancer patients. *European Journal of Cancer, 28A*(10), 1680–1686.

Cyranowski, J. M., & Andersen, B. L. (2000). Evidence of self-schematic cognitive processing in women with differing sexual self-views. *Journal of Social and Clinical Psychology, 19(4)*, 519–543.

Daker-White, G. (2002). Reliable and valid self-report outcomes measures in sexual (dys)function: A systematic review. *Archives of Sexual Behavior, 31*(2), 197–209.

Das, A. (2007). Masturbation in the United States. *Journal of Sex & Marital Therapy, 33*(4), 301–317.

Dennerstein, L., Anderson-Hunt, M., & Dudley, E. (2002). Evaluation of a short scale to assess female sexual functioning. *Journal of Sex and Marital Therapy, 28*(5), 389–397.

Dennerstein, L., & Lehert, P. (2004). Modeling mid-aged women's sexual functioning: A prospective, population-based study. *Journal of Sex and Marital Therapy, 30*(3), 173–183.

Derogatis, L. R. (1997). The Derogatis interview for sexual functioning (DISF/DISF-SR): An introductory report. *Journal of Sex & Marital Therapy, 23*(4), 291–304.

Derogatis L. R., & Lopez, M. C. (1983). *PAIS and PAIS-SR scoring manual 1.* Baltimore, MD: Johns Hopkins University, School of Medicine.

Derogatis, L. R., Rosen, R., Leiblum, S., Burnett, A., & Heiman, J. (2002). The female sexual distress scale (FSDS): Initial validation of a standardized scale for assessment of sexually related personal distress in women. *Journal of Sex and Marital Therapy, 28*(4), 317–330.

Fenichel, O. (1945). *The psychoanalytic theory of neurosis.* New York, NY: W. W. Norton.

Fergus, K., Gray R., & Fitch, M. (2002). Sexual dysfunction and the preservation of manhood: Experiences of men with prostate cancer. *Journal of Health Psychology, 7*(3), 303–316.

Fisher, T. D. (2007). Sex of experimenter and social norm effects on reports of sexual behavior in young men and women. *Archives of Sexual Behavior, 36*(1), 89–100.

Fisher, T. D. (2009). The impact of socially conveyed norms on the reporting of sexual behavior and attitudes by men and women. *Journal of Experimental Social Psychology, 45*(3), 567–572.

Flynn, K. E., Jeffery, D. D., Keefe, F. J., Porter, L. S., Shelby, R. A., Fawzy, M. R., … Weinfurt, K. P. (2011). Sexual functioning along the cancer continuum: Focus group results from the Patient-Reported Outcomes Measurement Information System (PROMIS®). *Psycho-Oncology, 20*(4), 378–386.

Fortune-Greeley, A. K., Flynn, K. E., Jeffery, D. D., Williams, M. S., Keefe, F. J., Reeve, B. B., … Weinfurt, K. P. (2009). Using cognitive interviews to evaluate items for measuring sexual functioning across cancer populations: Improvements and remaining challenges. *Quality of Life Research, 18*(8), 1085–1093.

Gamel, C., Hengeveld, M., & Davis, B. (2000). Informational needs about the effects of gynaecological cancer on sexuality: A review of the literature. *Journal of Clinical Nursing, 9*, 678–688.

Ganz, P. A., Rowland, J. H., Desmond, K., Meyerowitz, B. E., & Wyatt, G. E. (1998). Life after breast cancer: Understanding women's health-related quality of life and sexual functioning. *Journal of Clinical Oncology, 16*, 501–514.

Gotay, C. C., & Muraoka, M. Y. (1998). Quality of life in long-term survivors of adult-onset cancers. *Journal of the National Cancer Institute, 90*(9), 656–667.

Havenga, K., Maas C. P., DeRuiter, M. C., Welvaart, K., & Trimbos, J. B. (2000). Avoiding long-term disturbance to bladder and sexual function in pelvic surgery, particularly with rectal cancer. *Seminars in Surgical Oncology, 18*(3), 235–243.

Heiman, J. R. (2002). Sexual dysfunctions: Overview of prevalence, etiological factors and treatments. *Journal of Sex Research, 39*, 73–78.

Helgeson, V., Snyder, P., & Seltman, H. (2004). Psychological and physical adjustment to breast cancer over 4 years: Identifying distinct trajectories of change. *Health Psychology, 23*(1), 3–15.

Hendren, S. K., O'Connor, B. I., Liu, M., Asano, T., Cohen, Z., Swallow, C. J., … McLeod, R. S. (2005). Prevalence of male and female sexual dysfunction is high following surgery for rectal cancer. *Annals of Surgery, 242*(2), 212–223.

Hordern, A. (1999). Sexuality in palliative care: Addressing the taboo subject. In S. Aranda & M. O'Connor (Eds.), *Palliative care nursing: A guide to practice* (pp. 197–211). Melbourne, Australia: Ausmed.

Hordern, A. (2000). Intimacy and sexuality for the woman with breast cancer. *Cancer Nursing, 23,* 230–236.

Horne, S. G., & Zimmer-Gembeck, M. J. (2006). The female sexual subjectivity inventory: Development and validation of a multidimensional inventory for late adolescents and emerging adults. *Psychology of Women Quarterly, 30*(2), 125–138.

Impett, E. A., & Peplau, L. A. (2003). Sexual compliance: Gender, motivational, and relationship perspectives. *Journal of Sex Research, 40*(1), 87–100.

Inna, N., Phianmongkhol, Y., & Charoenkwan, K. (2009). Sexual function after loop electrosurgical excision procedure for cervical dysplasia. *Journal of Sexual Medicine, 7*(3), 1291–1297.

Jaarsma, T., Dracup, K., Walden, J., & Stevenson, L. W. (1996). Sexual function in patients with advanced heart failure. *Heart and Lung: Journal of Acute and Critical Care, 25*(4), 262–270.

Jeffery, D. D., Tzeng, J. P., Keefe, F. J., Porter, L. S., Hahn, E. A., & Flynn, K. E., ... Weinfurt, K. P. (2009). Initial report of the cancer Patient-Reported Outcomes Measurement Information System (PROMIS) sexual function committee: Review of sexual function measures and domains used in oncology. *Cancer, 115*(6), 1142–1153.

Jensen, P. T., Groenvold, M., Klee, M. C., Thranov, I., Petersen, M. A., & Machin, D. (2003). Longitudinal study of sexual function and vaginal changes after radiotherapy for cervical cancer. *International Journal of Radiation Oncology, 56*(4), 937–949.

Jones, L. R. A. (2002). The use of validated questionnaires to assess female sexual dysfunction. *World Journal of Urology, 20*(2), 89–92.

Kaplan, H. S. (1974). *The new sex therapy: Active treatment of sexual dysfunctions.* New York, NY: Brunner/Mazel.

Kaplan, H. S. (1979). *Disorders of sex desire.* New York: Brunner/Mazel.

Kaschak, E., & Tiefer, L. (Eds.). (2001). *A new view of women's sexual problems.* New York, NY: Haworth Press.

Kiefer, A. K., & Sanchez, D. T. (2007). Scripting sexual passivity: A gender role perspective. *Personal Relationships, 14*, 269–290.

Killackey, M. A. (2000). Avoidance of female genital tract complications in relation to pelvic surgery for cancer. *Seminars in Surgical Oncology, 18*(3), 229–234.

Kinsey, A. C., Pomeroy, W. B., & Martin, C. E. (1948). *Sexual behavior in the human male.* Bloomington, IA: Indiana University Press.

Kinsey, A. C., Pomeroy, W. B., Martin, C. E., & Gebhard, P. H. (1953). *Sexual behavior in the human female.* Bloomington, IA: Indiana University Press.

Lemieux, L., Kaiser, S., Pereira, J., & Meadows, L. M. (2004). Sexuality in palliative care: Patient perspectives. *Palliative Medicine, 18*, 630–637.

Lenahan, P. M. (2004). Sexual health and chronic illness. *Clinics in Family Practice, 6*(4), 955–973.

Levant, R., & Richmond, K. (2007). A review of research on masculinity ideologies using the male role norms inventory. *Journal of Men's Studies, 15*(2), 130–146.

Levant, R., Richmond, K., Cook, S., House, A. T., & Aupont, M. (2007). The femininity ideology scale: Factor structure, reliability, convergent and discriminant validity, and social contextual variation. *Sex Roles, 57*, 373–383.

Lindau, S. T., Schumm, L. P., Laumann, E. O., Levinson, W., O'Muircheartaigh, C. A., & Waite, L. J. (2007). A study of sexuality and health among older adults in the United States. *New England Journal of Medicine, 357*(8), 762–774.

Litwin, M. S., Hays, R. D., Fink, A., Ganz, P. A., Leake, B., & Brook, R. H. (1998). The UCLA prostate cancer index: Development, reliability, and validity of a health-related quality of life measure. *Medical Care, 36*, 1002.

Lucas, T., & Parkhill, M. R. (2009). Strategic impression management: Audience sex and response anonymity affect sex differences in perceived extra-pair paternity. *Journal of Evolutionary Psychology, 7*(1), 49–63.

Lue, T. F., Guiliano, F., Montorsi, F., Rosen, R. C., Andersson, K. E., Althof, S., ... Wagner, G. (2004). Summary of the recommendations on sexual dysfunctions in men. *Journal of Sexual Medicine, 1*(1), 6–23.

Lund-Nielsen, B. (2005). Malignant wounds in women with breast cancer: Feminine and sexual perspectives. *Journal of Clinical Nursing, 14*(1), 56–64.

Lykins, A. D., Janssen, E., & Graham, C. A. (2006). The relationship between negative mood and sexuality in heterosexual college women and men. *Journal of Sex Research, 43*, 136–143.

Machado, A., & Silva, F. J. (2007). Toward a richer view of the scientific method: The role of conceptual analysis. *American Psychologist, 62*(7), 671–681.

Majerovitz, S. D., & Revenson, T. A. (1994). Sexuality and rheumatic disease the significance of gender. *Arthritis Care and Research, 7*(1), 29–34.

Maliski, S. L., Rivera, S., Connor, S., Lopez, G., & Litwin, M. S. (2008). Renegotiating masculine identity after prostate cancer treatment. *Qualitative Health Research, 18*, 1609.

Manderson, L. (1999). Gender, normality and the post-surgical body. *Anthropology & Medicine, 6*(3), 381–394.

Mansfield, P. K., Koch, P. B., & Voda, A. M. (1998). Qualities midlife women desire in their sexual relationships and their changing sexual response. *Psychology of Women Quarterly, 22*, 285–303.

Marriott, C., & Thompson, A. R. (2008). Managing threats to femininity: Personal and interpersonal experience of living with vulval pain. *Psychology & Health*, *23*(2), 243–258.

Masters, W. H., & Johnson, V. E. (1966). *Human sexual response*. Toronto, Quebec, Canada: Bantam Books.

Masters, W. H., & Johnson, V. E. (1970). *Human sexual inadequacy*. Toronto, Quebec, Canada: Bantam Books.

McCabe, J. M., Tanner, A. E., & Heiman, J. R. (2010). The impact of gender expectations on meanings of sex and sexuality: Results from a cognitive interview study. *Sex Roles, 62*(3–4), 252–263.

McClelland, S. I. (2010). Intimate justice: A critical analysis of sexual satisfaction. *Social and Personality Psychology Compass, 4*(9), 663–680.

Meston, C. M., & Derogatis, L. R. (2002). Validated instruments for assessing female sexual function. *Journal of Sex and Marital Therapy*, *28*(s), 155–164.

Meuleman, E. J., & van Lankveld, J. J. (2005). Hypoactive sexual desire disorder: An underestimated condition in men. *BJU International*, *95*(3), 291–296.

Meyerowitz, B. E., Desmond, K. A., & Rowland, J. H. (1999). Sexuality following breast cancer. *Journal of Sex & Marital Therapy*, *25*(3), 237–250.

Moynihan, R. (2003). The making of a disease: Female sexual dysfunction. *BMJ*, *326*, 45–47.

National Cancer Institute (NCI). (2004). Living beyond cancer: Finding a new balance. Retrieved from http://deainfo.nci.nih.gov/ADVISORY/pcp/pcp03-04rpt/Survivorship.pdf

Oliffe, J. (2005). Constructions of masculinity following prostatectomy-induced impotence. *Social Science & Medicine*, *60*(10), 2249–2259.

Oliver, M. B., & Hyde, J. S. (1993). Gender differences in sexuality: A meta-analysis. *Psychological Bulletin*, *114*(1), 29–51.

Penson, R., Wenzel, L., Vergote, I., & Cella, D. (2006). Quality of life considerations in gynecologic cancer. *International Journal of Gynecology & Obstetrics, 95*, S247–S257.

Petersen, J. L., & Hyde, J. S. (2010). A meta-analytic review of research on gender differences in sexuality, 1993–2007. *Psychological Bulletin*, *136*(1), 21–38.

Pikler, V., & Winterowd, C. (2003). Racial and body image differences in coping for women diagnosed with breast cancer. *Health Psychology*, *22*(6), 632–637.

Pluhar, E. (2007). Childhood sexuality. In M. S. Tepper & A. F. Owens (Eds.), *Sexual health: Vol. 1. Psychological foundations* (pp. 155–181). Westport, CT: Praeger.

Pocard, M., Zinzindohoue, F., Haab, F., Caplin, S., Parc, R., & Tiret, E. (2002). A prospective study of sexual and urinary function before and after total mesorectal excision with autonomic nerve preservation for rectal cancer. *Surgery*, *131*(4), 368–372.

Potts, A. (2000). "The essence of the hard on": Hegemonic masculinity and the cultural construction of "erectile dysfunction." *Men & Masculinities*, *3*(1), 85–103.

Potts, A., Grace, V., Gavey, N., & Vares, T. (2004). "Viagra stories": Challenging "erectile dysfunction." *Social Science and Medicine*, *59*(3), 489–499.

Range, L. M., & Jenkins, S. R. (2010). Who benefits from Pennebaker's expressive writing paradigm? Research recommendations from three gender theories. *Sex Roles, 63*(3–4), 149–164.

Raphael, D., Rukholm, E., Brown, I., Hill-Bailey, P., & Donato, E. (1996). The quality of life profile—Adolescent version: Background, description, and initial validation. *Journal of Adolescent Health*, *19*(5), 366–375.

Rees, P. M., Fowler, C. J., & Maas, C. P. (2007). Sexual function in men and women with neurological disorders. *Lancet*, *369*, 512–525.

Robinson, J. W., Saliken, J. C., Donnelly, B. J., Barnes, P., & Guyn, L. (2000). Quality-of-life outcomes for men treated with cryosurgery for localized prostate carcinoma. *Cancer*, *86*(9), 1793–1801.

Rosen, R. C. (2002). Assessment of female sexual dysfunction: Review of validated methods. *Fertility and Sterility*, *77*(4), 89–93.

Rosen, R. C., Brown, C., Heiman, J., Leiblum, S., Meston, C., & Shabsigh, R., … D'Agostino, R., Jr. (2000). The Female Sexual Function Index (FSFI): A multidimensional self-report instrument for the assessment of female sexual function. *Journal of Sex and Marital Therapy*, *26*, 191–208.

Rosen, R. C., Riley, A., Wagner, G., Osterloh, I. H., Kirkpatrick, J., & Mishra, A. (1997). The International Index of Erectile Function (IIEF): A multidimensional scale for assessment of erectile dysfunction. *Urology*, *49*, 822–830.

Rostosky, S., Dekhtyar, O., Cupp, P., & Anderman, E. (2008). Sexual self-concept and sexual self-efficacy in adolescents: A possible clue to promoting sexual health? *Journal of Sex Research*, *45*(3), 277–286.

Sanchez, D. T., Crocker, J., & Boike, K. R. (2005). Doing gender in the bedroom: Investing in gender norms and the sexual experience. *Personality and Social Psychology Bulletin, 31,* 1445–1455.

Schmidt, E. Z., Hofmann, P., Niederwieser, G., Kapfhammer, H. P., & Bonelli, R. M. (2005). Sexuality in multiple sclerosis. *Journal of Neural Transmission*, *112*(9), 1201–1211.

Schneidewind-Skibbe, A., Hayes, R. D., Koochaki, P. E., Meyer, J., & Dennerstein, L. (2008). The frequency of sexual intercourse reported by women: A review of community-based studies and factors limiting their conclusions. *Journal of Sexual Medicine*, *5*(2), 301–335.

Schover L. R., Fouladi R. T., Warneke, C. L., Neede, L., Klein, E. A., Zippe, C., & Kupelian, P. A. (2002). Defining sexual outcomes after treatment for localized prostate cancer. *Cancer*, *95*, 1773–1778.

Schover, L., Fouladi, R., Warneke, C., Neese, L., Klein, E., Zippe, C., & Kupelian, P. A. (2004). Seeking help for erectile dysfunction after treatment for prostate cancer. *Archives of Sexual Behavior*, *33*(5), 443–454.

Schover, L. R., & Jensen, S. B. (1988). *Sexuality and chronic illness: A comprehensive approach.* New York, NY: Guilford Press.

Scott, J. L., Halford, W. K., & Ward, B. G. (2004). United we stand? The effects of a couple-coping intervention on adjustment to early stage breast or gynecological cancer. *Journal of Consulting and Clinical Psychology*, *72*(6), 1122–1135.

Sorrell, J. H., & Brown, J. R. (2006). Sexual functioning in patients with end-stage liver disease before and after transplantation. *Liver Transplantation*, *12*(10), 1473 – 1477.

Sprangers, M. A., Cull, A., Groenvold, M., Bjordal, K., Blazeby, J., & Aaronson, N. K. (1998). The European Organization for Research and Treatment of Cancer approach to developing questionnaire modules: An update and overview. EORTC Quality of Life Study Group. *Quality of Life Research, 7,* 291–300.

Sprangers, M. A., Groenvold, M., Arraras, J. I., Franklin, J., te Velde, A., & Muller, M., … Aaronson, N. K. (1996). The European Organization for Research and Treatment of Cancer breast cancer–specific quality-of-life questionnaire module: First results from a three-country field study. *Journal of Clinical Oncology*, *14*(10), 2756–2768.

Sprangers, M. A., Taal, B. G., Aaronson, N. K., & te Velde, A. (1995). Quality of life in colorectal cancer. Stoma vs. nonstoma patients. *Diseases of the Colon and Rectum*, *38*(4), 361–369.

Stanton, A. L. (2006). Psychosocial concerns and interventions for cancer survivors. *Journal of Clinical Oncology*, *24*(32), 5132–5137.

Stanton, A. L., Revenson, T. A., & Tennen, H. (2007). Health psychology: Psychological adjustment to chronic disease. *Annual Reviews in Psychology*, *58*, 565–592.

Stausmire, J. M. (2004). Sexuality at the end of life. *American Journal of Hospice and Palliative Medicine*, *21*(1), 33–39.

Syrjala, K. L., Roth-Roemer, S. L., Abrams, J. R., Scanlan, J. M,, Chapko, M. K., Visser, S., & Sanders, J. E. (1998). Prevalence and predictors of sexual dysfunction in long-term survivors of marrow transplantation. *Journal of Clinical Oncology, 16*(9), 3148–3157.

Talcott, J. A., Manola, J., Clark, J. A., Kaplan, I., Beard, C. J., Mitchell, S. P., … D'Amico, A. V. (2003). Time course and predictors of symptoms after primary prostate cancer therapy. *Journal of Clinical Oncology*, *21*(21), 3979–3986.

Taylor, J. F., Rosen, R. C., & Leiblum, S. R. (1994). Self-report assessment of female sexual function: Psychometric evaluation of the brief index of sexual functioning for women. *Archives of Sexual Behavior*, *23*(6), 627–643.

Thompson, E. H., & Pleck, J. H. (1986). The structure of male role norms. *American Behavioral Scientist*, *29*, 531–543.

Tiefer, L. (1996). The medicalization of sexuality: Conceptual, normative, and professional issues. *Annual Review of Sex Research*, *7*, 252.

Tiefer L. (2004). *Sex is not a natural act & other essays* (2nd ed.). Boulder, CO: Westview Press.

Tolman, D. L., & Porche, M. V. (2000). The adolescent femininity ideology scale: Development and validation of a new measure for girls. *Psychology of Women Quarterly*, *24*, 365–376.

Tolman, D. L., & Szalacha, L. A. (1999). Dimensions of desire. *Psychology of Women Quarterly*, *23*(1), 7–39.

Tomic, D., Gallicchio, L., Whiteman, M., Lewis, L., Langenberg, P., & Flaws, J. (2006). Factors associated with determinants of sexual functioning in midlife women. *Maturitas, 53*(2), 144–157.

Tristano, A. G. (2009). The impact of rheumatic diseases on sexual function. *Rheumatology International*, *29*(8), 853–860.

Van Berlo, W. T. M., van de Wiel, H. B. M., Taal, E., Rasker, J. J., Weijmar Schultz, W. C. M., & van Rijswijk, M. H. (2007). Sexual functioning of people with rheumatoid arthritis: A multicenter study. *Clinical Rheumatology*, *26*(1), 30–38.

Verschuren, J. E. A., Enzlin, P., Dijkstra, P. U., Geertzen, J. H. B., & Dekker, R. (2010). Chronic disease and sexuality: A generic conceptual framework. *Journal of Sex Research*, *47*(2), 153–170.

Waite, L. J., Laumann, E. O., Das, A., & Schumm, L. P. (2009). Sexuality: Measures of partnerships, practices, attitudes, and problems in the national social life, health and aging study. *Journals of Gerontology: Social Sciences, 64B*(Suppl. 1), i56–i66.

West, S. L., Vinikoor, L. C., & Zolnoun, D. (2004). A systematic review of the literature on female sexual dysfunction prevalence and predictors. *Annual Review of Sex Research, 15*, 40–172.

Wilmoth, M. C. (2001). The aftermath of breast cancer: An altered sexual self. *Cancer Nursing, 24*, 278–286.

Wilmoth, M. C., & Spinelli, A. (2000). Sexual implications of gynecologic cancer treatments. *Journal of Obstetric, Gynecologic, & Neonatal Nursing, 29*(4), 413–421.

Wilson, G. D. (2010). Measurement of sex fantasy. *Sexual and Relationship Therapy, 25*(1), 57–67.

Wolpe, J. (1958). *Psychotherapy by reciprocal inhibition.* Stanford, CA: Stanford University Press.

Yost, K. J., & Cella, D. (2003). Health-related quality of life and colorectal cancer. *Colorectal Cancer Index & Review, 4*(4), 4–7.

Yurek, D., Farrar, W., & Andersen, B. L. (2000). Breast cancer surgery: Comparing surgical groups and determining individual differences in postoperative sexuality and body change stress. *Journal of Consulting and Clinical Psychology, 68*(4), 697–709.

Zemishlany, Z., & Weizman, A. (2008). The impact of mental illness on sexual dysfunction. *Advances in Psychosomatic Medicine, 29*, 89–106.

12 Patient Adherence to Treatment Regimen

Jacqueline Dunbar-Jacob, Elizabeth Schlenk, and Maura McCall
University of Pittsburgh School of Nursing

Although attention has been given to identifying and intervening on poor adherence to treatment regimen for more than 35 years, the problem remains a significant one in health care. In an environment struggling to contain health care costs, billions of dollars are wasted treating the consequences of poor adherence. This chapter will address the impact of poor adherence on health care costs as well as on clinical outcomes and will update information on the magnitude of the problem as well as the efforts to predict, remediate, or prevent it. The confounding influence of multiple definitions and measurement methods will also be addressed.

IMPACT OF POOR ADHERENCE ON HEALTH CARE COSTS

There is little doubt that a major contributor to health care costs is the failure of patients to adhere satisfactorily to a treatment regimen. More than 15 years ago, estimates were that nonadherence resulted in health care costs of $100 billion (Grahl, 1994). A more recent estimate indicates that the number may be closer to $300 billion (DiMatteo, 2004). Although research on the overall economic impact of nonadherence is sparse, studies of specific conditions have afforded a glimpse of potential resulting costs. More specifically, estimated costs attributed to a nonadherent patient's chronic bronchitis antibiotic treatments were reportedly $141 more than the patient's adherent counterparts (Sorenson et al., 2009). According to claims data, nonadherent transplant patients incurred approximately $33,000 more health care costs after three years than those with excellent adherence (Pinsky et al., 2009), and adherent ulcerative colitis patients incur almost 50% less overall health care costs (Kane & Shaya, 2008). Although no significant cost savings were found for patients adherent with their congestive heart failure and hypertensive medications, overall health costs were significantly reduced with adherence to diabetes and cholesterol medicines (Sokol, McGuigan, Verbrugge, & Epstein, 2005). Costs of nonadherence to other forms of treatment (e.g., diet, exercise, smoking cessation, and dialysis) are more challenging to estimate; but given their contribution to disease management, they yield costs over and above those resulting from poor adherence to prescribed medication. When considering both direct and indirect costs, such as time away from work, the financial consequences of nonadherence become evident.

Failure to adhere satisfactorily to a treatment regimen also leads to the necessity to treat the complications or progression of varied diseases. As complications or disease progression appear, the cost of care rises. For example, the person with hypertension who adheres poorly to treatment may progress to a stroke, resulting in hospitalization and rehabilitation. The poorly adherent person with diabetes may develop neuropathy, retinopathy, cardiovascular disease, and/or renal disease, each requiring some form of treatment. Even in life-threatening conditions, poor adherence has been observed. For example, poor adherence to treatment accounts for 25% of graft failures in organ transplantation (Rovelli et al., 1989) and a 43%–46% increased risk of failure in kidney transplantation (Takemoto et al., 2007). Such patients may require retransplantation. Indeed, poor adherence to treatment has been linked to unnecessary complications, as well as to disease progression in multiple diseases (Dunbar-Jacob & Schlenk, 1996). In each case, health care costs rise.

The rising cost of poor adherence is also found in preventive services. For example, in primary prevention, immunization rates are less than optimal in both the pediatric and geriatric groups. The failure to immunize leads to excess cases of such conditions as measles in childhood (Mason, 1992), alarming increases in the prevalence of such preventable diseases as pertussis, which may reach its greatest number of reported cases in California since 1958 (Winter et al., 2010), and pneumonia among the elderly (Nichol, Margolis, Wuorenma, & Von Sternberg, 1994). Recent public health campaigns have focused on adult immunization promotion. Each case of preventable disease, however, leads to an increase in health care costs.

IMPACT ON CLINICAL OUTCOMES

Cost is only one negative outcome of poor adherence. As noted earlier, adherence is a mediator of clinical outcome. DiMatteo, Giordani, Lepper, and Croghan (2002) conducted a meta-analysis of 63 articles and found that treatment adherence decreases the overall risk of a poor outcome by 26% (95% CI 20%, 32%) and that an adherent patient is 2.88 times more likely to have a better outcome than a nonadherent patient (95% CI 2.33, 3.73). However, there is a paucity of knowledge about the amount of adherence to a prescribed treatment that is required to produce a desired clinical outcome. Only a few studies have investigated the amount of medication adherence required to produce a desired clinical outcome (DeGeest, 1996; Haynes et al., 1976). No studies have investigated the amount of adherence to behavioral treatment required for a desired clinical outcome.

The relations between the three adherence behaviors of medication taking, following a therapeutic diet, and following an exercise program and clinical outcomes are discussed. The clinical outcomes reported in the literature include relapse, sign and symptom relief, health status, hospitalization, morbidity, and mortality.

MEDICATION ADHERENCE AND CLINICAL OUTCOMES

Most of the research on the relationship between adherence and clinical outcomes has been conducted in the area of pharmacological treatment. Better medication adherence has generally been linked to better outcomes. Better medication adherence was related to prevention of relapse in tuberculosis (Dupon & Raynaud, 1992; Shin et al., 2010), epilepsy (Cramer, Mattson, Prevey, Scheyer, & Ouellette, 1989; Reynolds, 1987), childhood leukemia (Klopovich & Trueworthy, 1985), schizophrenia (Leff et al., 1989; Mantonakis, Jemos, Christodoulou, & Lykouras, 1982), and alcoholism (Fawcett et al., 1987; Fawcett et al., 1984; Pisani, Fawcett, Clark, & McQuire, 1993). In addition, treatment adherence in hypercholesterolemia, hypertension, intestinal disease, and sleep apnea were all significantly related to outcomes (DiMatteo et al., 2002). Likewise, hypertensive patients who reported forgetting their medicine were significantly more likely to have a cardiovascular event (M. R. Nelson, Reid, Ryan, Willson, & Yelland, 2006). In a systematic review of adherence intervention studies, Kripalani, Yao, and Haynes (2007) reported that 11 of 37 trials showed improvement in at least one clinical outcome, though this improvement was not necessarily related to adherence rates. Interestingly, adherence to antibiotics, measured by urinary assay, for otitis media was not related to decreased reoccurrence (Reed, Lutz, Zazove, & Ratcliffe, 1984). In addition, adherence to ocular treatments produced mixed results concerning its impact on visual fields and intraocular pressure (Olthoff, Schouten, van de Borne, & Webers, 2005).

Better medication adherence has also been associated with sign and symptom relief in a number of conditions. For example, improvement was found among persons with hypertension (Fletcher, Deliakis, Schoch, & Shapiro, 1979; Haynes, Gibson, Taylor, Bernholz, & Sackett, 1982; McKenny, Munroe, & Wright, 1992), peptic esophageal stenosis (Starlinger, Appel, Schemper, & Schiessel, 1985), chronic bronchitis (Dompeling et al., 1992), schizophrenia (Verghese et al., 1989), manic depression (Connelly,

Davenport, & Nurnberger, 1982), and chronic pain (Berndt, Maier, & Schutz, 1993). However, adherence is not always related to clinical outcome—a complication in examining the effectiveness of adherence interventions. For example, medication adherence was not related to symptom relief in asthma (Dompeling et al., 1992) or open-angle glaucoma (Granstrom, 1985).

Better medication adherence has been associated with dimensions of health status in a few studies. In hypertension, medication adherence was related to clinical health status and perceived health status but not functional status (Given, Given, & Simoni, 1979). In rheumatoid arthritis, self-reported medication adherence was not related to health status or functional status (Taal, Rasker, Seydel, & Weigman, 1993) but was related to reduced pain (Dunbar-Jacob, Kwoh, et al., 1996). Because self-report tends to overestimate medication adherence, measurement errors may have obscured the relationship between adherence and health status.

Medication nonadherence has been associated with higher rates of hospitalization and/or costs of hospitalization. Higher hospitalization rates with poorer adherence were found for hypertension (Maronde et al., 1989), manic depression (Connelly et al., 1982; Lehmann & Rabins, 2006), schizophrenia (Gaebel & Pietzcker, 1985), and alcoholism (Fawcett et al., 1987). Good adherence in ulcerative colitis led to 62% lower hospitalization costs (Kane & Shaya, 2008).

Medication nonadherence was related to morbidity across acute and chronic disorders as well as preventive regimens. Adherence to antibiotics was related to resolution of acute urinary tract infections in the elderly (Cheung et al., 1988). In chronic bronchitis, medication nonadherence was related to poorer pulmonary function test results (Dompeling et al., 1992). In psychiatric disorders, such as depression in the elderly (Cole, 1985; Lin et al., 2004), and manic depression (Connelly et al., 1982), medication nonadherence was related to a worse clinical course. Medication nonadherence among renal transplant recipients resulted in return to dialysis (Kalil, Heim-Duthoy, & Kasiske, 1992), renal insufficiency during pregnancy (O'Donnell et al., 1985), and organ rejection (Pinsky et al., 2009; Rovelli et al., 1989; Schweizer et al., 1990). Similarly, heart transplant recipients, who had minor departures in immunosuppressive medications, exhibited organ rejection and other adverse occurrences (DeGeest, 1996), and adherence plays a key role in outcomes (Owen, Bonds, & Wellisch, 2006). Nonadherence to medications taken for preventive purposes was related to higher morbidity as well. Nonadherence to antihypertensive medications was related to an increased risk for coronary heart disease (Psaty, Koepsell, Wagner, LoGerfo, & Inui, 1990). Similarly, nonadherence to preventive medications for tuberculosis (Nolan, Aitken, Elarth, Anderson, & Miller, 1986; Shin et al., 2010) and malaria (Wetsteyn & deGeus, 1993; Yeboah-Antwi et al., 2001) was related to higher occurrence of these respective disorders.

Death is also a consequence of poor adherence. Medication nonadherence was related to mortality in patients with epilepsy (Lip & Brodie, 1992; Davis, Candrilli, & Edin, 2008), asthma (Robertson, Rubinfeld, & Bowes, 1992; Strandbygaard, Thomsen, & Backer, 2010), and organ transplantation (Lanza, Cooper, Boyd, & Barnard, 1984; Pinsky et al., 2009; Schweizer et al., 1990). Similarly, medication adherence was related to survival among patients with hematologic malignancies (Richardson, Shelton, Krailo, & Levine, 1990).

As noted earlier, poor adherence has also been associated with the development of treatment-resistant organisms in infectious disease. The resurgence of tuberculosis from 1985 to 1992 has been linked in part to variable adherence and/or to early cessation of antituberculosis medications (Bloom & Murray, 1992; Gibbons, 1992; Nolan et al., 1986). A recent study noted a 17% increased risk of developing an extensively drug-resistant tuberculosis organism for each month of <80% adherence (Shin et al., 2010). The current U.S. plan to combat the disease includes promoting medication adherence and treatment completion (LoBue, Sizemore, & Castro, 2009). Similarly, poor adherence to antibiotic therapies has been associated with treatment resistance among children with otitis media (DeLalla, 1998) and has been suspected in a portion of disease-resistant staphylococcal and streptococcal infections (Schwarzmann, 1998). There are indications where even slight deviations from prescribed directions may lead to the development of drug-resistant strains, for example, antiretroviral medications in treatment of HIV (Vanhove, Schapiro, Winters, Merigan, & Blaschke, 1996).

In fact, an adherence of ≥95% is recommended for optimal virologic outcome, and those patients with adherence levels of less than 80% may increase risk of treatment failure by 14 times when compared to the ≥95% group (Paterson et al., 2000). Unfortunately, these drug-resistant viruses are themselves transmissible.

In summary, nonadherence to prescribed medication has been associated with poorer clinical outcomes across a wide variety of disorders. The outcomes range from progression of disease, complications, reduced health status, increased symptom presentation, hospitalization, death, and the development of treatment-resistant organisms. The costs of nonadherence are high in terms of patient health, health care utilization, and even death.

DIETARY ADHERENCE AND CLINICAL OUTCOMES

Dietary prescriptions are also a common recommended treatment, particularly in a variety of chronic diseases. They also influence clinical outcomes. Nonadherence to low-fat diets was related to mortality (Singh, Niaz, Ghosh, Singh, & Rastogi, 1993; Swank & Dugan, 1990) and cardiac events (Singh et al., 1993). Nonadherence to diabetic diets was related to diabetic ketoacidosis (Mulrow, Bailey, Sonksen, & Slavin, 1987; White, Kolman, Wexler, Polin, & Winter, 1984) and to hospitalizations and emergent visits (H. A. Fishbein, 1985; White et al., 1984), but not to such measures of diabetic control as weight and glycosylated hemoglobin (Mulrow et al., 1987). Given that multiple factors influence diabetic control in conjunction with medication adherence, it may be difficult to impact these specific clinical measures. More recently, elderly who adhered to a Mediterranean diet and exercise had a decreased risk of developing Alzheimer's disease (Scarmeas et al., 2009). In addition, greater adherence to the Mediterranean diet was associated with lower glycosylated hemoglobin and postprandial glucose levels (Esposito, Maiorino, Di Palo, & Giugliano, 2009).

EXERCISE ADHERENCE AND CLINICAL OUTCOMES

Exercise prescriptions are made for general health as well as a component of treatment for multiple acute and chronic conditions. Nonadherence to prescribed exercise in postsurgical patients was related to lower range of motion, joint extension, functional status, and higher relapse (R. B. Hawkins, 1989; R. J. Hawkins & Switlyk, 1993; Rives, Gelberman, Smith, & Carney, 1992). In older women, adherence to group exercise improved change in sway (Lichtenstein, Shields, Shiavi, & Burger, 1989). In a systematic review of studies delivering an exercise regimen to hospitalized patients, de Morton, Keating, and Jeffs (2007) noted a slight decrease of approximately $300 per stay for those receiving exercise during their hospitalization. In summary, exercise adherence has been associated with clinical outcomes.

MAGNITUDE OF THE PROBLEM

As noted, the problem of poor adherence to treatment regimen has a significant impact on the outcomes of care and subsequently on health care costs. Unfortunately, nonadherence to health care regimens is a prevalent problem that cuts across disorders, treatment regimens, ages, gender, and ethnic and socioeconomic groups (Burke & Dunbar-Jacob, 1995; Dunbar-Jacob, Burke, & Puczynski, 1995). Using medication possession ratios, Thier and colleagues (2008) determined overall medication adherence rates were an alarming 26%; whereas Claxton, Cramer, and Pierce (2001) reviewed electronic-monitor data from 14 studies revealing an overall average adherence of 59%, indicating that adherence rates have not improved significantly over the years.

There is some indication that persons with life-threatening conditions may adhere somewhat better than others (Sullivan et al., 2007; Tessema et al., 2010). But in these conditions (e.g., cancer, AIDS, and transplantation), there is a burgeoning body of evidence to suggest that even modest deviations have significant clinical impact (DeGeest, 1996; M. Nelson et al., 2010). In addition, there is some evidence that persons participating in clinical trials may also have better adherence (Hall & Most, 2005; Schron et al., 1995). Even in these situations, adherence is far from perfect. Nonadherence varies over the course of treatment, with steeper declines in adherence noted earlier in treatment. For example, from 16% to 50% of patients with hypertension discontinue their medication within the first 12 months (Flack, Novikov, & Ferrario, 1996; Jones, Gorkin, Lian, Staffa, & Fletcher, 1995), and 50% of patients in cardiac rehabilitation programs drop out in the first 12 months (Oldridge, 1984). Over the long run, adherence continues to decrease, but at a less marked rate than observed at the outset of treatment. For example, in the Lipid Research Clinic–Coronary Primary Prevention Trial (LRC-CPPT), reductions in dietary fat and cholesterol began to show reversals at 12 months that continued over the seven-year clinical trial (Lipid Research Clinics Program, 1984a, 1984b). The importance of treatment persistence has been recognized and is being studied with greater frequency (e.g., Gallagher, Leighton-Scott, & van Staa, 2009; Hasford, Uricher, Tauscher, Bramlage, & Virchow, 2010; McHorney, Victor Spain, Alexander, & Simmons, 2009).Thus, interventions to promote adherence necessitate a focus on initial adherence as well as maintenance of adherence.

Medication Adherence

Studies have shown that from 20% to 80% of persons do not adhere to medication prescriptions to the extent of gaining therapeutic benefit (Dunbar-Jacob et al., 1995). Among persons with chronic disorders, from 50% to 90% do not adhere to medication prescriptions (Cramer, Scheyer, & Mattson, 1990). A systematic review of ocular medication adherence reported rates between 4.6% and 80% (Olthoff et al., 2005). Medication nonadherence rates vary depending on the method and time of measurement. A review of antihypertensive medication adherence found that adherence by self-report was 75%, whereas adherence by pill count was 52% (Dunbar-Jacob, Dwyer, & Dunning, 1991). Dunbar-Jacob, Burke, et al. (1996) compared self-report, pill count, and electronic monitors in subjects taking a lipid-lowering drug and found poor correspondence among the measures with self-report by seven-day recall at 97%, pill count at 94%, and electronic monitors at 84%. Thus, adherence rates vary by measurement method. Using electronic monitors in subjects with epilepsy, Cramer et al. (1990) reported mean adherence rates of 88% during the five days before the clinic visit, 86% during the five days after the clinic visit, and only 67% during a five-day period one month later. A similar phenomenon was observed in glaucoma patients (Okeke et al., 2009). Thus, it appears as though daily adherence declines between clinic visits and rebounds just before and after planned clinical contact. Estimates of adherence at clinic visits may actually overestimate patient behavior.

Dietary Adherence

Dietary recommendations often accompany medication prescriptions for chronic-disorder regimens, for example, hypertension, diabetes, and hyperlipidemia. Modifying long-standing dietary habits and maintaining newly established eating plans can be difficult. Adherence with low-fat, low-cholesterol diets ranges from 13% to 76% (Glanz, 1979), whereas long-term adherence with weight-reducing diets is less than 50%, with few persons maintaining the weight loss (Glanz, 1979). According to a review, adherence to fluid restriction in end-stage renal-disease patients range from 30% to 74% (Denhaerynck, Manhaeve, et al., 2007). The rates, then, appear similar to those for medication.

Exercise Adherence

Exercise adherence is a problem across healthy and chronic-disorder populations, with 50% dropping out of exercise during the first three to six months and a leveling off of the dropout rate between

55% and 75% by one year (Carmody, Senner, Malinow, & Matarazzo, 1980). Indeed, adherence to exercise recommendations hovers at 40% (Berrigan, Dodd, Troiano, Krebs-Smith, & Barbash, 2003). An exercise regimen can be time consuming, inconvenient, and expensive, all of which are barriers to adherence. For persons managing chronic disorders, additional exercise barriers exist, among them fatigue and pain. For example, in fibromyalgia, exercise nonadherence was high at 44%. Reasons reported for missing exercise included finding time when facing changes in routine (85.2%) and presence of such fibromyalgia symptoms as fatigue and pain (44.4%; Schlenk, Okifuji, Dunbar-Jacob, & Turk, 1996).

In 1996, the U.S. surgeon general released a report on physical activity and health that recommended 30 minutes or more of moderate-intensity physical activity on all, or most, days of the week (U.S. Department of Health and Human Services, 1996). This physical activity can be accumulated during the course of the day (Pate et al., 1995). Despite this recommendation, over 60% of U.S. adults are not regularly active, and 25% of U.S. adults are not active at all. Only 22% of U.S. adults engage in sustained physical activity of any intensity five times weekly for 30 minutes (U.S. Department of Health and Human Services, 1996). In fact, U.S. adherence to all five healthy lifestyle choices fell significantly from an already low 15% to 8% between 1988 and 2006 (D. E. King, Mainous, Carnemolla, & Everett, 2009). Poor adherence has also been a significant problem in rehabilitation where performance of therapeutic exercise looks similar to efforts to follow drug regimen (Dunbar-Jacob, 1998).

DEFINITIONS OF ADHERENCE

One factor that influences the degree of poor adherence found in research and clinical populations is the definition of adherence that is selected. Adherence can be defined in at least two general ways. The first is through the pattern of adherence displayed by the patient. The second is by the quantitative assessment that is made.

PATTERNS OF ADHERENCE

There are at least six behavior patterns that constitute problematic adherence. These consist of failure to adopt the regimen, early stoppage of treatment, reduction in levels of treatment, overtreatment, variability in the conduct of the regimen, and dosage interval errors. Several of these could occur within the same patient.

Adoption of the treatment regimen is the first step in adherence. Yet the problem of adoption is fairly significant. There are some data to suggest that as many as 20% of persons fail to fill medication prescriptions (Burns, Sneddon, Lovell, McLean, & Martin, 1992). A review of surveys on cost-related prescription underuse found that rates ranged from 1.6% to 22% (Kirking, Lee, Ellis, Briesacher, & McKercher, 2006). In a study of 71 patients taking statins, half (51%) tried dietary modification and 73% persisted six months or less (Mann et al., 2007). An adherence rate of less than 50% exercise-class attendance may be considered nonadherence for cardiac rehabilitation. Sharp and Freeman (2009) noted that 35% of their sample conveyed no intention of participating in cardiac rehabilitation exercise classes. The proportion of persons who simply fail to start dietary or exercise regimens has been less well studied but is estimated to be significant. These individuals are rarely described in studies of adherence.

For those individuals who initiate treatment, there is the problem of early stoppage. These persons are often referred to as dropouts or as nonadherers. There is considerable variation in the proportion of persons who drop out of treatment, with the lowest rates seen in clinical trials and the highest in exercise regimen. Indeed, 50% of persons who initiate exercise programs for cardiac rehabilitation are found to terminate early (Oldridge, 1984, 1988), and over one third of those who indicated interest in classes were considered nonadherent with less than 50% attendance (Sharp & Freeman, 2009). Mann et al. (2007) found that of those patients who tried dietary modification,

73% persisted for six months or less. In the clinical trials arena, the rates of dropout are estimated to average between 5% and 25% (Dunbar & Knoke, 1986). Several researchers found significant withdrawal from treatment in the first six months (Chapman et al., 2005; Donnelly, Doney, Morris, Palmer, & Donnan, 2008; Perreault et al., 2005). One of the difficulties in defining dropping out of treatment is that some portion of these persons may drop back in to treatment at a later point in time or with a different care provider.

For those individuals who stay in treatment, several patterns may be found. First among those patterns is alterations in treatment dosing. This alteration may include both reductions in the dose or increases in the dose that has been prescribed. For example, the patient may reduce or increase the dose of medication that is taken or the number of exercise regimens performed per week. Self-reported adherence to duration of exercise was found to be greater than adherence to frequency (Medina-Mirapeix et al., 2009). Underdosing may occur, for example, in response to cost, to side effects, to spacing-out inadequate quantities of medication, or to a belief that a lower dose is preferable. Overdosing occurs in at least two ways. Patients may miss medication and "double up" to achieve the requisite number of doses. Or individuals may decide that extra doses are called for to combat symptoms. In either case, the risks of overdosing and of untoward side effects are high. Research has found these patterns in patients with rheumatoid arthritis and for those with hyperlipidemia, symptomatic and asymptomatic disorders, respectively, as well as among posttransplant patients. Both patterns may be found within the same individual.

The second pattern found among those patients who stay in treatment is variability in adherence. This pattern may be the most common form of adherence problem found. In this instance, the individual follows the medication, dietary, and/or exercise regimen to varying degrees over time. Typically, the regimen may be missed at episodic intervals. Whole days or specific doses may be missed for varying intervals. When the regimen is missed for a period of several days and then resumed seemingly spontaneously, the period is referred to as a "regimen holiday" (Urquhart & Chevalley, 1988). Women being treated for pelvic inflammatory disease, for example, took a drug holiday from their treatment approximately 22% of the time (Dunbar-Jacob, Sereika, Foley, Bass, & Ness, 2004).

The third type of problem found among those who stay in treatment is that of dosing interval errors. This pattern is particularly the case for medication taking but also may be seen with exercise regimen. In the case of medication taking, individuals may consume doses too close together or too far apart. For example, asthma patients have been found to consume puffs of inhaled medication too close together to support efficacy (Berg, Dunbar-Jacob, & Rohay, 1995). Similarly, patients with rheumatoid arthritis have been found to take doses as close as two hours apart as well as more than 36 hours apart (Dunbar-Jacob et al., 1992). Claxton and colleagues (2001) reviewed timing adherence in studies using electronic monitors and found a range of 40% adherence for four-times-per-day dosing to 74% for once-a-day dosing. Adherence to immunizations requiring a schedule of two or three doses is low, with few patients completing the doses and long intervals among those who do complete the series (J. C. Nelson et al., 2009). Renal transplant patients' mean dose interval adherence was 91.9% with a range of 18%–100% (Denhaerynck, Steiger, et al., 2007).

There are, therefore, numerous patterns of poor adherence or nonadherence. Typically, these have been treated as equivalent in studies of adherence with the term *adherence* defined as the total dosage consumed divided by the total prescribed over some period of time. This definition obscures the nature of the adherence problem. Thus, the first consideration in defining poor adherence is the specification of the type of adherence problem or problems that are of interest.

QUANTITATIVE ASSESSMENT OF ADHERENCE

Another approach to defining poor adherence relates to the level of data used. The proportion of the prescribed regimen that is carried out can be examined. This yields a percentage adherence score. For a group, then, the average (mean or median) adherence is reported. Related to this, and often not clearly specified in the literature, is a report of the proportion of persons who meet some adherence criterion, that is, defining a group's adherence by the proportion of persons who achieve or fail to achieve some preestablished level of adherence. The convention has been 80% for most investigations since the landmark study of adherence to antihypertensive medications by Haynes et al. (1976). Although logic suggests that the level of adherence set would be related to the level necessary to achieve therapeutic benefit, little data are available on the relationship between level of adherence and achievement of clinical benefit. In HIV/AIDS adherence research, emphasis on timing of medication taking brings the recommended adherence level at or above 95%, though this may be called into question (Rosenblum, Deeks, van der Laan, & Bangsberg, 2009). In contrast, exercise adherence has used 50% or above as a determination of acceptable adherence. Other methods of defining adherence include a determination of the proportion of persons who have attained clinical benefit, a desired outcome of good adherence, but not the equivalent; the clinical judgment of level of adherence; and the level of attainment of performance of multiple components of a treatment regimen. Each of these definitions influences the rate of adherence reported.

MEASURES OF ADHERENCE

An examination of the research on adherence shows that just as there are multiple definitions of adherence, there are multiple methods of assessment. These include such strategies as self-report (interview or questionnaire or daily diaries), clinician reports, pill counts, biological indicators, clinical outcome, medical claims data, medication possession ratios, and electronic event monitoring. Each yields somewhat different information about the patient's behavior with regard to regimen as well as different reports of adherence. Thus, the selection of a strategy to measure adherence requires careful attention to the limitations of each method and ideally requires a well-specified definition of adherence. There is no gold standard for assessment of adherence (Cramer et al., 1989), though electronic event monitors provide the most complete and timely data on adherence (Dunbar-Jacob, Sereika, Rohay, & Burke, 1998). Measures should, in general, provide accurate, relevant, specific, and objective data and be economically feasible, practical, and easy to administer (Westfall, 1986).

One of the major differences between measurement methods is the difference in reported adherence that may be obtained between methods, even when the same regimen in the same person is assessed (Bangsberg, Hecht, Charlebois, Chesney, & Moss, 2001; Hamilton, 2003). The variation in reported adherence by different measurement methods was first reported by Mattson and Friedman (1984) based on data from the Aspirin Myocardial Infarction Study. In this study, subjects were randomly assigned to aspirin or to placebo. Adherence was measured by pill count, platelet aggregation, and salicylate levels. Adherence ranged from 81% to 97% in the drug group and from 78% to 97% in the placebo group depending on the strategy examined, with adherence highest for the behavioral (pill count) method. These variations are likely dependent on characteristics of the measures. Salicylate levels would be fairly short lived and would reflect adherence just prior to the clinic visit. Work by a number of investigators indicates that adherence is at its peak just before and just after a clinic visit (Cramer et al., 1989; Kass, Meltzer, Gordon, Cooper, & Goldberg, 1986; Norell, 1981; Olthoff et al., 2005). Thus, the salicylate levels would reflect adherence just prior to the visit. Platelet aggregation would have a longer impact but would not provide information on the degree of adherence over time. Individual variations in drug metabolism and other related biological factors would affect the level of platelet aggregation identified. The pill count, while estimating the amount of medication consumed over the measurement period, would also be affected by the subjects' willingness to return all unused medication as well as their memory to do so.

Similar differences in adherence by measurement method have been reported by others (e.g., Burke et al., 1992; Dunbar, Dunning, Dwyer, Burke, & Snetselaar, 1991; Dunbar-Jacob, Burke, Rohay, Sereika, & Muldoon, 1997; Dunbar-Jacob, Burke, et al., 1996; Hyman et al., 1982; Norell, 1981; Petitti, Friedman, & Kahn, 1981; Rand & Wise, 1994; Rudd, Ahmed, Zachary, Barton, & Bonduelle, 1990; Stone, Shiffman, Schwartz, Broderick, & Hufford, 2003; Wilson & Endres, 1986).

Typically, self-report measures overestimate adherence when compared with other measures. This is not unexpected because the self-report measures rely on memory and willingness to report. Given the difficulties in remembering recurring behaviors, the tendency is to rely on recent events as indicators of longer term events. Coupled with peak adherence at the time of assessment at a clinic visit, this basis for estimation of adherence would lead to a personal overrating of longer term adherence behaviors. The diaries are more accurate than interviews or questionnaires, but they are also limited by the willingness of the patient to record daily and accurately. Work suggests that group averages may approximate those seen with electronic monitoring, but sensitivity to poor adherence is low (Dunbar-Jacob, Sereika, & Burke, 1998). Stone and colleagues (2003), however, demonstrated the high level of error in diary recording when compared with unobtrusive electronic monitoring.

The electronic measures tend to report the lowest levels of adherence. These methods record onto microprocessor chips the exact time and date that an event occurred. (For a fuller discussion, see Dunbar-Jacob, Sereika, Rohay, et al., 1998.) Thus, patterns of poor adherence can be identified. Monitors are available for medication taking, exercise, and cued diary entries. The major limitation is sensitivity to actual regimen conduct. Experience with electronic monitoring of medication taking over as much as a 12-month period suggests that the effort to manipulate the monitor at the prescribed time day after day without taking medication is an unlikely expenditure. Deception with the monitor may be estimated with the addition of relevant biological assays.

No matter the method of assessment, however, the distribution of adherence data for medication consumption and for appointment keeping appears to assume a J-curve, which is robust and resistant to transformation (Dunbar-Jacob, Sereika, Rohay, & Probstfield, 1994). Thus, the analysis of adherence data does not lend itself to traditional parametric approaches. Unfortunately, many analyses do just that—not attending to the distribution of the data. Less information is available on the distribution of adherence data for exercise or for diet. Information on these distributions would be valuable.

PREDICTORS OF POOR ADHERENCE

In general, the literature over the past three decades has examined poor adherence as a solitary construct. Most predictors that have been identified have accounted for small proportions of variance in adherence and, furthermore, have not been consistently supported in studies. Perhaps the most consistent predictors have included self-efficacy, initial adherence, complexity of the regimen, and disruptive schedules (e.g., Chapman et al., 2005; Dunbar-Jacob, 1998; Dunbar-Jacob, Schlenk, Burke, & Matthews, 1998). Numerous other factors have been identified, but they have not been consistently related to adherence across studies. These factors include age, social support, mood, income, system of care, clinician–patient communication, comorbid conditions, race, and beliefs (e.g., Dunbar-Jacob, Schlenk, et al., 1998; Harrold et al., 2009; Sullivan et al., 2007; Unni & Farris, 2011).

Predictor studies and intervention studies have typically not discriminated between the various patterns of poor adherence. Nor have the predictor studies distinguished between varying models of adherence. Yet poor adherence can take multiple forms. Thus, it makes intuitive sense that predictors and interventions might vary between these forms. There are a number of dimensions that appear to separate adherence behaviors into independent categories or models, with the probability of identifying differing predictor variables and differing effectiveness in interventions. Two of these important dimensions include whether poor compliance is intentional or unintentional and whether it reflects a lack of capability. Unfortunately, little research on predictors of adherence has separated out factors that may predict a decision not to adhere versus unintentional nonadherence episodes versus a lack of capability to adhere.

Much of the literature on adherence treats adherence problems as intentional decisions or a failure of motivation on the part of patients. Thus, patients may make decisions based on numerous factors. One of these important factors is beliefs: These may be beliefs about treatment, about capability to carry out treatment, or about the effectiveness of treatment. Several theories have addressed adherence from this perspective, including the self-efficacy theory (Bandura, 1997), health belief model (Janz & Becker, 1984; Rosenstock, 1974), theory of reasoned action/theory of planned behavior (Ajzen, 1991; M. Fishbein & Ajzen, 1975), and the commonsense model of illness (Leventhal, Meyer, & Nerenz, 1980). More recently, the motivational interviewing approach has been used (Konkle-Parker, 2001; Ogedegbe et al., 2007; Rubak, Sandbaek, Lauritzen, & Christensen 2005). A second factor, which relates to an intentional decision model of adherence, is the evaluation of the burden of adherence. In this case, such factors as the personal costs associated with care, the stigma that may be encountered from having treatment witnessed, the impact on quality of life, and the effort associated with managing treatment all may influence the decision to follow treatment.

An examination of the patient reports of poor adherence reveals that the most commonly reported reason for failing to adhere to a prescribed regimen is forgetting (Cooper et al., 2007; Dunbar-Jacob, 1997; Fransen, Mesters, Janssen, Knottnerus, & Muris, 2009; Sullivan et al., 2007). Research (Morell, Park, Kidder, & Martin, 1997) suggests that busy and/or disruptive schedules may also contribute to poor adherence. Forgetting and disruption would be related to nonintentional nonadherence episodes. Research has suggested that it is not unusual for patients to report intending to take a dose of medication but something interrupted them (a phone call, a visitor, etc.) and then they became distracted and forgot to return to the medication when the distraction ended. Similarly, patients who report business travel or vacations where daily schedules are disrupted also report higher missed doses of treatment (Dunbar-Jacob, 1997; Schlenk et al., 1996). In depressed patients, almost one third indicated that they sometimes or often forgot to take their medicine (Shigemura, Ogawa, Yoshino, Sato, & Nomura, 2010), and just over 56% of pediatric renal transplant patients report forgetting as the main barrier to adherence (Zelikovsky, Schast, Palmer, & Meyers, 2008). Although such reports are offered by patients, there has been little systematic research in this area.

A third model of poor adherence addresses the patient's capability to carry out the regimen. A variety of factors are at play here. These factors include whether the patient has adequate knowledge to carry out the treatment, whether the skills are present, and whether the patient has the cognitive and/or physical capability to engage in the treatment. Studies identifying the proportion of poor adherence that was related to lack of adequate knowledge were conducted in the mid-1970s (e.g., Boyd, Covington, Stanaszek, & Coussons, 1974) but have not been examined more recently. Low health literacy's effect on adherence has been mixed (Muir et al., 2006; Paasche-Orlow et al., 2006; Wolf et al., 2007). Mood, namely, depression, has been associated with adherence in some studies (Morris et al., 2006; Siegel, Lopez, & Meier, 2007), but not in others (Schweitzer, Head, & Dwyer, 2007; Shemesh et al., 2004). Studies examining cognitive or physical capability have also been limited. Park, Willis, Morrow, Diehl, and Gaines (1994) suggested that those dimensions tapped by standard neuropsychological tests have not been associated with adherence. Personality traits have been examined, and conscientiousness was a predictor of cholesterol medication adherence (Stilley, Sereika, Muldoon, Ryan, & Dunbar-Jacob, 2004). The impact of coping styles, optimism, anxiety, emotional distress, and hostility on adherence has been studied, but much work remains to be done in these dimensions.

In addition to the failure to examine determinants of or predictors of adherence from the perspective of either patterns of adherence or models of poor adherence, multiple methods of measurement of adherence have been used in these studies. Different measures of adherence classify different persons as adherent or nonadherent. It is likely, therefore, that predictor variables will behave differently in different studies. Research supports this notion, suggesting that different measurement methods lead to different predictor variables in the same population on the same regimen (Dunbar-Jacob, Sereika, Rohay, Burke, & Kwoh, 1995).

INTERVENTIONS TO PROMOTE ADHERENCE

Interventions to promote adherence across medication, dietary, and exercise regimens have tended to focus on behavioral strategies or education plus behavioral strategies. Cochrane reviews report on 78 randomized controlled trials (RCT) of medication adherence interventions (Haynes, Ackloo, Sahota, McDonald, &Yao, 2008) and 42 RCT and quasi-experimental trials for exercise adherence interventions (Jordan, Holden, Mason, & Foster, 2010). Interestingly, there are numerous Cochrane reviews for various diets; however, a Cochrane review specifically addressing adherence to dietary recommendations alone could not be found. This may be because other lifestyle changes are linked with dietary change, for example, exercise in weight loss or fluid restriction in kidney failure. Modest improvements have been shown in some studies, but few randomized, controlled clinical trials have been undertaken. The strategies that have been shown to be successful in improving adherence include some combination of self-monitoring, counseling, stimulus control or cueing, positive reinforcement, self-efficacy enhancement, and social support enhancement.

Self-monitoring of blood pressure and/or medication taking (Edmonds et al., 1985; Haynes et al., 1976; Logan, Milne, Achber, Campbell, & Haynes, 1979) and exercise (Atkins, Kaplan, Timms, Reinsch, & Lofback, 1984; A. C. King, Taylor, Haskell, & DeBusk, 1988; Rogers et al., 1987) improved regimen adherence. Counseling promoted adherence with medication taking (Bailey et al., 1990; Colcher & Bass, 1972; Peterson, McLean, & Millingen, 1984), dietary management in large clinical trials (Dolecek et al., 1986; Glueck, Gordon, Nelson, Davis, & Tyroler, 1986; Simkin-Silverman et al., 1995), and exercise (Belisle, Roskies, & Levesque, 1987; A. C. King & Frederiksen, 1984; A. C. King et al., 1988). Stimulus control or cueing improved adherence to medication taking (Haynes et al., 1976; Logan et al., 1979) and exercise (Atkins et al., 1984; Keefe & Blumenthal, 1980). Positive reinforcement promoted adherence to medications (Bailey et al., 1990; Haynes et al., 1976; Logan et al., 1979) and exercise (Atkins et al., 1984; Keefe & Blumenthal, 1980). Self-efficacy enhancement, based on social cognitive theory (Bandura, 1997), has been used successfully to promote dietary adherence (McCann, Follette, Driver, Brief, & Knopp, 1988). Social support enhancement promoted adherence to medication taking (Kirscht, Kirscht, & Rosenstock, 1981; Morisky et al., 1983) and dietary prescriptions (Barnard, Scherwitz, & Ornish, 1992; Bovbjerg et al., 1995).

An accumulation of adherence research over time has resulted in numerous systematic reviews. Patient reminders helped to increase immunization rates (Jacobson Vann & Szilagyi, 2005). Contracts between patients and health care personnel have yielded limited results (Bosch-Capblanch, Abba, Prictor, & Garner, 2007). A review of interventions to improve ocular medication adherence drew no conclusions because of the design and methodological quality of the studies, though there were interventions showing some improvement to adherence (Gray, Orton, Henson, Harper, & Waterman, 2009). Design and methodological quality is a persistent problem throughout these reviews. A review of reminder packaging produced positive but limited results (Heneghan, Glasziou & Perera, 2006), as did a reviews of patient reminders and late-patient tracers for tuberculosis treatments (Liu et al., 2008), reinforcement and reminding for those individuals taking cholesterol medications (Schedlbauer, Davies, & Fahey, 2010), patient support and education for HIV/AIDS treatments (Rueda et al., 2006), and interventions to improve exercise adherence in patients with chronic musculoskeletal pain (Jordan et al., 2010). No conclusions could be drawn in a review of adherence interventions for Type 2 diabetes patients (Vermeire et al., 2009). Haynes and colleagues (2008) noted that though there is some positive evidence (less than half of the reviewed studies) for simple interventions in the short term, long-term interventions for chronic conditions are more complex and not as effective. Similarly, Schroeder, Fahey, and Ebrahim (2008) noted that simplifying the hypertensive patients' daily dosing may be helpful, but the jury is out for motivational strategies and other complex interventions. Most of the aforementioned reviews demonstrate and acknowledge the need for larger, high-quality studies of adherence interventions.

In summary, these studies suggest that regimen adherence may be improved by behavioral interventions. However, interventions shown to be effective tend to be multicomponent and tend to have modest effects (Haynes et al., 2008). Future efforts should be focused on the development and testing of new treatments addressing specific patterns of poor adherence.

CONCLUSION

Adherence to a treatment regimen poses a significant problem in medical care both in terms of the patient's clinical status as well as financial burden. Efforts to intervene have been limited. Thus, there is minimal information that can be relied on with confidence in efforts to improve adherence within either a clinical or research setting. Clearly, there is a need for randomized, controlled studies evaluating interventions.

As the clinical outcomes associated with poor adherence have become more salient and the costs have had an impact on a cost-conscious health care system, the interest in adherence has increased. The newer measurement technologies permit a more refined and specific assessment of adherence problems and patterns, which is contributing toward a finer understanding of this significant problem in health care. The limited studies detailing the problems of adherence, the paucity of intervention studies, and the variability created by the coarser view of adherence that has characterized research in the field all point to the need for further focused research in this difficult problem affecting all aspects of health care.

Thus, considerable work is continuing to develop a deeper understanding of patient adherence and strategies to improve it. Yet 35 years after the first randomized controlled trial of an adherence intervention (Haynes et al., 1976), we continue to have adherence rates that parallel those of the 1970s and 1980s. The impact of poor adherence on clinical outcomes and health care costs is too great to allow one half of patients to fail to benefit from care. We need to consider how to accelerate the pace of research.

As noted earlier, about one half of the adherence intervention studies have been positive but have generally shown modest improvements in adherence, not always resulting in changes in clinical outcomes (Haynes et al., 2008). Furthermore, the interventions that have been successful have been complex, with multiple components within the intervention. One of the difficulties is that interventions have addressed a variety of problems under the adherence umbrella. That umbrella includes such behaviors as lack of willingness to accept the regimen; failure to initiate the regimen, including the failure to fill prescriptions as well as the failure to initiate treatment despite filling the regimen; reduction in the prescription; planned skipped doses; episodic missed doses; extra dosing; and early cessation of the regimen. Moreover, the problems themselves have varied from lack of understanding, memory problems, cost, failure to monitor behavior, motivation, difficulties with self-management, and multiple other issues. It is quite likely that each of these behaviors and related problems has its own precipitants, which might be influenced by specific interventions. As long as multicomponent interventions are required to address multiple behaviors and multiple etiologies, we are unlikely to see significant improvements of any magnitude. Future research might better address the influences and interventions for separate adherence behaviors and separate contributing factors. This way, we may better learn how to educate for adherence, how to develop and sustain self-monitoring, how to compensate for memory difficulties, and so on.

Just as multiple behaviors comprising adherence pose complexities, so too do multiple definitions of what constitutes good adherence. It may take quite different interventions to bring a patient to 80% adherence, a common cut point, than to bring blood pressure under control. The question arises as to whether better information can be obtained about specific drug regimen that would permit the establishment of adherence levels necessary to obtain clinical effect among the average population with the condition of relevance. It would also be helpful to provide quantitative reports on adherence rather than the more qualitative assessments often seen. Within the quantitative definitions of adherence is the need to specify the nature of the data being examined. Is the information related to the proportion of doses taken, the proportion of days accurate doses were taken, the proportion of days accurate doses were taken on time, the proportion of persons who accurately took doses over a time period, or the clinician's judgment of what the patient has done? Depending on which definition was used, adherence has been shown to range, for example, from 35% to 88% for the same drug and the same behavior in the same time period in the same persons (Dunbar-Jacob, 2005). It would be useful for each study to have data available that would permit the post hoc comparison of adherence with other studies using standardized definitions of adherence. Although different definitions may be important for different regimen, the collection of standardized data would permit examination of adherence outcomes under different definitions. Standardization across studies would then permit pooled analysis or meta-analysis. In this way, interventions could be evaluated more robustly.

Variability also exists in the measurement of adherence. Most of the studies have used self-report, a measure that has been shown in numerous studies to overestimate adherence. Other studies have used pharmacy fill rates, with a variety of methods of calculation, clinical outcomes, pill counts, and electronic monitors, among others. The variability in outcomes in intervention research is likely to be related to the variability in measurement methods. Although cost factors complicate an accurate assessment of adherence, it is important to gain a more valid outcome measure.

With variability in adherence reports related to multiple measurement methods, variety in definitions of adherence, and numerous behaviors comprising the umbrella of adherence, it is no wonder that the predictors of adherence have been weak and have varied from study to study. Yet many of the interventions chosen are based on the presumption that the predictors would influence adherence if chosen as targets for intervention. Some of these have been associated with the system of delivery of treatment, the education of patients, and the level of motivation of patients. Strong data do not exist to indicate that these predictors are, indeed, causative in producing low adherence. Further, the many predictors examined have not been studied in relation to a specific phase in the adherence process—acceptance of treatment, filling prescriptions, initiating the regimen accurately, remembering to carry out the regimen on time, or planning and sustaining the regimen.

Before we reach another decade without significant improvement in the rates of adherence to treatment, we need to step back to review what we have done. We need to determine how we can best reduce the multiple variabilities within the research and strive to understand the problem that has been lingering for decades. What specific causes lead to specific poor adherence behaviors? What specific causes can be modified to produce improvement? How can we come together on standardization of measurement and definitions? Until these issues are resolved, we are unlikely to improve adherence in the populations of patients where poor adherence is limiting effective treatment.

REFERENCES

Ajzen, I. (1991). The theory of planned behavior. *Organizational behavior and human decision processes, 50*(2), 179–211.

Atkins, C. J., Kaplan, R. M., Timms, R. M., Reinsch, S., & Lofback, K. (1984). Behavioral exercise programs in the management of chronic obstructive pulmonary disease. *Journal of Consulting and Clinical Psychology, 52*(4), 591–603.

Bailey, W. C., Richards, J. M., Jr., Brooks, C. M., Soong, S. J., Windsor, R. A., & Manzella, B. A. (1990). A randomized trial to improve self-management practices of adults with asthma. *Archives of Internal Medicine, 150*(8), 1664–1668.

Bandura, A. (1997). *Self-efficacy: The exercise of control.* New York, NY: Freeman.

Bangsberg, D. R., Hecht, F. M., Charlebois, E. D., Chesney, M., & Moss, A. (2001). comparing objective measures of adherence to HIV antiretroviral therapy: Electronic medication monitors and unannounced pill counts. *AIDS and Behavior, 5*(3), 275–281.

Barnard, N. D., Scherwitz, L. W., & Ornish, D. (1992). Adherence and acceptability of a low-fat, vegetarian diet among patients with cardiac disease. *Journal of Cardiopulmonary Rehabilitation, 12*(6), 423–431.

Belisle, M., Roskies, E., & Levesque, J. M. (1987). Improving adherence to physical activity. *Health Psychology, 6*(2), 159–172.

Berg, J., Dunbar-Jacob, J., & Rohay, J. (1995). Assessing inhaler medication adherence using an electronic monitoring device. *Annals of Behavioral Medicine, 17S.*

Berndt, S., Maier, C., & Schutz, H. W. (1993). Polymedication and medication compliance in patients with chronic non-malignant pain. *Pain, 52*(3), 331–339.

Berrigan, D., Dodd, K., Troiano, R. P., Krebs-Smith, S. M., & Barbash, R. B. (2003). Patterns of health behavior in U.S. adults. *Preventive Medicine, 36*(5), 615–623.

Bloom, B. R., & Murray, C. J. L. (1992). Tuberculosis: Commentary on a reemergent killer. *Science, 257*(5073), 1055–1064.

Bosch-Capblanch, X., Abba, K., Prictor, M., & Garner, P. (2007). Contracts between patients and healthcare practitioners for improving patients' adherence to treatment, prevention and health promotion activities [Electronic version]. *Cochrane Database of Systematic Reviews, 2007*. Retrieved from http://onlinelibrary.wiley.com/o/cochrane/clsysrev/articles/CD004808/frame.html

Bovbjerg, V. E., McCann, B. S., Brief, D. J., Follette, W. C., Retzlaff, B. M., Dowdy, A. A., … Knopp, R. H. (1995). Spouse support and long-term adherence to lipid-lowering diets. *American Journal of Epidemiology, 141*(5), 451–460.

Boyd, J. R., Covington, T. R., Stanaszek, W. F., & Coussons, R. T. (1974). Drug defaulting: I. Determinants of compliance. *American Journal of Hospital Pharmacy, 31*(4), 362–367.

Burke, L. E., & Dunbar-Jacob, J. (1995). Adherence to medication, diet, and activity recommendations: From assessment to maintenance. *Journal of Cardiovascular Nursing, 9*(2), 62–79.

Burke, L. E., Dunbar-Jacob, J., Glaister, C., McCall, M., Sereika, S., Dwyer, K., … Starz, T. W. (1992, May). *Influence of question type on self-reported medication compliance in rheumatoid arthritis patients.* Paper presented at the Sigma Theta Tau International Nursing Research Conference, Columbus, OH.

Burns, J. M., Sneddon, I., Lovell, M., McLean, A., & Martin, B. J. (1992). Elderly patients and their medication: A post-discharge follow-up study. *Age and Ageing, 21*(3), 178–181.

Carmody, T. P., Senner, J. W., Malinow, M. R., & Matarazzo, J. D. (1980). Physical exercise rehabilitation: Long-term dropout rate in cardiac patients. *Journal of Behavioral Medicine, 3*(2), 163–168.

Chapman, R. H., Benner, J. S., Petrilla, A. A., Tierce, J. C., Collins, S. R., Battleman, D. S., … Schwartz, J. S. (2005). Predictors of adherence with antihypertensive and lipid-lowering therapy. *Archives of Internal Medicine, 165*(10), 1147–1152.

Cheung, R., Sullens, C. M., Seal, D., Dickins, J., Nicholson, P. W., Deshmukh, A. A., … Dobbs, S. M. (1988). The paradox of using a 7 day antibacterial course to treat urinary tract infections in the community. *British Journal of Clinical Pharmacology, 26*(4), 391–398.

Claxton, A. J., Cramer, J., & Pierce, C. (2001). A systematic review of the associations between dose regimens and medication compliance. *Clinical Therapeutics, 23*(8), 1296–1310.

Colcher, I. S., & Bass, J. W. (1972). Penicillin treatment of streptococcal pharyngitis: A comparison of schedules and the role of specific counseling. *Journal of the American Medical Association, 222*(6), 657–659.

Cole, M. G. (1985). The course of elderly depressed out-patients. *Canadian Journal of Psychiatry, 30*(3), 217–220.

Connelly, C. E., Davenport, Y. B., & Nurnberger, J. I., Jr. (1982). Adherence to treatment regimen in a lithium carbonate clinic. *Archives of General Psychiatry, 39*(5), 585–588.

Cooper, C., Bebbington, P., King, M., Brugha, T., Meltzer, H., Bhugra, D., … Jenkins, R. (2007). Why people do not take their psychotropic drugs as prescribed: Results of the 2000 National Psychiatric Morbidity Survey. *Acta Psychiatrica Scandinavica, 116*(1), 47–53.

Cramer, J. A., Mattson, R. H., Prevey, M. L., Scheyer, R. D., & Ouellette, V. L. (1989). How often is medication take as prescribed? A novel assessment technique. *Journal of the American Medical Association, 261*(22), 3273–3277.

Cramer, J. A., Scheyer, R. D., & Mattson, R. H. (1990). Compliance declines between clinic visits. *Archives of Internal Medicine, 150*(7), 1509–1510.

Davis, K. L., Candrilli, S. D., & Edin, H. M. (2008). Prevalence and cost of nonadherence with antiepileptic drugs in an adult managed care population. *Epilepsia, 49*(3), 446–454.

DeGeest, S. (1996, March). Assessment of adherence in heart transplant recipients. In J. Dunbar-Jacob (Chair), *Adherence in chronic disease.* Symposium presented at the Fourth International Congress of Behavioral Medicine, Washington, DC.

DeLalla, F. (1998). Cefixime in the treatment of upper respiratory tract infections and otitis media. *Chemotherapy, 44*(Suppl. 1), 19–23.

De Morton, N. A., Keating, J. L., & Jeffs, K. (2007). Exercise for acutely hospitalised older medical patients [Electronic version]. *Cochrane Database of Systematic Reviews, 2007*. Retrieved from http://onlinelibrary.wiley.com/o/cochrane/clsysrev/articles/CD005955/frame.html

Denhaerynck, K., Manhaeve, D., Dobbels, F., Garzoni, D., Nolte, C., & De Geest, S. (2007). Prevalence and consequences of nonadherence to hemodialysis regimens. *American Journal of Critical Care, 16*(3), 222–235.

Denhaerynck, K., Steiger, J., Bock, A., Schäfer-Keller, P., Köfer, S., Thannberger, N., … De Geest, S. (2007). Prevalence and risk factors of non-adherence with immunosuppressive medication in kidney transplant patients. *American Journal of Transplantation, 7*(1), 108–116.

DiMatteo, M. R. (2004). Variations in patients' adherence to medical recommendations: A quantitative review of 50 years of research. *Medical Care, 42*(3), 200–209.

DiMatteo, M. R., Giordani, P. J., Lepper, H. S., & Croghan, T. W. (2002). Patient adherence and medical treatment outcomes: A meta-analysis. *Medical Care, 40*(9), 794–811.

Dolecek, T. A., Milas, N. C., Van Horn, L. V., Farrand, M. E., Gorder, D. D., Duchene, A. G., ... Randall, B. L. (1986). A long-term nutrition intervention experience: Lipid responses and dietary adherence patterns in the Multiple Risk Factor Intervention Trial. *Journal of the American Dietetic Association, 86*(6), 752–758.

Dompeling, E., van Grunsven, P. M., van Schayck, C. P., Folgering, H., Molema, J., & van Weel, C. (1992). Treatment with inhaled steroids in asthma and chronic bronchitis: Long-term compliance and inhaler technique. *Family Practice, 9*(2), 161–166.

Donnelly, L. A., Doney, A. S. F., Morris, A. D., Palmer, C. N. A., & Donnan, P. T. (2008). Long-term adherence to statin treatment in diabetes. *Diabetes Medicine, 25*(7), 850–855.

Dunbar, J., Dunning, E. J., Dwyer, K., Burke, L., & Snetselaar, L. (1991, March). *Influence of question type on self-reported compliance with dietary regimen.* Paper presented at the 12th annual meeting of the Society of Behavioral Medicine, Washington, DC.

Dunbar, J., & Knoke, J. (1986, May). *Prediction of medication adherence at one year and seven years: Behavioral and psychological factors.* Paper presented at the Society for Clinical Trials Seventh Annual Conference, Montreal, Canada.

Dunbar-Jacob, J. (1997, November). *Understanding the reasons for patient's noncompliance and how these reasons impact therapeutic regimens and outcomes of care.* Paper presented at a workshop, Pharmaceutical Care Programs: Their Role in Medication Compliance by EMMG, Kansas City, KS.

Dunbar-Jacob, J. (1998, December). *Challenges in rehabilitation clinical trials: Adherence to intervention regimens.* Paper presented at the Workshop on Clinical Trials in Rehabilitation by the National Advisory Board on Medical Rehabilitation Research, Bethesda, MD.

Dunbar-Jacob, J. (2005). Public policy: Chronic disease: A patient-focused view. *Journal of Professional Nursing: Official Journal of the American Association of Colleges of Nursing, 21*(1), 3–4.

Dunbar-Jacob, J., Burke, L. E., & Puczynski, S. (1995). Clinical assessment and management of adherence to medical regimens. In P. M. Nicassio & T. W. Smith (Eds.), *Managing chronic illness: A biopsychosocial perspective* (pp. 313–349). Washington, DC: American Psychological Association.

Dunbar-Jacob, J., Burke, L. E., Rohay, J. M., Sereika, S., & Muldoon, M. F. (1997, November). *How comparable are self-report, pill count, and electronically monitored adherence data*? Poster presented at the 70th scientific session of the American Heart Association, Orlando, FL.

Dunbar-Jacob, J., Burke, L. E., Rohay, J. M., Sereika, S., Schlenk, E. A., Lipello, A., & Muldoon, M. F. (1996). Comparability of self-report, pill count, and electronically monitored adherence data. *Controlled Clinical Trials, 17*(Suppl. 2), 80S.

Dunbar-Jacob, J., Dwyer, K., & Dunning, E. J. (1991). Compliance with antihypertensive regimen: A review of the research in the 1980s. *Annals of Behavioral Medicine, 13*(1), 31–39.

Dunbar-Jacob, J., Kwoh, C. K., Rohay, J. M., Burke, L. E., Sereika, S., & Starz, T. (1996, March). *Medication adherence and functional outcomes in rheumatoid arthritis.* Poster presented at the Fourth International Congress of Behavioral Medicine, Washington, DC.

Dunbar-Jacob, J., Kwoh, C. K., Starz, T. W., Sereika, S., McCall, M., Glaister, C., ... Holmes, J. (1992, July). *Adherence to arthritis medication.* Poster presented at the International Congress of Behavioral Medicine, Hamburg, Germany.

Dunbar-Jacob, J., & Schlenk, E. A. (1996). Treatment adherence and clinical outcome: Can we make a difference? In R. J. Resnick & R. H. Rozensky (Eds.), *Health psychology through the life span: Practice and research opportunities* (pp. 323–343). Washington, DC: American Psychological Association.

Dunbar-Jacob, J., Schlenk, E. A., Burke, L. E., & Matthews, J. T. (1998). Predictors of patient adherence: Patient characteristics. In S. A. Shumaker, E. Schron, J. Ockene, & W. L. McBee (Eds.), *Handbook of health behavior change* (2nd ed., pp. 491–511). New York, NY: Springer.

Dunbar-Jacob, J., Sereika, S., & Burke, L. E. (1998, August). *Use of daily diaries in assessing compliance.* Paper presented at the Fifth International Congress of Behavioral Medicine, Copenhagen, Denmark.

Dunbar-Jacob, J., Sereika, S. M., Foley, S. M., Bass, D. C., & Ness, R. B. (2004). Adherence to oral therapies in pelvic inflammatory disease. *Journal of Women's Health, 13*(3), 285–291.

Dunbar-Jacob, J., Sereika, S., Rohay, J., & Burke, L. E. (1998). Electronic methods in assessing adherence to medical regimens. In D. S. Kranz & A. Baum (Eds.), *Technology and methods in behavioral medicine* (pp. 95–113). Mahwah, NJ: Erlbaum.

Dunbar-Jacob, J., Sereika, S., Rohay, J. M., Burke, L. E., & Kwoh, C. K. (1995). Predictors of adherence: Differences by measurement method. *Annals of Behavioral Medicine, 17S*, S196.

Dunbar-Jacob, J., Sereika, S., Rohay, J. M., & Probstfield, J. (1994). J-shaped compliance distribution revisited. *Controlled Clinical Trials*, *15*(3S), 120.

Dupon, M., & Raynaud, J. M. (1992). Tuberculosis in patients infected with human immunodeficiency virus 1: A retrospective multicentre study of 123 cases in France. *Quarterly Journal of Medicine*, *85*(306), 719–730.

Edmonds, D., Foester, E., Groth, H., Greminger, P., Siegenthaler, W., & Vetter, W. (1985). Does self-measurement of blood pressure improve patient compliance in hypertension? *Journal of Hypertension*, *3*(Suppl. 1), S31–S34.

Esposito, K., Maiorino, M. I., Di Palo, C., & Giugliano, D. (for the Campanian Postprandial Hyperglycemia Study Group). (2009). Adherence to a Mediterranean diet and glycaemic control in type 2 diabetes mellitus. *Diabetic Medicine*, *26*(9), 900–907.

Fawcett, J., Clark, D. C., Aagesen, C. A., Pisani, V. D., Tilkin, J. M., Sellers, D., … Gibbons, R. D. (1987). A double-blind, placebo-controlled trial of lithium carbonate therapy for alcoholism. *Archives of General Psychiatry*, *44*(3), 248–256.

Fawcett, J., Clark, D. C., Gibbons, R. D., Aagesen, C. A., Pisani, V. D., Tilkin, J. M., … Stutzman, D. (1984). Evaluation of lithium therapy for alcoholism. *Journal of Clinical Psychiatry*, *45*(12), 494–499.

Fishbein, H. A. (1985). Precipitants of hospitalization in insulin-dependent diabetes mellitus (IDDM): A statewide perspective. *Diabetes Care*, *8*(Suppl. 1), 61–64.

Fishbein, M., & Ajzen, I. (1975). *Belief, attitude, intention, and behavior: An introduction to theory and research.* Reading, MA: Addison-Wesley.

Flack, J. M., Novikov, S. V., & Ferrario, C. M. (1996). Benefits of adherence to antihypertensive drug therapy. *European Heart Journal*, *17*(Suppl. A), 16–20.

Fletcher, S. W., Deliakis, J., Schoch, W. A., & Shapiro, S. H. (1979). Predicting blood pressure control in hypertensive patients: An approach to quality-of-care assessment. *Medical Care*, *17*(3), 285–292.

Fransen, G. A. J., Mesters, I., Janssen, M. J. R., Knottnerus, J. A., & Muris, J. W. M. (2009). Which patient-related factors determine self-perceived patient adherence to prescribed dyspepsia medication? *Health Education Research*, *24*(5), 788–798.

Gaebel, W., & Pietzcker, A. (1985). One-year outcome of schizophrenic patients: The interaction of chronicity and neuroleptic treatment. *Pharmacopsychiatry*, *18*(3), 235–239.

Gallagher, A. M., Leighton-Scott, J., & van Staa, T. P. (2009). Utilization characteristics and treatment persistence in patients prescribed low-dose buprenorphine patches in primary care in the United Kingdom: A retrospective cohort study. *Clinical Therapeutics*, *31*(8), 1707–1715.

Gibbons, A. (1992). Exploring new strategies to fight drug-resistant microbes. *Science*, *257*(5073), 1036–1038.

Given, B., Given, C. W., & Simoni, L. E. (1979). Relationships of processes of care to patient outcomes. *Nursing Research*, *28*(2), 85–93.

Glanz, K. (1979). Dietitians' effectiveness and patient compliance with dietary regimens: A pilot study. *Journal of the American Dietetic Association*, *75*(6), 631–636.

Glueck, C. J., Gordon, D. J., Nelson, J. J., Davis, C. E., & Tyroler, H. A. (1986). Dietary and other correlates of changes in total and low-density lipoprotein cholesterol in hypercholesterolemic men: The lipid research clinics coronary primary prevention trial. *American Journal of Clinical Nutrition*, *44*(4), 489–500.

Grahl, C. (1994). Improving compliance: Solving a $100 billion problem. *Managed HealthCare*, S11–S13.

Granstrom, P. A. (1985). Progression of visual field deficits in glaucoma: Relation to compliance with pilocarpine therapy. *Archives of Ophthalmology*, *103*(4), 529–531.

Gray, T. A., Orton, L. C., Henson, D., Harper, R., & Waterman, H. (2009). Interventions for improving adherence to ocular hypotensive therapy [Electronic version]. *Cochrane Database of Systematic Reviews, 2009.* Retrieved from http://onlinelibrary.wiley.com/o/cochrane/clsysrev/articles/CD006132/frame.html

Hall, D. M., & Most, M. M. (2005). Dietary adherence in well-controlled feeding studies. *Journal of the American Dietetic Association*, *105*(8), 1285–1288.

Hamilton, G. (2003). Measuring adherence in a hypertension clinical trial. *European Journal of Cardiovascular Nursing*, *2*(3): 219–228.

Harrold, L., Andrade, S., Briesacher, B., Raebel, M., Fouayzi, H., Yood, R., … Ockene, I. S. al. (2009). Adherence with urate-lowering therapies for the treatment of gout. *Arthritis Research & Therapy*, *11*(2), R46.

Hasford, J., Uricher, J., Tauscher, M., Bramlage, P., & Virchow, J. C. (2010). Persistence with asthma treatment is low in Germany especially for controller medication—A population based study of 483,051 patients. *Allergy*, *65*(3), 347–354.

Hawkins, R. B. (1989). Arthroscopic stapling repair for shoulder instability: A retrospective study of 50 cases. *Arthroscopy: The Journal of Arthroscopic and Related Surgery, 5*(2), 122–128.

Hawkins, R. J., & Switlyk, P. (1993). Acute prosthetic replacement for severe fractures of the proximal humerus. *Clinical Orthopaedics and Related Research, 289,* 156–160.

Haynes, R., Ackloo, E., Sahota, N., McDonald, H. P., & Yao, X. (2008). Interventions for enhancing medication adherence [Electronic version]. *Cochrane Database of Systematic Reviews, 2008.* Retrieved from http://www.mrw.interscience.wiley.com/cochrane/clsysrev/articles/CD000011/frame.html

Haynes, R. B., Gibson, E. S., Taylor, D. W., Bernholz, C. D., & Sackett, D. L. (1982). Process versus outcome in hypertension: A positive result. *Circulation, 65*(1), 28–33.

Haynes, R. B., Sackett, D. L., Gibson, E. S., Taylor, D. W., Hackett, B. C., Roberts, R. S., & Johnson, A. L. (1976). Improvement of medication compliance in uncontrolled hypertension. *Lancet, 1,* 1265–1268.

Heneghan, C., Glasziou, P., & Perera, R. (2006). Reminder packaging for improving adherence to self-administered long-term medications (Publication No. 0.1002/14651858.CD005025.pub2). Retrieved from http://onlinelibrary.wiley.com/o/cochrane/clsysrev/articles/CD005025/frame.html

Hyman, M. D., Insull, W., Jr., Palmer, R. H., O'Brien, J., Gordon, L., & Levine, B. (1982). Assessing methods for measuring compliance with a fat-controlled diet. *American Journal of Public Health, 72*(2), 152–160.

Jacobson Vann, J. C., & Szilagyi, P. (2005). Patient reminder and recall systems to improve immunization rates [Electronic version]. *Cochrane Database of Systematic Reviews, 2005.* Retrieved from http://onlinelibrary.wiley.com/o/cochrane/clsysrev/articles/CD003941/pdf_fs.html

Janz, N. K., & Becker, M. H. (1984). The health belief model: A decade later. *Health Education Quarterly, 11*(1), 1–47.

Jones, J. K., Gorkin, L., Lian, J. F., Staffa, J. A., & Fletcher, A. P. (1995). Discontinuation of and changes in treatment after start of new courses of antihypertensive drugs: A study of a United Kingdom population. *British Medical Journal, 311*(7000), 293–295.

Jordan, J., Holden, M., Mason, E., & Foster, N. (2010). Interventions to improve adherence to exercise for chronic musculoskeletal pain in adults [Electronic version]. *Cochrane Database of Systematic Reviews, 2010 (Issue 1, Art. No. CD005956).* Retrieved from http://www.mrw.interscience.wiley.com/cochrane/clsysrev/articles/CD005956/frame.html

Kalil, R. S. N., Heim-Duthoy, K. L., & Kasiske, B. L. (1992). Patients with a low income have reduced renal allograft survival. *American Journal of Kidney Diseases, 20*(1), 63–69.

Kane, S., & Shaya, F. (2008). Medication non-adherence is associated with increased medical health care costs. *Digestive Diseases and Sciences, 53*(4), 1020–1024.

Kass, M. A., Meltzer, D. W., Gordon, M., Cooper, D., & Goldberg, J. (1986). Compliance with topical pilocarpine treatment. *American Journal of Ophthalmology, 101*(5), 515–523.

Keefe, F. J., & Blumenthal, J. A. (1980). The life fitness program: A behavioral approach to making exercise a habit. *Journal of Behavior Therapy and Experimental Psychology, 11*(1), 31–34.

King, A. C., & Frederiksen, L. W. (1984). Low-cost strategies for increasing exercise behavior: Relapse preparation training and social support. *Behavior Modification, 8*(1), 3–21.

King, A. C., Taylor, C. B., Haskell, W. L., & DeBusk, R. F. (1988). Strategies for increasing early adherence to and long-term maintenance of home-based exercise training in healthy middle-aged men and women. *American Journal of Cardiology, 61*(8), 628–632.

King, D. E., Mainous Iii, A. G., Carnemolla, M., & Everett, C. J. (2009). Adherence to healthy lifestyle habits in US adults, 1988–2006. *American Journal of Medicine, 122*(6), 528–534.

Kirking, D. M., Lee, J. A., Ellis, J. J., Briesacher, B., & McKercher, P. L. (2006). Patient-reported underuse of prescription medications: A comparison of nine surveys. *Medical Care Research and Review, 63*(4), 427–446.

Kirscht, J. P., Kirscht, J. L., & Rosenstock, I. M. (1981). A test of interventions to increase adherence to hypertensive medical regimens. *Health Education Quarterly, 8*(3), 261–272.

Klopovich, P. M., & Trueworthy, R. C. (1985). Adherence to chemotherapy regimens among children with cancer. *Topics in Clinical Nursing, 7*(1), 19–25.

Konkle-Parker, D. J. (2001). A motivational intervention to improve adherence to treatment of chronic disease. *Journal of the American Academy of Nurse Practitioners, 13*(2), 61–68.

Kripalani, S., Yao, X., & Haynes, R. B. (2007). Interventions to enhance medication adherence in chronic medical conditions: A systematic review. *Archives of Internal Medicine, 167*(6), 540–549.

Lanza, R. P., Cooper, D. K. C., Boyd, S. T., & Barnard, C. N. (1984). Comparison of patients with ischemic, myopathic, and rheumatic heart diseases as cardiac transplant recipients. *American Heart Journal, 107*(1), 8–12.

Leff, J., Berkowitz, R., Shavit, N., Strachan, A., Glass, I., & Vaughn, C. (1989). A trial of family therapy v. a relatives group for schizophrenia. *British Journal of Psychiatry, 154*, 58–66.

Lehmann, S. W., & Rabins, P. V. (2006). Factors related to hospitalization in elderly manic patients with early and late-onset bipolar disorder. *International Journal of Geriatric Psychiatry, 21*(11), 1060–1064.

Leventhal, H., Meyer, D., & Nerenz, D. (1980). The common-sense representation of illness danger. In S. Rachman (Ed.), *Medical psychology* (pp. 7–30). New York, NY: Pergamon.

Lichtenstein, M. J., Shields, S. L., Shiavi, R. G., & Burger, C. (1989). Exercise and balance in aged women: A pilot controlled clinical trial. *Archives of Physical Medicine and Rehabilitation, 70*(2), 138–143.

Lin, E. H. B., Katon, W., Von Korff, M., Rutter, C., Simon, G. E., Oliver, M., … Young, B. (2004). Relationship of depression and diabetes self-care, medication adherence, and preventive care. *Diabetes Care, 27*(9), 2154–2160.

Lip, G. Y. H., & Brodie, M. J. (1992). Sudden death in epilepsy: An avoidable outcome? *Journal of the Royal Society of Medicine, 85*(10), 609–611.

Lipid Research Clinics Program. (1984a). The Lipid Research Clinics Coronary Primary Prevention Program Trial results: I. Reduction in incidence of coronary heart disease. *Journal of the American Medical Association, 251*(3), 351–364.

Lipid Research Clinics Program. (1984b). The Lipid Research Clinics Coronary Primary Prevention Program Trial results: II. The relationship of reduction in incidence of coronary heart disease to cholesterol lowering. *Journal of the American Medical Association, 251*(3), 365–374.

Liu, Q., Abba, K., Alejandria, M., Balanag, V., Berba, R., & Lansang, M. (2008). Reminder systems and late patient tracers in the diagnosis and management of tuberculosis [Electronic version]. *Cochrane Database of Systematic Reviews, 2008*. Retrieved from http://onlinelibrary.wiley.com/o/cochrane/clsysrev/articles/CD006594/frame.html

LoBue, P., Sizemore, C., & Castro, K. (2009). Plan to combat extensively drug-resistant tuberculosis recommendations of the Federal Tuberculosis Task Force. *Morbidity and Mortality Weekly Report, 58*(RR03), 1–43.

Logan, A. G., Milne, B. J., Achber, C., Campbell, W. P., & Haynes R. B. (1979). Work site treatment of hypertension by specially trained nurses. *Lancet, 2*(8153), 1175–1178.

Mann, D. M., Allegrante, J. P., Natarajan, S., Montori, V. M., Halm, E. A., & Charlson, M. (2007). Dietary indiscretion and statin use. *Mayo Clinic Proceedings, 82*(8), 951–953.

Mantonakis, J. E., Jemos, J. J., Christodoulou, G. N., & Lykouras, E. P. (1982). Short-term social prognosis of schizophrenia. *Acta Psychiatrica Scandinavica, 66*(4), 306–310.

Maronde, R. F., Chan, L. S., Larsen, F. J., Strandberg, L. R., Laventurier, M. F., & Sullivan, S. R. (1989). Underutilization of antihypertensive drugs and associated hospitalization. *Medical Care, 27*(12), 1159–1166.

Mason, J. O. (1992). Addressing the measles epidemic. *Public Health Reports, 107*(3), 241–242.

Mattson, R. H., & Friedman, R. B. (1984). Medication adherence assessment in clinical trials. *Journal of Controlled Clinical Trials, 5*(4), 488–496.

McCann, B. S., Follette, W. C., Driver, J. L., Brief, D. J., & Knopp, R. H. (1988, August). *Self-efficacy and adherence in the dietary treatment of hyperlipidemia*. Paper presented at the American Psychological Association 96th Annual Convention, Atlanta, GA.

McHorney, C. A., Victor Spain, C., Alexander, C. M., & Simmons, J. (2009). Validity of the adherence estimator in the prediction of 9-month persistence with medications prescribed for chronic diseases: A prospective analysis of data from pharmacy claims. *Clinical Therapeutics, 31*(11), 2584–2607.

McKenney, J. M., Munroe, W. P., & Wright, J. T., Jr. (1992). Impact of an electronic medication compliance aid on long-term blood pressure control. *Journal of Clinical Pharmacology, 32*(3), 277–283.

Medina-Mirapeix, F., Escolar-Reina, P., Gascón-Cánovas, J. J., Montilla-Herrador, J., Jimeno-Serrano, F. J., & Collins, S. M. (2009). Predictive factors of adherence to frequency and duration components in home exercise programs for neck and low back pain: An observational study [Electronic version]. *BMC Musculoskeletal Disorders, 10*, from http://www.biomedcentral.com/1471-2474/10/155

Morell, R. W., Park, D. C., Kidder, D. P., & Martin, M. (1997). Adherence to antihypertensive medications across the life span. *Gerontologist, 37*(5), 609–619.

Morisky, D. E., Levine, D. M., Green, L. W., Shapiro, S., Russell, R. P., & Smith, C. R. (1983). Five-year blood pressure control and mortality following health education for hypertensive patients. *American Journal of Public Health, 73*(2), 153–162.

Morris, A. B., Li, J., Kroenke, K., Bruner-England, T. E., Young, J. M., & Murray, M. D. (2006). Factors associated with drug adherence and blood pressure in patients with hypertension. *Pharmacotherapy, 26*, 483–492.

Muir, K. W., Santiago-Turla, C., Stinnett, S. S., Herndon, L. W., Allingham, R. R., Challa, P., & Lee, P. P. (2006). Health literacy and adherence to glaucoma therapy. *Ophthalmology, 142*, 223–226.

Mulrow, C., Bailey, S., Sonksen, P. H., & Slavin, B. (1987). Evaluation of an audiovisual diabetes education program: Negative results of a randomized trial of patients with non-insulin-dependent diabetes mellitus. *Journal of General Internal Medicine, 2*(4), 215–219.

Nelson, J. C., Bittner, R. C. L., Bounds, L., Zhao, S., Baggs, J., Donahue, J. G., ... Jackson, L. A. (2009). Compliance with multiple-dose vaccine schedules among older children, adolescents, and adults: Results from a vaccine safety datalink study. *American Journal of Public Health, 99*(S2), S389–397.

Nelson, M., Girard, P.-M., DeMasi, R., Chen, L., Smets, E., Sekar, V., & Lavreys, L. (2010). Suboptimal adherence to darunavir/ritonavir has minimal effect on efficacy compared with lopinavir/ritonavir in treatment-naive, HIV-infected patients: 96 week ARTEMIS data. *Journal of Antimicrobial Chemotherapy, 65*(7), 1505–1509.

Nelson, M. R., Reid, C. M., Ryan, P., Willson, K., & Yelland, L. (on behalf of the ANBP2 Management Committee). (2006). Self-reported adherence with medication and cardiovascular disease outcomes in the Second Australian National Blood Pressure Study (ANBP2) [Electronic version]. *Medical Journal of Australia, 185* (9), 487–489. Retrieved from http://www.mja.com.au/public/issues/185_09_061106/nel10178_fm.html

Nichol, K. L., Margolis, K. L., Wuorenma, J., & Von Sternberg, T. (1994). The efficacy and cost effectiveness of vaccination against influenza among elderly persons living in the community. *New England Journal of Medicine, 331*, 778–784.

Nolan, C. M., Aitken, M. L., Elarth, A. M., Anderson, K. M., & Miller, W. T. (1986). Active tuberculosis after isoniazid chemoprophylaxis of Southeast Asian refugees. *American Review of Respiratory Disease, 133*(3), 431–436.

Norell, S. E. (1981). Monitoring compliance with pilocarpine therapy. *American Journal of Ophthalmology, 92*(5), 727–731.

O'Donnell, D., Sevitz, H., Seggie, J. L., Meyers, A. M., Botha, J. R., & Myburgh, J. A. (1985). Pregnancy after renal transplantation. *Australian and New Zealand Journal of Medicine, 15*(3), 320–325.

Ogedegbe, G., Schoenthaler, A., Richardson, T., Lewis, L., Belue, R., Espinosa, E., ... Charlson, M. E. (2007). An RCT of the effect of motivational interviewing on medication adherence in hypertensive African Americans: Rationale and design. *Contemporary Clinical Trials, 28*(2), 169–181.

Okeke, C. O., Quigley, H. A., Jampel, H. D., Ying, G.-S., Plyler, R. J., Jiang, Y., & Friedman, D. S. (2009). Adherence with topical glaucoma medication monitored electronically: The travatan dosing aid study. *Ophthalmology, 116*(2), 191–199.

Oldridge, N. B. (1984). Compliance and dropout in cardiac exercise rehabilitation. *Journal of Cardiac Rehabilitation, 4*(5), 166–177.

Oldridge, N. B. (1988). Cardiac rehabilitation exercise programme: Compliance and compliance-enhancing strategies. *Sports Medicine, 6*(1), 42–55.

Olthoff, C. M. G., Schouten, J. S. A. G., van de Borne, B. W., & Webers, C. A. B. (2005). Noncompliance with ocular hypotensive treatment in patients with glaucoma or ocular hypertension: An evidence-based review. *Ophthalmology, 112*(6), 953–961.e957.

Owen, J. E., Bonds, C. L., & Wellisch, D. K. (2006). Psychiatric evaluations of heart transplant candidates: Predicting post-transplant hospitalizations, rejection episodes, and survival. *Psychosomatics, 47*(3), 213–222.

Paasche-Orlow, M. K., Cheng, D. M., Palepu, A., Meli, S., Fabel, V., & Samet, J. H. (2006). Health literacy, antiretroviral adherence and HIV-RNA suppression: A longitudinal perspective. *Journal of General Internal Medicine, 21*, 835–840.

Park, D. C., Willis, S. L., Morrow, D., Diehl, M., & Gaines, C. L. (1994). Cognitive function and medication usage in older adults. *Journal of Applied Gerontology, 13*(1), 39–57.

Pate, R. R., Pratt, M., Blair, S. N., Haskell, W. L., Macera, C. A., Bouchard, C., ... Wilmore, J. H. (1995). Physical activity and public health: A recommendation from the Centers for Disease Control and Prevention and the American College of Sports Medicine. *Journal of the American Medical Association, 273*(5), 402–407.

Paterson, D. L., Swindells, S., Mohr, J., Brester, M., Vergis, E. N., Squier, C., ... Singh, N. (2000). Adherence to protease inhibitor therapy and outcomes in patients with HIV infection. *Annals of Internal Medicine, 133*(1), 21–30.

Perreault, S., Lamarre, D., Blais, L., Dragomir, A., Berbiche, D., Lalonde, L., ... Collin, J. (2005). Persistence with treatment in newly treated middle-aged patients with essential hypertension. *Annals of Pharmacotherapy, 39*(9), 1401–1408.

Peterson, G. M., McLean, S., & Millingen, K. S. (1984). A randomized trial of strategies to improve patient compliance with anticonvulsant therapy. *Epilepsia, 25*(4), 412–417.

Petitti, D. B., Friedman, G. D., & Kahn, W. (1981). Accuracy of information on smoking habits provided on self-administered research questionnaires. *American Journal of Public Health, 71*(3), 308–311.

Pinsky, B. W., Takemoto, S. K., Lentine, K. L., Burroughs, T. E., Schnitzler, M. A., & Salvalaggio, P. R. (2009). Transplant outcomes and economic costs associated with patient noncompliance to immunosuppression. *American Journal of Transplantation, 9*(11), 2597–2606.

Pisani, V. D., Fawcett, J., Clark, D. C., & McGuire, M. (1993). The relative contributions of medication adherence and AA meeting attendance to abstinent outcome for chronic alcoholics. *Journal of Studies on Alcohol, 54*(1), 115–119.

Psaty, B. M., Koepsell, T. D., Wagner, E. H., LoGerfo, J. P., & Inui, T. S. (1990). The relative risk of incident coronary heart disease associated with recently stopping the use of beta-blockers. *Journal of the American Medical Association, 263*(12), 1653–1657.

Rand, C. S., & Wise, R. A. (1994). Measuring adherence to asthma medication regimens. *American Journal of Respiratory and Critical Care Medicine, 149*(2, Pt. 2), S69–S76.

Reed, B. D., Lutz, L. J., Zazove, P., & Ratcliffe, S. D. (1984). Compliance with acute otitis media treatment. *Journal of Family Practice, 19*(5), 627–632.

Reynolds, E. H. (1987). Early treatment and prognosis of epilepsy. *Epilepsia, 28*(2), 97–106.

Richardson, J. L., Shelton, D. R., Krailo, M., & Levine, A. M. (1990). The effect of compliance with treatment on survival among patients with hematologic malignancies. *Journal of Clinical Oncology, 8*(2), 356–364.

Rives, K., Gelberman, R., Smith, B., & Carney, K. (1992). Severe contractures of the proximal interphalangeal joint in Dupuytren's disease: Results of a prospective trial of operative correction and dynamic extension splinting. *Journal of Hand Surgery, 17*(6), 1153–1159.

Robertson, C. F., Rubinfeld, A. R., & Bowes, G. (1992). Pediatric asthma deaths in Victoria: The mild are at risk. *Pediatric Pulmonology, 13*(2), 95–100.

Rogers, F., Juneau, M., Taylor, C. B., Haskell, W. L., Kraemer, H. C., Ahn, D. K., & DeBusk, R. F. (1987). Assessment by a microprocessor of adherence to home-based moderate-intensity exercise training in healthy, sedentary middle-aged men and women. *American Journal of Cardiology, 60*(1), 71–75.

Rosenblum, M., Deeks, S. G., van der Laan, M., & Bangsberg, D. R. (2009). The risk of virologic failure decreases with duration of HIV suppression, at greater than 50% adherence to antiretroviral therapy [Electronic version]. *PLoS ONE, 4*, e7196. Retrieved from http://www.ncbi.nlm.nih.gov/pmc/articles/PMC2747009/

Rosenstock, I. M. (1974). The historical origins of the health belief model. *Health Education Monographs, 2*, 328–335.

Rovelli, M., Palmeri, D., Vossler, E., Bartus, S., Hull, D., & Schweizer, R. (1989). Noncompliance in organ transplant recipients. *Transplantation Proceedings, 21*(1, Pt. 1), 833–834.

Rubak, S., Sandbaek, A., Lauritzen, T., & Christensen, B. (2005). Motivational interviewing: A systematic review and meta-analysis. *British Journal of General Practice, 55*, 305–312.

Rudd, P., Ahmed, S., Zachary, V. Barton, C., & Bonduelle, D. (1990). Improved compliance measures: Applications in an ambulatory hypertensive drug trial. *Clinical Pharmacology and Therapeutics, 48*(6), 676–685.

Rueda, S., Park-Wyllie, L. Y., Bayoumi, A. M., Tynan, A. M., Antoniou, T. A., Rourke, S. B., & Glazier, R. H. (2006). Patient support and education for promoting adherence to highly active antiretroviral therapy for HIV/AIDS [Electronic version]. *Cochrane Database of Systematic Reviews, 2006*. Retrieved from http://onlinelibrary.wiley.com/o/cochrane/clsysrev/articles/CD001442/frame.html

Scarmeas, N., Luchsinger, J. A., Schupf, N., Brickman, A. M., Cosentino, S., Tang, M. X., & Stern, Y. (2009). Physical activity, diet, and risk of Alzheimer's disease. *JAMA, 302*(6), 627–637.

Schedlbauer, A., Davies, P., & Fahey, T. (2010). Interventions to improve adherence to lipid lowering medication. [Electronic version]. *Cochrane Database of Systematic Reviews, 2010*. Retrieved from http://onlinelibrary.wiley.com/o/cochrane/clsysrev/articles/CD004371/frame.html

Schlenk, E. A., Okifuji, A., Dunbar-Jacob, J. M., & Turk, D. C. (1996). Exercise adherence in fibromyalgia. *Arthritis and Rheumatism, 39*(9, Suppl.), S221.

Schroeder, K., Fahey, T., & Ebrahim, S. (2008). Interventions for improving adherence to treatment in patients with high blood pressure in ambulatory settings [Electronic version]. *Cochrane Database of Systematic Reviews, 2004*. Retrieved from http://onlinelibrary.wiley.com/o/cochrane/clsysrev/articles/CD004804/frame.html

Schron, E. B., Hamilton, G., Rand, C., Friedman, R., Dunbar-Jacob, J., & Sereika, S. (1995, May). *Adherence in clinical trials: Ancillary studies of strategies to improve adherence.* Paper presented at a workshop at the 16th annual meeting of the Society for Clinical Trials, Seattle, WA.

Schwarzmann, S. W. (1998). Novel cost-effective approaches to the treatment of community-acquired infections. *Annals of Pharmacotherapy*, *32*(1), S27–S30.

Schweitzer, R. D., Head. K., & Dwyer, J. W. (2007). Psychological factors and treatment adherence behavior in patients with chronic heart failure. *Journal of Cardiovascular Nursing*, *22*, 76–83.

Schweizer, R. T., Rovelli, M., Palmeri, D., Vossler, E., Hull, D., & Bartus, S. (1990). Noncompliance in organ transplant recipients. *Transplantation*, *49*(2), 374–377.

Sharp, J., & Freeman, C. (2009). Patterns and predictors of uptake and adherence to cardiac rehabilitation. *Journal of Cardiopulmonary Rehabilitation and Prevention*, *29*(4), 241–247.

Shemesh. E., Yehuda. R., Milo, O., Dinur. I., Rudnick. A., Vered Z., & Cotter, G. (2004). Posttraumatic stress, nonadherence, and adverse outcome in survivors of a myocardial infarction. *Psychosomatic Medicine*, *66*, 521–526.

Shigemura, J., Ogawa, T., Yoshino, A., Sato, Y., & Nomura, S. (2010). Predictors of antidepressant adherence: Results of a Japanese Internet-based survey. *Psychiatry and Clinical Neurosciences*, *64*(2), 179–186.

Shin, S. S., Keshavjee, S., Gelmanova, I. Y., Atwood, S., Franke, M. F., Mishustin, S. P., … Cohen, T. (2010). Development of extensively drug-resistant tuberculosis during multidrug-resistant tuberculosis treatment. *American Journal of Respiratory and Critical Care Medicine*, *182*(3), 426–432.

Siegel, D., Lopez, J., & Meier, J. (2007). Antihypertensive medication adherence in the Department of Veterans Affairs. *The American Journal of Medicine, 120*(1), 26–32.

Simkin-Silverman, L., Wing, R. R., Hansen, D. H., Klem, M. L., Pasagian-Macaulay, A. P., Meilahn, E. N., & Kuller, L. H. (1995). Prevention of cardiovascular risk factor elevations in healthy premenopausal women. *Preventive Medicine*, *24*(5), 509–517.

Singh, R. B., Niaz, M. A., Ghosh, S., Singh, R., & Rastogi, S. S. (1993). Effect on mortality and reinfarction of adding fruits and vegetables to a prudent diet in the Indian experiment of infarct survival (IEIS). *Journal of the American College of Nutrition*, *12*(3), 255–261.

Sokol, M., McGuigan, K., Verbrugge, R. R., & Epstein, R. S. (2005). Impact of medication adherence on hospitalization risk and healthcare cost. *Medical Care*, *43*(6), 521–530.

Sorensen, S. V., Baker, T., Fleurence, R., Dixon, J., Roberts, C., Haider, D., & Hughes, D. (2009). Cost and clinical consequence of antibiotic non-adherence in acute exacerbations of chronic bronchitis. *International Journal of Tuberculosis and Lung Disease*, *13*(8), 945–954.

Starlinger, M., Appel, W. H., Schemper, M., & Schiessel, R. (1985). Long-term treatment of peptic esophageal stenosis with dilation and cimetidine: Factors influencing clinical result. *European Surgical Research*, *17*(4), 207–214.

Stilley, C. S., Sereika, S., Muldoon, M. E, Ryan, C. M., & Dunbar-Jacob, J. (2004). Psychological and cognitive function: Predictors of adherence with cholesterol lowering treatment. *Annals of Behavioral Medicine*, *27*, 117–124.

Stone, A. A., Shiffman, S., Schwartz, J. E., Broderick, J. E., & Hufford, M. R. (2003). Patient compliance with paper and electronic diaries. *Controlled Clinical Trials*, *24*(2), 182–199.

Strandbygaard, U., Thomsen, S. F., & Backer, V. (2010). A daily SMS reminder increases adherence to asthma treatment: A three-month follow-up study. *Respiratory Medicine*, *104*(2), 166–171.

Sullivan, P. S., Campsmith, M. L., Nakamura, G. V., Begley, E. B., Schulden, J., & Nakashima, A. K. (2007). Patient and regimen characteristics associated with self-reported nonadherence to antiretroviral therapy. *PLoS ONE*, *2*(6), e552.

Swank, R. L., & Dugan, B. B. (1990). Effect of low saturated fat diet in early and late cases of multiple sclerosis. *Lancet*, *336*(8706), 37–39.

Taal, E., Rasker, J. J., Seydel, E. R., & Weigman, O. (1993). Health status, adherence with health recommendations, self-efficacy and social support in patients with rheumatoid arthritis. *Patient Education and Counseling*, *20*(2–3), 63–76.

Takemoto, S. K., Pinsky, B. W., Schnitzler, M. A., Lentine, K. L., Willoughby, L. M., Burroughs, T. E., & Bunnapradist, S. (2007). A retrospective analysis of immunosuppression compliance, dose reduction and discontinuation in kidney transplant recipients. *American Journal of Transplantation*, *7*, 2704–2711.

Tessema, B., Biadglegne, F., Mulu, A., Getachew, A., Emmrich, F., & Sack, U. (2010). Magnitude and determinants of nonadherence and nonreadiness to highly active antiretroviral therapy among people living with HIV/AIDS in Northwest Ethiopia: A cross-sectional study. *AIDS Research and Therapy*, *7*(1), 2.

Thier, S. L., Yu-Eisenberg, K. S., Leas, B. F., Cantrell, C. R., DeBussey, S., Goldfarb, N. I., & Nash, D. B. (2008). In chronic disease, nationwide data show poor adherence by patients to medication and by physicians to guidelines. *Managed Care*, *17*(2), 48–52, 55–47.

Unni, E. J., & Farris, K. B. (2011). Unintentional non-adherence and belief in medicines in older adults. *Patient Education and Counseling, 83*(2), 265–268.

Urquhart, J., & Chevalley, C. (1988). Impact of unrecognized dosing errors on the cost and effectiveness of pharmaceuticals. *Drug Information Journal, 22,* 363–378.

U.S. Department of Health and Human Services. (1996). *Physical activity and health: A report of the Surgeon General Executive Summary.* Rockville, MD: Author.

Vanhove, G. F., Schapiro, J. M., Winters, M. A., Merigan, T. C., & Blaschke, T. F. (1996). Patient compliance and drug failure in protease inhibitor monotherapy. *Journal of the American Medical Association, 276*(24), 1955–1956.

Verghese, A., John, J. K., Rajkumar, S., Richard, J., Sethi, B. B., & Trivedi, J. K. (1989). Factors associated with the course and outcome of schizophrenia in India: Results of a two-year multicentre follow-up study. *British Journal of Psychiatry, 154,* 499–503.

Vermeire, E. I. J. J., Wens, J., Van Royen, P., Biot, Y., Hearnshaw, H., & Lindenmeyer, A. (2009). Interventions for improving adherence to treatment recommendations in people with type 2 diabetes mellitus [Electronic version]. *Cochrane Database of Systematic Reviews, 2005.* Retrieved from http://onlinelibrary.wiley.com/o/cochrane/clsysrev/articles/CD003638/frame.html

Westfall, U. E. (1986). Methods for assessing compliance. *Topics in Clinical Nursing, 7*(4), 23–30.

Wetsteyn, J. C. F. M., & deGeus, A. (1993). Comparison of three regimens for malaria prophylaxis in travelers to east, central, and southern Africa. *British Medical Journal, 307*(6911), 1041–1043.

White, K., Kolman, M. L., Wexler, P., Polin G., & Winter, R. J. (1984). Unstable diabetes and unstable families: A psychosocial evaluation of diabetic children with recurrent ketoacidosis. *Pediatrics, 73*(6), 749–755.

Wilson, D. P., & Endres, R. K. (1986). Compliance with blood glucose monitoring in children with type I diabetes mellitus. *Journal of Pediatrics, 108*(6), 1022–1024.

Winter, K., Harriman, K., Schechter, R., Yamada, E., Talarico, J., & Chavez, G. (2010). Notes from the field: Pertussis—California, January–June 2010. *Morbidity and Mortality Weekly Report 59*(26), 815.

Wolf, M. S., Davis, T. C., Osborn, C. Y., Skripkauskas, S., Bennett, C. L., & Makoul, G. (2007). Literacy, self-efficacy, and HIV medication adherence. *Patient Education and Counseling, 5,* 253–260.

Yeboah-Antwi, K., Gyapong, J. O., Asare, I. K., Barnish, G., Evans, D. B., & Adjei, S. (2001). Impact of pre-packaging antimalarial drugs on cost to patients and compliance with treatment. *Bulletin of the World Health Organanization, 79*(5), 394–399.

Zelikovsky, N., Schast, A. P., Palmer, J., & Meyers, K. E. (2008). Perceived barriers to adherence among adolescent renal transplant candidates. *Pediatric Transplantation, 12*(3), 300–308.

13 Caregiving and Care Receiving in Later Life

Health Effects and Promising Interventions

Lynn M. Martire
Pennsylvania State University

Richard Schulz
University of Pittsburgh

The provision of ongoing care to an impaired older friend or relative is often a stressful experience that impacts the mental and physical health of the caregiver. Because caregiving sometimes has severe consequences for the health of the caregiver, and because these individuals are an invaluable resource to the rapidly growing population of older adults, in the past decade research on the health effects of caregiving has become both more common and more rigorously conducted. Many of the advances made in understanding the consequences of caregiving have resulted from the application of theoretical models and methodologies borrowed from health psychology.

In this chapter, we first describe the nature of informal caregiving to older adults and provide recent statistics regarding the prevalence of caregiving. In the second and third sections of the chapter, we review recent evidence for the effects of caregiving on the individual who provides care and on the older adult who receives that care, respectively. Finally, we highlight findings from studies testing recent psychosocial interventions for caregivers or caregiver–care recipient dyads. Throughout this chapter, in order to describe research published since the first edition of the *Handbook of Health Psychology* (see Martire & Schulz, 2001), we emphasize original research and reviews of the literature that have been published in the past decade.

INFORMAL CAREGIVING TO OLDER ADULTS: RECENT TRENDS

One unfortunate consequence of growing older is the increased difficulty in carrying out such everyday activities as driving, shopping, and preparing meals (instrumental activities of daily living, IADLs), or even such personal care activities as bathing and dressing (activities of daily living, ADLs). For many older adults, this difficulty stems from such illnesses as arthritis, heart disease, and diabetes, the most chronic health problems of older men and women. Such difficulty with everyday activities, often referred to as functional disability, eventually progresses to the point where the older adult needs assistance from others.

Although the likelihood of becoming disabled increases with age, the functional ability of the older adult population is actually characterized by much variability. Of the 95% of U.S. adults from age 65 to 74 who live in noninstitutionalized settings, only 11% are ADL or IADL impaired. This percentage rises to 27% for those from age 75 to 84, and 60% of those over age 85 experience some amount of disability (Manton, Corder, & Stallard, 1997). Investigations utilizing several different national data sets have shown that between 1982 and 1994, the proportion of the population age 65 and older that was disabled decreased slightly (Crimmins, Saito, & Reynolds, 1997; Manton et al., 1997). Despite the relatively low rates of disability before age 85 and the modest improvements in the physical functioning of older adults in general, the contrasting dramatic growth in the proportion of the population that is older will result in a predictable increase in the number of disabled older adults in the future. Thus, as the number of older adults continues to grow, so will the number of older adults who have difficulty with everyday activities and who need and receive assistance from informal caregivers.

Some amount of functional disability in the older adult population is attributable to disease that results in cognitive impairment, particularly Alzheimer's disease. Current estimates indicate that 5 million adults age 65 or older are cognitively impaired, and this number is projected to rise to 7.7 million by the year 2030 (Alzheimer's Association, 2008). The majority of these individuals reside in the community with the support of a family caregiver.

National household surveys show that families continue to be the primary sources of care and support for older adults. Prevalence estimates vary widely depending on definitions used and populations sampled. For example, at one extreme, there are estimates that 21.2% of the U.S. adult population, or 48.9 million Americans, provided unpaid care to an adult relative in 2009, with the majority (72%) of this care being delivered to persons age 50 years or older (NAC and AARP Survey, 2009). At the other extreme, data from the National Long-Term Care Survey suggest that as few as 3.5 million caregivers provided IADL or ADL assistance to persons age 65 and over. These differences are in part attributable to when the data were collected, to the age range of the potential caregiver and care-recipient populations targeted, but most important to the definition of caregiving. Thus, the high-end estimates are largely a result of the broad and inclusive definitions of caregiving, and the low-end estimates are generated by first confirming the presence of functional disability in an older person who might require assistance and then following up to ascertain the presence of a caregiver who provides ADL or IADL assistance (e.g., Wolff & Kasper, 2006).

Most older adults who need care receive assistance from their spouses. But when the spouse is no longer alive or is unavailable to provide assistance, adult children usually step in to help. Adult daughters and daughters-in-law are more likely than sons and sons-in-law to provide routine assistance with household chores and personal care over long periods of time (e.g., Horowitz, 1985), and they also spend more hours per week in providing assistance (e.g., Montgomery, 1992). Although caregiving tasks are sometimes divided among several family members or friends, the more typical scenario is that the majority of care is provided by one family member.

EFFECTS OF PROVIDING ONGOING CARE TO AN ILL OLDER RELATIVE

Our model of the health effects of elder caregiving (Martire & Schulz, 2001) is a modification of a stress-process model linking environmental demands to health outcomes (Cohen, Kessler, & Gordon, 1995; see Figure 13.1). As applied to caregiving, environmental demands include providing instrumental assistance and emotional support in response to the older adult's disability. If individuals perceive these demands as threatening and also view their coping resources as inadequate, they perceive themselves as under stress (e.g., Lazarus & Folkman, 1984). The appraisal of stress is presumed to trigger physiological, affective, behavioral, or cognitive responses that place the individual at increased risk for mental and physical health problems. Physiological responses include altered immune and endocrine function, as well as cardiovascular reactivity. Affective responses may include changes in positive or negative mood, whereas behavioral responses include such things as preventive health behaviors, among them exercise, proper diet, and mammograms (e.g., did not find time for exercise, had inadequate rest, did not take enough time to rest when sick, and forgot to take medications). Examples of cognitive responses to caregiving stress include an enhanced or eroded sense of control or mastery over events occurring in life.

This model allows for the possibility that individuals may feel they have the capacity to deal with caregiving demands and thus appraise these demands positively (Kramer, 1997; Lawton, Kleban,

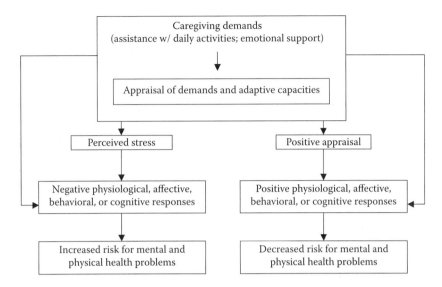

FIGURE 13.1   A model of the health effects of elder caregiving. (Adapted from Cohen, S., Kessler, R. C., & Gordon, L. U., in *Measuring Stress: A Guide for Health and Social Scientists*, 3–26, Oxford University Press, New York, 1995.)

Moss, Rovine, & Glicksman, 1989). This appraisal may in turn lead to positive physiological, affective, behavioral, or cognitive responses and decreased risk for mental and physical health problems. It is important to note that this second pathway has less empirical support than the first but has also received less attention.

NEGATIVE EFFECTS OF CAREGIVING

In addition to seminal reviews of research on family caregiving that were published in the 1990s (e.g., Schulz, O'Brien, Bookwala, & Fleissner, 1995; Wright, Clipp, & George, 1993), there have been important quantitative reviews in the past decade (Pinquart & Sorensen, 2003, 2005, 2006; Vitaliano, Zhang, & Scanlan, 2003). In this section, we describe findings from these reviews as well as specific studies that illustrate the latest methodologies in this area. Many studies continue to examine the effects of providing care to an older adult with Alzheimer's disease or other types of dementia; however, family also play an important role in adjustment to and management of such other illnesses as cancer (Kim & Given, 2008), diabetes (Gonder-Frederick, Cox, & Ritterband, 2002), musculoskeletal disorders (Keefe et al., 2002), and spinal cord injury (Dreer, Elliott, Shewchuk, Berry, & Rivera, 2007). Relatedly, there is increased recognition that caregiving is a broad set of activities that encompasses not only physical assistance with activities of daily living but also emotional support, advice, and problem solving in regard to navigating the health care system, managing medication, and changing health behaviors (e.g., diet and exercise).

Mental Health

Evidence for the negative impact of caregiving on family members' psychological health continues to accumulate. In a recent meta-analysis of 84 studies, Pinquart and Sorensen (2003) found that caregivers were more stressed and depressed and had lower levels of subjective well-being (e.g., life satisfaction, positive affect) and self-efficacy than did noncaregivers. The strongest negative effects of caregiving were observed for clinician-rated depression (e.g., the Hamilton Depression Rating Scale [Hamilton, 1967]). Overall, the size of the differences between the groups was small to medium, but larger effects were found in studies comparing dementia caregivers to noncaregivers; spousal caregivers to adult child caregivers; and female caregivers to male caregivers.

As depicted in Figure 13.1, the negative effects of caregiving are typically attributed to a variety of patient illness–related factors, including the care demands engendered by the patient's illness and functional disability. Our recent conceptual and empirical work has explored the question of whether past research has ignored a key aspect of the caregiving experience—patient suffering— that is harmful to caregivers' mental health (Schulz et al., 2007). We believe that patient suffering is distinct from illness and disability because not all illnesses entail suffering, and individuals vary widely in the extent to which they experience and express their suffering in response to a given health problem. In a recent analysis of data from the Resources for Enhancing Alzheimer's Caregiver Health (REACH) study, we found that emotional and existential aspects of patient suffering are distinct from such other attributes of Alzheimer's disease as physical and cognitive disability and are independently associated with caregiver depression. Specifically, caregivers of patients who showed increased emotional and existential distress over time became more depressed even after controlling for a host of other factors related to patient illness, including such factors as physical and cognitive disability and the amount of care provided (Schulz et al., 2008). We believe that this type of research may tell us why some family members are more affected by caregiving than others and may suggest new strategies for intervention.

Another recent shift in the past decade of caregiver research can be seen in the increased attention to change in caregivers' mental health after placement of the older relative in a long-term-care setting. Perhaps not surprisingly, dementia caregivers continue to report symptoms of depression and anxiety 18 months after placement that are as high as when they were in-home caregivers, especially if they are spouses and if they visit the patient often (Schulz et al., 2004). There has also been an increased focus in recent years on change in caregivers' mental health after death of their older relative (e.g., Taylor, Kuchibhatla, Ostbye, Plassman, & Clipp, 2008; Tweedy & Guarnaccia, 2007–2008). A key factor to examine in this type of research is the nature of care provided prior to patient death. One study showed that spouses who reported caregiver strain prior to patient death did not become more depressed over a four-year follow-up, whereas nonstrained caregivers did show increased depressive symptomatology similar to a bereavement effect (Schulz et al., 2001). A second study of dementia caregivers showed that within three months of the older relative's death, caregivers had clinically significant declines in depressive symptoms; and within one year, symptomatology was less than that experienced during caregiving (Schulz, Mendelsohn, et al., 2003). Taken together, these studies suggest that bolstered by the knowledge that they provided care when it was needed, caregivers experience some amount of relief when the suffering of their loved one ends.

There continues to be empirical interest in possible moderators of the caregiver stress process. A recent meta-analysis of 116 studies of family caregivers to older adults (with or without dementia) showed that African American caregivers had lower levels of caregiver burden and depression than did White caregivers, but Hispanic and Asian American caregivers were more depressed than White non-Hispanics. All groups of minority caregivers reported poorer perceived health or more physical symptoms than did White caregivers (Pinquart & Sorensen, 2005). Overall, these ethnic differences were small and were explained not by differences in stressors but, rather, by resources, coping processes, and background variables. Another meta-analysis by the same authors, focused on 229 studies, concluded that gender differences in caregiver psychological and physical health have been overestimated in the scientific community (Pinquart & Sorensen, 2006). That is, statistically controlling for the higher level of stressors and lower levels of social support in women caregivers resulted in very small gender differences in depression and perceived health in these studies.

Work and Financial Well-Being

Despite relatively small differences in the impact of caregiving on men versus women, caregiving does take a greater toll on women's work life. Middle-aged women at the peak of their earning power, many of whom are employed, provide much of the care to disabled older relatives (Wolff & Kasper, 2006). These caregivers often rearrange their work schedules to manage caregiving demands (e.g., Doty, Jackson, & Crown, 1998). And although low levels of caregiving demand can be absorbed by employed caregivers with little impact on their work life, heavy demands (e.g., 20 hours or more of caregiving per week) result in significant work adjustment. Recently two waves of data from the National Survey of Families and Households were used to show that the initiation of parental caregiving led to a substantial reduction in women's weekly hours worked and annual earnings (Wakabayashi & Donato, 2005). A subsequent study showed that being a caregiver in 1991 increased women's risks of living in households with incomes below the poverty threshold, receiving public assistance, and being covered by Medicaid in 1999 (Wakabayashi & Donato, 2006).

Caregiving can also impact the quality of work life for women. Women caregivers with multiple social roles (e.g., wife, mother to children living at home, and employee) have reported that the work role conflicts the most with caregiving (Stephens, Townsend, Martire, & Druley, 2001). Working women report problematic interactions with work associates that stem from the demands of juggling elder caregiving and work. These caregivers report that supervisors and coworkers are sometimes insensitive about their attempts to juggle parent care and work, or these colleagues fail to understand the difficulties of providing parent care. Women who had more such problematic interactions have less positive affect and greater depressive symptoms, even after controlling for the amount of time they work and the stress experienced in their caregiving and work roles. In addition, women who have more problematic interactions with work associates have poorer physical health in terms of self-rated global health and health-related limitations (Atienza & Stephens, 2000).

Physical Health and Mortality

Perhaps the area of greatest advancement in the past decade of caregiving research has occurred in the area of physical health outcomes of caregiving. One recent review focused on dementia caregivers from 23 different samples comprising a total of 1,594 caregivers and 1,478 noncaregivers (Vitaliano et al., 2003). This meta-analysis aggregated findings for self-reported health outcomes (e.g., global perceived health and physical symptoms) as well as physiological indicators (e.g., stress hormones, lymphocyte counts, and antibodies). Compared to noncaregivers, caregivers had a 23% higher level of stress hormones (e.g., growth hormone expression; Wu et al., 1999), a 16% lower level of global self-rated health (e.g., Rose-Rego, Strauss, & Smyth, 1998), and a 15% lower level of antibody response (e.g., immunoglobin response to influenza vaccination; Vedhara et al., 1999). As noted by the authors, these findings are especially striking because caregivers were 65 years of age on average and likely to be at greater risk than younger individuals for such illnesses as hypertension, diabetes, and influenza.

Studies published since the review by Vitaliano and colleagues (2003) have added substantially to the evidence base in this area, and we provide a few examples here. High levels of caregiving burden for ill spouses have been shown to increase the risk of coronary heart disease (CHD) among women. In a study of 54,412 women from the Nurses' Health Study, caregiving for a disabled or ill spouse for more than nine hours per week was associated with increased risk of CHD over a four-year follow-up (i.e., nonfatal cases of myocardial infarction, and CHD deaths), controlling for such factors as age, smoking, exercise, alcohol intake, body mass index, hypertension, and diabetes mellitus (Lee, Colditz, Berkman, & Kawachi, 2003). Greater depressive symptoms in dementia caregivers specifically has been shown to predict a diagnosis of cardiovascular disease over an 18-month follow-up (Mausbach, Patterson, Rabinowitz, Grant, & Schulz, 2007). Other work on cardiovascular outcomes includes a study linking patient dementia severity and laboratory-induced stress with higher levels of hypercoagulability (i.e., procoagulant factor D-dimer) in older spousal caregivers (Aschbacher et al., 2006).

Damjanovic and colleagues (2007) have recently demonstrated that the impaired immune functioning seen in Alzheimer's caregivers is in turn associated with loss of telomeres, the region of repetitive DNA that is found at the end of chromosomes and protects them from destruction. Another line of research has shown that caregiving negatively impacts sleep (Creese, Bedard, Brazil, & Chambers, 2008; Kochar, Fredman, Stone, & Cauley, 2007; von Kanel et al., 2006) and such health behaviors as physical activity (Fredman, Bertrand, Martire, Hochberg, & Harris, 2006).

Perhaps reflecting these effects of caregiving on physiological functioning and health behaviors, our research has shown that strained spousal caregivers are 62% more likely than nonstrained caregivers to die over a four-year follow-up (Schulz & Beach, 1999).

POSITIVE EFFECTS OF CAREGIVING

In contrast to the focus of the vast majority of caregiver research, family caregiving is not always a negative experience. In studies of caregiving based on large population-based samples, a significant proportion of caregivers report neither strain nor negative health effects (Schulz et al., 1997). This is particularly true for caregivers in the early stages of a caregiving career (Burton. Zdaniuk, Schulz, Jackson, & Hirsch, 2003; Hirst, 2005). Even when caregiving demands become more intense, resulting in high levels of distress and depression, caregivers at the same time acknowledge positive aspects of the caregiving experience. They report that it makes them feel good about themselves, makes them feel useful and needed, gives meaning to their lives, enables them to learn new skills, and strengthens relationships with others. Because research on positive aspects of caregiving is relatively new, we know little about how these experiences may have direct effects on health (see Figure 13.1) or whether they moderate the effects of stress on health.

Researchers have known for some time that individuals in supportive social relationships are happier, healthier, and live longer than those who are socially isolated (Brown, 2007; House, Landis, & Umberson, 1988). Recent findings suggest that giving support or helping others may be just as beneficial to health as receiving support. After controlling for baseline health status, one study found that individuals who reported providing instrumental support to friends, relatives, and neighbors, and individuals who provided emotional support to their spouses, had lower five-year mortality rates than did individuals who did not help others or did not support their spouses (Brown, Nesse, Vinokur, & Smith, 2003). This research is complemented by a recent study of benefit finding in the cancer caregiving experience. In that study, greater acceptance and increased appreciation for new relationships with others was associated with greater life satisfaction and fewer depressive symptoms in caregivers (Kim, Schulz, & Carver, 2007).

To summarize this section, there is consistent evidence of the negative effects of caregiving on mental health, and researchers are beginning to study caregivers as they experience such important transitions as institutionalization or death of their older relative. Research on the role of race and ethnicity in caregiving indicates that minority status can be either an advantage or a disadvantage with regard to caregiver health, and differences vary across ethnic groups. There is now strong evidence that caregiving has the potential to profoundly affect the financial well-being of women. There also is compelling evidence for the harmful effects of caregiving on objective physical health outcomes, and dementia caregiving continues to be a useful chronic stress paradigm in this regard. The health effects of caregiving may be less pronounced in studies that do not focus on dementia caregivers. However, population-based studies with representative samples may underestimate the negative impact of caregiving as a result of the common approach of defining caregiving as a minimal level of assistance with activities of daily living or merely share a residence with an older relative (Fredman et al., 2004; Schulz et al., 1997). Finally, we need a better understanding of different types of caregiver helping experiences and their effects on health. Although providing help that fails to enhance the quality of patient life leads to frustration, resignation, and negative health effects in the caregiver, it is likely that providing help that significantly addresses the needs and desires of a patient is uplifting to the caregiver and contributes to positive health effects.

EFFECTS ON OLDER ADULTS OF RECEIVING FAMILY CARE

In our model of the health effects of care receiving (Martire & Schulz, 2001), receipt of assistance with daily activities (i.e., instrumental support) and illness-specific emotional support are conceptualized as experiences that are appraised by the care recipient as either helpful or unhelpful, depending

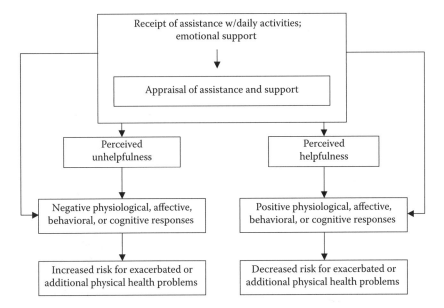

FIGURE 13.2 A model of the health effects of elder care receiving. (Adapted from Cohen, S., Kessler, R. C., & Gordon, L. U., in *Measuring Stress: A Guide for Health and Social Scientists*, 3–26, Oxford University Press, New York, 1995.)

on whether or not such support fits the recipient's needs or preferences (see Figure 13.2). Similar to the caregiving model, the appraisal of assistance as unhelpful is presumed to result in negative physiological, affective, behavioral, or cognitive responses that place the older adult at increased risk for exacerbated or additional mental and physical health problems (Newsom, 1999). Alternatively, assistance from others may be perceived as helpful and thus lead to positive responses associated with a decreased risk for exacerbated or additional mental and physical health problems.

A likely indicator of mental health to be affected by the quality of instrumental and emotional support from others is the recipient's experience of depressive symptoms. An aspect of physical health that is likely to reflect the effects of receiving support is the older adult's level of functional disability. That is, the extent to which assistance is helpful or unhelpful is likely to affect older adults' future ability to carry out daily activities on their own or with minimal help from others (Baltes & Wahl, 1992).

Cognitive responses have been proposed as likely mediators of the relationship between receipt of care and such mental health problems as depressive symptomatology. It has been suggested that emotional support and instrumental assistance contain self-relevant messages for recipients that may apply generally to their life or to coping with illness. Specifically, self-evaluations of domain-specific efficacy may explain to older adults the positive or negative effects of support on their mental health. Responses that may mediate the relationship between receipt of care and disability are most likely to be cognitive or behavioral in nature and include following a proper diet, using assistive devices, and obtaining medical care. It seems especially plausible that assistance received from informal caregivers has an impact on the extent to which older adults take care of their own health. As noted by others, family members often serve as a source of motivation and advice regarding health behaviors and also play an important role in terms of interactions with the health care system (e.g., Prohaska, 1998).

Negative Effects of Care Receiving

There continues to be less research attention to the effects on older adults of receiving family care than to the experiences of family caregivers. The greater focus on the caregiver in past research is in part because many studies have focused on caregiving to older adults who are cognitively impaired, and it is challenging to assess the perspective of these care recipients. Similar to our review of recent caregiver research, we emphasize recent findings regarding negative effects of care receiving because positive, personal effects of receiving care from family are rarely subjected to empirical investigation.

Our chapter in the first edition of this handbook (see Martire & Schulz, 2001) described research showing that actions or communications that caregivers intend to be supportive may backfire and have negative rather than positive effects on the care recipient. Studies published in the past decade have added to this small literature. For example, older adults who feel that they have little control over the assistance they receive from their spouses, or who feel less competent in carrying out tasks on their own as a result of this assistance, experience more depressive symptoms and less life satisfaction (Martire et al., 2002). In a second study focused on perceptions of the amount, manner, and timing of spousal care, there were no gender differences overall, but female care recipients were significantly less satisfied than male recipients with the manner in which assistance was provided. Furthermore, care recipients who perceived poorer quality of care from their spouses were more depressed and had a lesser sense of mastery in life one year later; these effects were observed even after controlling for the care recipient's sociodemographic characteristics, physical disability, marital quality, and strain from receiving care, as well as the caregiver's well-being (Martire, Schulz, Wrosch, & Newsom, 2003).

Of course, negative consequences of care receiving also occur when an older adult's family caregiver is critical or hostile in actions or communications, or even abusive. We next provide an overview of this area of research.

Potentially Harmful Caregiver Behavior and Elder Mistreatment

Greater depressive symptomatology in the caregiver (Williamson & Shaffer, 2001) and resentment of the older care recipient (Williamson et al., 2005) are factors that are associated with such potentially harmful behavior as screaming or yelling, using a harsh tone of voice, and insulting the care recipient. One study found that physical forms of harmful behavior (e.g., hitting or slapping, handling roughly) were reported by only 1% of care recipients, but negative verbal interactions were reported by 22%. Potentially harmful caregiver behaviors were more likely when the caregiver was the spouse rather than an adult son or daughter, as well as when the caregiver was in poor physical or mental health (Beach et al., 2005).

The potentially harmful behaviors that have been examined in recent caregiver research can be viewed as precursors to the elder mistreatment that sometimes occurs when caregivers are pushed to a breaking point. A recent survey indicates that few older adults (0.2%) report physical mistreatment from family members, with 0.9% reporting verbal mistreatment and 3.5% reporting financial mistreatment (Laumann, Leitsch, & Waite, 2008). Risk factors for elder neglect include caregiver characteristics (i.e., functional status, childhood trauma, and personality) and care-recipient characteristics (i.e., cognitive and functional status, depression, social support, childhood trauma, and personality; Fulmer et al., 2005).

Although the prevalence of elder mistreatment from family members appears to be quite low, it is important to explore new methodologies for assessing mistreatment that will better ensure honest reporting by care recipients. Our recent work has used an experimental design to determine the feasibility of different survey methods, including automated computer-assisted self-interviews (A-CASI) and interactive voice response (IVR). We found that A-CASI offered the most promising approach and was perceived as increasing privacy to a greater extent than IVR. Using A-CASI, six-month prevalence rates for psychological and financial mistreatment were 16.4% and 7.3%, respectively, whereas the ability of either A-CASI or IVR to assess physical mistreatment was less clear (Beach et al., 2010).

To summarize this section, further evidence has accumulated over the past decade with regard to the occasional negative impact of emotional support and task assistance from family caregivers. Findings from this small group of studies are consistent with the broader health psychology literature documenting the impact of the social environment on adults with chronic health conditions (e.g., Baker et al., 1999; Weihs, Enright, & Simmens, 2008). For the purposes of both description and intervention, it is important to determine why well-intended actions of family caregivers are unhelpful. It also is important to identify correlates of elder mistreatment. These issues will become even more important as our population ages, especially for those families who do not have the financial resources to purchase paid care or to take advantage of emerging technologies that enable older adults to be more independent of family care.

PROMISING PSYCHOSOCIAL INTERVENTION APPROACHES

The dynamic, cyclical nature of the caregiving–care-receiving process, and the potentially negative effects of elder caregiving on both the family caregiver and the care recipient, provide a strong argument for psychosocial or behavioral intervention at either the caregiver level or the dyad level. In this section, we highlight recent reviews and selected studies in these two areas.

CAREGIVER INTERVENTIONS

Recent reviews of the literature indicate small to medium effect sizes of psychosocial interventions for family caregivers, for such outcomes as psychological burden, depressive symptoms, subjective well-being, and knowledge (Martire, Lustig, Schulz, Miller, & Helgeson, 2004; Sorensen, Pinquart, & Duberstein, 2002). These two reviews also found that interventions for dementia caregivers achieved smaller effects than did interventions for other types of elder caregivers, likely reflecting that the former group is faced with increasingly uncontrollable stressors over time that are difficult to counteract. Spousal caregivers also seem to benefit less from intervention than do adult children. Psychotherapeutic and psycho-educational interventions show the most consistent effects (Sorensen et al., 2002).

Given the public health impact of Alzheimer's disease and related disorders, most interventions for caregivers to older adults have been targeted at dementia populations (Brodaty, Green, & Koschera, 2003; Schulz et al. 2002). In contrast to a sole focus on the statistical significance of intervention effects, one recent review examined the practical significance of dementia caregiver interventions in terms of change in psychiatric symptoms, quality of life, social significance (e.g., residential-care placement), and social validity (e.g., caregiver satisfaction with intervention; Schulz et al., 2002). This review found that interventions show promise of achieving clinically significant outcomes in improving caregivers' depressive symptoms and, to a lesser degree, in reducing anxiety, anger, and hostility. Although the ability thus far to improve overall quality of life for caregivers appears to be limited, there is evidence that such specific components of quality of life as caregiver burden, mood, and perceived stress are responsive to interventions. Some impressive and clinically meaningful effects have been demonstrated for delayed institutionalization of the care recipient. Finally, most of the studies reviewed met criteria for social validity; that is, caregivers consistently rated the interventions as beneficial, helpful, or valuable.

The most ambitious caregiver intervention trial to date, the REACH study, tested several different social and behavioral interventions designed to enhance family caregiving for Alzheimer's disease and related disorders, with total N equal to 1,222 dyads (Schulz, Belle, et al., 2003; Wisniewski et al., 2003). Although different interventions were carried out at different sites, all sites used the same measurement protocol, enabling the researchers to carry out preplanned meta-analysis to assess the effects of active treatments versus control conditions, as well as to conduct hierarchical linear modeling to identify key elements of interventions that contributed most to positive caregiver outcomes. The results showed that among all caregivers combined, active treatments were superior to control conditions in reducing caregiver burden. In particular, less-educated women (those with high school or lower) who were in active treatment reported significantly lower burden than did similar individuals in control conditions. Caregivers in active interventions who were Hispanic, those who were nonspouses, and those who had less than high school education reported lower depression scores than did those with the same characteristics who were in control conditions. Interventions that emphasized behavioral-skills training had the greatest impact in reducing caregiver depression (Belle et al., 2003; Gitlin et al., 2003).

Based on findings from Phase 1 of REACH, a new intervention that combined the most promising elements of the Phase 1 trial was developed. The strategy used in Phase 2 was to assess caregiver risk in five domains: safety, social support, health and self-care, emotional well-being, and care-recipient problem behaviors. The intervention addressed all five domains, but at varying doses, depending on the risk profile of the caregiver; and the outcome was a quality-of-life indicator comprising caregiver depression, burden, self-care, social support, and care-recipient problem behaviors at a six-month follow-up. Results from the primary analyses showed that Hispanic and White caregivers who received the intervention experienced significantly greater improvement in quality of life than did those in the control condition, and Black spousal caregivers also improved significantly more. In addition, prevalence of clinical depression was lower among caregivers in the intervention group (Belle et al., 2006).

DYADIC INTERVENTIONS

The effects of family caregiving on both the caregiver and the care recipient argue for a truly dyadic approach to psychosocial or behavioral intervention. In fact, Brodaty and colleagues (2003) found that dementia caregiver interventions were more successful if the patient also was involved in some way. However, dyadic interventions for chronic illness are more feasible and thus more common in studies focused on nonneurological disorders that are behaviorally driven and affected by the social environment. Studies in this area have compared a dyadic psychosocial intervention, that is, one

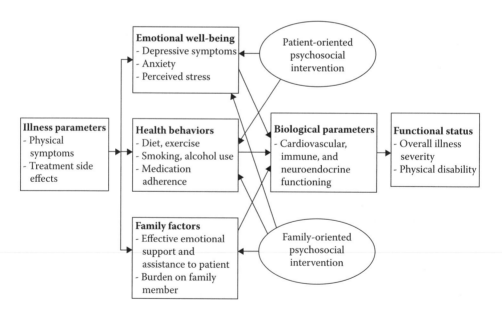

FIGURE 13.3   A model depicting the potential added benefit of family-oriented intervention for chronic illness as compared to patient-oriented intervention, due to its effects on an additional domain of functioning (i.e., family factors; Martire & Schulz, 2007). The type of family-oriented intervention depicted in this model includes standard content (e.g., education regarding illness etiology and cognitive-behavioral skills training for illness management) and incorporates a close family member by treating that individual as a collaborator in the patient's intervention and/or by addressing his or her personal concerns, burden, and supportiveness of the patient. Examples of specific constructs are provided for each domain of functioning.

usually focused on the patient and spousal caregiver, to a similar intervention that is targeted at only the patient or caregiver (Martire, 2005); or they have compared a dyadic intervention to usual medical care for the patient (Martire et al., 2004). A heuristic model depicting the potential advantage of dyadic, or family-oriented, psychosocial intervention over patient-oriented psychosocial intervention is presented in Figure 13.3 (Martire & Schulz, 2007). As depicted in this model, both types of intervention approaches may improve the emotional well-being and health behaviors of either individual, but dyadic intervention has greater potential because of its effects on such factors as effective support seeking and support provision within the dyad.

We reviewed 12 studies comparing dyadic and patient-focused interventions through a randomized controlled-trial design (Martire, 2005). Patients and family caregivers in these studies were in their late 50s or early 60s on average and were coping with heart disease, chronic pain, arthritis, or Type 2 diabetes. Approximately half of the studies reported a statistically significant advantage of dyadic intervention or, in the absence of differences between the two approaches, showed significant improvements over time for those individuals receiving a dyadic intervention. One study found an unexpected advantage for the patient-focused intervention, and the remaining studies found that the more efficacious approach for patients depended on such factors as patient gender and specific type of intervention (i.e., educational vs. behavioral approach). Despite the dyadic approach used in these studies, caregiver outcomes were rarely assessed.

CONCLUSION

Awareness of the public health significance of providing care to an older family member has come to the forefront as the Baby Boomers enter their later years. As we have tried to illustrate in this chapter, family caregiver research continues to become more methodologically sophisticated and focused on physical health consequences. The experience of needing and receiving care and the ways to maintain independence without the help of family members also are important issues but have received much less research attention.

Evidence for the negative effects of informal caregiving on family caregivers, as well as subsequent risks to the mental and physical well-being of their care recipients, suggests that psychosocial interventions should target both the family caregiver and the care recipient. There is not yet strong evidence for the efficacy of dyadic intervention, but relatively few studies have been designed to answer this question. Future research on late-life chronic illness should explore a dyadic approach to both psychosocial intervention and evaluation of outcomes.

ACKNOWLEDGMENTS

Preparation of this chapter was supported in part by National Institute of Health grants R01 AG026010 and R24 HL076852-076858 (Pittsburgh Mind-Body Center).

REFERENCES

Alzheimer's Association. (2008). Alzheimer's disease: Facts and figures. *Alzheimer's & Dementia*. Chicago, IL: Alzheimer's Association.

Aschbacher, K., von Kanel, R., Dimsdale, J., Patterson, T., Mills, P., Mausbach, B., … Grant, I. (2006). Dementia severity of the care receiver predicts procoagulant response in Alzheimer caregivers. *American Journal of Geriatric Psychiatry*, *14*, 694–703.

Atienza, A. A., & Stephens, M. A. P. (2000). Social interactions at work and the well-being of daughters involved in parent care. *Journal of Applied Gerontology*, *19*(3), 243–263.

Baker, B., Helmers, K., O'Kelly, B., Sakinofsky, I., Abelsohn, A., & Tobe, S. (1999). Marital cohesion and ambulatory blood pressure in early hypertension. *American Journal of Hypertension*, *12*, 227–230.

Baltes, M. M., & Wahl, H. W. (1992). The dependency-support script in institutions: Generalization to community settings. *Psychology & Aging*, *7*, 409–418.

Beach, S. R., Schulz, R., Degenholtz, H. B., Castle, N. G., Rosen, J., Foz, A. R., & Morycz, R. K. (2010). Using audio computer-assisted self-interviewing and interactive voice response to measure elder mistreatment in older adults: Feasibility and effects on prevalence estimates. *Journal of Official Statistics, 26*, 507–533.

Beach, S. R., Schulz, R., Williamson, G. M., Miller, L. S., Weiner, M. F., & Lance, C. E. (2005). Risk factors for potentially harmful informal caregiver behavior. *Journal of the American Geriatrics Society, 53*, 255–261.

Belle, S. H., Burgio, L., Burns, R.. Coon, D., Czaja, S. J., Gallagher-Thompson, D., … Zhang, S. (2006). Enhancing the quality of life of dementia caregivers from different ethnic or racial groups: A randomized, controlled trial. *Annals of Internal Medicine, 145*, 727–738.

Belle, S. H., Czaja, S. J., Schulz, R., Zhang, S., Burgio, L. D., Gitlin, L. N., … Ory, M. G. (for the REACH Investigators). (2003). Using a new taxonomy to combine the uncombinable: Integrating results across diverse interventions. *Psychology & Aging, 18*, 396–405.

Brodaty, H., Green, A., & Koschera, A. (2003). Meta-analysis of psychosocial interventions for caregivers of people with dementia. *Journal of the American Geriatrics Society, 51*, 657–664.

Brown, S. L. (2007). Health effects of caregiving: Studies of helping behavior needed! *Alzheimer's Care Today, 8*, 235–246.

Brown, S. L., Nesse, R. M., Vinokur, A. D., & Smith, D. M. (2003). Providing social support may be more beneficial than receiving it: Results from a prospective study of mortality. *Psychological Science, 14*, 320–327.

Burton, L. C., Zdaniuk, B., Schulz, R., Jackson, S., & Hirsch, C. (2003). Transitions in spousal caregiving. *Gerontologist, 43*, 230–241.

Cohen, S., Kessler, R. C., & Gordon, L. U. (1995). Strategies for measuring stress in studies of psychiatric and physical disorders. In S. Cohen, R. C. Kessler, & L. U. Gordon (Eds.), *Measuring stress: A guide for health and social scientists* (pp. 3–26). New York, NY: Oxford University Press.

Creese, J., Bedard, M., Brazil, K., & Chambers, L. (2008). Sleep disturbances in spousal caregivers of individuals with Alzheimer's disease. *International Psychogeriatrics, 20*, 149–161.

Crimmins, E. M., Saito, Y., & Reynolds, S. L. (1997). Further evidence on recent trends in the prevalence and incidence of disability among older Americans from two sources: The LSOA and the NHIS. *Journal of Gerontology: Social Sciences, 52B*, S59–S71.

Damjanovic, A. K., Yang, Y., Glaser, R., Kiecolt-Glaser, J. K., Nguyen, H., Laskowski, B., … Weng, N. (2007). Accelerated telomere erosion is associated with a declining immune function of caregivers of Alzheimer's disease patients. *Journal of Immunology, 179*, 4249–4254.

Doty, P., Jackson, M. E., & Crown, W. (1998). The impact of female caregivers' employment status on patterns of formal and informal elder care. *Gerontologist, 38*, 331–341.

Dreer, L. E., Elliott, T. R., Shewchuk, R., Berry, J. W., & Rivera, P. (2007). Family caregivers of persons with spinal cord injury: Predicting caregivers at risk for probable depression. *Rehabilitation Psychology, 52*, 351–357.

Fredman, L., Bertrand, R. M., Martire, L. M., Hochberg, M., & Harris, E. L. (2006). Leisure-time exercise and overall physical activity in older women caregivers and non-caregivers from the Caregiver-SOF Study. *Preventive Medicine, 43*, 226–229.

Fredman, L., Tennstedt, S., Smyth, K. A., Kasper, J. D., Miller, B., Fritsch, T., … Harris, E. L. (2004). Pragmatic and internal validity issues in sampling in caregiver studies: A comparison of population-based, registry-based, and ancillary studies. *Journal of Aging & Health, 16*, 175–203.

Fulmer, T., Paveza, G., VandeWeerd, C., Fairchild, S., Guadagno, L., Bolton-Blatt, M., & Norman, R. (2005). Dyadic vulnerability and risk profiling for elder neglect. *Gerontologist, 45*, 525–534.

Gitlin, L. N., Belle, S. H., Burgio, L. D., Czaja, S. J., Mahoney, D., Gallagher-Thompson, D., … Ory, M. G. (for the REACH investigators). (2003). Effect of multicomponent interventions on caregiver burden and depression: The REACH multisite initiative at 6-month follow-up. *Psychology and Aging, 18*, 361–374.

Gonder-Frederick, L. A., Cox, D. J., & Ritterband, L. M. (2002). Diabetes and behavioral medicine: The second decade. *Journal of Consulting and Clinical Psychology, 70*, 611–625.

Hamilton, M. (1967). Development of a rating scale for primary depressive illness. *British Journal of Social and Clinical Psychology, 6*, 278–296.

Hirst, M. (2005). Carer distress: A prospective, population-based study. *Social Science and Medicine, 61*, 697–708.

Horowitz, A. (1985). Sons and daughters as caregivers to older parents: Differences in role performance and consequences. *Gerontologist, 25*, 612–617.

House, J. S., Landis, K. R., & Umberson, D. (1988). Social relationships and health. *Science, 241*, 540–545.

Keefe, F. J., Smith, S. J., Buffington, A. L. H., Gibson, J., Studts, J. L., & Caldwell, D. (2002). Recent advances and future directions in the biopsychosocial assessment and treatment of arthritis. *Journal of Consulting and Clinical Psychology, 70*, 640–655.

Kim, Y., & Given, B. A. (2008). Quality of life of family caregivers of cancer survivors: Across the trajectory of illness. *Cancer, 112*, 2556–2568.

Kim, Y., Schulz, R., & Carver, C. (2007). Benefit finding in the cancer caregiving experience. *Psychosomatic Medicine, 69*, 283–291.

Kochar, J., Fredman, L., Stone, K. L., & Cauley, J. A. (for the Study of Osteoporotic Fractures). (2007). Sleep problems in elderly women caregivers depend on the level of depressive symptoms: Results of the Caregiver Study of Osteoporotic Fractures. *Journal of the American Geriatrics Society, 55*, 2003–2009.

Kramer, B. J. (1997). Gain in the caregiving experience: Where are we? What next? *Gerontologist, 37*, 218–232.

Laumann, E. O., Leitsch, S. A., & Waite, L. J. (2008). Elder mistreatment in the United States: Prevalence estimates from a nationally representative study. *Journal of Gerontology: Social Sciences, 63B*, S248–S254

Lawton, M. P., Kleban, M. H., Moss, M., Rovine, M., & Glicksman, A. (1989). Measuring caregiving appraisal. *Journal of Gerontology: Psychological Sciences, 46*, P181–P189.

Lazarus, R. S., & Folkman, S. (1984). *Stress, appraisal, and coping.* New York, NY: Springer.

Lee, S., Colditz, G. A., Berkman, L. F., & Kawachi, I. (2003). Caregiving and risk of coronary heart disease in U.S. women: A prospective study. *American Journal of Preventive Medicine, 24*, 113–119.

Manton, K. G., Corder, L., & Stallard, E. (1997). Chronic disability trends in elderly United States populations, 1982–1994. *Proceedings of the National Academy of Sciences: Medical Sciences, 94*, 2593–2598.

Martire, L. M. (2005). The "relative" efficacy of involving family in psychosocial interventions for chronic illness: Are there added benefits to patients and family members? *Families, Systems & Health, 23*, 312–328.

Martire, L. M., Lustig, A. P., Schulz, R., Miller, G. E., & Helgeson, V. S. (2004). Is it beneficial to involve a family member? A meta-analytic review of psychosocial interventions for chronic illness. *Health Psychology, 23*, 599–611.

Martire, L. M., & Schulz, R. (2001). Informal caregiving to older adults: Health effects of providing and receiving care. In A. Baum, T. Revenson, & J. Singer (Eds), *Handbook of health psychology.* (pp. 477–493). Mahwah, NJ: Erlbaum.

Martire, L. M., & Schulz, R. (2007). Involving family in psychosocial interventions for chronic illness. *Current Directions in Psychological Science, 16*, 90–94.

Martire, L. M., Schulz, R., Wrosch, C., & Newsom, J. T. (2003). Perceptions and implications of received spousal care: Evidence from the Caregiver Health Effects Study. *Psychology and Aging, 18*, 593–601.

Martire, L. M., Stephens, M. A. P., Druley, J. A., Berthoff, M. A., Fleisher, C. L., & Wojno, W. C. (2002). Older women coping with osteoarthritis: Negative reactions to spousal support. *Health Psychology, 21*, 167–176.

Mausbach, B., Patterson, T., Rabinowitz, Y., Grant, I., & Schulz, R. (2007). Depression and distress predict time to cardiovascular disease in dementia caregivers. *Health Psychology, 26*, 539–544.

Montgomery, R. J. (1992). Gender differences in patterns of child–parent caregiving relationships. In J. W. Dwyer & R. T. Coward (Eds.), *Gender, families, and elder care* (pp. 65–83). Newbury Park, CA: Sage.

National Alliance for Caregiving (NAC) and American Association of Retired Persons (AARP). (2009). *Caregiving in the U.S.* Washington, DC: National Alliance for Caregiving.

Newsom, J. T. (1999). Another side to caregiving: Negative reactions to being helped. *Current Directions in Psychological Science, 8*, 183–187.

Pinquart, M., & Sorensen, S. (2003). Differences between caregivers and noncaregivers in psychological health and physical health: A meta-analysis. *Psychology and Aging, 18*, 250–267.

Pinquart, M., & Sorensen, S. (2005). Ethnic differences in stressors, resources, and psychological outcomes of family caregiving: A meta-analysis. *Gerontologist, 45*, 90–106.

Pinquart, M., & Sorensen, S. (2006). Gender differences in caregiver stressors, social resources, and health: An updated meta-analysis. *Journal of Gerontology: Psychological Sciences, 61B*, P33–P45.

Prohaska, T. (1998). The research basis for the design and implementation of self-care programs. In M. G. Ory & G. H. DeFriese (Eds.), *Self-care in later life: Research, program, and policy issues* (pp. 62–84). New York, NY: Springer.

Rose-Rego, S. K., Strauss, M. E., & Smyth, K. A. (1998). Differences in the perceived well-being of wives and husbands caring for persons with Alzheimer's disease. *Gerontologist, 38*, 224–230.

Schulz, R., & Beach, S. R. (1999). Caregiving as a risk factor for mortality: The Caregiver Health Effects Study. *Journal of the American Medical Association, 282*, 2215–2219.

Schulz, R., Beach, S. R., Lind, B., Martire, L. M., Zdaniuk, B., Hirsch, C., ... Burton, L. (2001). Involvement in caregiving and adjustment to death of a spouse: Findings from the Caregiver Health Effects Study. *Journal of the American Medical Association, 285,* 3123–3129.

Schulz, R., Belle, S., Czaja, S. J., Gitlin, L. N., Wisniewski, S. R., & Ory, M. G., (for the REACH investigators). (2003). Introduction to the special section on Resources for Enhancing Alzheimer's Caregiver Health (REACH). *Psychology & Aging, 18,* 357–360.

Schulz, R., Belle, S. H., Czaja, S. J., McGinnis, K. A., Stevens, A., & Zhang, S. (2004). Long-term care placement of dementia patients and caregiver health and well-being. *Journal of the American Medical Association, 292,* 961–967.

Schulz , R., Hebert, R. S., Dew, M. A., Brown, S. L., Scheier, M. F., Beach, S. R., ... Nichols, L. (2007). Patient suffering and caregiver compassion: New opportunities for research, practice, and policy. *Gerontologist, 47,* 4–13.

Schulz, R., McGinnis, K. A., Zhang, S., Martire, L. M., Hebert, R. S., Beach, S. R., ... Belle, S. H. (2008). Dementia patient suffering and caregiver depression. *Alzheimer's disease and Associated Disorders, 22,* 170–176.

Schulz, R., Mendelsohn, A. B., Haley, W. E., Mahoney, D., Allen, R. S., Zhang, S, ... Belle, S. H. (2003). End-of-life care and the effects of bereavement on family caregivers of persons with dementia. *New England Journal of Medicine, 349,* 1936–1942.

Schulz, R., Newsom, J., Mittelmark, M., Burton, L., Hirsch, C., & Jackson, S. (1997). Health effects of caregiving: The caregiver health effects study: An ancillary study of the cardiovascular health study. *Annals of Behavioral Medicine, 19,* 110–116.

Schulz, R., O'Brien, A., Bookwala, J., & Fleissner, K. (1995). Psychiatric and physical morbidity effects of dementia caregiving: Prevalence, correlates, and causes. *Gerontologist, 35,* 771–791.

Schulz, R, O'Brien, A., Czaja, S., Ory, M., Norris, R., Martire, L. M., ... Stevens, A. (2002). Dementia caregiver intervention research: In search of clinical significance. *Gerontologist, 42,* 589–602.

Sorensen, S., Pinquart, M., & Duberstein, P. (2002). How effective are interventions with caregivers? An updated meta-analysis. *Gerontologist, 42,* 356–372.

Stephens, M. A. P., Townsend, A. L., Martire, L. M., & Druley, J. A. (2001). Balancing parent care with other roles: Interrole conflict of adult daughter caregivers. *Journal of Gerontology: Psychological Sciences, 56B,* P24–P34.

Taylor, D. H., Kuchibhatla, M., Ostbye, T., Plassman, B. L., & Clipp, E. C. (2008). *Aging & Mental Health, 12,* 100–107.

Tweedy, M. P., & Guarnaccia, C. A. (2007–2008). Change in depression of spousal caregivers of dementia patients following patient's death. *Omega—Journal of Death & Dying, 56,* 2007–2008.

Vedhara, K., Cox, N. K., Wilcock, G. K., Perks, P., Hunt, M., Anderson, S., ... Shanks, N. M. (1999). Chronic stress in elderly carers of dementia patients and antibody response to influenza vaccination. *Lancet, 353,* 627–631.

Vitaliano, P. P., Zhang, J., & Scanlan, J. M. (2003). Is caregiving hazardous to one's physical health? A meta-analysis. *Psychological Bulletin, 129,* 946–972.

Von Kanel, R., Dimsdale, J. E., Ancoli-Israel, S., Mills, P. J., Patterson, T. L., McKibbin, C., ... Grant, I. (2006). Poor sleep is associated with higher plasma proinflammatory cytokine interleukin-6 and procoagulant marker fibrin D-dimer in older caregivers of people with Alzheimer's disease. *Journal of the American Geriatrics Society, 54,* 431–437.

Wakabayashi, C., & Donato, K. M. (2005). The consequences of caregiving: Effects on women's employment and earnings. *Population Research and Policy Review, 24,* 467–488.

Wakabayashi, C., & Donato, K. M. (2006). Does caregiving increase poverty among women in later life? Evidence from the health and retirement survey. *Journal of Health and Social Behavior, 47,* 258–274.

Weihs, K. L., Enright, T. M., & Simmens, S. J. (2008). Close relationships and emotional processing predict decreased mortality in women with breast cancer: Preliminary evidence. *Psychosomatic Medicine, 70,* 117–124.

Williamson, G. M., Martin-Cook, K., Weiner, M. F., Svetlik, D. A., Saine, K., Hynan, L. S., ... Schulz, R. (2005). Caregiver resentment: Explaining why care-recipients exhibit problem behavior. *Rehabilitation Psychology, 50,* 215–223.

Williamson, G. M., & Shaffer, D. R. (2001). Relationship quality and potentially harmful behaviors by spousal caregivers: How we were then, how we are now. *Psychology and Aging, 16,* 217–226.

Wisniewski, S. R., Belle, S. H., Coon, D. W., Marcus, S. M., Ory, M. G., Burgio, L. D., ... Schulz, R. (for the REACH investigators). (2003). The Resources for Enhancing Alzheimer's Caregiver Health (REACH): Project design and baseline characteristics. *Psychology & Aging, 18,* 375–384.

Wolff, J. L., & Kasper, J. D. (2006). Caregivers of frail elders: Updating a national profile. *Gerontologist, 46,* 344–356.

Wright, L. K., Clipp, E. C., & George, L. K. (1993). Health consequences of caregiver stress. *Medicine, Exercise, Nutrition, and Health, 2,* 181–195.

Wu, H., Wang, J., Cacioppo, J. T., Glaser, R., Kiecolt-Glaser, J. K., & Malarkey, W. (1999). Chronic stress associated with spousal caregiving of patients with Alzheimer's dementia is associated with down regulation of B-lymphocyte GH mRNA. *Journals of Gerontology: Biological Sciences and Medical Sciences, 54,* M212–M215.

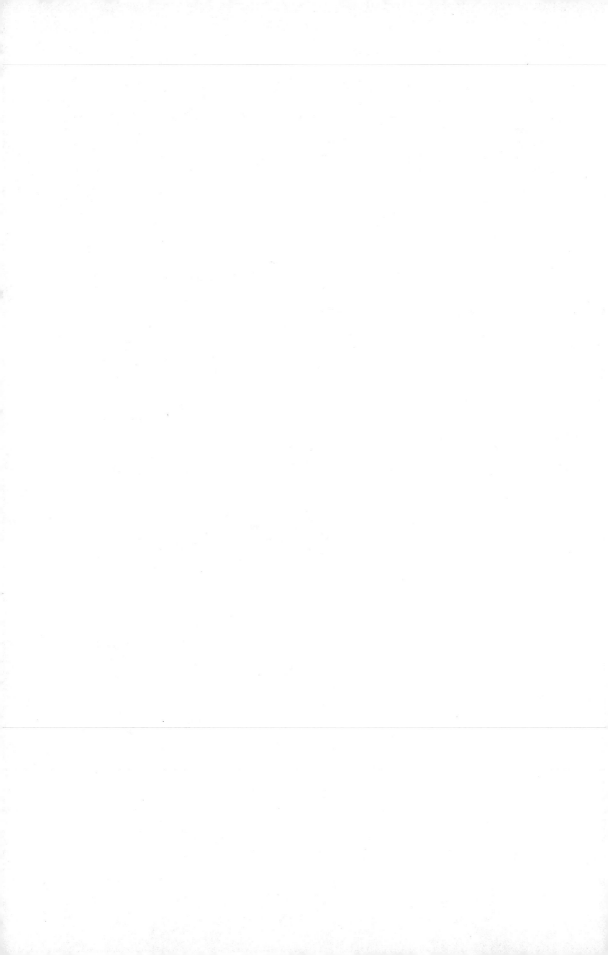

Section III

Risk and Protective Factors

14 Tobacco Use
Psychology, Neurobiology, and Clinical Implications

Neil E. Grunberg, Sarah Shafer Berger,
and Amy K. Starosciak
Uniformed Services University of the Health Sciences

Tobacco use is like entering a dark house that is occupied by a psychotic murderer in a movie thriller. We all know that we should not go in, but something draws the risk-takers in us and among us. For those who enter, risks are compounded the more time that is spent in the house of danger and the deeper they wander into the house and away from escape routes. To make matters worse, the victims-to-be typically separate from anyone who entered the house with them so that they are on their own trying to survive. Once-bold adventurers become trembling and disoriented pawns of the murderer. Frustrated observers must wonder: Why did they enter the house? Why did they separate? Why don't they turn on the lights or use flashlights to see the dangers before it is too late? Why didn't they bring protective gear or relevant weapons to fight the murderer?

This chapter tells the story of the dangerous "house of tobacco use," giving current information about who enters, what happens to them, why it happens, and how to get out. Knowledge about this house of horrors has grown so much since the last edition of this volume that this chapter is but a synopsis. It provides information to explain why one should avoid the house of tobacco use, what happens inside, why it is so difficult to get out, and what to do for those people who enter. This chapter addresses psychology, neurobiology, and clinical issues relevant to tobacco use. It presents epidemiology of tobacco use, health effects, why people smoke cigarettes and self-administer nicotine, interactions with other drugs, cessation effects, treatment recommendations, and issues relevant to special populations.

EPIDEMIOLOGY

NATIONAL STATISTICS

Tobacco is the leading cause of preventable death and illness in the United States. In the United States alone, tobacco use is associated with almost one-half million deaths per year. Yet 20% (45.3 million) of American adults continue to smoke cigarettes (Centers for Disease Control, 2007). According to the 2006 National Health Interview Survey, smoking prevalence is higher among men (23.9%) than women (18.0%). Across ethnic groups, American Indians and Alaskan Natives have the highest prevalence (32.4%), followed by non-Hispanic Blacks (23.0%), non-Hispanic Whites (21.9%), Hispanics (15.2%), and Asians (10.4%). Smoking is inversely related to level of education and socioeconomic status.

Cigarette smoking in the United States declined from the mid-1990s until 2004 but has remained stable over the past five years. The Centers for Disease Control and Prevention (CDC) attributes this asymptote to a 20% decrease in funding for state tobacco prevention and control programs since 2002 and to a $13 billion increase in tobacco company marketing since 1998 (CDC, 2007).

The marketing strategies, including two-for-one coupons, discounts, and merchandising, soften the blow of increased tobacco prices, which have been raised to discourage smoking initiation and maintenance.

Global Statistics

The American Cancer Society (Shafey, Dolwick, & Guindon, 2003) estimates that 1.3 billion people use tobacco worldwide, and that three quarters of those people are men. Worldwide, more than 5.4 million annual deaths are attributed to cigarette smoking. Across major world regions, the Western Pacific region has the highest average prevalence of adult smokers (30.7%), followed by Europe (27.6%), Southeast Asia (27.1%), Eastern Mediterranean (25.3%), Africa (24.3%), and Pan-America (21.9%). The range within each of these broad regions is large, and the difference between male and female smokers is substantial, with males usually showing more tobacco use than do females (World Health Organization, 2008b).

With regard to the prevalence of child and adolescent smoking, every day more than 4,000 children under the age of 18 begin smoking in the United States (CDC, 2003) and more than one third of high school students smoke at least once a month and another 17% of high school students report smoking almost every day (American Legacy Foundation, 2001). Globally, the Western Pacific has the highest prevalence (19.4%), followed by Pan-America (19.0%), Africa (17.3%), Eastern Mediterranean (12.9%), Europe (12.5%), and Southeast Asia (9.5%). As with adult prevalence, child and adolescent prevalence varies widely among countries and between males and females (WHO, 2008b).

Global Tobacco Control

Tobacco control programs vary widely across the globe. Many underdeveloped countries have no tobacco regulation. Even in more developed areas, tobacco control is often limited and ineffective. In 2005, the World Health Organization (WHO) instituted a treaty that outlined tobacco control issues based on the Framework Convention on Tobacco Control (FCTC). This treaty includes many tobacco control approaches, including smoking bans, campaigns against tobacco advertising, restrictions on the sale and distribution of tobacco products, more effective warning labels on tobacco products, and better regulations to reduce the toxicity and addictiveness of tobacco products (WHO, 2008b). Other important issues that parties of the FCTC address include finding alternative crops for regions that rely on tobacco farming and gaining control over illicit tobacco trade (WHO, 2008b). More than 160 countries have ratified this treaty, but the United States has not (WHO, 2008a).

HEALTH EFFECTS OF TOBACCO SMOKING

Cigarette smoking is the single most important factor contributing to premature mortality and morbidity in the United States. The annual American death toll from tobacco use is greater than the total number of American soldiers killed in all five years of World War II. Put another way, the number of American tobacco deaths is similar to the death toll of 9/11 occurring almost three times each week all year around. Tobacco kills 440,000 Americans each year, accounting for one out of five deaths. Globally, tobacco use accounts for more than 5 million annual deaths, and it is estimated that this number will reach 8 million by the year 2030 (WHO, 2008b). This preventable, premature death and illness is primarily the result of cardiovascular diseases (CVD), cancers, and chronic obstructive pulmonary diseases (COPD).

The overall premature mortality ratio (or relative risk ratio) for all smokers of cigarettes is about 2.0 compared to nonsmokers. Smokers have a 100% greater chance than nonsmokers to die prematurely, and smokers die an average of 13–14 years earlier than nonsmokers. Overall mortality ratios increase with the amount smoked and are proportional to duration of cigarette smoking. Historically, men had greater disease and mortality rates caused by smoking than did women, but that difference is disappearing as smoking behavior becomes similar among men and women. Mortality risk is similar for men and women (after menopause) who have smoked or who continue to smoke (CDC, 2006).

Coronary heart disease is the chief contributor to the mortality associated with cigarette smoking. Other CVDs caused by smoking include myocardial infarction, sudden cardiac death, atherosclerosis, and hypertension. Lung cancer is the second leading contributor to mortality associated with cigarette smoking. In fact, every part of the body that comes in contact with tobacco smoke can develop cancer, including the lung, larynx, oral cavity, nasal passages, esophagus, stomach, bladder, kidney, and pancreas. Tobacco smoke constituents (especially polycyclic aromatic hydrocarbons and nitrosamines) are the main cause of cancers. The third leading contributor to mortality associated with cigarette smoking and tobacco smoking, COPD leads to lung damage and decreased pulmonary function (CDC, 2006).

Passive smoking (also called environmental tobacco smoke or secondhand smoke) is also dangerous, especially in confined places with poor ventilation, and can lead to the same diseases causes by direct, voluntary smoking. Approximately 40,000 nonsmoking Americans die annually from secondhand smoke. Spouses of heavy smokers have a greater likelihood of respiratory problems and lung cancer. Children of heavy smokers have higher incidence of respiratory problems, including asthma and bronchitis, and infections. There also is an increased risk for sudden infant death syndrome in households filled with tobacco smoke (U.S. Department of Health and Human Services [USDHHS], 2006).

Tobacco use is comorbid with psychopathology, including anxiety, mood, and thought disorders. Nearly half of all cigarettes sold in the United States are sold to people with mental illness. Men and women with mental disorders are twice as likely as the general public to smoke. When illnesses are asymptomatic for one year or more, the rates of smoking are similar between individuals with or without a psychiatric history (Breslaue, Novak, & Kessler, 2004). It has been suggested that tobacco use is a form of self-medication for the psychological disorders in many of these cases (see discussion of possible medicinal uses of nicotine, later). Unfortunately, tobacco smoking causes the physical health problems identified here. Therefore, it is wise to help all smokers abstain from tobacco use and to treat any mental health conditions with psychological and pharmacological treatments other than tobacco use per se.

WHY PEOPLE SMOKE

Considering the devastating health effects of tobacco use, it is a wonder that so many people smoke. This odd juxtaposition of facts—that tobacco use leads to illnesses and death, yet thousands of young people in the United States alone take up smoking every day—raises the important question: Why do people use tobacco products? This question has been the inspiration for decades of research inside and outside the tobacco industry. Conceptually, it is valuable to break this question into several questions: Why do people start using tobacco products? Why do people keep using tobacco products? Why is it so difficult to abstain from tobacco use? What happens when people abstain from tobacco use? Or, more simply, what contributes to tobacco initiation, maintenance, and cessation? Initiation and maintenance will be discussed next, and cessation will be discussed in detail later in the chapter.

INITIATION

There are many reasons for tobacco initiation that can be categorized as social reasons, beliefs, motivations, and biological variables. Social reasons include social pressure; imitation of peers, family members, and adult role models; influences of advertising and tobacco promotion. Beliefs include misconceptions concerning health risks of tobacco use; belief that one can stop smoking whenever desired; and belief that one may be immune to health hazards. Motivations for initiation of tobacco use include adolescent rebellion, antisocial tendencies, and desire for perceived "benefits" of tobacco use (e.g., weight control, mood modulation, or cognitive enhancement). Relevant biological variables include individual susceptibility to tobacco addiction and prenatal/early-life exposure that may have altered sensitivity to tobacco use (Levin et al., 2006; Shram, Funk, Li, & Lê, 2008).

Various theoretical frameworks have been offered to explain tobacco initiation and may be relevant to tobacco prevention or treatment. Briefly, with regard to major psychological theories and likelihood of tobacco use: Psychoanalytic theory emphasizes psychosexual development and fixation during the oral gratification period of development to enhance the likelihood of tobacco initiation later in adolescence or adulthood (Freud, 1905/1949). Psychosocial development emphasizes the importance of experiences during late childhood (6–11 years of age) and adolescence (12–18 years of age), when struggles to overcome inferiority and to establish personal identity are especially important (Erikson, 1963). Social learning theory emphasizes the importance of reinforcing social influences that exit in each individual's social world or are presented through the contrived world of advertising (Dollard, Doob, Miller, Mowrer, & Sears, 1939; Bandura, 1986). The arousal model argues that individual differences in resting physiological states (coinciding with such personality differences as introversion and extraversion) and the drive to reach optimal states of arousal largely determine who will initiate the use of certain drugs, including tobacco (Eysenck & Eysenck, 1963). The adolescent deviant behavior view holds that problem behaviors, including tobacco use, are a special case of transition through adolescence that are used by certain individuals (Chassin, Presson, & Sherman, 1984; Jessor & Jessor, 1977). Alternatively, biological theories of initiation have argued that nicotine in tobacco is reinforcing and that exposure to nicotine will result in addiction (e.g., Jarvik, 1977; Russell, 1971). Other variations on these themes and integrations across psychology and biology include rational choice theory, behavioral economics, opponent process theory satisfaction of appetitive behaviors, self-medication, and genetic susceptibility (USDHHS, 1988). Several of these ideas and principles are particularly relevant to maintenance of tobacco use.

MAINTENANCE

All the psychological and biological reasons for tobacco initiation also apply to maintenance of tobacco use behavior. The maintenance of tobacco use is, however, particularly powerful because it involves actions of the addictive drug nicotine. Here, we provide information about nicotine and then follow with a discussion of psychobiological mechanisms involved in nicotine use.

Chemical and Physical Properties of Nicotine

Nicotine, or 3-(1-methyl-2-pyrrolidinyl)-pyridine, is a liquid alkaloid found in the tobacco plant and is the addictive component of cigarettes and other tobacco products (USDHHS, 1988). Nicotine is a bicyclic compound with pyridine and pyrrolidine rings. The compound possesses one asymmetric carbon, so it may exist in two enantiomeric forms. In nature, however, nicotine exists in the S-shape, or levorotary form. The base is colorless and odorless, with a dissociation constant (pK_a) of approximately 8.0. Nicotine is hydrophilic and lipophilic and is absorbed through the skin, mucous membranes, lungs, and gastrointestinal tract. Nicotine has a half-life ($t_{1/2}$) of approximately two hours, and the majority of it is metabolized to cotinine by the liver (Benowitz, 1988; Taylor, 2006). The relatively short $t_{1/2}$ is one of the reasons for frequent smoking by people who are addicted to nicotine.

Nicotine Receptors

Nicotine acts at receptors located throughout the body, which partially explains its wide-ranging effects. Nicotine is an agonist at nicotinic acetylcholine receptors (nAChRs) in the central and peripheral nervous systems ($nAChR_N$), but it has little or no effect at similar nicotinic acetylcholine receptors in the muscle ($nAChR_M$). The receptors are presynaptic ligand-gated ion channels that are composed of five subunits. There are several classes of subunits (including α and β), each of which has several different subtypes (e.g., α2-10, β2-4). Alpha subunits are differentiated from the β subunits because they have two adjacent cysteine residues that are necessary for the binding of acetylcholine. The fact that nicotine's effects in humans and animals vary with physiological states, psychological states, and environmental conditions may be partially explained by the fact that sub-unit combinations result in different responses (e.g., mood-altering effects, cognitive enhancing effects). Nicotine receptors are found on dopaminergic (α4β2, α6β2, α6β3 [Mineur & Picciotto, 2008; Mugnaini et al., 2006]), glutamatergic (α4β2 [Alkondon, Rocha, Maelicke, & Albuquerque, 1996; Lambe, Picciotto, & Aghajanian, 2003], α7 [McGehee, Heath, Gelber, Devay, & Role, 1995; Radcliffe & Dani, 1998]), GABAergic (α4β2 [Dani & Bertrand, 2007]), adrenergic (α3β2, α7 [Vizi & Lendvai, 1999]), and cholinergic (α3β4 [Léna et al., 1999]) nerve terminals. The receptors are located in such areas of the brain as the substantia nigra pars compacta (SNc), ventral tegmental area (VTA), nucleus accumbens (NAcc), midbrain tegmentum, striatum, and various regions of the cerebral cortex (Feldman, Meyer, & Quenzer, 1997). Because the receptors are located presyn-aptically in the brain, nicotine binding increases depolarization of the nerve terminal, leading to an influx of Ca^{2+}, ultimately enhancing neurotransmission at that terminal, thereby increasing the actions of the drug. Stimulation of nAchRs in the VTA, for example, enhances dopamine release in the NAcc, an area responsible for the reinforcing effects of many drugs (Feldman et al., 1997).

Nicotine in the Nervous System

The central nervous system (CNS) is made up of the brain and the spinal cord, and the peripheral nervous system (PNS) is comprised of the somatic and autonomic nervous system (ANS). Nicotine acts at many sites in the CNS and PNS, including the brain and the autonomic nervous system. Sites in the brain that have the highest affinity for nicotine include the medial habenula, interpeduncular nucleus (Clarke, Schwartz, Paul, Pert, & Pert, 1985; Härfstrand et al., 1988), SNc, and the VTA (Clarke et al., 1985; Grinevich et al., 2005; Härfstrand et al., 1988; Mugnaini et al., 2006). These sites are relevant to many of nicotine's physical (movement), cognitive (attention), and motivational (reinforcement and reward) actions and are relevant to therapeutic effects of nicotine (e.g., to treat schizophrenia, dementia, or Parkinson's disease).

The ANS has nAchRs located in nerve terminals of the sympathetic and parasympathetic branches. Nicotine induces the release of norepinephrine in the sympathetic branch and acetylcho-line in the parasympathetic branch. Because the two branches have opposing actions, nicotine can exert differential effects depending on which branch of the ANS is more activated. These opposing effects may help to explain why nicotine (through tobacco use) can be stimulating or relaxing. In the somatic nervous system, nicotine acts at different receptors to exert a broad range of physiologic actions. For example, nicotine increases respiratory rate through receptors in the aortic arch and carotid body, induces vomiting and nausea through receptors in the emetic trigger zone in the area postrema of the midbrain (which is why first-time smokers often feel sick), and induces vasopressin secretion by acting in the supraoptic nucleus of the hypothalamus (Taylor, 2006).

Nicotine Self-Administration

Careful empirical studies using human and animal subjects have reported that nicotine is self-administered (Perkins, 1999b; Rose & Corrigall, 1997; USDHHS, 1988). The fact that any drug is self-administered suggests that it has reinforcing properties. There are several types of human nico-tine self-administration studies: smoking topography in laboratory settings; smoking topography in natural settings in which the nicotine yield is manipulated; machine-measured smoking topography in laboratory settings; nicotine self-administration simultaneous with nicotine administration by means of a separate source (e.g., intravenous infusion); smoking topography when nicotine excre-tion is manipulated (e.g., by manipulation of urinary pH); and intravenous self-administration (e.g.,

Chandra, Shiffman, Scharf, Dang & Shadel, 2007; Donny, Houtsmuller, & Stitzer, 2007; Goldfarb, Jarvik, & Glick, 1970; Henningfield & Goldberg, 1983, 1988; Jarvik, Glick, & Nakamura, 1970; Kalman & Smith, 2005; Schachter, Kozlowski, & Silverstein, 1977; Shahab et al., 2008; Pomerleau, Fertig, Seyler, & Jaffe, 1983; Russell, Wilson, Patel, Feyerabend, & Cole, 1975). There also are several types of animal laboratory studies of nicotine self-administration: intravenous nicotine self-administration, intracranial nicotine self-administration, inhalation of tobacco smoke, and oral liquid self-administration (Clarke & Kumar, 1984; Corrigall & Coen, 1989, 1991; Cox, Goldstein, & Nelson, 1984; Donny, Caggiula, Knopf, & Brown, 1995; Hanson, Ivester, & Morton, 1979; Kenny & Markou, 2006; O'Dell & Koob, 2007; Shoaib, Schindler, & Goldberg, 1997; Valette et al., 2003). Humans and animals self-administer nicotine because it is rewarding and this behavior follows well-established principles of psychology (Hull, 1943; Koffka, 1925; Köhler, 1925; Pavlov, 1927; Skinner, 1938; Thorndike, 1911; Watson & Raynor, 1920), which will be discussed in detail in the next section.

REWARD AND ADDICTION

Addiction includes compulsive seeking and consumption of a drug, inability to control drug consumption, and feelings of dysphoria and negative affect after abstaining from the drug (Koob & Le Moal, 1997). Addiction is also a key reason for drug maintenance because drugs produce positively reinforcing effects (i.e., those that increase behaviors that induce pleasant effects). In addition, acute withdrawal from nicotine causes unpleasant effects, including increased appetite, dysphoria, irritability, anxiety, reduction in motivation, and disrupted attention and concentration. These pleasurable and uncomfortable effects that are a part of addiction involve the interaction of psychological and biological processes. Psychological processes will be reviewed first, followed by a transition into more biologically focused processes involved in addiction.

Psychological learning principles are central to the role of nicotine self-administration and addiction. Nicotine's effects to reduce appetite and modulate stress, tension, and anxiety involve positive and negative reinforcement effects. Operant conditioning or instrumental learning occurs when the consequences of a behavior come to increase or decrease the likelihood of a given behavior (e.g., nicotine self-administration). Reinforcement occurs because nicotine has effects that result in increased nicotine self-administration. Positive reinforcement operates in that nicotine results in specific effects that are found to be pleasant and desirable and thereby maintain and increase nicotine self-administration. These positive reinforcing actions include specific neurochemical changes that result in euphoria; neuroendocrine changes that modulate reward and regulate physiological processes; control of appetite and body weight; alterations in attention; and psychosocial rewards (e.g., imitation of role models, acceptance of peers). Negative reinforcement operates in that nicotine offsets specific actions that are found to be undesirable (which accompany abstinence from nicotine self-administration after consistent exposure). These negatively reinforcing effects of nicotine self-administration include offsetting the unpleasantness of classic withdrawal symptoms (e.g., craving, irritability) as a result of nicotine abstinence and offsetting other undesired effects of nicotine abstinence (e.g., body weight gain, attentional difficulties, sleep disturbances). Nicotine also serves as a negative reinforcer because it can remove perceived pain or stress that an individual experiences.

Other psychological variables and actions that contribute to nicotine self-administration include classical conditioning; spatial and temporal paired associations; cue reactivity; and reinforcer enhancement. Classical or Pavlovian conditioning refers to the phenomenon in which stimuli that initially do not elicit a given response (neutral stimuli, NS) do eventually come to elicit those responses (conditional or conditioned responses, CR) when paired repeatedly with a stimulus that normally elicits the given response (unconditional or unconditioned response, US). In Pavlov's classic studies of digestive physiology in dogs, a tone (NS) was repeatedly paired with food (US) until eventually the presentation of the tone alone—now a conditional or conditioned stimulus (CS)—resulted in salivation (CR). Paired associationism was a concept studied by Gestaltist psychologists that referred to the phenomenon by which stimuli "associated" in time or space (e.g., experienced close together chronologically or spatially) come to be psychologically joined and bound together. For example, the co-occurrence of visual stimuli near each other results in a perception and memory of these stimuli together.

These psychological principles operate with the biological effects of nicotine to reinforce tobacco use. The multiplicity of the drug's effects are reflected in the variety of reasons that people report for smoking: to control appetite and reduce body weight; to enhance attention and decrease distraction; to manage negative affect; to relax; to relieve boredom; and to alleviate or cope with stress (Rugkåsa et al., 2001; Scales, Monahan, Rhodes, Roskos-Ewoldsen, & Johnson-Turbes, 2009; USDHHS, 1988). Further, individuals who fail to maintain tobacco cessation report that body weight gain, altered attention, negative affect, feelings of anxiety, and the inability to cope with stress are major reasons for relapse (Hughes, Stead, & Lancaster, 2005; Jarvis, 2004; Shiffman, 1982, 1986; USDHHS, 1988). Many of these effects of nicotine have been reported in experimental settings, using humans and animals as subjects (e.g., Acri, Grunberg, & Morse, 1991; Acri, Morse, Popke, & Grunberg, 1994; Epstein & Collins, 1977; Grunberg, 1982, 1986; Grunberg, Winders, & Wewers, 1991; Heishman, Snyder, & Henningfield, 1993; Klesges, et al., 1997; Rose, Ananda, & Jarvik, 1983; Spilich, June, & Renner, 1992). The many psychological reasons for nicotine self-administration and tobacco use work in combination with the biological actions of nicotine.

Regions of the brain that mediate reward are phylogenetically old and respond to natural stimuli, addictive drugs, and electrical stimulation. Stimuli that evoke dopamine release in the mesocorticolimbic pathway act in the VTA and project to the NAcc and the prefrontal cortex (PFC). This neurotransmission is associated with such behaviors essential to survival as feeding, sexual behavior, birth, and care of offspring, as well as some social behaviors. Cellular and molecular changes in these same areas that occur after repeated self-administration of an addictive drug (like nicotine) may contribute to drug dependence and addiction (Balfour, 1994; Koob & Bloom, 1988; Koob & Swerdlow, 1988).

MOLECULAR BASIS OF REWARD AND ADDICTION

There are at least a dozen subunits (α2-α10, β2-β4) of the nAchRs that combine in different ways to exert different functions. Mice with the β2 (Lambe et al., 2003; Picciotto et al., 1998) or the α4 (Marubio et al., 2003) subunit "knocked out" do not show an increase in dopamine in response to nicotine, and they do not maintain nicotine self-administration. These data suggest that the α4β2 receptor is necessary for this dopamine release in the NAcc and necessary for maintenance of nicotine self-administration. Tapper and colleagues (2004) created a "knock-in" mouse with a mutation in the α4 subunit and reported that the α4 subunit was necessary and sufficient for nicotine sensitization, reward, and tolerance. The α7 subunit seems to be involved in axogenesis (Chan & Quik, 1993) and neuroprotection (Hejmadi, Dajas-Bailador, Barns, Jones, & Wonnacott, 2003). Slotkin, Cousins, and Seidler (2004) identified a potential susceptibility of the α7 receptor subunit to nicotine's effects in adolescence. Knowledge of these subunits could aid in the development of novel pharmaceutical treatments for nicotine dependence.

Pathways

The mesolimbic and mesocortical dopaminergic pathways are critical for reward and addiction. The major dopaminergic neurons of both pathways originate in the VTA and project to the NAcc, pallidum, hippocampus, amygdala, and medial prefrontal cortex in the mesolimbic circuit, or to other areas of the frontal cortex in the mesocortical pathway (Pierce & Kumaresan, 2006). The mesocorticolimbic pathways are involved in reinforcing effects of pleasurable experiences or activities (e.g., sexual activity, feeding, drug use). For example, when a smoker experiences reward after smoking a cigarette, dopamine levels in the NAcc increase (Dani & Heinemann, 1996).

New Developments

Recently Naqvi, Rudrauf, Damasio, and Bechara (2007) have discovered that the insula, sometimes called the "fifth lobe" of the brain, and which is involved in conscious urges, may be intricately involved in maintenance of nicotine self-administration and smoking. Cigarette smokers with damage to the insula quit smoking with relative ease after the injury, did not smoke again after quitting, and felt no urges to smoke again. This fascinating report suggests that pharmaceutical or other interventions that "silence" the insula may be a novel way to help smokers abstain.

INTERACTIONS WITH OTHER DRUGS

Tobacco smoke consists of about 4,000 different chemicals and compounds, each of which may interact with other drugs. Some of the chemicals in tobacco smoke interact with the enzymes that metabolize nicotine and alter the distribution of nicotine within the body. Other chemicals in smoke affect the metabolism of other drugs that may be ingested (e.g., licit and illicit drugs, medications). Two types of interactions are discussed in this section: pharmacokinetic (effects on drug absorption, distribution, metabolism, and clearance) and pharmacodynamic (drug effects on the body). These interactions are relevant to the intake of prescription or over-the-counter medications by smokers because the interactions may alter the psychobiological and pathophysiological effects of each drug that people take into the body.

INTERACTIONS WITH NICOTINE METABOLISM

The liver is the main site for drug and toxin metabolism, and the cytochrome P450 (CYP) enzymes are the key drivers of this action. Nicotine is primarily metabolized by the CYP2A6 and 2B6 enzymes into the nicotine imminium ion and then into the primary metabolite cotinine by aldehyde oxidase (Ring et al., 2007). There are many chemicals found in tobacco smoke (e.g., γ-heptalactone) that inhibit CYP2A6, thereby slowing the metabolism of nicotine in the body and maintaining higher blood levels of the drug (Rabinoff, Caskey, & Park, 2007). Acute alcohol inhibits the actions of some CYP enzymes, so the metabolism of nicotine is slowed during acute alcohol consumption but not by chronic alcohol use (Fleming, Mihic, & Harris, 2006). This effect suggests that smokers should smoke less while drinking (acute drinking, that is) because they would have more nicotine in the body. However, the opposite happens. People tend to smoke more while drinking (e.g., Friedman, Sieglaub, & Seitzer, 1974; Koslowski et al., 1993). If the enzymatic alterations are involved, then perhaps nicotine becomes more reinforcing in this situation.

Pharmacokinetic Interactions

Polycyclic aromatic hydrocarbons (PAHs), chemicals that are formed during combustion, are carcinogenic compounds in cigarette smoke and induce specific CYP enzymes, including 1A1, 1A2, and 2E1 (Zevin & Benowitz, 1999). Induction of the enzymes results in faster metabolism and clearance of the substrates. Therefore, a smoker who is taking drugs that are metabolized by these enzymes may need larger doses of the drug or may need to take the drug more often to achieve desired effects. For example, some widely used prescription and over-the-counter drugs are metabolized in part by CYP1A2, including clozapine and olanzapine (antipsychotics), fluvoxamine (SSRI), tacrine (infrequently used to treat Alzheimer's disease), theophylline (infrequently used to treat asthma or COPD, naturally found in tea), and caffeine (Kroon, 2007). Caffeine interactions are particularly interesting because smokers often light up with a cup of coffee or other sources of caffeine even when it is not their first cigarette of the day.

Other chemicals in tobacco smoke interact with other pharmacokinetic processes (e.g., absorption, distribution, clearance). For example, decreased plasma concentration, decreased half-life, and increased clearance of drugs occur with many drugs in cigarette smokers (e.g., alprazolam, haloperidol, propranolol, tricyclic antidepressants). Therefore, alteration of the pharmacokinetics of these drugs may require an increase in the dose or decrease in dosing intervals to maintain appropriate effects. These dosage considerations often are not addressed by physicians.

Pharmacodynamic Interactions

Many pharmacodynamic interactions occur between tobacco smoke and medications, and these interactions have important health implications for patients that are not always considered by physicians. For example, hormonal contraceptives and tobacco smoke synergistically increase risk for myocardial infarction, ischemic stroke, and thromboembolisms in women over 35. Asthmatic patients who use inhaled corticosteroids and smoke cigarettes may experience a reduced efficacy of the asthma drug and may experience less symptomatic relief than do nonsmoker asthmatics using the same drug (Kroon, 2007). In patients receiving cancer treatment, smokers are more likely to experience reduced efficacy and greater toxicity to radiation therapy, and they have a poorer survival rate. Smokers also have poorer healing of wounds after surgical removal of tumors (Gritz, Dresler, & Sarna, 2005).

Interactions With Smoking Cessation

There are several considerations to take into account when a patient decides to quit smoking. Because dosages of some medications may have been increased to compensate for interaction with tobacco smoke, effects should be closely monitored and dosages adjusted after smoking cessation. When prescribing a nicotine replacement therapy (NRT) or another smoking cessation medication (e.g., varenicline, bupropion), it is important that the patient not continue to smoke. If the patient continues smoking while using an NRT, then nicotine overdose is a possibility.

SMOKING CESSATION

More than 80% of individuals who smoke express a desire to stop smoking (American Psychiatric Association [APA], DSM-IV-TR, 2000; Hughes, Huggins, & Hatsukami, 1990), but abstinence is difficult because the withdrawal symptoms can be powerful. Smoking withdrawal can cause clinical distress and impairment and interfere with the ability to quit smoking (Hughes, 2007a). Significant withdrawal symptoms reportedly occur in at least half of smokers when they try to quit (Hughes, 2007a).

SYMPTOMS OF WITHDRAWAL

Abstinence from consistent tobacco use or nicotine self-administration usually results in withdrawal symptoms (APA, 2001). Nicotine withdrawal includes dysphonic or depressed mood; insomnia; irritability, frustration, or anger; anxiety; difficulty concentrating; restlessness or impatience; decreased heart rate; and increased appetite or weight gain (APA, DSM-IV-TR, 2001). Other features of nicotine withdrawal include intense cravings, a desire for sweets, a dry or productive cough, constipation, dizziness, increased dreaming, mouth ulcers, or drowsiness (Hughes, 2007b). In clinical settings, nicotine withdrawal can resemble other substance withdrawal syndromes, caffeine intoxication, anxiety, mood or sleep disorders, or medication-induced akathisia (APA, 2001). Therefore, it is important for practitioners to make differential diagnoses to determine if particular mental health symptoms are the result of tobacco cessation, underlying psychological problems, or both.

Withdrawal symptoms often begin within the first one to two days after cessation, peak within the first week and last for two to four weeks, with the majority lasting for about 10 days. Depression is a common symptom of drug withdrawal (Hughes, 2007b). One symptom of cessation that is of great concern to smokers, especially women, is weight gain. Individuals who quit smoking often gain 7–14 pounds over the first year (APA, 2001) because of increased consumption of sweet and high-caloric foods and some decreased metabolic rate (Grunberg, 1992; APA, DSM-IV-TR, 2001). Some tobacco advertisements have taken advantage of this phenomenon and entice women to smoke to control body weight and appetite.

Sleep disturbance is another commonly reported symptom of nicotine withdrawal (Colrain, Trinder, & Swan, 2004). Nocturnal awakening occurs in about 40% of individuals in nicotine withdrawal (Hughes, Higgins, & Bickel, 1994). Frequency of night awakenings during the first month of abstinence is a strong predictor of relapse within the first six month (Persico, 1992). Nicotine withdrawal can lead to insomnia, sleep fragmentation, nighttime nicotine craving, depression (which in turn affects sleep), and abnormal dreams (Htoo, Talwar, Feinsilver, & Greenberg, 2004). Some treatments for smoking cessation, such as nicotine replacement therapy, also may affect sleep (Colrain et al., 2004).

PSYCHOBIOLOGY OF WITHDRAWAL

The "opponent process" model (Solomon & Corbit, 1973; Koob & Le Moal, 2001) hypothesizes that drug addiction involves the pairing of pleasure with emotions associated with withdrawal. Initially, there are high levels of pleasure (known as the A process) and low levels of withdrawal (known as the B process). With repeated drug use, the levels of pleasure from the drug decrease and the levels of withdrawal result from not taking the drug. This increased B process serves as a motivator for increased drug use.

Neurochemical explanations for withdrawal postulate that there is a decrease in dopaminergic activity that leads to negative affect and decreased reward, thereby creating unpleasant symptoms. Alternatively, it has been hypothesized that receptor changes occur in nicotine withdrawal, but the exact changes have not been identified (Hughes, 2007a). Other physiological effects of withdrawal include decreased muscle response and decreased catecholamine and cortisol release (APA, 2001). There also may be cognitive changes, including changes in attention, concentration, or memory. Having a better understanding of neurochemical explanations for withdrawal can lead to better pharmacological treatments for nicotine withdrawal or medication that can be used to offset withdrawal symptoms.

INDIVIDUAL DIFFERENCES IN WITHDRAWAL

There are several reports that withdrawal differs with sex, age, and ethnicity. Women report more withdrawal symptoms, greater severity of withdrawal symptoms, and less success abstaining from tobacco than do men (Hughes et al., 1994; Shiffman, 1979; Perkins, 2001; Pomerleau, Tate, Lumley, & Pomerleau, 1994). Age also may be relevant to tobacco/nicotine withdrawal symptoms. Animal studies suggest that adolescents have fewer withdrawal behaviors than do adult rats (O'Dell, Bruijnzeel, Ghozland, Markou, & Koob, 2004; O'Dell, Torres, Natividad, & Tejeda, 2006). There also may be cultural differences in withdrawal. For example, reported tobacco withdrawal rates are 76% in the United States compared with 40% in Germany and Japan (Hughes, 2007a). As with neurochemical explanations, a better understanding of individual differences in withdrawal can help clinicians better assist their patients with tobacco cessation.

CLINICAL IMPLICATIONS OF WITHDRAWAL SYMPTOMS

Many smokers attempting to quit will relapse shortly after their cessation attempt. The discomfort of nicotine withdrawal is likely to contribute to this relapse. Therefore, it is useful to assess nicotine withdrawal in clinical settings. Health care practitioners helping smokers to abstain should assess distress, daily functioning, and the extent to which withdrawal symptoms undermine smoking cessation and contribute to relapse (see Hughes, 2007a). Distress, daily functioning, and perception are key areas for psychosocial interventions for patients experiencing withdrawal symptoms.

TREATMENT RECOMMENDATIONS

The U.S. Department of Health and Human Services 2008 *Guide for Treating Tobacco Use and Dependence* points out that tobacco use creates an interesting confluence of events—it is a major health threat for which there are effective interventions, and yet many health care professional are reticent to intervene. This section briefly summarizes effective treatments available for nicotine cessation and addresses relevant issues.

ROLE OF MOTIVATION IN TREATMENT

People who want to abstain from tobacco use are more likely to succeed than are those who do not want to stop smoking but must. For example, some smokers may need to quit for immediate health reasons (e.g., serious asthma, lung disease, cancer) even though their motivation to quit is low. As a result, it is important to recognize that motivation level affects success of abstinence and that it may need to be addressed and encouraged (USDHHS, 2008). For the patient willing to quit, the health professional should assist and arrange for follow-up that reinforces abstinence or progress toward abstinence (i.e., reduction of use). Health care professionals can help the smoker develop a quit plan; recommend behavioral, cognitive, and pharmaceutical strategies; provide practical counseling (e.g., problem-solving skills training); recommend intratreatment social support (e.g., hotlines or support groups); and provide educational and other supportive materials. A quit plan includes STAR: setting a quit date (ideally within two weeks); telling family, friends, and coworkers about quitting and request understanding and support; anticipating challenges (e.g., withdrawal symptoms) to the upcoming quite attempt, especially during the first few weeks; and removing tobacco products from the environment. For patients unwilling to quit, time should be spent promoting motivation. Possible reasons for decreased motivation include lack of information about harmful effects of tobacco, lack of financial resources, fears about quitting, or unsuccessful prior quit attempts (Donze, Ruffieux, & Cornuz, 2007; Fagan et al., 2007; Rundmo, Smedslund, & Gotestam, 1997). Motivational interviewing (MI), a directive, patient-centered counseling intervention, can effectively increase motivation to quit. The techniques in MI can be summarized by the five *R*s: relevance, risks, rewards, roadblocks, and repetition. Relevance refers to getting the patient to express personally relevant reasons for wanting to quit (e.g., health or family). Risks include health risks, and rewards involve having the patient identify potential benefits of quitting. Roadblocks are potentials barriers to quitting (e.g., times of stress, having a spouse that still smokes). Repetition includes repeating MI techniques at every visit (including postcessation to help maintenance of cessation).

COUNSELING AND BEHAVIORAL TECHNIQUES

A variety of counseling and behavioral techniques are useful in smoking cessation. The most effective techniques are providing practical counseling (e.g., problem-solving skill training) and support (USDHHS, 2008). Practical counseling is an effective intervention for smoking cessation when it focuses on problem-solving skills training. Some of the topics addressed in skills training include identifying what helped and did not help in previous quit attempts, anticipating triggers or challenges in an upcoming attempt and how the individual will overcome them (e.g., avoiding triggers, altering routines, considering limited alcohol use, handling other smokers in the household). Providing support also helps with smoking cessation. Proactive telephone counseling, group counseling, and individual counseling all are effective. Quit lines have a broad reach, are relatively inexpensive, and have been shown to be quite effective. Also useful is cognitive behavioral therapy.

MEDICATIONS

Pharmaceutical agents available for smoking cessation include first- and second-line treatments that have been approved by the U.S. Food and Drug Administration (FDA) except in the presence of contraindications. The current first-line medications are bupropion SR (Wellbutrin® or Zyban®), nicotine gum, nicotine inhaler, nicotine lozenge, nicotine nasal spray, nicotine patch, and varenicline (Chantix®). Bupropion SR was the first non-nicotine medication shown to be effective for smoking cessation. It is presumed to work by a blockade of neuronal reuptake of dopamine and/or norepineph-rine. Nicotine gum is available over the counter. It is has been reported that regular-course and long-term nicotine gum increases the likelihood of long-term abstinence by about 50% compared with placebo (Silagy et al., 2004). The 2-mg dosage of nicotine gum is recommended for patients smoking <25 cigarettes per day, whereas the 4-mg gum is recommended for patients smoking 25+ cigarettes per day. It is recommended that ≤24 pieces of nicotine gum per day be used for ≤12 weeks (USDHHS, 2008). Nicotine inhalers are currently available only by prescription. Nicotine inhalers almost double smoker's likelihood of long-term abstinence from tobacco compared with placebo (Silagy et al., 2004). Nicotine lozenges are available over the counter. A randomized controlled trial reported that the 2-mg lozenge for low-dependent smokers and the 4-mg lozenge for highly dependent smokers almost dou-bled the odds of abstinence at six months postquit compared with placebo (Shiffman, DiMarino, & Pillitteri, 2005). Nicotine nasal spray is available only by prescription and also has been reported to nearly double the likelihood of long-term abstinence from tobacco (Silagy et al., 2004). Nicotine patches have similar effectiveness to other nicotine replacement products. Varenicline (Chantix®) is the newest non-nicotine medication shown to be effective for smoking cessation approved by the FDA (in 2006). It is assumed it works by serving as a partial nicotine receptor agonist and a nicotine recep-tor antagonist. It has recently been reported that varenicline increases the odds of quitting over that of bupropion SR (Bullen, Whittaker, Walker, & Wallace-Bell, 2006). There have been some recent case reports of side effects (e.g., sleep difficulty) that need further investigation.

Side effects of the first-line medications vary based on the medication. None of the medications are recommended for women who are pregnant or breastfeeding. Care also must be used in patients with certain cardiovascular diseases because nicotine replacement products can aggravate certain CVDs and bupropion can increase hypertension. The side effects for the nicotine replacement ther-apy are generally mild and depend on the mode of administration. The most common side effects of bupropion include dry mouth and insomnia. Reported side effects for varenicline include nausea, trouble sleeping, and abnormal or vivid dreams.

Second-line medications have evidence for treating tobacco dependence, but they have not been approved by the FDA or there are more concerns about the side effects. The second-line medications include clonidine (Catapres®) and nortriptyline (Aventyl®, Pamelor®). Clonidine is primarily used as an antihypertensive medication. It has been reported to approximately double absence rates when com-pared to placebo. The concern is that clonidine is effective in promoting smoking cession, but promi-nent side effects of dry mouth, drowsiness, dizziness, sedation, and constipation can occur. These side effects appear to limit the drug's usefulness (Gourlay, Stead, & Benowitz, 2004). Nortriptyline is mainly used as a tricyclic antidepressant. It has been reported to almost double a smoker's likelihood of achieving long-term abstinence from tobacco as compared to placebo. There also is some concern that the side-effect profile of nortriptyline may outweigh the use of this mediation as a valuable drug for tobacco cessation (Hughes, Stead, & Lancaster, 2005). Side effects include weight gain, sedation, dry mouth, blurred vision, urinary retention, lightheadedness, and shaky hands.

The issue of combining medications has been debated over the years. There is some evidence that com-bining certain first-line treatments may be effective. These combinations include long-term (> 14 weeks) nicotine patch with other nicotine replacement therapies (e.g., gum), the nicotine patch and the nicotine inhaler, or the nicotine patch and bupropion. The combination of medication may suppress tobacco with-drawal symptoms more than does a single medication (Bohadana, Nilsson, Rasmussen, & Martinet, 2000; Schnieder et al., 2006; Sweeney, Fant, Fagerstrom, McGovern, & Henningfield, 2001), but patient preference should be considered because combination treatments may produce more side effects than does a single medication (Croghan et al., 2003; Jamerson et al., 2001; Schneider et al., 2006).

ADDRESSING WEIGHT GAIN CONCERNS

The concern of many smokers when quitting smoking is weight gain, especially among women (Borrelli, Spring, Niaura, Hitsman, & Papandonatos, 2001; Meyers et al., 1997; Pomerleau,

Zucker, & Stewart, 2001). This concern is reasonable because most smokers who quit gain weight, ranging from a few pounds up to 30 pounds (Eisenberg & Quinn, 2006; Klesges et al., 1998). Women gain slightly more than men; African Americans, people under age of 55, and heavy smokers (more than 25 cigarettes per day) are at the highest risk for weight gain after quitting smoking (Froom, Melamed, & Benbassat, 1998; Klesges et al., 1998; Williamson et al., 1991). Postcessation weight gain is likely caused by increased intake of certain foods and by metabolic changes (Filozof, Fernandez Pinilla, & Fernandez-Cruz, 2004; Grunberg, 1992; Pisinger & Jorgensen, 2007). Weight concerns also may affect relapse (Copeland, Martin, Geiselman, Rash, & Kendzor, 2006). Therefore, it is important to remind patients that the health threat of gaining weight is small compared with the risk of continued smoking (Eisenberg & Quinn, 2006; USDHHS, 1988). Practitioners should recommend increased physical activity and a healthy diet, encouraging avoidance of highly caloric and sweet-tasting foods to control weight. It is noteworthy that nicotine gum has been able to curb postcessation weight gain (Allen, Hatsukami, Brintnell, & Bade, 2005; Jorenby, 2002). Practitioners can help the patient with weight control after the patient has successfully quit smoking. It is important to note that counseling interventions specifically designed to alleviate weight gain during cessation attempts have not been effective (Cooper et al., 2005; Copeland et al., 2006). There is also evidence that counseling for healthy eating and smoking cessation should be sequential and not concurrent (Cooper et al., 2005; Copeland et al., 2006; Perkins et al., 2001).

POTENTIAL NEW TREATMENTS

There are several new treatments in the works for potential use in the future. These treatments are in various stages of trials or development. One option is a nicotine vaccine. A nicotine vaccine (compared with nicotine replacement therapies) would induce sufficient nicotine-specific antibodies and prevent activation of nicotine receptors in the brain. The hope is that the rewarding effects of tobacco would be eliminated or greatly attenuated. The vaccine has passed through animal and human testing and is likely to receive increased research and public attention soon (Maurer & Bachmann, 2006). Another medication under development is rimonabant, a cannabinoid CB-1 receptor antagonist. There is some thought that nicotine's actions are partially mediated by neurochemical receptors and mechanisms that are shared with actions of cannabis and Δ^9-tetrahydrocannibinol (active ingredients in marijuana). Therefore, medications that act on these receptors may offer additional help modifying actions of nicotine and craving for nicotine (e.g., Parolaro & Rubino, 2008). This possibility is currently under study.

CONCLUSIONS REGARDING CURRENT TREATMENTS

Over the past 30 years, increased understanding that tobacco use is a psychobiological phenomenon has resulted in multifaceted treatment approaches that include motivational, cognitive, behavioral, and pharmacological facets. There now are many available strategies and new medications appearing every year. It is important to remember that smokers need to be encouraged to give up tobacco, that social support from practitioners, friends, and family is vital, and that if a particular medication or psychological approach does not work, then there is another one to try. The challenge for smokers and for health care practitioner is to find the optimal strategy to achieve long-lasting tobacco abstinence and to recognize that the most effective treatment may depend on the individual.

SPECIAL POPULATIONS

Certain populations may be particularly vulnerable to the addictive effects of tobacco and the health consequences of smoking. These populations include, but are not limited to, women, children and adolescents, and ethnic minorities.

WOMEN

Women make up 20% of smokers worldwide, but the gender gap in tobacco use is small in developed countries and, ironically, narrows as countries become more developed. As a result, women's share of tobacco-related diseases has risen dramatically over the last 60 years. For example, lung cancer accounted for only 3% of all female cancer deaths in 1950, but it accounted for almost 25% in 2000 (Ries et al., 2000). Moreover, the World Health Organization estimates that the number of women who smoke will almost triple over the next generation. Because women provide an unsaturated market for tobacco products, they are targeted by tobacco-marketing strategies. Of great concern for women is that women may have a harder time with cessation (Grunberg, Winders, & Wewers, 1991; Perkins, 1999a, 2001; Reichert, Seltzer, Efferen, & Kohn, 2004). Smoking by women can lead to disrupted tubal and ovulatory function, oocyte depletion, and premature menopause. Estrogen appears to induce CYP2A6 enzymes, so premenopausal women metabolize nicotine faster than peri- and postmenopausal women and faster than men; women who use oral contraceptives metabolize nicotine faster than those who do not (Benowitz, Lessov-Schlaggar, Swan, & Jacob, 2006). There also can be a dangerous synergistic effect for CVD in women who smoke and use oral contraceptives (USDHHS, 1983).

Furthermore, smoking during pregnancy has large risks for the woman and the developing fetus. It can result in increased risk of ectopic pregnancy, spontaneous abortion, perinatal mortality, low birth weight, and premature birth.

Practitioners helping women smokers to abstain should consider restrictions of NRT and other medications in pregnant women, emphasis on social support and other psychological techniques to maintain abstinence, and the possibility that environmental cues may be especially influential in smoking behavior among women (Perkins et al., 2001).

CHILDREN AND ADOLESCENTS

Ninety percent of adult smokers begin smoking before the age of 18 (Gilpin, Choi, Berry, & Pierce, 1999). Worldwide, one in five teens smokes, with the highest youth smoking rates in Central and Eastern Europe, sections of India, and some Western Pacific islands. In the United States, one in three teens reported smoking at least once a month, and another 17% reported smoking almost every day (American Legacy Foundation, 2001). Fifty percent of young people who continue to smoke will die from smoking-related diseases (WHO, 2008b), and many will go on to abuse other drugs, including alcohol, marijuana, cocaine, or heroin (Kandel, 2002).

The behavioral, cognitive, and emotional effects of tobacco and nicotine use in adults have been extensively researched. It is clear that tobacco and nicotine use elevates mood, decreases body weight and food consumption, alters attention, modulates stress, and so on, in adults; but it is not clear whether these effects are identical, greater, or lesser in adolescents and children (Elliott, Faraday, Phillips, & Grunberg, 2004; Faraday, Elliott, & Grunberg, 2001; Faraday, Elliott, Phillips, & Grunberg, 2003; Kassel, Stroud, & Patronis, 2003; USDHHS, 1988; Wilmouth & Spear, 2004). Adolescents and children are not just miniadults when it comes to nicotine responses. In fact, some researchers have found striking differences between adults and adolescents in nicotine responses, including reports that adolescents may experience more reward from nicotine self-administration and fewer such negative effects as withdrawal (O'Dell, Bruijnzeel, Ghozland, Markou, & Koob, 2004; Breslaue et al., 2004). Adolescents also should not be considered mini-adults when it comes to treatment recommendations. Practitioners should routinely assess for tobacco use in children and adolescents, particularly because 82% of 11–19-year-olds who smoke are thinking about quitting and 77% have made a serious quite attempt in the past year (Hollis, Polen, Lichtenstein, & Whitlock, 2003). Extra attempts to offer assistance may increase the success of these quit attempts. Counseling interventions can be effective, whether they are group, one-on-one, or telephone interventions, but such interventions should be developmentally appropriate across the adolescent lifespan (e.g., early adolescence compared with late adolescence; USDHHS, 2008). Such medications as bupropion SR and NRT appear to be safe in adolescents, but efficacy research is lacking. Therefore, pharmacological treatments are not currently recommended for cessation intervention in adolescent populations (K. Hanson, Allen, Jensen, & Hatsukami, 2003; Houtsmuller, Henningfield, & Stitzer, 2003; Moolchan et al., 2005; Niederhofer & Huber, 2004).

ETHNICITY, SOCIOECONOMIC STATUS, AND OTHER DEMOGRAPHICS

Health disparities are marked by differences in ethnicity, socioeconomic status (SES), and other demographics (USDHHS, 2008). For example, African Americans have higher mortality rates for cancers, CVDs, and other diseases that are affected by tobacco use (Abidoye, Ferguson, Salgia, 2007; Kurian & Cardarelli, 2007). American Indian and Alaska Native peoples have high infant mortality rates from sudden infant death syndrome, which is affected by tobacco use (Iyasu et al., 2002). There are differences in tobacco use prevalence and cessation depending on ethnicity and SES (Anderson & Burns, 2000; Chae, Gavin, & Takeuchi, 2006; Levinson, Perez-Stable, Espinoza, Flores, & Byers, 2004; Watson et al., 2003). When individuals do try to abstain from tobacco use, success rates are lower among some ethnic groups perhaps because less effective treatments are used (Levinson et al., 2004). Because there are differences in tobacco use and disease vulnerability among subgroups of the population, it is important to consider these differences with regard to treatment recommendations. Unfortunately, little research attention has focused on this important issue, so there remains a need for effective and perhaps specialized treatments within various subgroups.

CONCLUSION

This chapter began with the analogy that tobacco use is like entering a dark house occupied by a murderer. The best way to avoid the danger is simply not to enter. People who do not try tobacco products do not fall prey to most of the risks (with the exception of exposure to secondhand tobacco smoke). Effective preventive medicine is clearly valuable to avoid disease and injury, and it is an important part of health psychology. This chapter focused on what happens "inside the house." The dangers are real and serious. The difficulties to escape the potential murderer are great. However, with eyes wide open about the dangers, strong social support, and currently available weapons of behavioral, cognitive, motivational, and pharmaceutical treatment, people can survive and escape the house of tobacco use. The call for help is well within reach—it just has to be used. Ever more protective weapons are becoming available, and health psychologists, including researchers and practitioners, continue to play central roles in developing, understanding, and utilizing these impressive weapons.

REFERENCES

Abidoye, O., Ferguson, M. K., & Salgia, R. (2007). Lung carcinoma in African Americans. *National Clinical Practice of Oncology, 4*, 118–129.

Acri, J. B., Grunberg, N. E., & Morse, D. E. (1991). The effects of nicotine on the acoustic startle reflex amplitude in rats. *Psychopharmacology, 104*, 244–248.

Acri, J. B., Morse, D. E., Popke, E. J., & Grunberg, N. E. (1994). Nicotine increases sensory gating measured as inhibition of the acoustic startle reflex in rats. *Psychopharmacology, 114*, 369–374.

Alkondon, M., Rocha, E., Maelicke, A., & Albuquerque, E. X. (1996). Alpha-bungarotoxin-sensitive nicotinic receptors in olfactory bulb neurons and presynaptic modulation of glutamate release. *J Pharmacology and Experimental Therapies, 278*, 1460–1471.

Allen, S. S., Hatsukami, D., Brintnell, D. M., & Bade, T. (2005). Effect of nicotine replacement therapy on post-cessation weight gain and nutrient intake: A randomized controlled trial of postmenopausal femal smokers. *Addictive Behaviors, 30*, 1273–1280.

American Legacy Foundation (2001). Cigarette smoking among youth: Results from the 2000 National Youth Tobacco Survey (Legacy First Look Report, 7). Washington, DC: American Legacy Foundation.

American Psychiatric Association. (2000). *Diagnostic and statistical manual of mental disorders* (DSM-IV-TR, 4th ed., text revised). Washington, DC: Author

Anderson, C., & Burns, D. M. (2000). Patterns of adolescent smoking initiation rates by ethnicity and sex. *Tobacco Control, 9* (Suppl. 2), 114–118.

Balfour, D. J. (1994). Neural mechanisms underlying nicotine dependence. *Addiction, 89*(11), 1419–1423.

Bandura, A. (1986). *Social foundations of thought and action: A social cognitive theory.* Englewood Cliffs, NJ: Prentice-Hall.

Benowitz, N. L. (1988). Pharmacokinetcs and pharmacodynamics of nicotine. In M. J. Rand & K. Thurau (Eds.), *The pharmacology of nicotine* (pp. 3–19). Oxford, England: ICSU Press.

Benowitz, N. L., Lessov-Schlaggar, C. N., Swan, G. E., & Jacob, P., III. (2006). Female sex and oral contraceptive use accelerate nicotine metabolism. *Clinical Pharmacology and Therapeutics, 79*(5), 480–488.

Bohadana, A., Nilsson, F., Rasmussen, T., & Martinet, Y. (2000). Nicotine inhaler and nicotine patch as a combination therapy for smoking cessation: A randomized, double-blind, placebo-controlled trial. *Archives of Internal Medicine, 160*, 3128–3134.

Borrelli, B., Spring, B., Niaura, R., Hitsman, B., & Papandonatos, G. (2001). Influences of gender and weight gain on short-term relapse to smoking in a cessation trial. *Journal of Clinical and Consulting Psychology, 69*, 511–515.

Breslaue, N., Novak, S. P., & Kessler, R. C. (2004). Psychiatric disorders and stages of smoking. *Biological Psychiatry, 55*, 69–76.

Bullen, C., Whittaker, R., Walker, N., & Wallace-Bell, M. (2006). Pre-quitting nicotine replacement therapy: Findings from a pilot study. *Tobacco Induced Diseases, 3*, 35–40.

Centers for Disease Control and Prevention (2003). Tobacco use among middle and high school students—United States, 2002. *Morbidity and Mortality Weekly Report (MMWR), 52*, 1096–1098.

Centers for Disease Control and Prevention. (2006). *Cigarette smoking-related mortality.* Retrieved from http://www.cdc.gov/tobacco/data_statistics/factsheets/ cig_smoking_mort.htm (accessed July 23, 2008).

Centers for Disease Control and Prevention. (2007). Cigarette smoking among adults—United States, 2006. *Mortality and Morbidity Weekly Report, 56*(44): 1157–1161.

Chae, D. H., Gavin, A. R., & Takeuchi, D. T. (2006). Smoking prevalence among Asian Americans: Findings from the National Latino and Asian American Study (NLAAS). *Public Health Representatives, 121*, 755–763.

Chan, J., & Quik, M. (1993). A role for the nicotinic alpha-bungarotoxin receptor in neurite outgrowth in PC12 cells. *Neuroscience, 56*(2), 441–451.

Chandra, S., Shiffman, S., Scharf, D. M., Dang, Q., & Shadel, W. G. (2007). Daily smoking patterns, their determinants, and implications for quitting. *Experimental and Clinical Psychopharmacology, 5*(1), 67–80.

Chassin, L., Presson, C. C., & Sherman, S. J. (1984). Cigarette smoking and adolescent psychosocial development. *Basic and Applied Social Psychology, 5*(4), 295–315.

Clarke, P. B., & Kumar, R. (1984). Some effects of nicotine on food and water intake in undeprived rats. *British Journal of Pharmacology, 82*(1), 233–239.

Clarke, P. B. S., Schwartz, R. D., Paul, S. M., Pert, C. B., & Pert, A. (1985). Nicotinic binding in rat brain: Autoradiographic comparison of [^{3}H]acetylcholine, [^{3}H]nicotine, and [^{125}I]-α-bungarotoxin. *Journal of Neuroscience, 5*(5), 1307–1315.

Colrain, I. M., Trinder, J., & Swan, G. E. (2004). The impact of smoking cessation on objective and subjective markers of sleep: Review, synthesis, and recommendations. *Nicotine & Tobacco Research, 6*, 913–925.

Cooper, T. V., Klesges, R. C., Debon, M. W., Zbikowski, S. M., Johnson, K. C., & Clemens, L. H. (2005). A placebo controlled randomized trial of the effects of phenylpropanolamine and nicotine gum on cessation rates and postcessation weight gain in women. *Addictive Behaviors, 20*, 61–75.

Copeland, A. L., Martin, P. D., Geiselman, P. J., Rash, C. J., & Kendzor, D. E. (2006). Smoking cessation for weight-concerned women: group vs. individually tailored, dietary, and weight-control follow-up sessions. *Addictive Behaviors, 31*, 115–127.

Corrigall, W. A., & Coen, K. M. (1989). Nicotine maintains robust self-administration in rats on a limited-access schedule. *Psychopharmacology, 99*(4), 473–478.

Corrigall, W. A., & Coen, K. M. (1991). Selective dopamine antagonists reduce nicotine self-administration. *Psychopharmacology, 104*(2), 171–176.

Cox, B. M., Goldstein, A., & Nelson, W. T. (1984). Nicotine self-administration in rats. *British Journal of Pharmacology, 83*(1), 49–55.

Croghan, G. A., Sloan, J. A., Croghan, I. T., Novotny, P., Hurt, R. D., DeKrey, W. L., … Loprinzi, C. (2003). Comparison of nicotine patch alone versus nicotine nasal spray alone versus a combination for treating smokers: A minimal intervention, randomized multicenter trial in a nonspecialized setting. *Nicotine and Tobacco Research, 5,* 181–187.

Cummings, K. M., Giovino, G., Jaen, C. R., & Emrich, L. J. (1985). Reports of smoking withdrawal symptoms over a 21 day period of abstinence. *Addictive Behaviors, 10,* 373–381.

Dani, J. A., & Bertrand, D. (2007). Nicotinic acetylcholine receptors and nicotinic cholinergic mechanisms of the central nervous system. *Annual Review of Pharmacology and Toxicology, 47,* 699–729.

Dani, J. A., & Heinemann, S. (1996). Molecular and cellular aspects of nicotine abuse. *Neuron, 16*(5), 905–908.

Dollard, J., Doob, L. W., Miller, N. E., Mowrer, O. H., & Sears, R. R. (1939). *Frustration and aggression.* New Haven, CT: Yale University Press.

Donny, E. C., Caggiula, A. R., Knopf, S., & Brown, C. (1995). Nicotine self-administration in rats. *Psychopharmacology, 122*(4), 390–394.

Donny, E. C., Houtsmuller, E., & Stitzer, M. L. (2007). Smoking in the absence of nicotine: Behavioral, subjective and physiological effects over 11 days. *Addiction, 102*(2), 324–334.

Donze, J., Ruffieux, C., & Cornuz, J. (2007). Determinants of smoking and cessation in older women. *Age and Ageing, 36,* 53–57.

Eisenberg, D., & Quinn, B. C. (2006). Estimating the effect of smoking cessation on weight gain: An instrumental variable approach. *Health Services Research, 41,* 2255–2266.

Elliott, B. M., Faraday, M. M., Phillips, J. M., & Grunberg, N. E. (2004). Effects of nicotine on elevated-plus maze and locomotor activity in male and female adolescent and adult rats. *Pharmacology Biochemistry & Behavior, 77,* 21–28.

Epstein, L., & Collins, F. (1977). The measurement of situational influences of smoking. *Addictive Behaviors, 2,* 47–53.

Erikson, E. H. (1963). *Childhood and society* (2nd ed.). New York: W. W. Norton.

Eysenck, H. J., & Eyesenck, S. B. G. (1963). *The Eysenck Personality Inventory.* San Diego, CA: Educational and Industrial Testing Service.

Fagan, P., Augustson, E., Backinger, C. L., O'Connell, M. E., Vollinger, R. E., Jr., Kaufman, A., & Gibson, J. T. (2007). Quit attempts and intention to quit cigarette smoking among young adults in the United States. *American Journal of Public Health, 97,* 1412–1420.

Faraday, M. M., Elliott, B. M., & Grunberg, N. E. (2001). Adult vs. adolescent rats differ in biobehavioral responses to chronic nicotine administration. *Pharmacology Biochemistry & Behavior, 70,* 475–489.

Faraday, M. M., Elliott, B. M., Phillips, J. M., & Grunberg, N. E. (2003). Adolescent and adult male rats differ in sensitivity to nicotine's activity effects. *Pharmacology Biochemistry & Behavior, 74,* 917–931.

Feldman, R. S., Meyer, J. S., & Quenzer, L. F. (Eds.). (1997). *Principles of neuropsychopharmacology* (pp. 591–611). Sunderland, MA: Sinauer.

Filozof, C., Fernandez Pinilla, M. C., & Fernandez-Cruz, A. (2004). Smoking cessation and weight gain. *Obesity Reviews, 5,* 95–103.

Fleming, M., Mihic, S. J., & Harris, R. A. (2006). Ethanol. In L. L. Brunton, J. S. Lazo, & K. L. Parker (Eds.), *Goodman & Gilman's The pharmacological basis of therapeutics* (11th ed., pp. 324–359). New York, NY: McGraw Hill.

Freud, S. (1949). *Three essays on the theory of sexuality* (J. Strachey, Trans.). London, England: Imago (Original work published 1905).

Friedman, G. D., Sieglaub, A. B., & Seitzer, C. C. (1974). Cigarettes, alcohol, coffee, and peptic ulcer. *New England Journal of Medicine, 290,* 469–473.

Froom, P., Melamed, S., & Benbassat, J. (1998). Smoking cessation and weight gain. *Journal of Family Practitioners, 46,* 460–464.

Gilpin, E. A., Choi, W. S., Berry, C., & Pierce, J. (1999). How many adolescents start smoking each day in the United States? *Journal of Adolescent Health, 25,* 248–255.

Goldfarb, T. L., Jarvik, M. E., & Glick, S. D. (1970). Cigarette nicotine content as a determinant of human smoking behavior. *Psychopharmacologia, 17*(1), 89–93.

Gourlay, S. G., Stead, L. F., & Benowitz, N. L. (2004). Clonidine for smoking cessation, *Cochrane Database Systematic Review,* CD000058.

Grinevich, V. P., Letchworth, S. R., Lindenberger, K. A., Menager, J., Mary, V., Sadieva, K. A., … Bencherif, M. (2005). Heterologous expression of human $\alpha6\beta4\beta3\alpha5$ nicotinic acetylcholine receptors: Binding properties consistent with their natural expression require quaternary subunit assembly including the $\alpha5$ subunit. *Journal of Pharmacology and Experimental Therapeutics, 312*(2), 619–626.

Gritz, E. R., Dresler, C., & Sarna, L. (2005). Smoking, the missing drug interaction in clinical trials: Ignoring the obvious. *Cancer Epidemiology, Biomarkers, & Prevention, 14*(10), 2287–2293.

Grunberg, N. E. (1982). The effects of nicotine and cigarette smoking on food consumption and taste preferences. *Addictive Behaviors, 7*, 317–331.

Grunberg, N. E. (1986). Nicotine as a psychoactive drug: Appetite regulation. *Psychopharmacology Bulletin, 22*, 875–881.

Grunberg, N. E. (1992). Cigarette smoking and body weight: A personal journey through a complex field. *Health Psychology, 11*(Suppl.), 26–31.

Grunberg, N. E., Winders, S. E., & Wewers, M. E. (1991). Gender differences in tobacco use. *Health Psychology, 10*(2), 143–153.

Hanson, H. M., Ivester, C. A., & Morton, B. R. (1979). Nicotine self-administration in rats. *NIDA Research Monograph, 23*, 70–90.

Hanson, K., Allen, S., Jensen, S., & Hatsukami, D. (2003). Treatment of adolescent smokers with the nicotine patch. *Nicotine & Tobacco Research, 5*, 515–526.

Härfstrand, A., Adem, A., Fuxe, K., Agnati, L., Andersson, K., & Nordberg, A. (1988). Distribution of nicotinic cholinergic receptors in the rat tel- and diencephalons: A quantitative receptor autoradiographical study using [^{3}H]acetylcholine, [α-^{125}I]-bungarotoxin and [^{3}H] nicotine. *Acta Physiol Scand, 132*, 1–14.

Heishman, S. J., Snyder, F. R., & Henningfield, J. E. (1993). Performance, subjective, and physiological effects of nicotine in non-smokers. *Drug and Alcohol Dependence, 34*, 11–18.

Hejmadi, M. V., Dajas-Bailador, F., Barns, S. M., Jones, B., & Wonnacott, S. (2003). Neuroprotection by nicotine against hypoxia-induced apoptosis in cortical cultures involves activation of multiple nicotinic acetylcholine receptor subtypes. *Molecular & Cellular Neuroscience, 24*(3), 779–786.

Henningfield, J. E., & Goldberg, S. R. (1983). Control of behavior by intravenous nicotine injections in human subjects. *Pharmacology, Biochemistry, and Behavior, 19*(6), 1021–1026.

Henningfield, J. E., & Goldberg, S. R. (1988). Pharmacologic determinants of tobacco self-administration by humans. *Pharmacology, Biochemistry, and Behavior, 30*(1), 221–226.

Hollis, J. F., Polen, M. R., Lichtenstein, E., & Whitlock, E. P. (2003). Tobacco use patterns and attitudes among teens being seen for routine primary care. *American Journal of Health Promotion, 17*, 231–239.

Houtsmuller, E. J., Henningfield, J. E., & Stitzer, M. L. (2003). Subjective effects of the nicotine lozenge: Assessment of abuse liability. *Psychopharmaocology, 167*, 20–27.

Htoo, A., Talwar, A., Feinsilver, S. H., & Greenberg, H. (2004). Smoking and sleep disorders. *Medical Clinics of North America, 88*, 1575–1591.

Hughes, J. R. (2007a). Effects of abstinence from tobacco: Etiology, animal models, epidemiology, and significance: A subjective review. *Nicotine & Tobacco Research, 9*, 329–339.

Hughes, J. R. (2007b). Effects of abstinence from tobacco: Valid symptoms and time course. *Nicotine & Tobacco Research, 9*, 315–327.

Hughes, J. R., Higgins, S. T., & Bickel, W. K. (1994). Nicotine withdrawal versus other drug withdrawal syndromes: Similarities and dissimilarities. *Addiction, 89*, 1461–1470.

Hughes, J. R., Higgins, S. T., & Hatsukami, D. K. (1990). Effects of abstinence from tobacco: A critical review. In L. T. Koszlowski, H. M. Annis, H. D. Cappell, F. B. Glaser, M. S. Goodstat, & Y. Israel (Eds.), *Research advances in alcohol and drug problems* (pp. 317–98). New York, NY: Plenum.

Hughes, J. R., Stead, L. F., & Lancaster, T. (2005). Nortriptyline for smoking cessation: A review. *Nicotine and Tobacco Research, 7*, 491–499.

Hull, C. L. (1943). *Principles of Behavior.* New York, NY: Appleton-Century.

Iyasu, S., Randall, L. L., Welty, T. K., Hsia, J., Kinney, H. C., & Mandell, F., … Willinger, M. (2002). Risk factors for sudden infant death syndrome among Northern Plains Indians. *JAMA, 288*, 2717–2723.

Jamerson, B. D., Nides, M., Jorenby, D. E., Donahue, R., Garrett, P., & Johnston, J. A., … Leischow, S. J. (2001). Late-term smoking cessation despite initial failure: An evaluation of bupropion sustained release, nicotine patch, combination therapy, and placebo. *Clinical Therapeutics, 23*, 744–752.

Jarvik, M. E. (1977). *Biological factors underlying the smoking habit*: NIDA Research Monograph No. 17. U.S. Department of Health, Education, and Welfare, Public Health Service, Alcohol, Drug Abuse, and Mental Health Administration, National Institute on Drug Abuse.

Jarvik, M. E., Glick, S. D., & Nakamura, R. K. (1970). Inhibition of cigarette smoking by orally administered nicotine. *Clinical Pharmacology and Therapeutics, 11*(4), 574–576.

Jarvis, M. J. (2004). Why people smoke. *BMJ, 328*(7434), 277–279.

Jessor, R., & Jessor, S. (1977). *Problem behavior and psychosocial development: A longitudinal study of youth.* New York, NY: Academic Press.

Jorenby, D. (2002). Clinical efficacy of bupropion in the management of smoking cessation. *Drugs, 62*(Suppl. 2), 25–35.

Kalman, D., & Smith, S. S. (2005). Does nicotine do what we think it does? A meta-analytic review of the subjective effects of nicotine in nasal spray and intravenous studies with smokers and nonsmokers. *Nicotine and Tobacco Research, 7*(3), 317–333.

Kandel, D. B. (2002). *Stages and pathways of drug involvement. Examining the Gateway Hypothesis.* New York, NY: Cambridge University Press.

Kassel, J. D., Stroud, L., & Patronis C. (2003). Smoking, nicotine, and stress: Correlation, causation, and context across stages of smoking. *Psychological Bulletin, 129*, 270–304.

Kenny, P. J., & Markou, A. (2006). Nicotine self-administration acutely activates brain reward systems and induces a long-lasting increase in reward sensitivity. *Neuropsychopharmacology, 31*(6), 1203–1211.

Klesges, R. C., Ward, K. D., Ray, J. W., Cutter, G., Jacobs, D. R., Jr., & Wagenknecht, L. E. (1998). The prospective relationships between smoking and weight in a young, biracial cohort: The coronary artery risk development in young adults study. *Journal of Consulting and Clinical Psychology, 66*, 987–993.

Klesges, R. C., Winders, S. E., Meyers, A. W., Eck, L. W., Ward, K. D., & Hultquist, C. M., … Shadish, W. R. (1997). How much weight gain occurs following smoking cessation? A comparison of weight gain using both continuous and point prevalence abstinence. *Journal of Consulting and Clinical Psychology, 65*, 286–291.

Koffka, K. (1925). *The growth of the mind.* New York, NY: Harcourt.

Kohler, W. (1925). *The mentality of apes.* New York, NY: Harcourt.

Koob, G. F., & Bloom, F. E. (1988). Cellular and molecular mechanisms of drug dependence. *Science, 242*(4879), 715–723.

Koob, G. F., & LeMoal, M. (1997). Drug abuse: Hedonic homeostatic dysregulation. *Science, 278*, 52–58.

Koob, G. F., & LeMoal, M. (2001). Drug addiction, dysregulation of reward, and allostasis. *Neuropsychopharmacology, 24*, 97–129.

Koob, G. F., & Swerdlow, N. R. (1988). The functional output of the mesolimbic dopamine system. *Annals of the New York Academy of Science, 537*, 216–227.

Koslowski, L. T., Henningfield, J. E., Keenan, R. M., Lei, H., Leigh, G., & Jelinek, L. C., … Haertzen, C. A. (1993). Patterns of alcohol, cigarette, and caffeine use in two drug-abusing populations. *Journal of Substance Treatment, 10*, 171–179.

Kroon, L. A. (2007). Drug interactions with smoking. *American Journal of Health-System Pharmacy, 64*, 1917–1921.

Kurian, A. K., & Cardarelli, K. M. (2007). Racial and ethnic differences in cardiovascular disease risk factors: A systematic review. *Ethnic Disparities, 17*, 143–152.

Lambe, E. K., Picciotto, M. R., & Aghajanian, G. K. (2003). Nicotine induces glutamate release from thalamocortical terminals in prefrontal cortex. *Neuropsychopharmaology, 28*(2), 216–225.

Léna, C., de Kerchove D'Exaerde, A., Cordero-Erausquin, M., Le Novère, N., del Mar Arroyo-Jimenez, M., & Changeux, J. P. (1999). Diversity and distribution of nicotinic acetylcholine receptors in the locus ceruleus neurons. *Proceedings of the National Academy of Sciences of the U.S.A., 96*(21), 12126–12131.

Levin, E. D., Lawrence, S., Petro, A., Horton, K., Seidler, F. J., & Slotkin, T. A. (2006). Increased nicotine self-administration following prenatal exposure in female rats. *Pharmacology, Biochemistry, & Behavior, 85*(3), 669–674.

Levinson, A. H., Perez-Stable, E. J., Espinoza, P., Flores, E. T., & Byers, T. E. (2004). Latinos report less use of pharmaceutical aids when trying to quit smoking. *American Journal of Preventative Medicine, 26*, 105–111.

Marubio, L. M., Gardier, A. M., Durier, S., David, D., Klink, R., Arroyo-Jimenez, M. M., … Changeux, J. P. (2003). Effects of nicotine in the dopaminergic system of mice lacking the alpha4 subunit of neuronal nicotinic acetylcholine receptors. *European Journal of Neuroscience, 17*, 1329–1337.

Maurer, P., & Bachmann, M. F. (2006). Therapeutic vaccines for nicotine dependence. *Current Opinion in Molecular Therapeutics, 8*(1), 11–16.

Maurer, P., & Bachmann, M. F. (2007). Vaccination against nicotine: An emerging therapy for tobacco dependence. *Expert Opinion on Investigational Drugs, 16*, 1775–1783.

McGehee, D. S., Heath, M. J. S., Gelber, S., Devay, P., & Role, L. W. (1995). Nicotine enhancement of fast excitatory synaptic transmission in the CNS by presynaptic receptors. *Science, 269*, 1692–1696.

Meyers, A. W., Klesges, R. C., Winders, S. E., Ward, K. D., Peterson, B. A., & Eck, L. H. (1997). Are weight concern predictive of smoking cessation? A prospective analysis. *Journal of Consulting and Clinical Psychology, 65*, 448–452.

Mineur, Y. S., & Picciotto, M. R. (2008). Genetics of nicotinic acetylcholine receptors: Relevance to nicotine addiction. *Biochemical Pharmacology, 75*(1), 323–333.

Moolchan, E. T., Robinson, M. L., Ernst, M., Cadet, J. L., Pickworth, W. B., & Heishman, S. J., & Schroeder, J. R. (2005). Safety and efficacy of the nicotine patch and gum for the treatment of adolescent tobacco addiction. *Pediatrics, 2005*, 115, e407–e414.

Mugnaini, M., Garzotti, M., Sartori, I., Pilla, M., Repeto, P., Heidbreder, C. A., & Tessari, M. (2006). Selective down-regulation of [(125)I]Y0-alpha-conotoxin MII binding in rat mesostriatal dopamine pathway following continuous infusion of nicotine. *Neuroscience, 137*(2), 565–572.

Naqvi, N. H., Rudrauf, D., Damasio, H., & Bechara, A. (2007). Damage to the insula disrupts addiction to cigarette smoking. *Science, 315*, 531–534.

Niederhofer, H., & Huber, M. (2004). Bupropion may support psychosocial treatment of nicotine-dependent adolescents: Preliminary results. *Pharmacothearpy, 24*, 1524–1528.

O'Dell, L. E., Bruijnzeel, A. W., Ghozland, S., Markou, A., & Koob, G. F. (2004). Nicotine withdrawal in adolescent and adult rats. *Annals of the New York Academy of Sciences, 1021*, 167–174.

O'Dell, L. E., & Koob, G. F. (2007). Nicotine deprivation effects in rats with intermittent 23-hour access to intravenous nicotine self-administration. *Pharmacolology, Biochemistry, & Behavior, 86*(2), 346–353.

O'Dell, L. E., Torres, O. V., Natividad, L. A., & Tejeda, H. A. (2006). Adolescent nicotine exposure produces less affective measures of withdrawal relative to adult nicotine exposure in male rats. *Neurotoxicology and Teratology, 29*, 17–22.

Parolaro, D., & Rabino, T. (2008).The role of endogenous cannabinoid system in drug addiction. *Drug News & Perspectives, 21*, 149–157.

Pavlov, I. P. (1927). *Conditioned reflexes.* New York, NY: Oxford University Press.

Perkins, K. A. (1999a). Nicotine discrimination in men and women. *Pharmacology Biochemistry and Behavior, 64*, 295–299.

Perkins, K. A. (1999b). Nicotine self-administration. *Nicotine and Tobacco Research, 1*(Suppl.), S133–S137.

Perkins K. A. (2001). Smoking Cessation in Women: Special Considerations. *CNS Drugs, 15*(5), 391–411.

Perkins, K. A., Marcus, M. D., Levine, M. D., D'Amico, D., Miller, A., Broge, M., … Shiffman, S. (2001). Cognitive-behavioral therapy to reduce weight concerns improves smoking cessation outcome in weight-concerned women. *Journal of Consulting and Clinical Psychology, 69*, 604–613.

Persico, A. M. (1992). Predictors of smoking cessation in a sample of Italian smokers. *International Journal of Addiction, 27*, 683–695.

Picciotto, M. R., Zoli, M., Rimondini, R., Léna, C., Marubio, L. M., Pich, E. M., … Changeux, J. P. (1998). Acetylcholine receptors containing the β2 subunit are involved in the reinforcing properties of nicotine. *Nature, 391*, 173–177.

Pierce, R. C., & Kumaresan, V. (2006). The mesolimbic dopamine system: The final common pathway for the reinforcing effect of drugs of abuse? *Neuroscience and Biobehavioral Reviews, 30*(2), 215–238.

Pisinger, C., & Jorgensen, T. (2007). Waist circumference and weight following smoking cessation in a general population: The Inter99 Study. *Preventive Medicine, 44*, 290–295.

Pomerleau, C. S., Tate, J. C., Lumley, M. A., & Pomerleau, O. F. (1994). Gender differences in prospectively versus retrospectively assessed smoking withdrawal symptoms. *Journal of Substance Abuse, 6*, 433–440.

Pomerleau, C. S., Zucker, A. N., & Stewart, A. J. (2001). Characterizing concerns about post-cessation weight gain: Results from a national survey of women smokers. *Nicotine and Tobacco Research, 3*, 51–60.

Rabinoff, M., Caskey, N., & Park., C. (2007). Pharmacological and chemical effects of cigarette additives. *American Journal of Public Health, 97*(11), 1981–1991.

Radcliffe, K. A., & Dani, J. A. (1998). Nicotinic stimulation produces multiple forms of increased glutamatergic synaptic transmission. *Journal of Neuroscience, 18*(18), 7075–7083.

Reichert, V. C., Seltzer, V., Efferen, L. S., & Kohn, N. (2004). Women and tobacco dependence. *Medical Clinics of North America, 88*, 1467–1481.

Ries, L. A., Wingo, P. A., Miller, D. S., Howe, H. L., Weir, H. K., Rosenberg, H. M., … Edwards, B. K. (2000). The annual report to the nation on the status of cancer, 1973–1997, with a special section on colorectal cancer. *Cancer, 88*, 2398–2424.

Ring, H. Z., Valdes, A. M., Nishita, D. M., Prasad, S., Jacob, P., III, Tyndale, R. F., … Benowitz N. L. (2007). Gene-gene interactions between CYP2B6 and CYP2A6 in nicotine metabolism. *Pharmacogenetics and Genomics, 17*(12), 1007–1015.

Rose, J. E., Ananda, S., & Jarvik, M. E. (1983). Cigarette smoking during anxiety-provoking and monotonous tasks. *Addictive Behaviors, 8*, 353–359.

Rose, J. E., & Corrigall, W. A. (1997). Nicotine self-administration in animals and humans: Similarities and differences. *Psychopharmacology, 130*(1), 28–40.

Rugkåsa, J., Knox, B., Sittlington, J., Kennedy, O., Treacy, M. P., & Abaunza, P. S. (2001). Anxious adults vs. cool children: Children's views on smoking and addiction. *Social Science & Medicine, 53*(5), 593–602.

Rundmo, T., Smedslund, G., & Gotestam, K. G. (1997). Motivation for smoking cessation among the Norwegian public. *Addictive Behaviors, 22*, 377–386.

Russell, M. A. (1971). Cigarette smoking: Natural history of a dependence disorder. *British Journal of Medical Psychology, 22*, 1–16.

Russell, M. A., Wilson, C., Patel, U. A., Feyerabend, C., & Cole, P. V. (1975). Plasma nicotine levels after smoking cigarettes with high, medium, and low nicotine yields. *British Medical Journal, 2*(5968), 414–416.

Scales, M. B., Monahan, J. L., Rhodes, N., Roskos-Ewoldsen, D., & Johnson-Turbes, A. (2009). Adolescents' perceptions of smoking and stress reduction. *Health Education & Behavior, 36*(4), 746–758.

Schachter, S., Kozlowski, L. T., & Silverstein, B. (1977). Studies on the interaction of psychological and pharmacological determinants of smoking. The effects of urinary pH on cigarette smoking. *Journal of Experimental Psychology, 106*(1), 13–19.

Schnieder, N. G., Koury, M. A., Cortner, C., Olmstead, R. E., Hartman, N., Kleinman, L., ... Leaf, D. (2006). Preferences among four combination nicotine treatments. *Psychopharmacology, 187*, 476–485.

Shafey, O., Dolwick, S., & Guindon, G. E. (Eds). (2003). *Tobacco control country profiles, 2003* (2nd ed.). Atlanta, GA: American Cancer Society.

Shahab, L., Hammond, D., O'Connor, R. J., Cummings, K. M., Borland, R., King, B., & McNeill, A. (2008). The reliability and validity of self-reported puffing behavior: Evidence from a cross-national study. *Nicotine and Tobacco Research, 10*(5), 867–874.

Shiffman, S. (1979). The tobacco withdrawal syndrome. *NIDA Research Monographs, 23*, 158–184.

Shiffman, S. (1982). Relapse following smoking cessation: A situational analysis. *Journal of Consulting & Clinical Psychology, 50*, 71–86.

Shiffman, S. (1986). A cluster-analytic classification of smoking relapse episodes. *Addictive Behaviors, 11*, 295–307.

Shiffman, S., DiMarino, M. E., & Pillitteri, J. L. (2005). The effectiveness of nicotine patch and nicotine lozenge in very heavy smokers. *Journal of Substance Abuse and Treatment, 28*, 49–55.

Shoaib, M., Schindler, C. W., & Goldberg, S. R. (1997). Nicotine self-administration in rats: Strain and nicotine pre-exposure effects on acquisition. *Psychopharmacology, 129*(1), 35–43.

Shram, M. J., Funk, D., Li, Z., & Lê, A. D. (2008). Nicotine self-administration, extinction responding and reinstatement in adolescent and adult male rats: Evidence against a biological vulnerability to nicotine addiction during adolescence. *Neuropsychopharmacology, 33*(4), 739–748.

Silagy, C., Lancaster, T., Stead, L., Mant, D., & Fowler, G. (2004). Nicotine replacement therapy for smoking cessation. *Cochrane Database Systematic Reviews*, CD00146.

Skinner, B. F. (1938). *The behavior of organisms*. New York, NY: Appleton-Century-Crofts.

Slotkin, T. A., Cousins, M. M., & Seidler F. J. (2004). Administration of nicotine to adolescent rats evokes regionally selective upregulation of CNS α7 nicotinic acetylcholine receptors. *Brain Research, 1030*, 159–163.

Solomon, R. L., & Corbit, J. D. (1973). An opponent-process theory of motivation: II. Cigarette addiction. *Journal of Abnormal Psychology, 81*(2), 158–171.

Spilich, G. J., June, L., & Renner, J. (1992). Cigarette smoking and cognitive performance. *British Journal of Addiction, 87*, 1313–1326.

Sweeney, C. T., Fant, R. V., Fagerstrom, K. O., McGovern, J. F., & Henningfield, J. E. (2001). Combination nicotine replacement therapy for smoking cessation: rationale, efficacy and tolerability. *CNS Drugs, 15*, 453–467.

Tapper, A. R., McKinney, S. L., Nashmi, R., Schwarz, J., Deshpande, P., Labarca, C., ... Lester, H. A. (2004). Nicotine activation of alpha4* receptors: Sufficient for reward, tolerance, and sensitization. *Science, 306*(5698), 1029–1032.

Taylor, P. (2006). Agents acting at the neuromuscular junction and autonomic ganglia. In L. L. Brunton, J. S. Lazo, & K. L. Parker (Eds.), *Goodman & Gilman's The pharmacological basis of therapeutics* (11th ed.) New York: McGraw-Hill.

Thorndike, E. L. (1911). *Animal intelligence: Experimental studies*. New York, NY: Macmillian.

U.S. Department of Health and Human Services. (1983). *The health consequences of smoking: Cardiovascular disease: A Report of the Surgeon General*. Atlanta, GA.

U.S. Department of Health and Human Services. (1988). *The health consequences of smoking, a report of the Surgeon General: Nicotine addiction*. Washington, DC: U.S. Government Printing Office. DHHS Publication No. (CD) 88-8406.

U.S. Department of Health and Human Services. (2006). *The health consequences of involuntary exposure to tobacco smoke: A report of the surgeon general.* Atlanta, GA.

U.S. Department of Health and Human Services. (2008). Treating tobacco use and dependence: 2008 update: U.S. Public Health Service Clinical Practice Guideline executive summary. *Respiratory Care, 53*(9), 1217–1222.

Valette, H., Bottlaender, M., Dollé, F., Coulon C., Ottaviani, M., & Syrota, A. (2003). Long-lasting occupancy of central nicotinic acetylcholine receptors after smoking: A PET study in monkeys. *Journal of Neurochemistry, 84*(1), 105–111.

Vizi, E. S., & Lendvai, B. (1999). Modulatory role of presynaptic nicotinic receptors in synaptic and non-synaptic chemical communication in the central nervous system. *Brain Research Reviews, 30*(3), 219–235.

Watson, J. B., & Rayner, R. (1920). Conditioned emotional reactions. *Journal of Experimental Psychology, 3*, 1–14.

Watson, J. M., Scarinci, I. C., Klesges, R. C., Murray, D. M., Vander Weg, M., DeBon, M., … McClanahan, B. (2003). Relationships among smoking status, ethnicity, socioeconomic indicators, and lifestyle variables in a biracial sample of women. *Preventive Medicine, 37*, 138–147.

Williamson, D. F., Madans, J., Anda, R. F., Kleinman, J. C., Giovino, G. A., & Byers, T. (1991). Smoking cessation and severity of weight gain in a national cohort. *New England Journal of Medicine, 324*, 739–745.

Wilmouth, C. E., & Spear, L. P. (2004). Adolescent and adult rats' aversion to flavors previously paired with nicotine. *Annals of the New York Academy of Sciences, 1021*, 462–464.

World Health Organization. (2008a). *Full list of signatories and parties to the WHO Framework Convention on Tobacco Control.* Retrieved from http://www.who.int/fctc/signatories_parties/en/index.html

World Health Organization. (2008b). *WHO Report on the global tobacco epidemic, 2008.* Retrieved from http://www.who.int/tobacco/mpower/2008/en

Zevin, S., & Benowitz, N. L. (1999). Drug interactions with tobacco smoking: An update. *Clinical Pharmacokinetics, 36*(6), 425–438.

15 Obesity

Rena R. Wing
The Miriam Hospital and the Warren Alpert Medical School,
Brown University

Suzanne Phelan
California Polytechnic State University

Obesity is a significant health problem in the United States (Flegal, Carroll, Ogden, & Curtin, 2010). It is a major cause of morbidity and mortality, both independently and through its association with hypertension and diabetes. Although genetic factors clearly play a role in obesity, this chapter focuses primarily on the behavioral factors associated with the development of obesity and lifestyle interventions that have been developed for the prevention and treatment of this major health problem.

DEFINING OBESITY

Obesity is most commonly quantified using *body mass index* (BMI), which is weight in kilograms divided by height in meters squared. The BMI is highly correlated with measures of body fat and predicts both morbidity and mortality, but it may be less accurate in minority populations, people who have unusually high or low muscle mass, or people under 5 feet tall (NHLBI, 1998). A BMI of 18.5–24.9 kg/m² is considered "normal" weight, a BMI of 25.0–29.9 kg/m² is "overweight," and obesity begins at a BMI of 30 kg/m², with "extreme" obesity defined as a BMI ≥ 40 kg/m² (NHLBI, 1998).

Other measures of body fatness are used primarily in research settings. These include measuring skin fold thickness with calipers, using bioelectric impedance machines, underwater weighing, or dual x-ray absorptiometry (Van Loan, 2003). Also, computerized tomography (CT) or magnetic resonance imaging (MRI) scans allow calculation of abdominal and visceral fat.

PREVALENCE

Obesity is a major health problem in the United States because of its prevalence and its association with morbidity and mortality. It is estimated that one of every three Americans is obese (BMI ≥ 30; Flegal et al., 2010). Obesity increases with age, peaking at about age 50, and occurs more commonly in women than in men, especially in minority women. Approximately 45% to 50% of African American women and Mexican American women are obese (see Figure 15.1).

The prevalence of obesity in adults increased steadily in the 1980s and 1990s from 25% to 33% (Flegal, Carroll, Kuczmarski, & Johnson, 1998), but since that time it appears to have leveled off (Flegal et al., 2010). Genetic factors clearly play a role in the development of obesity (French, Story, & Jeffery, 2001; Hill, Wyatt, Reed, & Peters, 2003; Weinsier, Hunter, Heine, Goran, & Sell, 1998), but the rapid rise in the prevalence of obesity is a result of environmental changes such as increases in calorie intake (Centers for Disease Control and Prevention, 2004), changes in the U.S. food supply (Gerrior, Bente, & Hiza, 2004), availability of high-fat and energy-dense foods (Brantley, Myers, & Roy, 2005), and physical inactivity (Heini & Weinsier, 1997).

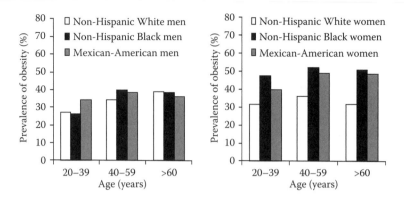

FIGURE 15.1   Unadjusted prevalence of overweight by age and race/ethnicity for men and women, U.S. population age 20 and older, 1999–2008. (Adapted from Flegal, K. M., Carroll, M. D., Ogden, C. L., and Curtin, L. R., *JAMA*, 303, 3, 2010.)

CAUSES OF THE OBESITY EPIDEMIC

GENETICS

Scientific research over the past 100 years has demonstrated that heredity plays a major role in the development of obesity (Bray & Bouchard, 1997). Reports have now confirmed that 7 to 10 specific genes contribute to common forms of obesity (Sabatti et al., 2009; Thorleifsson et al., 2009; Willer et al., 2009), including FTO (Frayling et al., 2007) and MC4R (Loos et al., 2008). However, it is nearly certain that many of the genes that influence appetite and expenditure have relatively small effects on obesity phenotypes and that expression depends, in large part, on environmental conditions. Bouchard et al. (1990) were one of the first to show that genetic variation interacts with environmental manipulations in determining weight change. These investigators overfed 12 pairs of monozygotic twins 1,000 kcal/day extra for 100 days. They found marked variability between twin pairs in the amount of weight gained with overfeeding, but a high degree of concordance within twin pairs; thus, weight gain in one twin predicted weight gain in the other. Similar findings were observed with exercise (Bouchard et al., 1994), suggesting that the effect of these behavior changes on body weight may be mediated by genetic factors.

Similarly, as native populations become Westernized, their risk of obesity rises dramatically. These changes are attributable to adoption of a Western diet and decreased physical activity. This connection is well illustrated by a study comparing Pima Indians who live in the United States with a group of Pimas from the same genetic background who live in a rural area of Mexico (Ravussin, Valencia, Esparza, Bennett, & Schultz, 1994). The Mexican Pimas, who have no electricity, maintain an agrarian lifestyle and consume a traditional Pima diet. Whereas 50% of American Pimas are overweight, with a mean BMI of 35.5, the Mexican Pimas have an average BMI of only 25.1. Such data suggest that genetic background may predispose some individuals to obesity or leanness, but environmental factors determine whether these predispositions will be manifested.

Of interest to researchers is that the majority of genes identified as contributors to obesity are expressed in the brain, emphasizing the role of the central nervous system in obesity predisposition (Willer et al., 2009). The recent upsurge in research has uncovered brain circuitries that regulate appetite, energy expenditure, and fat deposition that are under the control of several neuropeptides, including, most notably, leptin and ghrelin (Kalra & Kalra, 2010). Chronic sleep disturbance—which affects millions of Americans—may result in alterations in these metabolism-regulating peptides and may, thus, increase the risk for obesity (Gimble et al., 2009). It is likely that the plethora of recent discoveries, including advent of a comprehensive human genetic linkage map, will lead to major advances in the understanding of the genetic, molecular, and physiological basis of obesity.

Environmental and Behavioral Factors

Body weight is regulated by the amount of energy taken in through eating and the amount of energy expended. When these two factors are in balance, weight is maintained. Energy imbalance will result in weight change. When there is an increase in calorie intake or a decrease in expenditure, weight gain occurs; with decreased calorie intake and/or increased expenditure, weight loss occurs. Factors that influence food intake and physical activity are described in the next sections.

Eating Behavior

Several eating behaviors have been strongly associated with weight gain, including frequent consumption of fast foods, sugar-sweetened beverages, foods prepared outside the home, and large portion sizes. These eating behaviors are influenced by a wide range of determinants, including the characteristics of the food supply, the social and cultural context in which the behavior occurs, and the knowledge, attitudes, emotional state, and experiences of the individual. Clearly, overconsumption occurs when food is more palatable than usual and when it is presented in energy-dense formulations (Rolls, 2009), as, for example, in the high-calorie, high-fat, and highly palatable foods so ubiquitous in the food supply of Western societies. Fast-food restaurants have exploded in number, most now with drive-through windows, breakfast, packaged meals, and massive serving sizes. Most service stations have been remodeled to have convenience-food markets. Malls have food courts, airports and train stations have fast-food franchises, and there are even cases of fast-food restaurants in the lobbies of children's hospitals and in schools.

With the rise in food supply, the number of different types of food available has also increased. Several studies have now shown that food intake is higher when a variety of foods is presented compared with a single food type (Raynor & Epstein, 2001). If only one type of food is available at a meal, people will eat some of this item and then gradually cease eating. If a new type of food is then introduced, however, consumption of the new food will increase, demonstrating a phenomenon called "sensory specific satiety" (Rolls, Hetherington, & Burley, 1988).

Such cues as the sight or smell of food or even social situations can also stimulate appetite and promote high food consumption and obesity. Large packages, plates, serving bowls, and even pantry arrangements can all increase how much a person serves and consumes by 15%–25% (Wansink, 2010). People eat more when in the company of others and will gauge how much they should eat or drink based on the consumption of their peers (Mattes, 1997). Recent research has documented the powerful influence a peer or family member can have in the development of obesity. A study conducted of a social network of 12,067 people as part of the Framingham Heart Study found that obesity spread through social ties (Christakis & Fowler, 2007). A person's chances of becoming obese increased by 57% if he or she had a friend who became obese; similar influences were found between spouses and other family members.

Food prices and attractive size and quantity discounts in restaurants also influence consumption. "Value meals" offering larger burgers, fries, and soft drinks for only a small increase in cost have continued to gain in popularity. Similarly, a 22-oz soft drink at a movie theatre may cost $3.50, whereas a drink twice the size (i.e., 44 oz) costs only 50 cents more. In addition, marketing data suggest that supersizing and multiple-unit pricing (i.e., "two for $1.00" instead of "50 cents each") translate into greater food consumption.

Stress and negative emotions may also trigger higher than normal food intake. Both laboratory and epidemiological studies (Adam & Epel, 2007; Wardle, Steptoe, Oliver, & Lipsey, 2000) suggest that depressive symptoms and stressful events motivate higher fat and higher calorie food choices. Most people, but women and binge eaters in particular, show a tendency to increase intake of sweet and fatty foods under stress, and doing this may be part of a coping response (Wardle, 2007).

Energy Expenditure

There are several components to energy expenditure. Resting metabolic rate (RMR) is the energy expended when resting in bed in order to maintain various body systems (e.g., body temperature).

In sedentary individuals, RMR accounts for approximately 60% to 70% of total energy expenditure and is primarily determined by the amount of lean body mass. Overweight individuals have more lean body mass, as well as more fat mass; thus, these individuals tend to have higher RMR than do less overweight people.

The second component of energy expenditure (accounting for about 10% of expenditure) is the thermic effect of food, or the energy cost involved in metabolizing food. There is inconsistency regarding differences between obese and lean in this component of energy expenditure; but even if differences do occur, they are small and represent an unlikely explanation for marked obesity.

The third component of energy expenditure is physical activity. This component is the most variable. Although it accounts for 20% to 30% of total energy expenditure in sedentary individuals, it represents a larger component in those people who are more active. Reductions in physical activity have, over time, been implicated in the rise in obesity prevalence rates. Daily physical activity decreased substantially as our nation changed from an agricultural to an industrial economy and, more recently, from a service to an information economy. Our increasing reliance on automobiles, elevators and escalators, cellular telephones, computers, and remote-control devices contributes to the development of obesity. Overweight individuals are less active than normal-weight individuals (Black, Coward, Cole, & Prentice, 1996) and not only spend less time engaging in physical activity but also spend more time involved in such inactive pursuits as watching TV. A number of studies have shown a direct association between hours of TV/day and prevalence of obesity (Parsons, Manor, & Power, 2008). Even the amount of nonvolitional muscle activity (e.g., fidgeting, muscle tone, or maintenance of posture) may be important in determining body weight (Levine, Eberhardt, & Jensen, 1999). The physical activity component of energy expenditure is clearly the most easily modified aspect of energy expenditure and is a primary target of lifestyle interventions for prevention and treatment of obesity.

IMPACT OF OBESITY AND WEIGHT LOSS

MEDICAL AND PSYCHOSOCIAL CONSEQUENCES OF OBESITY

Obesity is a strong risk factor for the development of several morbidities, including coronary heart disease, diabetes, and cancer, as well as liver and kidney disease, osteoarthritis, sleep apnea, and urinary incontinence (Pi-Sunyer, 2009). Obesity is also strongly associated with an increased risk of all-cause mortality and cardiovascular and cancer mortality (Pi-Sunyer, 2009). Some of these negative influences of obesity are dependent on the regional distribution of the adipose tissue. Upper body fat distribution, particularly visceral adipose tissue, is strongly associated with an increased risk of cardiovascular disease, insulin resistance, Type 2 diabetes, and stroke. Abdominal obesity is seen most commonly in men, and in overweight individuals it also appears to be associated with high dietary fat intake, low exercise, and smoking. Furthermore, there appears to be a genetic contribution to body fat distribution (Gao, 2008; Wannamethee, Shaper, & Whincup, 2006). Abdominal obesity is also one of a group of specific risk factors, including high triglyceride levels and high fasting blood glucose levels, which make up the metabolic syndrome—a strong independent risk factor for developing diabetes and heart disease.

The psychosocial consequences of obesity are also well documented. Social marginalization and stigmatization of obesity in adults is common, with evidence that obese individuals face social disadvantages in nearly every domain of living, including employment, education, health care, and interpersonal relationships (Puhl, Andreyeva, & Brownell, 2008; Puhl, Moss-Racusin, Schwartz, & Brownell, 2008). Moreover, the bias against overweight people begins at an early age. In several studies, elementary school children have described obese individuals as more likely to be "lazy, dirty, stupid," and "dumb," compared to lean individuals (Hansson, Karnehed, Tynelius, & Rasmussen, 2009; Latner & Stunkard, 2003). Physicians and health practitioners have similarly described their obese patients as "weak-willed, ugly, and awkward" (Harris, Hamaday, & Mochan, 1999). Obese people are less likely to seek medical help for a given condition than are people without weight problems, failing to seek help in part because of embarrassment, shame, and fear of being criticized. Income and earning power are suppressed in overweight people, and such untoward social conditions as absence of romantic relationships are more common (Puhl & Latner, 2007).

Studies examining the moderating role of stigmatizing experiences on psychological functioning and health behaviors suggest that weight bias may contribute to psychological distress in obese individuals and increase vulnerability to depression, low self-esteem, poor body image, and other psychiatric disorders (Puhl & Heuer, 2009). However, this science is still in its infancy. In studies examining the global relationship between psychological distress and obesity, findings have generally been mixed. An association between obesity and major depressive disorder has been recognized, but a causal association remains to be determined (Atlantis & Baker, 2008). Overall, however, most of the recognized psychological effects of obesity seem to be very specific to obesity, including dissatisfaction with body shape and problems with binge eating. *Binge eating disorder* (BED), which was included in the appendix of *Diagnostic and Statistical Manual of Mental Disorders* (DSM-IV; APA, 1994), is characterized by periods of eating large amounts of food and a feeling of loss of control. As many as 20% to 30% of individuals who seek weight reduction have been found to suffer from binge eating disorder or comorbid depression (Marcus, 1993).

BENEFITS OF WEIGHT LOSS

Weight loss is known to improve most obesity-related morbidities, including blood pressure, total and LDL cholesterol, HDL cholesterol, triglycerides, glycemic control, and osteoarthritis pain (Maggio & Pi-Sunyer, 1997). Weight loss with lifestyle intervention has also been associated with a significant reduction in the prevalence of abdominal obesity (Ilanne-Parikka et al., 2008), sleep apnea (Grunstein et al., 2007), and urinary incontinence (Subak et al., 2009). Although most studies have examined only the short-term benefits of weight loss, recent evidence has also documented long-term benefits. Long-term weight loss was associated with a reduction in the risk of Type 2 diabetes in the Diabetes Prevention Program (Fujimoto et al., 2007) and improved diabetes control in the Look AHEAD (Action for Health in Diabetes) Study. The Diabetes Prevention Program (DPP) was a major multicenter clinical research study that examined whether modest weight loss through dietary changes and increased physical activity could prevent or delay the onset of Type 2 diabetes in 3,234 overweight and obese prediabetics (Knowler et al., 2002). The lifestyle intervention produced a 5.6-kg weight loss and reduced the risk of developing diabetes by 58%; the intervention also reduced high blood pressure and metabolic syndrome. Look AHEAD is a randomized trial of intensive lifestyle intervention versus diabetes support and education (control group) in 5,145 patients with Type 2 diabetes and BMI > 25 kg/m^2. At one year, the intensive group lost 8.6% of body weight compared with 0.7% in the control group (P < .00001), which was associated with improved diabetes control and reduction in CVD risk factors and medication use (Pi-Sunyer et al., 2007). At four years, the intensive lifestyle intervention group continues to have greater improvements in weight, fitness, glycemic control, blood pressure, and most lipid parameters (Wing et al., 2010). Look AHEAD will continue to follow these patients to determine whether intentional weight loss has positive effects on cardiovascular morbidity and mortality. Studies of patients undergoing gastric bypass surgery for morbid obesity have demonstrated a significant reduction in mortality with substantial weight loss (Sjostrom et al., 2007), but the association between more modest weight loss and long-term mortality remains to be determined.

There are also positive effects of weight loss on psychosocial variables. Behavioral weight control programs that assess mood before, during, and after participation in treatment show reductions in depression and anxiety over the course of the program (Wadden & Stunkard, 1993); in addition, larger reductions in depressive symptoms are generally observed in obese individuals with binge eating disorder (Gladis et al., 1998). Body image also improves in obese individuals who lose weight with behavioral weight control (Foster, Wadden, & Vogt, 1997).

Unfortunately, approximately two thirds of individuals who try to lose weight will experience initial success followed subsequently by weight regain (Phelan, Wing, Loria, & Lewis, 2010). However, the behavioral consequences of volitional weight loss and regain was reviewed by the National Task Force (National Task Force on the Prevention and Treatment of Obesity, 2000) and determined to have no negative effects. When overweight individuals lose weight and then subsequently return to baseline, their lipids and blood pressure also return but do not overshoot baseline. Weight cycling also does not negatively affect resting metabolic rate, the ease or difficulty of future weight loss efforts, or body fat distribution. Fewer studies have assessed psychological parameters, but these too do not appear to differ consistently between weight cyclers and non–weight cyclers (Foster, Wadden, Kendall, Stunkard, & Vogt, 1996; Venditti, Wing, Jakicic, Butler, & Marcus, 1996).

Importantly, many of the positive effects of weight loss on medical and psychosocial variables occur after just a modest amount of weight loss. Although larger weight losses produce greater benefits, small weight losses of 5%–10% in even very overweight persons will produce significant improvement in health parameters. Thus, markedly overweight individuals do not need to reduce to ideal body weight to experience health benefits; rather, such individuals should be encouraged to lose 10% of their weight (20 lb in a 200-lb person) and then maintain this weight loss as a way of improving their health.

TREATMENT

Since the 1970s, behavioral approaches have been the treatment of choice for mild to moderate obesity. The basic premise of behavioral approaches is to help patients change their eating and exercise behaviors by providing clear goals and ways to monitor these behaviors and then teaching patients how to rearrange the antecedents (cues) and consequences (reinforcers) that control these behaviors. Behavioral programs are typically delivered in a closed-group format, where all patients start treatment at the same time. Meetings are held weekly for approximately six months, followed by less frequent contact. At each meeting, participants are weighed individually, self-monitoring records are collected and reviewed, and a lecture is presented and discussed. Typical topics of lectures and discussions include nutrition and exercise information (e.g., low-fat eating, eating in restaurants, or exercise in different weather conditions) and behavioral topics (e.g., self-monitoring of eating and exercise behavior, stimulus control, or assertiveness).

The weight losses obtained during the initial phase of behavioral treatment programs have improved over the past 25 years. Initially, in the 1970s, participants lost 3.8 kg during an eight- to 10-week behavioral program. Now most programs achieve average weight loss of 7–10 kg (7% to 10% of initial body weight) at six months. Most of this weight loss is maintained through 12 months, but subsequently there is a gradual regain. In such larger, longer behavior trials as the Diabetes Prevention Program (Fujimoto et al., 2007) and Look AHEAD (Wing et al., 2010), weight losses of 4% to 5% or 4–5 kg have been observed at three- to four-year follow-ups.

The basic behavioral techniques used in standard behavioral weight control programs are described next, and new approaches being used to produce longer lasting changes in diet, exercise, and body weight are highlighted.

Dietary Prescriptions

Participants in behavioral weight loss programs are given calorie and fat-gram goals designed to produce a weight loss of about 2 lb per week. To determine an appropriate calorie goal for weight loss, current intake may be estimated by assuming that the individual consumes 12 kcal/lb of body weight. Thus a 200-lb person would be estimated to be eating 2,400 kcal/day to maintain weight. In order to promote a weight loss of 2 lb/week, this intake must be reduced by 1,000 kcal/day or 7,000 kcal/week. Typically, behavioral programs use calorie goals of 1,000 kcal/day to 1,800 kcal/day, with the higher goal reserved for individuals who weigh more than 200 lb. The fat goal may range from 20% to 30% of calories from fat and is usually prescribed to participants in grams per day to facilitate self-monitoring. If an individual was assigned a 1,000-kcal goal with 20% as fat, then 200 calories would be from fat; because one gram of fat has nine calories, the participant would be given a fat-gram goal of 22 grams of fat.

The dietary prescriptions used in current behavioral programs have been derived from a large number of research studies comparing different degrees of caloric restriction and different macronutrient distributions.

Calorie Goals

Most current behavioral weight loss programs recommend diets of 1,000 kcal/day to 1,800 kcal/day. However, in the 1980s, there was tremendous interest in the use of very low-calorie diets (VLCDs), which were diets with < 800 kcal/day, usually consumed as liquid formula. The simplicity of drinking several cans of liquid each day and removing food entirely from the diet makes such regimens effective for many individuals. In fact, VLCDs were shown to produce weight losses of approximately 20 lb in 12 weeks (Wadden, Stunkard, & Brownell, 1983). However, the problem was that the weight was often regained when foods were reintroduced to the diet. Efforts to combine VLCDs, for initial weight loss, with behavioral strategies to improve maintenance were not successful; in the long term, patients treated with programs that combined behavior modification with VLCDs had weight loss comparable to that achieved by patients in behavioral programs with balanced diets of 1,000 kcal/day to 1,500 kcal/day throughout (Wing et al., 1994; Wadden, Foster, & Letizia, 1994). Thus, the field has tended to move away from VLCDs to these higher calorie regimens.

Macronutrient Distribution

Initially, behavioral treatment programs focused primarily on calorie restriction, with the recognition that "a calorie is a calorie." More recently, there has been greater interest in the types of foods consumed. Typically in behavioral weight loss programs, participants are given goals for calorie and fat intake and asked to monitor and modify both aspects of their behavior. This increased emphasis on restricting dietary fat intake is in part a result of the evidence that overweight individuals have higher consumption of fat (Rolls & Shide, 1992; Tucker & Kano, 1992). Moreover, fat is energy dense compared to other macro nutrients (i.e., fat has 9 kcal/gram, and carbohydrate and protein have only 4 kcal/gram), and thus it is easy to overeat when consuming a high-fat diet. Several studies (Pascale, Wing, Butler, Mullen, & Bononi, 1995; Schlundt et al., 1993) found that better weight losses were achieved when subjects were given goals for both calories and fat. Consequently, most behavioral treatment programs now focus on reducing calorie intake as well as fat intake.

Others have argued that limiting carbohydrates (rather than fat) may promote better weight loss. Several studies have been conducted comparing low-carbohydrate diets (e.g., the Atkins diet) with low-fat regimens (Foster et al., 2010; Hauner, 2004; Ornish et al., 2008; Samaha et al., 2003; Wycherley et al., 2010). These studies have found that in the long-term, the weight losses are similar across these different types of regimens. In a two-year study of 307 obese participants who were randomly assigned to a low-carbohydrate or a low-fat diet, weight losses averaged 11 kg (11%) at year 1 and 7 kg (7%) at year 2 and did not differ between the two dietary regimens (Foster et al., 2010).

What appears to affect weight loss in these studies is not the macronutrient distribution but the level of adherence to the regimen (and ultimately the number of calories that are consumed). Although weight losses achieved with very different macronutrient diets appear to be similar, those participants who adhere better to any of the diets lose more weight than do those who adhere less well (Dansinger, Gleason, Griffith, Selker, & Schaefer, 2005).

Promoting Adherence to Dietary Recommendations

The key issue for long-term weight loss does not appear to be the number of calories or the composition of the diet prescribed; rather, it is how best to promote long-term adherence to dietary changes.

Behaviorists learned something important from the experience with the VLCDs, described earlier. They recognized that the advantage of these diets, which were typically provided as liquid formula, may be a result not of their extreme restriction of calories but of the high degree of structure they provide. Thus, current programs have attempted to increase the amount of structure given to participants. Rather than simply telling patients to eat 1,200 to 1,500 calories per day, researchers have shown that incorporating frozen entrees or liquid formula for some of the meals may help to improve adherence to the calorie goals and consequently improve weight loss outcomes. Wadden and Frey (1997) utilized a 900-kcal/day diet that consisted of four servings daily of liquid meal replacement (150 kcal each) and a prepackaged dinner entree (about 300 kcal) with salad. Subjects utilizing this diet as part of an intensive behavioral program lost 14.5 kg after 17 weeks and maintained the weight loss at one year (Wadden & Frey, 1997). Similarly, subjects participating in a 10-center clinical trial of cardiovascular risk factor management who were given prepackaged foods lost more weight over 10 weeks than did subjects who were allowed to select their own diets according to the American Heart Association (AHA) Step 1 and Step 2 guidelines: 4.5 kg versus 3.5 kg for men; 4.8 kg versus 2.8 kg for women (McCarron et al., 1997). Jeffery et al. (1993) and Wing et al. (1996) also showed that providing subjects with food or prescribing a meal-by-meal eating plan improved weight losses. These more structured regimens led to greater changes in the types of food stored in the home, and participants reported a more regular pattern of meal eating and less difficulty with estimating portion size, finding time to plan meals, and controlling eating when not hungry.

EXERCISE PRESCRIPTIONS

In order to lose weight, it is necessary to produce negative energy balance, that is, a situation where calories taken in are below calories expended. To maximize weight loss, behavioral programs focus on both sides of the energy balance equation; behavioral programs help participants not only to reduce their calorie intake but also to increase their caloric expenditure. Caloric expenditure is the sum of the calories burned in resting metabolism, thermic effect of food, and physical activity. Because the calories burned in physical activity is the only component that is under an individual's control, behavioral weight loss programs target this aspect of energy expenditure. Bouchard and Katzmarzyk's book *Physical Activity and Obesity* (2000) provides further information related to this topic.

Increasing exercise alone, without also changing dietary intake, has been shown to produce very modest weight losses, typically 1–2 kg. Similarly, the short-term effect of adding physical activity to a diet program is not very pronounced. However, randomized trials comparing diet alone, exercise alone, and the combination of diet and exercise consistently show that long-term weight losses are better with the combination (Pronk, Wing, & Jeffery, 1994). Correlational studies also indicate that the single-best predictor of long-term maintenance of weight loss is exercise. Exercise may improve long-term weight loss by both psychological and physiological mechanisms. Exercise increases caloric expenditure and may also minimize loss of lean body mass, thereby lessening the reduction in resting energy expenditure observed with weight loss. In addition, exercise has been shown to influence mood state and may maintain or even suppress appetite, thereby making it easier for patients to adhere to their diet in the long term.

Behavioral weight loss programs typically recommend walking as the preferred type of exercise because it is easy and requires minimal equipment. A good rule of thumb is that one mile of walking expends 100 calories; thus, 1,000 kcals can be expended by walking two miles on five days each week. More detailed energy expenditure charts that take into account current body weight and indicate calories expended in a variety of other activities are often used in behavioral programs.

Exercise Goals

In order to increase physical activity, it is important to start slowly and gradually increase the level of activity. However, an important question in the field has been how much activity to ultimately recommend. Several studies have shown that the higher the level of exercise achieved in a weight loss program, the better the weight losses and maintenance. Jakicic, Winters, Lang, and Wing (1999) showed that women who reported having done 200 minutes of physical activity at 6, 12, and 18 months as part of a behavioral weight loss program had better weight losses and maintenance than did those reporting lesser amounts. Jeffery, Wing, Sherwood, and Tate (2003) examined this experimentally by randomizing some participants to a 1,000-kcal/week goal and others to a 2,500-kcal/week goal. The higher exercise goal led to better weight losses at 12 and 18 months. Moreover, those individuals who continued to adhere to this exercise goal at 30 months achieved excellent maintenance, but few were able to maintain this high level (Tate, Jeffery, Sherwood, & Wing, 2007).

Types of Exercise

Aerobic activity, particularly walking, is usually recommended in weight loss programs. However, there has been increased interest in including at least some resistance training within these programs. Resistance training improves strength and can thus be beneficial to individuals; however, there is little evidence that resistance training increases fat loss or prevents the decrease in metabolic rate that occurs with weight loss (Hansen, Dendale, Berger, van Loon, & Meeusen, 2007).

Similarly, several studies have compared the effects of supervised exercise programs, where the participant exercises as part of a class, versus home-based or lifestyle programs (Perri, Martin, Leermakers, Sears, & Notelovitz, 1997). The two approaches appear to produce comparable initial weight losses, but long-term results are better in the home-based models. The additional time and effort required traveling to the exercise facility and the decreased flexibility in the timing of the exercise may create barriers to long-term adherence to supervised exercise.

Promoting Adherence to Exercise

Higher levels of physical activity are related to better maintenance of weight loss, so the issue becomes how best to encourage overweight individuals to adopt and maintain a higher level of physical activity. One approach may be to encourage more flexible exercise routines. Jakicic, Wing, Butler, and Robertson (1992) hypothesized that encouraging overweight women to exercise in several 10-minute bouts might be more effective than the usual 30- to 40-minute-bout prescription. In this study, all women received the same diet, the same behavioral program, and the same exercise goals. However, the long-bout group did their exercise in one 40-minute bout, whereas the short-bout group was instructed to exercise in four 10-minute bouts. Thus, members of the short-bout group could take a brief walk after each meal or whenever they found a free 10 minutes. The short-bout exercise prescription led to better exercise adherence; these subjects were more likely to exercise on any given day and completed more minutes of exercise over the course of the program. Their weight losses were also somewhat better. Interesting to researchers was that the short- and long-bout groups had comparable improvements in cardiovascular fitness.

Another way to improve exercise adherence is to focus more on the environmental cues for exercise. Jakicic, Wing, Butler, and Robertson (1999) found that providing subjects with a home treadmill led to increased physical activity and better weight losses compared to the same exercise prescriptions without the treadmills. Epstein et al. (1995), in their work with overweight children, compared the effectiveness of increasing physical activity (as done in the aforementioned studies) with the effectiveness of decreasing sedentary activities (e.g., watching TV and using computers). A treatment focusing on decreasing sedentary activities was found to produce greater weight losses, better dietary adherence, and increased liking for high-intensity activities in children.

SELF-MONITORING

The cornerstone of behavior change is self-monitoring, in which patients track their progress toward calorie, fat, and exercise goals. Patients are asked to keep a diary of their eating and exercise behaviors and are required to fill it out throughout the day, rather than retrospectively. They are instructed to list everything they eat and drink, using food labels or a book of food composition to estimate calories and/or fat. Each type of exercise is also listed, as are the time spent exercising and the number of calories expended. The patients are then taught to use the diary to evaluate their current behavior, identify problems, and select specific behaviors to target for change.

Such technologies as the Internet, PDAs, and smartphones may make the task of self-monitoring easier for patients (Burke et al., 2010). Patients are able to look up the calories in a database and save the data to an online record. Similarly, a variety of instruments that can provide objective measures of the level of physical activity is now available. These instruments may not only make self-monitoring easier but also provide a way for therapists to monitor patients' behavior in real time and provide important guidance and support (Harvey-Berino, Pintauro, Buzzell, & Gold, 2004).

GOAL SETTING

After identifying a target behavior, goal setting is used to specify the desired change. Although the overall goals for weight loss are quite general (e.g., eat 1,500 kcal/day, < 20% from fat, and exercise 1,000 kcal/week), the use of specific goals serves to break the behavior change into small, achievable steps. Thus, individuals whose diaries show they are exceeding their fat goal are more likely to succeed if they set a small, specific goal (e.g., use jam instead of margarine on toast at breakfast), rather than such a general goal as to continue to lower fat intake.

STIMULUS CONTROL

Stimulus control techniques are a powerful tool for reorganizing the environment to support the desired behaviors. Patients are taught that it is difficult to consistently make good eating and exercise choices in an environment that does not support the desired behavior. Thus, they are instructed to reduce or eliminate cues that encourage overeating and high-fat eating (e.g., do not allow chips, desserts, or other tempting foods in the house) and to make it as easy as possible to make good choices (e.g., leave exercise equipment in a highly visible area or have low-fat snacks readily available in refrigerator).

COGNITIVE TECHNIQUES

Behavioral programs also teach patients to identify and change the maladaptive thoughts and emotions that can contribute to overeating and inactivity. Patients are taught to identify dichotomous thinking ("If I can't eat healthy at every meal, I might as well not do it at all") and rationalizations ("I've had a hard day, I deserve a piece of pie") and to replace these negative thoughts with more positive self-statements. Similarly, they are taught to use problem-solving techniques to overcome the barriers to their behavior change.

SOCIAL SUPPORT

Social support is also an important determinant of long-term adherence to new eating and exercise behavior. In an interesting study, Gorin et al. (2008) showed that there is a "ripple effect" of participating in a weight loss program; not only do participants in a weight loss program lose weight but so do their spouses, even though the spouse attends no meetings. Moreover, the greater the weight loss of the participant, the greater the weight loss in the spouse. Based on such findings as this, a common treatment strategy has been to ask spouses to actually participate in the weight loss program along with the participant and to make the same changes in eating and exercise behavior. A meta-analysis of this literature showed a small positive effect of spouse involvement (Black, Gleser, & Kooyers, 1990), but results have been inconsistent.

Other researchers have begun to investigate support from a wider group, including coworkers, other participants, or friends. Wing and Jeffery (1999) compared the weight loss outcomes of participants who were recruited either as individuals or in groups of four acquaintances and then were randomly assigned to either a weight loss intervention designed to increase social support through team-building activities and group competitions or to a standard weight loss intervention. They found the best weight losses in those individuals who were recruited with friends and provided with the social support intervention. Worksite interventions that include team competitions have also been shown to improve long-term weight loss (Hennrikus & Jeffery, 1996). These data suggest that efforts to increase social support may be effective in improving both initial weight loss and long-term weight loss.

RELAPSE PREVENTION

Based on Marlatt and Gordon's relapse prevention model (1985), an effort has been made to identify specific situations that might pose problems for dieters and to determine whether coping skills are related to success in dealing with such relapse crises. Three types of high-risk situations for dieters have been identified: situations involving food cues (e.g., being in a restaurant, during a family meal), situations involving affective cues (e.g., anger, depression), and situations involving boredom or transition (e.g., watching TV). These three high-risk situations are quite similar to those identified by smokers. Moreover, performance of a coping response appears to be related to surviving the relapse crisis. Grilo, Shiffman, and Wing (1989) showed that behavioral coping strategies (e.g., leaving the room) and cognitive coping responses (e.g., devaluing the food) were equally effective in preventing lapses but that the combination of a behavioral and cognitive strategy was most effective.

Providing participants with training in relapse prevention and with continued therapist contact improves long-term weight maintenance (Perri, Shapiro, Ludwig, Twentyman, & McAdoo, 1984). Relapse prevention training was provided to one group during the last six weeks of the treatment program; these participants were taught about the process of relapse, and they practiced skills needed to identify and cope with high-risk situations and to recover from acute lapses. Then, during the first six months after treatment, half of the participants were asked to maintain weekly contact with therapists by mailing in postcards with information about their progress; receipt of the postcards was followed by a telephone call from the therapist. The group that received both relapse prevention training and continued therapist contact had significantly better weight maintenance than did any other group.

MAINTENANCE OF WEIGHT LOSS

Because relatively few participants in clinical weight loss programs are successful in losing significant amounts of weight and maintaining their weight losses long term, some researchers have begun to recruit and study individuals who have successfully lost weight and maintained the weight loss. Wing and Hill (2001) developed a national registry of individuals who have successfully lost 30 lb (regardless of method) and maintained the loss for at least a year; registry members are recruited primarily through media coverage (i.e., magazine, radio, newspaper). Although this population is not a representative sample of all successful losers, the registry provides a rare opportunity to study weight maintenance. The initial cohort of 784 individuals in the registry reported an average weight loss of 66 lb, which they had kept off for five years. Nearly all the registry members used both diet and exercise to lose weight and to maintain their weight loss (Klem, Wing, McGuire, Seagle, & Hill, 1997). Reported calorie and fat intake were low (averaging 1,380 kcal/day with 24% as fat) and exercise levels were very high (2,800 kcal/week). These data suggest the continued importance of these two behavioral strategies for long-term weight control. The successful weight loss maintainers also reported frequent self-weighing, typically daily (Butryn, Phelan, Hill, & Wing, 2007), consistency in their diet across weekdays, weekends, and holidays (Gorin, Phelan, Wing, & Hill, 2004), and low levels of TV viewing (Raynor, Phelan, Hill, & Wing, 2006). When these behaviors were not maintained over time, the risk of regaining weight was dramatically increased.

Other researchers have examined behavioral strategies that may improve weight loss maintenance. After completing an initial behavioral weight loss program, participants are randomly assigned to different treatment maintenance approaches, and the long-term results are compared. Using this type of experimental design, Perri, Nezu, Patti, and McCann (1989) showed that the most important feature was the provision of ongoing contact. Participants in 40-week programs achieved significantly greater weight losses than did those in 20-week programs, and participants who were seen more biweekly between months 6 and 18 did better than those who were not offered ongoing treatment. The nature of the treatment sessions, whether they focused on problem solving, exercise, or social support appeared less important than the ongoing contact.

More recently, Internet approaches have been examined as a way to maintain the treatment contact. In the Weight Loss Maintenance Trial (Svetkey et al., 2008), participants who had lost at least 4 kg during the initial six-month program were randomly assigned to either an interactive technology–based maintenance program, a personal contact intervention (monthly phone contacts and quarterly in-person sessions), or a minimal contact control. The in-person program produced the best long-term results, with no difference between the other two conditions.

Face-to-face contact was also most effective in STOP Regain (Wing, Tate, Gorin, Raynor, & Fava, 2006). This trial was unique in that participants were recruited after they had lost weight, either on their own or through any type of program. They were then offered a program designed to help them maintain their weight losses over the next 18 months. The program was based on self-regulation and taught participants to weigh daily and to use the information from the scale to determine if adjustments in diet and activity were needed. Those participants who were randomly assigned to receive the program through monthly face-to-face meetings had better outcomes than did those who received the program over the Internet, with the poorest results in participants in the control group.

OTHER TREATMENT OPTIONS

In recent years, there has been tremendous interest in the pharmacologic treatment of obesity (Mayer, Hocht, Puyo, & Taira, 2009). This interest is spurred by the fact that long-term results of behavioral programs continue to be disappointing. There is also increased recognition that obesity is a chronic problem, requiring chronic ongoing therapy. Thus, investigator are beginning to consider long-term (perhaps lifelong) drug treatment for obesity, as would occur with hypertension or other chronic diseases. Currently, orlistat, which is a pancreatic lipase inhibitor, is the only approved medication for weight. Sibutramine, which is a norepinephrine and serotonin reuptake inhibitor, was formerly approved by the FDA but was withdrawn from the market in 2010 due to potential excess cardiovascular risk. Orlistat appears to be modestly effective, producing weight losses of about 5%, and has relatively few risks in carefully selected patients under 65 years of age. In general, obesity medications are typically considered adjuncts to behavioral lifestyle interventions, and the combination of behavioral approaches and medications is most effective (Wadden et al., 2005).

Another treatment option, particularly for those with a BMI > 40 or a BMI > 35 with obesity-related comorbidities, is bariatric surgery. A variety of different surgical approaches have been developed to produce weight loss by either restricting the size of the stomach, creating malabsorption, or combining the two approaches. These procedures are associated with very marked weight losses, with patients losing 50% to 70% of their excess weight. Of particular note are the dramatic effects of these procedures on Type 2 diabetes. In the Swedish Obese Subject (SOS) Trial, the largest and longest trial of surgical approaches, patients in the surgical subgroup lost 20% to 30% of their body weight at years 1 to 2 (depending on the type of surgery) and maintained a weight loss of 14% to 25% of body weight at 10-year follow-up (Sjostrom et al., 2004). Surgery was associated with improvements in cardiovascular risk factors, sleep apnea, joint pain, and improved quality of life (Sjostrom et al., 2004); surgery also led to a 24% reduction in overall mortality at 10 years relative to matched controls (Sjostrom et al., 2007).

PEDIATRIC OBESITY

Even more startling than the epidemic of obesity in adults has been the dramatic increase in the prevalence of obesity in children and adolescents. Approximately 17% of children and adolescents are obese, defined as having a BMI ≥ 95% for their age and gender (Ogden, Carroll, & Flegal, 2008). Pediatric obesity is of concern for a large number of reasons (Jelalian, Hart, & Rhee, 2009). First, obesity in childhood is associated with obesity in adulthood; the older the child, the stronger the association between childhood weight status and adult weight status. Second, childhood obesity is associated with the same health consequences as adult obesity, in particular with increased risk of hypertension and diabetes. Overweight children also are more likely to have asthma and sleep apnea. Several recent studies (Baker, Olsen, & Sorensen, 2007; Franks et al., 2010) have shown that obesity in childhood is also associated with risk of coronary heart disease and premature death. The psychosocial consequences are also of concern. Overweight children and adolescents report poorer quality of life and poorer self-concept; and in some studies, they have higher rates of depression and anxiety. Many overweight adolescents report weight-related teasing and victimization (Puhl & Latner, 2007).

There are a wide variety of causes of the increasing rates of child and adolescent obesity. Clearly, genetic factors pay a large role in the development of obesity, but genetics alone cannot explain the sharp rise in obesity. It is suggested that genes and environment may interact to determine obesity. In considering putative environmental causes of obesity in children and adolescents, much attention has focused on the time spent watching television, videotapes, and videogames and on excessive calorie intake from sweetened beverages and fruit juice. Amount of television viewing and having a television in the bedroom have both been related to the development of obesity. Children who watch more hours of television report more dietary fat and higher overall calorie intake than those who watch less television; they also have lower levels of activity and fitness. Thus, TV viewing may impact body weight by influencing both sides of the energy balance equation. Robinson (1999) conducted a school-based intervention in which some third- and fourth-grade students were helped to decrease their television and videogame watching. Compared to students in control schools, those students who decreased television and video viewing had significant reductions in BMI.

The last few decades have seen a variety of other changes in diet that could also be related to the increased risk of obesity in children. These include increased frequency of soft-drink consumption, eating out, especially in fast-food restaurants, supersizing of meals, and decreased emphasis on family dinners.

Prevention of obesity in children has become a major area of interest. The majority of these programs have been conducted in schools. Although some school-based interventions have focused on changing only the diet or the level of physical activity, most have been more comprehensive in their scope. A recent review (Brown & Summerbell, 2009) suggests that about half of the comprehensive programs have demonstrated significant effects in the intervention versus control conditions, whereas others conclude that these programs have had more limited success (Birch & Ventura, 2009). Some researchers have argued that school age is too late to begin intervention (Birch & Ventura, 2009); others note that programs must include not only the school setting but also the parents and the community at large; and yet others have suggested that broader policy changes are critical (Economos & Irish-Hauser, 2007).

As with adults, the most common approach to treatment of obesity in children and adolescents is lifestyle or behavioral interventions. There are a number of excellent reviews of this literature (Jelalian & Hart, 2009; Jelalian & Saelens, 1999; Wilfley, Tibbs, et al., 2007). Many of the treatment programs target overweight or obese children ages 8 to 12; these youngsters are typically treated as a group, with some level of parent involvement (Epstein, Valoski, Wing, & McCurley, 1994). The programs focus on changing both diet and physical activity and incorporate a variety of such behavioral techniques as self-monitoring, goal setting, and contingency management. These programs produce 5% to 20% reductions in obesity, and excellent long-term outcomes have been observed. Wilfley, Stein, et al. (2007) examined maintenance of weight loss in a group given a behavioral-skills maintenance program, a group given a social-facilitation maintenance program, or a control condition. Both maintenance approaches were helpful in increasing the maintenance of weight loss in these 7- to 11-year-old children.

Behavioral interventions with adolescents have had more variable results. The role of the parent in these programs is less clear, and peer groups may play a greater role. In one study, Jelalian et al. (2010) randomized overweight and obese adolescents to group programs that included either a peer-enhanced adventure therapy or a supervised aerobic-exercise approach. Both interventions let to average reductions of 1.75 BMI units. A review of the adolescent treatment studies concludes that comprehensive programs, with diet, exercise, and behavioral components, are helpful in reducing obesity (Tsiros, Sinn, Coates, Howe, & Buckley, 2008).

CONCLUSION

This chapter has broadly reviewed obesity, with a focus on areas relevant to health psychology. Obesity has long been a focus of health psychologists because behavior plays such an important role in the etiology and treatment of this highly prevalent disorder, which is associated with poor health outcomes, including heart disease and diabetes. Although there are widely varying areas of obesity research, we have identified three key areas where attention is clearly needed: prevention, maintenance, and dissemination. The following sections touch on these important areas.

PREVENTION

There are several promising areas to pursue for the primary prevention of obesity in at-risk groups. New developments in nutrition, exercise, and behavioral science are needed to maximize prevention efforts in children and young adults. Given the high prevalence of obesity in minority populations, development and dissemination of effective interventions for underserved populations is also critical. Some church-based and culturally tailored approaches have shown promise (Thompson, Berry, & Nasir, 2009), but more research is needed to examine the effectiveness of culturally adapted weight loss approaches taking into consideration the ways in which minority populations interact with the health care system, school system, and other community settings.

The time surrounding pregnancy is another understudied and potentially powerful "teachable moment" for obesity prevention (Phelan, 2010). Ideally, efforts to promote weight control would start before pregnancy and then be carried over during pregnancy (to prevent excessive gestational weight gain) and the postpartum period (to prevent high postpartum weight retention). However, limited research has been conducted in ways to reduce prepregnancy obesity. More research has been done during pregnancy, and initial findings suggests that helping women gain the recommended amount during pregnancy through healthy eating and physical activity could make a major contribution to preventing postpartum weight retention, partiuclarly in normal-weight women (Olson, Strawderman, & Reed, 2004; Polley, Wing, & Sims, 2002). However, more randomized controlled trials with larger sample sizes are needed to identify the most effective and disemminatable interventions during pregnancy, particularly for the obese. Similarly, efforts to promote postpartum weight loss in high weight retainers have met with some success (Leermakers, Anglin, & Wing, 1998; Lovelady, Garner, Moreno, & Williams, 2000), but research is needed to target the postpartum populations most at risk, such as low-income women, and to identify innovative ways to prevent high treatment attrition, as frequently seen during postpartum interventions.

MAINTENANCE

Weight loss is clearly effective in preventing and treating a variety of health problems. Over the past several decades, our ability to help overweight and obese patients to lose weight has clearly improved. As noted in the foregoing sections, the average participant in a lifestyle intervention now typically achieves a 7 to 10 kg weight loss (or 7% to 10% of initial body weight). However, over time, there is a gradual regain of weight, with an average weight loss of 4 to 5 kg at three- to four-year follow-up. It is critical that we better understand the environmental, physiological, and psychological factors that make it difficult to maintain weight loss long term and lead to this gradual regain. Efforts to overcome these barriers with new behavioral approaches may lead to better long-term outcomes.

Dissemination

Lifestyle programs can have important health benefits, but they are still not readily available to many overweight or obese individuals. Further research is needed to determine how best to disseminate these programs more widely. Of particular interest is the role of technology in expanding the audience who could participate. Whether these programs should be covered by insurance programs is an important public health issue. Efforts are also needed to document the outcomes that participants experience in commercial weight loss programs, including both face-to-face and Internet approaches, in order to determine what role these programs can play in combating the obesity epidemic. Recent studies using such ongoing programs as available in the YMCAs (Ackermann & Marrero, 2007) show promise as ways to reach a broader audience.

It is vitally important that health psychologists continue to work with scientists and practitioners in these fields, together using a multidisciplinary approach to further understand the determinants of obesity and how best to prevent and treat this condition.

REFERENCES

Ackermann, R. T., & Marrero, D. G. (2007). Adapting the Diabetes Prevention Program lifestyle intervention for delivery in the community: The YMCA model. *Diabetes Educator, 33*(1), 69–78.

Adam, T. C., & Epel, E. S. (2007). Stress, eating and the reward system. *Physiology & Behavior, 91*(4), 449–458.

American Psychiatric Association (APA). (1994). *Diagnostic and statistical manual of mental disorders* (DSM-IV, 4th ed.). Washington, DC: American Psychiatric Press.

Atlantis, E., & Baker, M. (2008). Obesity effects on depression: Systematic review of epidemiological studies. *International Journal of Obesity (London), 32*(6), 881–891.

Baker, J. L., Olsen, L. W., & Sorensen, T. I. (2007). Childhood body-mass index and the risk of coronary heart disease in adulthood. *New England Journal of Medicine, 357*(23), 2329–2337.

Birch, L. L., & Ventura, A. K. (2009). Preventing childhood obesity: What works? *International Journal of Obesity (London), 33*(Suppl. 1), S74–S81.

Black, A. E., Coward, W. A., Cole, T. J., & Prentice, A. M. (1996). Human energy expenditure in affluent societies: An analysis of 574 doubly-labeled water measurements. *European Journal of Clinical Nutrition, 50*(2), 72–92.

Black, D. R., Gleser, L. J., & Kooyers, K. J. (1990). A meta-analytic evaluation of couples weight-loss programs. *Journal of Health Psychology, 9*(3), 330–347.

Bouchard, C., & Katzmarzyk, P. T. (2000). *Physical activity and obesity*. Champaign, IL: Human Kinetics.

Bouchard, C., Tremblay, A., Despres, J., Nadeau, A., Lupien, P. J., Theriault, G., … Fournier, G. (1990). The response to long-term overfeeding in identical twins. *New England Journal of Medicine, 322*, 1477–1482.

Bouchard, C., Tremblay, A., Despres, J. P., Theriault, G., Nadeau, A., Lupien, P. J., … Fournier, G. (1994). The response to exercise with constant energy intake in identical twins. *Obesity Research, 2*, 400–410.

Brantley, P. J., Myers, V. H., & Roy, H. J. (2005). Environmental and lifestyle influences on obesity. *Journal of the Louisiana State Medical Society, 156*, S19–S27.

Bray, G., & Bouchard, C. (1997). Genetics of human obesity: Research directions. *FASEB, 11*(12), 937–945.

Brown, T., & Summerbell, C. (2009). Systematic review of school-based interventions that focus on changing dietary intake and physical activity levels to prevent childhood obesity: An update to the obesity guidance produced by the National Institute for Health and Clinical Excellence. *Obesity Reviews, 10*(1), 110–141.

Burke, L. E., Conroy, M. B., Sereika, S. M., Elci, O. U., Styn, M. A., Acharya, S. D., … Glanz, K. (2010). The effect of electronic self-monitoring on weight loss and dietary intake: A randomized behavioral weight loss trial. *Obesity (Silver Spring), 19*, 338–344.

Butryn, M. L., Phelan, S., Hill, J. O., & Wing, R. R. (2007). Consistent self-monitoring of weight: A key component of successful weight loss maintenance. *Obesity (Silver Spring), 15*(12), 3091–3096.

Centers for Disease Control and Prevention. (2004). Trends in intake of energy and macronutrients—United States, 1971–2000. *Morbidity and Mortality Weekly Report, 53*(04), 80–82.

Christakis, N. A., & Fowler, J. H. (2007). The spread of obesity in a large social network over 32 years. *New England Journal of Medicine, 357*(4), 370–379.

Dansinger, M. L., Gleason, J. A., Griffith, J. L., Selker, H. P., & Schaefer, E. J. (2005). Comparison of the Atkins, Ornish, Weight Watchers, and Zone diets for weight loss and heart disease risk reduction: A randomized trial. *JAMA, 293*(1), 43–53.

Economos, C. D., & Irish-Hauser, S. (2007). Community interventions: A brief overview and their application to the obesity epidemic. *Journal of Law, Medics, & Ethics, 35*(1), 131–137.

Epstein, L. H., Valoski, A. M., Vara, L. S., McCurley, J., Wisniewski, L., Kalarchian, M. A., … Shrager, L. R. (1995). Effects of decreasing sedentary behavior and increasing activity on weight change in obese children. *Journal of Health Psychology, 14*(2), 109–115.

Epstein, L. H., Valoski, A., Wing, R. R., & McCurley, J. (1994). Ten-year outcomes of behavioral family-based treatment for childhood obesity. *Journal of Health Psychology, 13*(5), 373–383.

Flegal, K. M., Carroll, M. D., Kuczmarski, R. J., & Johnson, C. L. (1998). Overweight and obesity in the United States: Prevalence and trends, 1960–1994. *International Journal of Obesity and Related Metabolic Disorders, 22*(1), 39–47.

Flegal, K. M., Carroll, M. D., Ogden, C. L., & Curtin, L. R. (2010). Prevalence and trends in obesity among US adults, 1999–2008. *JAMA, 303*(3), 235–241.

Foster, G. D., Wadden, T. A., Kendall, P. C., Stunkard, A. J., & Vogt, R. A. (1996). Psychological effects of weight loss and regain: A prospective evaluation. *Journal of Consulting and Clinical Psychology, 64*(4), 752–757.

Foster, G. D., Wadden, T. A., & Vogt, R. A. (1997). Body image in obese women before, during, and after weight loss treatment. *Journal of Health Psychology, 16*(3), 226–229.

Foster, G. D., Wyatt, H. R., Hill, J. O., Makris, A. P., Rosenbaum, D. L., Brill, C., … Klein, S. (2010). Weight and metabolic outcomes after 2 years on a low-carbohydrate versus low-fat diet: A randomized trial. *Annals of Internal Medicine, 153*(3), 147–157.

Franks, P. W., Hanson, R. L., Knowler, W. C., Sievers, M. L., Bennett, P. H., & Looker, H. C. (2010). Childhood obesity, other cardiovascular risk factors, and premature death. *New England Journal of Medicine, 362*(6), 485–493.

Frayling, T. M., Timpson, N. J., Weedon, M. N., Zeggini, E., Freathy, R. M., Lindgren, C. M., … McCarthy, M. I. (2007). A common variant in the FTO gene is associated with body mass index and predisposes to childhood and adult obesity. *Science, 316*(5826), 889–894.

French, S. A., Story, M., & Jeffery, R. W. (2001). Environmental influences on eating and physical activity. *Annual Review of Public Health, 22*, 309–335.

Fujimoto, W. Y., Jablonski, K. A., Bray, G. A., Kriska, A., Barrett-Connor, E., Haffner, S., … PiSunyer, F. X. (2007). Body size and shape changes and the risk of diabetes in the diabetes prevention program. *Diabetes, 56*(6), 1680–1685.

Gao, W. (2008). Does the constellation of risk factors with and without abdominal adiposity associate with different cardiovascular mortality risk? *International Journal of Obesity (London), 32*(5), 757–762.

Gerrior, S., Bente, L., & Hiza, H. (2004). *Nutrient content of the U.S. food supply, 1909–2000: A summary report.* Washington, DC: U.S. Department of Agriculture, Center for Nutrition Policy and Promotion.

Gimble, J. M., Ptitsyn, A. A., Goh, B. C., Hebert, T., Yu, G., Wu, X., … Floyd, Z. E. (2009). Delta sleep-inducing peptide and glucocorticoid-induced leucine zipper: Potential links between circadian mechanisms and obesity? *Obesity Reviews, 10*(Suppl. 2), 46–51.

Gladis, N. M., Wadden, T. A., Vogt, R., Foster, G., Kuehnel, R. H., & Bartlett, S. J. (1998). Behavioral treatment of obese binge eaters: Do they need different care? *Journal of Psychosomatic Research, 44*, 375–384.

Gorin, A. A., Phelan, S., Wing, R. R., & Hill, J. O. (2004). Promoting long-term weight control: Does dieting consistency matter? *International Journal of Obesity and Related Metabolic Disorders, 28*(2), 278–281.

Gorin, A. A., Wing, R. R., Fava, J. L., Jakicic, J. M., Jeffery, R., West, D. S., … Dilillo, V. G. (2008). Weight loss treatment influences untreated spouses and the home environment: Evidence of a ripple effect. *International Journal of Obesity (London), 32*(11), 1678–1684.

Grilo, C. M., Shiffman, S., & Wing, R. R. (1989). Relapse crises and coping among dieters. *Journal of Consulting and Clinical Psychology, 57*(4), 488–495.

Grunstein, R. R., Stenlof, K., Hedner, J. A., Peltonen, M., Karason, K., & Sjostrom, L. (2007). Two-year reduction in sleep apnea symptoms and associated diabetes incidence after weight loss in severe obesity. *Sleep, 30*(6), 703–710.

Hansen, D., Dendale, P., Berger, J., van Loon, L. J., & Meeusen, R. (2007). The effects of exercise training on fat-mass loss in obese patients during energy intake restriction. *Sports Medicine, 37*(1), 31–46.

Hansson, L. M., Karnehed, N., Tynelius, P., & Rasmussen, F. (2009). Prejudice against obesity among 10-year-olds: A nationwide population-based study. *Acta Paediatrica, 98*(7), 1176–1182.

Harris, J. E., Hamaday, V., & Mochan, E. (1999). Osteopathic family physicians' attitudes, knowledge, and self-reported practices regarding obesity. *Journal of the American Osteopathic Association, 99*(7), 358–365.

Harvey-Berino, J., Pintauro, S., Buzzell, P., & Gold, E. C. (2004). Effect of Internet support on the long-term maintenance of weight loss. *Obesity Research, 12*(2), 320–329.

Hauner, H. (2004). [Low-carbohydrate or low-fat diet for weight loss—Which is better?]. *MMW Fortschr Med, 146*(41), 33–35, 37.

Heini, A. F., & Weinsier, R. L. (1997). Divergent trends in obesity and fat intake patterns: The American paradox. *American Journal of Medicine, 102*, 259–264.

Hennrikus, D. J., & Jeffery, R. W. (1996). Worksite intervention for weight control: A review of the literature. *American Journal of Health Promotion, 10*(6), 471–498.

Hill, J. O., Wyatt, H. R., Reed, G. W., & Peters, J. C. (2003). Obesity and the environment: Where do we go from here? *Science, 299*(7), 853–855.

Ilanne-Parikka, P., Eriksson, J. G., Lindstrom, J., Peltonen, M., Aunola, S., Hamalainen, H., … Tuomilehto, J. (2008). Effect of lifestyle intervention on the occurrence of metabolic syndrome and its components in the Finnish Diabetes Prevention Study. *Diabetes Care, 31*(4), 805–807.

Jakicic, J. M., Wing, R. R., Butler, B. A., & Robertson, R. J. (1995). Prescribing exercise in multiple short bouts versus one continuous bout: Effects on adherence, cardiorespiratory fitness, and weight loss in overweight women. *International Journal of Obesity, 19*(12), 893–901.

Jakicic, J. M., Winters, C., Lang, W., & Wing, R. R. (1999). Effects of intermittent exercise and use of home exercise equipment on adherence, weight loss, and fitness in overweight women: A randomized trial. *JAMA, 282*(16), 1554–1560.

Jeffery, R. W., Wing, R. R., Sherwood, N. E., & Tate, D. F. (2003). Physical activity and weight loss: Does prescribing higher physical activity goals improve outcome? *American Journal of Clinical Nutrition, 78*(4), 684–689.

Jeffery, R. W., Wing, R. R., Thorson, C., Burton, L. R., Raether, C., Harvey, J., & Mullen, M. (1993). Strengthening behavioral interventions for weight loss: A randomized trial of food provision and monetary incentives. *Journal of Consulting and Clinical Psychology, 61*(6), 1038–1045.

Jelalian, E., & Hart, C. N. (2009). In M. C. Roberts & Ric G. Steele (Eds.), *Handbook of pediatric psychology* (4th ed., 446–463). New York, NY: Guilford Press.

Jelalian, E., Hart, C., & Rhee, K. E. (2009). Treatment of pediatric obesity. *Medicine & Health/Rhode Island, 92*, 48–49.

Jelalian, E., Lloyd-Richardson, E. E., Mehlenbeck, R. S., Hart, C. N., Flynn-O'Brien, K., Kaplan, J., … Wing, R. R. (2010). Behavioral weight control treatment with supervised exercise or peer-enhanced adventure for overweight adolescents. *Journal of Pediatrics, 157*(6), 923–928.

Jelalian, E., & Saelens, B. E. (1999). Empirically supported treatments in pediatric psychology: Pediatric obesity. *Journal of Pediatric Psychology, 24*(3), 223–248.

Kalra, S. P., & Kalra, P. S. (2010). Neuroendocrine control of energy homeostasis: Update on new insights. *Progress in Brain Research, 181*, 17–33.

Klem, M. L., Wing, R. R., McGuire, M. T., Seagle, H. M., & Hill, J. O. (1997). A descriptive study of individuals successful at long-term maintenance of substantial weight loss. *American Journal of Clinical Nutrition, 66*, 239–246.

Knowler, W. C., Barrett-Connor, E., Fowler, S. E., Hamman, R. F., Lachin, J. M., Walker, E. A., & Nathan, D. M. (2002). Reduction in the incidence of type 2 diabetes with lifestyle intervention or metformin. *New England Journal of Medicine, 346*(6), 393–403.

Latner, J. D., & Stunkard, A. J. (2003). Getting worse: The stigmatization of obese children. *Obesity Research, 11*(3), 452–456.

Leermakers, E. A., Anglin, K., & Wing, R. R. (1998). Reducing postpartum weight retention through a correspondence intervention. *International Journal of Obesity, 22*, 1103–1109.

Levine, J. A., Eberhardt, N. L., & Jensen, M. D. (1999). Role of nonexercise activity thermogenesis in resistance to fat gain in humans. *Science, 283*(5399), 212–214.

Loos, R. J., Lindgren, C. M., Li, S., Wheeler, E., Zhao, J. H., Prokopenko, I., … Mohlke, K. L. (2008). Common variants near MC4R are associated with fat mass, weight and risk of obesity. *Nature Genetics, 40*(6), 768–775.

Lovelady, C. A., Garner, K. E., Moreno, K. L., & Williams, J. P. (2000). The effect of weight loss in overweight, lactating women on the growth of their infants. *New England Journal of Medicine, 342*(7), 449–453.

Maggio, C., & Pi-Sunyer, F. X. (1997). The prevention and treatment of obesity: Application to type 2 diabetes. *Diabetes Care, 20*(11), 1744–1766.

Marcus, M. D. (1993). Binge eating in obesity. In C. G. Fairburn & G. T. Wilson (Eds.), *Binge eating: Nature, assessment, and treatment* (pp. 77–96). New York, NY: Guilford Press.

Marlatt, G. A., & Gordon, J. R. (1985). *Relapse prevention: Maintenance strategies in addictive behavior change.* New York, NY: Guilford.

Mattes, R. D. (1997). Physiologic responses to sensory stimulation by food: Nutritional implications. *Journal of American Diet Association, 97*(4), 406–413.

Mayer, M. A., Hocht, C., Puyo, A., & Taira, C. A. (2009). Recent advances in obesity pharmacotherapy. *Current Clinical Pharmacology, 4*(1), 53–61.

McCarron, D. A., Oparil, S., Chait, A., Haynes, R. B., Kris-Etherton, P., Stern, J. S., … Pi-Sunyer, F. X. (1997). Nutritional management of cardiovascular risk factors: A randomized clinical trial. *Archives of Internal Medicine, 157*(2), 169–177.

National Task Force on the Prevention and Treatment of Obesity. (2000). Dieting and the development of eating disorders in overweight and obese adults. *Archives of Internal Medicine, 160*, 2581–2589.

NHLBI. (1998). Clinical guidelines on the identification, evaluation, and treatment of overweight and obesity in adults: The evidence report. *Obesity Research, 6*, 51S–210S.

Ogden, C. L., Carroll, M. D., & Flegal, K. M. (2008). High body mass index for age among US children and adolescents, 2003–2006. *JAMA, 299*(20), 2401–2405.

Olson, C. M., Strawderman, M. S., & Reed, R. G. (2004). Efficacy of an intervention to prevent excessive gestational weight gain. *American Journal of Obstetrics & Gynecology, 191*(2), 530–536.

Ornish, D. (2008). Weight loss with a low-carbohydrate, Mediterranean, or low-fat diet. *New England Journal of Medicine, 359*(20), 2171–2172.

Parsons, T. J., Manor, O., & Power, C. (2008). Television viewing and obesity: A prospective study in the 1958 British birth cohort. *European Journal of Clinical Nutrition, 62*(12), 1355–1363.

Pascale, R. W., Wing, R. R., Butler, B. A., Mullen, M., & Bononi, P. (1995). Effects of a behavioral weight loss program stressing calorie restriction versus calorie plus fat restriction in obese individuals with NIDDM or a family history of diabetes. *Diabetes Care, 18*(9), 1241–1248.

Perri, M. G., Martin, A. D., Leermakers, E. A., Sears, S. F., & Notelovitz, M. (1997). Effects of group- versus home-based exercise in the treatment of obesity. *Journal of Consulting and Clinical Psychology, 65*(2), 278–285.

Perri, M. G., Nezu, A. M., Patti, E. T., & McCann, K. L. (1989). Effect of length of treatment on weight loss. *Journal of Consulting and Clinical Psychology, 57*(3), 450–452.

Perri, M. G., Shapiro, R. M., Ludwig, W. W., Twentyman, C. T., & McAdoo, W. G. (1984). Maintenance strategies for the treatment of obesity: An evaluation of relapse prevention training and posttreatment contact by mail and telephone. *Journal of Consulting and Clinical Psychology, 52*(3), 404–413.

Phelan, S. (2010). Pregnancy: A "teachable moment" for weight control and obesity prevention. *American Journal of Obstetrics & Gynecology, 202*(2), 135, e131–138.

Phelan, S., Wing, R. R., Loria, C., & Lewis, C. (2010). Prevalence and predictors of weight loss maintenance in a bi-racial cohort: Results from the CARDIA Study. *American Journal of Preventative Medicine, 39*(6), 546–554.

Pi-Sunyer, X. (2009). The medical risks of obesity. *Postgraduate Medicine, 121*(6), 21–33.

Pi-Sunyer, X., Blackburn, G., Brancati, F. L., Bray, G. A., Bright, R., Clark, J. M., … Yanovski, S. Z. (2007). Reduction in weight and cardiovascular disease risk factors in individuals with type 2 diabetes: One-year results of the Look AHEAD Trial. *Diabetes Care, 30*(6), 1374–1383.

Polley, B. A., Wing, R. R., & Sims, C. J. (2002). Randomized controlled trial to prevent excessive weight gain in pregnant women. *International Journal of Obesity and Related Metabolic Disorders, 26*(11), 1494–1502.

Pronk, N. P., Wing, R. R., & Jeffery, R. W. (1994). Effects of increasing stimulus control for exercise through use of a personal trainer. Poster presented at the 15th meeting of the Society of Behavioral Medicine, Boston, MA, April 1994.

Puhl, R. M., Andreyeva, T., & Brownell, K. D. (2008). Perceptions of weight discrimination: Prevalence and comparison to race and gender discrimination in America. *International Journal of Obesity (London), 32*(6), 992–1000.

Puhl, R. M., & Heuer, C. A. (2009). The stigma of obesity: A review and update. *Obesity (Silver Spring), 17*(5), 941–964.

Puhl, R. M., & Latner, J. D. (2007). Stigma, obesity, and the health of the nation's children. *Psychological Bulletin, 133*(4), 557–580.

Puhl, R. M., Moss-Racusin, C. A., Schwartz, M. B., & Brownell, K. D. (2008). Weight stigmatization and bias reduction: Perspectives of overweight and obese adults. *Health Education Research, 23*(2), 347–358.

Ravussin, E., Valencia, M. E., Esparza, J., Bennett, P. H., & Schultz, L. O. (1994). Effects of a traditional lifestyle on obesity in Pima Indians. *Diabetes Care, 17,* 1067–1074.

Raynor, D. A., Phelan, S., Hill, J. O., & Wing, R. R. (2006). Television viewing and long-term weight maintenance: Results from the National Weight Control Registry. *Obesity (Silver Spring), 14*(10), 1816–1824.

Raynor, H. A., & Epstein, L. H. (2001). Dietary variety, energy regulation, and obesity. *Psychological Bulletin, 127*(3), 325–341.

Robinson, T. N. (1999). Reducing children's television viewing to prevent obesity: A randomized controlled trial. *JAMA, 282*(16), 1561–1567.

Rolls, B. J. (2009). The relationship between dietary energy density and energy intake. *Physiology & Behavior, 97*(5), 609–615.

Rolls, B. J., Hetherington, M., & Burley, V. J. (1988). Sensory stimulation and energy density in the development of satiety. *Physiology & Behavior, 44*(6), 727–733.

Rolls, B. J., & Shide, D. J. (1992). The influence of dietary fat on food intake and body weight. *Nutrition Reviews, 50*(10), 283–290.

Sabatti, C., Service, S. K., Hartikainen, A. L., Pouta, A., Ripatti, S., Brodsky, J., … Peltonen, L. (2009). Genome-wide association analysis of metabolic traits in a birth cohort from a founder population. *Nature Genetics, 41*(1), 35–46.

Samaha, F. F., Iqbal, N., Seshadri, P., Chicano, K. L., Daily, D. A., McGrory, J., … Stern, L. (2003). A low-carbohydrate as compared with a low-fat diet in severe obesity. *New England Journal of Medicine, 348*(21), 2074–2081.

Schlundt, D. G., Hill, J. O., Pope-Cordle, J., Arnold, D., Virts, K. L., & Katahn, M. (1993). Randomized evaluation of a low fat ad libitum carbohydrate diet for weight reduction. *International Journal of Obesity and Related Metabolic Disorders, 17*(11), 623–629.

Sjostrom, L., Lindroos, A. K., Peltonen, M., Torgerson, J., Bouchard, C., Carlsson, B., … Wedhel, H. (2004). Lifestyle, diabetes, and cardiovascular risk factors 10 years after bariatric surgery. *New England Journal of Medicine, 351*(26), 2683–2693.

Sjostrom, L., Narbro, K., Sjostrom, C. D., Karason, K., Larsson, B., Wedel, H., … Carlsson, L. M. S. (2007). Effects of bariatric surgery on mortality in Swedish obese subjects. *New England Journal of Medicine, 357*(8), 741–752.

Subak, L. L., Wing, R., West, D. S., Franklin, F., Vittinghoff, E., Creasman, J. M., … Grady, D. (2009). Weight loss to treat urinary incontinence in overweight and obese women. *New England Journal of Medicine, 360*(5), 481–490.

Svetkey, L. P., Stevens, V. J., Brantley, P. J., Appel, L. J., Hollis, J. F., Loria, C. M., … Aicher, K. (2008). Comparison of strategies for sustaining weight loss: The weight loss maintenance randomized controlled trial. *JAMA, 299*(10), 1139–1148.

Tate, D. F., Jeffery, R. W., Sherwood, N. E., & Wing, R. R. (2007). Long-term weight losses associated with prescription of higher physical activity goals. Are higher levels of physical activity protective against weight regain? *American Journal of Clinical Nutrition, 85*(4), 954–959.

Thompson, E., Berry, D., & Nasir, L. (2009). Weight management in African-Americans using church-based community interventions to prevent type 2 diabetes and cardiovascular disease. *Journal of the National Black Nurses Association, 20*(1), 59–65.

Thorleifsson, G., Walters, G. B., Gudbjartsson, D. F., Steinthorsdottir, V., Sulem, P., Helgadottir, A., … Stefansson, K. (2009). Genome-wide association yields new sequence variants at seven loci that associate with measures of obesity. *Nature Genetics, 41*(1), 18–24.

Tsiros, M. D., Sinn, N., Coates, A. M., Howe, P. R., & Buckley, J. D. (2008). Treatment of adolescent overweight and obesity. *European Journal of Pediatrics, 167*(1), 9–16.

Tucker, L. A., & Kano, M. J. (1992). Dietary fat and body fat: A multivariate study of 205 adult females. *American Journal of Clinical Nutrition, 56*(4), 616–622.

Van Loan, M. D. (2003). Body composition in disease: What can we measure and how can we measure it? *Acta Diabetologica, 40*(Suppl. 1), S154–S157.

Venditti, E. M., Wing, R. R., Jakicic, J. M., Butler, B. A., & Marcus, M. D. (1996). Weight cycling, psychological health, and binge eating in obese women. *Journal of Consulting and Clinical Psychology, 64*(2), 400–405.

Wadden, T. A., Berkowitz, R. I., Womble, L. G., Sarwer, D. B., Phelan, S., Cato, R. K., … Stunkard, A. J. (2005). Randomized trial of lifestyle modification and pharmacotherapy for obesity. *New England Journal of Medicine, 353*(20), 2111–2120.

Wadden, T. A., Foster, G. D., & Letizia, K. A. (1994). One-year behavioral treatment of obesity: Comparison of moderate and severe caloric restriction and the effects of weight maintenance therapy. *Journal of Consulting and Clinical Psychology, 62*(1), 165–171.

Wadden, T. A., & Frey, D. L. (1997). A multicenter evaluation of a proprietary weight loss program for the treatment of marked obesity: A five-year follow-up. *International Journal of Eating Disorders, 22*(2), 203–212.

Wadden, T. A., & Stunkard, A. J. (1993). Psychosocial consequences of obesity and dieting: Research and clinical findings. In A. J. Stunkard & T. A. Wadden (Eds.), *Obesity: Theory and therapy* (2nd ed., pp. 163–179). New York, NY: Raven Press.

Wadden, T. A., Stunkard, A. J., & Brownell, K. D. (1983). Very low calorie diets: Their efficacy, safety, and future. *Annals of Internal Medicine, 99*(5), 675–684.

Wannamethee, S. G., Shaper, A. G., & Whincup, P. H. (2006). Modifiable lifestyle factors and the metabolic syndrome in older men: Effects of lifestyle changes. *Journal of the American Geriatrics Society, 54*(12), 1909–1914.

Wansink, B. (2010). From mindless eating to mindlessly eating better. *Physiology & Behavior, 100*, 454–463.

Wardle, J. (2007). Eating behaviour and obesity. *Obesity Reviews, 8*(Suppl. 1), 73–75.

Wardle, J., Steptoe, A., Oliver, G., & Lipsey, Z. (2000). Stress, dietary restraint and food intake. *Journal of Psychosomatic Research, 48*(2), 195–202.

Weinsier, R. L., Hunter, G. R., Heine, A. F., Goran, M. I., & Sell, S. M. (1998). The etiologoy of obesity: Relative contribution of metabolic factors, diet, and physical activity. *American Journal of Medicine, 105*, 145–150.

Wilfley, D. E., Stein, R. I., Saelens, B. E., Mockus, D. S., Matt, G. E., Hayden-Wade, H. A., … Epstein, L. H. (2007). Efficacy of maintenance treatment approaches for childhood overweight: A randomized controlled trial. *JAMA, 298*(14), 1661–1673.

Wilfley, D. E., Tibbs, T. L., Van Buren, D. J., Reach, K. P., Walker, M. S., & Epstein, L. H. (2007). Lifestyle interventions in the treatment of childhood overweight: A meta-analytic review of randomized controlled trials. *Journal of Health Psychology, 26*(5), 521–532.

Willer, C. J., Speliotes, E. K., Loos, R. J., Li, S., Lindgren, C. M., Heid, I. M., … Hirschhorn, J. N. (2009). Six new loci associated with body mass index highlight a neuronal influence on body weight regulation. *Nature Genetics, 41*(1), 25–34.

Wing, R. R. (2010). Long-term effects of a lifestyle intervention on weight and cardiovascular risk factors in individuals with type 2 diabetes mellitus: Four-year results of the Look AHEAD Trial. *Archives of Internal Medicine, 170*(17), 1566–1575.

Wing, R. R., Blair, E. H., Bononi, P., Marcus, M. D., Watanabe, R., & Bergman, R. N. (1994). Caloric restriction per se is a significant factor in improvements in glycemic control and insulin sensitivity during weight loss in obese NIDDM patients. *Diabetes Care, 17*(1), 30–36.

Wing, R. R., & Hill, J. O. (2001). Successful weight loss maintenance. *Annual Review of Nutrition, 21*, 323–341.

Wing, R. R., & Jeffery, R. W. (1999). Benefits of recruiting participants with friends and increasing social support for weight loss and maintenance. *Journal of Consulting and Clinical Psychology, 67*(1), 132–138.

Wing, R. R., Jeffery, R. W., Burton, L. R., Thorson, C., Nissinoff, K. S., & Baxter, J. E. (1996). Food provision vs structured meal plans in the behavioral treatment of obesity. *International Journal of Obesity and Related Metabolic Disorders, 20*(1), 56–62.

Wing, R. R., Tate, D. F., Gorin, A., Raynor, H. A., & Fava, J. L. (2006). A self-regulation program for maintenance of weight loss. *New England Journal of Medicine, 346*, 393–403.

Wycherley, T. P., Brinkworth, G. D., Keogh, J. B., Noakes, M., Buckley, J. D., & Clifton, P. M. (2010). Long-term effects of weight loss with a very low carbohydrate and low fat diet on vascular function in overweight and obese patients. *Journal of Internal Medicine, 267*(5), 452–461.

16 Health-Enhancing Physical Activity

Glenn S. Brassington
Sonoma State University and Stanford University School of Medicine

Eric B. Hekler, Zachary Cohen, and Abby C. King
Stanford University School of Medicine

> Lack of activity destroys the good condition of every human being, while movement and methodical physical exercise save it and preserve it.
>
> **—Plato**

Physical activity holds great promise for improving the quality of life of virtually every person in the world, regardless of age, sex, race, or health status. Over the past 40 years, researchers from a variety of academic disciplines (e.g., public health, exercise science, and psychology) have provided data on the powerful positive effects of physical activity on every system in the human body (e.g., cardiovascular, respiratory, immune, and muscular) and the detrimental health effects of inactivity. In this chapter, we will discuss the current research on key topics related to the health-enhancing effects of physical activity and the most promising factors associated with its promotion. To do this, our chapter is divided into six sections: (1) epidemiology of and national guidelines for health-enhancing physical activity (HEPA), (2) physical and mental effects of HEPA, (3) using psychosocial variables to promote HEPA, (4) using state-of-the-art technology to promote HEPA, (5) effects of built environment on HEPA, and (6) conclusions and future directions. The breadth of research in the field of physical activity precludes the possibility of exhaustively reviewing each of the topics in this chapter. Hence, a greater emphasis is placed on the use of technology and the built environments to promote HEPA because these areas hold great promise for increasing HEPA in the United States as well as internationally.

EPIDEMIOLOGY OF AND NATIONAL GUIDELINES FOR HEPA

A number of terms have been used to define physical activity in the public health literature. The terms most relevant to this chapter are *physical activity, exercise*, and *health-enhancing physical activity*. The 2008 U.S. Department of Health and Human Services (USDHHS) *Physical Activity Guidelines Report* (Physical Activity Guidelines Committee, 2008) uses definitions of physical activity and exercise previously described by Casperson, Powell, and Christenson (1985) and used in the 1996 *Surgeon General's Report on Physical Activity* (U.S. Department of Health and Human Services, 1996):

> Physical activity is any bodily movement produced by the contraction of skeletal muscle that increases energy expenditure above a basal level.... Physical activity can be categorized according to mode, intensity, and purpose.... Exercise is a subcategory of physical activity that is planned, structured, repetitive and purposive in the sense that the improvement or maintenance of one or more components of physical fitness is the objective. (Physical Activity Guidelines Committee, 2008, p. C-1)

Health-enhancing physical activity, or HEPA, as mentioned earlier, is a more current term being used by public health researchers to describe any physical activity sufficient to enhance health. Common categorizations of physical activity by purpose include occupational, utilitarian (i.e., to accomplish daily tasks), recreational, and fitness- or sport-oriented (Marttila, Laitakari, Nupponen, Miilunpalo, & Paronen, 1998). Several types of physical activity have been categorized by their effects on the human body; among these categories are increased flexibility, increased muscular strength, increased aerobic capacity, and mind-body integration, the latter a goal of tai chi and yoga training. Although it may seem that being inactive is simply at the low end of the continuum of being physically active, recent research suggests that inactivity (e.g., sitting for long periods of time) is independently associated with risk of such diseases as diabetes (Ford & Li, 2006) and should be considered as a risk factor for disease (Hamilton, Hamilton, & Zderic, 2007; Owen, Bauman, & Brown, 2009; Salmon, Dunstan, & Owen, 2008) and as a target of intervention development in its own right (Church & Blair, 2009).

Government agencies have been monitoring physical activity trends in the United States for several decades. The majority of available data come from four national surveys and capture participation in primarily structured, leisure-time activities in high school students and adults; however, no survey has consistently quantified such overall daily physical activity as may be accrued at work or home or consistently collected physical activity in very young children. Notably, in recent years the National Health and Nutrition Examination Survey (NHANES) has collected objective physical activity data by means of accelerometry from a representative sample of the U.S. population ages 6 years and older that better captures physical activity across the day (Troiano et al., 2008). These data spotlight the generally low levels of daily physical activity obtained regularly by a significant proportion of the U.S. population (Troiano et al., 2008). Information about each of these government surveys can be found on their respective Web sites: Behavioral Risk Factor Surveillance System (BRFSS; http://www.cdc.gov/brfss), Youth Risk Behavior Surveillance System (YRBSS; http://www.cdc.gov/HealthyYouth/yrbs), National Health and Nutrition Examination Survey (NHANES; http://www.cdc.gov/nchs/nhanes.htm), and National Health Interview Survey (NHIS; http://www.cdc.gov/nchs/nhis.htm).

The national surveillance data collected over the past 20 years indicate that a substantial proportion of U.S. children and adults are not meeting national physical activity recommendations (Centers for Disease Control and Prevention, 2007; U.S. Department of Health and Human Services, 1996), with 20% to 30% of adults reporting no leisure-time physical activity (Centers for Disease Control and Prevention, 2005). According to these survey data, levels of physical activity are generally higher in younger adults, men, non-Hispanic Whites, and high school graduates.

In relation to youth, it was estimated in 2005 that only 35.8% of high school students meet the national guidelines of 60 minutes of moderate physical activity five days per week (Centers for Disease Contro and Prevention, 2007). As with adults, boys are generally more likely to meet the guidelines than girls (43.8% versus 27.8%), and White non-Hispanic students are more likely to meet the guidelines than are their underrepresented peers. Approximately 10% of high school students have reported not participating in any moderate physical activity (Centers for Disease Control and Prevention, 2008).

As noted, recent attempts to quantify population physical activity levels using objective assessment tools (accelerometry) have occurred in children, adolescents, and adults (Troiano et al., 2008). Based on accelerometry data, Troiano and colleagues (2008) reported recently that men are generally more active than women and that physical activity levels are lower with increasing age, beginning in adolescents, with 42% of children, 8% of adolescents, and 5% of adults obtaining 30 minutes per day of moderate activity. These accelerometer-measured physical activity data suggest that levels of physical activity may be lower than previously thought based on self-report survey data, although some researchers have pointed out that accelerometry data may provide an overly conservative estimate of true populationwide physical activity levels. Even so, the authors suggest that care be taken when interpreting self-report data about absolute levels of HEPA.

Inactivity is associated with increased chronic disease, decreased quality of life, and great economic costs (DeVol et al., 2007; Pratt, Macera, & Wang, 2000). It is estimated that the economic costs of inactivity are approximately $76 billion (in year 2000 dollars) per year (Pratt, et al., 2000) and that if 10% of sedentary adults began a regular walking program, $5.6 billion (in 1994 dollars) could be saved from coronary heart disease costs alone (Jones & Eaton, 1994). Thus, it has been increasingly argued that investments in populationwide approaches to physical activity promotion are strongly indicated (Fulton et al., 2009).

The U.S. government published its first formal set of physical activity guidelines for Americans in 2008 (Physical Activity Guidelines Committee, 2008). The 683-page report can be found at http://www.health.gov/paguidelines/default.aspx. A summary of the key recommendations is contained in Table 16.1.

The guidelines encourage every American to engage in at least moderate-intensity physical activity on most days of the week and, if physical disability precludes this level of exercise, then to be as physically active as possible while avoiding extensive periods of inactivity. Although the basic recommendations are associated with substantial health benefits, additional improvements can be achieved with greater participation, given that there is a dose-response effect (Haskell, Blair, & Hill, 2009). The guidelines also indicate that aerobic physical activity (e.g., jogging, brisk walking, bicycling, or swimming, which all involve repetitive movement of large muscles groups) obtained in as low as 10-minute bouts provides substantial health benefits (DeBusk, Hakansson, Sheehan, & Haskell, 1990; Murphy, Blair, & Murtagh, 2009).

TABLE 16.1
Physical Activity Guidelines for Americans

Age Group	Physical Activity Associated With Substantial Health Benefits	Physical Activity Associated With Additional Health Benefits
Children and adolescents (6–17 yrs)	• Engage daily in 60 minutes or more of moderate- or vigorous-intensity aerobic physical activity. • As part of their daily physical activity, do 3 days per week of muscle- and bone-strengthening activity.	
Adults (18–65 yrs)	• Engage in150 minutes of moderate-intensity or 75 minutes of high-intensity aerobic physical activity per week or an equivalent combination of both in episodes of at least 10 minutes, preferably spread throughout the week. • Do muscle-strengthening activities involving all muscle groups on 2 or more days per week.	• Engage in 300 minutes of moderate-intensity or 150 minutes of vigorous-intensity aerobic activity per week or an equivalent combination of both.
Older adults (65+ yrs)	• Follow adult guidelines. • If not possible, be as active as possible. • Engage in physical activity that maintains or improves balance. • Avoid inactivity.	
People with disabilities	• Follow adult guidelines. • If not possible, be as active as possible. • Avoid inactivity.	

Source: Adapted from U.S. Department of Health and Human Services, Physical Activity Guidelines Committee, 2008.

PHYSICAL AND MENTAL HEALTH EFFECTS OF HEPA

The physical and mental health effects of HEPA were recently assessed by an advisory committee of scientists appointed by the USDHHS secretary as part of developing the national physical activity guidelines (Physical Activity Guidelines Committee, 2008). The task of the committee was to thoroughly review the scientific literature in order to provide federal guidelines on physical activity, fitness, and health for Americans. The advisory committee focused on studies examining the relationship between physical activity and nine health-related outcomes: all-cause mortality, cardiorespiratory health, metabolic health, energy balance, musculoskeletal health, functional health, cancer, and mental health. A summary of the central findings from the USDHHS's 2008 *Advisory Committee Report* is provided in Table 16.2 (physical health) and Table 16.3 (mental health); the findings demonstrate the positive benefits of regular physical activity across a range of physical and mental health conditions and diseases. Also, see Dunn and Jewell (2010) for a more recent review of the effects of physical activity on mental health.

The mechanisms by which physical activity decreases morbidity and increases mortality (e.g., insulin resistance in diabetes) are beginning to be understood and involve a very complex set of interactions among numerous systems of the human body ranging from gene expression to overall organ functioning. The primary mechanisms currently being explored to explain the physical health effects of physical activity involve organ functioning, immune system responses, metabolism, inflammation, oxidation, muscular-skeletal strength, and gene expression (Alexander, 2010; Handschin & Spiegelman, 2008; Kemi & Wisloff, 2010). For example, physical activity may protect against cardiovascular disease by preserving heart function through increased cardiac capacity, improved endothelial cell activity, reduced coronary artery thickening, and decreased inflammation (Ashrafian, Frenneaux, & Opie 2007; Handschin & Spiegelman, 2008). The primary mechanisms being explored to explain mental health effects of physical activity are less well understood than those for physical health and include neurotransmitter, endorphin, neurotrophic, thermogenic, distraction, cognitive, affective, and allostatic load. For example, depression may be decreased and memory enhanced by physical activity's ability to increase the brain-derived neurotrophic factor responsible for neurogenesis and modulating several brain neurotransmitters (Sylvia, Ametrano, & Nierenberg, 2010). Physical activity may at the same time reduce allostatic load (i.e., the physiological burden of stress) by making one less reactive to stressful events (Sylvia et al., 2010). For further reviews of mechanisms thought to explain the relationship between exercise and mental health, see Dishman et al. (2006), Dishman and O'Connor (2009), and van Praag (2009).

USING PSYCHOSOCIAL VARIABLES TO PROMOTE HEPA

Over the past three decades, researchers have examined the relationships among a large number of variables in the search for factors related to participation in physical activity (Bauman, Sallis, Dwewaltowski, & Owen, 2002; Dishman & Sallis, 1994). Determinants research in this field has increasingly benefited from a multilevel social ecological perspective (Sallis & Owen, 1997). These variables are demographic (e.g., age, gender, ethnicity, education, income, employment status, marital status), biological (e.g., health status, body weight), cognitive/affective (e.g., self-efficacy, health beliefs, depressive symptoms), social (e.g., modeling of physical activity, family and friend support), behavioral (e.g., time management, smoking status), and environmental (e.g., access to facilities, neighborhoods where one can safely walk, climate). Table 16.4 provides a summary of the evidence for the association of each variable with HEPA, whether a particular variable can be changed by health promotion interventions, and whether changing a particular variable is associated with changes in HEPA.

In addition to exploring the associations between physical activity and such variables, researchers have applied a range of psychological theories, originally developed for other areas, which have incorporated a number of these variables in an attempt to explain or predict participation

TABLE 16.2
Association Between Physical Activity and Physical Health Outcomes

Physical Health Outcome	Conclusions
All-cause mortality	• Strong support exists for an inverse association between physical activity and all-cause mortality. • There is a 30% decreased risk. • Effects observed in the United States and abroad. • Effect are not moderated by age, ethnicity, or disability.
Cardiorespiratory health	• Strong support exists for an inverse association between physical activity and coronary heart disease and cardiovascular disease morbidity and mortality. • As compared to being sedentary, moderate activity is associated with 20% lower risk, whereas higher activity or intensity is associated with 30% lower risk. • Effects are not moderated by age, race, or ethnicity.
Metabolic health	• Regular physical activity is associated with reduced risk of syndrome. • Regular physical activity is associated with significantly decreased risk of developing Type 2 diabetes. • Insufficient data exists to determine how much physical activity is needed to achieve these effects. • Insufficient data exists to determine whether physical activity prevents diabetes in African American, Hispanic, and Asian groups. • There is strong support for physical activity's role in reducing risk of cardiovascular events and mortality in Type 2 diabetics. • Preliminary data suggest that physical activity may prevent diabetic neuropathy.
Energy balance	• Regular participation in physical activity (150 min/week) is associated with weight stability. • Regular participation in physical activity (350 min/week) is associated with preventing weight regain following weight loss. • Insufficient data exist to determine whether these effects differ by age, sex, and ethnicity.
Musculoskeletal health	• Physical activity can increase or reduce the loss of bone mineral density in spine and hip regions of the body by about 1%–2% compared to sedentary control groups over a one-year period. • Physical activity is inversely associated with risk of fractures of the femur, with greater protection afforded at higher levels of activity. • There is sparse evidence that physical activity may reduce risk of hip and knee osteoarthritis. • Aerobic and strengthening physical activity do not exacerbate or worsen osteoarthritis or rheumatic conditions. • Strength-training physical activities can preserve and increase skeletal muscle mass, strength, and power.
Functional health	• Strong observational evidence indicates that physical activity is associated with a 30% reduced risk of functional limitations in midlife and older adults. • Older adults with functional limitations can improve their functional ability with physical activity. • Clear evidence exists that physical activity can decrease risk of falls but not injurious falls. Physical activity interventions that include balance training and muscle strengthening such as tai chi may provide protection from falls.
Cancer	• Strong observational evidence indicates that moderate physical activity is associated with a 30% reduced risk of colon cancer and a 20% to 40% reduced risk of breast cancer. • Active people have a reduced risk of lung (20%), endometrial (30%), and ovarian (20%) cancers compared to sedentary people. • Randomized controlled trials (RCT) data indicated that physical activity is associated with markers of cancer risk (e.g., sex hormones, insulin, and cytokines). • Support was not found for prostate or rectal cancers.

Source: Adapted from U.S. Department of Health and Human Services, Physical Activity Guidelines Committee, 2008.

TABLE 16.3
Association Between Physical Activity and Mental Health Outcomes

Mental Health Effects	Conclusions
Depression	• There is strong evidence that regular physical activity reduces the risk of developing symptoms of depression and major depressive disorder. • Randomized controlled trial (RCT) data indicated that physical activity programs reduce symptoms of depression in people with a diagnosis of depression, healthy adults, and medical patients.
Anxiety	• Physical activity is associated with reduce risk of developing anxiety symptoms and disorders. • RCT data indicated that physical activity programs reduce symptoms of anxiety in anxiety disorder patients.
Distress and well-being	• Prospective cohort study data indicated a small-to-moderate association between physical activity and feelings of distress and enhanced well-being. • RCT data indicated that physical activity has a small impact on feelings of distress and enhanced well-being comparable to placebo control conditions.
Chronic fatigue	• Prospective population-based cohort studies reported that physical activity is associated with a reduced risk of experiencing feelings of fatigue or low energy. • Five relatively small RCTs reported a positive effect of exercise training on symptoms of chronic fatigue syndrome.
Self-esteem	• Meta-analysis of 50 RCTs (mostly small sample sizes) indicated a 0.25 SD average increase in self-esteem after participating a variety of exercises.
Cognitive function and dementia	• Prospective cohort study data indicated that participating in physical activity delays the onset of dementia and the cognitive decline associated with aging. • RCT data indicated that physical activity improves cognitive function and reduced symptoms of dementia in older adults and people with Alzheimer's disease or other dementias.
Sleep	• Participating in regular physical activity improves symptoms of poor sleep and sleep quality.

Source: Adapted from U.S. Department of Health and Human Services, Physical Activity Guidelines Committee, 2008.

in physical activity. To date, the major theories applied to physical activity behavior in the scientific literature include theory of reasoned action (Hausenblas, Carron, & Mack, 1997), theory of planned behavior (Ajzen, 1985), health belief model (Janz & Becker, 1984), transtheoretical model (Prochaska & DiClemente, 1984), social cognitive theory (Bandura, 1997, 2001), self-determination theory (Wilson, 2008), and control theory (Carver & Scheier, 1981). Unfortunately, even after three decades of research, these theories have changed little and have typically been found to explain only a small percentage of the variability in physical activity behavior (Weinstein & Rothman, 2005). This lack of success may be attributable to the ineffectiveness of the theories themselves or to the methods (e.g., assessments and interventions) used to test the theories. A suggested remedy for this lack of progress may be to develop more explicit and detailed methods for testing theories. Michie and Prestwich (2010) recently proposed a systematic method for evaluating how well theories are being tested in intervention studies to promote health behavior change. Their theory coding scheme contains 19 items (e.g., theory/model of behavior mentioned, theory/predictors used to tailor intervention techniques, and all theory-relevant constructs/predictors are explicitly linked to at least one intervention technique) designed to assess how well a theory has been applied to developing and evaluating behavior change interventions. It remains to be seen whether such systematic coding schemes provide the type of heuristic that can help to advance theory building and testing in this, as well as other, health behavior fields.

TABLE 16.4
Variables Associated With Physical Activity Participation

Variable	Association With Theory	Correlation With Physical Activity	Change Associated With Intervention	Change Associated With Physical Activity
		Demographics		
Age	—	– –	—	—
Blue-collar occupation	—	–	—	—
Childlessness	—	+	—	—
Education	—	++	—	—
Gender (male)	—	++	—	—
Gender (female)	—	++	—	—
High risk for heart disease	—	–	—	—
Income/SES	—	++	—	—
Injury history	SCT	+	—	—
Marital status	—	–	—	—
Overweight or obesity	—	00	—	—
Race/ethnicity (non-White)	—	– –	—	—
		Psychological, cognitive, and emotional factors		
Attitudes	HBM, TPB	0	+	+
Barriers to physical activities (PA): Cons	HBM, TPB, TTM	– –	+	—
Control over PA	TPB	+	—	—
Enjoyment of PA	SCT	++	+	—
Outcome expectations	SCT, TTM	++	+	+
Health locus of control	SDT	0	—	—
Intention to PA	TPB	++	+	+
Knowledge of health & PA	HBM	00	+	+
Lack of time	—	–	—	—
Mood disturbance	—	– –	+	—
Normative beliefs	TPB	00	—	—
Perceived health and fitness	—	++	++	++
Dispositional variables	—	+	—	—
Perceived competence	SDT	+	+	—
Autonomy	SDT	+	—	—
Poor body image	—	—	+	—
Psychological health	—	+	—	—
Self-efficacy	SCT, TPB, TTM	++	++	++
Self-motivation	—	++	—	—
Self-schemata for exercise	—	++	—	—
Motivational processes of change	TTM	++	++	++
Stages of change	TTM	—	++	—
Perceived stress		+	+	+
Susceptibility to illness/ seriousness of illness	HBM	00	—	—
Value of exercise outcomes	TPB	+	+	+

(Continued)

TABLE 16.4 (Continued)
Variables Associated With Physical Activity Participation

Variable	Association With Theory	Correlation With Physical Activity	Change Associated With Intervention	Change Associated With Physical Activity
Behavioral attributes and skills				
Activity history during childhood	—	00	—	—
Activity history during adulthood	SCT	++	—	—
Alcohol	—	0	—	—
Dietary habits	—	++	—	—
Past exercise program	—	+	—	—
Motivational processes of change	TTM	++	++	+
School sports	—	00	—	—
Skills for coping with barriers	SCT, TTM	+	—	—
Smoking	—	00	—	—
Sports media use	—	0	—	—
Type A behavior pattern	—	+	—	—
Decision balance sheet	TTM	+	+	+
Social and cultural factors				
Exercise models	SCT	0	—	—
Past family influences	SCT	0	—	—
Physician influence	SCT	++	+	+
Social isolation	—	–	—	—
Social support from friends & peers	SCT	++	++	+
Social support from spouse & family	SCT	++	++	+
Physical environment				
Access to facilities: actual	Eco	+	—	—
Access to facilities: perceived	Eco	00	—	—
Climate or season	Eco	– –	—	—
Cost of program	SCT, Eco	0	—	—

Source: Adapted from Brassington, G. S. and King, A. C., in *Health Enhancing Physical Activity*, 321–426, Meyer & Meyer Sport, New York, NY, 2004; and Bauman, A., Sallis, J. F., Dwewaltowski, D. A., and Owen, N., *American Journal of Preventive Medicine*, 23, 2, 5–14, 2002.

++, repeated positive association; +, weak or mixed evidence of positive association; 00, repeatedly documented lack of association; 0, weak or mixed evidence of no association; – –, repeatedly documented negative association; –, weak or mixed evidence of negative association; —, no data available; HBM, health beliefs model; TPB, theory of planned behavior; TTM, transtheoretical model; SCT, social cognitive theory; SDT, self-determination theory; Eco, ecological model.

Intervention programs directed toward individual behavior change based on the cognitive, behavioral, and social psychological theories described in the foregoing discussion have generally result in a 10%–25% increase in the amount of physical activity being performed by participants (Dishman & Buckworth, 1996; Marcus et al., 2000). In addition to these behavioral and social areas of influence, research in the field has also targeted informational efforts as well as environmental and policy approaches to physical activity promotion. The U.S. Task Force on Community Preventive Service (Task Force), under the auspices of the Centers for Disease Control and Prevention (CDC), conducted a systematic review of the effectiveness of intervention research in these three areas (Kahn et al., 2002). The results will be briefly discussed later.

Setting-specific and broader scale informational approaches are thought to increase HEPA by motivating and enabling people to change their behavior through applying relevant contextual information and resources as well as correcting misconceptions related to physical activity. These interventions generally include information about the health benefits of physical activity as well as challenging negative attitudes. Simple informational approaches have generally been tested by means of "point-of-decision" prompts (e.g., signs posted encouraging the use of stairs); communitywide mass media education campaigns, conducted through television, radio, newspapers, direct mailing, and trailers in movie theaters, directed to a general audience, and often combined with some type of social support (e.g., self-help groups, risk-factor screening); and classroom-based health education that provides students with skills for making rational decisions about health behaviors. The Task Force found strong support for the effectiveness of point-of-decision prompts and communitywide mass media campaigns but inconsistent results among studies for classroom-based health education focused on giving children information about the benefits of physical activity (Kahn et al., 2002).

Behavioral and social approaches focus on teaching behavioral management skills and providing social support for physical activity. These interventions may involve group meetings and facilitate involvement and support by family and friends. Of the interventions reviewed, school-based physical education enhancements increased physical activity. In contrast, classroom-based health instruction focused on reducing the use of television and video games and, though efficacious in maintaining healthful weight among youth, appeared in general to have less of a direct effect on physical activity levels. In terms of social support, strong evidence was found to support the positive impacts of community-based social support (e.g., through use of buddy systems and similar networks), but not necessarily family support enhancements on increasing physical activity. Also found to be effective were individually adapted health behavior change programs that utilized behavioral modification and related strategies that built behavioral skills (Kahn et al., 2002). Such individually adapted programs have been shown to be delivered successfully through a range of delivery channels and sources, including face-to-face and telephone contact, print services, interactive voice response systems, the Internet, and trained volunteers (Beaudoin, Fernandez, Wall, & Farley, 2007; King et al., 2007; King, Satariano, Marti, & Zhu, 2008; Marcus, Ciccolo, & Sciamanna, 2009).

Environmental and policy approaches focus on creating opportunities to engage in physical activity by modifying the built environment. Much of the research in this area remains observational, with relatively few systematic attempts to evaluate how changes in the built environment impact levels of physical activity. This limitation notwithstanding, the Task Force reported that the available evidence supports the potential effectiveness of creating and enhancing access to places for physical activity combined with informational outreach activities (Kahn et al., 2002). The Task Force has published a more extensive report exclusively on environmental and policy approaches focused on transportation policy, infrastructure changed to promote nonmotorized transit, and urban planning (Task Force on Community Preventive Services, 2002), which will be discussed in a later section of the chapter dedicated to the environment and physical activity.

A relatively small number of studies have examined such interventions in underrepresented populations (Pekmezi & Jennings, 2009). Pekmezi and Jennings (2009) suggest that point-of-decision prompts might be especially relevant to African Americans because they report using the stairs less frequently than do European Americans (Brownell, Stunkard, & Albaum, 1980). However, African Americans do not appear to respond in the same way as European Americans do to generic signs encouraging stair use. In two studies, generic "Try the stairs" signs were associated with lower levels of stair use among African Americans after the signs were put in place, ranging from 2%

to 17% (Andersen, Franckowiak, Snyder, Bartlett, & Fontaine, 1998; Andersen et al., 2006). After their first point-of-decision study, Andersen et al. (2006) conducted a focus group with African Americans to determine what type of message this group would find most motivating. The group members reported that they would find seeing a fit black role model motivating. They also reported that not having enough time was the biggest barrier they faced to participating in physical activity. Hence, a new culturally relevant sign was created containing a fit African American woman and the words "No time for exercise? Try the stairs." This sign increased stair use from 10.3% to 16.4% ($N = 8,477$). The results from this investigation provide support for the utility of community participatory approaches in developing contextually appropriate interventions for specific target audiences (Horowitz, Robinson, & Seifer, 2009).

Mass media campaigns that have been evaluated using quasi-experimental designs have also been shown to be potentially useful intervention tools with African Americans (Beaudoin et al., 2007). The campaign undertaken by Beaudoin et al. (2007) involved advertising with African American characters in mainstream social situations and encouraged fitting physical activity into existing daily activities. This campaign resulted in improved attitudes about physical activity but not increased physical activity behavior. Communitywide neighborhood campaigns have been conducted with African Americans and have shown increases in physical activity behavior (Plescia, Herrick, & Chavis, 2008). For example, the Charlotte REACH (Racial and Ethnic Approaches to Community Health) Project (Plescia et al., 2008) was implemented in 14 neighborhoods in a predominantly (89%) African American region of Charlotte, North Carolina. The campaign significantly increased physical activity from pre- to posttest by developing a community coalition and health center, lay health advisor program, and community environmental change strategies (e.g., extending YMCA physical activity programs into the local community).

Individually adapted health behavior change programs (Pekmezi et al., 2009) and social support interventions have shown some success in increasing physical activity with African American (Yancey, Lewis, et al., 2006; Yancey, McCarthy, et al., 2006) and Latino adults (Clarke et al., 2007; Hovell et al., 2008; Larkey, 2006). The authors recommend that such interventions be tailored to the cultural preferences and beliefs of the target group in order to avoid delivering interventions that are not effective in these communities. It is suggested that focus groups and other types of formative evaluation be conducted with potential participants before designing and implementing intervention (Horowitz et al., 2009).

Another group of researchers (Abraham & Michie, 2008) has been identifying and evaluating a taxonomy of behavior change techniques derived from the transtheoretical model (Prochaska, DiClemente, & Norcross, 1992), interventions to reduce weight gain (Hardeman, Griffin, Johnston, Kinmonth, & Wareham, 2000), and a meta-analysis of interventions to increase physical activity (Conn, Valentine, & Cooper, 2002). Abraham and Michie (2008) conducted three systematic reviews of interventions designed to increase physical activity in order to identify the behavior change techniques used in the interventions. They identified 26 discrete techniques that were used to increase physical activity. Examples of the techniques are as follows: Provide general information, set graded tasks, model or demonstrate behavior, prompt review of goals, prompt practice, plan social support for change, and time management. Subsequently, the authors and their colleagues assessed the effectiveness of all behavior change techniques used in a sample of 101 health behavior intervention studies using metaregression analysis (Michie, Abraham, Whittington, McAteer, & Gupta, 2009). The overall effect size for the interventions was 0.32. Their data indicate that 60% of the interventions prompted intention formation, 50% provided feedback on performance, 22% prompted specific goal setting, and 16% prompted review of behavioral goals. Overall, the most effective health behavior change interventions included self-monitoring combined with at least one of four other self-regulatory techniques derived from control theory (i.e., prompt intention formation, prompt specific goal setting, provide feedback on performance, prompt self-monitoring of behavior, prompt review of behavioral goals). The continued development and evaluation of the body of evidence in this manner may spur advances in theory-based intervention development in the field.

USING STATE-OF-THE-ART TECHNOLOGIES TO PROMOTE HEPA

Technology-based interventions for physical activity promotion—that is, interventions that utilize such communication technologies as computers, the Internet, automated telephone services, personal digital assistants (PDAs), and mobile telephones—have become a popular area of research (Fjeldsoe, Marshall, & Miller, 2009; Krishna, Boren, & Balas, 2009; Marcus et al., 2009; Neville, O'Hara, & Milat, 2009; Portnoy, Scott-Sheldon, Johnson, & Carey, 2008). Traditional health promotion delivery sources and channels (e.g., health educators delivering advice and information face to face) are often difficult to disseminate, and behavior change is often difficult to achieve (Brownson & Jones, 2009; Marcus et al., 2000). Technology-based interventions are well suited for improving dissemination and longer term participation in programs. For example, technology-based interventions do not necessarily need to rely on a health specialist to deliver the service. Therefore, they may be lower in cost and easier to disseminate than traditional programs, particularly among populations with time or travel constraints, as well as among rural and lower income individuals with limited access to health care facilities. Technology-based interventions are easily tailored to individuals, thereby potentially improving their overall efficacy beyond traditional health education programs (Abrams, Mills, & Bulger, 1999).

Technology-based interventions offer new opportunities for maintaining participation over time because these technologies can plausibly be used indefinitely and, in the case of mobile devices, can offer feedback in real time. Beyond dissemination and participation, technology-based interventions may be useful for improving assessment over time. For example, such mobile technologies as mobile telephones or PDAs allow data to be gathered throughout the day in a person's specific environmental contexts, which reduces memory problems and allows for more refined methods of testing underlying mechanisms and theories (e.g., ecological momentary assessment). Further, pedometers and accelerometers offer an easy complement for gathering objective data on physical activity that can be incorporated into tailored-intervention feedback. Finally, assessment through technology-based interventions can also be used to complement more traditional health promotion interventions by gathering more accurate data for health professionals to use as part of programs.

INTERNET- AND COMPUTER-BASED INTERVENTIONS

Internet-based interventions are attractive for promoting health behavior change for several reasons. Internet-based interventions can be accessed at any time and are relatively anonymous. They can gather information and provide tailored feedback, with easy use of rich graphic interfaces. Initial development costs are high and variable, but after setup, costs are often greatly reduced (Bennett & Glasgow, 2009). The Internet offers a potentially large global reach. Current estimates indicate that 74% of adults in the United States use the Internet at least occasionally (Rainie, 2010). Further, current estimates suggest that approximately 24.7% (approximately 1.7 billion people) of the global population use the Internet, with rapid growth observed in such underdeveloped areas as Africa (1,359.9% growth since 2000) and the Middle East (1,360.2% growth since 2000; Internet World Stats, 2009).

A recent meta-analysis of 75 health promotion interventions delivered over computer (some Internet-based, others not) suggests that computer-based interventions are efficacious at promoting short-term small- to medium-effect improvements in nutrition, smoking, sexual behavior, eating disorders, and general health but not physical activity (Portnoy et al., 2008). Computer-based interventions tended, in general, to be more effective at changing behavior among younger adults and when more frequent contact was targeted.

Unfortunately, results from this meta-analysis suggested that there is insufficient evidence currently demonstrating that physical activity can be promoted in a sustained fashion using the computer or Internet (Portnoy et al., 2008). This general conclusion has been reiterated by others based on qualitative review techniques (Bennett & Glasgow, 2009; Marcus et al., 2009; Neville et al.,

2009), although several studies supporting its utility have been published since these reviews were conducted (Block et al., 2008; Carr et al., 2008; Dunton & Robertson, 2008; Ferney, Marshall, Eakin, & Owen, 2009; Sternfeld et al., 2009). To the best of the authors' knowledge, 10 randomized controlled trials have been conducted comparing an Internet-based intervention to promote physical activity to a nonactive control group (e.g., assessment-only control, wait-list control). Of those 10, 5 found significant improvements in the Internet-based arms relative to an assessment-only control (Block et al., 2008; Dunton & Robertson, 2008; Hurling et al., 2007; Napolitano et al., 2003; Spittaels, De Bourdeaudbuij, & Vandelanotte, 2007; Sternfeld et al., 2009), and 4 found no differences between an Internet-only intervention and an assessment-only control group (Carr et al., 2008; Kypri & McAnally, 2005; Oenema, Brug, Dijkstra, de Weerdt, & de Vries, 2008; Winett, Anderson, Wojcik, Winett, & Bowden, 2007). Vandelanotte, De Bourdeaudhuij, Sallis, Spittaels, and Brug (2005) found differences between computer-based intervention arms and a wait-list control group for promoting physical activity across a 26-week period; but it should be noted that, despite randomization, the control arm consistently reported more physical activity relative to the intervention arms at all stages of the study, thus limiting the interpretability of these results.

Eleven studies have been conducted in adults comparing an Internet-based intervention to some other active treatment, most commonly print-based tailored messages. Of these studies, the majority found no significant differences between the two active forms of intervention (Booth, Nowson, & Matters, 2008; Bosak, Yates, & Pozehl, 2010; Cook, Billings, Hersch, Back, & Hendrickson, 2007; Hageman, Walker, & Pullen, 2005; Marcus et al., 2007; Marshall et al., 2003; Rovniak, Hovell, Wojcik, Winett, & Martinez-Donate, 2005; Spittaels, De Bourdeaudhuij, & Brug, 2007; Spittaels, De Bourdeaudhuij, & Vandelanotte, 2007; Steele, Mummery, & Dwyer, 2007). One study found significant differences between two active forms of intervention (Ferney et al., 2009). In this study, a neighborhood-focused Web site that was updated often resulted in significantly improved physical activity participation over a 26-week period relative to a nontailored motivationally focused Web site (Ferney et al., 2009).

Those interventions that worked better than assessment-only control arms utilized e-mail messaging in addition to a Web site (Block et al., 2008; Dunton & Robertson, 2008; Hurling et al., 2007; Sternfeld et al., 2009) and were based on social cognitive theory, the transtheoretical model, or other self-regulatory theories (Block et al., 2008; Booth et al., 2008; Hurling et al., 2007; Sternfeld et al., 2009). The one study that found significant differences between two active forms of intervention for physical activity participation suggested that Web site utility was improved if the Web site was updated frequently and focused on such very specific neighborhood-level contextual issues as local maps about access to good walking paths (Ferney et al., 2009).

Several studies in this area had greater than 20% of participants drop out (Block et al., 2008; Marshall et al., 2003; Napolitano et al., 2003; Spittaels, De Bourdeaudhuij, Brug, & Vandelanotte, 2007; Spittaels, De Bourdeaudhuij, & Vandelanotte, 2007; Sternfeld et al., 2009). High attrition is common in Internet-based interventions (Eysenbach, 2005). As suggested by Eysenbach (2005), more research is needed to better understand the often high rates of attrition observed in this specific type of intervention because it seems that once the novelty of Internet-based approaches wears off, many participants do not continue to use the program. Eysenbach (2005) suggested that "push reminders" (e.g., e-mail and postcards), incentives (e.g., raffles, point systems, and giveaways), self-monitoring, managing participant expectations prior to trial enrollment, minimizing usability challenges, and providing personal contact and positive feedback are useful for improving continued use. Despite these limitations, the current evidence suggests that continued research in this intervention area is warranted.

AUTOMATED TELEPHONE-LINKED COMPUTER SYSTEMS

Beyond computer and Internet-based interventions, there is increasing interest in promoting improved health outside the confines of a clinical setting such as a doctor's office. Indeed, recent work suggests that telephone-based interventions delivered by humans can be widely disseminated and result in improved physical activity (Eakin, Lawler, Vandelanotte, & Owen, 2007; Wilcox et al., 2008). Increasingly, researchers have started to explore the use of automated telephone-linked computer systems, also known as interactive voice response (IVR) systems, as a health care tool (Lee, Friedman, Cukor, & Ahern, 2003; Oake, Jennings, van Walraven, & Forster, 2009). These systems are of high potential value because they can be used for such simple tasks as appointment reminders and such complicated tasks as delivering fully automated advice and feedback about physical activity as well as other health behaviors. A recent meta-analysis of IVR telephone systems found that these automated calls were effective at promoting improved processes of care (e.g., coming to appointments) and disease states (e.g., improved glycemic control; Oake et al., 2009).

Although limited research has been conducted examining the utility of IVR systems for promoting physical activity, the current results are promising (Biem, Turnell, & D'Arcy, 2003; King et al., 2007; Pinto et al., 2002). For example, the most rigorous study to date examining the utility of IVR telephone systems found that an automated phone system was more effective than an attention control condition at promoting physical activity for 12 months and was equally as effective as a human-delivered telephone counseling program (King et al., 2007).

Because IVR systems are still relatively new, several qualitative studies have been conducted to understand factors that improve engagement with the systems (Farzanfar, Frishkopf, Migneault, & Friedman, 2005; Goldman et al., 2008; Kaplan, Farzanfar, & Friedman, 2003). One perceived barrier to using this technology is the perception that the IVR is a telemarketer (Goldman et al., 2008). In addition, participants in one study stated that the IVR was repetitive, did not understand statements from the participants, and talked too long (Farzanfar et al., 2005). Providing participants with a detailed description of the IVR system prior to its use resulted in improved acceptability of the technology (Goldman et al., 2008; King et al., 2007). Further, effective systems provided the chance to contact a human if problems arose with the program (Goldman et al., 2008; King et al., 2007). On a positive note, ethnographic work focused on understanding participants' reactions to IVR telephone systems found that some participants exhibited a strong emotional reaction to the computer system, with some individuals expressing a strong affinity for the automated voice akin to that for a mentor or close friend (Kaplan et al., 2003). This finding suggests that automated voices can be imbued with humanlike characteristics (Kaplan et al., 2003). This qualitative work collectively offers potential insights for the development of future IVR systems and other communication technology-based interventions in the physical activity field.

MOBILE TECHNOLOGIES

Utilizing mobile telephones as an agent of health promotion is a rapidly growing research area (Fjeldsoe et al., 2009; Krishna et al., 2009). This interest is in part based on the increasing mobile telephone usage across socioeconomic and age strata in the United States, a usage that has grown at a staggering rate, with 302.9 million wireless subscriber connections in 2010. This is one subscription for 96% of the U.S. population, up from 69% in 2005 (CTIA, 2011). Beyond the possibility of reaching a wide segment of the population, the advent of mobile communication technologies has created a vast potential for both collecting and delivering time- and context-sensitive health information. Mobile telephones have many capabilities that can be harnessed for promoting health (Patrick, Griswold, Raab, & Intille, 2008). On the most basic level, mobile telephones provide two-way communication by means of voice or text messaging. In addition, many telephones have built-in cameras, allow information to be stored on the phone, and can transmit data to outside networks. Next-generation telephones or "smart phones" have additional capabilities, including global positioning systems (GPS), built-in accelerometers, connectivity to WiFi, and wireless communication with external devices through blue-tooth (e.g., heart rate monitors, external accelerometers). Based on these technical characteristics, mobile telephones have the potential to transform health promotion research because the mobile telephone has the ability to assess behaviors, connect to outside sources for gathering and sharing information, and provide customized, content-relevant feedback about behaviors. These general capabilities can be used for simple tasks (e.g., appointment reminders) as well as such complicated tasks as fully automated services that promote increased health (Patrick et al., 2008; Patrick et al., 2009).

The vast majority of studies that have examined mobile telephone–based interventions have focused on diabetes management through improved assessment, by connectivity with clinicians, or as a reminder tool (Fjeldsoe et al., 2009; Krishna et al., 2009). Results of these studies generally suggest that mobile telephone interventions, in particular short-messaging services (SMS; also known as text messaging), were effective at improving diabetes management and smoking cessation, and they may be helpful for promoting such other preventive health behaviors as vitamin C use (Fjeldsoe et al., 2009; Krishna et al., 2009). These studies have been conducted in several different countries across four continents, suggesting the potential global reach of mobile telephones (Krishna et al., 2009).

Far fewer studies have examined mobile telephone interventions for physical activity promotion. Current evidence suggests that mobile telephones coupled with Internet services can promote increased physical activity (Hurling et al., 2007), and text messaging services are generally accepted by participants as an effective way to help increase physical activity (Gerber et al., 2009). Although not mobile telephones, PDAs share many positive characteristics with mobile telephones because they are portable, can assess activity within an individual's daily context, and can provide contextually relevant feedback. One randomized study examining the utility of a PDA-based physical activity intervention found that the intervention significantly improved physical activity over eight weeks relative to an assessment-only control (King, Ahn, et al., 2008).

Technologies to Promote HEPA: Future Directions

Although results generally suggest great promise with regard to technology-based interventions, much work still needs to be done. Future research should take into account the strengths and limitations of these modalities when designing interventions. For example, mobile telephones have several, as of yet, untapped strengths that can be harnessed for health promotion. As described in the foregoing section, a growing number of smart phones have accelerometers built in. This feature allows researchers to passively monitor physical activity and provide feedback directly from the telephone. However, there are important limitations to mobile telephones that must be kept in mind. For example, mobile telephones, even smart phones such as iPhones or Google-based Android phones, have relatively small screens. Therefore, surveys may be difficult to complete. Indeed, lengthy instructions with long statements about beliefs—as is common in many validated measures of such key constructs as perceived stress, social support, or self-efficacy—will likely need to be shortened to accommodate the limitations of this modality, thus creating the need for new validated measures that are appropriate for mobile devices. Short-message service (SMS) messaging customarily has a 160-character limit on texts, further suggesting the need to keep information brief.

This explosion of technology-based content and ideas makes it difficult for researchers to test technologies before they become obsolete. Indeed, although PDAs have been shown to be effective at improving physical activity (King, Ahn, et al., 2008), they have, in many ways, been replaced by mobile phones. Thus, scientific investigation may have difficulty keeping up with the technology and may need to embrace different scientific methods and approaches than what have traditionally been used in this field to date. For example, researchers may need to shift their emphasis from experimental designs and content generation to naturalistic experiments.

EFFECTS OF THE BUILT ENVIRONMENT ON PARTICIPATION IN PHYSICAL ACTIVITY

Urban planners have long recognized the relationship between the built environment and the modes of transportation individuals choose (Frank & Kavage, 2008). Some built environments naturally promote more car use (e.g., suburbia), whereas other community designs promote increased walking and other activity (e.g., such dense cities as New York City). Beyond transportation behavior, urban designers have also recognized that access to areas such as parks and green spaces has an impact on physical activity engagement (Frank & Kavage, 2008). Proximity to local destinations and street connectivity allowing an easy way to walk or bicycle to such destinations have been identified in the urban design and planning literature to be environmental attributes that are influential in affecting physical activity levels, particularly walking and bicycling for transportation purposes (Saelens, Sallis, & Frank, 2003). Proximity, the straight-line distance between two points of interest (e.g., home to work), is largely determined by density (e.g., how close homes are to one another) and land-use mix, that is, the mixture of residential and commercial land uses. It is generally suggested that areas with high density and high land-use mix are often more supportive of walking for transportation, whereas areas with low density and low land-use mix generally support more transportation by means of automobiles. Connectivity refers to the ease of access between destinations. For example, city designs that utilize a grid pattern offer several different ways to get to the same location, whereas suburban designs have limited connectivity because the roads use a branching model (e.g., cul de sacs) and provide fewer routes in or out of housing developments. Transportation research generally suggests that neighborhoods with higher connectivity and lower proximity between points of interest tend to facilitate more walking/cycling trips (Saelens et al., 2003).

Beyond such urban-planning concepts is an expanded ecological model predicting walking and cycling has been suggested that incorporates the importance of individual characteristics (e.g., car ownership, income, age, and psychosocial variables); along with elements of the neighborhood, including actual and perceived safety, access to bike lanes, sidewalks, trails, parks, community centers and other areas where residents may be active; and neighborhood aesthetics (see, Saelens et al., 2003, for a graphic depiction of this model). This and similar social ecological models have been supported in several recent observational studies in the field (Sallis, Bowles, et al., 2009; Sallis, Saelens, et al., 2009).

"Walkability" and similar constructs of a built environment can be assessed through objective means—by using geographical information systems (GIS), for example—as well as through self-report. Increasing evidence indicates that a number of these objective and perceived environmental constructs may be generalized across countries. For example, a recent study conducted within 11 countries, including Belgium, Colombia, Canada, New Zealand, and Japan, examined perceived neighborhood characteristics as a predictor sample percentage that was meeting physical activity recommendations of 150 minutes per week of moderate-intensity activity based on self-report (Sallis, Bowles, et al., 2009). Results suggested that five of seven perceived attributes thought to contribute to a walkable neighborhood (i.e., sidewalks on most streets, transit stops in the neighborhood, many shops nearby, bicycle facilities, and low-cost recreational facilities) were in fact associated with the increased likelihood of individuals meeting physical activity recommendations. In addition, the results suggested that there was a linear relationship between the number of perceived neighborhood walkability attributes and the percentage of the population meeting physical activity guidelines (Sallis, Bowles, et al., 2009).

Work examining the associations between objectively measured neighborhood characteristics and physical activity has also shown significant relationships (Sallis, Saelens, et al., 2009). For example, the results from a recently completed study undertaken around Seattle, Washington, and Baltimore, Maryland, suggested that residents living in 'high walkable" neighborhoods (based on GIS-determined characteristics) engaged in approximately 30 minutes more moderate-intensity physical activity per week (based on accelerometry) compared to residents living in "lower walkable" neighborhoods. The study results also suggested that although neighborhood walkability had a stronger relationship with physical activity levels in higher income areas, residents in lower income areas still benefited from being in a highly walkable area (Sallis, Saelens, et al., 2009). This same design was recently replicated among a sample of older adults aged 66 and over, with primary analyses currently being conducted by King and colleagues. Preliminary results indicate the same relationships between walkable neighborhoods and increased physical activity levels irrespective of neighborhood income.

Intervention research that takes into account factors relating to the built environment is still in its infancy but is of growing importance and concern. For instance, recent work suggests that the built environment (in particular, pedestrian safety concerns) moderates the efficacy of physical activity promotion interventions across different population groups (King et al., 2006). One promising study of promoting physical activity (Ferney et al., 2009) compared a neighborhood-focused Web site, where participants were given area maps that showed them acceptable places to walk in their neighborhoods, to a motivation-focused Web site that offered a more traditional, personal-level intervention. Results indicated that the neighborhood-focused Web site was better at promoting physical activity participation (Ferney et al., 2009). Although few studies have experimentally manipulated policy-level decisions (e.g., urban design, zoning, and transportation) to determine their influence on physical activity, there is some evidence, mostly from cross-sectional research, suggesting that policy-level factors can impact physical activity among neighborhood residents (Heath et al., 2006).

Future research in this area should examine different approaches to promoting walkability, among them policy changes, advocacy training, and changes in perceptions of the built environment, all of which may have an impact on either enabling physical activity or at minimum decreasing the environment's potentially deleterious effects on people living in low-walkable areas. In addition, important advances in computer-modeling technologies and statistical approaches should be used that allow for a more nuanced exploration of the relationship between people, places, and time (King, Satariano, et al., 2008). Beyond this, the definitions of "walkable neighborhood" are still evolving. Additional research focused on using audit tools to examine microlevel neighborhood factors (e.g., building architecture, curb cuts, the social environment) should be examined to further understand factors that may impact physical activity within a given area (Hoehner, Brennan Ramierez, Elliott, Handy, & Brownson, 2005). Examination of objectively measured microlevel factors that affect physical activity will likely be helpful in identifying aspects of the built environment that are potentially more amenable to local interventions than are such macrolevel factors as street connectivity and proximity to destinations. Finally, further exploration of rural walkable environments is also of vital importance for future research, given that rural population are less active than their urban counterparts (Shores, West, Theriault, & Davison, 2009).

CONCLUSION

Although progress has been made in understanding the complex set of individual, social, environmental, and policy factors that influence participation in HEPA, a great deal of work still needs to be done to increase the physical activity of a significant portion of the world. A number of central questions still need to be more fully answered and should be the focus of future research. First, what are the most effective behavior change techniques for individuals from a variety of ethnic and cultural backgrounds, and how can these techniques most effectively be taught? Second, what are the most effective social, environmental, and policy interventions for increasing physical activity across a broad sector of society? Third, how can the power of technology be leveraged to deliver tailored interventions to populations diverse in age, gender, ethnicity, and other ways? In the next decade, answering these questions and implementing solutions will require an interdisciplinary focus among professionals in disciplines as diverse as psychology, public health, urban planning, political science, and health economics in order to promote sustainable, physically active lifestyles that can improve the health and quality of life of persons of all ages.

REFERENCES

Abraham, C., & Michie, S. (2008). A taxonomy of behavior change techniques used in interventions. *Health Psychology*, *27*(3), 379–387.

Abrams, D. B., Mills, S., & Bulger, D. (1999). Challenges and future directions for tailored communication research. *Annals of Behavioral Medicine*, *21*, 299–306.

Ajzen, I. (1985). From intentions to actions: A theory of planned behavior. In J. Kuhl & J. Beckman (Eds.), *Action-control: From cognition to behavior* (pp. 11–39). Heidelberg, Germany: Springer.

Alexander, R. W. (2010). President's address: Common mechanisms of multiple diseases: Why vegetables and exercise are good for you. *Transactions of the American Clinical and Climatological Association*, *121*, 1–20.

Andersen, R. E., Franckowiak, S. C., Snyder, J., Bartlett, S. J., & Fontaine, K. R. (1998). Can inexpensive signs encourage the use of stairs? Results from a community intervention. *Annals of Internal Medicine*, *129*, 363–369.

Andersen, R. E., Franckowiak, S. C., Zuzak, K. B., Cummings, E. S., Bartlett, S. J., & Crespo, C. J. (2006). Effects of a culturally sensitive sign on the use of stairs in African American commuters. *International Journal of Public Health*, *51*(6), 373–380.

Ashrafian, H., Frenneaux, M. P., & Opie, L. H. (2007). Metabolic mechanisms in heart failure. *Circulation*, *116*, 434–448.

Bandura, A. (1997). *Self-efficacy: The exercise of control*. New York, NY: Freeman.

Bandura, A. (2001). Social cognitive theory: An agentic perspective. *Annual Reviews of Psychology*, *52*, 1–26.

Bauman, A., Sallis, J. F., Dwewaltowski, D. A., & Owen, N. (2002). Toward a better understanding of the influences on physical activity: The role of determinants, correlated, causal variables, mediators, moderators, and confouders. *American Journal of Preventive Medicine*, *23*(Suppl. 2), 5–14.

Beaudoin, C. E., Fernandez, C., Wall, J. L., & Farley, T. A. (2007). Promoting healthy eating and physical activity: Short-term effects of a mass media campaign. *American Journal of Preventive Medicine*, *32*(3), 217–223.

Bennett, G. G., & Glasgow, R. E. (2009). The delivery of public health interventions via the internet: Actualizing their potential. *Annual Review of Public Health*, *30*, 273–292.

Biem, H. J., Turnell, R. W., & D'Arcy, C. (2003). Computer telephony: Automated calls for medical care. *Clinical and Investigative Medicine*, *26*(5), 259–268.

Block, G., Sternfeld, B., Block, C. H., Block, T. J., Norris, J., Hopkins, D., … Clancy, H. A. (2008). Development of Alive! (A Lifestyle Intervention Via Email), and its effect on health-related quality of life, presenteeism, and other behavioral outcomes: Randomized controlled trial. *Journal of Medical Internet Research*, *10*(4), 18.

Booth, A. O., Nowson, C. A., & Matters, H. (2008). Evaluation of an interactive, Internet-based weight loss program: A pilot study. *Health Education Research*, *23*(3), 371–381.

Bosak, K. A., Yates, B., & Pozehl, B. (2010). Effects of an Internet physical activity intervention in adults with metabolic syndrome. *Western Journal of Nursing Research*, *32*(1), 5–22.

Brassington, G. S., & King, A. C. (2004). Theoretical considerations for physical activity promotion. In P. Poja & J. Borms (Eds.), *Health enhancing physical activity* (pp. 321–426). New York, NY: Meyer & Meyer Sport.

Brownell, K. D., Stunkard, A. J., & Albaum, J. M. (1980). Evaluation and modification of exercise patterns in the natural environment. *American Journal of Psychiatry*, *137*, 1540–1545.

Brownson, R. C., & Jones, E. (2009). Bridging the gap: Translating research into policy and practice. *Preventive Medicine*, *49*(4), 313–315.

Carr, L. J., Bartee, R. T., Dorozynski, C., Broomfield, J. F., Smith, M. L., & Smith, D. T. (2008). Internet-delivered behavior change program increases physical activity and improves cardiometabolic disease risk factors in sedentary adults: Results of a randomized controlled trial. *Preventive Medicine*, *46*(5), 431–438.

Carver, C. S., & Scheier, M. F. (1981). *Attention and self-regulation: A control theory to human behavior*. New York, NY: Springer-Verlag.

Caspersen, C. J., Powell, K. E., & Christenson, G. M. (1985). Physical activity, exercise, and physical fitness: Definitions and distinctions for health-related research. *Public Health Report*, *100*(2), 126–131.

Centers for Disease Control and Prevention. (2005). Trends in leisure-time physical inactivity by age, sex, and race/ethnicity—United States, 1994–2004. *Morbidity and Mortality Weekly Reports*, *54*(39), 991–994.

Centers for Disease Control and Prevention. (2007). Physical activity among adults—United States, 2001 and 2005. *Morbidity and Mortality Weekly Report*, *56*, 1209–1212.

Centers for Disease Control and Prevention. (2008, April). Data 2010: The healthy people, 2010 database. Retrieved from http://wonder.cdc.gov/data2010

Church, T. S., & Blair, S. N. (2009). When will we treat physical activity as a legitimate medical therapy . . . even though it does not come in a pill? *British Journal of Sports Medicine*, *43*(2), 80–81.

Clarke, K. K., Freeland-Graves, J., Klohe-Lehman, D. M., Milani, T. J., Nuss, H. J., & Laffrey, S. (2007). Promotion of physical activity in low-income mothers using pedometers. *Journal of the American Dietetic Association*, *107*(6), 962–967.

Conn, V. S., Valentine, J. C., & Cooper, H. M. (2002). Interventions to increase physical activity among aging adults: A meta analysis. *Annals of Behavioral Medicine*, *24*, 190–200.

Cook, R. F., Billings, D. W., Hersch, R. K., Back, A. S., & Hendrickson, A. (2007). A field test of a Web-based workplace health promotion program to improve dietary practices reduce, stress, and increase physical activity: Randomized controlled trial. *Journal of Medical Internet Research*, *9*(2), e17.

CITA. (2011). *U.S. wireless quick facts.* Retrieved from http://www.ctia.org/advocacy/research/index.cfm/AID/10323

DeBusk, R. F., Hakansson, U., Sheehan, M., & Haskell, W. L. (1990). Training effects of long vs. short bouts of exercise. *American Journal of Cardiology*, *65*, 1010–1013.

DeVol, R., Bedroussian, A., Charuworn, A., Chatterjee, A., Kim, I. K., Soojung, K., & Klowden, K. (2007). *An unhealthy America: The economic burden of chronic disease—Charting a new course to save lives and increase productivity and economic growth*. Santa Monica, CA: Milkin Institute.

Dishman R. K., Berthoud, H. R., Booth, F. W., Cotman, C. W., Edgerton, R., Fleshner, M. R., … Zigmond, M. J. (2006). Neurobiology of exercise. *Obesity*, *14*, 345–356.

Dishman, R. K., & Buckworth, J. (1996). Increasing physical activity: A quantitative synthesis. *Medicine and Science in Sports and Exercise*, *28*, 706–719.

Dishman, R. K, & O'Connor, P. J. (2009) Lesson in exercise neurobiology: The case of endorphins. *Mental Health and Physical Activity 2*, 4–9.

Dishman, R. K., & Sallis, J. F. (1994). Determinants and interventions for physical activity and exercise. In C. Bouchard, R. J. Shephard, & T. Stephens (Eds.), *Physical activity, fitness, and health: International proceedings and consensus statement* (pp. 214–238). Champaign, IL: Human Kinetics Publishers.

Dunn, A. L., & Jewell, J. S. (2010). The effect of exercise on mental health. *Current Sports Medicine Reports*, *9*(4), 202–207.

Dunton, G. F., & Robertson, T. P. (2008). A tailored Internet-plus-email intervention for increasing physical activity among ethnically-diverse women. *Preventive Medicine*, *47*(6), 605–611.

Eakin, E. G., Lawler, S. P., Vandelanotte, C., & Owen, N. (2007). Telephone interventions for physical activity and dietary behavior change: A systematic review. *American Journal of Preventive Medicine*, *32*(5), 419–434.

Eysenbach, G. (2005). The law of attrition. *Journal of Medical Internet Research*, *7*(1), e11.

Farzanfar, R., Frishkopf, S., Migneault, J., & Friedman, R. (2005). Telephone-linked care for physical activity: A qualitative evaluation of the use patterns of an information technology program for patients. *Journal of Biomedical Informatics*, *38*(3), 220–228.

Ferney, S. L., Marshall, A. L., Eakin, E. G., & Owen, N. (2009). Randomized trial of a neighborhood environment-focused physical activity Website intervention. *Preventive Medicine*, *48*(2), 144–150.

Fjeldsoe, B. S., Marshall, A. L., & Miller, Y. D. (2009). Behavior change interventions delivered by mobile telephone short-message service. *American Journal of Preventive Medicine*, *36*(2), 165–173.

Ford, E. S., & Li, C. (2006). Physical activity or fitness and the metabolic syndrome. *Expert review of cardiovascular therapy*, *4*(6), 897–915.

Frank, L. D., & Kavage, S. (2008). Urban planning and public health: A story of separation and reconnection. *Journal of Public Health Management and Practice*, *14*(3), 214–220.

Fulton, J. E., Dai, S., Steffen, L. M., Grunbaum, J. A., Shah, S. M., & Labarthe, D. R. (2009). Physical activity, energy intake, sedentary behavior, and adiposity in youth. *American Journal of Preventive Medicine*, *37*(Suppl. 1), S40–S49.

Gerber, B. S., Stolley, M. R., Thompson, A. L., Sharp, L. K., & Fitzgibbon, M. L. (2009). Mobile phone text messaging to promote healthy behaviors and weight loss maintenance: A feasibility study. *Health Informatics Journal*, *15*(1), 17–25.

Goldman, R. E., Sanchez-Hernandez, M., Ross-Degnan, D., Piette, J. D., Trinacty, C. M., & Simon, S. R. (2008). Developing an automated speech-recognition telephone diabetes intervention. *International Journal for Quality in Health Care, 20*(4), 264–270.

Hageman, P. A., Walker, S. N., & Pullen, C. H. (2005). Tailored versus standard internet-delivered interventions to promote physical activity in older adults. *Journal of Geriatric Physical Therapy, 28,* 28–33.

Hamilton, M. T., Hamilton, D. G., & Zderic, T. W. (2007). Role of low energy expenditure and sitting in obesity, metabolic syndrome, type 2 diabetes, and cardiovascular disease. *Diabetes, 56*(11), 2655–2667.

Handschin, C., & Spiegelman, B. M. (2008). The role of exercise and PGC1α in inflammation and chronic disease. *Nature 2008, 454*(7203), 463–469.

Hardeman, W., Griffin, S., Johnston, M., Kinmonth, A. L., & Wareham, N. J. (2000). Interventions to prevent weight gain: A systematic review of psychological models and behaviour change methods. *International Journal of Obesity and Related Metabolic Disorders, 24*(2), 131–143.

Haskell, W. L., Blair, S. N., & Hill, J. O. (2009). Physical activity: Health outcomes and importance for public health policy. *Preventive Medicine, 49*(4), 280–282.

Hausenblas, H. A., Carron, A. V., & Mack, D. E. (1997). Application of the theories of reasoned action and planned behavior to exercise behavior: A meta-analysis. *Journal of Sport & Exercise Psychology, 19,* 36–51.

Heath, G. W., Brownson, R. C., Kruger, J., Miles, R., Powell, K. E., & Ramsey, L. T. (2006). The effectiveness of urban design and land use and transport policies and practices to increase physical activity: A systematic review. *Journal of Physical Activity and Health, 3*(Suppl. 1), S55–S76.

Hoehner, C. M., Brennan Ramirez, L. K., Elliott, M. B., Handy, S. L., & Brownson, R. C. (2005). Perceived and objective environmental measures and physical activity among urban adults. *American Journal of Preventive Medicine, 28*(Suppl. 2), 105–116.

Horowitz, C. R., Robinson, M., & Seifer, S. (2009). Community-based participatory research from the margin to the mainstream: Are researchers prepared? *Circulation, 119*(19), 2633–2642.

Hovell, M. F., Mulvihill, M. M., Buono, M. J., Liles, S., Schade, D. H., Washington, T. A., … Sallis, J. F. (2008). Culturally tailored aerobic exercise intervention for low-income Latinas. *American Journal of Health Promotion, 22*(3), 155–163.

Hurling, R., Catt, M., Boni, M. D., Fairley, B. W., Hurst, T., Murray, P., … Sodhi, J. S. (2007). Using internet and mobile phone technology to deliver an automated physical activity program: Randomized controlled trial. *Journal of Medical Internet Research, 9*(2), e7.

Internet World Stats. (2009, November). World Internet Usage Statistics News and World Population Stats. Retrieved from http://www.internetworldstats.com/stats.htm

Janz, N. K., & Becker, M. (1984). The health belief model: A decade later. *Health Education Quarterly, 11,* 1–47.

Jones, T. F., & Eaton, C. B. (1994). Cost-benefit analysis of walking to prevent coronary heart disease. *Archives of Family Medicine, 3*(8), 703–710.

Kahn, E. B., Ramsey, L. T., Brownson, R. C., Heath, G. W., Howze, E. H., Powell, K. E., … Corso, P. (2002). The effectiveness of interventions to increase physical activity: A systematic review. *American Journal of Preventive Medicine, 22,* 73–106.

Kaplan, B., Farzanfar, R., & Friedman, R. H. (2003). Personal relationships with an intelligent interactive telephone health behavior advisor system: A multimethod study using surveys and ethnographic interviews. *International Journal of Medical Informatics, 71*(1), 33–41.

Kemi, O. J., & Wisloff, U. (2010). Mechanisms of exercise-induced improvements in the contractile apparatus of the mammalian myocardium. *Acta Physiologica, 199*(4), 425–439.

King, A. C., Ahn, D. K., Oliveira, B. M., Atienza, A. A., Castro, C. M., & Gardner, C. D. (2008). Promoting physical activity through hand-held computer technology. *American Journal of Preventive Medicine, 34*(2), 138–142.

King, A. C., Friedman, R., Marcus, B. H., Castro, C., Napolitano, M., & Ahn, D. (2007). Ongoing physical activity advice by humans versus computers: The Community Health Advice by Telephone (CHAT) trial. *Health Psychology, 26*(6), 718–727.

King, A. C., Satariano, W. A., Marti, J., & Zhu, W. (2008). Multilevel modeling of walking behavior: Advances in understanding the interactions of people, place, and time. *Medicine and Science in Sports and Exercise, 40*(Suppl. 7), S584–S593.

King, A. C., Toobert, D., Ahn, D., Resnicow, K., Coday, M., Riebe, D., … Sallis, J. F. (2006). Perceived environments as physical activity correlates and moderators of intervention in five studies. *American Journal of Health Promotion, 21*(1), 24–35.

Krishna, S., Boren, S. A., & Balas, E. A. (2009). Healthcare via cell phones: A systematic review. *Telemedicine Journal and E-Health, 15*(3), 231–240.

Kypri, K., & McAnally, H. M. (2005). Randomized controlled trial of a Web-based primary care intervention for multiple health risk behaviors. *Preventive Medicine*, *41*(3–4), 761–766.

Larkey, L. (2006). Las mujeres saludables: Reaching Latinas for breast, cervical and colorectal cancer prevention and screening. *Journal of Community Health*, *31*(1), 69–77.

Lee, H., Friedman, M. E., Cukor, P., & Ahern, D. (2003). Interactive voice response system (IVRS) in health care services. *Nursing Outlook*, *51*(6), 277–283.

Marcus, B. H., Ciccolo, J. T., & Sciamanna, C. N. (2009). Using electronic/computer interventions to promote physical activity. *British Journal of Sports Medicine*, *43*(2), 102–105.

Marcus, B. H., Dubbert, P. M., Forsyth, L. H., McKenzie, T. L., Stone, E. J., Dunn, A. L., & Blair, S. N. (2000). Physical activity behavior change: Issues in adoption and maintenance. *Health Psychology*, *19*(Suppl. 1), S32–S41.

Marcus, B. H., Napolitano, M. A., King, A. C., Lewis, B. A., Whiteley, J. A., Albrecht, A., ... Papandonatos, G. D. (2007). Telephone versus print delivery of an individualized motivationally tailored physical activity intervention: Project STRIDE. *Health Psychology*, *26*(4), 401–409.

Marshall, A. L., Leslie, E. R., Bauman, A. E., Marcus, B. H., & Owen, N. (2003). Print versus website physical activity programs: A randomized trial. *American Journal of Preventive Medicine*, *25*(2), 88–94.

Marttila, J., Laitakari, J., Nupponen, R., Miilunpalo, S., & Paronen, O. (1998). The versatile nature of physical activity—On the psychological, behavioural and contextual characteristics of health-related physical activity. *Patient Education and Counseling*, *33*(Suppl. 1), S29–S38.

Michie, S., Abraham, C., Whittington, C., McAteer, J., & Gupta, S. (2009). Effective techniques in healthy eating and physical activity interventions: A meta-regression. *Health Psychology*, *28*(6), 690–701.

Michie, S., & Prestwich, A. (2010). Are interventions theory-based? Development of a theory coding scheme. *Health Psychology*, *29*(1), 1–8.

Murphy, M. H., Blair, S. N., & Murtagh, E. M. (2009). Accumulated versus continuous exercise for health benefit: A review of empirical studies. *Sports Medicine*, *39*(1), 29–43.

Napolitano, M. A., Fotheringham, M., Tate, D., Sciamanna, C., Leslie, E., Owen, N., ... Marcus, B. (2003). Evaluation of an Internet-based physical activity intervention: A preliminary investigation. *Annals of Behavioral Medicine*, *25*(2), 92–99.

Neville, L. M., O'Hara, B., & Milat, A. (2009). Computer-tailored physical activity behavior change interventions targeting adults: A systematic review. *International Journal of Behavioral Nutrition and Physical Activity*, *6*, 12.

Oake, N., Jennings, A., van Walraven, C., & Forster, A. J. (2009). Interactive voice response systems for improving delivery of ambulatory care. *American Journal of Managed Care*, *15*(6), 383–391.

Oenema, A., Brug, J., Dijkstra, A., de Weerdt, I., & de Vries, H. (2008). Efficacy and use of an Internet-delivered computer-tailored lifestyle intervention, targeting saturated fat intake, physical activity and smoking cessation: A randomized controlled trial. *Annals of Behavioral Medicine*, *35*(2), 125–135.

Owen, N., Bauman, A., & Brown, W. (2009). Too much sitting: A novel and important predictor of chronic disease risk? *British Journal of Sports Medicine*, *43*(2), 81–82.

Patrick, K., Griswold, W. G., Raab, F., & Intille, S. S. (2008). Health and the mobile phone. *American Journal of Preventive Medicine*, *35*(2), 177–181.

Patrick, K., Raab, F., Adams, M. A., Dillon, L., Zabinski, M., Rock, C. L., ... Norman, G. J. (2009). A text message-based intervention for weight loss: Randomized controlled trial. *Journal of Medical Internet Research*, *11*(1). doi: 10.2196/jmir.1100

Pekmezi, D. W., & Jennings, E. (2009). Physical activity interventions in minority populations *Current Cardiovascular Risk Reports*, *3*(4), 275–280.

Pekmezi, D. W., Neighbors, C. J., Lee, C. S., Gans, K. M., Bock, B. C., Morrow, K. M., ... Marcus, B. (2009). A culturally adapted physical activity intervention for Latinas: A randomized controlled trial. *American Journal of Preventive Medicine*, *37*(6), 495–500.

Physical Activity Guidelines Committee. (2008). *Physical activity guidelines advisory committee report*. Washington, DC: U.S. Deparment of Health and Human Services.

Pinto, B., Friedman, R., Marcus, B. H., Kelley, H., Tennstedt, S., & Gillman, M. W. (2002). Effects of a computer-based, telephone-counseling system on physical activity. *American Journal of Preventive Medicine*, *23*(2), 113–120.

Plescia, M., Herrick, H., & Chavis, L. (2008). Improving health behaviors in an African American community: The Charlotte racial and ethnic approaches to community health project. *American Journal of Public Health*, *98*(9), 1678–1684.

Portnoy, D. B., Scott-Sheldon, L. A. J., Johnson, B. T., & Carey, M. P. (2008). Computer-delivered interventions for health promotion and behavioral risk reduction: A meta-analysis of 75 randomized controlled trials, 1988–2007. *Preventive Medicine*, *47*(1), 3–16.

Pratt, M., Macera, C. A., & Wang, G. (2000). Higher direct medical costs associated with physical inactivity. *Physician and Sportsmedicine, 28*, 63–70.

Prochaska, J. O., & DiClemente, C. C. (1984). *The transtheoretical approach: Crossing traditional boundaries of change.* Homewood, IL: Dorsey Press.

Prochaska, J. O., DiClemente, C. C., & Norcross, J. C. (1992). In search of how people change. *American Psychologist, 47*, 1102–1114.

Rainie, L. (2010). *Internet, broadband, and cell phone statistics.* Pew Research Center. Retrieved from http://www.pewinternet.org/Reports/2010/Internet-broadband-and-cell-phone-statistics.aspx

Rovniak, L. S., Hovell, M. F., Wojcik, J. R., Winett, R. A., & Martinez-Donate, A. P. (2005). Enhancing theoretical fidelity: An e-mail-based walking program demonstration. *American Journal of Health Promotion, 20*(2), 85–95.

Saelens, B. E., Sallis, J. F., & Frank, L. D. (2003). Environmental correlates of walking and cycling: Findings from transportation, urban design, and planning literatures. *Annals of Behavioral Medicine, 25*(2), 80–91.

Sallis, J. F., Bowles, H. R., Bauman, A., Ainsworth, B. E., Bull, F. C., Craig, C. L., … Bergman, P. (2009). Neighborhood environments and physical activity among adults in 11 countries. *American Journal of Preventive Medicine, 36*(6), 484–490.

Sallis, J. F., & Owen, N. (1997). Ecological models. In K. Glanz, F. M. Lewis, & B. K. Rimer (Eds.), *Health behavior and health education: Theory, research, and practice* (3rd ed., pp. 462–484). San Francisco, CA: Jossey-Bass.

Sallis, J. F., Saelens, B. E., Frank, L. D., Conway, T. L., Slymen, D. J., Cain, K. L., … Kerr, J. (2009). Neighborhood built environment and income: Examining multiple health outcomes. *Social Science & Medicine, 68*(7), 1285–1293.

Salmon, J., Dunstan, D., & Owen, N. (2008). Should we be concerned about children spending extended periods of time in sedentary pursuits even among the highly active? *International Journal of Pediatric Obesity, 3*(2), 66–68.

Shores, K. A., West, S. T., Theriault, D. S., & Davison, E. A. (2009). Extra-individual correlates of physical activity attainment in rural older adults. *Journal of Rural Health, 2*, 211–218.

Spittaels, H., De Bourdeaudbuij, I., Brug, J., & Vandelanotte, C. (2007). Effectiveness of an online computer-tailored physical activity intervention in real-life setting. *Health Education Research, 27*, 385–396.

Spittaels, H., De Bourdeaudhuij, I., & Vandelanotte, C. (2007). Evaluation of a Website-delivered computer-tailored intervention for increasing physical activity in the general population. *Preventive Medicine, 44*, 209–217.

Steele, R., Mummery, W. K., & Dwyer, T. (2007). Using the Internet to promote physical activity: A randomized trial of intervention delivery modes. *Journal of Physical Activity & Health, 4*, 245–260.

Sternfeld, B., Quesenberry, C. P., Block, T. J., Block, C. H., Husson, G., Norris, J., … Block, G. (2009). Improving diet and physical activity with ALIVE (A Lifestyle Intervention Via Email): Results from a worksite randomized trial. *American Journal of Preventive Medicine, 36*(6), 475–483.

Sylvia, L. G., Ametrano, R. M., & Nierenberg, A. A. (2010). Exercise treatment for bipolar disorder: Potential mechanisms of action mediated through increased Neurogenesis and decreased allostatic load. *Psychotherapy and Psychosomatic, 79*, 87–96.

Task Force on Community Preventive Services. (2002). Task force on community preventive services. *American Journal of Preventive Medicine, 22*(Suppl. 4), S67–S72.

Troiano, R. P., Berrigan, D., Dodd, K. W., Masse, L. C., Tilert, T., & McDowell, M. (2008). Physical activity in the United States measured by accelerometer. *Medicine and Science in Sports and Exercise, 40*(1), 181–188.

U.S. Department of Health and Human Services. (1996). *Physical activity and health: A report of the surgeon general.* Atlanta, GA: U.S. Department of Health and Human Services, Centers for Disease Control and Prevention, National Center for Chronic Disease Prevention and Health Promotion.

Van Praag H. (2009). Exercise and the brain: Something to chew on. *Trends in Neuroscience, 32*, 283–290.

Vandelanotte, C., De Bourdeaudhuij, I., Sallis, J. F., Spittaels, H., & Brug, J. (2005). Efficacy of sequential or simultaneous interactive computer-tailored interventions for increasing physical activity and decreasing fat intake. *Annals of Behavioral Medicine, 29*(2), 138–146.

Weinstein, N. D., & Rothman, A. J. (2005). Commentary: Revitalizing research on health behavior theories. *Health Education Research: Theory and Practice, 20*(3), 294–297.

Wilcox, S., Dowda, M., Leviton, L. C., Bartlett-Prescott, J., Bazzarre, T., Campbell-Voytal, K., … Wegley, S. (2008). Active for Life—Final results from the translation of two physical activity programs. *American Journal of Preventive Medicine, 35*(4), 340–351.

Wilson, P. M. (2008). Understanding motivation for exercise: A self-determination theory perspective. *Canadian Psychology*, *49*(3), 250–256.

Winett, R. A., Anderson, E. S., Wojcik, J. R., Winett, S. G., & Bowden, T. (2007). Guide to health: Nutrition and physical activity outcomes of a group-randomized trial of an Internet-based intervention in churches. *Annals of Behavioral Medicine*, *33*(3), 251–261.

Yancey, A. K., Lewis, L. B., Guinyard, J. J., Sloane, D. C., Nascimento, L. M., Galloway-Gilliam, L., … McCarthy, W. J. (2006). Putting promotion into practice: The African Americans building a legacy of health organizational wellness program. *Health Promotion Practice*, *7*(Suppl. 3), S233–S246.

Yancey, A. K., McCarthy, W. J., Harrison, G. G., Wong, W. K., Siegel, J. M., & Leslie, J. (2006). Challenges in improving fitness: Results of a community-based, randomized, controlled lifestyle change intervention. *Journal of Women's Health*, *15*(4), 412–429.

17 Personality and Health
Current Issues and Emerging Perspectives

Timothy W. Smith
University of Utah

Linda C. Gallo, Smriti Shivpuri, and Addie L. Brewer
San Diego State University

The contribution of personality characteristics to the development and course of physical illness is a central topic within both personality science and health psychology. In the former, evidence that personality traits predict longevity and other important health outcomes has done much to answer long-standing criticism that personality concepts and measures have limited utility (Mischel, 1968), and in this way it has contributed to the resurgence in personality psychology in recent decades (Roberts, Kuncel, Shiner, Caspi, & Goldberg, 2007). Within the latter, the hypothesis that stable individual differences in cognition, emotion, and behavior influence the pathophysiology of disease has been a cornerstone of the field since its inception (Cohen, 1980). Research on the association between personality and health has steadily matured, with mounting evidence of robust associations from methodologically sophisticated studies. This evidence has the potential to guide the development of risk-reducing interventions. However, unanswered questions, limitations in this research, and continuing controversies fuel both skepticism and the need for continuing improvements in methodological rigor. If insufficiently addressed, such limitations could ultimately limit the applied value of this work.

In this chapter, we provide an update of our prior review of the literature addressing the relationship between personality and health (Smith & Gallo, 2001; see also Smith & MacKenzie, 2006). Conceptual and methodological issues are discussed first, inasmuch as they continue to be essential as a guide to both the current state of this literature and the refinements needed in the next generation of research. Next, we review the specific personality traits that provide the best evidence of prospective associations with subsequent health. We then review the evidence regarding the mechanisms that might account for such associations and conclude with a brief discussion of emerging topics that will figure prominently in the coming years. Space precludes an exhaustive review, but we hope to illustrate the current challenges, vitality, and future promise of this long-standing research area.

METHODOLOGICAL AND CONCEPTUAL ISSUES

Despite its apparent simplicity, the hypothesis that various aspects of personality confer risk and resilience for important physical health outcomes has frequently been difficult to translate into definitive methodologies. Three critical issues have complicated this process. First, the personality variables studied as risk factors are sometimes conceptualized imprecisely, and the related measures are often lacking in one or more critical respects. Second, health outcomes are sometimes assessed in ways that contribute to difficulties in interpretation. Finally, design and analytic approaches used to examine associations between personality predictors and health outcomes are often the source of additional limitations.

CONCEPTUALIZING AND MEASURING PERSONALITY

At times in the history of the study of personality and health, basic measurement issues have received insufficient attention. In many cases, the reliability, structure, and construct validity of personality scales used in this research are not well established. Critically, scale labels based on item content are sometimes accepted as adequate evidence that the scale measures the intended construct, and in some instances scales with similar labels are interpreted as assessing similar constructs even without formal evidence of *convergent validity*. These are examples of what Block (1995) described as the "jingle fallacy" in personality measurement in which scales with similar names are interpreted as measuring similar constructs. This can result in a misleading heterogeneity of findings across studies. Rather than showing weak or inconsistent effects of a given personality trait on health, these mixed results could actually reflect a lack of convergence among quite distinct scales that are intended to be multiple measures of a single trait.

A related limitation, the "jangle fallacy" (Block, 1995) occurs when scales with different labels are interpreted as assessing distinct constructs, even in the absence of formal evidence of *discriminant validity*. As a result, well-established constructs are sometimes inadvertently studied using new scales intended to measure novel constructs. This makes the field prone to two additional worrisome limitations: the reinvention of previously identified traits under new labels (Holroyd & Coyne, 1987), and the failure to identify basic dimensions of risk within what erroneously seems to be a great variety of health-relevant aspects of personality. Even when the scales used have some evidence of convergent and discriminant validity, the potentially overlapping effects of correlated dimensions of personality are rarely examined, a less severe form of the jangle fallacy. Even rarer still are efforts to examine the potentially overlapping effects of personality risk factors and aspects of the social environment related to these dimensions of personality, such as social support versus isolation (Gallo & Smith, 1999).

These limitations in the measurement of personality variables in studies of health can be addressed through the more routine use of basic concepts and methods in personality science. First, formal studies of the convergent and discriminant validity of the scales used in this research are a necessity, especially when novel concepts and measures are introduced. The process of construct validation should always begin with detailed conceptual definitions of the domain the scale is intended to assess, including a description of the trait's structure (e.g., unidimensional vs. multifaceted) and its predicted associations with conceptually related but distinct traits as well as less closely related traits (McFall, 2005; West & Finch, 1997). This careful conceptual effort can guide evaluations of the structure and construct validity of personality measures used in studies of health in a theory-driven manner (Smith, 2007).

Using a common frame of reference in the development and evaluation of personality traits to be used in health research can facilitate the development of a more systematic literature by identifying similarities and differences among these concepts and scales. Comparisons with well-established trait concepts and measures help researchers to avoid the "reinvention" of old traits under new labels, as well as facilitates the identification of broad dimensions of risk. As presented in Table 17.1, the five-factor model (FFM) of personality is a widely accepted taxonomy of basic traits and their components (Costa & McCrae, 1992; Digman, 1990), and it can serve these essential functions in health research (Marshall et al., 1994; Smith & Williams, 1992). When assessed with well-validated measures (e.g., Costa & McCrae, 1992), the five main domains and their components provide a nomological net (Cronbach & Meehl, 1955), with both comprehensive breadth and considerable detail in documenting the similarities and differences among traits and measures used to study health.

TABLE 17.1
Elements of the Five-Factor Model of Personality

Trait	Opposite Pole	Facets
Neuroticism	Emotional stability	Anxiety, angry hostility, depression, self-consciousness, impulsiveness, vulnerability
Extraversion	Introversion	Warmth, gregariousness, assertiveness, activity, excitement-seeking, positive emotion
Openness	Closed-mindedness	Fantasy, aesthetics, feelings, actions, ideas, values
Agreeableness	Antagonism	Trust, straightforwardness, altruism, compliance, modesty, tender-mindedness
Conscientiousness	Unreliability	Competence, order, dutifulness, achievement-striving, self-discipline, deliberation

Source: Adapted from Costa, P. T., Jr. and McCrae, R. R., *Professional Manual: Revised NEO Personality Inventory (NEO-PI-R) and the NEO Five-Factor Inventory (NEO-FFI)*, Psychological Assessment Resources, Odessa, FL, 1992.

A second perspective in personality theory and research can facilitate the integration of personality traits with risk factors that are interpreted as reflecting aspects of the social environment. A central element of the interpersonal tradition (Horowitz, 2004; Kiesler, 1996; Pincus & Ansell, 2003) is a structural model of social behavior—the interpersonal circumplex (IPC), as depicted in Figure 17.1 (Kiesler, 1983). The two FFM traits most closely related to social behavior—extraversion (vs. introversion) and agreeableness (vs. antagonism)—are rotational equivalents of the two main dimensions of the IPC: affiliation (warmth vs. hostility) and control (dominance vs. submissiveness). Extraversion reflects somewhat warm dominance in the IPC, whereas agreeableness reflects somewhat submissive friendliness or warmth (McCrae & Costa, 1989; Traupman et al., 2009). The IPC is useful in comparing, contrasting, and ultimately organizing personality risk factors for

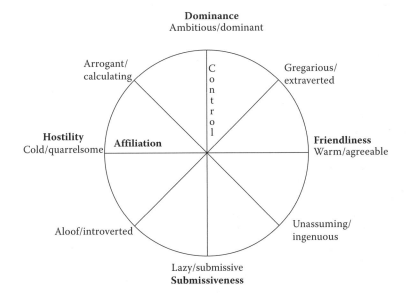

FIGURE 17.1 The interpersonal circumplex.

disease, especially those that involve social behavior (e.g., Gallo & Smith, 1998; Smith, Traupman, Uchino, & Berg, 2010). IPC-based scales that are supplemented by measures of the other FFM traits (i.e., neuroticism, conscientiousness, openness) can provide comprehensive frameworks for construct validation (e.g., Trapnell & Wiggins, 1990; Traupman et al., 2009).

The IPC has an additional important advantage, however. Its two main dimensions can also be used to describe psychosocial risk factors typically seen as reflecting such aspects of the social environment as social support (Trobst, 2000) and conflict or strain in close relationships (Smith et al., 2010). The opportunity to describe personality and interpersonal risk factors in a common conceptual space becomes more important in light of an additional major component of the interpersonal perspective—namely, the principle of complementarity (Horowtiz, 2004; Kiesler, 1996). In this view of social interactions, the behavior of an actor invites or tends to evoke behavioral responses from the interaction partner that are similar along the affiliation dimension of the IPC and opposite on the control dimension. That is, warmth invites warm responses from others, whereas hostility invites hostility in return. In contrast, dominant behavior invites, or communicates the expectation of, submissiveness in return. The complementary behavior of interaction partners has the effect of maintaining the actor's initial tendency to be warm, hostile, or dominant. Hence, the principle of complementarity provides a conceptual foundation for predictions about associations between risk factors typically seen as aspects of personality and those seen as reflecting the social environment. For example, hostile personality traits should be associated with low levels of positive social relations (e.g., low social support) and high levels of negative interactions (e.g., interpersonal conflict) at home and work. It also leads to the prediction that such risk factors should continue to be correlated over time.

In the interpersonal perspective, the process underlying complementarity in social interaction is described in the transactional cycle (Kiesler, 1996), as depicted in Figure 17.2. Various intraindividual variables (e.g., goals, expectations) guide the actor's overt behaviors, which in turn restrict the interaction partner's appraisals of and covert reactions to the actor. The partner is then likely to respond in ways that confirm the actor's original expectation, as when the warm behavior of trusting individuals evokes warmth in return. Hence, the IPC provides a framework for the description of both personality and social-environmental risk factors, the principle of complementarity provides a theory-based account of expected patterns of the correlations among personality and social-environmental risk factors, and the transactional cycle provides an explanatory framework for understanding the mechanisms through which personality and social-environmental risk factors are related. As such, the interpersonal perspective encourages a broadly integrative approach (Gallo & Smith, 1999; Smith & Cundiff, 2010; Smith, Glazer, Ruiz, & Gallo, 2004).

The active reciprocal processes through which individuals influence and are influenced by aspects of the social situations they encounter is quite consistent with another main perspective in current personality science—the social-cognitive perspective (Mischel, 2004; Mischel & Shoda, 1998). Whereas the FFM largely describes personality as characteristics individuals have, the social-cognitive approach describes personality largely in terms of things people do (Cantor, 1990). There is no widely accepted set of social-cognitive elements of personality analogous to the FFM taxonomy of traits, but highly informative lists have been described (Mischel, 2004; Mischel & Shoda, 1998). These include mental representations of the self, others, and social interaction sequences (i.e., schemas and scripts); such motivational variables as expectancies, goals, personal projects, and life tasks; attention, encoding, appraisals, and attributions regarding people and situations; coping and self-regulation processes; and competencies, strategies, and tactics in the pursuit of goals. These social-cognitive "middle units" of personality (McAdams, 1995) can be located within the transactional cycle described in the interpersonal perspective (see Figure 17.2).

The social-cognitive perspective describes personality not only through the content of these characteristics but also through their organization. Hence, individual differences in hostility are evident not only in the tendency to appraise the ambiguous actions of others as reflecting hostile intent; it is also evident in the process in which such appraisals rapidly and consistently activate a script involving the necessity of vigilance, defensiveness, and aggressive behavior. The social-cognitive

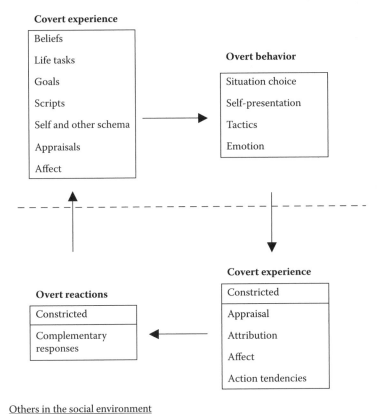

Individual

FIGURE 17.2 The transactional cycle. (Adapted from Kiesler, D. J., ed., *Contemporary Interpersonal Theory and Research: Personality, Psychopathology, and Psychotherapy*, New York, NY, Wiley, 1996.)

perspective also suggests that personality is not best seen in broad patterns of cross-situational consistencies in behavior. Rather, personality is evident in contextualized behavior, or "if-then" patterns of situation-response profiles or "behavioral signatures" (Mischel, 2004). Both the situational input (i.e., the "if") and the behavioral output or response (i.e., "then") can be described as locations on the IPC (Fournier, Moskowitz, & Zuroff, 2008). For example, despite the general tendency to display complementary behavior, one individual might be characterized by the tendency to respond with hostile dominance to dominant behavior from others and with warmth to submissiveness. A second person might display warm deference in response to dominant behavior from others and respond to submissiveness with hostile dominance. Even if these patterns resulted in the same aggregate level of hostile behavior across situations, they imply quite distinct personalities regarding resistance to power or authority versus abuse of power or authority.

Together, these three perspectives in personality science promote the integrative study of psychosocial risk for physical illness. The FFM provides the concepts and methodological tools for the development of a detailed understanding of the similarities and differences among these traits. The interpersonal perspective similarly facilitates comparisons among personality risk factors by examining their associations with the dimensions of the IPC. In that way it also promotes theoretical and empirical analysis of co-occurring personality and social-environmental risk factors. Finally, the transactional cycle within the interpersonal perspective and the elements and assumptions of the social-cognitive approach articulate the mechanisms through which such risk factors influence daily life in ways that ultimately confer risk and resilience.

In addition to useful methods for construct validation and integration of measures used to assess these risk factors, personality science also provides useful background in the selection of methods used to assess them. By far, most studies of personality and subsequent health have used self-report measures of personality. The resulting robust associations provide important evidence of their predictive utility (Roberts et al., 2007). However, self-reports and ratings by others are often modestly correlated and are often differentially related to outcomes of interest (Oltmanns & Turkheimer, 2006). More important is that interview-based behavioral ratings and ratings by significant others are often better predictors of health outcomes than are self-reports (Miller et al., 1996; Smith et al., 2008). This finding could reflect the fact that individuals are unwilling or unable to give completely accurate self-reports regarding potentially undesirable traits. Alternatively, behavioral ratings and ratings by others could reflect a combination of both the trait of interest and the individual's ability to modulate related expressive behavior. For example, spouse ratings of anxiety could reflect the target individual's level of emotional distress and his or her level of difficulty managing anxious affect. Self-reports would typically capture only the former individual difference. It is important that the few studies including both self-reports and other methods suggest that the reliance on self-reports of personality could have produced an underestimate of associations with health outcomes (e.g., Smith et al., 2008).

MEASURING HEALTH

Many of the health outcomes studied in this literature are straightforward. Longevity and the onset of objectively assessed disease (e.g., myocardial infarction, cancer, diabetes, hypertension) are relatively easily quantified; and even for complex conditions, well-established and widely accepted medical criteria can be used. However, personality traits have also been linked to such more subjective health outcomes as symptom reports, utilization of health care, and self-rated health. Most of these indicators of physical health are associated with more objective outcomes such as longevity (Idler & Benyamini, 1997). Further, physical symptoms, self-reported health status, and other subjective outcomes are important components of comprehensive definitions of health (Ryff & Singer, 1998), and utilization of health care has obvious practical importance in a climate of worrisome increases in health expenditures.

However, these more subjective health indicators cannot be interpreted as measures of health, per se, given that each of them reflects illness behavior—things people often do when actually ill—rather than the illness itself. The imperfect correspondence between measures of illness behavior and actual disease is evident in both the stoic's minimization and the excessive complaints of the "worried well." When health is measured in these ways, relationships with personality could reflect associations with objective disease, the discrepancy between reported and actual illness, or some combination of the two. Thus, although subjective health outcomes, health care utilization, and other illness behaviors are important outcomes in and of themselves, they are ambiguous proxies at best when studying associations between personality and disease.

TESTING ASSOCIATIONS: DESIGN AND ANALYSIS

The most informative designs testing associations between personality and health are prospective, because associations in cross-sectional designs could easily reflect effects of serious illness on psychological functioning, rather than effects of personality on the onset or course of disease (Cohen & Rodriguez, 1995). One recently emerging exception to this general assertion involves noninvasive assessments of asymptomatic or preclinical levels of disease. For example, coronary calcification can be assessed through CT scans in outwardly healthy individuals with no prior indications of coronary heart disease. Associations between personality and this index of atherosclerosis are unlikely to reflect responses to disease, given that the individual is unlikely to be aware of the presence or severity of the underlying disease. Similarly useful outcomes include ultrasound studies of carotid artery disease (i.e., atherosclerosis in arteries supplying blood to the brain) and endothelial dysfunction, an early and typically asymptomatic marker of atherosclerosis. Prospective studies of these outcomes are inherently more informative than cross-sectional designs, but reverse causality is not as likely a threat to validity as in cross-sectional studies comparing individuals with and without clinically apparent disease.

By necessity, studies of personality as risk factors are nonexperimental, observational designs. The results of such work might eventually guide randomized controlled trials intended to modify psychosocial risks, but those are typically undertaken only after many observational studies have suggested an important link between personality and health. Given their nonexperimental, observational nature, studies in this area have well-established limitations.

Most troublesome, personality risk factors are likely to be associated with many "third variables" that could contribute to artifactual associations. Such confounding factors are typically managed through statistical control that, though invaluable in such applications, has three potentially serious limitations. First, even if a comprehensive set of potential confounding factors can be identified, the factors are likely to be measured with less than ideal reliability and validity. Hence, there is likely to be residual confounding because imperfect measures cannot exhaust the variance in a confounding construct (Phillips & Davey Smith, 1991). Second, if associations between measures of personality risk factors and potential confounding factors are large and substantive (e.g., an association between depressive symptoms and difficulties in close relationships), statistical adjustments that force these variables to be independent can result in predictors with reduced resemblance to the original constructs of interest (Lynam, Hoyle, & Newman, 2006). That is, a predictor variable shorn of its overlapping variance with a closely related confounding factor may or may not still capture the construct originally assessed by that scale. Third, many confounders could actually be elements within a causal chain linking the personality trait with important health outcomes. For example, if statistical control of smoking attenuates the association between neuroticism and longevity, this is perhaps better seen as indicating a potential mediator of the effects of neuroticism on health, rather than the identification and elimination of a pesky confound.

Each of these issues in the analysis of observational designs with many likely complex, imperfectly measured, and confounded predictors underscores the value of conceptually driven analysis. Rather than reflexively controlling all possible overlapping predictors, analyses should be guided by clear, theory-based questions (Christenfeld, Sloan, Carroll, & Greenland, 2004; Smith, 2010). Any given analysis is likely to suffer from at least one limitation; hence, often the best approach involves multiple analyses carefully guided by well-articulated questions.

ASSOCIATIONS BETWEEN PERSONALITY AND HEALTH

Type A Behavior Pattern and Beyond

The Type A behavior pattern (TABP), originally defined by Friedman and Rosenman (1959), is characterized by a competitive and sustained drive for achievement and recognition, time urgency, easily provoked hostility, and a loud, rapid, and vigorous vocal style. This pattern of behavior has received considerable attention as a possible coronary risk factor for more than four decades (Friedman & Rosenman, 1959, 1974; Rosenman et al., 1964). The Western Collaborative Group Study (WCGS) found that over an eight-year period, Type A men were twice as likely to exhibit clinical manifestations of coronary heart disease (CHD) relative to Type B men (Brand, 1978; Rosenman et al., 1975). Findings from the WCGS and subsequent studies prompted a review panel, sponsored by the National Heart, Lung, and Blood Institute, to declare TABP an independent risk factor for CHD (Cooper, Detre, & Weiss, 1981).

Since the panel's conclusions, a large body of inconsistent findings has generated skepticism regarding the link between TABP and CHD. An extended follow-up to the WGCS revealed no association between TABP and 22-year CHD mortality (Ragland & Brand, 1988). Negative findings reported in the Aspirin Myocardial Infarction Study (Shekelle, Gale, & Norusis, 1985), Multiple Risk Factor Intervention Trial (Shekelle, Hulley, et al., 1985), and meta-analytic studies (Booth-Kewley & Friedman, 1987; Friedman & Booth-Kewley, 1987; Matthews, 1988) added to the uncertainty. Further, Gallacher, Sweetnam, Yarnell, Elwood, and Stansfeld (2003) identified TABP as a predictor of when a coronary event will occur rather than if it will occur. Specifically, this study suggested that TABP increases exposure to potential triggers, rather than affecting the underlying process of atherosclerosis itself.

Although many of the failures to replicate the association between TABP and CHD have been attributed to methodological issues (Miller, Turner, Tindale, Posavac, & Dugoni, 1991), the inconsistent results prompted attempts to disaggregate TABP and investigate the health implications of its components. Among the various Type A traits, anger and hostility were identified as significant predictors of CHD incidence and became the focus of subsequent research (Dembroski, MacDougall, Costa, Jr., & Grandits, 1989; Siegman, 1994). Although some inconsistent results emerged, reviewers found behavioral and self-report measures of anger and hostility to be significantly associated with CHD and premature mortality (Gallo & Matthews, 2003; Kop, 1999; Miller, Smith, Turner, Guijarro, & Hallet, 1996; Rozanski, Blumenthal, & Kaplan, 1999; Smith et al., 2004), and a recent quantitative review confirmed this conclusion (Chida & Steptoe, 2009).

Hostility is characterized as a "negative attitude toward others, consisting of enmity, denigration, and ill will" (Smith, 1994, p. 26), and trait anger, or frequent and pronounced episodes of "an unpleasant emotion ranging in intensity from irritation or annoyance to fury or rage" (Smith, 1994). As such, these characteristics reflect the FFM trait of antagonism (i.e., low agreeableness) and also a component of neuroticism. They also reflect the horizontal or affiliation axis of the IPC. Research suggests that these characteristics influence various stages of CHD (Smith et al., 2004). These traits are associated with early indications of atherosclerosis (Gottdiener et al., 2003; Harris, Matthews, Sutton-Tyrrell, & Kuller, 2003), more advanced but still asymptomatic atherosclerosis (Iribarren et al., 2000; Matthews, Owens, Kuller, Sutton-Tyrrell, & Jansen-McWilliams, 1998; Raikkonen, Matthews, Sutton-Tyrrell, & Kuller, 2004), and the development of clinically apparent cardiovascular disease (for reviews, see Smith et al., 2004; Smith & MacKenzie, 2006), as well as the recurrence of coronary events and cardiovascular death among patients with established CHD (e.g. Chaput et al., 2002; Matthews, Gump, Harris, Haney, & Barefoot, 2004). Hostility and anger also predict the development of hypertension and stroke (e.g., Everson et al., 1999; Rutledge & Hogan, 2002; J. E. Williams, Nieto, Sanford, Couper, & Tyroler, 2002; Yan et al., 2003).

Research has shown that additional components of the TABP may be predictors of CHD, independent of hostility and traditional risk factors. A reanalysis of the WCGS data found that individuals who exhibit a specific style of verbal behavior characterized by vigorous and interruptive speech are at increased risk for CHD (Houston, Chesney, Black, Cates, & Hecker, 1992). This set of behaviors, termed *social dominance* and closely resembling the vertical axis of the IPC described previously, also predicted mortality in the longer 22-year follow-up of the WCGS participants (Houston, Babyak, Chesney, Black, & Ragland, 1997). The association between social dominance and increased risk for CHD has been replicated in studies using self-report measures of dominance (Siegman et al., 2000; Whiteman, Deary, Lee, & Fowkes, 1997), in spouse ratings of partner dominance (Smith et al., 2008), and in animal research (Kaplan & Manuck, 1998). The current state of this literature suggests that studies of the globally defined TABP are no longer warranted. Instead, one of its components—anger and hostility—appears to be a robust risk factor for the development and course of CHD and also predicts all-cause mortality and reduced longevity. A second Type A risk component—social dominance—is less well established as a risk factor for CHD and reduced longevity, but preliminary support suggests further studies are warranted.

INDIVIDUAL DIFFERENCES IN NEGATIVE AFFECT: NEUROTICISM, DEPRESSION, AND ANXIETY

Neuroticism, or negative affectivity, describes the propensity to experience negative emotions (e.g., anxiety, sadness) and related cognitive and behavioral tendencies (McCrae & John, 1992). An early and frequently cited review concluded that negative affectivity should be considered an independent risk factor for poor physical health outcomes (Booth-Kewley & Friedman, 1987); however, the review was subsequently criticized for including studies with subjective health endpoints in addition to objectively documented morbidity and mortality (e.g., Matthews, 1988). Because neuroticism is associated with greater expression of somatic complaints in the absence of underlying disease, the estimated association may have been inflated by capturing illness behavior as well as objective outcomes. However, more recent methodologically rigorous studies suggest that several subdimensions of neuroticism (i.e., depression, anxiety, and anger), as well as the overarching trait, relate prospectively to risk of premature mortality and such verified disease outcomes as CHD (Suls & Bunde, 2005).

Unraveling the unique versus overlapping influence of the facets of neuroticism may be difficult, given that they represent correlated aspects of a multicomponent construct (Smith, 2010; Suls & Bunde, 2005). Nonetheless, a large body of research has examined specific features, with most studies focusing on depression, anxiety, and related psychological disorders. In addition, as described earlier, considerable research has examined the health effects of anger, which also overlap with the broader construct of neuroticism or negative affectivity and correlate consistently with such other facets of neuroticism as depression and anxiety.

Several recent reviews have synthesized findings from studies concerning the association between depression and objective health outcomes, with most emphasizing premature mortality and cardiovascular disease (CVD) incidence or progression. Generally, these reviews have concluded that depression poses a health risk both in initially healthy persons and in patient populations, independent of behavioral risk factors (e.g., smoking), baseline health, and other confounding factors (Barth, Schumacher, & Herrmann-Lingen, 2004; Carney, Freedland, & Jaffe, 2001; Nicholson, Kuper, & Hemingway, 2006; Rutledge, Reis, Linke, Greenberg, & Mills, 2006; Wulsin & Singal, 2003; Wulsin, Vaillant, & Wells, 1999). For example, a review and meta-analysis of 11 well-designed prospective cohort studies concluded that both depressive symptoms and clinically diagnosable depression predicted an increased risk of incident heart disease, independent of numerous covariates (Rugulies, 2002). Larger effect sizes were observed in relation to a major depression diagnosis (RR = 2.70) than depressed mood (RR = 1.50), suggesting a possible dose-response relationship. Additional work has identified a relationship between depression and other outcomes, including HIV progression (Leserman, 2008), longevity in stroke survivors (Everson, Roberts, Goldberg, & Kaplan, 1998), incident diabetes (Knol et al., 2006), and hypertension (Rutledge & Hogan, 2002). On the other hand, many mixed or null findings have appeared in the literature, and a number of robust studies have failed to identify an association between depression and endpoints, including CHD (Dickens et al., 2004; Lane, Carroll, Ring, Beevers, & Lip, 2001; McCusker et al., 2006). Methodological limitations, such as variability in the conceptualization and measurement of depression, and inconsistent control for behavioral risk factors and baseline health may contribute to variable findings and suggest the need for further research (Nicholson et al., 2006).

In addition to studies examining depression is a growing body of research that has evaluated the health implications of anxiety. Early research examined psychiatric-patient populations and emphasized cardiovascular outcomes. In general, these studies were characterized by mixed findings and serious methodological flaws (Fleet, Lavoie, & Beitman, 2000). However, more recent reviews and methodologically robust studies link various aspects of anxiety (e.g., anxious cognition, phobic anxiety, and general symptoms) with incident CHD and suggest a graded, or dose-response, association (for reviews, see Kubzansky & Kawachi, 2000; Kubzansky, Kawachi, Weiss, & Sparrow, 1998; Rozanski et al., 1999; for examples of recent studies, see Eaker, Sullivan, Kelly-Hayes, D'Agostino, Sr., & Benjamin, 2005; Walters, Rait, Petersen, Williams, & Nazareth, 2008). Limited research also suggests that anxiety is associated with poorer prognosis in CHD patient populations (Shibeshi, Young-Xu, & Blatt, 2007; Szekely et al., 2007), with one study showing that patients with high anxiety were nearly five times as likely to experience complications or death following myocardial infarction (Moser & Dracup, 1996). Moreover, anxiety has been associated with incident hypertension in some research (Rutledge & Hogan, 2002). As for depression, the evidence base is not entirely consistent, and some well-designed studies have identified no relationship between anxiety and all-cause mortality (Mykletun et al., 2007) and health outcomes in CHD patients (Lane et al., 2001).

Overall, the weight of the evidence suggests that higher levels of neuroticism and, in particular, such specific features as depression and anxiety have deleterious health implications. Nonetheless, null and mixed findings identified in methodologically robust studies are puzzling. Furthermore, intervention trials targeting depression and other negative affects in patient populations have generally failed to improve longevity (Berkman et al., 2003; Rees, Bennett, West, Davey, & Ebrahim, 2004), which would be expected if these variables are causally related to health. It is important to note, however, that stress management interventions have been found to reduce risk of recurrent coronary events among CHD patients (Linden, Phillips, & Leclerc, 2007; Orth-Gomér et al., 2009), suggesting that reducing general negative affect may be useful. Many questions remain unanswered (Dickens et al., 2007; Smith, 2010), among them questions concerning the timing with which depression and anxiety affect negative health outcomes and whether clinical or subclinical levels of negative emotion, or both, predict health and disease outcomes. These inconsistencies and outstanding questions suggest the need for large, prospective-cohort studies that include heterogeneous populations, adequate follow-up periods, and well-validated measures.

Conscientiousness

Although relatively limited, some research has also shown that the FFM trait *conscientiousness*—or the tendency to be organized, persistent, and disciplined and to maintain self-perceptions of competence—relates to health. Higher levels of conscientiousness predict greater longevity among healthy persons and longer survival in patient populations (Chapman, Lyness, & Duberstein, 2007; Iwasa et al., 2008; Weiss & Costa, 2005; Wilson, de Leon, Bienias, Evans, & Bennett, 2004). For example, a study that followed more than 2,000 healthy individuals across five decades estimated that every one standard deviation increase in conscientiousness led to a 27% reduction in risk of death (Terracciano, Lockenhoff, Zonderman, Ferrucci, & Costa, Jr., 2008). Kern and Friedman (2008) conducted a meta-analysis of 20 independent studies and found a robust positive association between conscientiousness and longevity, with stronger relationships observed for the *achievement* and *order* subdimensions of the construct. Additional research in nationally representative samples links conscientiousness with decreased risk for physical illnesses, including diabetes, tuberculosis, bone and joint problems, and hypertension (Goodwin & Friedman, 2006), as well as to slower disease progression in individuals with HIV/AIDS (O'Cleirigh, Ironson, Weiss, & Costa, 2007). One prospective study found teacher-rated childhood conscientiousness to predict better self-rated health and lower body mass index (BMI) in women 40 years later (Hampson, Goldberg, Vogt, & Dubanoski, 2006). The salubrious effects of conscientiousness may reflect increased medication adherence and self-discipline, more active health care–related decision-making styles, or more adaptive coping in those with higher conscientiousness (Flynn & Smith, 2007; O'Cleirigh et al., 2007; Vollrath, Landolt, Gnehm, Laimbacher, & Sennhauser, 2007).

Openness to Experience

Some research has considered the health effects of *openness to experience*, or the FFM domain encompassing the tendency to prefer variety and to be imaginative, curious, and attentive to internal feelings. The literature that is available reveals mixed findings. For example, a study in Japan (Iwasa et al., 2008) found that higher openness related to decreased all-cause mortality over a five-year follow-up period after controlling for demographic and other risk factors (i.e., living alone, presence of psychiatric problems, presence of chronic diseases). However, two prospective studies with U.S. samples reported no association between openness to experience and longevity (Weiss & Costa,

2005; Wilson et al., 2004), and another study showed that openness failed to predict physician-rated morbidity in an elderly sample of primary-care patients (Goodwin & Friedman, 2006). A recent study of CHD patients found that specific facets of openness (i.e., openness to actions and feelings) related to decreased risk for cardiovascular and all-cause mortality over 15 years, whereas the overall domain of openness did not predict outcomes (Jonassaint et al., 2007). Finally, some research has supported a link between increased openness and such better dietary habits as fruit and vegetable consumption (Brummett, Siegler, Day, & Costa, 2008; de Bruijn, Kremers, van Mechelen, & Brug, 2005). Overall, the limited available research and variable findings prohibit definitive conclusions, but they do suggest the potential value of additional research on openness and health.

EXTRAVERSION

The FFM domain of *extraversion* describes individual differences in such characteristics as sociability and assertiveness. In their study of a Japanese community population, Iwasa and colleagues (2008) found that higher extraversion related to positive health outcomes, including decreased all-cause mortality. After controlling for demographic risk factors, another study conducted with a healthy community population showed that a one standard deviation increase in the *general activity* subfacet of extraversion (i.e., rapid tempo, vigorous movement, sense of energy, and need to keep busy) led to a 13% reduction in risk of death (Terracciano et al., 2008). However, other studies have shown no association between extraversion and mortality in either initially healthy or patient populations (Christensen et al., 2002; Korten et al., 1999; Mroczek & Spiro, 2007; Shipley, Weiss, Der, Taylor, & Deary, 2007; Weiss & Costa, 2005). Behaviorally, extraversion has been associated with increased sports-related physical activity (de Bruijn et al., 2005). Conversely, extraversion has been linked to such risky health behaviors as smoking and sexual promiscuity (Gute & Eshbaugh, 2008; Munafo, Zetteler, & Clark, 2007), as well as increased risk of overweight (Kakizaki et al., 2008). Therefore, if a relationship exists between extraversion and health, it may be because of behavioral changes resulting from increased socialization; but whether this effect overall is positive or negative remains unclear. The mixed findings regarding health effects of extraversion could reflect the fact that it combines high dominance and high affiliation in the IPC. As described, these dimensions of social behavior tend to have opposite associations with health. Low levels of warmth and social contact might place introverts at increased risk, whereas the tendency to exert influence and control over others might place extroverts at risk.

OPTIMISM/PESSIMISM

Optimism, or the stable tendency to hold positive expectations about the future, has been shown to have salutary health effects in some research. For example, a study by Kubzansky, Sparrow, Vokanas, & Kawachi (2001) showed that older men with high levels of optimism were less than half as likely as their more pessimistic counterparts to develop CHD over a 10-year follow-up period, even after control for health behaviors and negative emotions such as depression and anger. More optimistic attitudes also predicted slower progression of atherosclerosis in initially health women (Matthews, Raikkonen, Sutton-Tyrrell, & Kuller, 2004). Other studies have shown that high levels of optimism predict longevity in general (Brummett, Helms, Dahlstrom, & Siegler, 2006; Giltay, Geleijnse, Zitman, Hoekstra, & Schouten, 2004; Maruta, Colligan, Malinchoc, & Offord, 2000) and lower risk of cardiovascular mortality in particular (Giltay et al., 2004). Research in medical populations has shown that patients reporting greater optimism recover more quickly and are less likely to be rehospitalized following coronary artery bypass graft (CABG) surgery (Scheier et al., 1989; Scheier et al., 1999), and they survive longer following diagnosis with head and neck cancer (Allison, Guichard, Fung, & Gilain, 2003).

The literature concerning optimism and health is characterized by a number of important conceptual questions. First, at least some research suggests that optimism and pessimism may represent unique factors, rather than polar ends of a single trait-continuum (Herzberg, Glaesmer, & Hoyer, 2006), and that the health implications of these factors may be unique (Kubzansky, Kubzansky, & Maselko, 2004). For example, higher levels of trait pessimism, but not lower optimism, predicted a lower survival rate in a study of cancer patients (though only in younger patients; Schulz, Bookwala, Knapp, Scheier, & Williamson, 1996). In addition, conceptualizations of optimism have differed across research programs, and the measures that stem from these operationalizations typically exhibit only modest correlations (Norem & Change, 2001), raising questions about whether they represent the same or distinct constructs. In addition, optimism overlaps conceptually with such other traits as hopelessness, which have likewise been associated with physical health outcomes— for example, longevity (Stern, Dhanda, & Hazuda, 2001) and cardiovascular and cancer mortality (Everson et al., 1996). The extent of confounding with negative or positive affect and the degree to which health effects of optimism may be explained by a shared association with trait affect is also largely unknown. Finally, it is important to note that the research findings are not entirely consistent, as some null results have appeared in the literature (Chida & Steptoe, 2008). Hence, although optimism/pessimism seems to be an important predictor of subsequent health, such issues suggest both caution and important directions for future research.

Other Traits

A number of additional individual characteristics have been examined in relationship to health. For example, researchers have evaluated the degree to which enduring tendencies to exhibit positive affect are health protective, with some studies suggesting that salubrious effects are distinct from the influence of negative affect (for reviews, see Chida & Steptoe, 2008; Cohen & Pressman, 2006). However, relative to the research base concerning neuroticism and its subcomponents, this work is in its formative stages and is also somewhat limited by the lack of available, well-validated measures of trait positive affect. Moreover, whether positive and negative affect are distinct influences on health remains an open research question (Reich, Zautra, & Davis, 2003; Russell & Carroll, 1999).

Other studies have examined the health implications of a *sense of coherence*, or individual differences in perceptions that one's life is meaningful and controllable. A strong sense of coherence was associated with a 30% reduction in mortality from all causes in a large, prospective community study conducted in the United Kingdom. Furthermore, this association remained consistent after control for demographic factors, baseline health, socioeconomic status, risk factors, and negative affect (Surtees, Wainwright, Luben, Khaw, & Day, 2003). A subsequent study in the same population showed an inverse association between sense of coherence and incident stroke (Surtees et al., 2007). Additional research suggests a link between this construct and lifestyle choices related to health (Wainwright et al., 2007) and indicates that these behavioral factors partially explain the association with mortality (Wainwright et al., 2008). Related adaptive individual-difference characteristics, including mastery or a sense of control over one's life, have also been associated with health outcomes (Taylor & Seeman, 1999), including mortality (Surtees, Wainwright, Luben, Khaw, & Day, 2006) and extent of atherosclerosis (Matthews, Owens, Edmundowicz, Lee, & Kuller, 2006). It is important to note that research concerning these constructs is relatively limited, and the degree of redundancy with previously established risk factors (e.g., depression, optimism) has not been fully elucidated.

Type D personality, or distressed personality, the tendency to exhibit a combination of negative affectivity and social inhibition, has been advanced as a unique health risk factor. This behavioral pattern has been associated with poor outcomes in CHD patient populations (for reviews, see Kupper & Denollet, 2007; Pedersen & Denollet, 2003); some evidence suggests that the effects of Type D are distinct from those of other psychosocial influences, including depression (Denollet & Pedersen, 2008; Schiffer, Pedersen, Widdershoven, & Denollet, 2008). Nonetheless, several researchers have expressed skepticism about the degree to which Type D personality is redundant with other psychosocial characteristics established as health risk factors (Smith & MacKenzie, 2006; Steptoe &

Molloy, 2007). In addition, some researchers have questioned whether Type D is indicative of progressive CVD, rather than representing a stable traitlike characteristic, though, recent studies suggest that Type D personality is both heritable (Kupper, Denollet, de Geus, Boomsma, & Willemsen, 2007) and stable across an 18-month period in heart disease patients (Martens, Kupper, Pedersen, Aquarius, & Denollet, 2007). Finally, the degree to which associations of Type D with subsequent health reflect the hypothesized interactive or synergistic effects of negative affectivity and social inhibition, simple additive effects of these two traits, or significant effects of only one of the dimensions cannot be determined from the manner in which associations of this construct with health are typically tested and reported (Smith & MacKenzie, 2006). Overall, additional research is needed to determine the specific and unique predictive utility of this construct.

CONCLUSIONS REGARDING ASSOCIATIONS

As even this brief review indicates, several personality characteristics (e.g., anger/hostility, negative affectivity and its components) have robust associations with such important objective health outcomes as longevity or the development and course of CHD. Smaller or somewhat inconsistent literatures suggest important areas for further research in other cases (e.g., optimism, dominance). Beyond making obviously important associations with longevity and survival, a majority of these studies examine cardiovascular health outcomes. Although this is perhaps understandable given the status of cardiovascular disease at the leading cause of death in most industrialized countries, it also suggests the need for expansion of the smaller literatures on other health outcomes in order to delineate the specific-versus-general effects of personality. Further, in nearly all cases of personality-health associations, it remains unclear if the association is relatively constant across the full personality dimension, if maladaptive characteristics (e.g., antagonism, negative affect, pessimism) confer risk, or if adaptive characteristics (e.g., high agreeableness, emotional stability and competence, optimism) actually confer protection or resilience. Refined personality measurement and quantitative methods (e.g., tests of nonlinear effects) could help address the personality risk-versus-protection issue, as it has important implications for the design and implementation of related interventions.

MECHANISMS

A key question concerns mechanisms responsible for these associations: How do stable aspects of emotion, cognition, and behavior influence the development and course of disease? Various mechanisms have been proposed as potential links between personality and health. Some of these models suggest quite different views of the association between personality and health, whereas others are not necessarily incompatible.

ILLNESS BEHAVIOR

Illness behavior (Mechanic, 1972) is a multifaceted construct referring to the perception and reporting of physical symptoms and to the responses to such perceived illnesses as seeking medical care, discussing health problems with family members, and limiting activities because of illness. Depending on the way health outcomes are assessed, associations between personality and health could reflect associations with illness behavior in the absence of actual illness, as discussed previously. This is clearly the case when health outcomes are assessed through self-reports of symptoms or physical limitations (i.e., disability). The fact that personality traits predict longevity and the onset of objectively assessed disease (e.g., myocardial infarctions as an index of coronary heart disease) indicates that this version of the illness behavior model of associations between personality and health outcomes is inadequate. However, some illness behaviors can influence actual health, as can adherence to medical regimens or ignoring early signs of disease. Although perhaps better seen as examples of the health behavior model described later, these latter illness behaviors are viable mechanisms even in studies of objective health outcomes.

CONSTITUTIONAL PREDISPOSITION

It is possible that associations between personality traits and objective indications of negative health outcomes reflect an underlying third variable—a genetic or constitutional predisposition to illness. In this model, personality factors and negative health outcomes are causally unrelated coeffects of an underlying biological factor, such as the high levels of limbic system activation that underlie negative emotionality or reduced functioning of prefrontal cortical structures and circuits that support self-regulation and emotional control. As we discuss later, recent advances in the neuroscience and genetics of personality support the plausibility of this view. However, the cognitive and behavioral aspects of personality could still play a role in linking such biological factors to subsequent health. For example, through the transactional processes described earlier, individuals with biological predispositions to excessive emotionality or limited self-regulation are likely to create more stressful social environments, which in turn would evoke unhealthy physiological responses especially among vulnerable individuals. Hence, advances in the underlying neuroscience and molecular genetics of personality and related links to the development of disease do not necessarily preclude a role for other aspects of personality.

HEALTH BEHAVIOR

Various personality traits are linked to a variety of aspects of health behavior, including smoking, physical activity levels, diet, and alcohol use. It is possible that these behaviors contribute to associations between personality traits and subsequent health. Although some studies find that such health behaviors as smoking account for the associations, many prospective studies find significant associations even when comprehensive sets of such behavioral risk factors are controlled. Hence, in general, health behaviors seem to be a potentially important but incomplete explanation for these associations.

STRESS MODERATION

Perhaps the most widely studied mechanism potentially linking personality and health has involved the psychophysiology of stress. In its most basic form, this hypothesis holds that personality influences the individual's overall level of physiological stress responses, and over time these responses hasten the development and progression of disease. The specific physiological responses involved are likely to vary across diseases, though some aspects of the stress response (e.g., heightened inflammatory activity) could influence the development and course of a variety of illnesses. Traditionally, this mechanism has involved the moderation of reactivity to stressful events and circumstances, but more recent conceptual analyses (P. G. Williams, Smith, & Cribbett, 2008; P. G. Williams, Smith, Gunn, & Uchino, 2009) have identified multiple aspects of the stress response as potential links.

Stress Exposure

As described in the interpersonal approach presented earlier, personality factors and environmental stressors are reciprocally related. Through the expressive aspects of their individual personality, people may be more or less likely to create or to find themselves in stressful circumstances. Individuals elect to enter some situations and not others, unintentionally evoke particular responses from others through expressive behavior, and intentionally manipulate the tone or focus of social interactions (Buss, 1987). Similar processes may influence the level of stress-reducing social support the individual enjoys. These stress exposures may take the form of such external events as "major life events" (e.g., divorce) or "daily hassles" (e.g., conflict with coworkers) and can also involve such cognitive processes as anticipation of stressful events (i.e., worry) and reimagined stressors (i.e., rumination).

There is growing evidence that personality characteristics are related to stress exposure. Within the FFM, neuroticism is the trait most consistently associated with greater stress exposure. Higher levels of neuroticism are associated with more frequent major life events, daily hassles, and such chronic stressors as family and relationship conflict (Bolger & Zuckerman, 1995; David, Green, Martin, & Suls, 1997; Gunthert, Cohen, & Armeli, 1999; Magnus, Diener, Fugita, & Pavot, 1993; Suls et al., 1998). Neuroticism is also associated with the tendency to worry and ruminate (Kotov, Watson, Robles, & Schmidt, 2007). Hostility, a facet of neuroticism as well as a central aspect of antagonism, is associated with social isolation, low levels of social support (Siegler et al., 2003), and higher levels of marital conflict (Baron et al., 2007).

Another FFM trait, *conscientiousness*, is associated with lower levels of stress exposure, such as lower rates of divorce (Roberts & Bogg, 2004). Conscientiousness is also associated with greater educational attainment and career success. Optimism is also associated with reduced stress exposure and negative social exchanges (Raikkonen et al., 1999), as well as with increased social support (Brissette, Scheier, & Carver, 2002).

Stress Reactivity

Personality can clearly influence the immediate emotional and physiological response to a potentially stressful event. The prevailing model of effects of psychological stress on the development and course of disease posits a central role for excessive and repeated activation of the sympathetic adrenomedullary (SAM) system and the hypothalamic-pituitary-adrenocortical (HPA) axis, central components of the physiological response to stress. Studies of personality and stress reactivity, therefore, often focus on cortisol responses, the primary hormone indicative of HPA axis activation, and cardiovascular reactivity (i.e., increases in heart rate and blood pressure), indicative of sympathetic activation of the cardiovascular system. More recently, changes in high-frequency heart rate variability (HF-HRV) or respiratory sinus arrhythmia (RSA) have been examined as an indication of parasympathetic aspects of the stress response. In addition, the variety of anatomical and neuroendocrine links between the nervous and immune systems indicates that physiological stress responses also include alterations in the immune system, including inflammatory processes that have widespread effects on health (Segerstom & Miller, 2004; Uchino, Smith, Holt-Lunstad, Campo, & Reblin, 2007).

Many aspects of these physiological responses to stress are associated with personality traits reflecting the experience of negative affect. Anger, hostility, and depression have been linked with increases in SAM and HPA system activation in response to stress (Smith & Ruiz, 2002). Associations between individual differences in hostility and cardiovascular reactivity to laboratory stressors are well documented (Smith et al., 2004), though the effects may be particular to interpersonal stress (Suls & Wan, 1993). A recent meta-analysis of laboratory studies found that that the constellation of related traits including anger, hostility, aggressiveness, or Type A behavior was significantly associated with cardiovascular reactivity. In contrast, anxiety, neuroticism, and negative affectivity were associated with decreased cardiovascular reactivity (Chida & Hamer, 2008). These negative affective traits have been found to be associated with various aspects of immune functioning (e.g., heightened inflammation; decreased cytotoxicity and proliferation), including acute response to stressors and more enduring levels of immune activity (Segerstrom & Smith, 2006).

Compared to traits involving chronic negative affect and antagonistic interpersonal behavior, the FFM trait *openness to experience* is less well studied, both as a predictor of health outcomes and as an influence of stress responses. However, recent studies suggest that openness predicts better health outcomes in chronically ill populations (Ironson, O'Cleirigh, Weiss, Schneiderman, & Costa, 2008; Jonaissant et al., 2007). Recent research also indicates that high-open individuals display lower sympathetic activation (i.e., increased blood pressure) and greater parasympathetic activation (i.e., HF-HRV) in response to stress, whereas low-open individuals evidence parasympathetic withdrawal and greater sympathetic reactivity (P. W. Williams, Rau, Cribbet, & Gunn, 2009).

One concern about research on associations between personality traits and physiological responses to laboratory stressors involves the extent to which they reflect real life. Ambulatory studies have demonstrated such associations for several traits. Optimism is associated with lower ambulatory blood pressure (Raikkonen et al., 1999), for example, whereas hostility has been associated with higher levels of blood pressure (Benotsch, Christensen, & McKelvey, 1997; Brondolo et al., 2003; Guyll & Contrada, 1998).

Stress Recovery

Individuals vary in the time required for their emotional or physiological arousal to return to normal after termination of a stressor. As an influence on physical health, the duration of stress-related cardiovascular responses may be as important as the magnitude of initial reactivity (Brosschot, Gerin, & Thayer, 2006; Schwartz et al., 2003). Consistent with this view, poor cardiovascular recovery has been associated with subsequent increases in blood pressure over a period of several years (Mosely & Linden, 2006; Stewart, Janicki, & Kamarck, 2006).

Trait hostility has been associated with poor recovery of cardiovascular responses following anger provocation (e.g., Anderson, Linden, & Habia, 2005). In the previously described meta-analysis, *neuroticism* and other anxiety-related traits were also associated with slower cardiovascular recovery following laboratory stressors (Chida & Hamer, 2008). In addition, individuals high in neuroticism tend to experience prolonged negative mood after aversive events (Suls & Martin, 2005).

Stress Restoration

After the experience of stress, restorative processes "refresh, buttress, and repair various forms of cellular damage" and return individuals to their typical baseline levels (Cacioppo & Berntson, 2007, p. 73). Sleep, wound healing, and humoral immunity are examples of these restorative processes. Although personality has been a less common focus of research compared to other aspects of the stress response, it is associated with restorative processes, especially sleep.

A small but growing body of evidence indicates that sleep quality predicts important health outcomes. Poor sleep, especially sleep deprivation, is related to reductions in immune functioning (Lange, Perras, Fehm, & Born, 2003) and increased risk of death (Dew et al., 2003). Sleep disruption also has negative effects on emotion regulation (Dinges et al., 1997; Yoo, Gujar, Hu, Jolesz, & Walker, 2007) and cognitive functioning (Van Dongen, Maislin, Mullington, & Dinges, 2003), perhaps indicating that poor sleep can trigger escalating stress-regulation difficulties.

Neuroticism and other anxiety-related personality constructs are consistently associated with poor sleep (Gray & Watson, 2002). Individuals with high trait anxiety take longer to fall sleep, have more frequent transitions to light sleep, and show lower REM density compared to persons with low trait anxiety (Fuller, Waters, Binks, & Anderson, 1997). Hostility is also associated with poor sleep, especially in response to interpersonal conflict (Brissette & Cohen, 2002). In contrast, high conscientiousness is associated with better sleep quality (Gray & Watson, 2002). Further, conscientiousness has been found to moderate the negative effects of neuroticism on sleep (P. W. Williams & Moroz, 2008).

PERSONALITY AS THE BUNDLING OF MULTIPLE MECHANISMS

Associations between personality traits and subsequent health may reflect the operation of multiple mechanisms, including multiple components of the stress response (i.e., exposure, reactivity, recovery, restoration), various health behaviors, and underlying constitutional vulnerabilities. Stable individual differences in thought, emotion, and behavior seem likely to affect these multiple processes, and perhaps the predictive utility of personality risk factors lies in their association with these bundled influences on health. Hence, future research on understanding mechanisms linking personality and health not only should pursue specific pathways but also should consider the possibility that multiple mechanisms are involved.

CONCLUSION

Even the brief foregoing review reveals several robust associations between personality traits and important health outcomes. It also provides preliminary support for plausible mechanisms underlying those associations. Yet, clearly, additional work is needed. In what follows, we discuss the directions and challenges in those future efforts.

SOCIOCULTURAL CONTEXT OF PERSONALITY AND HEALTH RESEARCH

To date, much of the research concerning the association between personality and health has adopted a main effects approach, without considering the possible moderating impact of the sociocultural context in which people live. To fully understand the health implications of personality, future research should consider how such factors as age, gender, race/ethnicity, culture, and socioeconomic status may shape personality, health, or their relationship.

From a developmental perspective, personality characteristics are relatively dynamic during childhood and adolescence and reach a moderate level of stability in adulthood (Roberts & DelVecchio, 2000). However, even during adulthood, normative changes occur in the levels of some personality variables (Roberts, Walton, & Viechbauer, 2006); consequently, the nature of associations among personality factors may also vary across time. Age can also modify the strength of association between a given personality predictor and health outcome. For example, a relationship could exist in early or middle adulthood, but not at older ages, given earlier mortality rates in vulnerable individuals. Supporting this assertion, one study found that age moderated the relationship between hostility and mortality in CHD patients, such that a significant relationship was identified only in younger individuals (Boyle et al., 2005). Overall, additional research that takes a life-span-development approach is needed to understand the various ways in which age shapes the association between personality and health (Smith & Spiro, 2002).

In addition to age, gender is a relevant contextual factor that deserves additional consideration in future studies. That sex and gender shape the nature of personality in important ways is well established. Indeed, sex differences exist for most of the personality characteristics considered to be health risk factors (P. G. Williams & Gunn, 2006). One well-established model of gender, personality, and health suggests that gender-related traits foster differential vulnerability to distinct stressor types in men and women. Specifically, given traditional feminine gender roles that emphasize nurturance and affiliation, women are believed to be more susceptible to communion-oriented stressors (e.g., those involving interpersonal relationships). In contrast, traditional male gender roles are characterized by accomplishment, dominance, and individual goals, and men may therefore be more susceptible to agentic, or achievement-related, stressors. A substantial body of research supports this perspective (Helgeson, 2003, Chapter 22 this volume). It is of interest, however, that the findings of a meta-analysis of studies concerning undergraduate profiles on measures of gender role traits found that women's scores on measures of agency (or masculinity) steadily increased between the years of 1973 and 1995, with markedly diminished gender differences during that time period (Twenge, 1997). In addition, research suggests that unmitigated agency and communion (i.e., high levels of either trait combined with low levels of the other) are associated with health risks for both men and women (Helgeson, 2003). Thus, researchers should consider the relative level and balance of gender-related characteristics within individuals. There are also gender differences in the nature and timing of various health conditions. For example, men tend to suffer from CHD about 10 years earlier than do women (American Heart Association, 2008). Because many prior studies concerning personality and health have examined men or women exclusively or have failed to report sex differences, additional research is needed to determine the ways in which sex moderates the relationship between personality and health.

Ethnicity, race, and culture also represent important contextual factors in the study of personality and health, and for a number of reasons. First, the nature of personality or of specific traits may differ across various ethnic and cultural groups. Most current models of personality are based in Western culture and incorporate the assumption that social behavior is driven by stable traits of the individual. Cultural theorists have argued that these models may not apply adequately to all cultures (Markus, 2004). In Asian cultures, for example, social behavior is viewed as strongly based in social context; examined from this perspective, specific traits would not be expected to be constant across all situations. Thus, individual traits may have greater or lesser relevance to health and well-being depending on the cultural context in which they exist.

Experiences specific to ethnic minority groups may also shape personality development in ways that affect health risk. Specifically, exposure to ethnic discrimination and socioeconomic hardships may foster a reduced sense of optimism or higher levels of cynical distrust. For instance, some studies have consistently shown higher levels of hostility and anger in African Americans relative to non-Hispanic Whites (Barefoot et al., 1991; Scherwitz, Perkins, Chesney, & Hughes, 1991). Such differences may contribute to cardiovascular and other health disparities observed in African American populations. A number of ethnic and culture-specific traits have also been proposed as potentially relevant to health and illness. For example, within the Latino culture, *familism* reflects a collective perspective where the needs and objectives of the family are placed over those of the individual and where strong value is placed on nuclear and extended familial attachments. Research suggests that Hispanics are more family oriented relative to such other ethnic groups as non-Hispanic Whites, and they have larger family networks characterized by connectedness, commitment, and reciprocity (Gaines, Jr., et al., 1997). Furthermore, familism has been related to better health behaviors, including seeking medical care when ill (Tamez, 1981) and obtaining mammography scans (Suarez, 1994). In the African American community, *John Henryism* is a culturally bound characteristic associated with active striving to manage environmental stressors (James, 1994). Some research suggests that African Americans who are higher in John Henryism evidence elevated blood pressure, possibly as a consequence of coping effort that is unsuccessful in the face of vast cultural and economic barriers (Dressler, Bindon, & Neggers, 1998). These and a variety of other cultural characteristics have been examined in relation to health. Unfortunately, the research concerning many of these variables is hampered by a lack of conceptual clarity and available well-validated measurement instruments. Moreover, the extent to which each of these characteristics is conceptually distinct from established personality risk or resilient factors remains unclear.

Finally, the socioeconomic context is an important consideration in the study of personality and health. Socioeconomic status shapes virtually every aspect of health risk, including many of the trait variables shown to be related to physical health outcomes. Higher socioeconomic status, characterized by educational attainment, income, and occupational status, has been related to lower levels of cynical hostility and anger, as well as to features of negative affectivity, including depression and anxiety (Gallo & Matthews, 2003). Additional research suggests that higher socioeconomic status is associated with lower levels of pessimism (Taylor & Seeman, 1999). As such, it has been suggested that individual-difference variables, including higher negative cognitive-emotional traits or lower intrapsychic resources, might contribute to the relationship between socioeconomic status and physical health outcomes, including cardiovascular disease and mortality from all causes (Gallo, Bogart, & Vranceanu, 2005; Gallo & Matthews, 2003). This research area would benefit from a consideration of how social contextual factors, including age, gender, ethnicity and culture, and socioeconomic status, might shape personality traits believed to be relevant to health or might alter the nature of associations between personality and health.

PERSONALITY WITHIN THE BIOPSYCHOSOCIAL MODEL

Throughout its history, health psychology has been guided by Engel's (1977) biopsychosocial model (Suls & Rothman, 2004). From this conceptual perspective, personality plays a key role in the processes through which both stressful and salubrious environments "get under the skin" (Taylor, Repetti, & Seeman, 1997, p. 411) to affect physical health. The health-relevant dimensions of those environments must in some way influence the individual's emotions, behavior, and related psychophysiological responses. It seems unlikely that those effects of environmental influences would be identical across individuals, and some of that variation likely reflects the role of personality. Hence, personality moderates the effects of environmental factors on health.

Further, in order to influence the often years-long pathophysiology of serious medical illness, exposure to those unhealthy social environments must be prolonged. In many cases, such prolonged exposures might involve imposed conditions that are independent of the individual's actions, such as low socioeconomic status or job stress. However, as described earlier, in those instances personality traits might moderate the impacts of those imposed environmental conditions. Perhaps more important is that other social environmental influences on health may be sufficiently stable to influence health because personality tends to prolong such exposures. That is, stable exposure to either healthy or unhealthy social environments likely reflects the effects of personality on those environments. As described, personality factors might contribute to the chronic levels of social isolation versus support the individual experiences, as well as the level of conflict in close relationships, through such transactional processes. Hence, personality plays an important role in the comprehensive biopsychosocial understanding of health and disease because it occupies a key place between social-environmental influences on health and the pathophysiology of disease.

BIOLOGICAL PERSPECTIVES

Other trends in personality science might also prove useful in understanding how individual differences in emotion, cognition, and behavior influence the physiological mechanisms ultimately causing disease. Specifically, developments in molecular genetics and other aspects of the neuroscience of personality (Canli, 2006) could contribute further to the biopsychosocial understanding of disease. Increasingly, neuroscience and behavioral genomics focus on identifying specific biological underpinnings of the complex cognitive, emotional, and social behaviors comprising personality. Such research explicates how individual differences in temperament and personality emerge and how such differences may confer vulnerability to poor stress regulation.

Temperament refers to basic individual differences in emotional, motor, and attentional responses and is often described as the substrates from which personality develops through interaction with experience (Rothbart, 2007). Identification of the neural networks underlying dimensions of temperament has become a focus of research (e.g., Posner & Rothbart, 2007), and the FFM has been characterized with respect to dimensions of temperament (Rothbart, 2007; Shiner & Caspi, 2003). Dimensions of temperament and FFM traits show significant heritability (e.g., Jang, McCrae, Angleitner, Riemann, & Livesley, 1998; Plomin et al., 1993), and in several cases the "candidate genes" underlying particular phenotypes (e.g., personality traits) have been identified, as have the genes controlling serotonin (e.g., 5-HT) that are related to individual differences in neuroticism, anxiety, and depression.

Neuroimaging studies of individuals with specific genetic variations as they respond to particular cognitive-emotional tasks also help explicate the associations of aspects of personality with stress responses. For example, those individuals with the 5-HTTLPR S allele exhibit greater amygdala activity while they process emotional information (Hariri et al., 2002), perhaps indicating that the negative emotionality associated with the short allele may reflect hyper-responsiveness of the amygdala to potentially stressful emotional external stimuli. Further, brain circuitry connecting the limbic system, particularly the amygdala, and the prefrontal cortex (PFC) appears to be important in emotion regulation. The PFC regions involved in top-down processing of emotion input are also key brain regions for executive functioning, a multifaceted neurocognitive construct comprising a number of basic processes, including conceptual reasoning, working memory, cognitive flexibility, response selection, inhibition, initiation, set formation, and set maintenance (Suchy, 2009). These processes underpin the ability to generate goals and plans, modify behavior in response to environmental changes, and follow through and execute actions needed to achieve those goals. Serotonergic functioning has been linked to both depressive vulnerabilities and impulsive aggressiveness, perhaps reflecting a common neurotransmitter system associated with executive functioning and related individual differences in self-regulation (Carver, Johnson, & Joormann, 2008).

These individual differences in executive functioning are also related to stress regulation (P. G. Williams, Suchy, & Rau, 2009). These same PFC circuits, for example, are associated with parasympathetic activity that dampens sympathetically mediated stress responses and mobilizes coping behavior (Porges, 2007; Thayer & Lane, 2000). Thus, some neural structures and circuits contribute to stress reactivity (e.g., amygdala), whereas others (e.g., underpinnings of executive functions in the PFC) influence the modulation of stress responses. Hence, executive functioning and related parasympathetic processes could influence stress exposure, reactivity, recovery, and restoration. This emerging understanding of neuropsychological underpinnings of personality, along with related associations with individual-difference executive functioning, may help clarify mechanisms linking personality and health.

IMPLICATIONS FOR INTERVENTIONS

Scientific understanding of the effects of such psychosocial factors as personality on the development and course of disease has intrinsic merit, given the age-old nature of speculation regarding links between mind and body. However, ultimately, the value of this work will be determined by the success of related interventions intended to reduce the risk of disease or improve its course. Concepts and methods of current personality science have much to offer in this regard, as well. The FFM and interpersonal perspectives can help clarify which risk factors should be addressed in such risk-reducing interventions, thereby helping identify who might benefit from such efforts. Other elements of the interpersonal and cognitive-social perspectives can be informative as to how such interventions should be structured. That is, the more dynamic accounts from these latter perspectives can help indentify specific targets for intervention by describing the potentially modifiable components of recurring person–environment transactions that otherwise contribute to unhealthy aspects of stress exposure, reactivity, recovery, and restoration. Hence, the conceptual perspectives and methodological approaches in current personality science can facilitate the development of a more accurate, complete, cumulative, and ultimately useful understanding of the influence of personality on physical health.

REFERENCES

Allison, P. J., Guichard, C., Fung, K., & Gilain, L. (2003). Dispositional optimism predicts survival status 1 year after diagnosis in head and neck cancer patients. *Journal of Clinical Oncology*, *21*, 543–548.

American Heart Association. (2008). Heart disease and stroke statistics—2008 Update. Dallas, TX: American Heart Association.

Anderson, J. C., Linden, W., & Habia, M. E. (2005). The importance of examining blood pressure reactivity and recovery in anger provocation research. *International Journal of Psychophysiology*, *57*, 159–163.

Barefoot, J. C., Peterson, B. L., Dahlstrom, W. G., Siegler, I. C., Anderson, N. B., & Williams, R. B., Jr. (1991). Hostility patterns and health implications: Correlates of Cook-Medley Hostility Scale scores in a national survey. *Health Psychology*, *10*, 18–24.

Baron, K. G., Smith, T. W., Butner, J., Nealey-Moore, J., Hawkins, M. W., & Uchino, B. N. (2007). Hostility, anger, and marital adjustment: Concurrent and prospective associations with psychosocial vulnerability. *Journal of Behavioral Medicine*, *30*, 1–10.

Barth, J., Schumacher, M., & Herrmann-Lingen, C. (2004). Depression as a risk factor for mortality in patients with coronary heart disease: A meta-analysis. *Psychosomatic Medicine*, *66*, 802–813.

Benotsch, E. G., Christensen, A. J., & McKelvey, L. (1997). Hostility, social support and ambulatory cardiovascular activity, *Journal of Behavioral Medicine*, *20*, 163–176.

Berkman, L. F., Blumenthal, J., Burg, M., Carney, R. M., Catellier, D., Cowan, M. J. … Schneiderman, N. (2003). Effects of treating depression and low perceived social support on clinical events after myocardial infarction: The Enhancing Recovery in Coronary Heart Disease Patients (ENRICHD) randomized trial. *JAMA*, *289*, 3106–3116.

Block, J. (1995). A contrarian view of the five-factor approach to personality description. *Psychological Bulletin, 117*, 187–215.

Bolger, N., & Zuckerman, A. (1995). A framework for studying personality in the stress process. *Journal of Personality and Social Psychology, 69*, 890–902.

Booth-Kewley, S., & Friedman, H. S. (1987). Psychological predictors of heart disease: A quantitative review. *Psychological Bulletin, 101*, 343–362.

Boyle, S. H., Williams, R. B., Mark, D. B., Brummett, B. H., Siegler, I. C., & Barefoot, J. C. (2005). Hostility, age, and mortality in a sample of cardiac patients. *American Journal of Cardiology, 96*, 64–66.

Brand, R. J. (1978). Coronary-prone behavior as an independent risk factor for coronary heart disease. In T. M. Dembroski, S. M. Weiss, H. L. Shields, S. G. Haynes, & M. Feinleib (Eds.), *Coronary-prone behavior* (pp. 11–24). New York, NY: Springer-Verlag.

Brissette, I., & Cohen, S. (2002). The contribution of individual differences in hostility to the association between daily interpersonal conflict, affect, and sleep. *Personality and Social Psychology Bulletin, 28*, 1265–1274.

Brissette, I., Scheier, M. F., & Carver, C. S. (2002). The role of optimism in social network development, coping, and psychological adjustment during a life transition. *Journal of Personality and Social Psychology, 82*, 102–111.

Brondolo, E., Rieppi, R., Erickson, S. A., Bagiella, E., Shapiro, P. A., McKinley, P., … Sloan, R. P. (2003). Hostility, interpersonal interactions, and ambulatory blood pressure. *Psychosomatic Medicine, 65*, 1003–1111.

Brosschot, J. F., Gerin, W., & Thayer, J. F. (2006). The perseverative cognition hypothesis: A review of worry, prolonged stress-related physiological activation, and health. *Journal of Psychosomatic Research, 60*, 113–124.

Brummett, B. H., Helms, M. J., Dahlstrom, W. G., & Siegler, I. C. (2006). Prediction of all-cause mortality by the Minnesota Multiphasic Personality Inventory Optimism–Pessimism Scale scores: Study of a college sample during a 40-year follow-up period. *Mayo Clinic Proceedings, 81*, 1541–1544.

Brummett, B. H., Siegler, I. C., Day, R. S., & Costa, P. T. (2008). Personality as a predictor of dietary quality in spouses during midlife. *Behavioral Medicine, 34*, 5–10.

Buss, D. M. (1987). Selection, evocation, and manipulation. *Journal of Personality and Social Psychology, 53*, 1214–1221.

Cacioppo, J. T., & Berntson, G. G. (2007). The brain, homeostasis, and health: Balancing demands of the internal and external milieu. In H. S. Friedman & R. Cohen Silver (Eds.), *Foundations of health psychology* (pp. 73–91). New York, NY: Oxford University Press.

Canli, T. (Ed.). (2006). *Biology of personality and individual differences*. New York, NY: Guilford Press.

Cantor, N. (1990). From thought to behavior: "Having" and "doing" in the study of personality and cognition. *American Psychologist, 45*, 735–750.

Carney, R. M., Freedland, K. E., & Jaffe, A. S. (2001). Depression as a risk factor for coronary heart disease mortality. *Archives of General Psychiatry, 58*, 229–230.

Carver, C. S., Johnson, S. C., & Joormann, J. (2008). Serotonergic function, two-mode models of self-regulation, and vulnerability to depression: What depression has in common with impulsive aggression. *Psychological Bulletin, 134*, 912–943.

Chapman, B. P., Lyness, J. M., & Duberstein, P. (2007). Personality and medical illness burden among older adults in primary care. *Psychosomatic Medicine, 69*, 277–282.

Chaput, L. A., Adams, S. H., Simon, J. A., Blumenthal, R. S., Vittinghoff, E., Lin, F., … Matthews, K. A. (2002). Hostility predicts recurrent events among postmenopausal women with coronary heart disease. *American Journal of Epidemiology, 156*, 1092–1099.

Chida, Y., & Hamer, M. (2008). Chronic psychosocial factors and acute physiological responses to laboratory-induced stress in healthy populations: A quantitative review of 30 years of investigations. *Psychological Bulletin, 134*, 829–884.

Chida, Y., & Steptoe, A. (2008). Positive psychological well-being and mortality: A quantitative review of prospective observational studies. *Psychosomatic Medicine, 70*, 741–756.

Chida, Y., & Steptoe, A. (2009). The association of anger and hostility with future coronary heart disease: A meta-analytic review of prospective evidence. *Journal of the American College of Cardiology, 53*, 774–778.

Christenfeld, N. J. S., Sloan, R. P., Carroll, D., & Greenland, S. (2004). Risk factors, confounding, and the illusion of statistical control. *Psychosomatic Medicine, 66*, 868–875.

Christensen, A. J., Ehlers, S. L., Wiebe, J. S., Moran, P. J., Raichle, K., Ferneyhough, K., & Lawton, W. J. (2002). Patient personality and mortality: A 4-year prospective examination of chronic renal insufficiency. *Health Psychology, 21*, 315–320.

Cohen, F. (1980). Personality, stress, and the development of physical illness. In G. C. Stone, F. Cohen, & N. E. Adler (Eds.), *Health psychology* (pp. 77–111). San Francisco, CA: Jossey-Bass.

Cohen, S., & Pressman, S. D. (2006). Positive affect and health. *Current Directions in Psychological Science, 15*, 122–125.

Cohen, S., & Rodriguez, M. (1995). Pathways linking affective disturbances and physical disorders. *Health Psychology, 14*, 374–380.

Cooper, T., Detre, T., & Weiss, S. M. (1981). Coronary-prone behavior and coronary heart disease: A critical review. [The review panel on coronary-prone behavior and coronary heart disease.] *Circulation, 63*, 1199–1215.

Costa, P. T., Jr., & McCrae, R. R. (1992). *Professional manual: Revised NEO Personality Inventory (NEO-PI-R) and the NEO Five-Factor Inventory (NEO-FFI).* Odessa, FL: Psychological Assessment Resources.

Cronbach, L. J., & Meehl, P. E. (1955). Construct validity in psychological tests. *Psychology Bulletin, 52*, 281–302.

David, J., Green, P., Martin, R., & Suls, J. (1997). Differential roles of neuroticism and extraversion and event desirability for mood in daily life: An integrative model of top-down and bottom-up influences. *Journal of Personality and Social Psychology, 73*, 149–159.

De Bruijn, G. J., Kremers, S. P. J., van Mechelen, W., & Brug, J. (2005). Is personality related to fruit and vegetable intake and physical activity in adolescents? *Health Education Research, 20*, 635–644.

Dembroski, T. M., MacDougall, J. M., Costa, P. T., Jr., & Grandits, G. A. (1989). Components of hostility as predictors of sudden death and myocardial infarction in the Multiple Risk Factor Intervention Trial. *Psychosomatic Medicine, 51*, 514–522.

Denollet, J., & Pedersen, S. S. (2008). Prognostic value of type D personality compared with depressive symptoms. *Archives of Internal Medicine, 168*, 431–432.

Dew, M. A., Hoch, C. C., Buysse, D. J., Monk, T. H., Begley, A. E., Houck, P. R., … Reynolds, C. F. (2003). Healthy older adults' sleep predicts all-cause mortality at 4 to 19 years of follow-up. *Psychosomatic Medicine, 65*, 63–73.

Dickens, C. M., McGowan, L., Percival, C., Douglas, J., Tomenson, B., Cotter, L., … Creed, F. H. (2004). Lack of a close confidant, but not depression, predicts further cardiac events after myocardial infarction. *Heart, 90*, 518–522.

Dickens, C., McGowan, L., Percival, C., Tomenson, B., Cotter, L., Heagerty, A., & Creed, F. H. (2007). Depression is a risk factor for mortality after myocardial infarction: Fact or artifact? *Journal of the American College of Cardiology, 49*, 1834–1840.

Digman, J. M. (1990). Personality structure: emergence of the five-factor model. *Annual Review of Psychology, 41*, 417–440.

Dinges, D. F., Pack, F., Williams, K., Gillen, K. A., Powell, J. W., Ott, G. E., … Pack, A. (1997). Cumulative sleepiness, mood disturbance, and psychomotor vigilance performance decrements during a week of sleep restricted to 4–5 hours per night. *Sleep, 20*, 267–277.

Dressler, W. W., Bindon, J. R., & Neggers, Y. H. (1998). John Henryism, gender, and arterial blood pressure in an African American community. *Psychosomatic Medicine, 60*, 620–624.

Eaker, E. D., Sullivan, L. M., Kelly-Hayes, M., D'Agostino, R. B., Sr., & Benjamin, E. J. (2005). Tension and anxiety and the prediction of the 10-year incidence of coronary heart disease, atrial fibrillation, and total mortality: The Framingham Offspring Study. *Psychosomatic Medicine, 67*, 692–696.

Engel, G. L. (1977). The need for a new medical model: A challenge for biomedicine. *Science, 196*, 129–136.

Everson, S. A., Goldberg, D. E., Kaplan, G. A., Cohen, R. D., Pukkala, E., Tuomilehto, J., & Salonen, J. T. (1996). Hopelessness and risk of mortality and incidence of myocardial infarction and cancer. *Psychosomatic Medicine, 58*, 113–121.

Everson, S. A., Kaplan, G. A., Goldberg, D. E., Lakka, T. A., Sivenius, J., & Salonen, J. T. (1999). Anger expression and incident stroke: Prospective evidence from the Kuopio Ischemic Heart Disease Study. *Stroke, 30*, 523–528.

Everson, S. A., Roberts, R. E., Goldberg, D. E., & Kaplan, G. A. (1998). Depressive symptoms and increased risk of stroke mortality over a 29-year period. *Archives of Internal Medicine, 158*, 1133–1138.

Fleet, R., Lavoie, K., & Beitman, B. D. (2000). Is panic disorder associated with coronary artery disease? A critical review of the literature. *Journal of Psychosomatic Research, 48*, 347–356.

Flynn, K. E., & Smith, M. A. (2007). Personality and health care decision-making style. *Journals of Gerontology: Series B: Psychological Sciences and Social Sciences, 62*, 261–267.

Fournier, M. A., Moskowitz, D. S., & Zuroff, D. C. (2008). Integrating dispositions, signatures, and the interpersonal domain. *Journal of Personality and Social Psychology, 94*, 531–545.

Friedman, H. S., & Booth-Kewley, S. (1987). Personality, type A behavior, and coronary heart disease: The role of emotional expression. *Journal of Personality and Social Psychology, 53*, 783–792.

Friedman, M., & Rosenman, R. H. (1959). Association of a specific overt behavior pattern with increases in blood cholesterol, blood clotting time, incidence of arcus senilis and clinical coronary artery disease. *JAMA, 169,* 1286–1296.

Friedman, M., & Rosenman, R. H. (1974). *Type A behavior and your heart.* New York, NY: Knopf.

Fuller, K. H., Waters, W. F., Binks, P. G., & Anderson, T. (1997). Generalized anxiety and sleep architecture: A polysomnographic investigation. *Sleep: Journal of Sleep Research & Sleep Medicine, 20,* 370–376.

Gaines, S. O., Jr., Marelich, W. D., Bledsoe, K. L., Steers, W. N., Henderson, M. C., Granrose, C. S., … Page, M. S. (1997). Links between race/ethnicity and cultural values as mediated by racial/ethnic identity and moderated by gender. *Journal of Personality & Social Psychology, 72,* 1460–1476.

Gallacher, J. E. J., Sweetnam, P. M., Yarnell, J. W. G., Elwood, P. C., & Stansfeld, S. A. (2003). Is type A behavior really a trigger for coronary heart disease events? *Psychosomatic Medicine, 65,* 339–346.

Gallo, L. C., Bogart, L. M., & Vranceanu, A. M. (2005). Socioeconomic status, resources, psychological experiences, and emotional responses: A test of the reserve capacity model. *Journal of Personality & Social Psychology, 88,* 386–399.

Gallo, L. C., & Matthews, K. A. (2003). Understanding the association between socioeconomic status and physical health: Do negative emotions play a role? *Psychological Bulletin, 129,* 10–51.

Gallo, L. C., & Smith, T. W. (1998). Construct validation of health-relevant personality traits: Interpersonal circumplex and five-factor model analyses of the Aggression Questionnaire. *International Journal of Behavioral Medicine, 5,* 129–147.

Gallo, L. C., & Smith, T. W. (1999). Patterns of hostility and social support: Conceptualizing psychosocial risk factors as characteristics of the person and the environment. *Journal of Research in Personality, 33,* 281–310.

Giltay, E. J., Geleijnse, J. M., Zitman, F. G., Hoekstra, T., & Schouten, E. G. (2004). Dispositional optimism and all-cause and cardiovascular mortality in a prospective cohort of elderly dutch men and women. *Archives of General Psychiatry, 61,* 1126–1135.

Goodwin, R. D., & Friedman, H. S. (2006). Health status and the five-factor personality traits in a nationally representative sample. *Journal of Health Psychology, 11,* 643–654.

Gottdiener, J. S., Kop, W. J., Hausner, E., McCeney, M. K., Herrington, D., & Krantz, D. S. (2003). Effects of mental stress on flow-mediated brachial arterial dilation and influence of behavioral factors and hypercholesterolemia in subjects without cardiovascular disease. *Americal Journal of Cardiology, 92,* 687–691.

Gray, E. K., & Watson, D. (2002). General and specific traits of personality and their relation to sleep and academic performance. *Journal of Personality, 70,* 177–206.

Gunthert, K. C., Cohen, L., & Armeli, S. (1999). The role of neuroticism in daily stress and coping. *Journal of Personality and Social Psychology, 77,* 1087–1100.

Gute, G., & Eshbaugh, E. M. (2008). Personality as a predictor of hooking up among college students. *Journal of Community Health Nursing, 25,* 26–43.

Guyll, M., & Contrada, R. J. (1998). Trait hostility and ambulatory cardiovascular activity: Responses to social interaction. *Health Psychology, 17,* 30–39.

Hampson, S. E., Goldberg, L. R., Vogt, T. M., & Dubanoski, J. P. (2006). Forty years on: Teachers' assessments of children's personality traits predict self-reported health behaviors and outcomes at midlife. *Health Psychology, 25,* 57–64.

Hariri, A. R., Mattay, V. S., Tessigore, A., Kolachana, B., Fera, F., Goldman, D., … Weinberger, D. R. (2002). Serotonin transporter genetic variation and the response of the human amygdala. *Science, 297,* 400–403.

Harris, K. F., Matthews, K. A., Sutton-Tyrrell, K., & Kuller, L. H. (2003). Associations between psychological traits and endothelial function in postmenopausal women. *Psychosomatic Medicine, 65,* 401–409.

Helgeson, V. S. (2003). Gender-related traits and health. In J.Suls & K. Wallston (Eds.), *Social psychological foundations of health and illness* (pp. 367–394). Oxford, England: Blackwell.

Herzberg, P. Y., Glaesmer, H., & Hoyer, J. (2006). Separating optimism and pessimism: A robust psychometric analysis of the revised Life Orientation Test (LOT-R). *Psychological Assessment, 18,* 433–438.

Holroyd, K. A., & Coyne, J. (1987). Personality and health in the 1980s: Psychosomatic medicine revisited? *Journal of Personality, 55,* 360–375.

Horowitz, L. M. (2004). *Interpersonal foundations of psychopathology.* Washington, DC. American Psychological Association.

Horowitz, L. M., Wilson, K. R., Turan, B., Zolotsev, P., Constantino, M. J., & Henderson, L. (2006). How interpersonal motives clarify the meaning of interpersonal behavior: A revised circumplex model. *Personality and Social Psychology Review, 10,* 67–86.

Houston, B. K., Babyak, M. A., Chesney, M. A., Black, G., & Ragland, D. R. (1997). Social dominance and 22-year all-cause mortality in men. *Psychosomatic Medicine, 59,* 5–12.

Houston, B. K., Chesney, M. A., Black, G. W., Cates, D. S., & Hecker, M. L. (1992). Behavioral clusters and coronary heart disease risk. *Psychosomatic Medicine, 54*, 447–461.

Idler, E. L., & Benyamini, Y. (1997). Self-rated health and mortality: A review of twenty-seven community studies. *Journal of Health and Social Behavior, 38*, 21–37.

Iribarren, C., Sidney, S., Bild, D. E., Liu, K., Markovitz, J. H., Roseman, J. M., & Matthews, K. (2000). Association of hostility with coronary artery calcification in young adults: The CARDIA Study. Coronary Artery Risk Development in Young Adults. *JAMA, 283*, 2546–2551.

Ironson, G. H., O'Cleirigh, C., Weiss, A., Schneiderman, N., & Costa, P. T., Jr. (2008). Personality and HIV disease progression: Role of NEO-PI-R openness, extraversion, and profiles of engagement. *Psychosomatic Medicine, 70(2)*, 245–253.

Iwasa, H., Masui, Y., Gondo, Y., Inagaki, H., Kawaai, C., & Suzuki, T. (2008). Personality and all-cause mortality among older adults dwelling in a Japanese community: A five-year population-based prospective cohort study. *American Journal of Geriatric Psychiatry, 16*, 399–405.

James, S. A. (1994). John Henryism and the health of African-Americans. *Culture, Medicine and Psychiatry, 18*, 163–182.

Jang, K. L., McCrae, R. R., Angleitner, A., Riemann, R., & Livesley, W. J. (1998). Heritability of facet-level traits in a cross-cultural twin sample: Support for a hierarchical model of personality. *Journal of Personality and Social Psychology, 74*, 1556–1565.

Jonassaint, C. R., Boyle, S. H., Williams, R. B., Mark, D. B., Siegler, I. C., & Barefoot, J. C. (2007). Facets of openness predict mortality in patients with cardiac disease. *Psychosomatic Medicine, 69*, 319–322.

Kakizaki, M., Kuriyama, S., Sato, Y., Shimazu, T., Matsuda-Ohmori, K., Nakaya, N., ... Tsuji, I. (2008). Personality and body mass index: A cross-sectional analysis from the Miyagi cohort study. *Journal of Psychosomatic Research, 64*, 71–80.

Kaplan, J. R., & Manuck, S. B. (1998). Monkeys, aggression, and the pathobiology of atherosclerosis. *Aggressive Behavior, 24*, 334.

Kern, M. L., & Friedman, H. S. (2008). Do conscientious individuals live longer? A quantitative review. *Health Psychology, 27*, 505–512.

Kiesler, D. J. (1983). The 1982 interpersonal circle: A taxonomy for complementarity in human transactions. *Psychology Review, 90*, 185–214.

Kiesler, D. J. (Ed.). (1996). *Contemporary interpersonal theory and research: Personality, psychopathology, and psychotherapy*. New York, NY: Wiley.

Knol, M. J., Twisk, J. W., Beekman, A. T., Heine, R. J., Snoek, F.J., & Pouwer, F. (2006). Depression as a risk factor for the onset of type 2 diabetes mellitus. A meta-analysis. *Diabetologia, 49*, 837–845.

Kop, W. J. (1999). Chronic and acute psychological risk factors for clinical manifestations of coronary artery disease. *Psychosomatic Medicine, 61*, 476–487.

Korten, A. E., Jorm, A. F., Jiao, Z., Letenneur, L., Jacomb, P. A., Henderson, A. S., ... Rodgers, B. (1999). Health, cognitive, and psychosocial factors as predictors of mortality in an elderly community sample. *Journal of Epidemiology and Community Health, 53*, 83–88.

Kotov, R., Watson, D., Robles, J. P., & Schmidt, N. B. (2007). Personality traits and anxiety symptoms: The multilevel trait predictor model. *Behaviour Research and Therapy, 45*, 1485–1503.

Kubzansky, L. D., & Kawachi, I. (2000). Going to the heart of the matter: Do negative emotions cause coronary heart disease? *Journal of Psychosomatic Research, 48*, 323–337.

Kubzansky, L. D., Kawachi, I., Weiss, S. T., & Sparrow, D. (1998). Anxiety and coronary heart disease: A synthesis of epidemiological, psychological, and experimental evidence. *Annals of Behavioral Medicine, 20*, 47–58.

Kubzansky, L. D., Kubzansky, P. E., & Maselko, J. (2004). Optimism and pessimism in the context of health: Bipolar opposites or separate constructs? *Personality & Social Psychology Bulletin, 30*, 943–956.

Kubzansky, L. D., Sparrow, D., Vokonas, P., & Kawachi, I. (2001). Is the glass half empty or half full? A prospective study of optimism and coronary heart disease in the Normative Aging Study. *Psychosomatic Medicine, 63*, 910–916.

Kupper, N., & Denollet, J. (2007). Type D personality as a prognostic factor in heart disease: Assessment and mediating mechanisms. *Journal of Personality Assessment, 89*, 265–276.

Kupper, N., Denollet, J., de Geus, E. J., Boomsma, D. I., & Willemsen, G. (2007). Heritability of type-D personality. *Psychosomatic Medicine, 69*, 675–681.

Lane, D., Carroll, D., Ring, C., Beevers, D. G., & Lip, G. Y. (2001). Mortality and quality of life 12 months after myocardial infarction: Effects of depression and anxiety. *Psychosomatic Medicine, 63*, 221–230.

Lange, T., Perras, B., Fehm, H. L., & Born, J. (2003). Sleep enhances the human antibody response to hepatitis A vaccination. *Psychosomatic Medicine, 65*, 831–835.

Lazarus, R. S., & Folkman, S. (1984). Stress, appraisal, and coping. New York, NY: Springer.

Leserman, J. (2008). Role of depression, stress, and trauma in HIV disease progression. *Psychosomatic Medicine*, *70*, 539–545.

Linden, W., Phillips, M. J., & Leclerc, J. (2007). Psychological treatment of cardiac patients: A meta-analysis. *European Heart Journal*, *28*(24), 2964–2966.

Lynam, D. R., Hoyle, R. H., & Newman, J. P. (2006). The perils of partialling: Cautionary tales from aggression and psychopathy. *Assessment*, *12*, 328–341.

Magnus, K., Diener, E., Fugita, F., & Pavot, W. (1993). Extraversion and neuroticism as predictors of objective life events: A longitudinal analysis. *Journal of Personality and Social Psychology*, *65*, 1046–1053.

Markus, H. R. (2004). Culture and personality: Brief for an arranged marriage. *Journal of Research in Personality*, *38*, 75–83.

Marshall, G. N., Wortman, C. B., Vickers, R. R., Kusulas, J. W., & Hervig, L. K. (1994). The five-factor model of personality as a framework for personality-health research. *Journal of Personality and Social Psychology*, *67*, 278–286.

Martens, E. J., Kupper, N., Pedersen, S. S., Aquarius, A. E., & Denollet, J. (2007). Type-D personality is a stable taxonomy in post-MI patients over an 18-month period. *Journal of Psychosomatic Resesearch*, *63*, 545–550.

Maruta, T., Colligan, R. C., Malinchoc, M., & Offord, K. P. (2000). Optimists vs pessimists: Survival rate among medical patients over a 30-year period. *Mayo Clinic Proceedings*, *75*, 140–143.

Matthews, K. A. (1988). Coronary heart disease and type A behaviors: Update on and alternative to the Booth-Kewley and Friedman (1987) quantitative review. *Psychological Bulletin*, *104*, 373–380.

Matthews, K. A., Gump, B. B., Harris, K. F., Haney, T. L., & Barefoot, J. C. (2004). Hostile behaviors predict cardiovascular mortality among men enrolled in the Multiple Risk Factor Intervention Trial. *Circulation*, *109*, 66–70.

Matthews, K. A., Owens, J. F., Edmundowicz, D., Lee, L., & Kuller, L. H. (2006). Positive and negative attributes and risk for coronary and aortic calcification in healthy women. *Psychosomatic Medicine*, *68*, 355–361.

Matthews, K. A., Owens, J. F., Kuller, L. H., Sutton-Tyrrell, K., & Jansen-McWilliams, L. (1998). Are hostility and anxiety associated with carotid atherosclerosis in healthy postmenopausal women? *Psychosomatic Medicine*, *60*, 633–638.

Matthews, K. A., Raikkonen, K., Sutton-Tyrrell, K., & Kuller, L. H. (2004). Optimistic attitudes protect against progression of carotid atherosclerosis in healthy middle-aged women. *Psychosomatic Medicine*, *66*, 640–644.

McAdams, D. P. (1995). What do we know when we know a person? *Journal of Personality*, *63*, 365–396.

McCrae R. R., & Costa, P. T., Jr. (1989). The structure of interpersonal traits: Wiggins circumplex and the five-factor model. *Journal of Personality and Social Psychology*, *56*, 586–595.

McCrae, R. R., & John, O. P. (1992). An introduction to the five-factor model and its applications. *Journal of Personality*, *60*, 175–215.

McCusker, J., Cole, M., Ciampi, A., Latimer, E., Windholz, S., & Belzile, E. (2006). Does depression in older medical inpatients predict mortality? *Journals of Gerontology: Series A. Biological Sciences and Medical Sciences*, *61*, 975–981.

McFall, R. M. (2005). Theory and utility—Key themes in evidence-based assessment: Comment on the special section. *Psychological Assessment*, *17*, 312–333.

Mechanic, D. (1972). Social psychological factors affecting the presentation of bodily complaints. *New England Journal of Medicine*, *286*, 1132–1139.

Miller, T. Q., Smith, T. W., Turner, C. W., Guijarro, M. L., & Hallet, A. J. (1996). A meta-analytic review of research on hostility and physical health. *Psychology Bulletin*, *119*, 322–348.

Miller, T. Q., Turner, C. W., Tindale, R. S., Posavac, E. J., & Dugoni, B. L. (1991). Reasons for the trend toward null findings in research on type A behavior. *Psychological Bulletin*, *110*, 469–485.

Mischel, W. (1968). *Personality and assessment*. New York, NY: Wiley.

Mischel, W. (2004). Toward an integrative science of the person. *Annual Review of Psychology*, *55*, 1–22.

Mischel, W., & Shoda, Y. (1998). Reconciling processing dynamics and personality dispositions. *Annual Review of Psychology*, *49*, 229–258.

Mosely, J. V., & Linden, W. (2006). Predicting blood pressure and heart rate change with cardiovascular reactivity and recovery: Results from a 3-year and 10-year follow-up. *Psychosomatic Medicine*, *68*, 833–843.

Moser, D. K., & Dracup, K. (1996). Is anxiety early after myocardial infarction associated with subsequent ischemic and arrhythmic events? *Psychosomatic Medicine*, *58*, 395–401.

Mroczek, D. K., & Spiro, A. I. (2007). Personality change influences mortality in older men. *Psychological Science*, *18*, 371–376.

Munafo, M. R., Zetteler, J. I., & Clark, T. G. (2007). Personality and smoking status: A meta-analysis. *Nicotine & Tobacco Research, 9*, 405–413.

Mykletun, A., Bjerkeset, O., Dewey, M., Prince, M., Overland, S., & Stewart, R. (2007). Anxiety, depression, and cause-specific mortality: The HUNT Study. *Psychosomatic Medicine, 69*, 323–331.

Nicholson, A., Kuper, H., & Hemingway, H. (2006). Depression as an aetiologic and prognostic factor in coronary heart disease: A meta-analysis of 6362 events among 146 538 participants in 54 observational studies. *European Heart Journal, 27*, 2763–2774.

Norem, J. K., & Change, E. C. (2001). A very full glass: Adding complexity to our applications of optimism and pessimism research. In E. C. Change (Ed.), *Optimism and pessimism: Implications for theory, research and practice* (pp. 347–367). Washington, DC: American Psychological Association.

O'Cleirigh, C., Ironson, G., Weiss, A., & Costa, P. T. J. (2007). Conscientiousness predicts disease progression (CD4 number and viral load) in people living with HIV. *Health Psychology, 26*, 473–480.

Oltmanns, T. E., & Turkheimer, E. (2006). Perceptions of self and others regarding pathological personality traits. In R. F. Krueger & J. L. Tackett (Eds.), *Personality and psychopathology* (pp. 71–111). New York, NY: Guilford Press.

Orth-Gomér, K., Schneiderman, N., Wang, H. X., Walldin, C., Blom, M., & Jernberg, T. (2009). Stress reduction prolongs life in women with coronary disease: The Stockholm Women's Intervention Trial for Coronary Heart Disease (SWITCHD). *Circulation: Cardiovascular Quality and Outcomes, 2*, 25–32.

Pedersen, S. S., & Denollet, J. (2003). Type D personality, cardiac events, and impaired quality of life: A review. *European Journal of Cardiovascascular Prevention & Rehabilitation, 10*, 241–248.

Phillips, A. N., & Davey Smith, G. (1991). Bias in relative odds estimation owing to imprecise measurement of correlated exposures. *Statistics in Medicine, 11*, 953–961.

Pincus, A. L., & Ansell, E. B. (2003). Interpersonal theory of personality. In T. Millon & M. J. Lerner (Eds.), *Handbook of psychology: Personality and social psychology* (Vol. 5, pp. 209–229). New York, NY: Wiley.

Plomin, R., Emde, R. N., Braungart, J. M., Campos, J., Corley, R., Fulker, D. W., … Zahn-Waxler, C. (1993). Genetic change and continuity from fourteen to twenty months: The MacArthur Longitudinal Twin Study. *Child Development, 64*, 1354–1376.

Porges, S. (2007). The polyvagal perspective. *Biological Psychology, 74*(2), 116–143.

Posner, M., & Rothbart, M. (2007). Research on attention networks as a model for the integration of psychological science. *Annual Review of Psychology, 58*, 1–23.

Ragland, D. R., & Brand, R. J. (1988). Type A behavior and mortality from coronary heart disease. *New England Journal of Medicine, 318*, 65–69.

Raikkonen, K., Matthews, K. A., Flory, J. D., Owens, J. F., & Gump, B. (1999). Effects of optimism, pessimism, and trait anxiety on ambulatory blood pressure and mood during everyday life. *Journal of Personality and Social Psychology, 76*, 104–113.

Raikkonen, K., Matthews, K. A., Sutton-Tyrrell, K., & Kuller, L. H. (2004). Trait anger and the metabolic syndrome predict progression of carotid atherosclerosis in healthy middle-aged women. *Psychosomatic Medicine, 66*, 903–908.

Rees, K., Bennett, P., West, R., Davey, S. G., & Ebrahim, S. (2004). Psychological interventions for coronary heart disease. Cochrane Database of Systematic Reviews, CD002902.

Reich, J. W., Zautra, A. J., & Davis, M. (2003). Dimensions of affect relationships: Models and their integrative implications. *Review of General Psychology, 7*, 66–83.

Roberts, B. W., & Bogg, T. (2004). A longitudinal study of the relationships between conscientiousness and the social-environmental factors and substance use behaviors that influence health. *Journal of Personality, 72*, 325–354.

Roberts, B. W., & DelVecchio, W. F. (2000). The rank-order consistency of personality traits from childhood to old age: A quantitative review of longitudinal studies. *Psychological Bulletin, 126*, 3–25.

Roberts, B. W., Kuncel, N. R., Shiner, R., Caspi, A., & Goldberg, L. R. (2007). The power of personality: The comparative validity of personality traits, socioeconomic status, and cognitive ability for predicting important life outcomes. *Perspectives in Psychological Science, 2*, 313–345.

Roberts, B. W., Walton, K. E., & Viechbauer, W. (2006). Patterns of mean-level change in personality traits across the life course: A meta-analysis of longitudinal studies. *Psychological Bulletin, 132*, 1–25.

Rosenman, R. H., Brand, R. J., Jenkins, D., Friedman, M., Straus, R., & Wurm, M. (1975). Coronary heart disease in Western Collaborative Group Study. Final follow-up experience of 8 1/2 years. *JAMA, 233*, 872–877.

Rosenman, R. H., & Friedman, M. (1974). Neurogenic factors in pathogenesis of coronary heart disease. *Medical Clinics of North America, 58*, 269–279.

Rosenman, R. H., Friedman, M., Straus, R., Wurm, M., Kositcheck, R., Hahn, W., & Werthessen, N. T. (1964). A predictive study of coronary heart disease. *JAMA, 189*, 15–22.

Rothbart, M. K. (2007). Temperament, development, and personality. *Current Directions in Psychological Science, 16*, 207–212.

Rozanski, A., Blumenthal, J. A., & Kaplan, J. (1999). Impact of psychological factors on the pathogenesis of cardiovascular disease and implications for therapy. *Circulation, 99*, 2192–2217.

Rugulies, R. (2002). Depression as a predictor for coronary heart disease: A review and meta-analysis. *American Journal of Preventive Medicine, 23*, 51–61.

Russell, J. A., & Carroll, J. M. (1999). On the bipolarity of positive and negative affect. *Psychological Bulletin, 125*, 3–30.

Rutledge, T., & Hogan, B. E. (2002). A quantitative review of prospective evidence linking psychological factors with hypertension development. *Psychosomatic Medicine, 64*, 758–766.

Rutledge, T., Reis, V. A., Linke, S. E., Greenberg, B. H., & Mills, P. J. (2006). Depression in heart failure: A meta-analytic review of prevalence, intervention effects, and associations with clinical outcomes. *Journal of the American College of Cardiology, 48*, 1527–1537.

Ryff, C. D., & Singer, B. (1998). The contours of positive human health. *Psychological Inquiry, 9*, 1–28.

Scheier, M. F., Matthews, K. A., Owens, J. F., Magovern, G. J., Sr., Lefebvre, R. C., Abbott, R. A., & Carver, C. S. (1989). Dispositional optimism and recovery from coronary artery bypass surgery: The beneficial effects on physical and psychological well-being. *Journal of Personality & Social Psychology, 57*, 1024–1040.

Scheier, M. F., Matthews, K. A., Owens, J. F., Schulz, R., Bridges, M. W., Magovern, G. J., & Carver, C. S. (1999). Optimism and rehospitalization after coronary artery bypass graft surgery. *Archives of Internal Medicine, 159*, 829–835.

Scherwitz, L., Perkins, L., Chesney, M., & Hughes, G. (1991). Cook-Medley Hostility Scale and subsets: Relationship to demographic and psychosocial characteristics in young adults in the CARDIA Study. *Psychosomatic Medicine, 53*, 36–49.

Schiffer, A. A., Pedersen, S. S., Widdershoven, J. W., & Denollet, J. (2008). Type D personality and depressive symptoms are independent predictors of impaired health status in chronic heart failure. *European Journal of Heart Failure, 10*, 922–930.

Schulz, R., Bookwala, J., Knapp, J. E., Scheier, M., & Williamson, G. M. (1996). Pessimism, age, and cancer mortality. *Psychology & Aging, 11*, 304–309.

Schwartz, A. R., Gerin W., Davidson, K. W., Pickering, T. G., Brosschot, J. F., Thayer, J. F.,... Linden, W. (2003). Toward a causal model of cardiovascular responses to stress and the development of cardiovascular disease. *Psychosomatic Medicine, 65*, 22–35.

Segerstrom, S. C., & Miller, G. E. (2004). Psychological stress and the human immune system: A meta-analytic study of 30 years of inquiry. *Psychological Bulletin, 130*, 601– 630.

Segerstrom, S. C., & Smith, T. W. (2006). Physiological pathways from personality to health: The cardiovascular and immune systems. In M. Vollrath (Ed.), *Handbook of personality and health* (pp. 175–194). New York, NY: Wiley.

Shekelle, R. B., Gale, M., & Norusis, M. (1985). Type A score (Jenkins Activity Survey) and risk of recurrent coronary heart disease in the Aspirin Myocardial Infarction Study. *American Journal of Cardiolology, 56*, 221–225.

Shekelle, R. B., Hulley, S. B., Neaton, J., Billings, J. H., Borhani, N. O., Gerace, T. A., ... Stamler, J. (1985). The MRFIT Behavior Pattern Study: II. Type A behavior and incidence of coronary heart disease. *American Journal of Epidemiology, 122*, 559–570.

Shibeshi, W. A., Young-Xu, Y., & Blatt, C. M. (2007). Anxiety worsens prognosis in patients with coronary artery disease. *Journal of the American College of Cardiology, 49*, 2021–2027.

Shiner, R., & Caspi, A. (2003). Personality differences in childhood and adolescence: Measurement, development, and consequences. *Journal of Child Psychology and Psychiatry, 44*, 2–32.

Shipley, B. A., Weiss, A., Der, G., Taylor, M. D., & Deary, I. J. (2007). Neuroticism, extraversion, and mortality in the UK Health and Lifestyle Survey: A 21-year prospective cohort study. *Psychosomatic Medicine, 69*, 923–931.

Siegler, I. C., Costa, P. T., Brummett, B. H., Helms, M. J., Barefoot, J. C., Williams, R. B., ... Rimer, B. K. (2003). Patterns of change in hostility from college to midlife in the UNC Alumni Heart Study predict high-risk status. *Psychosomatic Medicine, 65*, 738–745.

Siegman, A. W. (1994). From type A to hostility and anger: Reflections on the history of coronary-prone behavior. In A. W. Siegman & T. W. Smith (Eds.), *Anger, hostility, and the heart* (pp. 1–22). Hillsdale, NJ: Erlbaum.

Siegman, A. W., Kubzansky, L. D., Kawachi, I., Boyle, S., Vokonas, P. S., & Sparrow, D. (2000). A prospective study of dominance and coronary heart disease in the Normative Aging Study. *American Journal of Cardiology, 86*, 145–149.

Smith, T. W. (1994). Concepts and methods in the study of anger, hostility, and health. In A. W. Siegman & T. W. Smith (Eds.), *Anger, hostility, and the heart* (pp. 23–42). Hillsdale, NJ: Erlbaum.

Smith, T. W. (2007). Measurement in health psychology research. In R. Silver, & H. S. Friedman (Eds.), *Foundations of health psychology*, (pp 19–51). New York, NY: Oxford University Press.

Smith, T. W. (2010). Conceptualization, measurement, and analysis of negative affective risk factors. In A. Steptoe (Ed.), *Handbook of behavioral medicine research: methods and applications* (pp. 155–168). New York, NY: Springer.

Smith, T.W., & Cundiff, J. M. (2010). Risk for coronary heart disease: An interpersonal perspective. In L. M. Horowitz & S. Strack (Eds.), *Handbook of interpersonal psychology: Theory, research, assessment, and therapeutic interventions.* Hoboken, NJ: Wiley.

Smith, T. W., & Gallo, L. C. (2001). Personality traits as risk factors for physical illness. In A. Baum, T. Revenson, & J. Singer (Eds.), *Handbook of health psychology* (pp. 139–172). Hillsdale, NJ: Erlbaum.

Smith, T. W., Glazer, K., Ruiz, J. M., & Gallo, L. C. (2004). Hostility, anger, aggressiveness and coronary heart disease: An interpersonal perspective on personality, emotion and health. *Journal of Personality, 72*, 1217–1270.

Smith, T. W., & MacKenzie, J. (2006). Personality and risk of physical illness. *Annual Review of Clinical Psychology, 2*, 435–467.

Smith, T. W., & Ruiz, J. M. (2002). Psychosocial influences on the development and course of coronary heart disease: Current status and implications for research and practice. *Journal of Consulting and Clinical Psychology, 70*, 548–568.

Smith, T. W., & Spiro, A., III. (2002). Personality, health, and aging: Prolegomenon for the next generation. *Journal of Research in Personality, 36*, 363–394.

Smith, T. W., Traupman, E., Uchino, B. N., & Berg, C. (2010). Interpersonal circumplex descriptions of psychosocial risk factors for physical illness: Application to hostility, neuroticism, and marital adjustment. *Journal of Personality, 78*, 1011–1036.

Smith, T. W., Uchino, B. N., Berg, C. A., Florsheim, P., Pearce, G., Hawkins, M., ...Yoon, H. C. (2008). Self-reports and spouse ratings of negative affectivity, dominance and affiliation in coronary artery disease: Where should we look and who should we ask when studying personality and health? *Health Psychology, 27*, 676–684.

Smith, T. W., & Williams, P. G. (1992). Personality and health: Advantages and limitations of the five-factor model. *Journal of Personality, 60*, 395–423.

Steptoe, A., & Molloy, G. J. (2007). Personality and heart disease. *Heart, 93*, 783–784.

Stern, S. L., Dhanda, R., & Hazuda, H. P. (2001). Hopelessness predicts mortality in older Mexican and European Americans. *Psychosomatic Medicine, 63*, 344–351.

Stewart, J. C., Janicki, D. L., & Kamarck, T. W. (2006). Cardiovascular reactivity and recovery from psychological challenge as predictors of 3-year change in blood pressure. *Health Psychology, 25*, 111–118.

Suarez, L. (1994). Pap smear and mammogram screening in Mexican-American women: The effects of acculturation. *American Journal of Public Health, 84*, 742–746.

Suchy, Y. (2009). Executive functioning: Overview, assessment, and research issues for non-neuropsychologists. *Annals of Behavioral Medicine, 37*, 106–116

Suls, J., & Bunde, J. (2005). Anger, anxiety, and depression as risk factors for cardiovascular disease: The problems and implications of overlapping affective dispositions. *Psychological Bulletin, 131*, 260–300.

Suls, J., & Martin, R. (2005). The daily life of the garden-variety neurotic: Reactivity, stressor exposure, mood spillover, and maladaptive coping. *Journal of Personality, 73*, 1–25.

Suls, J., Martin, R., & David, J. (1998). Person-environment fit and its limits: Agreeableness, neuroticism and emotional reactivity to interpersonal conflict. *Personality and Social Psychology Bulletin, 24*, 88–98.

Suls, J., & Rothman, A. J. (2004). Evolution of the psychosocial model: Implications for the future of health psychology. *Health Psychology, 23*, 119–125.

Suls, J., & Wan, C. K. (1993). The relationship between trait hostility and cardiovascular reactivity: A quantitative review. *Psychophysiology, 30*, 615–626.

Surtees, P., Wainwright, N., Luben, R., Khaw, K. T., & Day, N. (2003). Sense of coherence and mortality in men and women in the EPIC-Norfolk, United Kingdom, Prospective Cohort Study. *American Journal of Epidemiology, 158*, 1202–1209.

Surtees, P. G., Wainwright, N. W., Luben, R., Khaw, K. T., & Day, N. E. (2006). Mastery, sense of coherence, and mortality: Evidence of independent associations from the EPIC-Norfolk Prospective Cohort Study. *Health Psychology, 25*, 102–110.

Surtees, P. G., Wainwright, N. W., Luben, R. L., Wareham, N. J., Bingham, S. A., & Khaw, K. T. (2007). Adaptation to social adversity is associated with stroke incidence: Evidence from the EPIC-Norfolk Prospective Cohort Study. *Stroke, 38*, 1447–1453.

Szekely, A., Balog, P., Benko, E., Breuer, T., Szekely, J., Kertai, M. D., … Thayer, J. F. (2007). Anxiety predicts mortality and morbidity after coronary artery and valve surgery: A 4-year follow-up study. *Psychosomatic Medicine, 69*, 625–631.

Tamez, E. G. (1981). Familism, machismo and child rearing practices among Mexican Americans. *Journal of Psychosocial Nursing & Mental Health Services, 19*, 21–25.

Taylor, S. E., Repetti, R. L., & Seeman, T. E. (1997). Health psychology: What is an unhealthy environment and how does it get under the skin? *Annual Review of Psychology, 48*, 411–447.

Taylor, S. E., & Seeman, T. E. (1999). Psychosocial resources and the SES-health relationship. In N. E. Adler, M. Marmot, B. S. McEwen, & J. Stewart (Eds.), *Socioeconomic status and health in industrial nations: Social, psychological, and biological pathways* (pp. 210–225). New York, NY: New York Academy of Sciences.

Terracciano, A., Lockenhoff, C. E., Zonderman, A. B., Ferrucci, L., & Costa, P. T., Jr. (2008). Personality predictors of longevity: Activity, emotional stability, and conscientiousness. *Psychosomatic Medicine, 70*, 621–627.

Thayer, J. F., & Lane, R. D. (2000). A model of neurovisceral integration in emotion regulation and dysregulation. *Journal of Affective Disorders, 61*(3), 201–216.

Thayer, J. F., & Lane, R. D. (2007). The role of vagal function in the risk for cardiovascular disease and mortality. *Biological Psychology, 74*(2), 224–242.

Trapnell, P. D., & Wiggins, J. S. (1990). Extension of the Interpersonal Adjective Scales to include the big five dimensions of personality. *Journal of Personality and Social Psychology, 59*, 781–790.

Traupman, E., Smith, T. W., Uchino, B. N., Berg, C. A., Trobst, K., & Costa, P. T. (2009). Interpersonal circumplex octant, dominance, and affiliation scales for the NEO-PI-R. *Personality and Individual Differences, 47*, 457–463.

Trobst, K. (2000). An interpersonal conceptualization and quantification of social support transactions. *Personality and Social Psychology Bulletin, 26*, 971–986.

Twenge, J. M. (1997). Changes in masculine and feminine traits over time: A meta-analysis. *Sex Roles, 36*, 305–325.

Uchino, B. N., Smith, T. W., Holt-Lunstad, J., Campo, R. A., & Reblin, M. (2007). Stress and illness. In J. T. Cacioppo, L. G. Tassinary, & G. G. Bertson (Eds.), *Handbook of psychophysiology* (pp. 608–632). New York, NY: Cambridge University Press.

Van Dongen, H. P. A., Maislin, G., Mullington, J. M., & Dinges, D. F. (2003). The cumulative cost of additional wakefulness: Dose-response effects on neurobehavioral functions and sleep physiology from chronic sleep restriction and total sleep deprivation. *Sleep, 26*(2), 117–126.

Vollrath, M. E., Landolt, M. A., Gnehm, H. E., Laimbacher, J., & Sennhauser, F. H. (2007). Child and parental personality are associated with glycaemic control in type 1 diabetes. *Diabetic Medicine, 24*, 1028–1033.

Wainwright, N. W., Surtees, P. G., Welch, A. A., Luben, R. N., Khaw, K. T., & Bingham, S. A. (2007). Healthy lifestyle choices: Could sense of coherence aid health promotion? *Journal of Epidiolology & Community Health, 61*, 871–876.

Wainwright, N. W., Surtees, P. G., Welch, A. A., Luben, R. N., Khaw, K. T., & Bingham, S. A. (2008). Sense of coherence, lifestyle choices and mortality. *Journal of Epidemiology & Community Health, 62*, 829–831.

Walters, K., Rait, G., Petersen, I., Williams, R., & Nazareth, I. (2008). Panic disorder and risk of new onset coronary heart disease, acute myocardial infarction, and cardiac mortality: Cohort study using the general practice research database. *European Heart Journal, 29*, 2981–2988.

Weiss, A., & Costa, P. T. J. (2005). Domain and facet personality predictors of all-cause mortality among Medicare patients aged 65 to 100. *Psychosomatic Medicine, 67*, 715–723.

West, S. G., & Finch, J. F. (1997). Personality measurement: Reliability and validity issues. In R. Hogan, J. Johnson, & S. Briggs (Eds.). *Handbook of personality psychology* (pp. 143–164). New York, NY: Academic Press.

Whiteman, M. C., Deary, I. J., Lee, A. J., & Fowkes, F. G. (1997). Submissiveness and protection from coronary heart disease in the general population: Edinburgh Artery Study. *Lancet, 350*, 541–545.

Williams, J. E., Nieto, F. J., Sanford, C. P., Couper, D. J., & Tyroler, H. A. (2002). The association between trait anger and incident stroke risk: The Atherosclerosis Risk in Communities (ARIC) Study. *Stroke, 33*, 13–20.

Williams, P. G., & Gunn, H. E. (2006). Gender, personality, and psychopathology. In J. C. Thomas & D. L. Siegl (Eds.), *Handbook of personality and psychopathology: Vol. 1. Personality and everyday functioning* (pp. 432–442). Hoboken, NJ: Wiley.

Williams, P. G., Smith, T. W., & Cribett, M. R. (2008). Personality and health: Current evidence, potential mechanisms, and future directions. In G. J. Boyle, G. Matthews, & D. H. Saklofske (Eds.), *Personality Theories and Models* (Vol. 1, pp. 635–658). Los Angeles, CA: Sage.

Williams, P. G., Smith, T. W., Gunn, H., & Uchino, B. N. (2011). Personality and stress: Individual differences in exposure, reactivity, recovery, and restoration. In R. Contrada & A. Baum (Eds.), *Handbook of stress science* (pp. 231–245). New York, NY: Springer.

Williams, P. G., Suchy, Y., & Rau, H. (2009). Individual differences in executive functioning: Implications for stress regulation. *Annals of Behavioral Medicine, 37,* 126–140.

Williams, P. W., & Moroz, T. L. (2008). *Personality vulnerability to stress-related sleep disruption: Pathways to adverse mental and physical health outcomes.* Manuscript submitted for publication.

Williams, P. W., Rau, H. K., Cribbet, M. R., & Gunn, H. E. (2009). Openness to experience and stress regulation. *Journal of Research in Personality, 43*(5), 777–784.

Wilson, R. S., de Leon, C. F. M., Bienias, J. L., Evans, D. A., & Bennett, D. A. (2004). Personality and mortality in old age. *Journals of Gerontology: Series B. Psychological Sciences and Social Sciences,* 110–116.

Wulsin, L. R., & Singal, B. M. (2003). Do depressive symptoms increase the risk for the onset of coronary disease? A systematic quantitative review. *Psychosomatic Medicine, 65,* 201–210.

Wulsin, L. R., Vaillant, G. E., & Wells, V. E. (1999). A systematic review of the mortality of depression. *Psychosomatic Medicine, 61,* 6–17.

Yan, L. L., Liu, K., Matthews, K. A., Daviglus, M. L., Ferguson, T. F., & Kiefe, C. I. (2003). Psychosocial factors and risk of hypertension: The Coronary Artery Risk Development in Young Adults (CARDIA) Study. *JAMA, 290,* 2138–2148.

Yoo, S., Gujar, N., Hu, P., Jolesz, F., & Walker, M. (2007). The human emotional brain without sleep: A prefrontal-amygdala disconnect? *Current Biology, 17,* R877–R878.

18 Meaning, Spirituality, and Growth

Protective and Resilience Factors in Health and Illness

Crystal L. Park
University of Connecticut

This chapter delineates pathways through which three protective and resilience-related resources—meaning, spirituality, and stress-related growth—promote health and well-being. Although the emphasis here is on physical health, literature regarding related mental health states is included as appropriate. In this chapter, the resources are each considered in turn, with the discussion reviewing the potential protective effects of their ongoing influence under ordinary circumstances and then reviewing their potential resilience effects on individuals confronting serious illness and other major life stressors. Specifically, this chapter reviews the empirical evidence regarding how these resources may (a) protect individuals' health by imbuing daily life with direction and positive emotional states and minimizing wear and tear, and (b) promote resilience in stressful situations by buffering stress and its resulting emotional and physiological strain. Suggestions for future research to better understand these important pathways and clinical implications conclude the chapter.

In reviewing this vast and growing literature, it is important to keep in mind that very little of this research has been conducted experimentally. Instead, most studies examining the potential health promotion and protection offered by meaning, spirituality, and growth have employed observational designs, precluding determination of causality. Further, many of these studies have been conducted cross-sectionally, measuring all the relevant variables simultaneously. More sophisticated work, conducted longitudinally, examines the ability of these factors to "predict," in a statistical sense, subsequent health; the better of these studies include and control for potential confounds and test alternative models, which, though still unable to establish causality among variables, can at least establish plausibility of such causal links. In spite of these severe limitations, many studies infer causality and describe their results in strong causal terms. For example, an intriguing analysis of data from the General Social Survey, a national probability sample of U.S. residents, found associations between fundamentalist religiousness and higher levels of health but lower levels of happiness (all self-report; Green & Elliott, 2010). The authors tentatively interpreted these findings as meaning that fundamentalist religions offer an optimistic worldview that reduces uncertainty while reducing the responsibility individuals take for their own health. Although the evaluation is plausible, there are many other possible reasons for these relationships. For example, people in ill health may turn to fundamentalist religion for comfort. Similar problems in interpreting the impact of growth on health should be noted; in particular, studies of growth rarely control for important third variables that might underlie the associations found (Park, 2009). This chapter describes the design of studies and avoids causal language except where warranted. Readers are urged to approach this literature cautiously and to be alert to potential alternative explanations.

MEANING

Meaning refers to a sense of understanding, significance, and purpose (Park & Folkman, 1997; see Park, 2010, and Klinger, in press). Meaning consists of both global and situational aspects (Park & Folkman, 1997). *Global meaning* refers to individuals' general orienting systems (Pargament, 1997), which allow them to observe their current reality, imagine alternative realities, interpret the past, anticipate the future, and then direct their behavior accordingly. As such, global meaning has a potent impact on health and emotional well-being in both ordinary times and times of crisis. In stressful encounters, global meaning informs the ways people appraise the significance of situations in terms of their relevance and implications (Lazarus & Folkman, 1984).

Global meaning systems encompass beliefs, goals, and subjective feelings of purpose or meaning in life (Dittman-Kohli & Westerhof, 2000; Park & Folkman, 1997). *Global beliefs*—also called "assumptive worlds," "personal theories," or "worldviews" (see Koltko-Rivera, 2004, for a review)—are the core schemas through which people interpret their experiences, including beliefs regarding fairness, justice, luck, control, predictability, coherence, benevolence, identity, and personal vulnerability. *Global goals* are internal representations of ultimate concerns (Emmons, 2005), one's desired long-term processes, events, or outcomes (Austin & Vancouver, 1996). Goals may be desired future states or states already possessed that one desires to maintain (Karoly, 1999; Klinger, 1998). Common global goals include relationships, health, work, wealth, knowledge, and achievement (Emmons, 2003). *Subjective sense of meaning* refers to feelings of "meaningfulness," direction, or purpose in life (Klinger, 1977; Reker & Wong, 1988). This sense of meaningfulness is derived from seeing one's actions as oriented toward or in the service of reaching a desired future state or goal (Steger, in press; Wrosch, Scheier, Miller, Schulz, & Carver, 2003; cf. King, Hicks, Krull, & Del Gaiso, 2006).

Relationships Between Global Meaning and Health and Well-Being

In support of the notion that global meaning exerts powerful influences on individuals' thoughts, actions, and emotional responses (Pargament, 1997; Park & Folkman, 1997), a fair amount of research has demonstrated links between global meaning (beliefs, goals, and sense of meaning) and general levels of physical health and psychological well-being.

Global Beliefs and Health

Although many global beliefs are related to health and well-being, the one receiving the most attention in this regard is control or *mastery*, referring to individuals' beliefs regarding their ability to control the circumstances of their lives (see Lachman, 2006, and Lachman & Firth, 2004, for reviews). Copious research has linked a sense of control or mastery with physical well-being. For example, several large-scale studies have demonstrated that mastery is associated with mortality and morbidity. A prospective epidemiologic study of English citizens (EPIC-Norfolk Prospective Cohort Study; Surtees, Wainwright, Luben, Khaw, & Day, 2006) found that during follow-up of up to six years, a strong sense of mastery was associated with lower rates of mortality from all causes, cardiovascular disease, and cancer, after adjusting for age, sex, and prevalent chronic physical disease. The association with all-cause mortality remained even after adjusting for cigarette smoking, social class, hostility, neuroticism, and extroversion (Surtees et al., 2006). In large, nationally representative samples in the United States and Germany, perceived control was related to fewer acute and chronic illnesses, higher functional status, and lower waist-hip ratio and body mass index (BMI; Lachman & Firth, 2004).

In addition to mastery beliefs, beliefs in a just world also appear to buffer the stressors of daily life. For example, just-world beliefs have been shown to moderate workplace stress and lead to less presenteeism, or coming to work when ill (Otto & Schmidt, 2007). Dealing with lab-based stressors, individuals high in just-world beliefs made more benign cognitive appraisals of the stress tasks, rated the tasks as less stressful, and had autonomic reactions more consistent with challenge (versus threat) than did those low in just-world beliefs (Tomaka & Blascovich, 1994).

Some studies, rather than focusing on a single belief such as mastery or just world, examine a range of global beliefs. The most commonly used scale for this purpose is the World Assumptions Scale (WAS; Janoff-Bulman, 1989), which taps eight global beliefs. Research with general population samples has produced inconsistent findings regarding relations with psychological well-being but generally shows a pattern of modest links between well-being and beliefs in luck, self-worth, and justice; whereas relations with control, self-control, and benevolence tend to be weaker or absent, and beliefs in randomness are related to poorer psychological well-being (e.g., Elklit, Shevlin, Solomon, & Dekel, 2007; Kaler et al., 2008; Solomon, Iancu, & Tyano, 1997; Tomich & Helgeson, 2002). Little research has examined the relations of the WAS scales with physical health (cf. Tomich & Helgeson, 2002).

The effects of these beliefs on health and well-being appear to operate through direct physiological and indirect behavioral pathways. For example, in a nationally representative sample of community-dwelling older adults who monitored their experiences of daily stressors, a high sense of personal mastery moderated their physical and psychological reactivity to a variety of daily stressors, including those related to work and interpersonal relationships (Neupert, Almeida, & Charles, 2007). Another study of healthy middle-aged women found that mastery was inversely related to aortic calcification (Matthews, Owens, Edmundowicz, Lee, & Kuller, 2006). In the nationally representative U.S. and German samples mentioned earlier, the relations of mastery with illness, functional status, and waist-hip ratio were mediated by the performance of health behaviors (Lachman & Firth, 2004). Beliefs in a just world have been shown to relate to fewer health complaints, mediated by better performance of health behaviors (Lucas, Alexander, Firestone, & Lebreton, 2008). Such links have also been reported in clinical samples. For example, in a sample of inner-city methadone-maintained patients, belief in a benevolent and meaningful world predicted sex-related, although not drug-related, HIV-preventive behavior (Avants, Marcotte, Arnold, & Margolin, 2006).

Goals and Health

Less research has been conducted linking goals with mental and physical well-being. Many dimensions of goals have been identified (e.g., structure, process, content, pursuit, attainment, maintenance, disengagement; Austin & Vancouver, 1996; Maes & Karoly, 2005), and preliminary research suggests that various dimensions have different relations with health.

One consistent finding is that individuals who feel they are making progress on their life goals are better off (Elliot, Sheldon, & Church, 1997). For example, in a sample of older adults, the individuals' sense of making progress on their goals was related to better physical health and less depression (Street, O'Connor, & Robinson, 2007). One study asked a large group of health care workers to describe their work goals (e.g., doing creative things, feeling as if they belonged, not being controlled by others, not being ill, and not being like everyone else) and the extent to which their work allowed them to fulfill these goals. Perceived nonfulfillment of work goals was a strong predictor of somatic complaints, burnout, anxiety, depression, and hostility (Maes & Gebhardt, 2000). In another work setting study, perceived setbacks in the pursuit of employees' self-set work goals predicted subsequent job dissatisfaction, burnout, depression, and somatic complaints (Pomaki, Maes & ter Doest, 2004).

Goal ambivalence and conflict are also related to well-being outside of work. For example, in a sample of undergraduates, goal ambivalence and conflict were associated with high levels of negative affect, depression, neuroticism, and psychosomatic complaints. Goal conflict was also associated with health center visits and illnesses over the past year. Further, baseline goal conflict and ambivalence ratings predicted subsequent psychosomatic complaints at one-year follow-up (Emmons & King, 1988).

Finally, some research has demonstrated that goal disengagement and reengagement are related to better health. A series of studies of adults and college students found that disengagement from goals perceived as unattainable was difficult for people to do, but was associated with better self-reported health and more normative patterns of diurnal cortisol secretion. Further, goal reengagement (towards goals perceived as more attainable) buffered some of the adverse effects of difficulty with goal disengagement (Wrosch, Scheier, & de Pontet, 2007).

Sense of Life Meaning and Health

A sense of life meaning can lead to clearer guidelines for living and continued motivation to take care of oneself and strive toward one's goals (Klinger, in press). Indeed, many studies have shown that a higher sense of meaning in life is related to higher levels of psychological well-being and physical health. For example, in a large, nationally representative sample in Hungary, a sense of life meaning was inversely related to cancer, cardiovascular, and total premature regional mortality rates after controlling for gender, age, and education. Further, life meaning scores were strongly associated with well-being and self-rated health, as well as with self-rated absence of depression and disability (Skrabski, Kopp, Rózsa, Réthelyi, & Rahe, 2005). Data from a nationwide survey of older people in the United States demonstrated that those individuals with a higher sense of meaning derived from important life roles enjoyed better health than did those with lower meaning in life (Krause & Shaw, 2003); further, a higher sense of meaning predicted lower subsequent mortality (Krause, 2009). Meaning in life also related to better self-rated health and health-related quality of life in a community sample of middle-aged women (Scheier et al., 2006) and in a sample of cardiac outpatients (Holahan, Holahan, & Suzuki, 2008).

There is evidence that having a strong sense of meaning in life can influence health and well-being through both direct and indirect pathways. For example, in experimental research, higher levels of meaning in life were related to better autonomic nervous system functioning (Ishida & Okada, 2006) and to lower mean heart rate and decreased heart rate reactivity (Edmondson et al., 2005). In addition, life meaning was associated with lower aortic calcification in a community sample of middle-aged women (Matthews et al., 2006) and to lower blood pressure in a representative sample of people in Chicago (Buck, Williams, Musick, & Sternthal, 2008). Meaning in life has been related to the performance of health-promoting activities in various samples, including Anglo women but not Hispanic women (Wells, Bush, & Marshall, 2002), Japanese adults (Seya, 2003), and cardiac outpatients (Holahan et al., 2008).

RELATIONS BETWEEN MEANING AND HEALTH AND WELL-BEING IN TIMES OF CRISIS AND ILLNESS

As influential as global meaning may be in dealing with daily life and its inevitable stresses and hassles, meaning seems to be even more relevant to health and well-being when individuals encounter *crises*—that is, highly stressful experiences perceived to entail a high probability of damage or loss. First, crises arise when individuals encounter situations they perceive to be highly discrepant with their global meaning, as, for example, when receiving a diagnosis of cancer. A cancer diagnosis is likely to violate one's beliefs in fairness, vulnerability, predictability, and benevolence of the world as well as to be discrepant with one's identity as a healthy person (Park, in press). In addition, goals of remaining vital and whole are violated, because cancer diagnosis and treatment typically disrupts many life routines and threatens long-term aspirations (Holland & Reznik, 2005). These violations can lead to a diminished sense of life meaning or purpose (Janoff-Bulman & Frantz, 1997; Simonelli, Fowler, Maxwell, & Andersen, 2008).

Global Beliefs and Health in Times of Crisis and Illness

Not only does global meaning, in its interaction with the environment, inform appraisals of a crisis, but it also determines individuals' responses to those crises. That is, global beliefs, goals, and a sense of meaning influence how individuals deal with and recover from highly stressful events. Research has shown that mastery beliefs are often quite helpful when facing life difficulties. In a large sample of older adults, a sense of mastery mediated the effects of both earlier and later life economic hardships on elders' current physical and mental health and also moderated the health impact of economic hardship (Pudrovska, Schieman, Pearlin, & Nguyen, 2005). Mastery is also helpful for those people dealing with serious illness. For example, in a sample of adults with rheumatoid arthritis, mastery predicted lower levels of pain, stress, fatigue, and blood pressure (Younger, Finan, Zautra, Davis, & Reich, 2008). Controlling for the effects of such other important covariates as gender, cancer site, stage of disease, and comorbidity, a longitudinal study of cancer patients undergoing chemotherapy found that patients with higher levels of mastery reported less severe pain and fatigue (Kurtz, Kurtz, Given, & Given, 2008). Some physiological pathways through which mastery operates in highly stressful situations have been identified. In a study of Alzheimer's caregivers, mastery moderated the effects of care-giving stress and life events on immune functioning (Mausbach et al., 2007), as well as on levels of plasminogen activator inhibitor (PAI)–1 antigen, implicated in the development of cardiovascular disease (Mausbach et al., 2008).

Other beliefs have been shown to relate to health in stressful times as well. For example, belief in a just world related to physical and psychological recovery following myocardial infarction (MI; Agrawal & Dalal, 1993); and in a sample of mothers whose children were undergoing bone marrow transplants, higher beliefs in chance were related to better physical health but unrelated to mental health (Rini et al., 2004). In a sample of symptomatic HIV/AIDS patients, beliefs in benevolence and luck were related to less distress and higher mental health–related quality of life, and beliefs in justice were related to higher physical health–related quality of life (Farber, Schwartz, Schaper, Moonen, & McDaniel, 2000).

These global beliefs may serve as important resources, leading individuals who possess high levels of mastery or just-world beliefs to make more adaptive appraisals of their stressful situations, perhaps framing them as challenges they can successfully meet, thus encouraging them to persist in their coping efforts (Aldwin, 2007; Folkman & Moskowitz, 2007). Perhaps some beliefs also allow individuals to maintain their views of the world as orderly and coherent, reducing the extent to which global meaning is disrupted (Park, 2010).

Global Goals and Health in Times of Crisis and Illness

Highly stressful situations may heighten the influence of global goals and their pursuit on well-being. One study of chronically ill patients found that goal discrepancies (the extent to which they appraised their goals as not feasible or not important) were associated with more anxiety and depressive symptoms and lower quality of life (Kuijer & De Ridder, 2003). Similarly, in adults living with HIV, the extent to which they perceived HIV as hindering important goals was related to lower quality of life and higher levels of depressive symptoms (van der Veek, Kraaji, van Koppen, Garnefski, & Joekes, 2007). A study of MI patients found that the extent to which the myocardial infarction was perceived to violate goals predicted increased depression and lower quality of life four months later (Boersma, Maes, & Van Elderen, 2005), and a study that assessed women with fibromyalgia multiple times per day over a one-month period found that the extent to which they perceived their pain and fatigue as hindering their health and fitness goals was related to subsequent deterioration of positive (but not negative) affect (Affleck et al., 1998).

These studies converge on the notion that such crises as serious illness are typically perceived as violating critically important goals, a highly stressful state, and that further, these violations are reflected in decrements in both physical and emotional well-being.

Sense of Meaning in Life and Health and Well-Being in Times of Crisis and Illness

Although important in everyday well-being, a sense of meaning in life seems to be particularly important in stressful times. Studies have illustrated how a strong commitment to core values or causes can buffer stress. An extreme example is torture survivors. One study found that tortured nonactivists had been subject to relatively less severe torture but showed higher levels of psychopathology and posttraumatic stress disorder symptoms compared with tortured political activists; this study concluded that having a strong sense of commitment to a cause greater than themselves helped these torture victims to better endure their ordeal (Basoglu et al., 1997).

Myriad studies have documented that higher levels of meaning in life are related to better self-rated health and health-related quality of life (Scheier et al., 2006), including in those individuals living with such serious illnesses as cancer (e.g., Simonelli et al., 2008) and heart failure (e.g., Park, Malone, Suresh, Bliss, & Rosen, 2008). Further, it appears that meaning in life mediates the relationship between social and physical functioning and distress in cancer survivors (Jim & Andersen, 2007). Studies have found that meaning in life was positively related to rate of recovery from knee surgery (Smith & Zautra, 2004); to pain, fatigue, and mental and physical health–related quality of life in rheumatoid arthritis patients (Verduin et al., 2008); and to perceived physical health in spousal caregivers of advanced-cancer patients (Stetz, 1989).

In sum, the literature relating all three aspects of global meaning—beliefs, goals, and subjective sense of purpose—are all linked to a vast array of health and well-being variables in a variety of samples ranging from general populations to people facing such high-magnitude stressors as chronic and life-limiting illness and care-giving. The findings suggest that these aspects of meaning can be an important protective factor on a daily basis as well as a resource on which to draw in times of heightened stress. However, most studies are suggestive rather than conclusive, given that the research is nearly all correlational. The studies that have demonstrated links with subsequent mortality as well as other such "hard endpoints" as aortic calcification are perhaps more convincing regarding a causal link, but it is possible that unmeasured but important third variables were not included in these studies. Thus, at this point, the research linking meaning and health and well-being may be considered as strongly suggestive of myriad helpful roles of meaning; conclusive evidence remains to be found.

SPIRITUALITY

Efforts to define the constructs of religion and spirituality and to distinguish between them have proliferated in recent years (e.g., Pargament & Zinnbauer, 2005; WHOQOL SRPB Group, 2006). Although consensus appears unlikely, one reasonable solution was advanced by Pargament and Zinnbauer (2005) in which *spirituality*, proposed to be the superordinate construct, is defined as "a personal or group search for the sacred" (p. 35). *Religiousness* is defined as a search for the sacred "that unfolds within a traditional sacred context" (p. 35); thus, spirituality is often, but not always, expressed through religiousness. In this chapter, the term *spirituality* is used to denote this broader search, although *religiousness* is used to describe constructs explicitly derived from traditional sacred contexts.

For many individuals, spirituality and religion are central to their global meaning system, influencing their global beliefs (McIntosh, 1995; Ozorak, 2005), goals (Emmons, 2005), and sense of meaning in life (Steger & Frazier, 2005). Research on general population samples reflects the high prevalence of religious beliefs and behaviors in the United States. For example, a recent poll of a nationally representative sample of Americans found that 92% believe in God or a universal spirit, 90% pray, 85% say religion is very or fairly important to them, and 41% attend religious services weekly or more often (Gallup, 2007; see Slattery & Park, in press–c). While studies conducted in other countries report lower levels of religion and spirituality than those found in the United States, they are still fairly high (e.g., Karsten, & Schaan, 2008; WHOQOL SRPB Group, 2006; Williams & Sternthal, 2007). Thus, although not all individuals are religious or spiritual, religion and spirituality appear to form a central part of the meaning systems of many individuals (Park, 2005; Silberman, 2005).

GENERAL INFLUENCES OF SPIRITUALITY ON HEALTH AND WELL-BEING

In recent years, researchers have become increasingly interested in the influence of religion and spirituality on physical health (for reviews, see George, Ellison, & Larson, 2002; Lee & Newberg, 2010; Powell, Shahabi, & Thoresen, 2003). Epidemiological studies have long demonstrated that higher levels of religiousness (assessed as service attendance) are related to lower mortality rates (e.g., Powell et al., 2003), even when taking into account such potential covariates as baseline health, social support, and health behaviors (Oman, Kurata, Strawbridge, & Cohen, 2002). More recently, recognizing the multidimensional nature of religiousness and spirituality, researchers have broadened their focus from attendance to additional aspects of religion and spirituality, including private religious behaviors, commitment, spiritual transcendence, and religious coping. Research has yielded generally positive though somewhat mixed findings (Powell et al., 2003). For example, some aspects of religiousness predict lower rates of disability and a range of illnesses, including alcoholism, cardiovascular disease, hypertension, and myocardial infarction (see Lee & Newberg, 2010; Miller & Thoresen, 2003).

Many pathways have been proposed to explain how religion and spirituality may exert salutary influences on well-being (Lee & Newberg, 2005; Levin & Vanderpool, 1989; Oman & Thoresen, 2005; Park, 2007). Among these are health-related behaviors and lifestyle, religious or spiritual social support; benefits of such religious practices as prayer and meditation, comfort provided by specific beliefs and interpretations, positive affect derived from certain spirituality-related states such as gratitude or compassion, and access to health promotion resources. The following section describes each of these pathways and presents relevant empirical findings. Note that some aspects of religion and spirituality may have a negative impact on well-being; these negative pathways are also detailed in this section.

Health-Related Behaviors

One pathway through which spirituality may influence health and well-being is through promoting a healthy lifestyle (i.e., behaviors that promote health). Large-scale epidemiological studies have demonstrated that health behaviors partially mediate the effects of service attendance on physical health, including mortality (e.g., L. B. Koenig & Vaillant, 2009; Strawbridge, Shema, Cohen, & Kaplan, 2001). Some religious denominations and traditions, in particular, promote health habits or other prescriptions or proscriptions that may promote health, such as prohibiting the use of alcohol or other intoxicants, prescribing a vegetarian diet, and forbidding sexual activity outside of marriage (Levin & Vanderpool, 1989).

In addition to explicit prescriptions and proscriptions, other aspects of religion and spirituality have been linked to health behaviors in many samples. For example, among the elderly, religiousness has been linked to lower levels of cigarette smoking (e.g., H. G. Koenig, George, Cohen, et al., 1998) and higher levels of preventive health behaviors (e.g., flu shots, cholesterol screening, breast self-exams, mammograms, pap smears, and prostate screening; Benjamins & Brown, 2004). Preventive health behaviors have also been linked to spirituality in many other samples, including a nationally representative sample of Presbyterian women (Benjamins, Trinitapoli, & Ellison, 2006), a statewide representative study of Texas residents (Hill, Ellison, Burdette, & Musick, 2007), and a sample of disenfranchised elderly African Americans (Aaron, Levine, & Burstin, 2003). Behaviors that reduce health risk have been related to diverse samples ranging from inner-city cocaine-using and methadone-maintained patients (Avants et al., 2006) to pregnant women in Appalachia (Jesse & Reed, 2006). Finally, some religious traditions promote higher fertility, thereby reducing risk of breast cancer (Gillum & Williams, 2009).

Social Support

Studies examining the attendance–mortality link often control for the influence of social support, the provision of resources by one's social network (see Wills and Ainette, Chapter 20, this volume). When the influence of social support is statistically controlled, the relationship between attendance and mortality often becomes substantially weaker (see George et al., 2002), indicating that social support mediates at least some of the effects of religion and spirituality on health. However, effects are inconsistent (George et al., 2002). It appears that social support is strongly related to mortality but that it often functions as an independent predictor rather than as a mediator. Those individuals who do not attend services regularly may seek out other sources of social support so that general levels of social support may not be related to religiousness. However, aspects of social support specific to religion may be qualitatively different from nonreligious social support (Krause, 2008) and may have more potent effects on health (Hayward & Elliott, 2011). In a nationally representative sample of older adults, congregational social support in particular led to a sense of belongingness and satisfaction with one's health (Krause & Wulff, 2005). Further, those individuals with higher anticipated congregational support experienced less decline in self-rated health across three years (Krause, 2006a).

Religious Practices

Studies on the effects of religious practices, such as prayer or meditation, on health and well-being have produced confusing, contradictory findings. Cross-sectionally, prayer is often related to more disability and pain (e.g., Hank & Schaan, 2008; Rippentrop, Altmaier, Chen, Found, & Keffala, 2005). Other studies, however, have demonstrated favorable links between prayer and health. For example, a longitudinal study of relatively healthy elderly adults found that such private religious behaviors as prayer were related to reduced mortality rates, controlling for many potential confounding variables, including demographics, health, health practices, and social support (Helm, Hays, Flint, Koenig, & Blazer, 2000). Negative relationships between prayer and health and well-being may, in part, be attributable to the fact that those who are ill and suffering turn to prayer as a way to deal with their distress (Rippentrop et al., 2005). In addition, there are many types of prayer, ranging from attunement to petition (Breslin & Lewis, 2008); different types of prayer may exert different effects on health outcomes (see Masters & Spielmans, 2007, for a review).

At this point, little is known about mechanisms through which prayer might influence health and health-relevant physiologic processes induced by different types of prayer. Breslin and Lewis (2008) outlined a number of potential pathways of prayer, including the placebo effect, correlates with health behaviors, attention diversion, supernatural intervention, and activation of such latent energies as chi. Wachholtz and Keefe (2006) speculated that daily prayer may reduce perceptions of pain in chronic pain patients through distraction and by generating positive emotions and a sense of relaxation. At this point, few clinical trials or experimental studies have examined the effects of prayer on health, and more definitive answers await further research.

Another private spiritual practice, meditation, may have a direct effect on health by calming the nervous system (Benson, 2000; see Cahn & Polich, 2006, for a review). Myriad studies have demonstrated that meditation can induce a sense of deep inner peace and calm, creating a shift from sympathetic nervous system arousal to parasympathetic nervous system relaxation (Yehuda & McEwen, 2004). There is evidence that those who meditate on a regular basis experience less stress and more positive affect as well as enhanced immune functioning and lower cardiovascular reactivity as well as more left-sided anterior activation (Davidson et al., 2003; Ditto, Eclache, & Goldman, 2006; Grossman, Niemann, Schmidt, & Walach, 2004). Meditation can be secular or spiritual, although spiritually based meditation may have more powerful effects on health than does meditation that is not spiritually based (Wachholtz & Pargament, 2008).

Specific Beliefs and Interpretations

Another way that spirituality may affect health is by providing beliefs that allow more benign interpretations of situations, minimizing exposure to negative affect and thus protecting against the daily wear and tear of stressors (Pargament, 1997; Slattery & Park, in press–b). For example, in a large national sample of American adults, an inverse relationship was found between belief in life after death and symptom severity on all six symptom clusters examined (i.e., anxiety, depression, obsession/compulsion, paranoia, phobia, and somatization) after controlling for demographic and other variables known to influence mental health (Flannelly, Koenig, Ellison, Galek, & Krause, 2006).

Positive Affect

Positive affect, feelings reflecting "pleasurable engagement with the environment, such as happiness, joy, excitement, enthusiasm, and contentment" (Cohen & Pressman, 2006, p. 122), is often associated with higher levels of religion and spirituality (Ellison & Fan, 2008; Saroglou, Buxant, & Tilquin, 2008; see Lewis & Cruise, 2006), positive affect is increasingly documented to favorably affect physical health as well as emotional well-being (see Pressman & Cohen, 2005, for a review). Thus, positive affect is a potentially important pathway through which religion and spirituality may influence health and well-being.

Religions often explicitly promote such spiritually relevant positive emotions as gratitude, compassion, optimism, and hope (Krause, 2002; Steffen & Masters, 2005), all of which have been proposed as leading to positive affect and thus to higher levels of positive physical well-being (Park, 2007; for research on optimism and health, see Scheier, Carver, & Armstrong, Chapter 4, this volume). Gratitude, the appreciation for the benefits or blessings which one has received, has been shown to be related to physical health in both correlational and experimental studies. For example, in a national sample of older adults, feeling more grateful to God buffered the chronic stresses of aging, effects that were stronger for women than for men (Krause, 2006b); and in an intervention study, having participants list their gratitudes on a daily basis led to better health and well-being compared to control groups (Emmons & McCullough, 2003).

Access to Health Promotion Activities

Lee and Newberg (2005, 2010) noted that members of religious groups may have better access to health care promotions and health-improvement programs (e.g., blood pressure screening, soup kitchens) sponsored by their congregation. One example of a religiously affiliated health promotion is the Weigh Down Workshops (Reicks, Mills, & Henry, 2004), which have recently been become very popular, although their effectiveness remains undemonstrated. Further, some religious organizations have substantial resources and prominent community positions, allowing them to exert positive influences on their followers by providing tangible resources (Lee & Newberg, 2005).

Negative Pathways

In addition to positive pathways of influence are aspects of religion and spirituality that have detrimental influences on health and well-being. Much of this influence involves spiritual strain or religious struggle, including feelings of anger, guilt, or doubts about the existence of God. For example, in a random sample of nearly two thousand Americans, having doubts about one's religious faith was related to poorer mental health, including depression, anxiety, hostility, and somatization (Galek, Krause, Ellison, Kudler, & Flannelly, 2007). An extrinsic religious orientation (i.e., one in which religion is considered a means to other ends) may have negative health concomitants. For example, several studies of older adults have found extrinsic religiousness to be related to exaggerated cardiac reactivity (Masters et al., 2004; Masters et al., 2005). In addition, religious communities can be a source of disagreement and dissension, creating negative emotional situations (Exline, 2002).

INFLUENCES OF SPIRITUALITY ON HEALTH AND WELL-BEING IN TIMES OF CRISIS AND ILLNESS

As with global meaning, the influence of spirituality on health and well-being, while pervasive in ordinary times, may be even more potent in times of major stress, including acute or chronic illness and physical suffering. These effects are primarily a result of the provision of spiritual and religious coping resources unavailable to those who are not spiritual or religious, including engaging in prayer and relying on one's congregation for support. In addition, religious beliefs can be comforting in the face of such major stressors as illness or bereavement (Wortmann & Park, 2008). Religiousness may also facilitate adherence to treatments, and religious traditions often promote forgiveness (McCullough & Worthington, 1999), which can help individuals who have suffered transgressions to move beyond them (McCullough, 2001). These potential pathways are discussed later. However, as will be reviewed, there are aspects of religion and spirituality that exert negative influences on physical and psychological well-being in high-stress situations.

Because most religions provide ways to understand, reinterpret, and even redeem suffering as well as ways to find the work of a loving or purposeful God within it (Park, 2005), individuals commonly turn to religion in their coping efforts (e.g., H. G. Koenig, George, & Siegler, 1998; Thune-Boyle, Stygall, Keshtgar, & Newman, 2006). Pargament, Koenig, and Perez (2000) have extensively studied and categorized the diversity of religious coping types and classified them broadly as positive and negative religious coping. Positive religious coping involves such activities as trusting in God's love, making benevolent religious reappraisals, using a collaborative approach with God in facing problems, seeking spiritual support, and seeking support from members of one's religious group. Religious individuals are more inclined to use religious coping (Pargament, 1997), which is often related to better psychological adjustment, including higher levels of life satisfaction and more stress-related growth as well as less depression and anxiety (Ai, Park, Huang, Rodgers, & Tice, 2007; Harrison, Koenig, Hays, Eme-Akwari, & Pargament, 2001; Pearce, Singer, & Prigerson, 2006; see Ano & Vasconcelles, 2005, for a review).

Given the positive links between religious coping and psychological aspects of well-being, it is perhaps surprising that little empirical evidence supports the notion that positive religious coping is related to better physical health outcomes following stressful experiences. A lack of significant effects has been reported in many longitudinal studies (e.g., Pargament, Koenig, Tarakeshwar, & Hahn, 2004; Sherman, Plante, Simonton, Latif, & Anaissie, 2009; Trevino et al., 2010). In fact, a number of studies have found positive religious coping related to poorer, rather than improved, health outcomes. For example, positive religious coping was related to poorer subsequent physical health in studies of both older adults' adjustment to illness (Gall, 2003) and advanced-cancer patients (Tarakeshwar et al., 2006). The use of prayer for serious illness specifically has also been shown to be related to poorer physical outcomes. For example, in a longitudinal study of a Swedish sample of persons with chronic pain, use of prayer as a coping strategy was positively associated with pain interference and impairment as well as anxiety and depression scores (Andersson, 2008). However, in a national sample of elders dealing with financial strain, praying for others (but not for one's self!) buffered the impact of stress on their self-reported health (Krause, 2003). As noted, the impact of prayer is complex, given the many types of prayer and variety of pathways through which it may affect health and well-being (Breslin & Lewis, 2008).

Forgiveness

The experience of physical and emotional injuries experienced at the hands of another is, perhaps, the worst kind of trauma (Frazier, Anders, et al., 2009), and it often leaves long-standing negative psychological and physical health sequelae in its wake (Krause, Shaw, & Cairney, 2004). Recovery from deliberate injury can be very difficult, but one pathway through and beyond is forgiveness (Worthington & Scherer, 2004). Forgiveness has been related to well-being in many studies. For example, in a national probability sample, forgiveness was related to better self-reported mental and physical health, especially for middle-aged and older adults (Toussaint, Williams, Musick, & Everson, 2001); and in lab-based research, forgiveness in response to an interpersonal transgression was associated with lower blood pressure, heart rate, and cardiac reactivity (Lawler et al., 2003). In a series of studies with middle-aged and older adults, Lawler-Row (2010) demonstrated that forgiveness mediated links between religion and a variety of health indicators, including not only self-reported health and symptoms but also medication use and sleep quality.

Religious and Spiritual Beliefs

Several studies have shown that particular beliefs are related to better physical health following highly stressful experiences. For example, religious beliefs were related to fewer complications and shorter hospital stays after coronary artery bypass graft surgery, even though prayer was unrelated to outcomes (Contrada et al., 2004), although a more recent study of the same population showed this belief measure to be related to higher levels of depression and anxiety (Contrada et al., 2008). In a study of Japanese elders, beliefs in an afterlife were related to lower blood pressure following bereavement (Krause et al., 2002). Not all studies have found favorable effects for religious beliefs, however. One longitudinal study of older adults' functional recovery following an acute myocardial infarction found that higher levels of self-defined spirituality led to poorer functional recovery. These findings remained after controlling for a range of covariates (Martin & Levy, 2006).

Self-rated spirituality is, however, related to life satisfaction and quality of life. A recent meta-analysis of 51 studies, many conducted with samples experiencing stressful events, found effects of moderate strength (Sawatzky, Ratner, & Chiu, 2005). In addition, spirituality has been linked to better physical health in a sample of women with metastatic breast cancer (i.e., greater numbers of circulating white blood cells and total lymphocyte counts; Sephton, Koopman, Schaal, Thoresen, & Spiegel, 2001). Also, in a sample of people recently diagnosed as HIV+, those who increased their self-ratings of religiousness and spirituality had greater preservation of CD4 cells over a four-year period and better control of viral load, results that held after controlling for a host of covariates (Ironson, Stuetzle, & Fletcher, 2006).

Treatment Adherence

Religiousness may facilitate adherence to treatment regimens (Park, 2007), which can substantially improve physical health (DiMatteo, 2004; DiMatteo & Haskard, 2006), but little research has tested this proposition. One recent study of congestive heart failure (CHF) patients found differential effects for different dimensions of religion and spirituality on different aspects of adherence. In particular, religious commitment predicted adherence to CHF-specific behaviors (e.g., weight monitoring) and advice regarding alcohol and tobacco use; religious social support also predicted self-reported adherence to advice regarding substance use. No religious or spiritual variables were related to adherence to diet (Park, Moehl, Fenster, Suresh, & Bliss, 2008), and neither positive nor negative religious coping was related to adherence to treatment. In a study of survivors of a variety of cancers, spiritual struggle, mediated through guilt, was related to poorer health behaviors and adherence; whereas daily spiritual experiences, mediated through a positive emotion, self-assurance, was related to better health behavior and adherence (Park, Edmondson, Hale-Smith, & Blank, 2009).

Negative Aspects of Religion or Spirituality

Life crises or trauma exposures can lead individuals to question their beliefs in a loving and omnipotent God, resulting in feelings of betrayal, anger, fear, and doubt (Gall & Grant, 2005; Park, 2005). The use of these negative types of religious coping with stressful events has been related to poorer physical as well as psychological health (Ano & Vasconcelles, 2005; Sherman et al., 2009). For example, a prospective cohort study of inpatients found that negative religious coping in the hospital (in particular, appraisals of the illness as a punishment from God and interpersonal religious discontent) was associated with subsequent declines in health and increased mortality rates of 19%–28% at the two-year follow-up, even controlling for relevant demographic and baseline characteristics (Pargament, Koenig, Tarakeshwar, & Hahn, 2001). Another study found that in a sample of medical rehabilitation patients, negative religious coping, particularly anger with God, was significantly related to lower levels of activities of daily living at a one-month follow-up (Fitchett, Rybarczyk, DeMarco, & Nicholas, 1999).

Thus, it appears that negative religious coping with highly stressful events, including serious illness, is consistently and fairly strongly related to poorer physical as well as psychological outcomes. These findings contrast with the relatively modest and inconsistent findings for other aspects of religiousness and spirituality and religious coping generally considered more positive. Some of these inconsistencies may be a result of the moderating influences of religiousness and spirituality; that is, they may be more or less effective depending on the particular person and circumstance (Pargament, 1997). Religious and spiritual coping may be more effective, for example, in situations that allow little control and that rouse existential concerns (Pargament, 1997). A religious outlook that is only moderately strongly held might be less protective than one that is firmly held (e.g., Wink & Scott, 2005). A reliance on faith when confronting an ongoing stressful life event may initially be helpful but eventually lead to negative attitudes toward faith for failing to provide relief (Exline & Rose, 2005; Gall, 2003; Gall & Cornblat, 2002). An intriguing study of maternal caregivers of chronically ill children found few relations of religious salience and prayer with quality of life and health symptoms. However, after education and income were taken into account, the relationships became statistically significant, such that prayer was associated with fewer health symptoms and better quality of life among less educated maternal caregivers but was unrelated to those with more education (Banthia, Moskowitz, Acree, & Folkman, 2007). Some research has also found that denomination may also influence relationships between religiousness and well-being (e.g., Tix & Frazier, 2005).

Taken together, the research on spirituality and health indicates that the links are complex, perhaps accounting for some of the inconsistency in the literature (Oman & Thoresen, 2005). Clearly, different dimensions of spirituality are differentially related to health and well-being. In particular, evidence appears strongest regarding forgiveness and negative religious coping. Forgiveness is increasingly recognized as closely linked with many indicators of health, and recent experimental research demonstrates at least short-term beneficial effects on health (e.g., Waltman et al., 2009). Negative religious coping has not been subjected to experimental work, but there is strong correlational evidence of its subsequent negative impact on well-being, including mortality (Pargament et al., 2001). Findings regarding the potential impact on health of other aspects of spirituality are less consistent. For example, prayer and positive religious coping are often found to lack associations with health (e.g., Sherman et al., 2009). Much more work is required to tease out the finer points of these aspects of spirituality.

GROWTH

Stress-related growth, the positive life changes that people report experiencing following stressful events, has garnered great research interest in recent years (see Tedeschi & Calhoun, 2006, for a review). Myriad studies have established that many people—in most studies, even the majority—report positive life changes after highly stressful experiences, including such illnesses as cancer (e.g., Tomich & Helgeson, 2004) and HIV (Bower, Kemeny, Taylor, & Fahey, 1998), sexual assault (Frazier, Tashiro, Berman, Steger, & Long, 2004), mass killing, plane crash, tornado (McMillen, Smith, & Fisher, 1997), childhood sexual abuse (McMillen, Zuravin, & Rideout, 1995), physical assault (Updegraff & Marshall, 2005), and such war experiences as combat (Elder & Clipp, 1989) and peacekeeping missions in military zones (Britt, Adler, & Bartone, 2001). These positive changes, variously labeled "posttraumatic growth," "perceived benefits," "adversarial growth," "benefit finding," and "stress-related growth," may occur in one's social relationships (e.g., becoming closer to family or friends), personal resources (e.g., developing patience or persistence), life philosophies (e.g., rethinking one's priorities), spirituality (e.g., feeling closer to God), coping skills (e.g., learning better ways to handle problems or manage emotions), and health behaviors or lifestyles (e.g., lessening stress and taking better care of one's self; Tedeschi & Calhoun, 2004; Park, 2009).

One of the most consistent findings emerging from this accumulating literature is that religion and spirituality are strongly related to growth (see Ano & Vasconcelles, 2005; and Shaw, Joseph & Linley, 2005, for reviews). This connection seems to go both ways in that religion and spirituality are major predictors of growth, and spiritual development and meaning are among the most commonly reported types of growth.

In spite of burgeoning research interest in recent years, stress-related growth remains poorly understood (Park, Lechner, Stanton, & Antoni, 2009; Park & Helgeson, 2006). For example, the processes through which growth arises (Park, 2009), the extent to which this growth is "real" or illusory (Frazier, Tennen, et al., 2009; Ransom, Sheldon, & Jacobsen, 2008), and the meaning of growth in terms of well-being (Helgeson, Reynolds, & Tomich, 2006) all are open questions. The following sections address this latter question and consider the implications of growth for physical health and well-being

GENERAL ASPECTS OF GROWTH

Unlike the potentially protective resources of meaning and spirituality, stress-related growth is not typically discussed in terms of everyday functioning. Instead, stress-related growth is by definition positive change that occurs in the aftermath of particular stressful experiences. Researchers conceptualize growth as a potentially important outcome in and of itself as well as a potential buffer of the negative effects of major stressors, including life-threatening and chronic illnesses (e.g., Morrill et al., 2008; Park, Chmielewski, & Blank, 2011). However, there are several ways in which stress-related growth may indeed influence well-being outside the specific context of highly stressful encounters. For example, Ryff (1989) described a personal growth orientation as openness to continued development and expansion and a sense of self-improvement over time in terms of self-knowledge and effectiveness. Considered an aspect of psychological well-being, personal growth is related to better physical health indices (Ryff et al., 2006).

In addition, the positive life changes that people experience following negative events are often lessons regarding themselves and their lives, which may feed forward to improve general life functioning. For example, such lessons may prevent future problems through proactive coping (Schwartzer & Taubert, 2002) and may also lead to development and maturity (Aldwin, Levenson, & Kelly, 2009). Some stress-related growth may also directly involve making healthy changes, among them improving one's diet or exercise regimen or taking specific steps to reduce stress (Andrykowski, Beacham, Schmidt, & Harper, 2006). In addition, stress-related growth might contribute to the performance of prosocial behavior, which has been demonstrated to have salubrious effects on physical well-being (e.g., Brown, Nesse, Vinokur, & Smith, 2003). Stress-related growth may contribute to the quantity and quality of one's social interactions, which may lead to subsequent increased well-being (e.g., Danoff-Burg & Revenson, 2005; see Algoe & Stanton, 2009). In all these ways, growth may feed forward to influence health in daily life.

GROWTH FROM MAJOR LIFE STRESSORS

Whether growth should be expected to be associated with physical and mental well-being following stressful life events is a matter of some dispute. That is, some theorists have argued that growth is a separate and important outcome in and of itself, and it is not necessarily related to other indices of adjustment (e.g., Tedeschi & Calhoun, 2004). Such a stance suggests that perceptions of growth are to be assessed and valued independently of other outcomes. In fact, it has been noted that stress-related growth might sometimes be expected to be related to more distress. For example, following a cancer diagnosis, individuals may feel they have a better and more accurate understanding of themselves and the world, an understanding they label growth, which includes a greater sense of vulnerability and awareness of their lack of control over important aspects of their lives (e.g., Tomich, Helgeson, & Vache, 2005), becoming "sadder but wiser" (Janoff-Bulman & Timko, 1987, p. 154). Nonetheless, many researchers have pursued the question of how stress-related growth relates to various aspects of mental and physical well-being.

Several recent literature reviews (Algoe & Stanton, 2009; Bower, Low, Moskowitz, Sepah, & Epel, 2008; Stanton, Bower, & Low, 2006) and a meta-analysis of 87 cross-sectional studies (Helgeson et al., 2006) provide useful summaries of the research to date on this question of the associations of growth and well-being. In general, stress-related growth has been found to relate often, but not consistently, to well-being across an array of studies diverse in samples and designs. In a meta-analysis of cross-sectional studies of growth following a wide range of stressors, Helgeson et al. (2006) found that growth was, in the aggregate, associated with less depression and more positive well-being but also with more intrusive and avoidant thoughts about the stressor. However, growth was unrelated to anxiety, global distress, quality of life, and subjective reports of physical health. Focusing on physical outcomes and potential physiological pathways, Bower et al. (2008) concluded, "Overall, the literature on benefit finding and health supports the hypothesis that individuals who are able to find benefit following stressful experiences show positive changes in various health-related outcomes, including decreases in morbidity and mortality and positive changes in immune and neuroendocrine function" (p. 226). For example, researchers have found that stress-related growth was related to higher levels of CD4 count in HIV+ adolescents (Milam, 2006) and reduced cortisol levels in early-stage breast cancer patients (Cruess et al., 2000). Regarding growth specifically from chronic illness, and reviewing only longitudinal studies, Algoe and Stanton (2009) concluded that the effects of growth were stronger and more consistently favorable for physical aspects of adjustment, especially those directly related to the illness (e.g., pain for those with arthritis) than for psychological outcomes (e.g., depressive symptoms).

Thus, findings suggest that relationships between growth and well-being are complex, inconsistent, and contingent on the particular aspect of well-being in question. Further, growth appears to be more strongly associated with aspects of physical health than of psychological well-being (cf., Helgeson et al., 2006). There are several caveats to these conclusions, however. First, many studies have reported findings contradictory to them. For example, numerous studies have found growth positively related to distress, especially anxiety and posttraumatic stress symptomatology (e.g., Park, Aldwin, Fenster, & Snyder, 2008; Updegraff & Marshall, 2005); whereas other studies have shown null results (e.g., Cordova, Cunningham, Carlson, & Andrykowski, 2001). Second, most studies have designs that preclude truly answering the question. That is, many studies utilized cross-sectional and retrospective designs, and most failed to control for potential confounding variables that might underlie the growth–health connection, such as optimism, mastery, and other personal and social characteristics that may more parsimoniously explain the links. Still, such findings are promising and suggest that growth is a topic deserving of continued study, particularly by researchers willing to employ more sophisticated and methodologically sound approaches (Park, 2009).

FUTURE RESEARCH DIRECTIONS AND APPLICATIONS

FUTURE RESEARCH DIRECTIONS

Research delving more deeply into the links between meaning, spirituality, and stress-related growth and outcomes such as psychological and physical health is proceeding apace. As knowledge accumulates, research that adds to our base of knowledge requires increasingly sophisticated approaches (Park, 2005; Park & Paloutzian, 2005). These approaches will involve diverse methods, including longitudinal and prospective designs, momentary assessment techniques, archival and epidemiological data, and multiple measurement tools, including psychometrically sound self-reports as well as behavioral and physiological indices (Hill, 2005; Hood & Belzen, 2005).

Among the research directions that appear most promising are the investigation of the specific structure and content of meaning systems and of the coherence among them. It is clear that assessing such broad constructs as meaning or spirituality will not yield the understanding or prediction that more fine-grained constructs will. In addition, it is important to study these aspects of meaning in the context of other variables that may serve as moderators. Some of the research reviewed in this chapter suggests that protective or resilient effects of meaning, spirituality, and growth are buffered by (i.e., interact with) such other variables as socioeconomic status and race (e.g., Banthia et al., 2007). Examining the conjoint influences of these variables will greatly increase our ability to understand the conditions under which they are relatively more—and less—potent influences. A further research direction clearly suggested by this review is that of delineating the pathways through which resilience and protection are conferred. Studies indicate that meaning, spirituality, and growth can influence health and well-being through both direct physiological and indirect behavioral pathways, but much remains to be learned.

Applications: Prevention and Intervention

Ideally, having a better understanding of these protective and resilience resources will lead to efforts not only to intervene with those who are suffering and experiencing poor health but also to head off or prevent problems in those who are yet well. For example, prevention efforts may attempt to build up aspects of global meaning that have been shown to be helpful in ordinary circumstances, such as a sense of mastery and a commitment to goals through which individuals connect with concerns larger than themselves, leading to a greater sense of meaning and fulfillment. Boosting these elements of global meaning would be expected to have a substantial impact on general health and well-being and would also serve as resilience resources when individuals encounter high-magnitude stressors. Some interventions to increase resilience resources at the community level are already being implemented for children (e.g., Penn Resiliency Project, 2008) and adults (e.g., American Psychological Association, 2011). If implemented on a broad scale, benefits could be affected population-wide, on the scale of public health efforts.

In addition to prevention, the constructs of meaning, spirituality, and growth have important clinical applications. Many therapeutic approaches have as their goals increasing adaptive beliefs and sources of meaning as well as the positive resolution of stressful encounter (Park & Slattery, 2008). An explicit focus on elements of global meaning that are particularly strongly related to higher levels of well-being may help guide therapists and provide specific targets for treatment (Slattery & Park, in press–a). Increasingly, therapists have been developing interventions that incorporate spirituality (e.g., Pargament, 2007), promote forgiveness (Waltman et al., 2009), focus on posttraumatic growth (Tedeschi & Calhoun, 2009), and address spiritual struggle (Murray-Swank & Pargament, 2005), including those interventions targeted to individuals with serious and life-threatening illnesses (Cole & Pargament, 1999). The literature linking these phenomena with psychological and physical well-being suggests that these foci are productive directions for intervention development.

In addition to using psychotherapy, health care providers may need to understand and intervene on these protective and resilience factors in other ways. Given the importance of these factors to patients, knowledgeable and competent health care treatment must take them into account. A literature on issues of spirituality in health care (e.g., discussions with patients, praying with patients) is growing (e.g., Magyar-Russell, Fosarelli, Taylor, & Finkelstein, 2008; Lundberg & Kerdonfag, 2010). At this point, less attention has been give to broader issues of global meaning and growth for health practitioners other than psychotherapists, but such attention is likely to grow as these factors become increasingly noted as important.

Some investigators have raised ethical questions regarding the promotion of spirituality by health care professionals (see Mills, 2002). That is, if spirituality is known to be related to better health, is it okay for physicians and others to promote it? For example, Jesse and Reed (2006) observed, "Increasing spiritual resources … during pregnancy offer(s) the potential to improve health promotion efforts in pregnancy with women from Appalachia" (p. 746). Further, Powell and colleagues (2003) concluded their review by declaring, "When one considers that attending religious services is an inexpensive but widely available resource in the community, this could be a very cost-effective way to maintain the health of elderly people with disability or chronic diseases" (p. 49). Hall (2006) noted how service attendance compares favorably to Lipitor for cardiovascular benefits on mortality in the general population. While cautioning that there are "ethical, theological, and methodological problems with this instrumental approach" (Hall, 2006, p. 107), he nonetheless suggested that the associations between attendance and other aspects of spirituality may have implications for medical practice.

Perhaps focusing on meaning as defined by individuals themselves is the best approach to these issues in intervention and prevention efforts. Although many or even most individuals may find and express their meaning through religious and spiritual means (Skrabski et al., 2005), not all do, and focusing on broader aspects of global meaning avoids the imposition of particular religious or spiritual perspectives on individuals. Nonetheless, it behooves therapists, physicians, nurses, counselors, and other interventionists to be familiar and comfortable with these various approaches to meaning in order to provide respectful and effective treatment.

CONCLUSION

This chapter delineates the multiple behavioral and physiological pathways through which the resources of meaning, spirituality, and stress-related growth may exert influences on many aspects of physical health. These resources have protective effects under ordinary circumstances by imbuing daily life with direction and positive emotional states and minimizing wear and tear. Perhaps more powerfully, they can promote resilience to stress when people are facing serious illness and other major life stressors. However, the research to date has many methodological limitations and much remains to be learned. Even at this stage of research, however, it is clear that meaning, spirituality, and stress-related growth are pervasive and important aspects of health and well-being.

REFERENCES

Aaron, K., Levine, D., & Burstin, H. (2003). African American church participation and health care practices. *Journal of General Internal Medicine, 18*, 908–913.

Affleck, G., Tennen, H., Urrows, S., Higgins, P., Abeles, M., Hall, C., … Newton, C. (1998). Fibromyalgia and women's pursuit of personal goals: A daily process analysis. *Health Psychology, 17*, 40–47.

Agrawal, M., & Dalal, A. K. (1993). Beliefs about the world and recovery from myocardial infarction. *Journal of Social Psychology, 13*, 385–394.

Ai, A., Park, C. L., Huang, B., Rodgers, W., & Tice, T. N. (2007). Psychosocial mediation of religious coping styles: A study of short-term adjustment following cardiac surgery. *Personality and Social Psychology Bulletin, 33*, 867–882.

Aldwin, C. M. (2007). *Stress, coping, and development* (2nd ed.). New York, NY: Guilford.

Aldwin, C. M., Levenson, M. R., & Kelly, L. L. (2009). Lifespan developmental perspectives on stress-related growth. In C. L. Park, S. Lechner, A. Stanton, & M. Antoni (Eds.), *Positive life changes in the context of medical illness: Can the experience of serious mental illness lead to transformation?* (pp. 87–104). Washington, DC: APA Press.

Algoe, S. B., & Stanton, A. L. (2009). Is benefit-finding good for individuals with chronic illness? In C. L. Park, S. Lechner, A. Stanton, & M. Antoni (Eds.), *Positive life change in the context of medical illness: Can the experience of serious illness lead to transformation* (pp. 173–193). Washington, DC: APA Press.

American Psychological Association (2011). *Road to resilience.* Retrieved July 7, 2011, from http://www.apa.org/helpcenter/road-resilience.aspx

Andersson, G. (2008). Chronic pain and praying to a higher power: Useful or useless? *Journal of Religion and Health, 47*, 176–187.

Andrykowski, M. A., Beacham, A. O., Schmidt, J. E., & Harper, F. W. K. (2006). Application of the theory of planned behavior to understand intentions to engage in physical and psychosocial health behaviors after cancer diagnosis. *Psycho-Oncology, 15*, 759–771.

Ano, G. G., & Vasconcelles, E. B. (2005). Religious coping and psychological adjustment to stress: A meta-analysis. *Journal of Clinical Psychology, 61*, 461–480.

Austin, J. T., & Vancouver, J. B. (1996). Goal constructs in psychology: Structure, process, and content. *Psychological Bulletin, 120*, 338–375.

Avants, S. K., Marcotte, D., Arnold, R., & Margolin, A. (2006). Spiritual beliefs, world assumptions, and HIV risk behavior among heroin and cocaine users. *Psychology of Addictive Behaviors, 17*, 159–162.

Banthia, R., Moskowitz, J. T., Acree, M., & Folkman, S. (2007). Socioeconomic differences in the effects of prayer on physical symptoms and quality of life. *Journal of Health Psychology, 12*, 249–260.

Basoglu, M., Mineka, S., Paker, M., Aker, T., Livanou, M., & Gok, S. (1997). Psychological preparedness for trauma as a protective factor in survivors of torture. *Psychological Medicine, 27*, 1421–1433.

Benjamins, M. R., & Brown, C. (2004). Religion and preventative health care utilization among the elderly. *Social Science and Medicine, 58*, 109–118.

Benjamins, M. R., Trinitapoli, J., & Ellison, C. G. (2006). Religious attendance, health maintenance beliefs, and mammography utilization: Findings from a nationwide survey of Presbyterian women. *Journal for the Scientific Study of Religion, 45*, 597–607.

Benson, H. (2000). *The relaxation response.* New York, NY: HarperCollins.

Boersma, S. N., Maes, S., & Van Elderen, T. (2005). Goal disturbance predicts health-related quality of life and depression 4 months after myocardial infarction. *British Journal of Health Psychology, 10*, 615–630.

Bower, J. E., Kemeny, M. E., Taylor, S. E., & Fahey, J. L. (1998). Cognitive processing, discovery of meaning, CD4 decline, and AIDS-related mortality among bereaved HIV-seropositive men. *Journal of Consulting and Clinical Psychology, 66*, 979–986.

Bower, J. E., Low, C. A., Moskowitz, J. T., Sepah, S., & Epel, E. (2008). Benefit finding and physical health: Positive psychological changes and enhanced allostasis. *Social and Personality Psychology Compass, 2*, 223–244.

Breslin, M. J., & Lewis, C. A. (2008). Spiritual practices such as prayer: Theoretical models of the nature of prayer and health: A review. *Mental Health, Religion & Culture, 11*, 9–21.

Britt, T. W., Adler, A. B., & Bartone, P. T. (2001). Deriving benefits from stressful events: The role of engagement in meaningful work and hardiness. *Journal of Occupational Health Psychology, 6*, 53–63.

Brown, S. L., Nesse, R. M., Vinokur, A. D., & Smith, D. M. (2003). Providing social support may be more beneficial than receiving it: Results from a prospective study of mortality. *Psychological Science, 14*, 320–327.

Buck, A. C., Williams, D. R., Musick, M. A., & Sternthal, M. J. (2008). An examination of the relationship between multiple dimensions of religiosity, blood pressure, and hypertension. *Social Science & Medicine, 68*, 314–322.

Cahn, B. R., & Polich, J. (2006). Meditation states and traits: EEG, ERP, and neuroimaging studies. *Psychological Bulletin, 132*, 180–211.

Cohen, S., & Pressman, S. D. (2006). Positive affect and health. *Current Directions in Psychological Science, 15*, 122–125.

Cole, B., & Pargament, K. I. (1999). Re-creating your life: A spiritual/psychotherapeutic intervention for people diagnosed with cancer. *Psycho-Oncology, 8*, 395–407.

Contrada, R. J., Boulifard, D. A., Hekler, E. B., Idler, E. L., Spruill, T. M., Labouvie, E. W., & Krause, T. J. (2008). Psychosocial factors in heart surgery: Presurgical vulnerability and postsurgical recovery. *Health Psychology, 27*, 309–319.

Contrada, R. J., Goyal, T. M., Caher, C., Rafalson, L., Idler, E. L., & Krause, T. J. (2004). Psychosocial factors in outcomes of heart surgery: The impact of religious involvement and depressive symptoms. *Health Psychology, 23*, 227–238.

Cordova, M. J., Cunningham, L. L., Carlson, C. R., & Andrykowski, M. A. (2001). Posttraumatic growth following breast cancer: A controlled comparison study. *Health Psychology, 20*, 176–185.

Cruess, D. G., Antoni, M. H., McGregor, B. A., Kilbourn, K. M., Boyers, A. E., Alferi, S. M., … Kumar, M. (2000). Cognitive-behavioral stress management reduces serum cortisol by enhancing benefit finding among women being treated for early stage breast cancer. *Psychosomatic Medicine, 62*, 304–308.

Danoff-Burg, S., & Revenson, T. A. (2005). Benefit-finding among patients with rheumatoid arthritis: Positive effects on interpersonal relationships. *Journal of Behavioral Medicine, 28*, 91–103.

Davidson, R. J., Kabat-Zinn, J., Schumacher, J., Rosenkranz, M., Muller, D., Santorellis, S. F., Urbanowski, F., … Sheridan, J. F. (2003). Alterations in brain and immune function produced by mindfulness meditation. *Psychosomatic Medicine, 65*, 564–570.

DiMatteo, M. R. (2004). Variations in patients' adherence to medical recommendations: A quantitative review of 50 years of research. *Medical Care, 42*, 200–209.

DiMatteo, M. R., & Haskard, K. B. (2006). Further challenges in adherence research: Measurements, methodologies, and mental health care. *Medical Care, 44*, 297–299.

Dittmann-Kohli, F., & Westerhof, G. J. (2000). The personal meaning system in a life-span perspective. In G. T. Reker & K. Chamberlain (Eds.), *Exploring existential meaning: Optimizing human development across the life span* (pp. 107–123). Thousand Oaks, CA: Sage.

Ditto, B., Eclache, M., & Goldman, N. (2006). Short-term autonomic and cardiovascular effects of mindfulness body scan meditation. *Annals of Behavioral Medicine, 32*, 227–234.

Edmondson, K. A., Lawler, K. A., Jobe, R. L., Younger, J. W., Piferi, R. L., & Jones, W. H. (2005). *Journal of Religion and Health, 44*, 161–171.

Elder, G. H., & Clipp, E. C. (1989). Combat experience and emotional health: Impairment and resilience in later life. *Journal of Personality, 57*, 311–341.

Elklit, A., Shevlin, M., Solomon, Z., & Dekel, R. (2007). Factor structure and concurrent validity of the World Assumptions Scale. *Journal of Traumatic Stress, 20*, 291–301.

Elliot, A. J., Sheldon, K. M., & Church, M. A. (1997). Avoidance personal goals and subjective well-being. *Personality and Social Psychology Bulletin, 23*, 915–927.

Ellison, C. G., & Fan, D. (2008). Daily spiritual experiences and psychological well-being among US adults. *Social Indicators Research, 88*, 247–271.

Emmons, R. A. (2003). Personal goals, life meaning, and virtue: Wellsprings of a positive life. In C. L. M. Keyes (Ed.), *Flourishing: The positive person and the good life* (pp. 105–128). Washington, DC: American Psychological Association.

Emmons, R. A. (2005). Striving for the sacred: Personal goals, life meaning, and religion *Journal of Social Issues, 61*, 731–745.

Emmons, R., & King, L. (1988). Conflict among personal strivings: Immediate and long-term implications for psychological and physical well-being. *Journal of Personality and Social Psychology, 54*, 1040–1048.

Emmons, R. A., & McCullough, M. E. (2003). Counting blessings versus burdens: An experimental investigation of gratitude and subjective well-being in daily life. *Journal of Personality and Social Psychology, 84*, 377–389.

Exline, J. J. (2002). Stumbling blocks on the religious road: Fractured relationships, nagging vices, and the inner struggle to believe. *Psychological Inquiry, 13*, 182–189.

Exline, J. J., & Rose, E. (2005). Religious and spiritual struggles. In R. F. Paloutzian & C. L. Park (Eds.), *Handbook of the psychology of religion and spirituality* (pp. 315–330). New York, NY: Guilford.

Farber, E. W., Schwartz, J. A. J., Schaper, P. E., Moonen, D. J., & McDaniel, J. S. (2000). Resilience factors associated with adaptation to HIV disease. *Psychosomatics; 41*, 140–146.

Fitchett, G., Rybarczyk, B. D., DeMarco, G. A., & Nicholas, J. J. (1999). The role of religion in medical rehabilitation outcomes: A longitudinal study. *Rehabilitation Psychology, 44*, 333–353.

Flannelly, K., Koenig, H. G., Ellison, C. G., Galek, K., & Krause, N. (2006). Belief in life after death and mental health: Findings from a national survey. *Journal of Nervous & Mental Disease, 194*, 524–529.

Folkman, S., & Moskowitz, J. T. (2007). Positive affect and meaning-focused coping during significant psychological stress. In M. Stroebe & H. Schut (Eds.), *The scope of social psychology: Theory and applications: Essays in honour of Wolfgang Stroebe* (pp. 193–208). New York, NY: Psychology Press.

Frazier, P., Anders, S., Perera, S., Tomich, P., Tennen, H., Park, C. L., & Tashiro, T. (2009). Potentially traumatic events among undergraduate students: Prevalence and associated symptoms. *Journal of Counseling Psychology, 56*, 450–460.

Frazier, P., Tashiro, T., Berman, M., Steger, M., & Long, J. (2004). Correlates of levels and patterns of positive life changes following sexual assault. *Journal of Consulting and Clinical Psychology, 72*, 19–30.

Frazier, P., Tennen, H., Gavian, M., Park, C. L., Tomich, P., & Tashiro, T. (2009). Does self-reported post-traumatic growth reflect genuine positive change? *Psychological Science, 20*, 912–919.

Galek, K., Krause, N., Ellison, C., Kudler, T., & Flannelly, K. (2007). Religious doubt and mental health across the lifespan. *Journal of Adult Development, 14*, 16–25.

Gall, T. L. (2003). The role of religious resources for older adults coping with illness. *Journal of Pastoral Care and Counseling, 57*, 211–224.

Gall, T. L., & Cornblat, M. W. (2002). Breast cancer survivors give voice: A qualitative analysis of spiritual factors in long-term adjustment. *Psycho-Oncology, 11*, 524–535.

Gall, T. L., & Grant, K. (2005). Spiritual disposition and understanding illness. *Pastoral Psychology, 53*, 515–533.

The Gallup Organization. (2007). *Americans more likely to believe in god than the devil, heaven more than hell.* Retrieved July 7, 2011, from http://www.gallup.com/poll/27877/Americans-More-Likely-Believe-God-Than-Devil-Heaven-More-Than-Hell.aspx

George, L., Ellison, C., & Larson, D. (2002). Explaining the relationships between religious involvement and health. *Psychological Inquiry, 13*, 190–200.

Gillum, F., & Williams, C. (2009). Associations between breast cancer risk factors and religiousness in American women in a national health survey. *Journal of Religion and Health, 48*, 178–188.

Green, M., & Elliott, M. (2010). Religion, health, and psychological well-being. *Journal of Religion and Health, 49*, 149–163.

Grossman, P., Niemann, L., Schmidt, S., & Walach, H. (2004). Mindfulness-based stress reduction and health benefits: A meta-analysis. *Journal of Psychosomatic Research, 57*, 35–43.

Hall, D. E. (2006). Religious attendance: More cost-effective than Lipitor? *Journal of the American Board of Family Medicine, 19*, 103–109.

Hank, K., & Schaan, B. (2008). Cross-national variations in the correlation between frequency of prayer and health among older Europeans. *Research on Aging, 30*, 36–54.

Harrison, M. O., Koenig, H. G., Hays, J. C., Eme-Akwari, A. G., & Pargament, K. I. (2001). The epidemiology of religious coping: A review of recent literature. *International Journal of Psychiatry, 13*, 86–93.

Hayward, R. D., & Elliott, M. (2011). Subjective and objective fit in religious congregations: Implications for well-being. *Group Processes & Intergroup Relations, 14*, 127–139.

Helgeson, V. S., Reynolds, K. A., & Tomich, P. L. (2006). A meta-analytic review of benefit finding and growth. *Journal of Consulting and Clinical Psychology, 74*, 797–816.

Helm, H. M., Hays, J. C., Flint, E. P., Koenig, H. G., & Blazer, D. G. (2000). Does private religious activity prolong survival? A six-year follow-up study. *Journals of Gerontology: Series A. Biological and Medical Science, 55*, 400–405.

Hill, P. (2005). Measurement in the psychology of religion and spirituality: Current status and evaluation. In R. F. Paloutzian & C. L. Park (Eds.), *Handbook of the psychology of religion and spirituality* (pp. 43–61). New York, NY: Guilford.

Hill, T. D., Ellison, C. G., Burdette, A. M., & Musick, M. A. (2007). Religious involvement and healthy lifestyles: Evidence from the survey of Texas adults. *Annals of Behavioral Medicine, 34*, 217–222.

Holahan, C. K., Holahan, C. J., & Suzuki, R. (2008). Purposiveness, physical activity, and perceived health in cardiac patients. *Disability & Rehabilitation, 30*, 1772–1778.

Holland, J. C., & Reznik, I. (2005). Pathways for psychosocial care of cancer survivors. *Cancer, 704*, 2624–2637.

Hood, R. W., Jr., & Belzen, J. A. (2005). Research methods in the psychology of religion. In R. F. Paloutzian & C. L. Park (Eds.), *Handbook of the psychology of religion and spirituality* (pp. 62–79). New York, NY: Guilford.

Ironson, G., Stuetzle, R., & Fletcher, M. A. (2006). An increase in religiousness/spirituality occurs after HIV diagnosis and predicts slower disease progression over 4 years in people with HIV. *Journal of General Internal Medicine, 21*, 62–68.

Ishida, R., & Okada, M. (2006). Effects of a firm purpose in life on anxiety and sympathetic nervous activity caused by emotional stress: Assessment by psycho-physiological method. *Stress & Health: Journal of the International Society for the Investigation of Stress, 22*, 275–281.

Janoff-Bulman, R. (1989). Assumptive worlds and the stress of traumatic events: Applications of the schema construct. *Social Cognition, 7*, 113–136.

Janoff-Bulman, R. (1992). *Shattered assumptions: Towards a new psychology of trauma*. New York, NY: Free Press.

Janoff-Bulman, R., & Frantz, C. M. (1997). The impact of trauma on meaning: From meaningless world to meaningful life. In M. Power & C. Brewin (Eds.), *The transformation of meaning in psychological therapies: Integrating theory and practice* (pp. 91–106). Sussex, England: Wiley.

Janoff-Bulman, R. & Timko, C. (1987). Coping with traumatic life events: The role of denial in light of people's assumptive worlds. In C. R. Snyder & C. E. Ford (Eds.), *Coping with negative life events: Clinical and social psychological perspectives* (pp. 135–159). New York, NY: Plenum.

Jesse, D. E., & Reed, P. G. (2006). Effects of spirituality and psychosocial well-being on health risk behaviors in Appalachian pregnant women. *Journal of Obstetric, Gynecologic, & Neonatal Nursing, 33*, 739–747.

Jim, H. S., & Andersen, B. L. (2007). Meaning in life mediates the relationship between social and physical functioning and distress in cancer survivors. *British Journal of Health Psychology, 12*, 363–381.

Kaler, M. E., Frazier, P. A., Anders, S. L., Tashiro, T., Tomich, P., Tennen, H., & Park, C. L. (2008). Assessing the psychometric properties of the World Assumptions Scale. *Journal of Traumatic Stress, 21*, 1–7.

Karoly, P. (1999). A goal systems–self-regulatory perspective on personality, psychopathology, and change. *Review of General Psychology, 3*, 264–291.

Karsten, H., & Schaan, B. (2008). Cross-national variations in the correlation between frequency of prayer and health among older Europeans. *Research on Aging, 30*, 36–54.

King, L. A., Hicks, J. A., Krull, J., & Del Gaiso, A. K. (2006). Positive affect and the experience of meaning in life. *Journal of Personality and Social Psychology, 90*, 179–196.

Klinger, E. (in press). The search for meaning in evolutionary perspective and its clinical implications. In P. T. P. Wong & P. S. Fry (Eds.), *The human quest for meaning: A handbook of psychological research and clinical applications* (2nd ed.). Mahwah, NJ: Erlbaum.

Klinger, E. (1977). *Meaning and void: Inner experience and the incentives in people's lives*. Minneapolis, MN: University of Minnesota Press.

Klinger, E. (1998). The search for meaning in evolutionary perspective and its clinical implications. In P. T. P. Wong & P. S. Fry (Eds.), *The human quest for meaning: A handbook of psychological research and clinical applications* (pp. 27–50). Mahwah, NJ: Erlbaum.

Koenig, H. G., George, L. K., Cohen, H. J., Hays, J. C., Larson, D. B., & Blazer, D. G. (1998). The relationship between religious activities and cigarette smoking in older adults. *Journals of Gerontology: Series A. Biological and Medical Sciences, 53*, 426–434

Koenig, H. G., George, L. K., & Siegler, I. (1998). The use of religion and other emotion-regulating coping strategies among older adults. *The Gerontologist, 38*, 303–310.

Koenig, L. B., & Vaillant, G. E. (2009). A prospective study of church attendance and health over the lifespan. *Health Psychology, 28*, 117–124.

Koltko-Rivera, M. (2004). The psychology of worldviews. *Review of General Psychology, 8*, 3–58.

Krause, N. (2002). Church-based social support and health in old age: Exploring variations by race. *Journals of Gerontology: Series B. Psychological Sciences & Social Sciences; 57B*, S332–S347.

Krause, N. (2003). Praying for others, financial strain, and physical health status in late life. *Journal for the Scientific Study of Religion, 42*, 377–391.

Krause, N. (2006a). Church-based social support and change in health over time. *Review of Religious Research; 48*, 125–140.

Krause, N. (2006b). Gratitude toward God, stress, and health in late life. *Research on Aging, 28*, 163–183.

Krause, N. (2008). The social foundation of religious meaning in life. *Research on Aging, 30*, 395–427.

Krause, N. (2009). Meaning in life and mortality. *Journals of Gerontology: Series B. Psychological Sciences and Social Sciences, 64B*(4), 517–527.

Krause, N., Liang, J., Shaw, B. A., Sugisawa, H., Kim, H. K., & Sugihara, Y. (2002). Religion, death of a loved one, and hypertension among older adults in Japan. *Journals of Gerontology. Series B. Psychological Sciences and Social Sciences, 57*, 96–107.

Krause, N., & Shaw, B. A. (2003). Role-specific control, personal meaning, and health in late life. *Research on Aging, 25*, 559–586.

Krause, N., Shaw, B. A., & Cairney, J. (2004). A descriptive epidemiology of lifetime trauma and the physical health status of older adults. *Psychology & Aging, 19*, 637–648.

Krause, N., & Wulff, K. M. (2005). Church-based social ties, a sense of belonging in a congregation, and physical health status. *International Journal for the Psychology of Religion, 15*, 73–93.

Kuijer, R. G., & De Ridder, D. T. D. (2003). Discrepancy in illness-related goals and quality of life in chronically ill patients: The role of self-efficacy. *Psychology & Health, 18*, 313–330.

Kurtz, M. E., Kurtz, J. C., Given, C. W., & Given, B. A. (2008). Patient optimism and mastery—Do they play a role in cancer patients" management of pain and fatigue? *Journal of Pain and Symptom Management, 36*, 1–10.

Lachman, M. E. (2006). Control: Perceived control over aging-related declines: Adaptive beliefs and behaviors. *Current Directions in Psychological Science, 15*, 282–286.

Lachman, M. E., & Firth, K. M. P. (2004). The adaptive value of feeling in control during midlife. In O. G. Brim, C. D. Ryff, & R. C. Kessler (Eds.), *How healthy are we? A national study on well-being at midlife* (pp. 320–349). Chicago, IL: University of Chicago Press.

Lawler, K. A., Younger, J. W., Piferi, R. L., Billington, E., Jobe, R., Edmondson, K., & Jones, W. H. (2003). A change of heart: Cardiovascular correlates of forgiveness in response to interpersonal conflict. *Journal of Behavioral Medicine, 26*, 373–393.

Lawler-Row, K. A. (2010). Forgiveness as a mediator of the religiosity–health relationship. *Psychology of Religion and Spirituality, 2*, 1–16.

Lazarus, R. S., & Folkman, S. (1984). *Stress, appraisal, and coping*. New York, NY: Guilford.

Lee, B. Y., & Newberg, A. B. (2005). Religion and health: A review and critical analysis. *Zygon, 40*, 443–468.

Lee, B. Y., & Newberg, A. B. (2010). The interaction of religion and health. In D. A. Monti & B. D. Beitman (Eds.), *Integrative psychiatry* (pp. 408–444). New York, NY: Oxford University Press.

Levin, J. S., & Vanderpool, H. Y. (1989). Is religion therapeutically significant for hypertension? *Social Science & Medicine, 29*, 69–78.

Lewis, C. A., & Cruise, S. M. (2006). Religion and happiness: Consensus, contradictions, comments and concerns. *Mental Health, Religion & Culture, 9*, 213–225.

Lucas, T., Alexander, S., Firestone, I., & Lebreton, J. M. (2008). Just world beliefs, perceived stress, and health behaviors: The impact of a procedurally just world. *Psychology & Health, 23*, 849–865.

Lundberg, P. C., & Kerdonfag, P. (2010). Spiritual care provided by Thai nurses in intensive care units. *Journal of Clinical Nursing, 19*, 1121–1128.

Maes, S., & Gebhardt, W. (2000). Self-regulation and health behavior: The health behavior goal model. In M. Boekaerts, M. Zeidner, & M. R. Pintrich (Eds.), *Handbook of self regulation* (pp. 343–368). San Diego, CA: Academic Press.

Maes, S., & Karoly, P. (2005). Self-regulation assessment and intervention in physical health and illness: A review. *Applied Psychology: An International Review, 54*, 267–299.

Magyar-Russell, G., Fosarelli, P., Taylor, H., & Finkelstein, D. (2008). Ophthalmology patients' religious and spiritual beliefs: An opportunity to build trust in the patient–physician relationship. *Archives of Opthalmology, 126*, 1262–1265.

Martin, K. M., & Levy, B. R. (2006). Opposing trends of religious attendance and religiosity in predicting elders' functional recovery after an acute myocardial infarction. *Journal of Religion and Health*, *45*, 440–451.

Masters, K. S., Hill, R. D., Kircher, J. C., Lensegrav-Benson, T. L., & Fallon, J. A. (2004). Religious orientation, aging, and blood pressure reactivity to interpersonal and cognitive stressors. *Annals of Behavioral Medicine*, *28*, 171–178.

Masters, K. S., Lensegrav-Benson, T. L., Kircher, J. C., & Hill, R. D. (2005). Effects of religious orientation and gender on cardiovascular reactivity among older adults. *Research on Aging*, *27*, 221–240.

Masters, K. S., & Spielmans, G. I. (2007). Prayer and health: Review, meta-analysis, and research agenda. *Journal of Behavioral Medicine*, *30*, 329–338.

Matthews, K. A., Owens, J. F., Edmundowicz, D., Lee, L., & Kuller, L. H. (2006). Positive and negative attributes and risk for coronary and aortic calcification in healthy women. *Psychosomatic Medicine*, *68*, 355–361.

Mausbach, B. T., Mills, P. J., Patterson, T. L., Aschbacher, K., Dimsdale, J. E., Ancoli-Israel, S., … Grant, I. (2007). Stress-related reduction in personal mastery is associated with reduced immune cell β_2-adrenergic receptor sensitivity. *International Psychogeriatrics*, *19*, 935–946.

Mausbach, B. T., von Känel, R., Patterson, T. L., Dimsdale, J. E., Depp, C. A., Aschbacher, K., … Grant, I. (2008). The moderating effect of personal mastery and the relations between stress and plasminogen activator inhibitor-1 (PAI-1) antigen. *Health Psychology*, *27*, S172–S179.

McCullough, M. E. (2001). Forgiveness: Who does it and how do they do it? *Current Directions in Psychological Science*, *10*, 194–197.

McCullough, M. E., & Worthington, E. L., Jr. (1999). Religion and the forgiving personality. *Journal of Personality*, *67*, 1141–1164.

McIntosh, D. N. (1995). Religion-as-schema, with implications for the relation between religion and coping. *International Journal for the Psychology of Religion*, *5*, 1–16.

McMillen, J. C., Smith, E. M., & Fisher, R. H. (1997). Perceived benefit and mental health after three types of disaster. *Journal of Consulting and Clinical Psychology*, *65*, 733–739.

McMillen, J. C., Zuravin, S., & Rideout, G. (1995). Perceived benefit from child sexual abuse. *Journal of Consulting and Clinical Psychology*, *63*, 1037–1043.

Milam, J. (2006). Posttraumatic growth and HIV disease progression. *Journal of Consulting and Clinical Psychology*, *74*, 817–827.

Miller, W. R., & Thoresen, C. E. (2003). Spirituality, religion, and health: An emerging research field. *American Psychologist*, *58*, 24–35.

Mills, P. J. (2002). Spirituality, religiousness, and health: From research to clinical practice. *Annals of Behavioral Medicine*, *24*, 1–2.

Morrill, E. F., Brewer, N. T., O'Neill, S. C., Lillie, S. E., Dees, E. C., Carey, L. A., & Rimer, B. K. (2008). The interaction of post-traumatic growth and post-traumatic stress symptoms in predicting depressive symptoms and quality of life. *Psycho-Oncology*, *17*, 948–953.

Murray-Swank, N. A., & Pargament, K. I. (2005). An empirically-based rationale for a spiritually-integrated psychotherapy. *Mental Health, Religion & Culture*, *8*, 191–203.

Neupert, S. D., Almeida, D. M., & Charles, S. T. (2007). Age differences in reactivity to daily stressors: The role of personal control. *Journal of Gerontology*, *62B*, P216–P225.

Oman, D., Kurata, J. H., Strawbridge, W. J., & Cohen, R. D. (2002). Religious attendance and cause of death over 31 years. *International Journal of Psychiatry in Medicine*, *32*, 69–89.

Oman, D., & Thoresen, C. (2005). Do religion and spirituality influence health? In R. F. Paloutzian & C. L. Park (Eds.), *Handbook of the psychology of religion and spirituality* (pp. 435–459). New York, NY: Guilford.

Otto, K., & Schmidt, S. (2007). Dealing with stress in the workplace: Compensatory effects of belief in a just world. *European Psychologist*, *12*, 272–282.

Ozorak, E. (2005). Cognitive approaches to religion. In R. F. Paloutzian & C. L. Park (Eds.), *Handbook of the psychology of religion and spirituality* (pp. 295–314). New York, NY: Guilford.

Pargament, K. I. (1997). *The psychology of religion and coping*. New York, NY: Guilford.

Pargament, K. I. (2007). *Spiritually integrated psychotherapy: Understanding and addressing the sacred*. New York, NY: Guilford.

Pargament, K. I., Koenig, H. G., & Perez, L. M. (2000). The many methods of religious coping: Development and initial validation of the RCOPE. *Journal of Clinical Psychology*, *56*, 519–543.

Pargament, K. I., Koenig, H. G., Tarakeshwar, N., & Hahn, J. (2001). Religious struggle as a predictor of mortality among medically ill elderly patients: A 2-year longitudinal study. *Archives of Internal Medicine*, *161*, 1881–1885.

Pargament, K. I., Koenig, H. G., Tarakeshwar, N., & Hahn, J. (2004). Religious coping methods as predictors of psychological, physical and spiritual outcomes among medically ill elderly patients: A two-year longitudinal study. *Journal of Health Psychology, 9*, 713–730.

Pargament, K. I., & Zinnbauer, B. J. (2005). Religiousness and spirituality. In R. F. Paloutzian & C. L. Park (Eds.), *Handbook of the psychology of religion and spirituality* (pp. 21–42). New York, NY: Guilford.

Park, C. L. (2005). Religion as a meaning-making framework in coping with life stress. *Journal of Social Issues, 61*, 707–730.

Park, C. L. (2007). Religiousness/spirituality and health: A meaning systems perspective. *Journal of Behavioral Medicine, 30*, 319–328.

Park, C. L. (2009). Overview of theoretical perspectives. In C. L. Park, S. Lechner, M. H. Antoni, & A. Stanton (Eds.), *Positive life change in the context of medical illness: Can the experience of serious illness lead to transformation?* (pp. 11–30). Washington, DC: American Psychological Association.

Park, C. L. (2010). Making sense of the meaning literature: An integrative review of meaning making and its effects on adjustment to stressful life events. *Psychological Bulletin, 136*, 257–301.

Park, C. L. (in press). Meaning making in cancer survivorship. In P. T. P. Wong (Ed.), *Handbook of meaning* (2nd ed.). Mahwah, NJ: Sage.

Park, C. L., Aldwin, C. M., Fenster, J. R., & Snyder, L. (2008). Coping with September 11th: Post-traumatic stress and post-traumatic growth in a national sample. *American Journal of Orthopsychiatry, 78*, 300–312.

Park, C. L., Chmielewski, J., & Blank, T. O. (2010). Post-traumatic growth: Finding positive meaning in cancer survivorship moderates the impact of intrusive thoughts on adjustment in younger adults. *Psycho-Oncology, 19*, 1139–1147.

Park, C. L., Edmondson, D., Hale-Smith, A., & Blank, T. O. (2009). Religiousness/spirituality and health behaviors in younger adult cancer survivors: Does faith promote a healthier lifestyle? *Journal of Behavioral Medicine, 32*, 582–591.

Park, C. L., & Folkman, S. (1997). The role of meaning in the context of stress and coping. *General Review of Psychology, 1*, 115–144.

Park, C. L., & Helgeson, V. S. (2006). Introduction to the special section: Growth following highly stressful life events—Current status and future directions. *Journal of Consulting and Clinical Psychology, 74*, 791–796.

Park, C. L., Lechner, S., Stanton, A., & Antoni, M. (Eds.). (2009). *Positive life changes in the context of medical illness* (pp. 87–104). Washington, DC: APA Press.

Park, C. L., Malone, M., Suresh, D. P., Bliss, D., & Rosen, R. (2008). Coping, meaning in life, and quality of life in congestive heart failure patients. *Quality of Life Research, 17*, 21–26.

Park, C. L., Moehl, B., Fenster, J. R., Suresh, D. P., & Bliss, D. (2008). Religiousness and adherence behavior in congestive heart failure patients. *Religion, Spirituality, & Aging, 20*, 249–266.

Park, C. L., & Paloutzian, R. F. (2005). One step toward integration and an expansive future. In R. F. Paloutzian & C. L. Park (Eds.), *Handbook of the psychology of religion and spirituality* (pp. 550–564). New York, NY: Guilford.

Park, C. L., & Slattery, J. M. (2008). Spirituality and case conceptualizations: A meaning system approach. In J. Aten & M. Leach (Eds.), *Spirituality and the therapeutic process: A guide for mental health professionals* (pp. 121–142). Washington, DC: American Psychological Association.

Pearce, M. J., Singer, J. L., & Prigerson, H. G. (2006). Religious coping among caregivers of terminally ill cancer patients: Main effects and psychosocial mediators. *Journal of Health Psychology, 11*, 743–759.

Penn Resiliency Project. (2008). Retrieved from http://www.ppc.sas.upenn.edu/prpsum.htm

Pomaki, G., Maes, S., & ter Doest, L. (2004). Work conditions and employees' self-set goals: Goal processes enhance prediction of psychological distress and wellbeing. *Personality and Social Psychology Bulletin, 30*, 685–694.

Powell, L. H., Shahabi, L., & Thoresen, C. E. (2003). Religion and spirituality: Linkages to physical health. *American Psychologist, 58*, 36–52.

Pressman, S. D., & Cohen, S. (2005). Does positive affect influence health? *Psychological Bulletin, 131*, 925–971.

Pudrovska, T., Schieman, S., Pearlin, L. I., & Nguyen, K. (2005). The sense of mastery as a mediator and moderator in the association between economic hardship and health in late life. *Journal of Aging and Health, 17*, 634–660.

Ransom, S., Sheldon, K. M., & Jacobsen, P. B. (2008). Actual change and inaccurate recall contribute to post-traumatic growth following radiotherapy. *Journal of Consulting and Clinical Psychology, 76*, 811–819.

Reicks, M., Mills, J., & Henry, H. (2004). Qualitative study of spirituality in a weight loss program: Contribution to self-efficacy and locus of control. *Journal of Nutrition Education and Behavior, 36,* 13–19.

Reker, G. T., & Wong, P. T. P. (1988). Aging as an individual process: Toward a theory of personal meaning. In J. E. Birren & V. L. Bengston (Eds.), *Emergent theories of aging* (pp. 214–246). New York, NY: Springer.

Rini, C., Manne, S., DuHamel, K. N., Austin, J., Ostroff, J., Boulad, F., & Redd, W. H. (2004). Mothers' perceptions of benefit following pediatric stem cell transplantation: A longitudinal investigation of the roles of optimism, medical risk, and sociodemographic resources. *Annals of Behavioral Medicine, 28,* 132–141.

Rippentrop, A., Altmaier, E., Chen, J., Found, E., & Keffala, V. (2005). The relationship between religion/spirituality and physical health, mental health, and pain in a chronic pain population. *Pain, 116,* 311–321.

Ryff, C. D. (1989). Happiness is everything, or is it? Explorations on the meaning of psychological well-being *Journal of personality and social psychology, 57,* 1069–1081.

Ryff, C. D., Love, G. D., Urry, H. L., Muller, D., Rosenkranz, M. A., Friedman, E. M., … Singer, B. (2006). Psychological well-being and ill-being: Do they have distinct or mirrored biological correlates? *Psychotherapy and Psychosomatics, 75,* 85–95.

Saroglou, V., Buxant, C., & Tilquin, J. (2008). Positive emotions as leading to religion and spirituality. *Journal of Positive Psychology, 3,* 165–173.

Sawatzky, R., Ratner, P. A., & Chiu, L. (2005). A meta-analysis of the relationship between spirituality and quality of life. *Social Indicators Research, 72,* 153–188.

Scheier, M. F., Wrosch, C., Baum, A., Cohen, S., Martire, L. M., Matthews, K. A., … Zdaniuk, B. (2006). The Life Engagement Test: Assessing purpose in life. *Journal of Behavioral Medicine, 29,* 291–298.

Schwarzer, R., & Taubert, S. (2002). Tenacious goal pursuits and striving toward personal growth: Proactive coping. In E. Frydenberg (Ed.), *Beyond coping: Meeting goals, visions and challenges* (pp. 19–35). London, England: Oxford University Press.

Sephton, S. E., Koopman, C., Schaal, M., Thoresen, C., & Spiegel, D. (2001). Spiritual expression and immune status in women with metastatic breast cancer: An exploratory study. *The Breast Journal, 7,* 345–353.

Seya, A. (2003). Life-style factors associated with perceived health status, life satisfaction and purpose in life. *Journal of the National Institute of Public Health, 52,* 242–244.

Shaw, A., Joseph, S., & Linley, P. A. (2005). Religion, spirituality, and posttraumatic growth: A systematic review. *Mental Health, Religion & Culture, 8,* 1–11.

Sherman, A. C., Plante, T. G., Simonton, S., Latif, U., & Anaissie, E. J. (2009). Prospective study of religious coping among patients undergoing autologous stem cell transplantation. *Journal of Behavioral Medicine, 32,* 118–128.

Silberman, I. (2005). Religion as a meaning system: Implications for the new millennium. *Journal of Social Issues, 61,* 641–663.

Simonelli, L. E., Fowler, J., Maxwell, G. L., & Andersen, B. L. (2008). Physical sequelae and depressive symptoms in gynecologic cancer survivors: Meaning in life as a mediator. *Annals of Behavioral Medicine, 35,* 275–284.

Skrabski, A., Kopp, M., Rózsa, S., Réthelyi, J., & Rahe, R. H. (2005). Life meaning: An important correlate of health in the Hungarian population. *International Journal of Behavioral Medicine, 12,* 78–85.

Slattery, J. M., & Park, C. L. (in press–a). Clinical approaches to discrepancies in meaning: Conceptualization, assessment, and treatment. In P. T. P. Wong (Ed.), *Handbook of meaning* (2nd ed.). Mahwah, NJ: Sage.

Slattery, J. M., & Park, C. L. (in press–b). Meaning making and spiritually-oriented interventions. In J. Aten, M. R. McMinn, & E. V. Worthington (Eds.), *Spiritually oriented interventions for counseling and psychotherapy.* Washington, DC: American Psychological Association.

Slattery, J. M., & Park, C. L. (in press–c). Religious and spiritual beliefs in psychotherapy: A meaning perspective. In J. Aten, K. O'Grady, & E. V. Worthington (Eds.), *The psychology of religion and spirituality for clinicians: Using research in your practice.* New York, NY: Routledge.

Smith, B. W., & Zautra, A. J. (2004). The role of purpose in life in recovery from knee surgery. *International Journal of Behavioral Medicine, 11,* 197–202.

Solomon, Z., Iancu, I., & Tyano, S. (1997). World assumptions following disaster. *Journal of Applied Social Psychology, 27,* 1785–1798.

Stanton, A. L., Bower, J. E., & Low, C. A. (2006). Posttraumatic growth after cancer. In L. G. Calhoun & R. G. Tedeschi (Eds.), *Handbook of posttraumatic growth: Research and practice* (pp. 138–175). Mahwah, NJ: Erlbaum.

Steffen, P. R., & Masters, K. S. (2005). Does compassion mediate the intrinsic religion-health relationship? *Annals of Behavioral Medicine, 30,* 217–224.

Steger, M. F. (in press). Meaning in life. In S. J. Lopez (Ed.), *Handbook of positive psychology* (2nd ed.). Oxford, England: Oxford University Press.

Steger, M. F., & Frazier, P. (2005). Meaning in life: One link in the chain from religion to well-being. *Journal of Counseling Psychology, 52,* 574–582.

Stetz, K. M. (1989). The relationship among background characteristics, purpose in life, and caregiving demands on perceived health of spouse caregivers. *Research and Theory for Nursing Practice, 3,* 133–153.

Strawbridge, W. J., Shema, S. J., Cohen, R. D., & Kaplan, G. A. (2001). Religious attendance increases survival by improving and maintaining good health practices, mental health, and stable marriages. *Annals of Behavioral Medicine, 23,* 68–74.

Street, H., O'Connor, M., & Robinson, H. (2007). Depression in older adults: Exploring the relationship between goal setting and physical health. *International Journal of Geriatric Psychiatry, 22,* 1115–1119.

Surtees, P., Wainwright, N., Luben, R., Khaw, K., & Day, N. (2006). Mastery, sense of coherence, and mortality: Evidence of independent associations from the EPIC-Norfolk Prospective Cohort Study. *Health Psychology, 25,* 102–110.

Tarakeshwar, N., Vanderwerker, L. C., Paulk, E., Pearce, M. J., Kasl, S. V., & Prigerson, H. G. (2006). Religious coping is associated with the quality of life of patients with advanced cancer. *Journal of Palliative Medicine, 9,* 646–657.

Tedeschi, R. G., & Calhoun, L. (2004). Posttraumatic growth: Conceptual foundations and empirical evidence. *Psychological Inquiry, 15,* 1–15.

Tedeschi, R. G., & Calhoun, L. (2006). *Handbook of posttraumatic growth.* Mahwah, NJ: Erlbaum.

Tedeschi, R. G., & Calhoun, L. (2009). The clinician as expert companion. In C. L. Park, S. Lechner, A. Stanton, & M. Antoni (Eds.), *Positive life changes in the context of medical illness* (pp. 215–235). Washington, DC: APA Press.

Thune-Boyle, I. C., Stygall, J. A., Keshtgar, M. R., & Newman, S. P. (2006). Do religious/spiritual coping strategies affect illness adjustment in patients with cancer? A systematic review of the literature. *Social Science & Medicine, 63,* 151–164.

Tix, A. P., & Frazier, P. A. (2005). Mediation and moderation of the relationship between intrinsic religiousness and mental health. *Personality and Social Psychology Bulletin, 31,* 295–306.

Tomaka, J., & Blascovich, J. (1994). Effects of justice beliefs on cognitive appraisal of and subjective physiological, and behavioral responses to potential stress. *Journal of Personality and Social Psychology, 67,* 732–740.

Tomich, P. L., & Helgeson, V. S. (2002). Five years later: A cross-sectional comparison of breast cancer survivors with healthy women. *Psycho-Oncology, 11,* 154–169.

Tomich, P. L., & Helgeson, V. S. (2004). Is finding something good in the bad always good? Benefit finding among women with breast cancer. *Health Psychology, 23,* 16–23.

Tomich, P. L., Helgeson, V. S., & Vache, E. J. N. (2005). Perceived growth and decline following breast cancer: A comparison to age-matched controls 5-years later. *Psycho-Oncology, 14,* 1018–1029.

Toussaint, L. L., Williams, D. R., Musick, M. A., & Everson, S. A. (2001). Forgiveness and health: Age differences in a U.S. probability sample. *Journal of Adult Development, 8,* 249–257.

Trevino, K. M., Pargament, K. I., Cotton, S., Leonard, A. C., Hahn, J., Caprini-Faigin, C. A., & Tsevat, J. (2010). Religious coping and physiological, psychological, social, and spiritual outcomes in patients with HIV/AIDS: Cross-sectional and longitudinal findings. *AIDS and Behavior, 14,* 379–389.

Updegraff, J. A., & Marshall, G. N. (2005). Predictors of perceived growth following direct exposure to community violence. *Journal of Social and Clinical Psychology, 24,* 58–560.

Van der Veek, S., Kraaij, V., van Koppen, W., Garnefski, N., & Joekes, K. (2007). Goal disturbance, cognitive coping and psychological distress in HIV-infected persons. *Journal of Health Psychology, 12,* 225–230.

Verduin, P. J. M., de Bock, G. H., Vlieland, T. P. M. V., Peeters, A. J., Verhoef, J., & Otten, W. (2008). Purpose in life in patients with rheumatoid arthritis. *Clinical Rheumatology, 27,* 899–908.

Wachholtz, A. B., & Keefe, F. J. (2006). What physicians should know about spirituality and chronic pain. *Southern Medical Journal, 99,* 1174–1175.

Wachholtz, A. B., & Pargament, K. I. (2008). Migraines and meditation: Does spirituality matter? *Journal of Behavioral Medicine, 31,* 351–366.

Waltman, M. A., Russell, D. C., Coyle, C. T., Enright, R. D., Holter, A. C., & Swoboda, C. M. (2009). The effects of a forgiveness intervention on patients with coronary artery disease. *Psychology & Health, 24,* 11–27.

Wells, J. N. B., Bush, H. A., & Marshall, D. (2002). Purpose-in-life and breast health behavior in Hispanic and Anglo women. *Journal of Holistic Nursing, 20,* 232–249.

WHOQOL SRPB Group. (2006). A cross-cultural study of spirituality, religion, and personal beliefs as components of quality of life. *Social Science & Medicine, 62*, 1486–1497.

Williams, D. R., & Sternthal, M. J. (2007). Spirituality, religion and health: Evidence and research directions. *Medical Journal of Australia, 186*, S47–S50.

Wink, P., & Scott, J. (2005). Does religiousness buffer against the fear of death and dying in late adulthood? Findings from a longitudinal study. *Journals of Gerontology: Series B. Psychological Sciences and Social Sciences, 60*, 207–214.

Worthington, E. L., & Scherer, M. (2004). Forgiveness is an emotion-focused coping strategy that can reduce health risks and promote health resilience: Theory, review, and hypotheses. *Psychology and Health, 19*, 385–405.

Wortmann, J., & Park, C. L. (2008). Religion and spirituality in adjustment following bereavement: An integrative review. *Death Studies, 32*, 703–736.

Wrosch, C., Scheier, M. F., & de Pontet, S. B. (2007). Giving up on unattainable goals: Benefits for health? *Personality and Social Psychology Bulletin, 33*, 251–265.

Wrosch, C., Scheier, M. F., Miller, G. E., Schulz, R., & Carver, C. S. (2003). Adaptive self-regulation of unattainable goals: Goal disengagement, goal reengagement, and subjective well-being. *Personality and Social Psychology Bulletin, 29*, 1494–1508.

Yehuda, R., & McEwen, B. S. (Eds.). (2004). Biobehavioral stress response: Protective and damaging effects. *Annals of the New York Academy of Sciences, 1032*.

Younger, J., Finan, P., Zautra, A., Davis, M., & Reich, J. (2008). Personal mastery predicts pain, stress, fatigue, and blood pressure in adults with rheumatoid arthritis. *Psychology & Health, 23*, 515–535.

19 Pregnancy and Birth Outcomes

A Multilevel Analysis of Prenatal Maternal Stress and Birth Weight

Christine Dunkel Schetter
University of California, Los Angeles

Marci Lobel
Stony Brook University

Not long ago, the study of pregnancy and birth was the sole domain of the field of medicine and the allied health professions. In recent decades, psychosocial and sociocultural factors have been increasingly incorporated into theory and research on pregnancy in order to improve our scientific understanding of the factors that elevate or reduce risk. When we began our work on pregnancy in the 1980s, it was recognized that even a complete analysis of medical risk factors did not account for much of the variation in rates of such adverse birth outcomes as preterm birth or low birth weight. However, approaches to the identification of psychosocial risk factors were still evolving in rigor and acceptance by biomedical scientists. In the intervening decades, psychosocial and interdisciplinary approaches to the study of pregnancy and birth have evolved considerably; they are not only accepted today but often welcomed. Many behavioral, sociological, cultural, and biomedical scientists now work together in collaboration to understand the complex interplay of multiple levels and types of concepts that contribute to maternal and child outcomes. Moreover, biopsychosocial integration is producing exciting findings and important insights that promise to improve future health outcomes for pregnant women and their offspring.

In this chapter, we provide brief background on the epidemiology of birth outcomes, especially focusing on low birth weight, and we outline a multilevel approach to understanding the etiology of low birth weight. We review the evidence regarding various types of prenatal maternal stress in the prediction of birth weight, and we focus on the theory and evidence on three modifiers of these effects—namely, medical risk, race and ethnicity, and social support. We explain the major mechanisms at physiological and behavioral levels, focusing in detail on research on smoking, physical activity, nutrition, and healthy lifestyles. Thereafter, there is a discussion of integrative models and we present a schematic diagram differing from others in its greater detail of psychological processes. Our conclusions offer suggestions for studying stress better in order to understand low birth weight. We propose studying health behaviors further as a set of mechanisms, and argue that we are not yet ready to intervene to reduce low birth weight with psychosocial approaches. A subtheme throughout the chapter is the importance of race and ethnicity as they pertain to disparities in birth outcomes and their understanding.

BACKGROUND ON BIRTH OUTCOMES

We use the term *adverse birth outcomes* broadly here to refer to preterm birth (PTB), low birth weight (LBW), infant mortality and related complications for the mother or infant at birth or shortly after. In this chapter, we build upon our earlier one entitled "Stress Processes in Pregnancy and Birth" (Dunkel Schetter, Gurung, Lobel, & Wadhwa, 2001), which appeared in the first edition of this handbook. Here, we focus on a broader range of issues but on only one outcome—LBW (low birth weight)—while still emphasizing stress, a primary area of our individual programs of research. Other recent reviews exist on stress and PTB (Dunkel Schetter & Glynn, 2010; Hobel, Goldstein, & Barrett, 2008), but none of which we are aware on stress and LBW. These two outcomes are objectively measured, and national and international data on population rates are published regularly. Although PTB and LBW are moderately correlated, the complex and multiple etiological pathways to them are increasingly distinguishable (Dunkel Schetter, 2010). Furthermore, disentangling these two outcomes and their precursors is critical to moving forward on national agendas to reduce rates of PTB, LBW, and infant mortality in high-risk populations.

RATES AND SIGNIFICANCE OF LBW

LBW is defined as infant weight at birth of less than 2,500 grams (5 pounds, 8 ounces). Fetal growth is the trajectory of growth, usually estimated through ultrasound examinations over the course of gestation. At 8.3%, the rate of LBW in the United States in 2006 was the highest in four decades (Martin, Hamilton, & Sutton, 2009) and higher than the rate for other industrialized countries. This high LBW rate reflects, in part, the growing number of multiple births in the United States (e.g., twins, triplets), more than half of which are LBW. However, the rate of LBW among singleton births is also considered high at 6.5% nationwide and has risen by approximately 10% in the last several years (Martin et al., 2009).

LBW co-occurs with PTB in one half to two thirds of cases. Babies born early are likely to weigh less; yet many babies born at full term (37 to 40 weeks) are LBW. Ultrasound and newborn exams are used to differentiate premature LBW from more mature growth-retarded LBW infants. Intrauterine growth restriction (IUGR) refers to a fetus not reaching its genetically predetermined size, based on population standards, usually as a result of pathological changes in the placenta (Marsal, 2002). A newborn that is *small for gestational age* (SGA) is below the 10th percentile of weight for gestational age at birth, a characteristic sometimes also referred to as *fetal growth retardation*, or FGR. These infants are at higher risk of abnormalities and risk of neonatal death compared to higher weight babies, and those babies below the fifth percentile are especially at risk of these outcomes.

Both underweight and preterm infants are at increased risk of infant mortality and other problems in infancy and childhood, including respiratory illness, impaired growth, cognitive deficits, and longer term neurological problems that may require special education (Hack, Klein, & Taylor, 1995; Newnham, 1998; Thompson et al., 1997). Research also suggests that LBW infants are at increased risk in adulthood for cardiovascular disease, noninsulin-dependent diabetes, obesity, and psychiatric conditions (Behrman & Stith Butler, 2007).

Studies of LBW examine both the clinically defined dichotomous outcome (i.e., normal vs. low birth weight) and the continuous variable of weight in grams at birth (ranging from 500 grams or less to more than 3,000 grams). LBW is further subdivided into *very low birth weight* (VLBW), defined as less than 1,500 grams at birth, and *extremely low birth weight* (ELBW), which is less than 1,000 grams at birth. Very large samples are needed to provide the statistical power to assess predictors of the categorical variables of LBW, VLBW, or ELBW; whereas studies with smaller samples can examine the correlates of the continuous birth weight variable with sufficient power. Both are valuable in understanding the effects of such psychosocial factors as stress. In fact, there is evidence that some child and adult health outcomes are influenced by small gradations in birth weight within the normal birth weight range (Breslau, Chilcoat, DelDotto, Andreski, & Brown, 1996; Matte, Bresnahan, Begg, & Susser, 2001; Richards, Hardy, Kuh, & Wadsworth, 2001; Sorensen et al., 1997). In addition, the effects of psychosocial variables on birth weight are often linear. Therefore, there is more than adequate justification, both empirically and clinically, for studying both birth weight variables. We believe that a focus on the etiology of LBW from a multilevel and, especially, psychosocial perspective is very valuable at this juncture.

RACIAL AND ETHNIC DISPARITIES IN LBW

LBW occurs disproportionately among ethnic groups within the United States. African Americans have approximately twice the LBW rate (14.0%) compared to non-Hispanic Whites (7.3%) and Hispanics (7.0%) and have a higher rate of LBW than other groups as well (Martin et al., 2009). African Americans also have higher rates of PTB. However, African American infants have a survival advantage at lower birth weights and younger gestational ages compared to European American infants (Alexander, Tompkins, & Hulsey, 2000; Wilcox & Russell, 1990). Furthermore, there is evidence suggesting that African American fetuses mature faster than European American fetuses (e.g., Alexander, Hulsey, Robillard, De Caunes, & Papiernik, 1994; Robillard et al., 1994). Thus, race-specific analyses are essential, and race-specific criteria for defining LBW may be needed.

In addition to the disparity between African Americans and other groups in LBW, there are differences among ethnic subgroups of Latinas. For instance, Puerto Rican women have higher rates of LBW (10% in 2003) than do other Latinas, and there is considerable variability within the Hispanic population as a function of socioeconomic status (SES) and acculturation. Campos and colleagues (2008) discussed two important and counterintuitive patterns within the Latina population that are relevant to studying pregnancy. First, Latino or Hispanic individuals of lower SES have better health outcomes in general, including pregnancy outcomes, than do Latinos of higher SES (Abraido-Lanza, Dohrenwend, Ng-Mak, & Turner, 1999; Hessol & Fuentes-Afflick, 2000). Second, more acculturated Latina women often have higher rates of adverse pregnancy outcomes than do less acculturated women. For example, in a study of nearly 1,100 poor minority women, two thirds of whom were of Mexican origin or descent and all of whom were having their first child, more acculturated women had lower birth weight infants and higher stress and substance use (Zambrana, Scrimshaw, Collins, & Dunkel-Schetter, 1997). They were also less enthusiastic about the pregnancy compared to women who were less acculturated.

In a similar study of a cohort of 1,064 Latina women (Campos, Dunkel Schetter, Walsh, & Schenker, 2007), two components of acculturation were distinguished, one involving use of English and contact with Anglos (labeled *Anglo orientation*), and the other involving immersion in Mexican and Spanish-speaking culture (labeled *Mexican orientation*). Although there were no associations of Mexican orientation with birth weight in this study, higher Anglo orientation was associated with lower infant birth weight (OR = 1.28, $p <. 01$). That is, Latina pregnant women who reported that they associated more often with Anglos and spoke, wrote, and thought more in English had lower birth weight babies, controlling for gestational age, compared to those who were lower on this factor.

Both of these studies suggest that increased involvement in Anglo culture poses pregnancy risk. Further consistent evidence comes from a recent study on racial and ethnic disparities in LBW in 2,412 unmarried mothers classified as non-Hispanic Black, non-Hispanic White, U.S.-born Mexican origin, and foreign-born Mexican origin, which found a Mexican-origin advantage in birth weight that was explained, in part, by better prenatal health and behaviors in Mexican-born women (Reichman, Hamilton, Hummer, & Padilla, 2008). Researchers are just beginning to understand the sometimes paradoxical differences among Latino subgroups in pregnancy. It appears that the Latina pregnant women most at risk may be those less likely to have cultural resilience factors such as larger social networks and stronger support, or highly valued family connections and mutual obligations (i.e., *familialism*), and they are less likely to highly value pregnancy and childbearing (Abdou et al., 2010; Campos et al., 2008; Campos et al, 2007).

Paradoxical findings also occur for African American women of higher SES. This group does not experience the lower rates of adverse birth outcomes that European American women of similar SES do (e.g., Din-Dzietham & Hertz-Picciotto, 1998). This may be partially because African American women with greater education or higher job status are less connected to a supportive community and more exposed to racism in ethnically integrated neighborhoods and places of work (Buka, Brennan, Rich-Edwards, Raudenbush, & Earls, 2003; Clark, Anderson, Clark, & Williams, 1999). The observation that higher SES Black women in the United States have poorer pregnancy outcomes on average than do poor White women points to critical interactions of SES, race, and ethnicity in pregnancy risk.

MULTILEVEL ANALYSES OF BIRTH OUTCOMES

Clearly, any comprehensive and useful understanding of LBW will involve thoughtful and detailed behavioral and sociocultural analyses, reaffirming that a complete understanding of pregnancy and birth outcomes requires interdisciplinary approaches. Many processes influence the rate of growth of a fetus and resultant birth weight of a baby. Table 19.1 contains a summary of a number of risk and resilience factors at each level that are known or commonly hypothesized to influence birth weight. Individual-level factors, interpersonal factors, sociocultural factors, and community factors all figure into the comprehensive prediction of LBW. Within these categories, there are further subcategories of variables that influence birth weight. These levels of analysis and specific factors have been examined in past research, although mostly in isolation rather than conjointly. There is increasing recognition that the prediction of birth outcomes is multifactorial, involving joint and interactive effects of many variables at several different levels. Thus, the taxonomy depicted in Table 19.1 may help to advance a comprehensive understanding of the processes that influence birth outcomes.

To expand on the multiple influences on birth outcomes, we note that medical, behavioral, and psychological factors all exert influence at the individual level. Medical risk factors include maternal history of disease, obstetric and gynecological risk factors including complications in prior pregnancies, and emerging symptoms and conditions in the present pregnancy. Behavioral risk factors of primary interest at the individual level include preconception and prenatal smoking, drug and alcohol use, nutrition, physical activity and fitness, and health care. Psychological factors at the individual level include exposure to stressors of many types, emotional and cognitive responses to stress, and personal resources that directly influence birth weight or modify effects of stressors on birth weight. In this chapter, we focus in greater detail on this level, that is, psychological factors and their incorporation into integrative predictive models, because this level involves areas of our unique past contributions and topics especially relevant to the field of health psychology.

At the interpersonal level, social integration, networks, support, and close relationship quantity and quality (e.g., with partner or baby's father) are all key factors, along with conflict and interpersonal violence in close relationships. Group- and sociocultural-level factors include race, ethnicity, nativity, acculturation, socioeconomic status, and social position. Community- and societal-level factors include community stressors and resources, neighborhood characteristics, and such institutional characteristics as systemic discrimination.

As can be seen in Table 19.1, it would be impossible to capture all these influences in a single study. However, in sum total, they represent the large array of established or likely influences on rate of fetal growth and resultant infant birth weight. Figure 19.1 is a simple schematic diagram of these multilevel categories of factors on birth weight. It depicts them as direct and equally important causal influences, although they may actually have different degrees of importance and, in some cases, are likely to interact in their effects.

TABLE 19.1
Multilevel Predictors, Mediators, and Moderators of Birth Weight

Level of Analysis	Risk and Resilience Factors
Individual: *Biological/medical*	Maternal medical history/risk factors
	Maternal pregnancy risk conditions and symptoms
	Preconception dysregulated HPA, immune, or other systems
	Genetic factors
Individual: *Behavioral*	Smoking in pregnancy
	Drug use in pregnancy
	Alcohol use in pregnancy
	Physical fitness
	Nutrition in pregnancy
	Vitamin use in pregnancy
	Health behaviors preconception
	Regular and preventive health care (immunizations, dental care)
	Prenatal care utilization
Individual: *Psychological*	Stress and emotion
	Major life events
	State anxiety
	Pregnancy anxiety/pregnancy distress
	Chronic stress
	Traumatic events
	Work stress
	Perceived racism
	Mental health indicators
	Depressed mood
	Anxiety disorders
	PTSD
	Personal resources
	Optimism
	Mastery
	Self-esteem
	Perceived available support
	Attitudes toward pregnancy
	Intendedness
	Coping style
	Approach/avoidance
	Positive emotions
	Religiosity/spirituality
Interpersonal: *Dyadic/familial/relational*	Social support received
	Social network properties
	Relationship characteristics of baby's father
	Family composition
	Quality of relationships
	Responsiveness
	Marital satisfaction
	Intergenerational factors
	Interpersonal violence (IPV)
Group: *Sociocultural*	Race/ethnicity
	Nativity
	Acculturation

continued

TABLE 19.1 (Continued)
Multilevel Predictors, Mediators, and Moderators of Birth Weight

Level of Analysis	Risk and Resilience Factors
Community: *Societal*	SES/social class
	Familism
	Collectivism
	Community stressors (e.g., noise, traffic, toxins, violence, pollution, crime, density of housing)
	Community cohesion, collectivism
	Neighborhood poverty
	Residential segregation
	Institutional discrimination
	Cultural norms and values

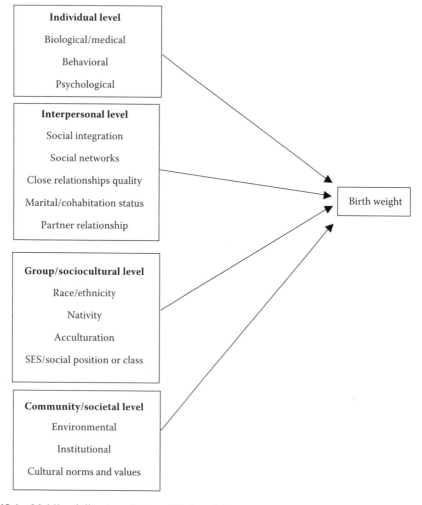

FIGURE 19.1   Multilevel direct predictors of birth weight.

Evidence Regarding Prenatal Maternal Stress and Birth Outcomes

The individual-level factor influencing birth outcomes that we have focused on most in a number of studies is stress. There is now compelling scientific evidence that prenatal maternal stress in various forms predicts PTB (Dunkel Schetter, 2009; Dunkel Schetter & Glynn, 2010), and there is also considerable evidence regarding LBW. For example, Beydoun and Saftlas (2008), who reviewed the human and animal evidence for prenatal maternal stress and adverse outcomes, indicate that 9 out of the 10 studies on LBW that they reviewed show significant effects. Stress has been operationalized in these studies in numerous ways, typically by measuring either major life events, perceived stress, general state anxiety, or pregnancy-specific anxiety or distress.

In our first study on this topic, we followed 130 women throughout their pregnancies with assessments of stress at every prenatal visit using multiple stress measures (Lobel, Dunkel-Schetter, & Scrimshaw, 1992). Using structural equation modeling to combine measures of perceived stress, state anxiety, and distress ensuing from life events, we tested whether the composite stress factor predicted time of delivery (weeks gestation) and birth weight (in grams) when controlling for medical risk factors and risk behaviors, including smoking. Women participating in this study were interviewed from four to 12 times in pregnancy in the public clinic where they received prenatal care. They were diverse in ethnicity and were mostly low income. Some were undocumented residents. Approximately half were interviewed in Spanish.

As hypothesized, we found that the composite stress factor was predictive of earlier delivery (i.e., younger gestational age at birth) and lower birth weight (see Figure 19.2). At that time, there was relatively little prospective evidence for the effects of stress on these outcomes. Stress assessment had been problematic in many prior studies that used measures of unknown reliability or validity (Lobel, 1994). Utilizing a composite stress factor and multivariate modeling techniques offered several statistical and conceptual advantages. However, these results called for replication. Furthermore, physicians and epidemiologists preferred to see the prediction of dichotomous outcomes and risk ratios for PTB and LBW in order to consider the findings clinically relevant.

In subsequent prospective studies, stress consistently predicted gestational age at birth (GA) or PTB. In particular, studies by Dunkel Schetter and colleagues (Dunkel Schetter, 1998, 2009, 2010; Rini, Dunkel-Schetter, Wadhwa, & Sandman, 1999; Roesch, Dunkel Schetter, Woo, & Hobel, 2004; Wadhwa, Sandman, Porto, Dunkel-Schetter, & Garite, 1993; Zambrana et al., 1997) have shown that pregnancy-related anxiety—that is, fears and concerns about this pregnancy and baby specifically—is a unique predictor of the timing of delivery (cf. Lobel, Cannella, et al., 2008). Furthermore, three large epidemiological studies in the United States and Canada (Dole et al., 2003; Kramer et al., 2009; Orr, Reiter, Blazer, & James, 2007) report odds ratios of 1.5 to 2 times greater risk of PTB among women with high pregnancy-linked anxiety during pregnancy.

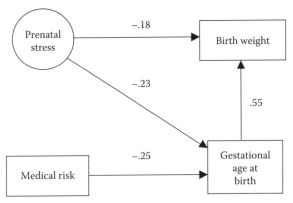

FIGURE 19.2 Effects of stress on birth outcomes. (Adapted from Lobel, M., Dunkel-Schetter, C., and Scrimshaw, S. C. M., *Health Psychology, 11*, 32–40, 1992.)

Thus, pregnancy-related anxiety appears to be a reliable and robust independent predictor of PTB. However, the effects of stress or anxiety on birth weight or LBW are less clear. For this reason, we believe that a review of the specific evidence about stress effects on birth weight and LBW is valuable in order to determine what forms of stress predict fetal growth outcomes and for whom.

EVIDENCE REGARDING STRESS AND LBW

Does prenatal (or prepregnancy) stress significantly influence infant birth weight independent of confounds including time of delivery (GA or PTB)? In order to examine this question, we systematically compiled available strong evidence on stress and birth weight or LBW published since 1990. Searches of relevant databases and citations in relevant articles yielded approximately 45–50 studies. The majority of the studies were prospective, a few utilized retrospective case-control designs, and a small group utilized state or national archives. Investigations were conducted in the United States and in several other countries including Brazil, Denmark, the Netherlands, Sweden, and New Zealand. We narrowed our review to investigations with at least 50 participants, but these studies usually had much larger samples sizes ranging up to 2,000 or more (Copper et al., 1996; Sable & Wilkinson, 2000), and in the archival studies, millions of births are involved (e.g., Khashan et al., 2008). Samples in the United States include teens, women of low-SES, African Americans, and residents from many regions of the country. Many of these investigations focused on the prediction of birth weight as the primary goal.

The assessment of stress varied greatly across studies which included measures of life events, depression, anxiety, general distress, and perceived stress and hassles, all of which are common measures. Still other approaches involve composite indices designed for pregnancy (e.g., Lobel, Canella, et al., 2008; Lobel, DeVincent, Kaminer, & Meyer, 2000; Pryor et al., 2003) or the examination of stress in the form of specific community events such as national tragedies in Sweden and the United States (Catalano & Hartig, 2001; Smits, Krabbendam, De Bie, Essed, & Van Os, 2006). Another form of stress studied is *racism*. These literatures virtually all measure stress at the individual level, in contrast to studies on neighborhoods that capture such stressful environmental conditions as neighborhood poverty (e.g. Collins, Wambach, David, & Rankin, 2009). A thorough review of evidence on neighborhood stressors and LBW is beyond the scope of this review, although it is necessary for any complete multilevel analysis.

The vast majority of studies that we reviewed found that measures of stress or emotion predicted either birth weight or the clinical outcome, LBW. Those studies that did not find such effects tended to have smaller samples, providing weak tests of the hypotheses, and had less rigorous study designs though a few exceptions to this rule exist. The nature of the measures used provides some clues to the patterns of findings, so we reviewed them by type of stress measure.

Several studies use the Perceived Stress Scale (PSS; Cohen, Kamarck, & Mermelstein, 1983) to study prenatal stress. This is a very general measure of stress reflecting inability to cope and being overwhelmed and not in control of stressful demands. A large prospective study in Sweden with 826 women giving birth for the first time found no effects of prenatal PSS scores on SGA births (i.e., births that are small for gestational age), although they included only four of the items on the original scale (Dejin-Karlsson et al., 2000). Similarly, a New Zealand case-control study of over 836 SGA births compared their PSS scores to those of 870 births that were average for gestational age and found no significant differences between the two groups (Pryor et al., 2003); this study does not report whether the researchers abbreviated the PSS or not. In contrast, Krabbendam et al. (2005) administered the full PSS to 5,511 Dutch women at 14 and 30 weeks of pregnancy and found that high perceived stress at 14 weeks increased risk of SGA but the effect was small after adjustment for education and smoking (OR = 1.16). Sable and Wilkinson (2000) conducted a retrospective case-control study of 2,378 pregnant women in Missouri, dividing them according to whether the infant was normal, low, or very low weight (with the latter, VLBW, defined as < 1500 g). They found that high perceived stress, reported retrospectively after birth, was associated with

1.5 times greater risk of a VLBW infant after adjusting for education, income, marital status, inadequate prenatal care, and smoking. A few other studies reported effects of stress on birth weight when the PSS was a part of a composite index (Dominguez, Dunkel Schetter, Mancuso, Rini, & Hobel, 2005; Lobel et al., 1992; Zambrana et al., 1997). However, others reported no effects of PSS as part of composite scores on birth weight (Rondo et al., 2003). Overall, stress as measured by the PSS does not seem to be a strong indicator of risk for LBW, especially when examined as the only stress measure.

The use of composite measures is one solution to stronger measurement in pregnancy (Lobel, 1994), and some studies suggest that this strategy increases predictive power (Herrera, Salmeron, & Hurtado, 1997; Lobel et al., 1992; Zambrana et al., 1997). For example, among 178 African American women studied prospectively beginning before 20 weeks' gestation, a composite of standardized prenatal stress variables accounted for 7% of the variance in birth weight adjusted for GA (Dominguez et al., 2005). However, composite stress variables have not always shown effects on birth weight (Lobel et al., 2000; Rini et al., 1999). Notably, these studies all included similar stress measures.

There is more consistent evidence that major life events contribute to LBW. Khashan et al. (2008) studied 1.38 million singleton Danish births over more than 20 years by merging birth data with records on specific severe life events. They found that the death of a relative during pregnancy, or in the six months prior to it, was associated with significantly higher risk of having small infants (RR = 1.17 for SGA; RR = 1.22 < 5th percentile). In another such study, Danish national databases were used to identify retrospectively 3,402 cases of LBW and 19,551 control cases (Precht, Andersen, & Olsen, 2007). Mothers exposed to severe life events before 32 weeks had twice the risk of SGA in these analyses. Another investigation showed that prepregnancy life events predicted birth weight after adjusting for controls in 100 low-educated, mostly White women studied prospectively (Pagel, Smilkstein, Regan, & Montano, 1990). In addition, a study of 92 mothers whose infants were LBW and 92 control women utilized objective coding of life events and chronic stress and found both were associated significantly with LBW, with some confounding variables controlled (Mutale, Creed, Maresh, & Hunt, 1991). A recent retrospective study examined 8,064 births in the South Carolina Pregnancy Risk Assessment and Monitoring System (PRAMS) and tested effects of life events in pregnancy reported after birth and of neighborhood poverty on both LBW and PTB (Nkansah-Amankra, Luchok, Hussey, Watkins, & Liu, 2010). In brief, they found significant effects of life events on LBW that were moderated in part by neighborhood context, with stronger effects for women in disadvantaged neighborhoods. Despite these findings, many of which involved strong measures and very large samples, a few studies have not found life event effects on birth weight (e.g., Hoffman & Hatch, 2000; McCormick et al., 1990).

Interesting results by Catalano and Hartig (2001) on Swedish birth data pertain to understanding communal life event stress and birth weight. They used time-series analyses to examine the effects of two national events that caused "communal bereavement:" a death of a national hero and a ship disaster that killed many people. The incidence of VLBW was higher in the months following the events compared to the months before. Similarly, Smits et al. (2006) found that pregnant women in the Netherlands exposed through the media to the September 11 attacks in New York City had lower birth weight infants (cf. Endara et al., 2009; Engels, Berkowitz, Wolff, & Yehuda, 2005; Eskenazi, Marks, Catalono, Bruckner, & Toniolo, 2007; Lederman et al., 2004). The possibility that community-wide tragedies pose risk of LBW is intriguing because pregnant women exposed to such events would be particularly amenable to intervention possibly in the context of prenatal care.

Investigators have also measured anxiety, depression, and general distress as predictors of LBW, birth weight, or related outcomes. General distress measured with the General Health Questionnaire (GHQ) during pregnancy was a significant risk factor for LBW in 865 Brazilian pregnant women (OR = 1.97; Rondo et al., 2003). Similarly, Hoffman and Hatch (2000) reported that depression measured with the Center for Epidemiological Studies Depression Scale (CES-D) at week 28 of pregnancy among 666 women was associated with smaller infants but only in the low SES group. A Dutch study of 396 first births found depressed mood posed significant risk for SGA after adjusting for smoking, education, weight, and height (Paarlberg et al., 1999), although the effect size was modest (OR = 1.12). However, Zimmer-Gembeck and Helfand (1996) reported that when adjusted for ethnicity, medical risk, and health behaviors, LBW was associated with negative mood in a sample of 3,073 low-income women (OR =1.65). Furthermore, a prospective study of 712 inner city pregnant teens and adults composed of mostly minority women (Steer, Scholl, Hediger, & Fischer, 1992) found that depression measured with the Beck Depression Inventory (BDI) predicted LBW and SGA with relatively large effect sizes (OR = 3.97; 3.02 respectively). Clearly, among the psychosocial stress factors studied, distress and depressed mood seem to be stronger risk factors for LBW relative to other stress measures, although at least a few epidemiological studies report no significant effects (Chung, Lau, Yip, Chiu, & Lee, 2001).

In addition to conducting studies of depressed mood, some investigators have looked at clinically significant diagnoses of depressive disorders. For example, LBW was predicted by depressive disorder in 1,100 pregnant women who were screened for psychiatric disorders during pregnancy, with an odds ratio of 1.82 (Rogal et al., 2007). In addition, Kelly et al. (2002) conducted a population-based retrospective cohort study of 521,490 California births using hospital discharge data and found that psychiatric diagnoses predicted normal birth weight and VLBW (OR = 2.0, 2.9) adjusted for marital status, ethnicity, and prenatal care adequacy. Thus, results of tests of psychiatric diagnoses with birth weight are consistent in size and direction with those results on depressed mood or symptomatology (cf. Berle et al., 2005).

Regarding anxiety, a study of 1,500 indigent pregnant women in Alabama found that trait anxiety in the second trimester significantly predicted IUGR (Goldenberg, Cliver, Cutter, & Hoffman, 1991). Although only marginally significant, depressed mood had a larger effect (OR = 1.47 trait anxiety; OR = 2.00 depressed mood). Another study of a smaller sample of 132 pregnant women studied prospectively found that highly anxious women were more likely to have an LBW infant (Field et al., 2008). However, the sample size precluded control of some confounds, among them medical risk. Furthermore, a number of studies reported no significant effects of anxiety or anxiety diagnoses as a predictor of LBW (e.g., Berle et al., 2005; Catov, Abatemarco, Markovic, & Roberts, 2010; Rondo et al., 2003). Rini et al. (1999) tested the effects of anxiety on GA and birth weight in a sample of 221 women followed during pregnancy and postpartum using multivariate techniques that enabled distinguishing predictors of each outcome and controlling for medical risk, ethnicity, and other confounds. What resulted was a clear pathway from anxiety to earlier delivery but no direct effect on birth weight, only an indirect effect through GA. Thus, evidence for the effects of anxiety on LBW is not compelling, especially compared to the consistency of the effects of prenatal anxiety on PTB (Dunkel Schetter & Glynn, 2010). In contrast, depression appears to be a more powerful affective state than anxiety with respect to fetal growth and LBW.

Still another approach to studying stress prenatally is to examine chronic stressors. For example, a study of 1,363 pregnant, low-income women in Illinois used multiple measures of stress tailored to this population and reported that LBW was associated with such chronic stressors as unemployment or crowding, with odds ratios of 2.7 to 3.8 (Borders, Grobman, Amsden, & Hall, 2007). Similarly, Orr et al. (1996) examined stressors in family, work, finances, neighborhood, and housing in a sample of 2,000 low-income women, the majority of whom were African American. They found that exposure to these chronic stressors predicted LBW adjusted for medical and behavioral risks (OR = 1.52). Similarly, a study of 480 Black and White women in Alabama who were prospectively assessed regarding job strain (perceived demands and control) showed that women with high-strain jobs had lower birth weight infants compared to those with lower strain and, with adjustment for many confounding variables, compared to those who were unemployed (Oths, Dunn, & Palmer, 2001). There was also an interaction with race such that the effects were stronger for Blacks. Finally, Pritchard and Teo (1994), in a study of 393 Scottish women who had given birth previously, measured perceived difficulties in their household roles at 20 and 30 weeks' gestation, finding that high difficulty predicted LBW after adjustment for SES and smoking (OR = 4.70). In sum, chronic stressors appear to be a robust predictor of LBW. Unfortunately, the studies of chronic stress do not generally measure mood to determine if the indirect effects of stress through a pregnant woman's mood states, particularly depression, might account for these effects.

EVIDENCE ON RACISM AND LBW

Another important body of evidence demonstrating effects of prenatal stress on birth weight consists of studies investigating racial discrimination in pregnant women of color, especially African Americans (e.g., Giscombé & Lobel, 2005; Rich-Edwards & Grizzard, 2005). Racial discrimination or racism has been defined as oppression, domination, and denigration of individuals by other individuals and by social and cultural institutions based on skin color or membership in a particular ethnic group (Clark et al., 1999; Jones, 2000; Krieger, Rowley, Herman, Avery, & Phillips, 1993; Utsey & Ponterotto, 1996). At least eight studies have investigated whether racial discrimination contributes to elevated risk of delivering a LBW infant, of which six focused specifically on explaining the high rate of LBW in African Americans. (The remaining two studies, of Latinas and Arab Americans, are discussed separately later.) Studies examining racism and LBW also differ in whether they are prospective or retrospective, in their measures of racism, and in whether they control for other predictors of LBW. Such differences hinder the ability to draw conclusions from these studies; nevertheless, several of these studies find associations between racism and LBW. We summarize the findings of these studies below.

Generally, studies of racism and LBW in African American women have employed two different study designs or approaches. One approach, namely a disparities analysis, involves measuring perceptions of racial discrimination and LBW in Black women compared to women of a different race (usually Whites), then examining whether group differences in discrimination accounted for disparities in LBW. One such study compared African American women to non-Hispanic White pregnant women using a measure of racism adapted from a widely used and well-validated instrument assessing experiences in such various life domains as employment, school, health care, and public settings (Dominguez, Dunkel Schetter, Glynn, Hobel, & Sandman, 2008). The measure was adapted to determine whether respondents had personally experienced racial discrimination or had witnessed others experiencing it and whether, for each of these, it occurred in childhood or as an adult. Prenatal reports by expecting mothers of both vicarious childhood exposure to racism and of lifetime exposure to racism predicted giving birth to infants of lower birth weight. These measures of perceived racism also accounted, in part, for differences in birth weight between African American and White women, with other predictors of birth weight, including gestational age at delivery, controlled.

In a retrospective study of African American and White women, perceptions of racial discrimination partially accounted for the difference in rates of LBW between these two groups of women (Mustillo et al., 2004). However, controlling for gestational age eliminated the association between racism and LBW, indicating that effects of racism on birth weight in this study were mediated fully by earlier delivery. Another comparative study of African American women and women of other racial backgrounds (Chinese, Dominican, Puerto Rican, Mexican, and White) asked study participants if they had "experienced one or more incidents of racial discrimination" during their pregnancy. The authors did not find a significant association between perceived racial discrimination experienced during pregnancy and birth weight (Shiono, Rauh, Park, Lederman, & Zuskar, 1997) after controlling for numerous other predictors. However, associations between discrimination and birth weight were not examined separately for each ethnic group in this study, and the measure of racism was of unknown reliability and validity. Potential interactive effects of discrimination and ethnicity were also not examined, although racial discrimination may have greater impact on some racial groups (e.g., African Americans) than on others (Dominguez et al., 2008).

The second design approach (within racial group analyses) involved studying African American women exclusively and testing whether women who perceive greater racism are more likely to deliver an LBW infant. Three studies utilized this approach. Two investigations used adapted versions of the Krieger (1990) discrimination measure administered to women after the birth of a normal-weight or VLBW infant (< 1500 g; Collins, David, Handler, Wall, & Andes, 2004; Collins et al., 2000). Either all or a majority of study participants were impoverished in these two samples. Both studies found that racism was associated with an increase in the likelihood that an African American woman would deliver a VLBW infant. In the first of the two studies, the variable examined was discrimination during pregnancy; the association of this variable with VLBW was strongest in women with other risk factors (e.g., late or no prenatal care; cigarette or alcohol use), suggesting interactive effects. In the latter study, lifetime exposure to discrimination showed strong, dose-response relationships with VLBW, but discrimination during pregnancy, which was not frequently experienced in this sample, was not associated with VLBW (Collins et al., 2004). The third study of low-income African American women did not find an association between racial discrimination and birth weight (Dailey, 2009), but this study used a different measure than the earlier studies and produced a complex set of findings.

Finally, two intriguing studies of groups other than African Americans have used indirect indicators of racism to examine association with birth weight. Landale and Oropesa (2005) used the darkness of skin tone among Puerto Rican women as an indicator of racism. These researchers found that among Puerto Rican women living in five eastern U.S. states, those with darker skin tones were more likely to deliver a LBW infant. This association remained significant after controlling for numerous other variables including socioeconomic background, current SES, health behaviors, and prenatal care utilization. Skin tone also predicted the continuous birth weight variable in this group of women; that is, darker skin tone was inversely associated with birth weight in a linear manner. However, skin tone was not associated with birth weight for Puerto Rican women living in their native country or those living in New York City. Because New York City has the largest concentration of Puerto Ricans in the United States and arguably has higher acceptance of immigrants, these results are consistent with an interpretation involving racism.

Another indirect indicator of racism was examined in a study that compared rates of LBW in Californian women with Arabic surnames (as listed on birth certificates) before and after the September 2001 terrorist attack on the United States, and in comparison to women of other ethnic backgrounds (Lauderdale, 2006). Prior to September 2001, Arabic-named women had rates of LBW that were equivalent to those of White women. In the six-month period following September 2001, women with Arabic names experienced a 34% increase in deliveries of LBW infants. This increase did not occur for women without Arabic names including White, Black, Hispanic, and Asian women. The authors document the widespread, extreme, and violent discrimination that Arab Americans experienced during the period following September 11, 2001. Pregnant women with Arab surnames clearly experienced or witnessed such discrimination or lived in fear of it during this time.

In sum, the available studies on racism and discrimination in pregnant women indicate likely effects on birth weight, but as discussed later in this chapter, more research is needed.

MODIFIERS OF STRESS EFFECTS ON LBW

A small number of studies have examined interactive effects of stress on birth weight. These studies examine three main modifiers of stress effects: (1) medical risk, (2) maternal ethnicity and race, and (3) social support. Medical risk is usually a count of the number of risk conditions a mother has from a total of two to as many as three dozen possible antenatal risk factors. Evidence for modification of stress effects on birth outcomes by medical risk appeared in our own prior work reviewed earlier (Lobel et al., 1992). Among the 130 women studied prospectively, there were significant interactions of medical risk and stress in effects on both PTB and LBW. That is, women who were high in both stress and medical risk were at much greater risk of LBW compared to those women with either high stress or high risk alone or low on both variables. These interactive effects also occurred in a similar pattern for GA. Given these interaction effects, we believe that interactions of stress with such specific medical risk factors as diabetes or hypertension may be important to test further, especially in populations that experience these conditions frequently. A recent study on stress and resting blood pressure in pregnant women (Hilmert et al., 2008) revealed that African American women who had a combination of high stress and high resting blood pressure (subclinical high levels) had infants of significantly lower-than-normal birth weight. These results are consistent with the notion that stress is more likely to contribute to an adverse outcome when it occurs in combination with medical risk conditions. However, most women in the study were not hypertensive; notably, high resting blood pressure values within normal range interacted with stress in effects on birth weight.

Another potentially important modifier of the effects of stress on birth outcomes is race or ethnicity, as alluded to earlier. Disparities in birth outcomes between African Americans and most other ethnic groups are integral to studies on stress and birth outcomes (Giscombé & Lobel, 2005; Hogue & Bremner, 2005). Two groups of researchers have examined interactive effects of prenatal stress and race on birth weight (Buka et al., 2003; Oths et al., 2001). In both studies, effects of stress on birth weight were greater in African American women than in European American women. Each study examined a different type of stress. Buka et al. (2003) found that the degree of poverty present in the neighborhood where a pregnant woman lived predicted lower birth weight in African American women but not in European American women. Oths et al. (2001) focused on job strain in pregnant women and found that it had a stronger inverse association with birth weight in African American women than in European American women. More attention to tests of interactions of stress in various forms with race is needed.

The third potential modifier of stress effects on birth weight is social support. Although most of the research on social support in pregnancy has examined only whether main effects on birth outcomes occur, the dominant hypothesis in the social support literature has been that support would interact with or modify effects of stress on health outcomes; that is, support would be expected to "buffer" effects of stress on birth outcomes. However, very few tests and little evidence of this exist. Turner, Grindstaff, and Phillips (1990), in one of the earliest and stronger studies of social support in pregnancy, found evidence of support moderation. This prospective study of 268 pregnant teenagers revealed that social support moderated effects of stress in the low-SES group but not in the higher SES group.

Collins, Dunkel-Schetter, Lobel, and Scrimshaw (1993) examined the role of social support in detail in predicting various birth outcomes, including birth weight. Among women who experienced high numbers of life events during pregnancy, those reporting higher quality social support delivered infants with higher birth weight, whereas women who had low levels of life events did not show the effect. Furthermore, whereas support quality was the only social support measure that had an interactive effect with stress, other aspects of support, including social network size, were directly associated with birth outcomes in this study. These findings indicate that researchers must assess various aspects of social support (e.g., quantity, quality, network) if they hope to understand social support processes in pregnancy (see Dunkel Schetter, 2010; Dunkel Schetter & Brooks, 2009; Rini, Dunkel Schetter, Hobel, Glynn, & Sandman, 2006). In addition, social support has shown benefits for only certain ethnic or racial subgroups in some studies suggesting interactions of race/ethnicity and social support on birth weight (Buka et al., 2003; Norbeck and Anderson, 1989; Sagrestano, Feldman, Killingsworth-Rini, Woo, & Dunkel-Schetter, 1999).

SUMMARY OF RESEARCH FINDINGS ON STRESS AND LBW

We observe that whereas research on stress and PTB has accumulated to a point where firmer conclusions can be drawn (Dunkel Schetter, 2009, 2010; Dunkel Schetter & Glynn, 2010; Savitz & Dunkel Schetter, 2006), the evidence regarding stress and lower birth weight lags behind. Altogether, available research findings indicate that stress in various forms including major and chronic stressors, emotional states, and perceived racism, predicts lower birth weight. However, a major problem with this literature is that the studies vary so much in design, sample, measures, and control of possible confounds that it is difficult to make sense of what the primary stressors are that pose risk and for whom. Nonetheless, the findings on depression, chronic stress, and stress composite indices are somewhat consistent; those on life events are uneven but, on balance, suggest effects of note; and results on anxiety in pregnancy and perceived stress are few or none.

Although small in number, the results of studies examining stress modifiers are particularly important for three reasons: (1) they demonstrate why tests of interactions should be conducted and reported more often; clearly, specific subgroups of women may be at greater risk of the effects of stress on birth outcomes; (2) existing research provides a strong rationale for measuring modifiers comprehensively, especially as medical risk, ethnicity and race, and social support; and (3) the studies suggest that stress may be especially important to assess in women with medical and demographic risk factors such as high blood pressure or low SES.

MECHANISMS: MULTILEVEL MEDIATING PROCESSES

In the past decade, many researchers have endeavored to study the predictors of birth outcomes, but only recently has attention been directed to the mechanisms involved. Some of the multilevel predictors shown in Table 19.1 may also mediate other factors' effects on birth weight and preterm birth. For example, the effects of community and cultural influences on health outcomes are often hypothesized to be mediated by such individual-level factors as health behavior or emotional states. Similarly, individual-level psychological factors undoubtedly influence birth outcomes through complex biological processes. However, our scientific knowledge of these multilevel pathways remains incomplete.

The mediating processes perhaps most studied are variants of stress pathways to birth outcomes. Stressors have been hypothesized to influence birth weight through both physiological and behavioral mechanisms (Dunkel Schetter et al., 2000). Stress causes dysregulation of the immune, cardiovascular, and neuroendocrine systems in nonpregnant women. In pregnancy, these processes become much more complex. Physiological mechanisms linking stress with earlier delivery and PTB have received a great deal of attention (Behrman & Stith Butler, 2007; Challis et al., 2009; Coussons-Read, Okun, & Simms, 2003; Dunkel Schetter & Glynn, 2010; Wadhwa et al., 2001), whereas the physiological pathways from stress to LBW have not been studied as often. For example, hormones that the placenta releases in response to stressors, such as corticotrophin-releasing hormone (CRH), seem to precipitate early delivery in animals and human, a phenomenon referred to as the "placental clock" (Hobel, Dunkel-Schetter, Roesch, Castro, & Arora, 1999; Majzoub et al., 1999; Sandman et al., 2006; Smith, Mesiano, & McGrath, 2002). Considerable research has been devoted to this topic and has resulted in important and interesting gains in scientific knowledge about PTB. However, stress can also impair a woman's motivation and ability to maintain healthy behavior in pregnancy, thereby contributing to adverse outcomes. We posit that this health behavioral pathway is implicated more in the etiology of LBW than that of PTB. In the remainder of our discussion of stress–birth weight mediation, we focus on these two sets of hypothesized processes: (1) physiological mediation, and (2) mediation involving various health behaviors.

PHYSIOLOGICAL MEDIATION OF STRESS: THE LBW LINK

A growth-restricted fetus is one that has not reached its growth potential at a given gestational age as a result of one or more causal factors (Lin & Santolaya-Forgas, 1998). Up to 70% of SGA infants who are are small simply because of constitutional factors determined by maternal weight, height, parity, and ethnicity. Normal fetal growth occurs in three stages. The first phase is during the first 16 weeks of pregnancy and involves cellular hyperplasia, or a rapid increase in cell number. The second phase at midgestation involves increase in cell number and size. The last phase is after 32 weeks and involves rapid increases in cell size. Patterns of fetal growth retardation differ depending on the causes, their duration, and the stage of gestation. In addition, growth restriction in the fetus can be symmetric or asymmetric, with the latter accounting for 79% to 80% of cases. *Asymmetric FGR* refers to greater decrease in size of the fetus's abdomen compared to the head. *Symmetric FGR* refers to growth patterns where head and abdomen are decreased proportionately. It is believed that symmetric FGR occurs when risks occur earlier in gestation, and that asymmetric FGR occurs when risks occur later.

A large number of fetal, placental, maternal, and other factors can lead to FGR. Fetal factors include chromosomal abnormalities, congenital malformations, and multiple gestations. Maternal factors include genetic or constitutional factors, obstetrical risk factors such as previous stillbirth, recurrent abortion, previous preterm births, and maternal diseases. They also include such environmental factors as altitude and, as noted earlier, such behavioral factors as nutrition, smoking, alcohol abuse, and drug use. The most common cause of FGR is chronic vascular disease related to hypertension, renal diseases, diabetes, and vascular diseases, especially when co-occurring with preeclampsia. Preeclampsia, a rapidly progressing condition related to pregnancy, is characterized by high blood pressure and the presence of protein in the urine. The fetus can be viewed as parasitic to the mother in that it depends on maternal supply of oxygen and nutrients. Although further detail is beyond the scope of this chapter, it is important to note that inadequate placental blood flow may lead to pregnancy-induced hypertension and to FGR.

One often discussed pathway from stress to LBW involves the vascular effects of stress. Specifically, chronic maternal stress can result in vasoconstriction, reduced uteroplacental perfusion, and hypoxia (reduced oxygen to the fetus), thereby contributing to fetal growth retardation and LBW (Cosmi, Luzi, Gori, & Chiodi, 1990; Shepherd & Kiel, 1992). However, evidence supporting this stress-to-birth-weight pathway is not extensive. Kurki, Hiilesmaa, Raitasalo, Mattila, and Ylikorkala (2000) studied 623 pregnancies at 10–17 weeks' gestation and at delivery. A small percentage developed preeclampsia, and both depression and anxiety predicted preeclampsia (OR = 3.1 for both together). Also, Teixeira, Fisk, and Glover (1999) found anxiety assessed at 32 weeks of pregnancy predicted uterine artery resistance, which is consistent with a vascular mechanism linking anxiety with fetal development or SGA (cf. Harville et al., 2008).

Hypothalamic pituitary adrenal (HPA) involvement as a pathway from stress to fetal growth has also been investigated. To begin with, there is evidence regarding stress hormones and growth or birth weight. For example, maternal CRH, the corticotrophin-releasing hormone released from the placenta into maternal blood as part of the HPA stress response, significantly differentiated those who later gave birth to LBW and normal birth weight infants in a sample of several hundred women (Wadhwa et al., 2004). In a more recent study, increases in plasma maternal cortisol at 15, 19, and 25 weeks and increases in placental CRH at 31 weeks in 158 pregnant women were significantly associated with lower infant maturation scores at birth using a standard clinical assessment after controlling for length of gestation, but the effects held only for male infants (Ellman, Dunkel Schetter, Hobel, Chicz-DeMet, Glynn, & Sandman, 2008). Further, a Dutch study of 2,820 women found that higher maternal cortisol levels at 13 weeks gestation predicted lower birth weight and higher SGA risk, but only among women who provided blood samples at 9 a.m. or earlier (Goedhart et al., 2010). These results are consistent with a stress-HPA-LBW meditational chain but not definitive without measuring stress explicitly.

Diego et al. (2006) utilized ultrasound data and collected first-morning urine samples to assess cortisol and norepinephrine, and obtained psychological stress measures in 98 women during midgestation (16 to 29 weeks). Daily hassles predicted higher urinary cortisol which significantly predicted lower fetal weight, controlling for gestational age at assessment and SES. There was also a significant direct effect of maternal distress (depressed and anxious mood) on fetal weight that was not mediated by cortisol, which may be a result of unmeasured behavioral mechanisms. Overall, 26% of the variance in fetal weight was explained in this study. As the authors discussed, unbound cortisol can cross the placenta and affect fetal development by dysregulation of placental CRH levels. This study is one of very few to include sociodemographic, biological, and psychosocial variables within a reasonably large sample and to predict fetal weight assessed by ultrasound (see also Diego, Field, Hernandez-Reif, Schanberg, Kuhn, & Gonzalez-Zuintero, 2009).

Of note, the techniques for obtaining biological samples, whether they are blood, urine, or saliva samples, and the details of how they are stored, processed, and assayed are critical to evaluating findings (Latendresse & Ruiz, 2008). In addition, preliminary evidence suggests that ethnic differences in HPA hormones during pregnancy may be important to consider in examining disparities in outcomes such as LBW (e.g. Glynn, Dunkel Schetter, Chicz-DeMet, Hobel, & Sandman, 2007). Very sophisticated multidisciplinary research on these HPA pathways is needed to replicate, extend, and clarify existing research.

Another set of physiological mechanisms likely to be involved in the associations between stress and LBW is the immune–inflammatory pathway. Prenatal stress has been linked to a greater likelihood of urogenital infection (Culhane et al., 2001) and infection is a known contributor to adverse birth outcomes. Much of this research has focused on the link between urogenital infection and PTB (Lu & Goldenberg, 2000; Newton, Piper, Shain, Perdue, & Peairs, 2001), although a few recent studies find an association between infections such as bacterial vaginosis and low birth weight (Svare, Schmidt, Hansen, & Lose, 2006; Thorsen et al., 2006; Vogel et al., 2006). We did not identify any published studies at time of writing linking stress, inflammation, and birth weight.

In sum, although the pathophysiology of fetal growth restriction is somewhat understood, it is quite complex. Furthermore, the ways in which stress is involved in these pathways has not been developed much in research.

HEALTH BEHAVIOR IN PREGNANCY AND LBW

Health behaviors represent an understudied and potent mechanism to explain any impact of prenatal stress on birth weight. In fact, LBW may be more behaviorally influenced than PTB. Many maternal behaviors influence the growth of the fetus; whereas fewer behaviors, mainly cocaine use and smoking, have clearly been documented to influence PTB (Savitz & Dunkel Schetter, 2006). The health behaviors known to contribute to LBW include smoking and substance use, diet and nutrition, and physical activity. As a result, women are advised by their health care providers to refrain from smoking and abusing substances and to eat a balanced diet at regular intervals during pregnancy. People experiencing high stress are, however, more likely to engage in various types of unhealthful behaviors that adversely affect birth weight, including poor eating habits, inadequate physical activity, cigarette smoking, and alcohol and other substance use (e.g., Ng & Jeffery, 2003; Stetson, Rahn, Dubbert, Wilner, & Mercury, 1997). Stress may also adversely influence women's attitudes toward their pregnancies, which in turn influence health behavior. For example, women who are unhappy about being pregnant seem to practice less optimal self-care during pregnancy compared to women who feel fortunate to be pregnant or feel that it is fulfilling a life goal (DeLuca & Lobel, 1995; Zambrana et al., 1997).

Despite the scientific plausibility of these behavioral mechanisms, surprisingly few studies have investigated the extent to which health behaviors mediate the impact of prenatal stress on birth weight. One exception is a recent study in which the impact of pregnancy-specific stress on birth weight was explained in part by its association with cigarette smoking using structural equation modeling techniques (Lobel, Canella, et al., 2008). An ethnically diverse sample of 279 women of moderate socioeconomic status was interviewed three times during early, mid-, and late pregnancy about various types of stress and health behaviors. Slightly more than a fifth of the study participants reported that they smoked during pregnancy. Those who were experiencing the greatest distress from such pregnancy-specific issues as their medical care, physical symptoms and bodily changes, concerns about becoming a parent, and worries about the baby's health were more likely to be smoking cigarettes during their pregnancy and, as a result, to deliver a LBW infant. Unhealthy eating, lack of physical activity, and other risky health behaviors did not mediate the association between stress and LBW but, as expected, were associated with pregnancy-specific stress. Thus, some health behaviors may mediate effects of stress on birth weight, whereas other health behaviors may not, and the patterns may be population-specific.

Although there is a dearth of research that simultaneously examines prenatal stress, health behaviors, and birth outcomes, studies that investigate the first link in the causal chain, that is, the associations of prenatal stress with health behaviors, are more common. Recent research on associations of stress in pregnancy with smoking, physical activity, and poor nutrition is reviewed next.

Stress, Cigarette Smoking, and Birth Weight

Cigarette smoking is a well-documented contributor to LBW (Crawford, Tolosa, & Goldenberg, 2008; Jaddoe et al., 2008; Phung et al., 2003; Windham, Hopkins, Fenster, & Swan, 2000), and there is some evidence that the impact of smoking in pregnancy may be greater in such otherwise vulnerable groups as older women and women of color (Windham et al., 2000). It is estimated that 20% to 30% of all LBW deliveries in the United States are attributable to maternal smoking during pregnancy (Crawford et al., 2008). Many female smokers do, however, abstain from cigarette smoking when they become pregnant out of concern for their baby's health or in response to health care provider recommendations (Crittenden, Manfredi, Cho, & Dolecek, 2007). However, approximately 10% of women continue to smoke during pregnancy (Crawford et al., 2008; Weaver, Campbell, Mermelstein, & Wakschlag, 2008).

Smoking during pregnancy has been shown to be associated with a variety of demographic factors including low education, low income, and non-Hispanic White ethnicity (Mathews, 2001). Smoking is also associated with various forms of stress, namely interpersonal violence, job strain, and low resources such as inadequate social support (Bullock, Mears, Woodcock, & Record, 2001; Crawford et al., 2008; Jesse, Graham, & Swanson, 2006; Song & Fish, 2006). In one of the more sophisticated analyses of the influence of prenatal stress on smoking, Weaver and colleagues (2008) found that low maternal education and low household income predicted persistent prenatal smoking (defined as smoking in at least two trimesters). Further, the number of cigarettes smoked was predicted by a latent psychosocial risk variable comprised of high numbers of stressful life events, dissatisfaction with social support, and little use of community resources. These authors suggest that the association between stress and smoking may be bidirectional; that is, women who smoke during pregnancy may feel distressed as a result of their smoking in addition to smoking in response to stress.

A recent study of 1,399 women living in an urban area of Russia examined the prospective prediction of birth weight in relation to prenatal stress, housing conditions, smoking, and alcohol consumption (Grjibovski, Bygren, Svartbo, & Magnus, 2004). Results indicated that smoking, living in a shared or crowded apartment, and perceived stress at work or at home were predictors of lower birth weight. Furthermore, smoking was correlated with lower education, being unmarried, living in a shared apartment, carrying an unplanned pregnancy, and perceived stress. Although mediational pathways were not examined in this study, the pattern of results suggests that such variables as stress and living in a shared apartment may have adversely affected birth weight through their association with smoking. Also notable in this study is that prenatal alcohol use was not correlated with any of the psychosocial variables examined, nor with smoking, and it did not predict LBW.

Stress, Physical Activity, and Birth Weight

Regular, moderately intense physical activity during pregnancy has been associated with higher birth weight (Clapp, Kim, Burciu, & Lopez, 2000; Lobel, DeVincent, Kaminer, & Meyer, 2000) and with other favorable pregnancy and labor outcomes, including fewer pregnancy-related discomforts (Horns, Ratcliffe, Leggett, & Swanson, 1996; Sternfeld, Quesenberry, Eskenazi, & Newman, 1995), less pain during labor (Varrassi, Bazzano, & Edwards, 1989), shorter duration of active labor (Clapp, 1990), shorter hospital stays (Hall & Kaufmann, 1987), and reduced likelihood of cesarean section (surgical) delivery in individual studies (Bungum, Peaslee, Jackson, &

Perez, 2000; Hall & Kaufmann, 1987). A meta-analysis of randomized controlled trials on aerobic exercise in pregnancy, however, found the available data insufficient to infer benefits for birth weight (Kramer & McDonald, 2009). They did, however, find effects of exercise on maternal fitness.

Furthermore, evidence is inconsistent about effects of physical activity from employment on birth outcomes. A recent meta-analysis of 29 studies (Mozurkewich, Luke, Avni, & Wolf, 2000) indicates that physically demanding work increases the likelihood of delivering a SGA infant (OR 1.37, 95% CI 1.30, 1.44). In another review (Clapp, 1996), two types of job-related activities that were most consistently linked to PTB and fetal growth restriction across studies involved "standing for long periods" and "working double-shifts," both activities that result in high fatigue and are thought to affect uterine blood flow and reduce oxygen and nutrients to the fetus. However, two other job-related activities, "heavy lifting" and "long periods of walking" were less consistently linked to PTB or restricted fetal growth (Clapp, 1996). The failure to differentiate between different types of job-related physical activities may help explain the contradictory pattern of findings that exists across studies on the effects of employment on pregnancy outcomes (see also Pompeii, Savitz, Evenson, Rogers, & McMahon, 2005). In addition, studies on employment typically fail to examine such characteristics of employment as the psychological demands (e.g., high strain, low control) that may help account for any adverse impact on birth outcomes in employed pregnant women (Woo, 1997).

Overall, research suggests that voluntary and moderate physical activity may have a direct and beneficial influence on birth weight, although more randomized controlled trials are needed to confirm this. In addition, this type of physical activity is associated with more favorable psychological and emotional states in pregnancy that may further influence birth weight positively. Moderate physical activity has been shown to be associated with lower stress and depression, better body image, and greater psychological well-being (Cannella, Lobel, & Monheit, 2008; Da Costa, Rippen, Dritsa, & Ring, 2003). Low-intensity activities like walking are also associated with improved psychological well-being in pregnancy (Da Costa et al., 2003; Sorensen, Williams, Lee, Dashow, Thompson, & Luthy, 2003). Conversely, in a variety of studies, reductions in physical activity during pregnancy have been linked to more negative mood (Poudevigne & O'Connor, 2006). However, the direction of these associations has not been definitively established. Associations between physical activity and prenatal psychological states may be bidirectional, thus requiring further prospective investigation.

It is of note that the prevalence of physical activity among women in the United States during pregnancy is low, consistent with larger trends of inactivity in women in general and particularly women of color (U.S. Department of Health and Human Services, 2008). It is estimated that 45% to 60% of pregnant women are sedentary (Leiferman & Evenson, 2003; Poudevigne & O'Connor, 2006; Zhang & Savitz, 1996). There has been little attention to the reasons for inactivity during pregnancy, but research in nonpregnant populations implicates the role of such stress-related factors as fatigue, lack of time, low income, lack of access to facilities, and insufficient tangible and emotional support (Albright, Maddock, & Nigg, 2005; King et al., 2000; Salmon, Owen, Crawford, Bauman, & Sallis, 2003). There may also be myths about exercising in pregnancy that motivate some women to rest more and reduce activity (Cannella, Lobel, & Monheit, 2010).

Stress, Poor Nutrition, and Birth Weight

There has been very little research examining the association between psychosocial factors and nutrition during pregnancy. However, it is well established that lower caloric consumption in pregnancy reduces fetal growth and contributes to lower birth weight (e.g., Scholl, 2008). Insufficient prenatal levels of such micronutrients as iron and folic acid also adversely influence birth weight (Haider & Bhutta 2006; Shah & Ohlosson, 2009). Shah and Ohlosson (2009) suggest a number of mechanisms that may explain how micronutrients affect fetal growth, including improved energy metabolism and better responses to stress. Other mechanisms, including enhanced immune function and decreased susceptibility to infection, are posited to explain the beneficial association between micronutrient levels and reduced incidence of PTB.

An insightful review by Hobel and Culhane (2003) documents that both stress and poor nutrition independently contribute to poorer birth outcomes, and these authors suggest that there may also be interactive effects. For example, a combination of high stress and poor diet may compound adverse effects on growth. Furthermore, Hobel and Culhane indicate that prenatal stress reduces maternal weight gain during pregnancy by means of metabolic changes that affect the conversion of dietary calories. This link suggests that nutrition may mediate the impact of prenatal stress on birth weight not merely through changes in highly stressed women's eating behaviors but also through physiological processes that are directly affected by nutrition (Hermann, Siega-Ritz, Hobel, Aurora, & Dunkel Schetter, 2001).

Stress may also have a direct effect on reduced appetite, leading to poor prenatal nutrition. Fasting and restricting calories is a known risk factor for fetal growth retardation (Lin & Santolaya-Forgas, 1998). Although there is some ability of the maternal system to adapt to minimal or even moderate changes in diet and calorie intake, severe restriction of calories because of loss of appetite would be a likely pathway to fetal growth retardation.

Stress, Healthy Lifestyle, and Birth Weight

Several studies have investigated associations between prenatal stress and combinations of various health behaviors during pregnancy, referred to as *healthy or unhealthy lifestyle*. This is a sensible approach, given that various health behaviors tend to be intercorrelated. For example, women who are physically active prenatally also tend to engage in other healthy behaviors in pregnancy, including better dietary and sleep habits (Cannella et al., 2008).

One study of more than 3,000 socioeconomically disadvantaged, mostly African American women examined the predictive validity of women's "psychosocial profile" and health practices in relation to LBW (Neggers, Goldenberg, Cliver, & Hauth, 2006). The psychosocial profile combined 28 items assessing low negative affect, worry and stress, and high positive affect, self-esteem, and mastery. Health practices were assessed with 11 items pertaining to vitamin use, exercise, alcohol and tobacco use, and preventive medical and dental care, all combined into one score. The psychosocial profile was significantly correlated with the health practices composite score such that lower psychosocial profiles co-occurred with poorer health practices. Further, LBW was significantly more common in women below the median on the psychosocial composite score compared to women above the median, but LBW was not associated with health practices. The latter finding is not surprising, given the variety of health practices combined in this measure and the unlikely association of some of these practices (e.g., flossing and pap smear use) with birth weight. Furthermore, the authors did not examine mediation by such specific health practices as cigarette smoking, despite their finding that cigarette smoking was significantly more common in women with below-median psychosocial scores.

In sum, much is known about the importance of health behaviors as contributors to optimal growth of the fetus, and there is a small but growing number of studies that examine how stress during pregnancy affects these health behaviors. Yet health psychologists are not as active in this domain as they might be. The expertise of health psychologists is highly valuable because of their theoretical models, established findings in other populations, and understanding of the motivational processes and possible interventions for changing unhealthy habits. We return to this topic at the end to suggest some research agendas.

FORMULATING INTEGRATIVE MODELS

Research on stress in pregnancy is beginning to integrate the multitude of operative factors into more comprehensive biopsychosocial models that can guide hypothesis generation, study design, and intervention. However, most of the models concentrate on PTB, and most focus on only a few of the levels or subsets of processes shown in Table 19.1 such as the biomedical level or the psychosocial level (Coussons-Read et al., 2003; Hobel et al., 2008; Hogue, Hoffman, & Hatch, 2001; Kramer et al., 2001; Lu & Halfon, 2003; Rutter & Quine, 1990; Wadhwa et al., 2001; Wang et al., 2001). This narrow focus probably reflects the fact that the research training of authors has been in specific disciplines rather than in interdisciplinary research.

A few researchers have provided conceptual models to guide research on LBW or a broader set of outcomes, each with a specific focus or theme. Such models provide useful broad or general frameworks that can be a starting point for identifying more specific mechanisms. For example, Misra, Guyer, and Allston (2003) propose a multiple-determinants model that takes a lifespan approach and incorporates preconception and interconception (between births) factors to improve perinatal health. Their model includes social, psychological, behavioral, environmental, and biological forces operating during pregnancy and influencing short- and long-term maternal and infant disease and complications, health, functioning, and well-being. As such, it is one of the most comprehensive models we have seen. Even larger in scope, Halbreich's model (2005) includes in one comprehensive framework, not only birth weight but also postpartum outcomes, offspring development, offspring long-term disorders, and next-generation vulnerability.

Culhane and Elo's (2005) conceptual framework includes neighborhood factors (e.g., social environment, physical characteristics) as well as individual-level factors (e.g., SES, other demographics), both hypothesized to predict another set of individual-level factors (e.g., psychosocial, support, behavior), stress physiology, and ultimately, birth outcomes, including LBW. The inclusion of neighborhood factors is an attractive feature; yet a weakness of the model is that different types of individual stressors are lumped together into one category labeled "psychosocial factors." As we have tried to illustrate in this chapter, differentiation of specific psychological concepts is needed to determine unique pathways to such specific outcomes as LBW.

These models all offer pieces of a valuable foundation to test multilevel, biopsychosocial hypotheses about the etiology of LBW in interdisciplinary teams. Nonetheless, there remains a need to integrate existing approaches into comprehensive biopsychosocial frameworks that represent existing data on LBW with equal emphasis on psychosocial, sociodemographic, sociocultural, and biological factors.

Figure 19.3 is a simple schematic of the multilevel factors hypothesized to influence stress processes in pregnancy and of the pathways most often thought to mediate effects of stress on birth weight. Both acute and chronic stress exposures are shown to influence infant birth weight through effects on emotional, cognitive, behavioral, and physiological responses to stress (Pathway B). These varied responses to stress are interrelated in complex and dynamic ways based on theory and research on stress in general. Stress responses influence the growth of the infant and resultant birth weight directly (Pathway C), but also by influencing the timing of delivery (Pathways D and E), consistent with the interrelationship of the two major birth outcomes and their overlapping and distinct etiologies. Medical risk conditions influence birth outcomes as well (Pathways H and I). Not shown is the possible effect of stress and stress responses on medical conditions or complications that could be hypothesized. In addition, this meditational model shows that such contextual effects as socioeconomic risk factors and social network resources influence both exposures to stress (Pathway A) and birth outcomes (Pathways F and G). However, possible pathways from these contextual factors to stress responses are not included in this diagram, nor are moderation effects depicted. Thus, this is a simplified model, though it conforms to existing data in many ways and it may be a useful guide for hypothesis generation and research design.

Many of the predictors of infant birth weight shown in Figure 19.3 may operate as modifiers of the effects of other predictors. In particular, interactions of stress, ethnicity, medical risk, and social support deserve attention, as discussed earlier. Although behavioral scientists often view interactions as more interesting and important than direct (main) effects, epidemiologists and health scientists in other disciplines are typically more interested in direct effects and in effect sizes. Given the predominant interest in identifying predictors and direct causes in research on

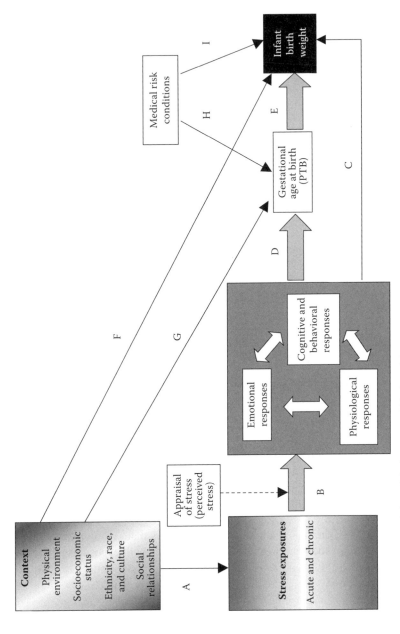

FIGURE 19.3 Multilevel biopsychosocial model of stress and birth weight.

pregnancy and birth, the study of moderation is not well developed, especially within interdisciplinary, multilevel analyses. Many studies do not test for interactions, and very few are designed to do this.

CONCLUSIONS AND THEMATIC ISSUES

We know much more today than we knew in 2001 when our chapter appeared in the first edition of this handbook. However, some of the observations we had then are still applicable today. For example, we suggested then that the psychosocial mechanisms linking stress to LBW might be different from those for PTB. This seems even more likely today since the two birth outcome literatures have grown immensely, and especially given the rapid growth of published research on PTB in recent years. This chapter's emphasis on LBW is intended to focus attention on the underdevelopment of the role of stress in fetal growth. Along with others, Brooks-Gunn (1991) pointed us in that direction long ago but, for various reasons, stress and birth weight research has not kept pace with research on stress and PTB, with a few important exceptions (Field, Diego, & Hernandez-Reif, 2006).

We highlighted in 2001 the need for multilevel analyses, a theme we continue as a focal point in this chapter. Without multilevel analysis, our understanding of LBW or any other birth outcome will not be advanced. We noted previously that behavioral mechanisms were important to examine, and there is now greater evidence that they are likely pathways linking stress to LBW. We emphasized the importance of social support and other potential moderators in our earlier chapter. Although there is only a little more research on support moderation of stress effects today, it remains a theoretically plausible and important topic for further investigation. Finally, almost 10 years ago we mentioned the importance of studying fathers as well as mothers, a call that has been echoed in the intervening years and is now gaining greater attention (Lu et al., 2010; Rini et al., 2006). In the remainder of this chapter, we highlight some conclusions on stress and birth weight in general and especially regarding African Americans. We further discuss health behavior mechanisms linking stress to birth weight. And, finally, we discuss why we may not be ready to intervene.

CONCLUSIONS REGARDING STRESS AND LBW

First, do we at present understand the role of stress in fetal growth or the etiology of LBW? In fact, conclusions are very difficult to draw. Researchers must continue to determine what forms of stress in pregnancy are the most significant risk factors for LBW and for whom. We hypothesize that chronic stress is especially harmful because it is most likely to have a sustained influence on biological mediating processes and on health behaviors or a healthy lifestyle. We expect that pregnant women who have chronically stressful jobs, troubled relationships or marriages, chaotic households, or adverse neighborhood environments are most likely to have aberrations in fetal growth, and there is some evidence to support this. Women who experience sudden, acute events that are not accompanied by a chronic aftermath may not be at risk of LBW because they are better able to manage the consequences of these short-lived events and because the human body may be better able to readjust to briefer stressors. There is some evidence suggesting that moderate and intermittent stress may even program the fetus for more optimal development (DiPietro et al., 2010).

Such major stressors as life events, community-level catastrophes, and chronic strain may all operate to influence birth outcomes through specific and distinguishable emotional effects. For example, depression appears to be a risk factor for LBW, whereas anxiety is linked more to PTB (Dunkel Schetter, 2010; Dunkel Schetter & Glynn, 2010). The effects of depression and anxiety may differ because of potentially distinct physiological processes. Evolving models of emotions and stress emphasize the functional properties of specific emotions and their distinct physiological correlates, at least under conditions of acute stress (Kemeny & Shestyuk, 2008; Moons, Eisenberger, & Taylor, 2010). This research has implications for studies of pregnancy that are untapped as yet.

Furthermore, such emotional states as depression or anxiety are rarely conceptualized as mediators of the effects of stress exposures on physiology or outcomes in pregnancy research, although this is a potentially valuable direction for research. In fact, state-of-the-art psychological theory and evidence on emotions generally is rarely integrated into the study of pregnancy. Yet, advances in emotion theory and research are highly relevant to the pregnant state and its influence on birth outcomes. In particular, we posit that the task of conceptualizing pathways from prenatal stress to such birth outcomes as LBW can benefit from advances in our understanding of the effects of specific emotions on physiology.

Stressors may be cumulative or interacting in their effects on birth outcome, and we can begin to understand them only if we find ways to conduct large-scale studies with multiple types and levels of stressors. For example, neighborhood and family stressors experienced together are likely to pose greater risk of adverse outcome than either alone; their interaction may be especially harmful. Health psychologists and psychological scientists who possess sophisticated measurement and statistical skills useful in formulating and testing multivariate models can help to improve the contributions of research on stress and birth outcomes.

CONCLUSIONS REGARDING STRESS AND BIRTH WEIGHT IN AFRICAN AMERICANS

Compared to other groups, African American women experience unique stressors, particularly personal and institutional racism. Although the findings are not completely consistent, evidence suggests that racism over one's lifetime, including childhood vicarious exposure to it, influences health outcomes in general and birth outcomes specifically. However, racial differences in LBW appear to persist even after accounting for the contribution of discrimination. Thus, racism is not a sufficient explanation for these group differences. Sexism and racism together have been hypothesized to create a "double jeopardy" in African American women (Woods-Giscombé & Lobel, 2008; Rosenthal & Lobel, 2011). Also, African American women are often the caretakers of their social network, creating additional responsibilities and stress for them, especially in communities where chronic strain and major life events are common and resources for coping with them are low.

The effects of racism are also compounded by low SES, possibly in a curvilinear fashion. That is, there is some evidence that both low and high SES appear to contribute additional risk for adverse birth outcomes beyond racial risks. For low-SES African American women, a source of stress may be living in a segregated community that is a target of institutional discrimination; high-SES African American women who work or live in integrated settings also incur stress exposure. It is very important for pregnancy research to disentangle SES from race and racism because these variables have often been confounded in previous studies. Among the studies of racial discrimination and birth weight in African Americans, only one that we identified used a sample of African Americans who were not predominantly low SES (Dominguez et al., 2008).

At present, we do not yet know what types of discrimination pose the greatest risk for pregnant women. We also have little data on the various ways that women of color cope with the threat of racism or its occurrence. Such behavioral responses as overeating, smoking, substance use, and alcohol consumption have been noted (Woods-Giscombé & Lobel, 2008). In general, responses to racism have been grouped into avoidant or direct action, but a more complete picture of the various behaviors and patterns of behavior that are used to manage the effects of exposure to personal racism and personal and institutional discrimination is needed to clarify their effects on pregnant women, as well as to identify the modifiers that may reduce or exacerbate these effects.

CONCLUSIONS REGARDING STRESS, HEALTH BEHAVIORS, AND BIRTH WEIGHT

As the studies reviewed in the foregoing sections indicate, there is ample evidence that stress and some related psychosocial factors are associated with poorer health behaviors during pregnancy, and separate evidence confirms that both stress and such health behaviors as cigarette smoking and inadequate nutrition predict LBW. This research provides a strong foundation for studies that simultaneously examine prenatal stress and the health behaviors that are likely mediators of birth weight (e.g., cigarette smoking and poor nutrition). Studies that examine stress and health behaviors should also investigate the interactive impact of stress and health behaviors. Detecting mediation through health behaviors does not preclude the possibility that stress also has direct effects on birth outcomes or other indirect effects. As we have noted throughout, effects of stress on birth weight, or any birth outcome, are likely to be explained by multiple mechanisms.

As with research on health behaviors in any population, an important challenge in pregnancy is identifying the best method of measurement. Most of the existing research on prenatal health behaviors uses self-report measures, yet there is a valid concern that women may be unusually reluctant to reveal to researchers that they are engaging in behaviors known to be harmful in pregnancy. However, there is some evidence that self-report measures of cigarette smoking during pregnancy are reliable and highly correlated with serum cotinine levels (McDonald, Perkins, & Walker, 2005; Okah, Cai, Dew, & Hoff, 2005). Similarly, physical activity recall measures show strong correlations with objective measures of activity in pregnant women (Lindseth & Vari, 2005; Timperio, Salmon, & Crawford, 2003). Further, there is some evidence that pregnant women accurately report their eating behaviors (Verbeke & De Bourdeaudhuij, 2007). Moreover, if such behaviors as cigarette smoking and poor eating habits are underreported by pregnant women, then studies using self-report measures that find effects may be underestimating the strength of those effects.

Another important challenge involves the difficulty in establishing causality among stress, health behaviors, and birth weight. There appear to be bidirectional associations between stress and some health behaviors. For example, negative correlations in cross-sectional research designs may mean that stress reduces the level of physical activity, but physical activity may also reduce stress (Cannella et al., 2008; Lobel, Hamilton, et al., 2008). Also, pregnant women are usually aware of the dangers of such behaviors as alcohol consumption, substance use, and cigarette smoking; therefore, those women who engage in harmful behaviors may have increased stress or worry as a result of their behavioral risk factors (Weaver et al., 2008). The frequency, pattern, and degree of engagement in specific health behaviors and the possibility of bidirectional associations with stress can be determined only through prospective, repeated and detailed assessments in observational studies or through experience-sampling methods.

Why We Are Not Ready to Intervene

Strong interventions are based on strong research findings and theory. In the study of stress and birth weight, researchers are not in a good position to design interventions because they lack strong theoretical and empirical bases for designing intervention at present. Results of observational research are just now accumulating a base of scientific knowledge to develop models of the pathways to LBW as distinct from those to PTB and that warrant interventions that target the modifiable components of these pathways. However, such interventions must be based in multilevel analysis taking into account sociocultural contexts, psychosocial processes, and biomedical and behavioral pathways. Until the science of prenatal risk and birth outcomes improves further, large-scale intervention studies are not, in our view, warranted. However, small-scale pilot investigations based on specific mechanisms influencing mediators may be valuable. For example, experimental studies might target one or more processes among the neuroendocrine, behavioral, and psychological processes that are hypothesized to affect birth weight. Then, having demonstrated effects on one or more of these mediating processes, a larger scale study targeting a birth outcome could follow. For example, small-scale randomized studies of the effects of social support enhancement or stress reduction on hypothesized behavioral or biological mediators may provide a basis for predicting larger scale effects on outcomes.

CONCLUSION

Our goal in this chapter has been to elucidate the state of research on psychosocial factors in pregnancy while focusing on processes leading to fetal growth and birth weight as distinct from the processes involved in other outcomes such as preterm birth. In doing so, a broader goal was to emphasize the value of a multilevel analysis of pregnancy and birth that incorporates more sophisticated and in-depth consideration of psychological factors. It is an exciting time for researchers working in this area because of advances on all fronts and transdisciplinary collaboration. With rigorous theory and research directed to the study of pregnancy and its outcomes, there should be important developments in our understanding of birth outcomes, especially low birth weight, to report when a third edition of this handbook appears.

REFERENCES

Abdou, C., Dunkel Schetter, C., Campos, B., Hilmert, C. J., Parker Dominguez, T., Hobel, C. J., ... Sandman, C. (2010). Communalism predicts prenatal affect, stress, and physiology better than ethnicity and socioeconomic status. *Cultural Diversity and Ethnic Minority Psychology, 16*(3), 395–403.

Abraido-Lanza, A. F., Dohrenwend, B. P., Ng-Mak, D. S., & Turner, J. B. (1999). The Latino mortality paradox: A test of the "salmon bias" and healthy migrant hypotheses. *American Journal of Public Health, 89*(10), 1543–1548.

Albright, C. L., Maddock, J. E., & Nigg, C. R. (2006). Physical activity before pregnancy and following childbirth in a multiethnic sample of healthy women in Hawaii. *Women and Health, 42*(3), 95–110.

Alder, J., Fink, N., Bitzer, J., Hosli, I., & Holzgreve, W. (2007). Depression and anxiety during pregnancy: A risk factor for obstetric, fetal and neonatal outcome? A critical review of the literature. *Journal of Maternal-Fetal and Neonatal Medicine, 20*(3), 189–209.

Alexander, G. R., Hulsey, T. C., Robillard, P. Y., De Caunes, F., & Papiernik, E. (1994). Determinants of meconium-stained amniotic fluid in term pregnancies. *Journal of Perinatology, 14*(4), 259–263.

Alexander, G. R., Tompkins, M. E., & Hulsey, T. C. (2000). Trends and racial differences in birth weight and related survival. *Maternal and Child Health Journal, 3*, 71–79.

Behrman, R. E., & Stith Butler, A. (Eds.). (2007). *Preterm birth: Causes, consequences, and prevention.* Washington, DC: National Academies Press.

Berle, J. O., Mykletun, A., Daltveit, A. K., Rasmussen, S., Holsten, F., & Dahl, A. A. (2005). Neonatal outcomes in offspring of women with anxiety and depression during pregnancy. *Archives of Women's Mental Health, 8*, 181–189.

Beydoun, H., and Saftlas, A. F. (2008). Physical and mental health outcomes of prenatal maternal stress in human and animal studies: A review of recent evidence. *Paediatric and Perinatal Epidemiology, 22*(5), 438–466.

Borders, A. E. B., Grobman, W. A., Amsden, L. B., & Holl, J. L. (2007). Chronic stress and low birth weight neonates in a low-income population of women. *Obstetrics & Gynecology, 109*(2), 331–338.

Breslau, N., Chilcoat, H., DelDotto, J., Andreski, P., & Brown, G. (1996). Low birth weight and neurocognitive status at six years of age. *Biological Psychiatry, 40*, 389–397.

Brooks-Gunn, J. (1991). Support and stress during pregnancy: What do they tell us about low birthweight? In H. Berendes, S. Kessel, & S. Yaffe (Eds.), *Advances in the prevention of low birthweight: An international symposium* (pp. 39–57). Washington, DC: National Center for Education in Maternal and Child Health.

Buka, S. L., Brennan, R. T., Rich-Edwards, J. W., Raudenbush, S. W., & Earls, F. (2003). Neighborhood support and the birth weight of urban infants. *American Journal of Epidemiology, 157*(1), 1–8.

Bullock, L. F. C., Mears, J. L. C., Woodcock, C., & Record, R. (2001). Retrospective study of the association of stress and smoking during pregnancy in rural women. *Addictive Behaviors, 26*(3), 405–413.

Bungum T. J., Peaslee, D. L., Jackson, A. W., & Perez, M. A. (2000). Exercise during pregnancy and type of delivery in nulliparae. *Journal of Obstetric, Gynecologic, and Neonatal Nursing, 29*(3), 258–264.

Campos, B., Dunkel Schetter, C., Abdou, C. M., Hobel, C. J., Glynn, L. M., & Sandman, C. A. (2008). Familism, social support, and stress: Positive implications for pregnant Latinas. *Cultural Diversity and Ethnic Minority Psychology, 14*(2), 155–162.

Campos, B., Dunkel Schetter, C., Walsh, J. A., & Schenker, M. (2007). Sharpening the focus on acculturative change: ARSMA-II, stress, pregnancy anxiety, and infant birthweight in recently immigrated Latinas. *Hispanic Journal of Behavioral Sciences, 29*(2), 209–224.

Cannella, D. T., Lobel, M., & Monheit, A. G. (2008). *Predictors of physical activity in pregnant women.* Presented at the annual meeting of the American Psychological Association, Boston, MA.

Cannella, D., Lobel, M., & Monheit, A. (2010). Knowing is believing: Information and attitudes towards physical activity during pregnancy. *Journal of Psychosomatic Obstetrics and Gynecology, 31*(4), 236–242.

Catalano, R., & Hartig, T. (2001). Communal bereavement and the incidence of very low birthweight in Sweden. *Journal of Health and Social Behavior, 42*(4), 333–341.

Catov, J. M., Abatemarco, D. J., Markovic, N., & Roberts, J. M. (2010). Anxiety and optimism associated with gestational age at birth and fetal growth, *Maternal and Child Health Journal, 14*(5), 758–764.

Challis, J. R., Lockwood, C. J., Myat, L., Norman, J. E., Strauss, J. F., III, & Petraglia, F. (2009). Inflammation and pregnancy. *Reproductive Science, 16*(2), 206–215.

Chung, T. K. H., Lau, T. K., Yip, A. S. K., Chiu, H. F. K., & Lee, D. T. S. (2001). Antepartum depressive symptomatology is associated with adverse obstetric and neonatal outcomes. *Psychosomatic Medicine, 63*, 830–834.

Clapp, J. F. (1990). The course of labor after endurance exercise during pregnancy. *American Journal of Obstetrics and Gynecology, 163*(6), 1799–1805.

Clapp, J. F. (1996). Pregnancy outcome: Physical activities inside versus outside the workplace. *Seminars in Perinatology, 20*(1), 70–76.

Clapp, J. F., Kim, H., Burciu, B., & Lopez, B. (2000). Beginning regular exercise in early pregnancy: Effect on fetoplacental growth. *American Journal of Obstetrics and Gynecology, 183*(6), 1484–1488.

Clark, R., Anderson, N. B., Clark, V. R., & Williams, D. R. (1999). Racism as a stressor for African Americans: A biopsychosocial model. *American Psychologist, 54*(10), 805–816.

Cohen, S., Kamarck, T., & Mermelstein, R. (1983). A global measure of perceived stress. *Journal of Health and Social Behavior, 24*, 385–396.

Collins, J. W., David, R. J., Handler, A., Wall, S., & Andes, S. (2004). Very low birthweight in African American infants: The role of maternal exposure to interpersonal racial discrimination. *American Journal of Public Health, 94*(12), 2132–2138.

Collins, J. W., David, R. J., Symons, R., Handler, A., Wall, S. N., & Dwyer, L. (2000). Low-income African-American mothers' perception of exposure to racial discrimination and infant birth weight. *Epidemiology, 11*(3), 337–339.

Collins, J. W., Wambach, J., David, R. J., & Rankin, K. M. (2009). Women's lifelong exposure to neighborhood poverty and low birth weight: A population-based study. *Maternal Child Health Journal, 13*(3), 326–333.

Collins, N. L., Dunkel-Schetter, C., Lobel, M., & Scrimshaw, S. C. M. (1993). Social support in pregnancy: Psychosocial correlates of birth outcomes and postpartum depression. *Journal of Personality and Social Psychology, 65*(6), 1243–1258.

Copper, R. L., Goldenberg, R. L., Das, A., Elder, N., Swain, M., Norman, G., … Meier, A. (1996). The preterm prediction study: Maternal stress is associated with spontaneous preterm birth at less than thirty five weeks' gestation. *American Journal of Obstetrics and Gynecology, 175*(5), 1286–1292.

Cosmi, E. V., Luzi, G., Gori, F., & Chiodi, A. (1990). Response of utero-placental fetal blood flow to stress situation and drugs. *European Journal of Obstetrics & Gynecology and Reproductive Biology, 36*(3), 239.

Coussons-Read, M., Okun, M., & Simms, S. (2003). The psychoneuroimmunology of pregnancy. *Journal of Reproductive and Infant Psychology, 21*(2), 103–112.

Crawford, J., Tolosa, J. E., & Goldenberg, R. L. (2008). Smoking cessation in pregnancy: Why, how, and what next. *Clinical Obstetrics and Gynecology, 51*(2), 419–435.

Crittenden, K. S., Manfredi, C., Cho, Y. I., & Dolecek, T. A. (2007). Smoking cessation processes in low-SES women: The impact of time-varying pregnancy status, health care messages, stress, and health concerns. *Addictive Behaviors, 32*(7), 1347–1366.

Culhane, J. F., & Elo, I. T. (2005). Neighborhood context and reproductive health. *American Journal of Obstetrics and Gynecology, 192*(5), S22–S29.

Culhane, J. F., Rauh, V., McCollum, K. F., Hogan, V. K., Agnew, K., & Wadhwa, P. D. (2001). Maternal stress is associated with bacterial vaginosis in human pregnancy. *Maternal and Child Health Journal, 5*(2), 127–134.

Da Costa, D., Rippen, N., Dritsa, M., & Ring, A. (2003). Self-reported leisure-time physical activity during pregnancy and relationship to psychological well-being. *Journal of Psychosomatic Obstetrics & Gynecology, 24*(2), 111–119.

Dailey, D. E. (2009). Social stressors and strengths as predictors of infant birth weight in low-income African American women. *Nursing Research, 58*(5), 340–347.

Dejin-Karlsson, E., Hanson, B. S., Ostergren, P. O., Lindgren, A., Sjöberg, N. O., & Marsal, K. (2000). Association of a lack of psychosocial resources and the risk of giving birth to small for gestational age infants: A stress hypothesis. *British Journal of Obstetrics and Gynecology, 107*(1), 89–100.

DeLuca, R. S., & Lobel, M. (1995). Conception, commitment, and health behavior practices in medically high-risk pregnant women. *Women's Health, 1*(3), 257–271.

Diego, M. A., Field, T., Hernandez-Reif, M., Schanberg, S., Kuhn, C., & Gonzalez-Quintero, V. H. (2009). Prenatal depression restricts fetal growth. *Early Human Development, 85*(1), 65–70.

Diego, M. A., Jones, N. A., Field, T., Hernandez-Reif, M., Schanberg, S., Kuhn, C., & Gonzalez-Garcia, A. (2006). Maternal psychological distress, prenatal cortisol, and fetal weight. *Psychosomatic Medicine, 68,* 747–753.

Din-Dzietham, R., & Hertz-Picciotto, I. (1998). Infant mortality differences between Whites and African Americans: The effect of maternal education. *American Journal of Public Health, 88*(4), 651–656.

DiPietro, J. A., Kivlighan, K. T., Costigan, K. A., Rubin, S. E., Shiffler, D. E., Henderson, J. L., & Pillion, J. P. (2010). Prenatal antecedents of newborn neurological maturation. *Child Development, 81*(1), 115–130.

Dole, N., Savitz, D. A., Hertz-Picciotto, I., Siega-Riz, A. M., McMahon, M. J., & Buekens, P. (2003). Maternal stress and preterm birth. *American Journal of Epidemiology, 157*(1), 14–24.

Dominguez, T. P., Dunkel Schetter, C., Glynn, L. M., Hobel, C., & Sandman, C. A. (2008). Racial differences in birth outcomes: The role of general, pregnancy, and racism stress. *Health Psychology, 27*(2), 194–203.

Dominguez, T. P., Dunkel Schetter, C., Mancuso, R., Rini, C. M., & Hobel, C. (2005). Stress in African-American pregnancies: Testing the roles of various stress concepts in prediction of birth outcomes. *Annals of Behavioral Medicine, 29*(1), 12–21.

Dunkel-Schetter, C. (1998). Maternal stress and preterm delivery. *Prenatal and Neonatal Medicine, 3,* 39–42.

Dunkel Schetter, C. (2009). Stress processes in pregnancy and preterm birth. *Current Directions in Psychological Science, 18*(4), 205–209.

Dunkel Schetter, C. (2010). Psychological science on pregnancy: Stress processes, biopsychosocial models, and emerging research issues. *Annual Review of Psychology.*

Dunkel Schetter, C., & Brooks, K. (2009). The nature of social support. In H. T. Reis and S. Sprecher (Eds.), *Encyclopedia of human relationships* (pp. 1565–1570). Thousand Oaks, CA: Sage Publications.

Dunkel Schetter, C., & Glynn, L. (2010). Stress in pregnancy: Empirical evidence and theoretical issue to guide interdisciplinary researchers. In R. Contrada & A. Baum (Eds.), *Handbook of stress* (2nd ed., pp. 321–343). New York, NY: Springer.

Dunkel Schetter, C., Gurung, R. A. R., Lobel, M., & Wadhwa, P. D. (2001). Stress processes in pregnancy and birth: Psychological, biological, and sociocultural influences. In A. Baum, T. A. Revenson, & J. E. Singer (Eds.), *Handbook of health psychology* (pp. 495–518). Hillsdale, NJ: Erlbaum.

Ellman, L. M., Dunkel Schetter, C., Hobel, C. J., Chicz-DeMet, A., Glynn, L. M., & Sandman, C. (2008). Timing of fetal exposure to stress hormones: Effects on newborn physical and neuromuscular maturation. *Developmental Psychobiology, 50*(3), 232–241.

Endara, S. M., Ryan, M. A. K., Sevick, C. J., Conlin, A. M. S., Macera, C. A., & Smith T. C. (2009). Does acute maternal stress in pregnancy affect infant health outcomes? Examination of a large cohort of infants born after the terrorist attacks of September 11, 2001. *BMC Public Health, 9,* 252–261.

Engel, S. M., Berkowitz, G. S., Wolff, M. S., & Yehuda, R. (2005). Psychological trauma associated with the World Trade Center attacks and its effect on pregnancy outcome. *Paediatric and Perinatal Epidemiology, 19*(5), 334–341.

Eskenazi, B., Marks, A. R., Catalano, R., Bruckner, T., & Toniolo, P. G. (2007). Low birthweight in New York City and upstate New York following the events of September 11th. *Human Reproduction, 22*(11), 3013–3020.

Field, T., Diego, M., & Hernandez-Reif, M. (2006). Prenatal depression effects on the fetus and newborn: A review. *Infant Behavior and Development, 29*(3), 445–455.

Field, T., Diego, M. A., Hernandez-Reif, M., Figueiredo, B., Ascencio, A., & Schanberg, S. (2008). Prenatal dysthymia versus major depression effects on maternal cortisol and fetal growth. *Depression and Anxiety, 25,* E11–E16.

Giscombé, C. L., & Lobel, M. (2005). Explaining disproportionately high rates of adverse birth outcomes among African Americans: The impact of stress, racism, and related factors in pregnancy. *Psychological Bulletin, 131*(5), 662–683.

Glynn, L. M., Dunkel Schetter, C., Chicz-DeMet, A., Hobel, C. J., & Sandman, C. A. (2007). Ethnic differences in adrenocorticotropic hormone, cortisol and corticotrophin-releasing hormone during pregnancy. *Peptides, 28*(6), 1155–1161.

Goedhart, G., Vrijkotte, T. G. M., Roseboom, T. J., van der Wal, M. F., Cuijpers, P., & Bonsel, G. J. (2010). Maternal cortisol and offspring birthweight: Results form a large prospective cohort study. *Psychoneuroendocrinology, 35*(5), 644–652.

Goldenberg, R. L., Cliver, S. P., Cutter, G. R., & Hoffman, H. J. (2001). Maternal psychological characteristics and intrauterine growth retardation. *Journal of Prenatal & Perinatal Psychology & Health, 6*(2), 129–134.

Grjibovski, A., Bygren, L. O., Svartbo, B., & Magnus, P. (2004). Housing conditions, perceived stress, smoking, and alcohol: Determinants of fetal growth in northwest Russia. *Acta Obstetricia et Gynecologica Scandinavica, 83*(12), 1159–1166.

Hack, M., Klein, N. K., & Taylor, H. G (1995). Long-term developmental outcomes of low birth weight infants. *The Future of Children, 5*(1), 176–196.

Haider B. A., & Bhutta Z. A. (2006). Multiple-micronutrient supplementation for women during pregnancy. *Cochrane Database of Systematic Reviews, 4*. Art. No.: CD004905. doi: 10.1002/14651858.CD004905. pub2

Halbreich, U. (2005). The association between pregnancy processes, preterm delivery, low birth weight, and postpartum depressions—The need for interdisciplinary integration. *American Journal of Obstetrics and Gynecology, 193*(4), 1312–1322.

Hall, D. C., & Kaufmann, D. A. (1987). Effects of aerobic and strength conditioning on pregnancy outcomes. *American Journal of Obstetrics and Gynecology, 157*(5), 1199–1203.

Harville, E. W., Savitz, D. A., Dole, N., Herrring, A. H., Thorp, J. M., & Light, K. C. (2008). Stress and placental resistance measured by Doppler ultrasound in early and mid-pregnancy. *Ultrasound Obstetrics and Gynecology, 32*(1), 23–30.

Herrera, J. A., Salmeron, B., & Hurtado, H. (1997). Prenatal biopsychosocial risk assessment and low birthweight. *Social Science & Medicine, 44*(8), 1107–1114.

Herrmann, T. S., Siega-Riz, A. M., Hobel, C. J., Aurora, C., & Dunkel Schetter, C. (2001). Prolonged periods without food intake during pregnancy increases risk for elevated maternal corticotropin-releasing hormone concentrations. *American Journal of Obstetrics and Gynecology, 185*(2), 403–412.

Hessol, N. A., & Fuentes-Afflick, E. (2000). The perinatal advantage of Mexican origin Latina women. *American Journal of Epidemiology, 10*(8), 516–523.

Hilmert, C. J., Dunkel Schetter, C., Parker Dominguez, T., Abdou, C., Hobel, C. J., Glynn, L. M., & Sandman, C. (2008). Stress and blood pressure during pregnancy: Racial differences and associations with birthweight. *Psychosomatic Medicine, 70*, 57–64.

Hobel, C., & Culhane, J. (2003). Role of psychosocial and nutritional stress on poor pregnancy outcome. *Journal of Nutrition, 133*(2), 1709–1717.

Hobel, C. J, Dunkel-Schetter, C., Roesch, S. C., Castro, L. C., & Arora, C. P. (1999). Maternal plasma corticotropin-releasing hormone associated with stress at 20 weeks' gestation in pregnancies ending in preterm delivery. *American Journal of Obstetrics and Gynecology, 180*(1), S257–S263.

Hobel, C. J., Goldstein, A., & Barrett, E. S. (2008). Psychosocial stress and pregnancy outcome. *Clinical Obstetrics and Gynecology, 51*(2), 333–348.

Hoffman, S., & Hatch, M. C. (2000). Depressive symptomatology during pregnancy: Evidence for an association with decreased fetal growth in pregnancies of lower social class women. *Health Psychology, 19*(6), 535–543.

Hogue, C. J. R., & Bremner, J. D. (2005). Stress model for research into preterm delivery among black women. *American Journal of Obstetrics and Gynecology, 192*(Suppl. 5), S47–S55.

Hogue, C. J. R., Hoffman, S., & Hatch, M. C (2001). Stress and preterm delivery: A conceptual framework. *Paediatric and Perinatal Epidemiology, 15*, 30–40.

Horns, P. N., Ratcliffe, L. P., Leggett, J. C., & Swanson, M. S. (1996). Pregnancy outcomes among active and sedentary primiparous women. *Journal of Obstetrics, Gynecology, and Neonatal Nursing, 25*(1), 49–54.

Jaddoe, V. W. V., de Ridder, M. A. J., van den Elzen, A. P. M., Hofman, A., Uiterwaal, C. S. P. M., & Whitteman, J. C. M. (2008). Maternal smoking in pregnancy is associated with cholesterol development in the offspring: A 27–years follow-up study. *Atherosclerosis, 196*(1), 42–28.

Jesse, E., Graham, D., & Swanson, M. (2006). Psychosocial and spiritual factors associated with smoking and substance use during pregnancy in African American and White low-income women. *Journal of Obstetric, Gynecologic, & Neonatal Nursing, 35*, 68–77. doi: 10.1111/j.1552-6909.2006.00010.x

Jones, C. P. (2000). Levels of racism: A theoretic framework and a gardener's tale. *American Journal of Public Health, 90*(8), 1212–1215.

Kelly, R. H., Russo, J., Holt, V. L., Danielsen, B. H., Zatzick, D. F., Walker, E., & Katon, W. (2002). Psychiatric and substance use disorders as risk factors for low birth weight and preterm delivery. *Obstetrics and Gynecology, 100*(2), 297–304.

Kemeny, M., & Shestyuk, A. (2008). Emotions, the neuroendocrine and immune systems, and health. In M. Lewis, J. M. Haviland-Jones, & L. F. Barrett (Eds.), *Handbook of emotions* (pp. 661–675). New York, NY: Guildford Press.

Khashan, A. S, McNamee, R., Abel, K. M., Pedersen, M. G., Webb, R. T., Kenny, L. C., ... Baker, P. N. (2008). Reduced infant birthweight consequent upon maternal exposure to severe life events. *Psychosomatic Medicine, 70*(6), 688–694.

King, A. C., Castro, C., Wilcox, S., Eyler, A. A., Sallis, J. F., & Brownson, R. C. (2000). Personal and environmental factors associated with physical inactivity among different racial-ethnic groups of U.S. middle-aged and older-aged women. *Health Psychology, 19*(4), 354–364.

Krabbendam, L., Smits, L., De Bie, R., Bastiaanssen, J., Stelma, F., & Van Os, J. (2005). The impact of maternal stress on pregnancy outcome in a well-educated Caucasian population. *Paediatric and Perinatal Epidemiology, 19*(6), 421–425.

Kramer, M. S., Goulet, L., Lydon, J., Seguin, L., McNamara, H., Dassa, C., ... Mortenson, P. B. (2001). Socio-economic disparities in preterm birth: Causal pathways and mechanisms. *Paediatric and Perinatal Epidemiology, 15*(2), 104–123.

Kramer, M. S., Lydon, J., Seguin, L., Goulet, L., Kahn, S. R., McNamara, H., ... Platt, R. W. (2009). Stress pathways to spontaneous preterm birth: The role of stressors, psychological distress, and stress hormones. *American Journal of Epidemiology, 169*(1), 1319–1326

Kramer, M. S., & McDonald, S. W. (2009). Aerobic exercise for women during pregnancy: A review. *Birth, 30*(4), 278–279.

Krieger, N. (1990). Racial and gender discrimination: Risk factors for high blood pressure? *Social Science & Medicine, 30*(12), 1273–1281.

Krieger, N., Rowley, D. L., Herman, A. A., Avery, B., & Phillips, M. T. (1993). Racism, sexism, and social class: Implications for studies of health, disease and well-being. *American Journal of Preventative Medicine, 9*(Suppl. 6), 82–122.

Kurki, T., Hiilesmaa, V., Raitasalo, R., Mattila, H., & Ylikorkala, O. (2000). Depression and anxiety in early pregnancy and risk for preeclampsia. *Obstetrics and Gynecology, 95*(4), 487–490.

Landale, N. S., & Oropesa, R. S. (2005). What does skin color have to do with infant health? An analysis of low birth weight among mainland and island Puerto Ricans. *Social Science & Medicine, 61*(2), 379–391.

Latendresse, G., & Ruiz, R. J. (2008). Bioassay research methodology: Measuring CRH in pregnancy. *Biological Research for Nursing, 10*(1), 54–62.

Lauderdale, D. S. (2006). Birth outcomes for Arabic-named women in California before and after September 11. *Demography, 43*(1), 185–201.

Lederman, S. A., Rauh, V., Weiss, L., Stein, J. L., Hoepner, L. A., Becker, M., & Perera, F. P. (2004). The effects of the World Trade Center event on birth outcomes among term deliveries at three lower Manhattan hospitals. *Environmental Health Perspective, 112*(17), 1772–1778.

Leiferman, J. A., & Evenson, K. R (2003). The effect of regular leisure physical activity on birth outcomes. *Maternal and Child Health Journal, 7*(1), 59–64.

Lin, C. C., & Santolaya-Forgas, J. (1998). Current concepts of fetal growth restriction: Part I. Causes, classification, and pathophysiology. *Obstetrics and Gynecology, 92*(6), 1044–1055.

Lindseth, V., & Vari, P. (2005). Measuring physical activity during pregnancy. *Western Journal of Nursing Research, 27*(6), 722–734.

Lobel, M. (1994). Conceptualizations, measurement, and effects of prenatal maternal stress on birth outcomes. *Journal of Behavioral Medicine, 17*(3), 225–272.

Lobel, M., Cannella, D. L., Graham, J. E., DeVincent, C., Schneider, J., & Meyer, B. A. (2008). Pregnancy-specific stress, prenatal health behaviors, and birth outcomes. *Health Psychology, 27*(5), 604–615.

Lobel, M., DeVincent, C., Kaminer, A., & Meyer, B. (2000). The impact of prenatal maternal stress and optimistic disposition on birth outcomes in medically high-risk women. *Health Psychology, 19*(6), 544–553.

Lobel, M., Dunkel-Schetter, C., & Scrimshaw, S. C. M. (1992). Prenatal maternal stress and prematurity: A prospective study of socioeconomically disadvantaged women. *Health Psychology, 11*(1), 32–40.

Lobel, M., Hamilton, J. G., & Cannella, D. L. (2008). Psychosocial perspectives on pregnancy: Prenatal maternal stress and coping. *Social and Personality Psychology Compass, 2*(4), 1600–1623.

Lu, G. C., & Goldenberg, R. L (2000). Current concepts on the pathogenesis and markers of preterm birth. *Clinics in Perinatology, 27*(2), 263–283.

Lu, M. C., & Halfon, N. (2003). Racial and ethnic disparities in birth outcomes: A life-course perspective. *Maternal and Child Health Journal, 7*(1), 13–30.

Lu, M. C., Jones, L., Bond, M. J., Wright, K., Pumpuang, M., Maidenberg, M., ... Rowley, D. L. (2010). Where is the F in MCH? Father involvement in African American families. *Ethnicity and Disease, 20*(Suppl. 2), S49–S61.

Majzoub, J. A., McGregor, J. A., Lockwood, C. J., Smith, R., Snyder Taggart, M., & Schulkin, J. (1999). A central theory of preterm and term labor: Putative role for corticotrophin-releasing hormone. *American Journal of Obstetrics and Gynecology, 180*(1, Suppl. 2), S232–S241.

Marsal, K. (2002). Intrauterine growth restriction. *Current Opinion in Obstetrics and Gynecology, 14*(2), 127–135.

Martin, J. A., Hamilton, B. E., Sutton, P. D., Ventura, S. J., Menacker, F., Kirmeyer, S., & Mathews, T. J. (2009). Births: Final data for 2006. *National Vital Statistics Reports* (Vol. 57, No. 7). Hyattsville, MD: National Center for Health Statistics.

Mathews, T. J. (2001). Smoking during pregnancy during the 1990s. *National Vital Statistics Reports* (Vol. 49, No. 7). Hyattsville, MD: National Center for Health Statistics.

Matte, T. D., Bresnahan, M., Begg, M. D., & Susser, E. (2001). Influence of variation in birth weight within normal range and within sibships on IQ at age 7 years: Cohort study. *British Medical Journal, 323*(7308), 310–314.

McCormick, M. C., Brooks-Gunn, J., Shorter, T., Holmes, J. H., Wallace, C. Y., & Heagarty, M. C. (1990). Factors associated with smoking in low-income pregnant women: Relationship to birth weight, stressful life events, social support, health behaviors and mental distress. *Journal of Clinical Epidemiology, 43*(5), 441–448.

McDonald, S. D., Perkins, S. L., & Walker, M. C. (2005). Correlation between self-reported smoking status and serum cotinine during pregnancy. *Addictive Behaviors, 30*(4), 853–857.

Misra, D. P., Guyer, B., & Allston, A. (2003). Integrated perinatal health framework: A multiple determinants model with a life span approach. *American Journal of Preventative Medicine, 25*(1), 65–75.

Moons, W. G., Eisenberger, N. I., & Taylor, S. E. (2010). Anger and fear responses to stress have different biological profiles. *Brain, Behavior and Immunity, 24*(2), 215–219.

Mozurkewich, E. L., Luke, B., Avni, M., & Wolf, F. M. (2000). Working conditions and adverse pregnancy outcome: A meta analysis. *Obstetrics and Gynecology, 95*(4), 623–635.

Mustillo, S., Krieger, N., Gunderson, E. P., Sidney, S., McCreath, H., & Kiefe, C. I. (2004). Self-reported experiences of racial discrimination and Black–White differences in preterm and low-birthweight deliveries: The CARDIA study of very low birthweight in African American infants: The role of maternal exposure to interpersonal racial discrimination. *American Journal of Public Health, 94*(12), 2125–2131.

Mutale, T., Creed, F., Maresh, M., & Hunt, L. (1991). Life events and low birthweight–Analysis by infants preterm and small for gestational age. *British Journal of Obstetrics and Gynecology, 98*(2), 166–172.

Neggers, Y., Goldenberg, R., Cliver, S., & Hauth, J. (2006). The relationship between psychological profile, health practices, and pregnancy outcomes. *Acta Obstetricia et Gynecologica, 85*, 277–285.

Newnham, J. (1998). Consequences of fetal growth restriction. *Current Opinion in Obstetrics and Gynecology, 10*(2), 145–149.

Newton, E. R., Piper, J. M., Shain, R. N., Perdue, S. T., & Peairs, W. (2001). Transactions of the nineteenth annual meeting of the American Gynecological and Obstetrical Society: Predictors of the vaginal microflora. *American Journal of Obstetrics and Gynecology, 184*(5), 845–855.

Ng, D. M., & Jeffery, R. W. (2003). Relationships between perceived stress and health behaviors in a sample of working adults. *Health Psychology, 22*(6), 638–642.

Nkansah-Amankra, S., Luchok, K. J., Hussey, J. R., Watkins, K., & Liu, X. (2010). Effects of maternal stress on low birth weight and preterm birth outcomes across neighborhoods of South Carolina, 2000–2003. *Maternal Child Health Journal, 14*, 215–226.

Norbeck, J. S., & Anderson, N. J. (1989). Psychosocial predictors of pregnancy outcomes in low-income, Black, Hispanic, and White women. *Nursing Research, 38*(4), 204–209.

Okah, F. A., Cai, J., Dew, P. C., & Hoff, G. L (2005). Are fewer women smoking during pregnancy? *American Journal of Health Behaviors, 29*(5), 456–461.

Orr, S. T., James, S. A., Miller, C. A., Barakat, B., Daikoku, N., Pupin, M., … Huggins, G. (1996). Psychosocial stressors and low birthweight in an urban population. *American Journal of Preventative Medicine, 12*(6), 459–466.

Orr, S. T., Reiter, J. P., Blazer, D. G., & James, S. A. (2007). Maternal prenatal pregnancy-related anxiety and spontaneous preterm birth in Baltimore, Maryland. *Psychosomatic Medicine, 69*(6), 566–570.

Oths, K. S., Dunn, L. L., & Palmer, N. S. (2001). A prospective study of psychosocial job strain and birth outcomes. *Epidemiology, 12*(6), 744–746.

Paarlberg, K. M., Vingerhoets, A. J. J. M., Passchier, J., Dekker, G. A., Heinen, A. G. J. J., & van Geijn, H. P. (1999). Psychosocial predictors of low birthweight: A prospective study. *British Journal of Obstetrics and Gynecology, 106*(8), 834–841.

Pagel, M. D., Smilkstein, G., Regen, H., & Montano, D. (1990). Psychosocial influences on new born outcomes: A controlled prospective study. *Social Science and Medicine, 30*(5), 597–604.

Phung, H., Bauman, A., Nguyen, T. V., Young, L., Tran, M., & Hillman, K. (2003). Risk factors for low birth weight in a socio-economically disadvantaged population: Parity, marital status, ethnicity and cigarette smoking. *European Journal of Epidemiology, 18*(3), 235–243.

Pompeii, L. A., Savitz, D. A., Evenson, K. R., Rogers, B., & McMahon, M. (2005). Physical exertion at work and the risk of preterm delivery and small-for-gestational- age birth. *Obstetrics and Gynecology, 106*(6), 1279–1288.

Poudevigne, M. S., & O'Connor, P. J. (2006). A review of physical activity patterns in pregnant women and their relationship to psychological health. *Sports Medicine, 36*(1), 19–38.

Precht, D. H., Andersen, P. R., & Olsen, J. (2007). Severe life events and impaired fetal growth: A nation-wide study with complete follow-up. *Acta Obstetricia et Gynecologica Scandinavica, 86*(3), 266–275.

Pritchard, C. W., & Teo Mfphm, P. Y. K. (1994). Preterm birth, low birthweight and the stressfulness of the household role for pregnant women. *Social Science and Medicine, 38*(1), 89–96.

Pryor, J. E., Thompson, J. M. D., Robinson, E., Clark, P. M., Becroft, D. M. O., Pattison, N. S., … Mitchell, E. A. (2003). Stress and lack of social support as risk factors for small-for-gestational-age birth. *Acta Pædiatrica, 92*(1), 62–64.

Reichman, N. E., Hamilton, E. R., Hummer, R. A., & Padilla, Y. C. (2008). Racial and ethnic disparities in low birthweight among urban unmarried mothers. *Maternal and Child Health Journal, 12*(2), 204–215.

Richards, M., Hardy, R., Kuh, D., & Wadsworth, M. E. J. (2001). Birthweight and cognitive function in the British 1946 birth cohort: Longitudinal population-based study. *British Medical Journal, 322*(7280), 199–203.

Rich-Edwards, J. W., & Grizzard, T. A. (2005). Psychosocial stress and neuroendocrine mechanisms in preterm delivery. *American Journal of Obstetrics and Gynecology, 192*(5), S30–S35.

Rini, C., Dunkel Schetter, C., Hobel, C. J., Glynn, L. M., & Sandman, C. A. (2006). Effective social support: Antecedents and consequences of partner support during pregnancy. *Personal Relationships, 13*(2), 207–229.

Rini, C. K., Dunkel-Schetter, C., Wadhwa, P. D., & Sandman, C. A. (1999). Psychological adaptation and birth outcomes: The role of personal resources, stress, and sociocultural context in pregnancy. *Health Psychology, 18*(4), 333–345.

Robillard, P. Y., Hulsey, T. C., Alexander, G. R., Sergenta, M. P., de Caunes, F., & Papiernikd, E. (1994). Hyaline membrane disease in Black newborns: Does fetal lung maturation occur earlier? *European Journal of Obstetrics & Gynecology and Reproductive Biology, 55*(3), 157–161.

Roesch, S. C., Dunkel Schetter, C., Woo, G., & Hobel, C. J. (2004). Modeling the types and timing of stress in pregnancy. *Anxiety, Stress, and Coping, 17*(1), 87–102.

Rogal, S. S., Poschman, K., Belanger, K., Howell, H. B., Smith, M. V., Medina, J., & Yonkers, K. A. (2007). Effects of posttraumatic stress disorder on pregnancy outcomes. *Journal of Affective Disorders, 102*(1–3), 137–143.

Rondo, P. H. C., Ferreira, R. F., Noguiera, F., Ribeiro, M. C. N., Lobert, H., & Artes, R. (2003). Maternal psychological stress and distress as predictors of low birth weight, prematurity, and intrauterine growth retardation. *European Journal of Clinical Nutrition, 57*, 266–272.

Rosenthal, L., & Lobel, M. (2011). Explaining racial disparities in adverse birth outcomes: Unique sources of stress for Black American women during pregnancy. *Social Science and Medicine, 72*, 977–983.

Rutter, D. R., & Quine, L. (1990). Inequalities in pregnancy outcome: A review of psychosocial and behavioural mediators. *Social Science and Medicine, 30*(5), 553–568.

Sable, M. R., & Wilkinson, D. S. (2000). Impact of perceived stress, major life events and pregnancy attitudes on low birth weight. *Family Planning Perspectives, 32*(6), 288–294.

Sagrestano, L. M., Feldman, P., Killingsworth-Rini, C., Woo, G., & Dunkel-Schetter, C. (1999). Ethnicity and social support during pregnancy. *American Journal of Community Psychology, 27*(6), 869–898.

Salmon, J., Owen, N., Crawford, D., Bauman, A., & Sallis, J. F. (2003). Physical activity and sedentary behavior: A population-based study of barriers, enjoyment, and preference. *Health Psychology, 22*(2), 178–188.

Sandman, C. A., Glynn, L. M., Dunkel Schetter, C., Wadhwa, P. D., Garite, T. J., Chicz-DeMet, A., & Hobel, C. (2006). Elevated maternal cortisol early in pregnancy predicts third trimester levels of placental corticotropin releasing hormone (CRH): Priming the placental clock. *Peptides, 27*(6), 1457–1463.

Savitz, D., & Dunkel Schetter, C. (2006). Behavioral and psychosocial contributors to preterm birth. In R. E. Behrman & A. S. Butler (Eds.), *Preterm birth: Causes, consequences and prevention* (pp. 87–123). Washington, DC: National Academy Press.

Scholl, T. O. (2008). Maternal nutrition before and during pregnancy. *Nestle Nutrition Workshop Pediatric Program, 61*, 79–89.

Shah, P. S., & Ohlosson, A. (2009). Effects of prenatal multimicronutrient supplementation on pregnancy outcomes: A meta-analysis. *Canadian Medical Association Journal, 180*(12), e99–e108.

Shepherd, A. P., & Kiel, J. W. (1992). A model of countercurrent shunting of oxygen in the intestinal villus. *American Journal of Physiology and Heart Circulation Physiology, 262*(4), 1136–1142.

Shiono, P. H., Rauh, V. A., Park, M., Lederman, S. A., & Zuskar, D. (1997). Ethnic differences in birthweight: The role of lifestyle and other factors. *American Journal of Public Health, 87*(5), 787–793.

Smith, R., Mesiano, S., & McGrath, S. (2002). Hormone trajectories leading to human birth. *Regulatory Peptides, 108*(2–3), 159–164.

Smits, L., Krabbendam, L., De Bie, R., Essed, G., & Van Os, O. (2006). Lower birth weights of Dutch neonates who were in utero at the time of the 9/11 attacks. *Journal of Psychosomatic Research, 61*(5), 715–717.

Song, H., & Fish, M. (2006). Demographic and psychosocial characteristics of smokers and nonsmokers in low-socioeconomic status rural Appalachian 2-parent families in southern West Virginia. *Journal of Rural Health, 22*(1), 83–87.

Sorensen, H. T., Sabroe, S., Olsen, J., Rothman, K. J., Gillman, M. W., & Fischer, P. (1997). Birth weight and cognitive function in young adult life: Historical cohort study. *British Medical Journal, 315*(7105), 401–403.

Sorensen, T. K., Williams, M. A., Lee, I. M., Dashow, E. E., Thompson, M. L., & Luthy, D. A. (2003). Recreational physical activity during pregnancy and risk of preeclampsia. *Hypertension, 41*(6), 1273–1280.

Steer, R. A., Scholl, T. O., Hediger, M. L., & Fischer, R. L. (1992). Self-reported depression and negative pregnancy outcomes. *Journal of Clinical Epidemiology, 45*(10), 1093–1099.

Sternfield, B., Quesenberry, C. P., Jr., Eskenazi, B., & Newman, L. A. (1995). Exercise during pregnancy and pregnancy outcome. *Medicine and Science in Sports and Exercise, 27*(5), 634–640.

Stetson, B. A., Rahn, J. M., Dubbert, P. M., Wilner, B. I., & Mercury, M. G. (1997). Prospective evaluation of the effects of stress on exercise adherence in community-residing women. *Health Psychology, 16*(6), 515–520.

Svare, J. A., Schmidt, H., Hansen, B. B., & Lose, G. (2006). Bacterial vaginosis in a cohort of Danish pregnant women: Prevalence and relationship with preterm delivery, low birthweight and perinatal infections. *British Journal of Obstetrics and Gynecology, 113*(12), 1419–1425.

Teixeira, J. M. A., Fisk, N. M., & Glover, V. (1999). Association between maternal anxiety in pregnancy and increased uterine artery resistance index: Cohort based study. *British Medical Journal, 318*, 153–157.

Thompson, R. J., Gustafson, K. E., Oehler, J. M., Catlett, A. T., Brazy, J. E., & Goldstein, R. P. (1997). Developmental outcome of very low birth weight infants at four years of age as a function of biological risk and psychosocial risk. *Journal of Developmental and Behavioral Pediatrics, 18*(2), 91–96.

Thorsen, P., Vogel, I., Olsen, J., Jeune, B., Westergaard, J. G., Jacobsson, B., & Møller, B. R. (2006). Bacterial vaginosis in early pregnancy is associated with low birth weight and small for gestational age, but not with spontaneous preterm birth: A population-based study on Danish women. *Journal of Maternal and Fetal Neonatal Medicine, 19*(1), 1–7.

Timperio, A., Salmon, J., & Crawford, D. (2003). Validity and reliability of a physical activity recall instrument among overweight and non-overweight men and women. *Journal of Science and Medicine in Sport, 6*(4), 477–491.

Turner, R. J., Grindstaff, C. F., & Phillips, N. (1990). Social support and outcome in teenage pregnancy. *Journal of Health and Social Behavior, 31*(1), 43–57.

United States Department of Health and Human Services. (2008). *Physical Activity Guidelines Advisory Committee report.* Retrieved from http://www.health.gov/PAGuidelines/Report/pdf/CommitteeReport.pdf

Utsey, S. O., & Ponterotto, J. G. (1996). Development and validation of the Index of Race-Related Stress (IRRS). *Journal of Counseling Psychology, 43*(4), 490–501.

Varrassi, G., Bazzano, C., & Edwards, W. T. (1989). Effects of physical activity on maternal plasma β-endorphin levels and perception of labor pain. *American Journal of Obstetrics and Gynecology, 160*(3), 707–712.

Verbeke, W., & De Bourdeaudhuij, I. (2007). Dietary behavior of pregnant versus non-pregnant women. *Appetite, 48*(1), 78–86.

Vogel, I., Thorsen, P., Hogan V. K., Schieve L. A., Jacobsson, B. O., & Ferre, C. D. (2006). The joint effect of vaginal *Ureaplasma urealyticum* and bacterial vaginosis on adverse pregnancy outcomes. *Acta Obstetrica et Gynecologica Scandinavica, 85*(7), 778–785.

Wadhwa, P. D., Culhane, J. F., Rauh, V., Barve, S. S., Hogan, V., Sandman, C. A., ... Glynn, L. (2001). Stress, infection and preterm birth: A biobehavioral perspective. *Paediatric and Perinatal Epidemiology, 15*(2), 17–29.

Wadhwa, P. D., Garite, T. J., Porto, M., Glynn, L., Chicz-DeMet, A., Dunkel Schetter, C., & Sandman, C. A. (2004). Placental corticotroprin-releasing hormone (CRH), spontaneous preterm birth and fetal growth restriction: A prospective investigation. *American Journal of Obstetrics and Gynecology, 191*(4), 1063–1069.

Wadhwa, P. D., Sandman, C. A., Porto, M., Dunkel-Schetter, C., & Garite, T. J. (1993). The association between prenatal stress and infant birth weight and gestational age at birth: A prospective investigation. *American Journal of Obstetrics and Gynecology, 169*(4), 858–865.

Wang, X., Zuckerman, B., Kaufman, G., Wise, P., Hill, M., Niu, T., ... Xu, X. (2001). Molecular epidemiology of preterm delivery: Methodology and challenges. *Paediatric and Perinatal Epidemiology, 15*(Suppl. 2), 63–77.

Weaver, K., Campbell, R., Mermelstein, R., & Wakschlag, L. (2008). Pregnancy smoking in context: The influence of multiple levels of stress. *Nicotine and Tobacco Research, 10*(6), 1065–1073.

Windham, G. C., Hopkins, B., Fenster, L., & Swan, S. H. (2000). Prenatal active or passive tobacco smoke exposure and the risk of preterm delivery or low birth weight. *Epidemiology, 11*(4), 427–433.

Woo, G. M. (1997). Daily demands during pregnancy, gestational age, and birthweight: Reviewing physical and psychological demands in employment and non-employment contexts. *Annals of Behavioral Medicine, 19*(4), 385–398.

Woods-Giscombé, C. L., & Lobel, M. (2008). Race and gender matter: A multidimensional approach to conceptualizing and measuring stress in African American women. *Cultural Diversity and Ethnic Minority Psychology, 14*(3), 173–182.

Zambrana, R. E., Scrimshaw, S. C. M., Collins, N., & Dunkel-Schetter, C. (1997). Prenatal health behaviors and psychosocial risk factors in pregnant women of Mexican origin: The role of acculturation. *American Journal of Public Health, 87*(6), 1022–1026.

Zhang, J., & Savitz, D. A. (1996). Exercise during pregnancy among U.S. women. *Annals of Epidemiology, 6*(1), 53–59.

Zimmer-Gembeck, M. J., & Helfand, M. (1996). Low birthweight in a public prenatal care program: Behavioral and psychosocial risk factors and psychosocial intervention. *Social Science and Medicine, 43*(2), 187–197.

20 Social Networks and Social Support

Thomas A. Wills
University of Hawaii Cancer Center

Michael G. Ainette
Dominican College

This chapter considers social networks and social support as predictive factors for health status. We cover the relation of social variables to morbidity, mortality, and recovery from illness. Over the past 30 years, research has shown that measures of social network structure, or perceived availability of supportive functions, are related to lower likelihood of morbidity or mortality, to higher levels of psychological well-being, and to lower levels of health-risk behavior (Cohen & Wills, 1985; Sandler, Miller, Short, & Wolchik, 1989; Seeman, 1996). Building on prior work (Wills & Filer, 2001), the present chapter includes research since 2000 on the relation of social support to health status. During this time there has been continued progress in understanding the breadth and nature of social support effects.

The theme of this chapter is how social support works. In recent years there has been more research in which social support is linked to such intermediate variables as positive affect, physiological intermediaries (e.g., blood pressure), or health-related behaviors (e.g., cigarette smoking), which are hypothesized to be the link between social processes and physical health outcomes (Berkman, Glass, Brissette, & Seeman, 2000; Kiecolt-Glaser, McGuire, Robles, & Glaser, 2002; Uchino, 2006). This approach is germane to health psychology because it represents the interface between psychological theories of emotion, stress/coping, and health behavior on the one hand, and physiological models of disease processes on the other. In this chapter we emphasize findings about the mechanisms of social support effects.

This chapter is organized by concepts and by areas. We first consider basic issues in the conceptualization and effects of social networks and social support, discuss methodological issues that are relevant for social support research, and outline theoretical models of support effects. We then consider how social support is involved in onset, progression, or recovery for cardiovascular disease, cancer, and several other chronic diseases. The next two sections consider the role of social support in two different types of health-related behavior, first with a focus on cigarette smoking and alcohol use, and then focusing on risk behavior for HIV/AIDS. A final section summarizes the findings and considers directions for further research.

CONCEPTUALIZATION AND EFFECTS OF SOCIAL SUPPORT

Social support is broadly defined as the extent of a person's social integration in the community (i.e., social network) and the resources provided by others that may be useful for helping to cope with problems (i.e., supportive functions). These perspectives on social support have produced different approaches, each with its own strengths and limitations.

STRUCTURAL VERSUS FUNCTIONAL MEASURES

Social support may be conceptualized as the number of social connections a person has. This exemplifies the sociological/epidemiological approach to the study of social relationships.

Structural measures give emphasis to assessing a person's social network and indexing the total number of linkages that person has with the community. This view assumes that regular social connections are important and suggests that the diversity of relationships, reflecting a person's connections throughout the community, may also be relevant. Structural measures typically include items asking about primary social relationships (e.g., being married, having children in the home) and may also tap frequency of visiting with neighbors and talking with friends and relatives on the telephone—or these days by Internet. Other items tap the existence of such defined social roles as belonging to a church, club, or other community organization. These items can be combined to produce indices for the total size of a person's network and the number of different social roles a person occupies, thereby providing a quantitative measure of the number of social connections a person has (Brissette, Cohen, & Seeman, 2000). Social integration measures are typically used in studies on mortality (House, Landis, & Umberson, 1988).

A comprehensive review by Uchino (2004) has considered the evidence from studies on social networks and health status. In the typical study, a social network measure is obtained from a large sample of participants from the general population, the sample is followed over a moderate-to-long time span (typically 5–10 years), and health status at follow-up is determined from interviews or death certificates. At present, more than 80 published studies have examined this question. Almost every study has shown that scores for network size or social integration are inversely related to mortality. Evidence is now available from large samples not only in the United States (e.g., Berkman & Syme, 1979; Blazer, 1982) but also in various European countries (Grand, Grosclaude, Bucquet, & Pous, 1990; B. S. Hanson, Isacsson, Janzon, & Lindell, 1989; Jylhä & Arö, 1989; Kaplan et al., 1988; Orth-Gomer & Johnson, 1987; Welin, Larsson, Svärdsudd, & Tibblin, 1992) and Asian countries (Ho, 1991; Sugisawa, Liang, & Liu, 1994). Alternative explanations of the protective effect for social integration have been ruled out by showing that the effect occurs with control for a number of demographic variables (e.g., gender, socioeconomic status) and by controlling for baseline health status so as to rule out reverse causation. Thus there is ample evidence for social integration as a protective factor with regard to health status, although there is still limited understanding of how this protective effect occurs.

Gradient Versus Threshold Effect

An issue in this research has been whether the effect of social networks represents a *threshold effect*, such that elevated mortality is found only for isolated persons with few social connections, or a *gradient effect*, with progressive reduction in mortality for each higher level of social integration. The literature is somewhat divided on this (House et al., 1988; Uchino, 2004). Some investigators have reported results that resemble a threshold effect, but other studies have shown a clear gradient effect, with a continuous reduction in mortality rates across increasing levels of network size (e.g., Kaplan et al., 1988; Williams et al., 1992; Welin et al., 1992). Current research continues this pattern (Ali, Medo, & Rosell, 2006; Rodriguez et al., 2006; Schmaltz, Southem, & Ghali, 2007; Steptoe, Owen, Kunz-Ebrecht, & Brydon, 2004). Although social isolation itself is a risk factor, findings of gradients suggest that the protective effect of social networks is not restricted to a small group of socially isolated persons.

FUNCTIONAL MEASURES

Social support may also be conceptualized as the level of supportive resources available to a person in time of need (irrespective of the number of connections). This exemplifies the clinical/psychological approach to social relationships. *Functional measures* are based on the assumption that social relationships provide supportive functions and that the quality of the support resources is important. Thus functional measures assess the extent to which supportive resources are perceived to be available if a person has a problem. In contrast to social network measures that establish the existence of relationships, functional measures ask about the extent to which a supportive function (e.g., confiding with somebody about problems) would be available if needed. These measures do not necessarily determine from whom the support comes but, rather, focus on the perceived availability of support from the relationships a person has. Scales for *emotional support* (also termed *appraisal or confiding support*) have items asking whether there are persons with whom you can share problems and worries and who make you feel understood and accepted. Scales for *instrumental support* (also termed *tangible or material support*) ask whether there are persons who could provide assistance with money, transportation, housework, or child care if needed. Scales for *informational support* (also termed *advice or guidance*) include items asking whether there are persons who could provide useful information about community resources and make helpful suggestions about solving problems. Scales for *companionship support* (also termed *belonging*) include items asking whether there are persons available for such leisure activities as going to movies, sporting events, theaters, or museums or going hiking. Scores for different dimensions of functional support typically are correlated; for example, individuals who report higher emotional support also tend to have higher scores for instrumental and informational support. Whether this correlation is attributable to the properties of support givers, to perceptual factors of the receiver, or to personality influences on the ability to garner support has not been entirely clarified (see Caspi, 2000; Coble, Gantt, & Mallinckrodt, 1996; Graves, Wang, Meade, Johnson, & Klag, 1998; Kendler, 1997; Lakey & Cohen, 2000; Shaw, Krause, Chatters, Connnell, & Ingersoll-Dayton, 2004).

Measures of supportive functions were not, historically, included in longitudinal studies of mortality. A number of shorter term studies with measures of depression/anxiety or physical symptomatology as criterion variables have shown measures of emotional, instrumental, or informational support to be related to higher levels of psychological well-being and lower levels of somatic symptoms (Cohen & Wills, 1985; Wills, 1991). These findings are independent of such demographic characteristics as gender and ethnicity. Personality characteristics (e.g., extraversion, neuroticism) are correlated with functional measures, but the protective effect of support typically remains significant when controlling for personality (e.g., Cohen, Sherrod, & Clark, 1986). A few studies on mortality have included functional measures. For example, B. S. Hanson et al. (1989) found that men with high emotional support had 2.5 times lower risk of mortality over the study period, controlling for demographic status and a variety of biomedical variables (cf. Lyyra & Heikkinen, 2006).

Correlation of Structural and Functional Measures

Several studies have shown that scores on structural and functional measures are not highly correlated. That is, the number of persons one knows is not strongly related to the availability of emotional and other types of support. Given that structural and functional measures are both related to health outcomes, the implication is that structural and functional aspects contribute to health status through different mechanisms. Theory has been formulated to search for answers to this question (Berkman et al., 2000; Cohen, Gottlieb, & Underwood, 2000; Uchino, 2006).

Main Effects Versus Buffering Effects

Because acute or chronic stress is a risk factor for a number of disease processes (Cohen, 2007; Kiecolt-Glaser et al., 2002), the question of whether social support acts to reduce the impact of stress (termed *stress-buffering*) or is beneficial irrespective of stress level (termed a *main-effect model*) has been addressed in considerable research. Studies testing for hypothesized buffering effects include both a measure of life stress and a measure of social support and test for a Stress X Support interaction effect, which if significant indicates that having a higher level of support reduces the impact of stress on symptomatology. Buffering effects have often been observed in studies that used functional measures; for example, having a high level of emotional support reduces the impact of stressors on symptomatology for adolescents (Wills, Mariani, & Filer, 1996) and for adults (Wills, 1991). Buffering effects have been found for other functions (e.g., instrumental support buffering the impact of financial stress; Pierce, Frone, Russell, & Cooper, 1996), but emotional support appears to be a useful function even in situations where one might not expect this (e.g., financial problems; Krause, 1987; Wills & Shinar, 2000).

Studies with structural measures have shown that persons with higher social integration have lower mortality rates, but these studies have generally not included stress measures. So it has been established that social integration is beneficial for physical health status (Uchino, 2004), but it is not clear whether this benefit depends on level of stress. There have been a few studies of mortality that have included stress measures; the ones that do have provided some evidence for buffering effects. Falk, Hanson, Isacsson, and Ostergren (1992) tested both structural and functional measures as possible buffers in relation to a measure of stress from job strain and found that having high emotional support reduced the impact of job stress on mortality. Social integration also had a buffering effect in this study, but the measures were not analyzed together. Rosengren, Orth-Gomer, Wedel, and Wilhelsen (1993) found that over four levels of life events, the range of mortality rates was 15.1 for men with low emotional support and 1.2 for men with high emotional support; these data indicate a buffering effect. For a social integration measure, no buffering effect was found. Thus there is some evidence that functional support has buffering effects with regard to mortality, but evidence for structural measures is not consistent.

RESEARCH DESIGN QUESTIONS

We now consider methodological issues for research on social support. We discuss questions about the point in the disease process where support acts, the statistical procedures used to analyze address support effects, and the mechanisms through which support may be related to health outcomes.

WHERE DOES SUPPORT ACT IN THE DISEASE PROCESS?

Given that social processes are related to mortality, the question is where in the disease process social support acts. Does social support act primarily to prevent development of risk factors among those who are healthy? Does having support retard onset of clinical-level disease among persons who have accumulated risk factors or promote recovery among persons who have had a disease episode (e.g., heart attack). Each of these three models is important from a health standpoint, but each suggests a quite different point for intervention; hence, studying where support acts is relevant for determining the crucial point for primary or secondary prevention.

Getting answers to each of these questions depends on different types of research designs, including longitudinal studies of large initially healthy populations, focused studies of higher risk samples, and clinical studies of persons who have suffered a significant disease episode. Longitudinal studies are necessary for conditions that take time to progress to clinical levels (e.g., heart disease), whereas shorter term studies are appropriate for conditions with a shorter disease course (e.g., upper respiratory infection). Longitudinal research and shorter term studies each have advantages and disadvantages, and the question of where support acts cannot be answered by any single study. Research conducted in recent years has enabled a fuller understanding of this question to emerge and has provided evidence for a significant role of social support at each point in various disease processes (Cohen, 2004; Gidron & Ronson, 2008; Lett et al., 2005).

TESTING INTERACTION MODELS

Is social support more relevant for persons with a high level of stress? Studying this question involves testing for an interaction between social support and life stress in relation to indices of mental or physical health, hypothesizing that the effect of stress differs according to one's level of support. This hypothesis has clinical implications because one wants to know whether social support interventions should be targeted to persons currently experiencing a high level of stress or should be directed at the whole population.

Testing interaction models can be done with analysis of variance using dichotomized predictors and testing for a Stress X Support interaction effect. Alternatively, questions about interaction can be tested in multiple regression using continuous predictors and testing the cross-product term for stress and support. In either case, the result of the analysis may indicate that support has a beneficial effect irrespective of stress level (Figure 20.1a). Alternatively, the analysis may indicate that support reduces the effect of stress on outcomes (Figure 20.1b) or completely eliminates the adverse impact of the risk factor (Figure 20.1c). The latter two results provide evidence for an interaction model, that is, a buffering effect of social support.

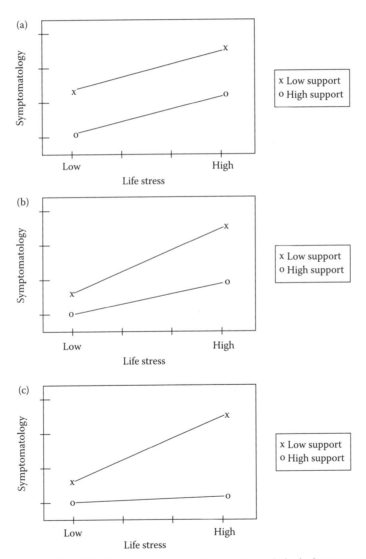

FIGURE 20.1 Theoretical models of stress-support relations, with psychological symptomatology as criterion variable. (a) Main-effect model: symptomatology is lower with high support level irrespective of stress level. (b) Partial-buffering model: support reduces effect of stress on symptomatology. (c) Full-buffering model: support eliminates effect of stress.

Interactions and Power

From the statistical standpoint, we should note that analyses using continuous variables are preferable because they typically increase statistical power. Though many studies have demonstrated buffering effects, it is good to keep in mind that testing interactions has more demanding power requirements than testing for main effects, hence, a study testing for buffering should have a sizable sample in order to have adequate power for detecting this type of interaction (Aiken & West, 1991).

TESTING FOR DIRECT AND INDIRECT EFFECTS

Another research question is whether the relationship of social support to health status involves intermediate processes. It is conceivable that some aspects of functional support or a large social network act directly on health status, but it is also possible that social variables act on intermediate processes that are, in turn, linked to health outcomes. In contrast to a *direct effect model*, which assumes no intervening processes between support and health status, the postulate that intermediate processes are involved is termed an indirect effect or *mediation model* (MacKinnon, 2006). Examples of the two types of models are presented in Figure 20.2. The first model is a pure direct effect (Figure 20.2a); the second, a pure mediation model in which all the protective effect of support is transmitted through an intermediate process (Figure 20.2b). The third panel in Figure 20.2 displays a situation in which part of the effect of support is direct and part goes through an intermediate process, which is possible in principle (Figure 20.2c). A mediation model is typically analyzed with a procedure such as structural equation modeling. In this procedure, a multivariate model specifies that social support is a predictor of one or more intermediate variables, which then are specified as predictors of the criterion variable (e.g., Wills, Resko, Ainette, & Mendoza, 2004). The adequacy of the model results is evaluated by determining whether relations between variables are significant and the significant paths fit the hypothesized pattern of relations.

Clinical Implications

The issue of direct versus indirect effects also has clinical implications. If social support acts directly on health, then an intervention would focus on increasing a person's level of support. However, if

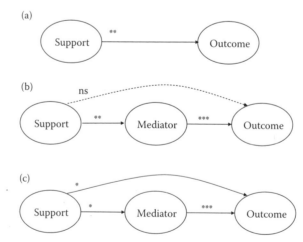

FIGURE 20.2 Theoretical models of how support operates, with illustrative effect sizes. (a) Pure direct-effect model: predictor acts directly on outcome with no intermediate process. (b) Pure mediation model: predictor acts on mediator with no significant direct effect to outcome. (c) Mixed model: significant mediation effect and significant direct effect both exist. *, smaller effect size; **, moderate effect size; ***, large effect size.

intermediate processes are involved, then an intervention researcher would want to find out what the intermediate processes are (e.g., self-esteem, perceived control, coping ability), consider how support is related to these, and measure whether intervention was successful in changing one or more of the intermediate processes (Mackinnon, 2006).

THEORETICAL MECHANISMS

What do we know about the mechanism of social support effects? Recent work has delineated several mechanisms through which social support may be related to health status. Here we outline six different mechanisms, which are diagrammed in Figure 20.3. It is important to note that the mechanisms are not mutually exclusive; it is possible that various aspects of social networks and social support influence health status through several of these mechanisms. This possibility should be considered in designing etiological and intervention studies.

Effect on Stable Attributes

Being embedded in a network could produce stable feelings of higher self-esteem or perceived control (Figure 20.3a). This feeling could be related to health status directly (Berkman et al., 2000), but intermediate processes are possible (Cohen & Lemay, 2007).

Reactivity Mechanism

Several investigators have proposed that having emotional or other support available reduces cardiac reactivity (i.e., variability in heart rate) to unpleasant or stressful conditions (Figure 20.3b). Sustained reactivity is believed to relate in the long term to hypertension, so support could in this way be related to likelihood of heart disease or stroke (Horsten, Mittleman, Wamala, & Scheck-Gustafsson, 1999; Raikkonen, Matthews, & Kuller, 2001; Rozanski, Blumenthal, & Kaplan, 1999). This relationship would likely take the form of a buffering effect.

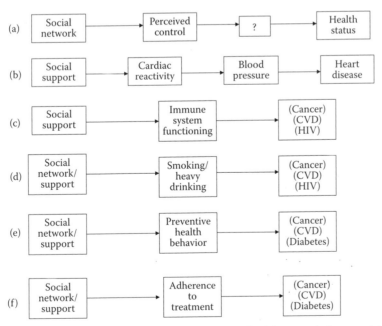

FIGURE 20.3 Theoretical mechanisms of support processes. (a) Social support influences stable psychological attribute relevant for health. (b) Support reduces cardiac reactivity. (c) Support is related to better immune system function. (d) Support reduces likelihood of substance use. (e) Support is linked to health-promoting behavior. (f) Support enhances adherence to treatment.

Immune System Function

Through influencing cognitive appraisal and emotional reactions to stress, social support could relate to better functioning of the immune system (Figure 20.3c). Better immune system functioning through social support could increase peripheral resistance to infectious diseases or internal surveillance for cancerous cells and could hence reduce risk for several types of disease (Kiecolt-Glaser et al., 2002). Immune system markers have also been related to arterial inflammatory processes that can bring about heart attacks or strokes (Uchino, 2006). Whether a relation of social support to inflammatory processes would occur as a main effect or buffering effect is not clear.

Substance Use

Several types of research have linked social variables to the likelihood of cigarette smoking and heavy alcohol use (Figure 20.3d). Both structural and functional aspects may be involved because the effect seems to occur in part through a normative mechanism (i.e., networks enforce social norms against substance use) and in part through a stress-buffering mechanism (i.e., functional support reduces the impact of stress on substance use). Both types of mechanisms have been studied (Wills, Gibbons, Gerrard, Murry, & Brody, 2003; Wills, Sandy, & Yaeger, 2002; Wills et al., 2004).

Health-Promoting Behavior

Some research suggests that social support encourages positive health behaviors (e.g., diet, exercise) and regular contact with the health care system for screening and physical examinations (Emmons, Barbewau, Gutheil, Stryker, & Stoddard, 2007; Honda & Kagawa-Singer, 2006; Tucker, Orlando, Elliott, & Klein, 2006). This health-promoting behavior could reduce risk for several types of disease through better physical status and early detection of developing disease conditions, probably as a main effect (Figure 20.3e).

Adherence to Treatment

Finally, having supportive persons available can influence the extent of adherence to medical treatment among persons who have suffered a disease episode (Figure 20.3f). Better adherence to treatment can reduce the likelihood of mortality or disease recurrence, and social support could have a health-protective effect in this way (DiMatteo, 2004).

SOCIAL SUPPORT IN CARDIOVASCULAR DISEASE AND CANCER

We now review evidence on how social support is involved in onset or recovery from diseases that are the two largest contributors to the disease burden in the United States and other countries: heart disease and cancer. We discuss studies with respect to the questions covered in the previous sections. We give attention to evidence on the mechanism of support effects when possible, though the various questions and issues have not been studied to the same extent for each disease condition. We should note that the research discussed here is only a part of the literature on social support and health; we select studies that address key issues in the area.

CARDIOVASCULAR DISEASE

A number of studies in Europe and the United States have found relations of structural and functional measures to heart disease and some have examined mechanisms for these (for reviews, see Rozanski et al., 1999; Uchino, 2006). In this section we discuss representative studies.

Onset of Heart Disease

Several studies have examined onset of heart disease among those initially disease free (i.e., incident disease). In a six-year study of Swedish men (Orth-Gomer, Rosengren, & Wilhelmsen, 1993), emotional support and social integration both were inversely related to incident heart disease, and analyses were conducted with biomedical controls. A study with a sample of HMO members by Vogt, Mullooly, Ernst, Pope, and Hollis (1992) covered a 15-year interval and used medical records to determine both prevalent and incident disease. Scores for connections with family, friend, and community networks were independent predictors of 15-year mortality. The strongest effect was for network diversity, with a relative risk for mortality of 6.7 for persons in the lower versus upper thirds of the distribution. For survival, data indicated that higher network scores predicted increased survival from heart disease, cancer, and stroke. Though results for incident disease were largely nonsignificant in this study, a project conducted in Sweden (Ali et al., 2006) did find that a social integration score predicted incident heart disease, and a recent study of women found that smaller networks predicted incident stroke (Rutledge et al., 2008).

Progression of Heart Disease

In a nine-year longitudinal study of a middle-aged female cohort, Raikkonen and colleagues (2001) found that decreases in functional support over time were related to development of hypertension. Angerer et al. (2000) found emotional support was related to less progression of coronary artery disease over a two-year period, as assessed by angiography, as did Wang, Mittleman, and Orth-Gomer (2005). Studies testing how social support might influence physiological mechanisms that affect disease progression have examined several pathways. A study of Swedish women found that higher functional support was related to lower levels on all four elements of the metabolic syndrome (central obesity, hypertension, dislipidemia, and elevated blood glucose), which is a general risk factor for heart disease (Horsten et al., 1999). Studies using ambulatory monitoring have shown social support related to blood pressure in daily situations; for example, Linden, Chambers, Maurice, and Lenz (1993) conducted a day of ambulatory blood pressure monitoring with college students and found that women who scored higher on available support showed lower aggregated systolic blood pressure in daily life. Studies in laboratory settings show that having support available is related to less reactivity under stress, whereas negative social interactions predict greater reactivity under stress (Uchino, 2006); and field studies have shown social support indices related to lower scores for allostatic load, a risk factor for several disease conditions (Karlamangla, Singer, & Seeman, 2006). Other studies have shown measures of loneliness or social support related to levels of C-reactive protein, a marker for arterial inflammation (Schnorpfeil et al., 2003); immune system measures implicated in inflammatory processes, including interleukin-6 and interleukin-8 (Loucks et al., 2006; Marsland, Sathanoori, Muldoon, & Manuck, 2007); and clotting factors such as fibrinogen (Loucks, Berkman, Gruenewald, & Seeman, 2005; Steptoe et al., 2004).

Recovery From Heart Attack

Several studies of marital status have found that survival times after myocardial infarction are longer for married individuals (e.g., Wiklund, Oden, Sanne, & Ulvenstam, 1988). A prospective study by Williams et al. (1992) followed a large sample of patients with coronary artery disease for an average of nine years after intake. Results showed that patients who were unmarried and without a confidant had a significantly lower survival rate (50%) compared with those having high support (82%); this effect was independent of medical risk and of the patient's economic resources. In an ongoing study of a large community sample, Berkman, Leo-Summers, and Horwitz (1992) found that persons with greater emotional support were more likely to survive over a one-year period after suffering a heart attack. The effect size for this support measure was comparable to the effects for several medical risk factors. Recent studies of patients with chronic heart disease (CHD) have been consistent with earlier findings, showing that measures of social participation and confidant availability related to lower likelihood of new disease episodes or mortality (e.g., Brummett et al., 2001; Dickens et al., 2004; Rodriguez et al., 2006). Measures of functional support were obtained by King, Reis, Porter, and Norsen (1993) in a sample of coronary artery surgery patients followed for one year after the operation. Esteem and companionship support were most consistently related to outcomes (i.e., less disability, fewer angina symptoms); some effects were also observed for instrumental support. Helgeson (1991) used structural and functional measures with myocardial infarction (MI) patients followed for three months to one year after the illness. Emotional support from spouse was inversely related to rehospitalization and positively related to perceived health; the structural measure was not significantly related to either criterion.

Conclusions Regarding Heart Disease

Significant relations of social support to heart disease have been found at all points in the disease process. Although evidence is less consistent for onset of heart disease, some studies have found relations to onset of disease for both structural measures and functional measures. Studies on progression have focused on mechanisms and linked social support measures to several physiological measures that are implicated in disease progression. Evidence is consistent in showing relations to survival time or recovery after a heart attack; this research dominated by functional measures, but findings for social participation scores have been noted. The effect sizes for social support are generally comparable to those of medical variables that are recognized predictors of outcome (Lett et al., 2005). These findings show social support to be an important protective factor for heart disease, though much remains to be learned about the mechanisms for this effect.

SOCIAL SUPPORT AND CANCER

Social support has been examined in relation to onset or progression of cancer (Gidron & Ronson, 2008) and to coping with cancer and other illnesses (Helgeson & Cohen, 1996; Stanton, Revenson, & Tennen, 2007). In the following section, we discuss examples of research in these areas.

Onset and Survival

For onset of cancer, several authors (e.g., Helgeson, Cohen, & Fritz, 1998; Uchino, 2006) have noted that data regarding the relationship of psychosocial factors to cancer onset are difficult to interpret because of the disease's heterogeneity and the long development time for most cancers. Data are most robust for survival after diagnosis. As noted earlier, the analysis of archival data by Vogt et al. (1992) found an effect of social network on survival. As well, several epidemiological studies have found larger social networks related to longer survival times (Ell, Nishimoto, Mediansky, & Mantell, 1992; Hislop, Waxler, Coldman, & Elwood, 1987; Reynolds & Kaplan, 1990; Waxler-Morrison, Hislop, Mears, & Kan, 1991; Welin et al., 1992), controlling for demographics and for such medical variables as stage at diagnosis. Controls for such variables as smoking sometimes reduce the effect, and this finding suggests an indirect-effect mechanism (i.e., social support discourages smoking and thereby increases survival from cancer). There is little evidence on functional measures, but Cousinne-Gelie, Bruchon-Sweitzer, Dilhuydy, and Jutand (2007) found that higher support availability predicted longer survival time in breast cancer patients. The consistency of findings on survival time suggests this as a promising area for further investigation (see Antoni & Lutgendorf, 2007; Helgeson et al., 1998).

Coping With Illness

Several studies have examined how support from family members and medical professionals is relevant for helping persons to cope with cancer. Similar to effects found for coping with other types of life stressors, social support has been shown in a number of studies to be related to indices of better adjustment to illness, such as reduced anxiety or increased self-esteem, and better functional ability (Helgeson & Cohen, 1996). In the few studies that compared different supportive functions, emotional support is the function most consistently related to adjustment, though effects for instrumental support are sometimes significant (e.g., Primomo, Yates, & Woods, 1990). Descriptive studies are informative in showing that emotional support is the function desired from family members, particularly with respect to discussing fears and concerns about the disease (Dakof & Taylor, 1990; Rose, 1990). In contrast, the data show that patients want informational support from medical professionals but do not want it from family members. However, emotional support may be inhibited in family settings through a reluctance of family members to talk about the disease because of fear that doing so will be upsetting to the patient. Perhaps for this reason, patients in these studies rate emotional support from family members as helpful but sometimes inadequate and report that they may keep their thoughts and feelings to themselves because other people do not really want to hear them.

Support and Recurrence

Research in recent years has suggested several ways in which support can affect susceptibility to recurrence of cancer. Research on immune system function is relevant because of the potential of negative emotions to exacerbate disease processes and suppress surveillance for malignant cells in the circulatory and lymphatic systems (Antoni & Lutgendorf, 2007; Uchino, 2006). Studies with animal models and human subjects have previously linked social affiliation and perceived support to such immune-function indices as greater T-cell proliferation and higher levels of natural killer (NK) cells (Kiecolt-Glaser et al., 2002). A mechanism has been suggested in which social support enhances emotional status, thereby affecting immune function; and several studies have found larger networks and higher functional support related to lower levels of cortisol, a marker for negative affect (Steptoe et al., 2004; Turner-Cobb, Sephton, Koopman, Blake-Mortimer, & Spiegel, 2000). Support measures have also been linked to levels of such cytokines as interleukin-2 and -6 and to tumor angiogenesis factors such as vascular endothelial growth factor (VEGF); for example, a study of patients with malignant tumors found that persons with greater social well-being had lower levels of VEGF (Lutgendorf et al., 2002). Significant findings have also been noted for NK cell activity, with measures of social networks and functional support related to higher circulating levels of NK cells (Lamkin et al., 2008; Lutgendorf et al., 2005; Steptoe et al., 2004). Some evidence has also suggested an adherence mechanism. Honda et al. (2006) found that family support (but not network size) was indirectly related to greater screening adherence through influencing norms about screening, whereas emotional support from friends had a direct relation to screening.

Conclusions Regarding Cancer

Evidence has consistently linked larger social networks to longer survival times among persons with cancer, though the mechanism of this effect remains largely unknown. A body of research has shown social support to be an important factor for helping persons cope with cancer; emotional and other types of support from family members are broadly useful functions, but informational support from medical professionals is also an important coping resource. Recent research has begun to clarify pathways through which social variables can help prevent recurrence of cancer. As in other areas, relations of social support variables to physiological measures are not always significant, but the amount of confirming evidence has suggested this as a promising direction (Antoni & Lutgendorf, 2007; Gidron & Ronson, 2008; Reblin & Uchino, 2008).

SOCIAL SUPPORT IN ARTHRITIS, DIABETES, AND KIDNEY DISEASE

We now discuss research on the role of social support for enhancing outcomes among persons with three chronic diseases, which involve both psychological distress and physical pain over considerable periods of time. Persons with diabetes and kidney disease also have a significant risk of mortality if treatment programs are not completely followed, so social support has considerable health relevance. Although the physical symptoms of these diseases are quite different, social relationships are important for adjustment to all these diseases.

ARTHRITIS

Arthritis involves unpredictability and interference with daily activities as well as recurrent pain. Supportive relationships, particularly with spouses, are relevant for facilitating adjustment, but negative aspects of relationships are also crucial (Manne & Zautra, 1989; Revenson, 1994). In descriptive research by Lanza, Cameron, and Revenson (1995), arthritis patients were interviewed about perceptions of recent support episodes. Instrumental support was most frequently reported as helpful (e.g., "Friend came and cleaned my whole house"), and emotional support (e.g., "Spouse understood how I felt") was second. For unhelpful episodes, lack of instrumental support was mentioned most often (e.g., "Husband expected me to do the laundry, which I couldn't"); critical remarks and lack of understanding were mentioned less often. Spouses were mentioned as most often providing helpful emotional support and physicians as providing useful instrumental support. Among arthritis patients, functional support is related to higher self-esteem, more positive affect, and greater life satisfaction (Affleck, Pfeiffer, Tennen, & Fifield, 1988; Fitzpatrick, Newman, Lamb, & Shipley, 1988; Smith, Dobbins, & Wallston, 1991). Longitudinal studies have also shown social support related to decreased depression over time (Brown, Wallston, & Nicassio, 1989; Fitzpatrick, Newman, Archer, & Shipley, 1991). Predictive effects are usually found for functional rather than structural measures (Goodenow, Reisine, & Grady, 1990), but exceptions can be noted (Revenson & Majerovitz, 1991). Positive and negative aspects of relationships were tested by Manne and Zautra (1989), who measured a 10-item composite of emotional and instrumental responses presumed to be helpful for persons with arthritis, together with responses predicted to be unhelpful (the number of critical remarks made by the spouse during an interview). Analyses indicated support was related to better adjustment whereas criticism was related to worse adjustment. Tests of an indirect-effect mechanism showed that support was related to more cognitive coping (which was related to better adjustment), whereas criticism was related to more avoidant coping (which was related to worse adjustment). A related study by Revenson, Schiaffino, Majerovitz, and Gibofsky (1991) showed opposite effects for supportive and problematic interaction behaviors; this study also found an interaction, with depressive symptoms particularly elevated among persons receiving fewer supportive behaviors and more problematic behaviors.

DIABETES

Diabetes is a chronic illness in which extensive self-care efforts are necessary, emotional distress may upset glucose metabolism, and failure to comply with the daily preventive regimen may lead to adverse physical complications. Zhang, Norris, Gregg, and Beckles (2007) found social integration significantly related to mortality in a sample of elderly persons with diabetes, net of a number of demographic and medical controls. A graded effect was found; compared to persons with low support, moderate support reduced mortality risk by 47% and high support reduced risk by 67%. Behavioral studies have indicated buffering effects. Littlefield, Rodin, Murray, and Craven (1990) examined buffering effects of social support on depression among a sample of individuals with Type 1 diabetes, using a measure of stress from disease-related disability. A functional index was obtained through an inventory for emotional and instrumental support. An interaction analysis indicated disability was strongly related to depression among persons with inadequate support, but the effect of disability was considerably reduced for persons with adequate support. Krause (1995) examined buffering effects of emotional support in a community sample of individuals 65 years of age or older. Stress was assessed in terms of the stressful life events in the preceding year. Findings indicated the risk of having diabetes increased with the number of undesirable life events, but high emotional support reduced the impact of life stress on diabetes. Griffith, Field, and Lustman (1990) tested buffering effects for social support and stressful life events with glucose control, assessed with a biochemical index, hemoglobin A1c (HbA1c), as the criterion. Under high stress, individuals with high levels of support satisfaction had better glucose control, but this result did not occur at a low level of stress. Vogelsang et al. (2007) found negative life events and inadequate emotional support increased the odds of having metabolic syndrome (including elevated blood glucose), adjusting for demographic and lifestyle factors. A study with diabetic adolescents by C. Hanson, Henggeler, and Burghen (1987) found that parental diabetes-specific support was correlated with better adherence, which in turn was correlated with better metabolic control indexed by HbA1c. Brody, Kogan, Murry, Chen, and Brown (2008) found that among rural African Americans, diabetes-specific support had an indirect effect on glycemic control through more frequent self-monitoring of blood sugar. Nakahara et al. (2006) also found an indirect effect of support on glycemic control, mediated through higher self-efficacy and better adherence. Thus, social support is related to better glycemic control and less risk of adverse outcomes; some findings suggest this effect is mediated through higher self-efficacy and better adherence to preventive regimens.

Kidney Disease

The health status of patients with kidney failure can be sustained through renal dialysis, a demanding procedure that involves continued effort by the patient and family. Strict compliance to a dietary regimen is also necessary to maintain electrolyte balance, and failure to do so carries medical risk (Ibarren, Jacos, Kiefe, & Lewis, 2005). Christensen and colleagues (Christensen et al., 1992; Christensen, Wiebe, Smith, & Turner, 1994) studied the role of family support in a sample of hemodialysis patients followed over an average 44-month period. Estimated five-year mortality rates were 18% for the high-support group and 52% for the low-support group. A subsequent study found support interacted with personality characteristics for predicting adjustment (Hoth, Christensen, Ehlers, & Raichle, 2007), and other studies have shown buffering effects for psychological distress among patients with renal failure (Ye et al., 2008) and renal cancer (Devine, Parker, Fouladi, & Cohen, 2003). Thus, evidence of several types has linked social support variables to better outcomes among patients with kidney disease.

Conclusions Regarding Arthritis, Diabetes, and Kidney Disease

Research on the role of social support in these chronic diseases has demonstrated several different facets of the area. For persons suffering from arthritis, emotional and instrumental support are shown to enhance adjustment, but negative aspects of social relationships (e.g., spousal criticism or failure to provide assistance when needed) can detract from adjustment. In diabetes, social support can be protective for the disease process through buffering against stress and facilitating adherence to preventive regimens. In both diabetes and kidney disease, structural and functional indices have been shown to be inversely related to disease-linked mortality.

SOCIAL SUPPORT AND HEALTH BEHAVIORS

Having discussed how social support is involved in diseases that are major causes of mortality, we now turn attention to how social support and social networks influence health-related behaviors that can increase or decrease persons' risk for disease. We focus on behaviors that have the largest attributable risk for health outcomes: cigarette smoking, heavy alcohol use, and healthy diet and exercise patterns. We note relations of support measures to other outcomes (e.g., mental health indices, adherence to treatment programs) when these were encompassed in the same studies.

Social Support in Children and Adolescents

Research on social support among children and adolescents contains a number of functional measures that index a combination of emotional and informational support from parents, sometimes with parallel measures for support from peers (see Grant et al., 2006; Wills & Shinar, 2000) or mentors (Barrera & Bonds, 2005). For example, a classic study by Newcomb and Bentler (1988) related a composite index of parental and peer support, measured in middle adolescence, to outcomes measured in young adulthood. The results indicated that support was a protective factor in relation to a range of mental health and behavioral outcomes (e.g., academic and vocational accomplishment, quality of interpersonal relationships), emphasizing that the impact of support is not restricted to a narrow domain. Research with adolescents has shown effects of social support mediated through higher self-esteem and self-efficacy (DuBois et al., 2002; Naar-King et al., 2006), more adaptive coping (Crean, 2004), and better academic performance (Schmeelk-Cone & Zimmerman, 2003). Also, adolescents with higher levels of support are more likely to seek professional help when they have a problem (Berdahl, Hoyt, & Whitbeck, 2005; Rickwood & Braithwaite, 1994; Sheffield, Fiorenza, & Sofronoff, 2004) and form better relationships with therapists when they do (Garner, Godley, & Funk, 2008).

Buffering effects have been demonstrated with substance use as well as mental health outcomes, particularly for parental support. Wills and Cleary (1996) showed in structural modeling that a buffering effect for parental support occurred through two different processes: one in which support reduced the impact of risk factors (e.g., negative life events) and another in which support increased the impact of protective factors (e.g., behavioral coping). Subsequent research has shown that social support buffers the effects of general negative life events (J. Hoffman & Su, 1998; Ostazewski & Zimmerman, 2006), child abuse (Esposito & Clum, 2002; Jun et al., 2008), or racial discrimination (Oppedal, Roysamb, & Sam, 2004; Scott & House, 2005). Protective effects of social support have also been found in relation to risk from exposure to political violence and terrorism (Bonnano, Galea, Bucciarelli, & Vlahov, 2007; La Greca, Silverman, Vernberg, & Roberts, 2002; Shamal & Kimhi, 2007); and buffering effects of social support have been found for the impact of community violence, a common stressor among urban minority youth (e.g., Hammack, Richards, Lo, Edlynn, & Roy, 2004; Kliewer, Murrelle, Mejia, Torres, & Angold, 2001; Rosario, Salzinger, Feldman, & Ng-Mak, 2008).

Negative as well as positive aspects of social relationships have been studied. Barrera, Chassin, and Rogosch (1993) studied the roles of support and strain. They found that support from parents was related to higher self-esteem and fewer externalizing behavior problems, whereas conflict with parents was related to lower self-esteem and more behavior problems. Similar effects were found for parental support and parent-child conflict by Wills et al. (2001). Prinstein, Boergers, and Spirito (2001) found that family dysfunction increased the impact of adverse peer influences on adolescents' substance use, aggressive behavior, and suicidality. Results in a high-risk population, adolescents having a parent with HIV/AIDS, indicated that persons who had more social support providers had lower levels of symptomatology, but negative role models (e.g., adults using illicit drugs) increased rates of problem behavior (Lee, Detels, Rotheram-Borus, & Duan et al., 2007).

Research with adolescents is theoretically complex because teens typically participate simultaneously in two different types of social networks, the family network and the peer network. Studies have found that the different networks can have opposite effects on outcomes (Wills, Mariani, & Filer, 1996) and that the balance of parent and peer support may have an interactive effect (DuBois et al., 2002; Dubow, Tisak, Causey, Hryshko, & Reid, 1991; Henrich et al., 2006). Studies with mental health outcomes (e.g., psychological distress) have shown protective effects for parental support, typically including stress-buffering effects, whereas effects for peer support are often nonsignificant (Farrell, Barnes, & Banerjee,1995; Forehand et al., 1991; Greenberg, Siegel, & Leitch, 1983; Hishinuma et al., 2004). A prospective study by DuBois, Felner, Meares, and Krier (1994) showed that a measure of family support was related to higher grade point average and less psychological distress and substance use. Interaction results were consistent with buffering effects, given that family support had stronger relationships to criterion variables among a high-disadvantage group compared with a low-disadvantage group. Buffering effects were found for support from school personnel as well as for support from family members. A mediation study by Wills et al. (2004) showed that parental support was related to more good self-control and less risk-taking tendency, whereas peer support was related to good self-control but also had indirect effects on substance use through paths to more impulsiveness, risk taking, and deviant peer affiliations, so its overall effect on substance use was positive. Thus, parental and peer support had complex effects that, in a sense, work against each other. Research on diet and physical activity has generally found both parent support and peer support for healthy behavior to be promotive, though the measures are somewhat different (Duncan, Duncan, & Strycker, 2005; Duncan, Duncan, Strycker, & Chaumeton, 2007; Kuo, Voorhees, Haythornthwaite, & Young, 2007; Motl, Dishman, Saunders, Dowda, & Pate, 2007; Neumark-Sztainer, Wall, Perry, & Story, 2003).

Social Support and Substance Use in Adults

Among adults, social support variables have been related to onset, cessation, or relapse after treatment (for review, see Moos, 2006). Most studies with adults show functional support measures related to decreased likelihood of substance use or lower amount of use (e.g., less heavy alcohol consumption). However, the composition of the social network is also important. Risk-promoting effects can occur when network members, even though perceived as emotionally supportive, are engaging in risky drug use or sexual behavior (De, Cox, Boivin, Platt, & Jolly, 2007; McCrady, 2006).

With regard to effects of social networks, Umberson (1987) found that persons who were married and/or had children showed lower rates of substance abuse as well as higher levels of health-protective behaviors. Data from other studies have shown indices of social integration and social support related to lower prevalence of cigarette smoking and heavy drinking (Brennan & Moos, 1990; B. S. Hanson, 1994; Perreira & Cortes, 2006; Romano, Bloom, & Syme, 1991; Sugisawa et al., 1994), even among persons with mental illness and/or substance abuse issues (Randolph et al., 2007; Warren, Stein, & Grella, 2007). B. S. Hanson, Isacsson, Janzon, & Lindell (1990) tested various structural measures and found that a measure reflecting formal and informal group memberships was related to a higher rate of quitting smoking. These findings have been interpreted as indicating the operation of a social control mechanism in which network members enforce norms about unhealthy behaviors (cf. Franks, Stephens, & Rook, 2006; Tucker, Elliott, & Klein, 2006), though it is also possible that persons with primary relationships feel more internal obligation to refrain from self-harmful behaviors.

With regard to buffering effects, a study of financial problems by Peirce and colleagues (1996) used scales for emotional, instrumental, and companionship support and found that high instrumental support reduced the relationship between life stress and problem drinking. Jenninson (1992) found that in a sample of older adults, several social network variables reduced the relationship between stress and drinking; these included church attendance, quality of marital relationship, number of close friends in the network, and support from siblings.

Studies of persons in treatment for substance abuse have identified social support as a factor that facilitated cessation of use or maintained abstinence after treatment (Moos, 2006; Moos, Finney, & Cronkite, 1990). Recent research has shown that effects of treatment programs are partly mediated though perceptions of support (Laudet, Cleland, Magura, Vogel, & Knight, 2004); however, some negative effects of social relationships were also found in that adverse outcomes were found among persons who had more close friends if the friends were engaging in heavy drinking or opiate use. With regard to smoking, Mermelstein, Cohen, Lichtenstein, and Kamarck (1986) followed persons from a clinic-based smoking cessation program and found that emotional support from spouse and friends facilitated quitting, but relapse after treatment was more likely if the spouse was a smoker. This finding is similar to results from B. S. Hanson et al. (1990), where a measure reflecting frequency of social contact was related to increase likelihood of relapse, probably because it indexed bar-going and partying where smoking models may occur. Other studies provide evidence that social integration and functional support may be promotive of cessation and protective for relapse, but drug use by network members is a significant risk factor both among adolescents in treatment (Godley, Kahn, Dennis, Godley, & Funk, 2005; Woodruff, Conway, & Edwards, 2008) and among adults (Havassey, Hall, & Wasserman, 1991; Longabaugh, Beattie, Noel, Stout, & Malloy, 1993; McSweeney, Zucker, Fitzgerald, Puttler, & Wong, 2005).

Conclusions Regarding Health Behaviors

Studies have shown that social support is just as relevant for adolescents as for adults, having a protective effect in relation to early smoking and alcohol use as well as other adverse outcomes. Stress-buffering effects, with substance use as the outcome, have been consistently demonstrated, and several studies have shown risk-promoting effects for negative aspects of social relationships, such as conflict with parents. Adolescent research has also shown that two types of social networks, the family network and the peer network, have different and sometimes opposite effects on adolescents' behavior. Similar conclusions are derived from studies of adults, which show functional support, as well as social integration, to be protective both for promoting cessation of substance use and for preventing relapse. However, the composition of the social network remains important, and adverse outcomes (e.g., relapse after treatment) may occur when network members are modeling smoking or alcohol use.

SOCIAL SUPPORT AND HIV/AIDS

In this area, measures of support are similar but the behaviors relevant for HIV infection, including risky sexual behavior (e.g., unprotected sex, multiple partners) and illicit drug use, can be fairly different (De et al., 2007; DiClemente et al., 2008). We discuss examples of research in this area to illustrate another aspect of how social support processes operate.

Social Support and HIV Risk Behavior

Among adolescents, emotional support from parents and strong connections with parents (vs. peers) is a general protective factor related to less substance use and less likelihood of precocious sexual behavior (Jessor et al., 2003; Mazzaferro et al., 2006; Wills et al., 2007). Research with a variety of samples has been consistent with this theme, but there are also some unique findings with regard to HIV risk behavior. For example, Springer, Parcel, Baumier, and Ross (2006) found parental support inversely related to a variety of risk behaviors, including sex, among high school students in El Salvador; and Randolph et al. (2007) found that larger social networks were related to less frequent sexual risk behavior in a sample of mentally ill women. However, some studies have found HIV-specific measures of support to be more consistently related to outcomes. For example, Naar-King et al. (2006) found that in a sample of HIV-positive youth, specific social support for reducing risk was related to higher self-efficacy, which in turn reduced unprotected sex, whereas general measures of support were less predictive. Findings on parent and peer support have also been more complex. For example, data from a representative national sample of adolescents showed that both connectedness with parents and supportive relationships with friends were protective factors against risky sexual behavior (Henrich, Brookmeyer, Shrier, & Shahar, 2006). However Lee et al. (2007) found that in a sample of adolescents having a parent with AIDS, family support was protective but negative role models in the network (e.g., a drug-using member) had adverse effects (cf. Gogineni, Stein, & Friedman, 2001). Findings on adjustment are also more complex. In a reversal of patterns found among general populations of adolescents, studies of adolescents and young adults who are HIV positive tend to show that support from friends is related to better adjustment but that family members are perceived as unsupportive if not hostile (Kalichman, DiMarco, Austin, Luke, & DiFonzo, 2003; Vandehey & Shuff, 2001). Moreover, studies on such high-risk behaviors as IV drug use and needle sharing have sometimes shown that emotional support from a partner increases high-risk behavior if the partner is an injecting drug user (De et al., 2007; Unger, Kipke, DeRosa, & Hyde, 2006). Thus, the context and nature of supportive relationships must be carefully defined along with the behavior of network members, particularly close ones.

Social Support and Adjustment to HIV/AIDS

Becoming HIV positive involves anxiety and uncertainty along with possible stigmatization and losses of network members. Hence, social support is an important factor for helping persons deal with this stressor. Research has shown various social support measures related to better adjustment among persons living with HIV/AIDS (e.g., Valverde et al., 2007). Furthermore, coping interventions with a support component may reduce HIV-risk behavior (Rotheram-Borus et al., 2001). Recent studies have linked emotional support not only to reduced depression and anxiety but also to the ability to employ cognitive coping to find benefits in the support available (Littlewood, Vanable, Carey, & Blair, 2008). A study by Deichert, Fekete, Boarts, and Druley (2008) found a mediation pathway with social support being related to less depression, which in turn was related to healthier lifestyle behaviors; another indirect pathway showed support related to more positive affect, a predictor of more active coping. Thus, social support may be useful not only for reducing negative affective states but also for encouraging active behavioral and cognitive approaches to coping.

Adherence to Treatment

Current treatments for HIV/AIDS require adherence to complex medication regimens, and social support concepts have been useful for studying factors that increase adherence to treatment in HIV-positive samples. Two studies (Atkinson, Schonnenesson, Williams, & Timpson, 2008; Nott, Vedhara, & Power, 1995) have found social support related to greater self-esteem and self-efficacy, which in turn are related to better treatment adherence. Gonzalez et al. (2004) found social support related to treatment adherence through more positive states of mind; Vyavaharkar et al. (2007) found that satisfaction with support was related to better adherence. Demas, Thea, Weedon, and McWayne (2005) found that participation in HIV support groups was related to better adherence, along with disclosure of HIV status to the participant's own mother. Simoni, Rick, and Huang (2006) found that support was related to less negative affect, which was related to greater self-efficacy to adhere to treatment and lower viral load at six months, with a partial replication by Power et al. (2003). Knowlton, Hua, and Latkin (2005) found that higher functional support was related to more consistent access to medical care. Thus, social support and social networks may enhance adherence to treatment in several ways. Whether better outcomes are mediated through an effect of social support on physiological variables that influence progression of disease remains unclear because literature on this topic includes null results as well as some positive findings (see Ironson & Hayward, 2008; Uchino, 2006).

Conclusions Regarding HIV/AIDS

Several aspects of social support are protective with regard to HIV/AIDS. This finding is true for reducing behavioral risk for HIV infection, enhancing adjustment to illness, and facilitating adherence to treatment regimens. In this area, HIV-specific measures of support are sometimes more useful than general ones, and family and peer networks may have different effects. Research has clarified some mechanisms of how support operates—for example, through affective pathways (e.g., less depression/anxiety) and through increasing coping ability (e.g., greater self-efficacy and cognitive coping). However, positive and negative aspects of social networks are both important because adverse behavior by network members (e.g., IV drug use) can increase risk for HIV infection.

CONCLUSION

This chapter has aimed to cover research on social networks and social support in relation to health outcomes. In broad outline, the basic findings in the field have been maintained, but the field has also changed over the past 10 years. There is more consideration given to negative as well of positive aspects of social relationships, and there is less emphasis on testing whether social support has buffering effects—because this relationship has now been observed in a large number of studies—and more attention is now focused on clarifying the behavioral and physiological mechanisms through which support exerts protective effects for disease onset or progression (e.g., Lett et al., 2005; Uchino, 2006). Because effects for structural and functional social measures have now been demonstrated in a variety of populations, there is more attention given to understanding cultural differences in social support processes (e.g., Kim, Sherman, & Taylor, 2008) and explicating the dynamics of support seeking and support giving in daily life (e.g., Bolger & Amarel, 2007; Wills & Gibbons, 2009). Also, protective effects for emotional and instrumental support have been consistently demonstrated in general populations, and there is now more attention given to studying how social relationships may protect against extreme stressors, including warfare (Alvarez, 2009; Bonnano, 2004; Charuvastra & Cloitre, 2008).

With regard to structural measures, the accumulated evidence shows that having more social connections is related to lower age-adjusted mortality rates. This finding has been observed in a considerable number of studies conducted with a wide variety of populations and has been obtained with statistical controls that rule out alternative explanations of the effect. Thus, one conclusion is that social integration is protective with regard to mortality. Evidence on the role of social integration for disease onset is mixed, but we believe the evidence supports a conclusion about protective effects of support for progression of cardiovascular disease and for recovery or survival time for heart disease and cancer. Investigators have often noted that effect sizes found for measures of social integration are comparable to those for medical variables, indicating thereby that social integration is a factor of importance from the public health standpoint.

Research with functional measures has consistently shown emotional support and other dimensions related to lower levels of depression/anxiety and higher levels of psychological well-being (e.g., positive affect). Findings of protective effects have occurred in a number of studies, where, again, significant effects obtained with a wide range of statistical controls. The details of the effect vary somewhat across populations and disease groups (e.g., parent vs. peer support for adolescents, friend vs. family relationships for HIV-positive persons), but a basic protective effect has been observed across different ages and disease conditions. It is also common to find buffering effects, such that stressors have less impact on persons with higher levels of support. Although exceptions can be noted (e.g., a significant main effect for support but a nonsignificant interaction), buffering effects have been observed with a variety of outcomes involving symptomatology and health behavior, and in a few studies with mortality as the outcome. Thus we conclude that functional support is a protective factor and a buffering agent, but there are still few studies directly comparing structural and functional measures.

Recent research has given more attention to intermediate processes in the relationship between social variables and health outcomes. Studies with psychosocial variables have shown functional support measures related to higher levels of self-esteem and self-efficacy, with these variables being proximal to reduced levels of mental health problems or risk behaviors. Studies with adolescents have also delineated pathways from parental emotional support (and sometimes friend support) to a variety of health-related behaviors, including substance use and sexual risk behavior; these pathways include mediation through academic competence, exposure to negative life events, and affiliation with deviant versus conventional peers. For physiological variables, evidence links supportive relationships to less cardiac reactivity, lower levels of physiological markers that indicate risk for cardiovascular disease (e.g., arterial occlusion, inflammatory processes, clotting factors), and indices of immune system functioning that could be protective for both heart disease and cancer (e.g., NK cells). Thus, more evidence is available on intermediate processes that can serve to inform and extend theory linking social relationships and health outcomes.

At present there is a need for more definitive types of studies to explicate the health effects of social support. For example, there is ample evidence that social integration is related to mortality, but studies testing for the pathways through which this effect occurs (e.g., through self-esteem and emotional states, through cigarette smoking and heavy alcohol use, through blood pressure or other physiological risk indices) remain to be conducted (Cohen & Lemay, 2007; Uchino, 2004). And at a basic level, there has been little research addressing the fact structural and functional measures are not highly correlated but both are related to health outcomes, which suggests that there are different mechanisms of effect. Mediation methods sufficient to address this question have been demonstrated (Richardson et al., 1987; Smith & Wallston, 1992; Wills et al. 2001; Wills et al., 2004) and methods for testing mediation are available (MacKinnon, 2006; MacKinnon, Taborga, & Morgan-Lopez, 2002). Understanding the pathways through which effects of social support occur remains one of the "big questions" in health psychology, so this seems a desirable next step.

An unresolved issue is the question of what was going on in intervention studies, which have tried—but predominantly failed—to increase social support. Discussions of this literature (Cohen & Janicki-Deverts, 2008; Helgeson, Cohen, Schulz, & Yasko, 2001; Reblin & Uchino, 2008) have suggested that the intervention methods employed in the studies were not tightly linked to previous theory and findings on social support. Promising results have been achieved by enhancing the ability of participants to utilize available support (Drentea, Clay, Roth, & Mittleman, 2006) and enlisting network members to improve adherence to treatment regimens (e.g., Barrera, Toobert, & Angell, 2006). Learning the best ways to implement interventions is an important area and can probably benefit from attention to the methodological issues raised in research about effects of psychotherapy for cancer patients (Boesen & Johansen, 2008; Coyne, Stefanek, & Palmer, 2007).

Another issue derives from the fact that although the great majority of studies have identified social connections or supportive functions as related to better physical or mental health, there are aspects of social relationships that may not always operate this way (Rook, 1990). For example, friendship networks can influence substance use (De et al., 2007; B. R. Hoffman, Sussman, Unger, & Valente, 2006), and social relationships involve elements of both support and strain, with level of support being protective and level of strain being a risk factor (Manne & Zautra, 1989; Revenson et al., 1991; Uchino, Holt-Lunstad, Smith, & Bloor, 2004). There is the possibility that transactions regarded as supportive by the giver may not always be perceived this way by the recipient (Coriell & Cohen, 1995; Gleason, Iida, Shrout, & Bolger, 2008; Newsom & Schulz, 1999), and providing support to a chronically ill family member may have an effect on the caregiver's health (Schulz & Beach, 1999). Recognizing that there are aspects of social relationships that may be risk-promoting for some persons at some times, we have concluded that on the balance, the effect of social support is a protective one. Understanding the balance of positive and negative aspects of relationships is a question of continuing interest for the field.

Finally, it should be recognized that the nature of social support itself is changing as face-to-face interactions are augmented or replaced by electronic communication over the Internet. This change may be particularly true for the new generation of adolescents (Greenfield & Yan, 2006) but is having an impact on persons of all ages. Support has been augmented in some ways through mobile phones (texting, video conferences, etc.), which can also be linked to the Internet through social network integration mobile features (e.g., access to Twitter exchanges, e-mail conversations, Facebook status). The fact that social networking sites have become an important venue for communication and that individuals may have a "virtual network" in addition to a concrete social network is raising questions about how the two networks overlap, whether Internet communications supplement existing relationships in a "rich get richer" model (Valkenburg & Peter, 2007), or whether heavy reliance on Internet communication detracts from the potential benefits of real social relationships (Leung, 2007; van den Eijnden, Meerkerk, Vermulst, Spijkerman, & Engels, 2008). As these questions are being studied, support interventions conducted over the Internet are proving feasible and, in some cases, effective (Mo & Coulson, 2008; Kalichman et al., 2006; Kalichman, Benotsch et al., 2003; McKay, Glasgow, & Feil, 2002). The role of electronic communication over the Internet seems likely to be a prominent area of social support research, with the potential to enhance intervention studies as well as basic research.

ACKNOWLEDGMENTS

This work was supported by grants R01 CA153154 from the National Cancer Institute and R01 DA021856 from the National Institute on Drug Abuse.

REFERENCES

Affleck, G., Pfeiffer, C., Tennen, H., & Fifield, H. (1988). Social support and psychosocial adjustment to rheumatoid arthritis. *Arthritis Care and Research, 1*, 71–77.

Aiken, L., & West, S. (1991). *Multiple regression: Testing and interpreting interactions.* Newbury Park, CA: Sage.

Ali, S., Medo, J., & Roswell, M. (2006). Social capital, traditionalism, and first time myocardial infarction: A study in southern Sweden. *Social Science and Medicine, 83*, 2204–2217.

Alvarez, L. (2009). Suicides of soldiers reach high of nearly 3 decades and army vows to bolster prevention. *New York Times*, January 30, 2009, p. A19.

Angerer, P., Siebert, U., Kothny, W., Muhlbauer, D., Mudra, H., & von Schacky, C. (2000). Impact of social support, cynical hostility, and anger expression on progression of coronary atherosclerosis. *Journal of the American College of Cardiology, 36*, 1781–1788.

Antoni, M., & Lutgendorf, S. (2007). Psychosocial factors and disease progression in cancer. *Current Directions in Psychological Science, 16*, 42–46.

Atkinson, J., Schonnenesson, L., Williams, M., & Timpson, S. (2008). Associations among correlates of schedule adherence to antiretroviral therapy. *AIDS Care, 20*, 260–269.

Barrera, M., & Bonds, D. (2005). Mentoring relationships and social support. In D. DuBois & J. Karcher (Eds.), *Handbook of youth mentoring* (pp. 133–142). Thousand Oaks, CA: Sage.

Barrera, M., Chassin, L., & Rogosch, F. (1993). Effects of social support and conflict on adolescent children. *Journal of Personality and Social Psychology, 64*, 602–612.

Barrera, M., Toobert, D., & Angell, R. E. (2006). Social support and ecological resources as mediators of intervention effects for type II diabetes. *Journal of Health Psychology, 11*, 483–495.

Berdahl, T., Hoyt, D., & Whitbeck, L. (2005). Predictors of first mental health service utilization among homeless and runaway adolescents. *Journal of Adolescent Health, 37*, 145–154.

Berkman, L. F., Glass, T., Brissette, I., & Seeman, T. E. (2000). From social integration to health. *Social Science and Medicine, 51*, 843–857.

Berkman, L. F., Leo-Summers, L., & Horwitz, R. (1992). Emotional support and survival after myocardial infarction. *Annals of Internal Medicine, 117*, 1003–1009.

Berkman, L. F., & Syme, S. L. (1979). Social networks, host resistance, and mortality: A nine-year follow-up study. *American Journal of Epidemiology, 109*, 186–204.

Blazer, D. G. (1982). Social support and mortality in an elderly community population. *American Journal of Epidemiology, 115*, 684–694.

Boesen, E., & Johansen, C. (2008). Impact of psychotherapy on cancer survival: Time to move one. *Current Opinion in Oncology, 20*, 372–379.

Bolger, N., & Amarel, D. (2007). Effects of support visibility on adjustment to stress. *Journal of Personality and Social Psychology, 92*, 458–475.

Bonnano, G. A. (2004). Loss, trauma, and human resilience: Have we underestimated the human capacity to adjust after extremely aversive events? *American Psychologist, 59*, 20–28.

Bonnano, G. A., Galea, S., Bucciarelli, A., & Vlahov, D. (2007). What predict psychological resilience after disaster? The role of demographics, resources, and life stress. *JCCP, 75*, 671–682.

Brennan, P. L., & Moos, R. H. (1990). Life stressors, social resources, and late-life problem drinking. *Psychology and Aging, 5*, 491–501.

Brissette, I., Cohen, S., & Seeman, T. (2000). Measuring social integration and social networks. In S. Cohen, L. Underwood, & B. Gottlieb (Eds.), *Social support measurement and intervention: Guide for health and social scientists* (pp. 53–85). New York, NY: Oxford University Press.

Brody, G. H., Kogan, S., Murry, V., Chen, Y., & Brown, A. (2008). Psychological functioning, support for self-management, and glycemic control among rural African American adults with diabetes. *Health Psychology, 27*(Suppl.), S83–S90.

Brown, G., Wallston, K., & Nicassio, P. (1989). Social support and depression in rheumatoid arthritis: A one-year prospective study. *Journal of Applied Social Psychology, 19*, 1164–1181.

Brummett, B., Barefoot, J., Siegler, I., Clapp-Channing, N. E., Lytle, B. L., Bosworth, H. B., … Mark, D. B. (2001). Characteristics of socially isolated patients with coronary artery disease at elevated risk for mortality. *Psychosomatic Medicine, 63*, 267–272.

Caspi, A. (2000). The child is father to the man: Personality continuities from childhood to adulthood. *Journal of Personality and Social Psychology, 78*, 158–172.

Charuvastra, A., & Cloitre, M. (2008). Social bonds and posttraumatic stress disorder. *Annual Review of Psychology, 59*, 301–328.

Christensen, A., Smith, T., Turner, C., Holman, J., Gregory, M., & Rich, M. (1992). Social support and adherence in dialysis: Examining main and buffering effects. *Journal of Behavioral Medicine, 15,* 313–325.

Christensen, A., Wiebe, J., Smith, T., & Turner, C. (1994). Predictors of survival among hemodialysis patients: Effect of perceived family support. *Health Psychology, 13,* 521–525.

Coble, H., Gantt, D., & Mallinckrodt, B. (1996). Attachment, social competency, and the capacity to use social support. In G. Pierce, B. Sarason, & I. Sarason (Eds.), *Handbook of social support and the family* (pp. 141–172). New York, NY: Plenum Press.

Cohen, S. (2004). Social relationships and health. *American Psychologist, 59,* 676–684.

Cohen, S. (2007). Psychological stress and disease. *Journal of the American Medical Association, 298,* 1685–1687.

Cohen, S., Gottlieb, B. H., & Underwood, L. G. (2000). Social relationships and health. In S. Cohen, L. Underwood, & B. Gottlieb (Eds.), *Social support measurement and intervention* (pp. 3–25). New York, NY: Oxford University Press.

Cohen, S., & Janicki-Deverts, D. (2008). Can we improve our physical health by altering our social networks? Manuscript submitted for publication.

Cohen, S., & Lemay, E. (2007). Why would social networks be linked to affect and health practices? *Health Psychology, 26,* 410–417.

Cohen, S., Sherrod, D. R., & Clark, M. S. (1986). Social skills and the stress-protective role of social support. *Journal of Personality and Social Psychology, 50,* 963–973.

Cohen, S., & Wills, T. (1985). Stress, social support, and the buffering hypothesis. *Psychological Bulletin, 98,* 310–357.

Coriell, M., & Cohen, S. (1995). Concordance in the face of an event: When do members agree that one supported the other? *Journal of Personality and Social Psychology, 69,* 289–299.

Cousinne-Gelile, F., Bruchon-Sweitzer, M., Dilhuydy, J. M., & Jutand, M. A. (2007). Do anxiety, body image, social support, and coping strategies predict survival in breast cancer? A ten–year follow-up study. *Psychosomatics, 48,* 211–216.

Coyne, J., Stefanek, M., & Palmer, S. (2007). Psychotherapy and survival in cancer: The conflict between hope and evidence. *Psychological Bulletin, 133,* 367–394.

Crean, H. (2004). Social support and adaptive coping strategies in Latino middle school students. *Journal of Adolescent Research, 19,* 657–676.

Dakof, G., & Taylor, S. (1990). Victims' perceptions of social support: What is helpful from whom? *Journal of Personality and Social Psychology, 58,* 80–89.

De, P., Cox, J., Boivin, J-F., Platt, R., & Jolly, A. (2007). The importance of social networks for drug equipment sharing among injection drug users: A review. *Addiction, 102,* 1730–1739.

Deichert, N., Fekete, E., Boarts, J., & Druley, J. (2008). Emotional support and affect: Associations with health behaviors and active coping efforts in men living with HIV. *AIDS and Behavior, 12,* 139–145.

Demas, P., Thea, D., Weedon, J., & McWayne, J. (2005). Adherence to zidovudine in HIV-infected pregnant women: Impact of social network factors and perceived treatment efficacy. *Women and Health, 42,* 99–115.

Devine, D., Parker, P., Fouladi, R., & Cohen, L. (2003). Association between social support, intrusive thoughts, and adjustment following cancer treatment. *Psycho-Oncology, 12,* 453–462.

Dickens, E., McGowan, L., Percival, C., Douglas, J., Tomenson, B., Cotter, L., … Creed, F. H. (2004). Lack of a close confidant predicts further cardiac events after myocardial infarction. *Heart, 90,* 518–522.

DiClemente, R., Crittenden, C., Rose, E., Sales, J., Wingood, G. M., Crosby, R. A., & Salazar, L. F. (2008). Psychosocial predictors of HIV-associated sexual behaviors and the efficacy of prevention interventions in adolescents. *Psychosomatic Medicine, 70,* 598–605.

DiMatteo, M. (2004). Social support and patient adherence to medical treatment: A meta-analysis. *Health Psychology, 23,* 207–218.

Drentea, P., Clay, O., Roth, D., & Mittleman, M. (2006). Predictors of improvement in social support in an intervention for spouses of patients with Alzheimer's disease. *Social Science and Medicine, 63,* 957–967.

DuBois, D. L., Burk-Braxton, C., Swenson, L., Tevendale, H., Lockerd, E. M., & Moran, B. L. (2002). Self-esteem and social support as resources during early adolescence. *Developmental Psychology, 38,* 822–839.

DuBois, D. L., Felner, R. D., Meares, H., & Krier, M. (1994). Prospective investigation of the effects of socioeconomic disadvantage, life stress, and social support on early adolescent adjustment. *Journal of Abnormal Psychology, 103,* 511–522.

Dubow, E. F., Tisak, J., Causey, D., Hryshko, A., & Reid, G. (1991). Stressful life events, social support, and problem-solving skills: Contributions to children's behavioral and academic adjustment. *Child Development, 62,* 583–599.

Duncan, S. C., Duncan, T. E., & Strycker, L. (2005). Sources and types of social support in youth physical activity. *Health Psychology*, *24*, 3–10.

Duncan, S. C., Duncan, T. E., Strycker, L. A., & Chaumeton, N. R. (2007). A cohort-sequential latent growth model of physical activity from ages 12 to 17 years. *Annals of Behavioral Medicine*, *33*, 80–89.

Ell, K., Nishimoto, R., Mediansky, L., & Mantell, J. (1992). Social relationships and survival among patients with cancer. *Journal of Psychosomatic Research*, *36*, 531–541.

Emmons, K., Barbewau, E., Gutheil, C., Stryker, J., & Stoddard, A. (2007). Social influences, social context, and health behaviors among working-class, multiethnic adults. *Health Education and Behavior*, *34*, 315–334.

Esposito, C., & Clum, G. (2002). Social support and problem solving as moderators of the relation between child abuse and suicidality. *Journal of Traumatic Stress*, *15*, 137–146.

Falk, A., Hanson, B., Isacsson, S. O., & Ostergren, P. O. (1992). Job strain and mortality in men: Social network and support as buffers. *American Journal of Public Health*, *82*, 1136–1139.

Farrell, M. P., Barnes, G. M., & Banerjee, S. (1995). Family cohesion as a buffer against the effects of problem-drinking fathers on psychological distress, deviant behavior, and heavy drinking in adolescents. *Journal of Health and Social Behavior*, *36*, 377–385.

Fitzpatrick, R., Newman, S., Archer, R., & Shipley, M. (1991). Social support, disability and depression: A longitudinal study of rheumatoid arthritis. *Social Science and Medicine, 33*, 605–611.

Fitzpatrick, R., Newman, S., Lamb, R., & Shipley, M. (1988). Social relationships and psychological well-being in rheumatoid arthritis. *Social Science and Medicine*, *27*, 399–403.

Forehand, R., Wierson, M., Thomas, A., Armistead, L., Kempton, T., & Neighbors, B. (1991). The role of family stressors and parent relationships on adolescent functioning. *Journal of the American Academy of Child and Adolescent Psychiatry*, *30*, 316–322.

Franks, M. M., Stephens, M. A. P., & Rook, K. S. (2006). Spouses' provision of health-related support and control. *Journal of Family Psychology*, *20*, 311–316.

Garner, B., Godley, S., & Funk, R. (2008). Predictors of therapeutic alliance among adolescents in substance abuse treatment. *Journal of Psychoactive Drugs*, *40*, 55–65.

Gidron, Y., & Ronson, A. (2008). Psychosocial factors, biological mediators, and cancer prognosis: A new look at an old story. *Current Opinion in Oncology*, *20*, 386–392.

Gleason, M., Iida, M., Shrout, P., & Bolger, N. (2008). Receiving support as a mixed blessing. *Journal of Personality and Social Psychology*, *94*, 828–838.

Godley, M., Kahn, J., Dennis, M., Godley, S., & Funk, R. (2005). Stability and impact of environmental factors on substance use and problems after adolescent outpatient treatment. *Psychology of Addictive Behaviors*, *19*, 62–70.

Gogineni, A., Stein, M., & Friedman, P. (2001). Social relationships and intravenous drug use among methadone maintenance patients. *Drug and Alcohol Dependence*, *64*, 47–53.

Gonzalez, J., Penedo, F., Antoni, M., Durgan, R., McPherson-Baker, S., Ironson, G., … Schneiderman, N. (2004). Social support, positive states of mind, and HIV treatment adherence. *Health Psychology*, *23*, 413–418.

Goodenow, C., Reisine, S., & Grady, K. (1990). Quality of social support and social and psychological functioning in women with rheumatoid arthritis. *Health Psychology*, *9*, 266–284.

Grand, A., Grosclaude, P., Bucquet, H., & Pous, J. (1990). Psychosocial factors and mortality among the elderly in a rural French population. *Journal of Clinical Epidemiology*, *43*, 773–782.

Grant, K., Compas, B., Thurm, A., McMahon, S., Gipson, P. Y., Campbell, A. J., … Westerholm, R. I. (2006). Stressors and child and adolescent psychopathology: Evidence for moderating and mediating effects. *Clinical Psychology Review*, *26*, 267–283.

Graves, P. L., Wang, N. Y., Mead, L., Johnson, J. V., & Klag, M. J. (1998). Early precursors of midlife social support. *Journal of Personality and Social Psychology*, *74*, 1329–1336.

Greenberg, M., Siegel, J., & Leitch, C. (1983). The nature and importance of relationships to parents and peers during adolescence. *Journal of Youth and Adolescence*, *12*, 373–386.

Greenfield, P., & Yan, Z. (2006). Children, adolescents, and the Internet: A new field of inquiry in developmental psychology. *Developmental Psychology*, *42*, 391–394.

Griffith, L., Field, B., & Lustman, P. (1990). Life stress and social support in diabetes: Association with glycemic control. *International Journal of Psychiatry in Medicine*, *20*, 365–372.

Hammack, P., Richards, N., Lo, Z., Edlynn, E., & Roy, K. (2004). Social support factors as moderators of community violence exposure among inner-city African-American young adolescents. *Journal of Clinical Child and Adolescent Psychology*, *33*, 450–462.

Hanson, C., Henggeler, S., & Burghen, G. (1987). Social competence and parental support as mediators of the link between stress and metabolic control in adolescents with insulin-dependent diabetes mellitus. *Journal of Consulting and Clinical Psychology*, *55*, 529–533.

Hanson, B. S. (1994). Social network, social support and heavy drinking in elderly men: A population study of men born in 1914, Malmö, Sweden. *Addiction, 89,* 725–732.

Hanson, B. S., Isacsson, J. T., Janzon, L., & Lindell, S. E. (1989). Social network and social support influence mortality in elderly men. *American Journal of Epidemiology, 130,* 100–111.

Hanson, B. S., Isacsson, S. O., Janzon, L., & Lindell, S. E. (1990). Social support and quitting smoking: Is there an association? Results from the population study "Men born in 1914," Malmo, Sweden. *Addictive Behaviors, 15,* 221–233.

Havassey, B., Hall, S., & Wasserman, D. (1991). Social support and relapse among alcoholics, opiate users, and cigarette smokers. *Addictive Behaviors, 16,* 235–246.

Helgeson, V. S. (1991). The effects of masculinity and social support on recovery from myocardial infarction. *Psychosomatic Medicine, 53,* 621–633.

Helgeson, V. S., & Cohen, S. (1996). Social support and adjustment to cancer: Reconciling descriptive, correlational, and intervention research. *Health Psychology, 15,* 135–148.

Helgeson, V. S., Cohen, S., & Fritz, H. L. (1998). Social ties and cancer. In J. C. Holland (Ed.), *Psycho-oncology* (pp. 99–109). New York, NY: Oxford.

Helgeson, V. S., Cohen, S., Schulz, R., & Yasko, J. (2001). Group support interventions for people with cancer: Benefits and hazards. In A. Baum & B. L. Andersen (Eds.), *Psychosocial interventions for cancer* (pp. 269–286). Washington, DC: American Psychological Association.

Henrich, C., Brookmeyer, K., Shrier, L., & Shahar, G. (2006). Supportive friendships and sexual risk behavior in adolescence. *Journal of Pediatric Psychology, 31,* 286–297.

Hishinuma, E., Johnson, R., Carlton, B., Andrade, N., Nishimura, S., Goebert, D. A., … Chang, J. Y. (2004). Demographic and social variables associated with psychiatric and school-related indicators for Asian / Pacific Islander adolescents. *International Journal of Social Psychiatry, 50,* 301–318.

Hislop, T., Waxler, N., Coldman A., & Elwood, J. M. (1987). The prognostic significance of psychosocial factors in women with breast cancer. *Journal of Chronic Diseases, 40,* 729–735.

Ho, S. C. (1991). Health and social predictors of mortality in an elderly Chinese cohort. *American Journal of Epidemiology, 133,* 907–921.

Hoffman, B. R., Sussman, S., Unger, J., & Valente, T. W. (2006). Peer influences on adolescent cigarette smoking: A theoretical review. *Substance Use and Misuse, 41,* 103–155.

Hoffman, J., & Su, S. (1998). Stressful life events and adolescent substance use and depression: Conditional and gender effects. *Substance Use and Misuse, 33,* 2219–2262.

Honda, K., & Kagawa-Singer, M. (2006). Cognitive mediators linking social support networks to colorectal cancer screening adherence. *Journal of Behavioral Medicine, 29,* 449–460.

Horsten, M., Mittleman, M. A., Wamala, S. P., & Scheck-Gustafsson, K. (1999). Social relations and the metabolic syndrome in women. *Journal of Cardiovascular Risk, 6,* 391–397.

Hoth, K., Christensen, A., Ehlers, S., & Raichle, K. (2007). A longitudinal study of social support and depressive symptoms in chronic kidney disease. *Journal of Behavioral Medicine, 30,* 69–76.

House, J. S., Landis, K. R., & Umberson, D. (1988). Social relationships and health. *Science, 241,* 540–545.

Ibarren, C., Jacos, D., Kiefe, C., & Lewis S. (2005). Causes and demographic, medical, lifestyle, and psychosocial predictors of premature mortality. *Social Science and Medicine, 60,* 4711–482.

Ironson, G., & Hayward, H. S. (2008). Do positive psychosocial factors predict disease progression in HIV-1? A review of the evidence. *Psychosomatic Medicine, 70,* 546–554.

Jennison, K. M. (1992). The impact of stressful life events and social support on drinking among older adults. *International Journal of Aging and Human Development, 35,* 99–123.

Jessor, R., Turbin, M. S., Costa, F. M., Dong, Q., Zhang, H., & Wang, C. (2003). Adolescent problem behaviors in China and the United States: A cross-national study of psychosocial protective factors. *Journal of Research on Adolescence, 13,* 329–360.

Jun, H. J., Rich-Edwards, J., Boynton-Jarrett, R., Austin, S. G., Frazier, A. L., & Wright, R. J. (2008). Child abuse and smoking among young women. *Journal of Adolescent Health, 41,* 55–63.

Jylha, M., & Arö, S. (1989). Social ties and survival among the elderly in Tampere, Finland. *International Journal of Epidemiology, 18,* 158–164.

Kalichman, S. C., Benotsch, E. G., Winhardt, L., Austin, J., Luke, W., & Cherry, C. (2003). Health-related Internet use, coping, social support, and health indicators in people with HIV/AIDS. *Health Psychology, 22,* 111–116.

Kalichman, S. C., Cherry, C., Cain, D., Pope, H., Kalichman, M., Eaton, L., … Benotsch, E. G. (2006). Internet-based health information consumer skills intervention for people living with HIV/AIDS. *Journal of Consulting and Clinical Psychology, 74,* 545–554.

Kalichman, S. C., DiMarco, M., Austin, J., Luke, W., & DiFonzo, K. (2003). Stress, social support, and HIV-status disclosure to family and friends among HIV positive men and women. *Journal of Behavioral Medicine, 26*, 315–332.

Kaplan, G. A., Salonen, J. T., Cohen, R. D., Brand, R. J., Syme, S. L., & Puska, P. (1988). Social connections and mortality in Finland. *American Journal of Epidemiology, 128*, 370–380.

Karlamangla, A., Singer, B., & Seeman, T. (2006). Reduction in allostatic load in older adults is associated with lower all-cause mortality risk. *Psychosomatic Medicine, 68*, 500–507.

Kendler, K. (1997). Social support: A genetic-epidemiologic investigation. *American Journal of Psychiatry, 154*, 1398–1404.

Kiecolt-Glaser, J., McGuire, L., Robles, T., & Glaser, R. (2002). Emotions, morbidity, and mortality: Perspectives from psychoneuroimmunology. *Annual Review of Psychology, 53*, 83–107.

Kim, H., Sherman, D. K., & Taylor, S. (2008). Culture and social support. *American Psychologist, 63*, 518–526.

King, K., Reis, H., Porter, L., & Norsen, L. (1993). Social support and long-term recovery from coronary artery surgery: Effects on patients and spouses. *Health Psychology, 12*, 56–63.

Kliewer, W., Murrelle, L., Mejia, R., Torres, G., & Angold, A. (2001). Exposure to violence against a family member and internalizing symptoms in Colombian adolescents: The protective effects of family support. *JCCP, 69*, 971–982.

Knowlton, A., Hua, W., & Latkin, C. (2005). Social support networks and medial service use among HIV positive injectio n drug users. *AIDS Care, 17*, 479–492.

Krause, N. (1987). Chronic financial strain, social support, and depressive symptoms among older adults. *Psychology and Aging, 2*, 185–192.

Krause, N. (1995). Stress and diabetes mellitus in later life. *International Journal of Aging and Human Development, 40*, 125–1433.

Kuo, J., Voorhees, C., Haythornthwaite, J., & Young, D. (2007). Association of family support and physical activity in urban adolescent girls. *American Journal of Public Health, 97*, 101–103.

La Greca, A. M., Silverman, W. K., Vernberg, E. M., & Roberts, M. C. (Eds.). (2002). *Helping children cope with disasters and terrorism*. Washington, DC: American Psychological Association.

Lakey, B. E., & Cohen, S. (2000). Social support theory and measurement. In S. Cohen, L. Underwood, & B. Gottlieb (Eds.), *Social support measurement and intervention: A guide for health and social scientists* (pp. 29–52). New York, NY: Oxford University Press.

Lamkin, D. M., Lutgendorf, S., McGinn, S., Dao, M., Maiseri, H., DeGeest, K., … Lubaroff, D. M. (2008). Positive psychosocial factors and NK cells in ovarian cancer patients. *Brain, Behavior, and Immunity, 22*, 65–73.

Lanza, A., Cameron, A., & Revenson, T. (1995). Perceptions of helpful and unhelpful support among individuals with rheumatic diseases. *Psychology and Health, 10*, 449–462.

Laudet, A., Cleland, C., Magura, S., Vogel, H., & Knight, E. (2004). Social support mediates the effects of dual-focus mutual aid groups on abstinence from substance use. *American Journal of Community Psychology, 34*, 175–185.

Lee, S. J., Detels, R., Rotheram-Borus, M. J., & Duan, N. (2007). Effects of social support on mental and behavioral outcomes among adolescents with parents with HIV/AIDS. *American Journal of Public Health, 97*, 1820–1826.

Lett, H., Blumenthal, J., Babyak, M., Strauman, T., Robins, C., & Sherwood, A. (2005). Social support and coronary heart disease: Evidence and implications for treatment. *Psychosomatic Medicine, 67*, 869–878.

Leung, L. (2007). Stressful life events, motives for internet use, and social support among digital kids. *CyperPsychology and Behaviour, 10*, 204–214.

Linden, W., Chambers, L., Maurice, J., & Lenz, J. (1993). Sex differences in social support, hostility, and ambulatory cardiovascular activity. *Health Psychology, 12*, 376–380.

Littlefield, C., Rodin, G., Murray, M., & Craven, J. (1990). Influence of social support on depressive symptoms in persons with diabetes. *Health Psychology, 9*, 737–749.

Littlewood, R., Vanable, P., Carey, M., & Blair, D. (2008). The association of benefit finding with psychosocial and behavioral adaptation among HIV positive men. *Journal of Behavioral Medicine, 31*, 145–155.

Longabaugh, R., Beattie, M., Noel, N., Stout, R., & Mallory, P. (1993). The effect of social investment on treatment outcome. *Journal of Studies on Alcohol, 54*, 465–478.

Loucks, E., Berkman, L., Gruenewald, T., & Seeman, T. (2005). Social integration is associated with fibrinogen concentration in elderly men. *Psychosomatic Medicine, 67*, 353–368.

Loucks, E., Sullivan, L. M., D'Agostino, R. B., Larson, M. G., Berkman, L. F., & Benjamin, E. J. (2006). Social networks and inflammatory markers in the Framingham Heart Study. *Journal of Biosocial Science, 38*, 845–852.

Lutgendorf, S. K., Johnsen, E. L., Cooper, B., Anderson, B., Sorosky, J. I., Buller, R. E., & Sood, A. K. (2002). Vascular endothelial growth factor and social support in patients with ovarian carcinoma. *Cancer, 95*, 808–815.

Lutgendorf, S. K., Sood, A. K., Anderson, B., McGinn, S., Maiseri, H., Dao, M., ... Lubaroff, D. M. (2005). Social support, psychological distress, and natural killer cell activity in ovarian cancer. *Journal of Clinical Oncology, 23*, 7105–7113.

Lyyra, T. M., & Heikkinen, R. L. (2006). Perceived social support and mortality in elderly people. *Journal of Gerontology: Series B. Psychology and Social Science, 61*, S147–S162.

MacKinnon, D. P. (2006). Mediation analysis. *Annual Review of Psychology, 58*, 593–614.

MacKinnon, D. P., Taborga, M. P., & Morgan-Lopez, A. A. (2002). Mediation designs for prevention research. *Drug and Alcohol Dependence, 68*(Suppl. 1), S69–S83.

Manne, S. L., & Zautra, A. J. (1989). Spouse criticism and support: Their association with coping and psychological adjustment among women with rheumatoid arthritis. *Journal of Personality and Social Psychology, 56*, 608–617.

Marsland, A. L., Sathanoori, R., Muldoon, M. F., & Manuck, S. B. (2007). Stimulated production of interleukin-8 covaries with psychosocial risk factors for inflammatory disease among middle-aged community volunteers. *Psychosomatic Medicine, 21*, 218–228.

Mazzaferro, K. E., Murray, P. J., Ness, R. B., Bass, D. C., Tyus, N., & Cook, R. L. (2006). Depression, stress, and social support as predictors of risky sexual behaviors in young women. *Journal of Adolescent Health, 39*, 601–603.

McCrady, B. (2006). Family and other close relationships. In W. R. Miller & K. M. Carroll (Eds.), *Rethinking substance abuse* (pp. 166–181). New York, NY: Guilford.

McKay, H., Glasgow, R., Feil., E., Boles, S. M., & Barrera, M. (2002). Internet-based diabetes self-management and support. *Rehabilitation Psychology, 47*, 31–48.

McSweeney, M., Zucker, R., Fitzgerald, H., Puttler, L, & Wong, M. (20005). Predictors of recovery from alcohol disorder in a community sample. *Journal of Studies on Alcohol, 66*, 220–228.

Mermelstein, R., Cohen, S., Lichtenstein, E., & Kamarck, T. (1986). Role of social support in smoking cessation and maintenance. *Journal of Consulting and Clinical Psychology, 54*, 447–453.

Mo, P., & Coulson, N. (2008). Social support in virtual communities: Content analysis of messages for an online HIV/AIDS support group. *CyperPsychology and Behaviour, 111*, 371–374.

Moos, R. H. (2006). The social context of substance use. In W. R. Miller & K. M. Carroll (Eds.), *Rethinking substance abuse* (pp. 182–200). New York, NY: Guilford Press.

Moos, R. H., Finney, J., & Cronkite, R. (1990). *Alcoholism treatment: Context, process, and outcome.* New York, NY: Oxford University Press.

Motl, R. W., Dishman, R. K., Saunders, R. P., Dowda, M., & Pate, R. R. (2007). Physical and social environmental variables as correlates of self-reported physical activity among adolescent girls. *Journal of Pediatric Psychology, 32*, 6–12.

Naar-King, S., Wright, K., Parsons, J., Frey, M., Templin, T., & Ondersma, S. (2006). Transtheoretical model and condom use in HIV-positive youths. *Health Psychology, 25*, 648–652.

Nakahara, R., Yoshiuchi, K., Kumano, H., Hara, Y., Sumatsu, H., & Kuboki, T. (2006). Prospective study on influence of psychosocial factors on glycemic control in Japanese patients with type II diabetes. *Psychosomatics, 47*, 240–246.

Neumark-Sztainer, D., Wall, M., Perry, C., & Story, M. (2003). Correlates of fruit and vegetable intake among adolescents: Data from Project EAT. *Preventive Medicine, 37*, 198–208.

Newcomb, M., & Bentler, P. (1988). Impact of adolescent drug use and social support on problems of young adults: A longitudinal study. *Journal of Abnormal Psychology, 97*, 64–75.

Newsom, J., & Schulz, R. (1999). Caregiving from the recipient's perspective: Negative reactions to being helped. *Health Psychology, 17*, 172–181.

Oppedal, B., Roysamb, E., & Sam, D. (2004). Effect of acculturation and social support on change in mental health among young immigrants. *International Journal of Behavioral Development, 28*, 481–494.

Orth-Gomer, K., & Johnson, J. V. (1987). Social network interaction and mortality: A 6-year follow-up study of a sample of the Swedish population. *Journal of Chronic Disease, 40*, 949–957.

Orth-Gomer, K., Rosengren, A., & Wilhelmsen, L. (1993). Lack of social support and incidence of heart disease in middle-aged Swedish men. *Psychosomatic Medicine, 55*, 37–43.

Ostazewski, K., & Zimmerman, M. (2006). The effects of cumulative risks and protective factors on urban adolescent alcohol and other drug use: A longitudinal study of resiliency. *American Journal of Community Psychology, 38*, 237–249.

Peirce, R. S., Frone, M. R., Russell, M., & Cooper, M. L. (1996). Financial stress, social support, and alcohol involvement: A longitudinal test of the buffering hypothesis in a general population survey. *Health Psychology, 15*, 38–47.

Perreira, K., & Cortes, K. (2006). Race/ethnicity differences in tobacco and alcohol use during pregnancy. *American Journal of Public Health, 96*, 1629–1636.

Power, R., Koopman, C., Volk, J., Israelski, D. M., Stone, L., Chesney, M. A., & Spiegel, D. (2003). Social support, substance use, and denial in relation to ART adherence among HIV-infected persons. *AIDS Patient Care and STDs, 17*, 245–252.

Primomo, J., Yates, B. C., & Woods, N. F. (1990). Social support for women during chronic illness. *Research in Nursing and Health, 13*, 153–161.

Prinstein, M., Boergers, J., & Spirito, A. (2001). Adolescents' and their friends' health-risk behavior: Factors that moderate peer influence. *Journal of Pediatric Psychology, 26*, 287–298.

Raikkonen, K., Matthews, K. A., & Kuller, L. H. (2001). Trajectory of psychological risk and incident hypertension in middle-aged women. *Hypertension, 38*, 798–802.

Randolph, M., Pinkerton, S., Somlai, A., Kelly, J. A., McAuliffe, T. L., Gibson, R. H., & Hackl, K. (2007). Mentally ill women's HIV risk: The influence of social support, substance use, and contextual risk factors. *Community Mental Health Journal, 43*, 33–47.

Reblin, M., & Uchino, B. (2008). Social and emotional support and its implications for health. *Current Opinion in Psychiatry, 21*, 201–205.

Revenson, T. A. (1994). Social support and marital coping with chronic illness. *Annals of Behavioral Medicine, 16*, 122–130.

Revenson, T. A., & Majerovitz, S. D. (1991). The effects of chronic illness on the spouse: Social resources as stress buffers. *Arthritis Care and Research, 4*, 63–72.

Revenson, T. A., Schiaffino, K. M., Majerovitz, S. D., & Gibofsky, A. (1991). The relation of positive and problematic support to depression among rheumatoid arthritis patients. *Social Science and Medicine, 33*, 807–813.

Reynolds, P., & Kaplan, G. A. (1990). Social connections and risk for cancer: Prospective evidence from the Alameda County Study. *Journal of Behavioral Medicine, 16*, 101–110.

Richardson, J., Marks, G., Johnson, C., Graham, J., Chan, K. K., Selser, J. N., … Levine, A. M. (1987). Path model of multidimensional compliance with cancer therapy. *Health Psychology, 6*, 183–207.

Rickwood, D. J., & Braithwaite, V. A. (1994). Social-psychological factors affecting help-seeking for emotional problems. *Social Science and Medicine, 39*, 563–572.

Rodriguez Artalejo, F., Guallar-Castillón, P., Herrera, M. C., Otero, C. M., Chiva, M. O., Ochoa, C. C., … Pascual, C. R. (2006). Social network as a predictor of hospital readmission and mortality among older patients with heart failure. *Journal of Cardiac Failure, 12*, 621–627.

Romano, P. S., Bloom, J., & Syme, S. L. (1991). Smoking, social support, and hassles in an urban African-American community. *American Journal of Public Health, 81*, 1415–1422.

Rook, K. S. (1990). Parallels in the study of social support and social strain. *Journal of Social and Clinical Psychology, 12*, 118–132.

Rosario, M., Salzinger, S., Feldman, R. S., & Ng-Mak, D. S. (2008). Intervening processes between youths' exposure to community violence and internalizing symptoms. *American Journal of Community Psychology, 41*, 43–62.

Rose, J. H. (1990). Social support and cancer: Adult patients' desire for support from family, friends, and health professionals. *American Journal of Community Psychology, 18*, 439–464.

Rosengren, A., Orth-Gomer, K., Wedel, H., & Wilhelmsen, L. (1993). Stressful life events, social support, and mortality in men born in 1933. *British Medical Journal, 307*, 102–105.

Rotheram-Borus, M., Lee, M., Murphy, D., Futterman, D., Duan, N., Birnbaum, J. M., … Lightfoot, M. (2001). Efficacy of a preventive intervention for HIV positive youths. *American Journal of Public Health, 91*, 400–405.

Rozanski, A., Blumenthal, J. A., & Kaplan, J. (1999). Impact of psychological factors on the pathogenesis of cardiovascular disease. *Circulation, 99*, 2192–2217.

Rutledge, T., Linke, S., Olsen, M,. Francis, J., Johnson, D. B., Bittner, V., … Merz, C. N. (2008). Social networks and stroke among women with suspected myocardial ischemia. *Psychosomatic Medicine, 70*, 282–287.

Sandler, I. N., Miller, P., Short, J., & Wolchik, S. A. (1989). Social support as a protective factor for children in stress. In D. Belle (Ed.), *Children's social networks and social supports* (pp. 277–307). New York, NY: Wiley.

Schmaltz, H. N., Southern, D., Ghali, W. A., Jelinski, S. E., Parsons, G. A., King, K. M., & Maxwell, C. J. (2007). Living alone, patient sex, and mortality after myocardial infarction. *Journal of General Internal Medicine, 22*, 572–578.

Schmeelk-Cone, K., & Zimmerman, M. (2003). A longitudinal analysis of stress in African American youth. *Journal of Youth and Adolescence, 32*, 419–430.

Schnorpfeil, P., Noll, A., Schulze, R., & Ehlert, U. (2003). Allostatic load and work conditions. *Social Science and Medicine, 57*, 647–656.

Schulz, R., & Beach, S. (1999). Caregiving as a risk factor for mortality. *Journal of the American Medical Association, 282*, 2215–2219.

Scott, L. D., & House, L. E. (2005). Coping with perceived racial discrimination among Black youth. *Journal of Adolescent Health, 31*, 254–272.

Seeman, T. E. (1996). Social ties and health: The benefits of social integration. *Annals of Epidemiology, 6*, 442–451.

Shamal, M., & Kimhi, S. (2007). Teenagers' response to threat of war and terror: Gender and the role of social systems. *Community Mental Health Journal, 43*, 358–374.

Shaw, B., Krause, N., Chatters, L., Connell, K., & Ingersoll-Dayton, B. (2004). Emotional support from parents early in life, aging, and health. *Psychology and Aging, 19*, 4–12.

Sheffield, J., Fiorenza, E., & Sofronoff, K. (2004). Adolescents' willingness to seek psychological help: Predictive factors. *Journal of Youth and Adolescence, 33*, 495–507.

Simoni, J., Rick, P., & Huang, B. (2006). Evaluation of a social support model of medication adherence among HIV positive men and women. *Health Psychology, 25*, 74–81.

Smith, C., Dobbins, C., & Wallston, K. (1991). Mediational role of perceived competence in adjustment to rheumatoid arthritis. *Journal of Applied Social Psychology, 21*, 1218–1247.

Smith, C., & Wallston, K. (1992). Adaptation in patients with chronic rheumatoid arthritis: Application of a general model. *Health Psychology, 11*, 151–162.

Springer, A., Parcel, G., Baumier, E., & Ross, M. (2006). Supportive relationships and health risk behavior among school students in El Salvador. *Social Science and Medicine, 62*, 1628–1640.

Stanton, A., Revenson, T., & Tennen, H. (2007). Health psychology: Adjustment to chronic disease. *Annual Review of Psychology, 58*, 565–592.

Steptoe, A., Owen, N., Kunz-Ebrecht, S. R., & Brydon, L. (2004). Loneliness and neuroendocrine, cardiovascular, and inflammatory stress responses in middle-aged men and women. *Psychoneuroendocrinology, 29*, 593–611.

Sugisawa, H., Liang, J., & Liu, X. (1994). Social networks, social support, and mortality among older people in Japan. *Journal of Gerontology: Social Sciences, 49*, S3–S13.

Tucker, J., Elliott, M., & Klein, D. (2006). Social control of health behavior. *Personality and Social Psychology Bulletin, 32*, 1143–1152.

Tucker, J., Orlando, M., Elliott, M., & Klein, D. (2006). Affective and behavioral responses to health-related social control. *Health Psychology, 25*, 715–722.

Turner-Cobb, J. M., Sephton, S. E., Koopman, C., Blake-Mortimer, J., & Spiegel, D. (2000). Social support and salivary cortisol in women with metastatic breast cancer. *Psychosomatic Medicine, 62*, 337–345.

Uchino, B. N. (2004). Social support and physical health: *Understanding the health consequences of relationships*. New Haven, CT: Yale University Press.

Uchino, B. N. (2006). Social support and health: A review of physiological processes potentially underlying links to disease outcomes. *Journal of Behavioral Medicine, 29*, 377–387.

Uchino, B. N., Holt-Lunstad, J., Smith, T. W., & Bloor, L. (2004). Heterogeneous social networks: Models linking relationships to health outcomes. *Journal of Social and Clinical Psychology, 23*, 123–139.

Umberson, D. (1987). Family status and health behaviors: Social control as a dimension of social integration. *Journal of Health and Social Behavior, 28*, 306–319.

Unger, J., Kipke, M., DeRosa, C., Hyde, J., Ritt-Olson, A., & Montgomery, S. (2006). Needle sharing among IV drug users and their social network members. *Addictive Behaviors, 31*, 1607–1618.

Valkenburg, P., & Peter, J. (2007). Adolescents' online communication and their closeness to friends. *Developmental Psychology, 43*, 267–277.

Valverde, E., Purcell, D., Waldrop-Valverde, D., Malow, R., Knowlton, A. R., Gomez, C. A., … Latka, M. H. (2007). Correlates of depression among HIV-positive women and men who inject drugs. *JAIDS: Journal of Acquired Immune Deficiency Syndromes, 46*(Suppl. 2), S86–S100.

Vandehey, M., & Shuff, M. (2001). HIV infection and stage of illness: A comparison of family, friend, and professional support providers over a 2-year period. *Journal of Applied Social Psychology, 31*, 2217–2229.

Van den Eijnden, R., Meerkerk, G-J., Vermulst, A., Spijkerman, R., & Engels, R. C. (2008). Online communication, compulsive internet use, and psychosocial well-being among adolescents. *Developmental Psychology, 44*, 655–665.

Vogelsang, N., Beekman, A. T. S., Kritchevsky, S. B., Newman, A. B., Pahor, M., Yaffe, K., … Penninx, B. W. (2007). Psychosocial risk factors and the metabolic syndrome in elderly persons. *Journal of Gerontology: Series A. Biological Sciences and Medical Sciences, 62A,* 563–569.

Vogt, T. M., Mullooly, J. P., Ernst, D., Pope, C. R., & Hollis, J. F. (1992). Social networks as predictors of ischemic heart disease, cancer, stroke and hypertension. *Journal of Clinical Epidemiology, 45,* 659–666.

Von Dras, D. D., & Siegler, I. C. (1997). Stability in extraversion and aspects of social support at midlife. *Journal of Personality and Social Psychology, 72,* 233–241.

Vyavaharkar, M., Moneyham, L., Tavakoli, A., Phillips, K. D., Murdaugh, C., Jackson, K., & Meding, G. (2007). Social support, coping, and medication adherence among HIV positive women. *AIDS Patient Care and STDs, 21,* 667–683.

Wang, H. X., Mittleman, M. A., & Orth-Gomer, K. (2005). Influence of social support on progression of coronary artery disease in women. *Social Science and Medicine, 60,* 599–607.

Warren, J., Stein J., & Grella, C. (2007). Role of social support and self0effiacacy in treatment outcomes among clients with co-occurring disorders. *Drug and Alcohol Dependence, 89,* 267–274.

Waxler-Morrison, N., Hislop, T. G., Mears, B., & Kan, L. (1991). Social relationships and survival for women with breast cancer. S*ocial Science and Medicine, 33,* 177–183.

Welin, L., Larsson, B., Svärdsudd, K., & Tibblin, B. (1992). Social network and activities in relation to mortality from cardiovascular disease, cancer and other causes. *Journal of Epidemiology and Community Health, 46,* 217–132.

Wiklund, I., Oden, A., Sanne, H., & Ulvenstam, G. (1988). Importance of somatic and social variables after a first myocardial infarction. *American Journal of Epidemiology, 128,* 786–795.

Williams, R., Barefoot, J., Califf, R., Haney, T., Saunders, W. B., Pryor, D. B., … Mark, D. B. (1992). Prognostic importance of social resources among patients with CAD. *Journal of the American Medical Association, 267,* 520–524.

Wills, T. (1991). Social support and interpersonal relationships. In M. Clark (Ed.), *Review of personality and social psychology* (Vol. 12, pp. 265–289). Newbury Park, CA: Sage.

Wills, T., & Cleary, S. (1996). How are social support effects mediated: Parental support and adolescent substance use. *Journal of Personality and Social Psychology, 71,* 937–952.

Wills, T., Cleary, S., Filer, M., Shinar, O., Mariani, J., & Spera, K. (2001). Temperament related to early-onset substance use: Test of a developmental model. *Prevention Science, 2,* 145–163.

Wills, T., & Filer, M. (2001). Social networks and social support. In A. Baum, T. Revenson, & J. Singer (Eds.), *Handbook of health psychology* (pp. 209–234). Mahwah, NJ: Erlbaum.

Wills, T. A., & Gibbons, F. X. (2009). Using psychological theory in help-seeking research. *Clinical Psychology Science and Practice, 16,* 440–444.

Wills, T., Gibbons, F., Gerrard, M., Murry, V., & Brody, G. (2003). Family communication and religiosity related to substance use and sexual behavior in early adolescence. *Psychology of Addictive Behaviors, 17,* 312–323.

Wills, T., Mariani, J., & Filer, M. (1996). The role of family and peer relationships in adolescent substance use. In G. Pierce, B. Sarason, & I. Sarason (Eds.), *Handbook of social support and the family* (pp. 521–549). New York, NY: Plenum Press.

Wills, T., Murry, V., Brody, G., Gibbons, F., Gerrard, M., Walker, C., & Ainette, M. G. (2007). Ethnic pride and self-control related to protective and risk factors. *Health Psychology, 26,* 50–59.

Wills, T., Resko, J., Ainette, M., & Mendoza, D. (2004). Parent and peer support in adolescent substance use: Mediated effects. *Psychology of Addictive Behaviors, 18,* 122–134.

Wills, T., Sandy, J. M., & Yaeger, A. M. (2002). Stress and smoking in adolescence: A test of directional hypotheses with latent growth analysis. *Health Psychology, 21,* 122–130.

Wills, T., & Shinar, O. (2000). Measuring perceived and received social support. In S. Cohen, L. Underwood, & B. Gottlieb (Eds.), *Social support measurement and intervention: A guide for health and social scientists* (pp. 86–135). New York, NY: Oxford University Press.

Woodruff, S., Conway, T., & Edwards, C. (2008). Predictors of smoking-related behavior change among high school smokers. *Addictive Behaviors, 33,* 354–358.

Ye, X. Q., Chen, W. Q., Lin, J. X., Wang, R. P., Zhang, Z. H., Yang, X., & Yu, X. Q. (2008). Effects of social support on depression in patients on peritoneal dialysis. *Journal of Psychosomatic Research, 65,* 157–164.

Zhang, X., Norris, S. L., Gregg, E. W., & Beckles, G. (2007). Social support and mortality among elderly persons with diabetes. *Diabetes Education, 33,* 273–281.

21 Health and Illness in the Context of the Family

Melissa A. Alderfer
Children's Hospital of Philadelphia and University
of Pennsylvania Perelman School of Medicine

Caroline M. Stanley
Wilmington College

The social nature of human beings almost invariably dictates that multiple people contribute to and are impacted by the health or illness of any given individual. We each exist within a series of social contexts (Bronfenbrenner, 1977), ranging from small networks such as family and friends to broad social constructions such national values, public policy, and socioeconomics. Although personal characteristics (e.g., gender, biological predispositions), thoughts, beliefs, and behaviors contribute greatly to individuals' health status, so too do individuals' interactions with others. Of course, for most individuals, the most immediate and important of these social contexts is the family system.

It is of interest that our most basic understanding of the family system originates in biologically based systems theory (Engle, 1980; von Bertalanffy, 1968). This theory holds that the family operates as an organized unit comprised of component members, their relationships with one another, and their rule-governed patterns of interaction. Because of the interdependencies within the system, change in one member or one aspect of the family is reciprocated by changes in other members or aspects of the system. Families also self-regulate. That is, as a unit they develop methods for maintaining stability while also accommodating change (Hoffman, 1981; Nichols & Schwartz, 2001; Wynne, 2003).

The purpose of this chapter is to introduce the reader to the conceptualization of health and illness in the context of the family. Literature on families and health emerges from various disciplines of psychology (e.g., pediatric psychology, health psychology), medicine (e.g., family medicine, behavioral medicine, nursing) and family studies, producing a diffuse research base. These literatures agree, however, that families are important to health and may contribute to a positive course and outcome or may place the individual at greater risk for poor outcomes (Weihs, Fisher, & Baird, 2002). They also recognize that the developmental stage of the ill family member (i.e., infant, child, adolescent, young adult, adult, elderly) and that individual's position within the family (e.g., child, sibling, parent, spouse) greatly influences both the reaction of the family system to the illness and the role the family plays in management. Because of the breadth of this literature, a comprehensive review of health and illness in the context of the family is beyond the scope of a single chapter. To best introduce health and illness in the context of the family, we focus primarily on work regarding families of ill children. But to illustrate the role of the family in health and illness across the lifespan, we also provide examples of research when an adult, spouse, or parent is diagnosed with illness. For a more comprehensive review of couples coping with illness, see Revenson and Delongis (2011).

We begin this chapter with an overview of some frameworks that describe how families react to illness and how they adapt to its challenges. We summarize these models, draw out their similarities, and provide empirical examples of the proposed effects. Next, we consider the pathways through which the family may directly influence health and illness, provide some empirical evidence for these models, and describe their clinical implications. Then, we briefly illustrate, through examples, the research regarding the utility of family-based interventions for improving management of health and illness. Finally, we summarize the main points of the chapter, discuss the challenges of researching health and illness in the context of the family, and provide suggestions for future work.

FAMILY REACTIONS AND ADAPTATION TO ILLNESS

Family theorists and researchers have proposed various models of the ways in which families adapt to extreme such stressors as the diagnosis of an illness. Here, we present an overview of some of these models as an introduction to the types of family-based constructs that have been deemed important when attempting to understand the ways in which families respond to a stressor such as illness.

THE CIRCUMPLEX MODEL OF MARITAL AND FAMILY SYSTEMS

The circumplex model (Olson & Gorall, 2003; Olson, Russel, & Sprenkle, 1983) proposes two important dimensions of family functioning: cohesion and flexibility. *Cohesion* refers to the emotional bonds between family members, and *flexibility* refers to adaptability in a family's leadership, roles, and relationship rules. Families very high in cohesion are described as enmeshed, whereas those very low are considered disengaged. Families very high in flexibility are considered chaotic, whereas those who are very low are described as rigid. Families falling at the extremes on these dimensions are considered poorly functioning or unbalanced, whereas those falling midrange are considered well functioning or balanced. A third component of the model—*communication*—is considered a facilitating dimension of family functioning that allows the family to effectively adapt to meet changing needs (Olson et al., 1983).

These dimensions of family functioning are not static. According to the circumplex model, family cohesion and flexibility change in predictable ways across the family lifespan, particularly under times of stress. In a hypothesized example, Olson (2000) describes expected changes in family functioning in response to a father's debilitating heart attack. In response to the crisis, the family members draw closer emotionally, moving toward enmeshment. To accommodate the demands of treatment, the family members make dramatic changes in their daily routines, which results in chaos. After the crisis phase resolves, the family remains enmeshed but rigidly adheres to the patterns and routines that have enabled its members to manage treatment. After mastering disease management, the family becomes balanced again, but perhaps more cohesive and structured than before.

FAMILY STRESS THEORY

Many different groups of researchers have applied stress and coping models to family systems. These various models, such as Hill's ABC-X model (Hill, 1949), the double ABCX model of family stress (McCubbin & Patterson, 1983), and the family adjustment and adaptation model (Patterson, 1988; Patterson & Garwick, 1994), have been classified under the general category of family stress theory (Hobfoll & Spielberger, 1992). Three basic elements are deemed important across these models: (1) the nature of the stressor, (2) the resources of the family, and (3) family perceptions and meaning.

Within the framework of family stress theory, a *stressor* is an environmental influence, such as illness, that threatens the family's well-being. The specific qualities of the threat determine, in part, its stressfulness and the type of demands it imposes on the family. To address these demands, families employ their *resources*, or their material (i.e., income), social (i.e., extended family), interpersonal (i.e., communication), and psychological (i.e., motivation) assets (Patterson & McCubbin, 1983). The strengths of individual family members, and of the family as a whole, contribute to family resources. Further, conceptualizations of the stressor and of the family's resources for managing it comprise family *perceptions* and *meaning* (Boss, 1988; Patterson & McCubbin, 1983). During a crisis, the family members cope by fitting their resources to the demands of the illness, seeking or developing more resources as needed, changing their perception of their circumstances, and/or removing some of the illness demands. Families experience repeated cycles of stable adjustment, crisis, and adaptation while managing the challenge.

THE FAMILY RESILIENCE APPROACH

Building upon the family stress theories, Walsh (2002, 2003, 2006) has proposed a family resilience framework that focuses on positive adaptation and the possibility for family and individual growth in response to such aversive life events as illness. Instead of proposing a model of how families respond to and meet challenges, this approach describes the characteristics of families who thrive in response to adversity and proposes a clinical pathway for helping families build resilience. Aversive life events are seen as catalysts or opportunities to discover new abilities and resources. Three aspects of family functioning are central to the family resilience approach: (1) the family belief system, (2) family organization patterns, and (3) family communication and problem-solving processes.

Resilient families tend to have *belief systems* that allow them to make meaning out of adversity, maintain a positive outlook, and connect to some sort of higher power or sense of purpose in life. In terms of *organizational patterns*, resilient families can more readily accept and adapt to change while maintaining some sort of stability and continuity in spite of disruptions. Family members provide support, collaboration, commitment, and nurturance for one another. Finally, the *communication patterns* of the resilient family are clear, open, and consistent; foster a climate of mutual trust, empathy, and acceptance of differences; and allow for appropriate sharing of a range of emotions and positive, pleasurable interactions even in times of stress. Resilient families are also capable of *collaborative problem solving*, in which they set clear goals and priorities and work toward them, building on successes, learning from failures, and managing conflicts as they arise.

FAMILY SYSTEMS HEALTH MODEL

The family systems health model (Rolland, 1984, 1987, 2003) describes complex mutual interactions between illness and the family. This model stresses that the "goodness of fit" between the family's style and the demands of disease determines adaptation and disease management over time as part of a developmental process. Factors influencing this goodness of fit include aspects of the illness, including such *illness attributes* as onset, course, outcome, and uncertainty. Different psychosocial challenges arise for the family depending on whether the onset is acute or gradual; whether the course is progressive, constant, or relapsing; and whether the outcome is death, shortened life expectancy, or disability. The specific *illness phase* (e.g., diagnosis, treatment initiation, illness stabilization) also influences this fit between the family and the illness.

Analogous to the specific characteristics and patterns of illnesses, family systems also have specific characteristics that influence the way they interact with illness, including *prior experiences* with illness, loss, and crisis, *health and illness beliefs,* and their own *developmental phases*. The prior experiences of individuals within the family and of the family as a whole give rise to beliefs. These beliefs, in turn, provide the framework from which such new and ambiguous situations as serious illness are approached. Families burdened by unresolved issues and dysfunctional patterns in relation to illness are less well equipped to adapt to the challenges presented by a serious medical condition. Also according to this model, two different forces manifest in the family at different points in development. *Centripetal forces* focus the family internally, weakening internal boundaries, allowing for greater collaboration among family members, and strengthening boundaries between the family and external agents. *Centrifugal forces,* on the other hand, push family members apart to allow for shifts in family structure and the emphasis on individual family members' lives outside of the family. Physical symptoms such as loss of function and the demands of shifting or acquiring new illness-related roles and responsibility, along with the fear of losing the ill member, are postulated to exert a centripetal pull on the family system. This centripetal pull of the disorder causes different normative strains on the family depending where the family is on the life cycle phase—that is, whether the family is in a centrifugal (e.g., launching of a teenager) or centripetal (e.g., birth of a baby) period of development.

SUMMARY

There are many similarities across the aforementioned models. All propose that the diagnosis of illness in a family member will result in some expected turmoil within the family. This turmoil impacts both the emotional climate and the organizational structure of the family. Across the models, the following family-level constructs emerge as important: cohesion (e.g., involvement and closeness); affective environment (e.g., expression of feelings and conflict); adaptability (e.g., flexibility in roles and responsibilities); problem-solving ability (e.g., goal-directed negotiation and task accomplishment); and organization (e.g., roles, leadership). Also, the individual and shared beliefs and perceptions of family members, ability to communicate clearly and directly, available resources, developmental stage of the family and its members, and specific characteristics of the illness are important factors in how the family responds to illness and mobilizes to manage it. These models also accept that adaptation to illness is a process that unfolds and shifts across time and development.

EMPIRICAL EVIDENCE

The aforementioned models put forth many tenets that are supported in the current empirical base. Although research on families of children with chronic illnesses dominates this body of research, example studies on the families of adults with medical conditions and on caregivers of older adults with disease or disability are also available and provided below.

IMPACT ON THE FAMILY: INDIVIDUAL DISTRESS

A wealth of research documents that the diagnosis of a health problem in a family member causes distress within the family. Generally this distress is greatest at the time of diagnosis and diminishes with time (e.g., Alderfer & Kazak, 2006; Northam, Anderson, Adler, Werther, & Warne, 1996), but it is moderated by numerous factors (e.g., course of illness; personal characteristics) and may linger long term for some families (e.g., Kazak, Alderfer, Rourke, et al., 2004; Northouse, 1989).

Qualitative interviews have revealed such intense negative emotions as anxiety, anguish, frustration, terror, panic, and depression among parents of children with such disorders as hemolytic uremic syndrome (Pollock, Duncan, & Cowden, 2009), as well as uncertainty, helplessness, and guilt among parents of children with asthma (Trollvik & Severinsson, 2004). Quantitative studies have documented that within one month of diagnosis, about 60% of parents of children with diabetes meet clinical cutoffs for depression and anxiety (Streisand et al., 2008) and 40%–50% of parents of children with cancer qualify for a diagnosis of acute stress disorder (Patiño-Fernández et al., 2008). Siblings of children diagnosed with illness are also at risk for psychological distress (P. D. Williams, 1997). This effect has been confirmed in meta-analysis (Sharpe & Rossiter, 2002) and has specifically been documented in reviews of research regarding siblings of children with traumatic brain injury (Sambuco, Brookes, & Lah, 2008), cystic fibrosis (Berge & Patterson, 2004), and cancer (Alderfer et al., 2010).

When an adult experiences a significant health event, spouses and children are greatly impacted. Partner distress in response to spousal illness has been well documented in the literature (e.g., Cochrane & Lewis, 2005; Cooper et al., 2006). For example, significant others of adults with diabetes or cancer report shock, anger, fear, worry, helplessness, and concern for their partners (Beverly, Penrod, & Wray, 2007; Hilton, Crawford, & Tarko, 2000; Stodberg, Sunvisson, & Ahlstrom, 2007), and their rates of anxiety and depressive symptoms are elevated (e.g., Hilton et al., 2000). Investigations particularly targeting caregivers of older adults with chronic disease or disability, be they spouses or adult children (see Martire & Schulz, Chapter 13, this volume), also reveal personal distress and burden, resulting in greater risk for psychological difficulties than found in the general population as demonstrated by meta-analysis (Pinquart & Sorensen, 2003). Feelings of sadness, worry, anger, and guilt are also common among young children of adults diagnosed with such medical conditions as inflammatory bowel disease (Mukherjee, Sloper, & Lewin, 2002), multiple sclerosis (Turpin, Leech, & Hackenberg, 2008), and cancer (Grabiak, Bender, & Puskar, 2007). Children of adults with cancer (Compas et al., 1994; Lewis & Hammond, 1996; Osborn, 2007) and HIV (Nostlinger, Bartoli, Gordillo, Roberfroid, & Colebunders, 2006) have also been found to be at risk for emotional or behavioral problems.

IMPACT ON THE FAMILY: THE EMOTIONAL DIMENSION

In addition to causing individuals within the family to experience distress, the illness of a family member impacts the affective climate of the family. It seems that a greater sense of emotional closeness or cohesion is evident in many samples of families dealing with illness in a child. For example, Blair, Freeman, and Cull (1995) found that families of children with cystic fibrosis were more emotionally involved compared to families with healthy children. Studies have also indicated that families of children with diabetes (Dashiff, 1993) and cancer (Varni, Katz, Colegrove, & Dolgin, 1996) show higher than average levels of cohesion shortly after diagnosis. Increased cohesion is a common theme in qualitative studies of families of children with cancer (e.g., Wiener et al., 2008); however, reports of sibling rivalry and family conflict have also emerged (e.g., Brown, Pikler, Lavish, Keune, & Hutto, 2008). In fact, a meta-analysis of the influence of pediatric cancer on family functioning revealed higher levels of maternal-reported conflict in these families compared to those families with healthy children (Pai et al., 2007). Similarly, Liakopoulou and colleagues (2001) observed mothers of children with diabetes to express more critical comments, hostility, and overinvolvement with their children. Greater difficulties in affect management, affective responsiveness, and affective involvement have been reported for families of children with diabetes (Piazza-Waggoner et al., 2008) and adolescent cancer survivors (Alderfer, Navsaria, & Kazak, 2009). In sum, although families of children with illness seem to be more emotionally connected, they experience difficulties managing appropriate levels of affective involvement and responsiveness and seem prone to conflict.

Although research on the emotional climate of the family when a parent is diagnosed with illness is scarce, the research that does exist suggests that cohesion may be impaired. Among families where a parent underwent coronary bypass surgery (van der Poel & Greeff, 2003) or with mothers with diabetes or chronic pain (Dura & Beck, 1988), lower cohesiveness was reported compared to families with no illness.

IMPACT ON THE FAMILY: THE ORGANIZATIONAL DIMENSION

Both qualitative and quantitative research suggests that families reorganize in response to an illness in a family member. For example, parents of children with hemolytic-uremic syndrome report on the illness's "impact on daily behavior" (Pollock et al., 2009, p. 267), and parents of children with asthma report a need for "adaptation to everyday life" (Trollvik & Severinsson, 2004, p. 96). Spouses of adults with chronic illness report "the struggle of everyday life" (Eriksson & Svedlund, 2006, p. 328). Children of parents with multiple sclerosis and cancer report changing roles and responsibilities (Grabiak et al., 2007; Turpin et al., 2008). Also, adults who have experienced a stroke report a "loss of role and identity" (Thompson & Ryan, 2009 p. 1807). Each of these examples describes how illness has changed routines, roles, and responsibilities of every family member and created a need to adjust daily life to accommodate the demands of the illness or its treatment. Quantitative studies have found that family members' roles are less clear and more difficult to establish and maintain when someone has an illness. These patterns have been documented in families of children with diabetes (Piazza-Waggoner et al., 2008), spina bifida (Ammerman et al., 1998), and cancer survivors (Alderfer et al., 2009). Families of adults with chronic obstructive pulmonary disease have also been found to have difficulties developing and maintaining roles within the family (Kanervisto, Paavilainen, & Heikkila, 2007).

There is also some evidence that families managing illness are dysregulated in terms of flexibility. Families of children with cancer have been found to be more likely than healthy families to be either chaotic (very high in flexibility) or rigid (very low in flexibility; Horwitz & Kazak, 1990; Madan-Swain et al., 1994). There is also some evidence that families of children with diabetes are more likely to be more rigid than is the norm (Lawler, Volk, Viviani, & Mengel, 1990) and to become less flexible across the first few months after diagnosis (Northam et al., 1996).

FAMILY FUNCTIONING AND MEDICAL OUTCOMES

Research has also accumulated demonstrating that the functioning of the family is related to medical outcomes. A review of research regarding family functioning and childhood asthma concludes that poorer parental psychological functioning (e.g., Shalowitz, Berry, Quinn, & Wolf, 2001) and a more conflictual and critical parent-child relationship (e.g., Schobinger, Florin, Reichbauer, Lindemann, & Zimmer, 1993) are associated with poorer asthma adherence, more asthma symptomatology, and greater health service utilization (Kaugars, Klinnert, & Bender, 2004). In addition, families of children with controlled asthma have been found to be higher in cohesion than are families of children with uncontrolled asthma (Meijer, Griffioen, van Nierop, & Oppenheimer, 1995), and families with poorer affective responsiveness have been found to have poorer asthma adherence (Bender, Milgrom, Rand, & Ackerson, 1998). Cohesive, open, and nonconflictual family relationships have been linked to better diabetes management (Naar-King, Podolski, Ellis, Frey, & Templin, 2006), metabolic control (e.g., Cohen, Lumley, Naar-King, Partridge, & Cakan, 2004; Marteau, Bloch, & Baum, 1987), and fewer episodes of ketoacidosis (Dumont et al., 1995; Geffken et al., 2008); whereas critical comments, hostility, emotional overinvolvement, and poorer affective responsiveness have been linked to poorer adherence and metabolic control (e.g., Leonard, Jang, Savik, & Plumbo, 2005; Lewin et al., 2006; Liakopoulou et al., 2001; Miller-Johnson et al., 1994; Swift, Chen, Hershberger, & Holmes, 2006). Relationship quality (happy, open, nonconflictual) and more emotional expressiveness among family members have also been found to predict adherence for children with cystic fibrosis (DeLambo, Ievers-Landis, Drotar, & Quittner, 2004; Patterson, Goetz, Budd, & Warwick, 1993).

Adults who have experienced strokes show better functional recovery when they receive emotional support that meets their needs (e.g., Evans & Northwood, 1983; Glass & Maddox, 1992) and better treatment adherence when their families have appropriate levels of affective involvement (Evans, Bishop, & Haselkorn, 1991). Better emotional management within families of adults with Type 2 diabetes, specifically the ability to effectively resolve conflicts, predicts better disease management across time (Chesla et al., 2003). Similarly, greater marital distress has been found to relate to poorer blood glucose levels for adults with diabetes (Trief et al., 2006). Also, one study using a combined measure of emotional and instrumental support for diabetes care (e.g., respect, understanding, help with self-care) predicted number of blood glucose tests for African American adults with Type 2 diabetes (Brody, Kogan, Murry, Chen, & Brown, 2008). For more information on this topic, see the recent chapter on dyadic coping with chronic illness by Revenson and DeLongis (2011).

In turning toward more organizational components of the family, it is clear that among families of children with medical needs, parents play a large role in structuring, managing, and overseeing treatment regimens. When responsibility for disease management tasks is unclear or parental oversight and monitoring are poor, adherence suffers for children with asthma, cancer, diabetes, and renal disease (Rapoff, 2009). Among families with children with diabetes, parental guidance and oversight has been related to better adherence and metabolic control (Gowers, Jones, Kiana, North, & Price, 1995; Lewin et al., 2006), as has better parent–adolescent collaboration around the diabetes regimen (Wiebe et al., 2005). Qualitative studies of adolescents with leukemia reveal that adolescents view their parents, particularly their mothers, as playing a substantial role in managing and organizing their medications, allowing for greater adherence (Malbasa, Kodish, & Santacroce, 2007). Quantitative studies have found that better family-based problem solving is associated with better adherence for children with sickle cell disease (Barakat, Smith-Whitley, & Ohene-Frempong, 2002) and cystic fibrosis (DeLambo et al., 2004).

For adults with illness, qualitative studies reveal that family members may be helpful or harmful to disease management. Developing a working organizational pattern to include required components of the treatment regimen may require new roles, responsibilities, and restrictions for all family members (see also Martire & Schulz, Chapter 13, this volume). If family members accept these changes and alter their own behaviors to support the patient, disease management is more easily achieved. For example, a qualitative study of men with prostate cancer and their wives revealed that wives needed to communicate directly with their husbands' physicians to maximize disease management because the men would disclose information to their wives but not their doctors (Gray, Fitch, Phillips, Labrecque, & Fergus, 2000). Furthermore, Beals, Wight, Aneshensel, Murphy, and Miller-Martinez (2006) demonstrated that HIV-positive patients displayed poorer medication compliance when their caregivers perceived more hassles regarding medication management. However, this dynamic has been most frequently examined in relation to prescribed dietary changes (e.g., Beverly, Miller, & Wray, 2008; Chesla, 1999; Jones et al., 2008; Paisley, Beanlands, Goldman, Evers, & Chappell, 2008), demonstrating that spousal support and alterations in their own behavior are important to success.

SUMMARY

The models reviewed specify ways in which the physical condition of one member impacts the family system and how the family comes to manage that condition. The empirical evidence supports the propositions of these models. Both emotional and organizational aspects of the family are challenged when a family member is diagnosed with a medical condition; at the same time, these aspects of the family seem to be related to medical outcomes. Families who are able to pull together emotionally yet appropriately manage their affect and resolve conflicts are better able to maintain health and manage disease. Similarly, families who can work together collaboratively, solve problems effectively, and establish workable routines ensure better adherence to medical regimens and better outcomes. Such observations have lead to models of mechanisms of the family's influence on health and illness.

MECHANISMS OF FAMILY INFLUENCE ON HEALTH AND ILLNESS

There are at least two proposed mechanisms by which families impact health and illness (Fisher & Weihs, 2000). First, the family may impact the self-care behaviors of the patient. Maintaining health while managing illness requires adherence to specific regimens of diet, exercise, and medication, for example. The family members can organize to promote these behaviors or they can undermine such efforts. Second, the emotional climate of the family may impact the patient's physiological functioning. Secure attachments and cohesion among family members may ease physiological reactivity, whereas conflict and hostility may disrupt or exacerbate it. Neuroendocrine, immunologic, and other biological systems have been implicated in such processes (McEwen & Stellar, 1993). Next, we discuss models exemplifying these proposed mechanisms, present some empirical evidence that support them, and provide implications of these models for intervention to improve health and disease management.

FAMILY ROUTINES, RITUALS, AND HEALTH

Although not presented as a specific model of family functioning per se, Fiese (2006, 2007) and Denham (2002, 2003) have conceptualized family routines and rituals as important structural and emotional components of the family that have direct implications for managing health and illness. Indeed, given that maintaining health and managing illness are greatly dependent on daily behavioral regimens (e.g., exercise, diet, medication), development of routines that accommodate these behavioral patterns is vital to health and illness management. Furthermore, creating positive meaning in these interactions, or avoiding negative perceptions, may be important to the well-being of family members. Examining family routines and rituals provides a window into the transactional nature of the individual's effect on the family and the family's effect on the individual (Fiese, 2006; Fiese et al., 2002).

Family *routines* are common interactions of daily life. They recur regularly, have a relatively clear beginning and end, follow a certain pattern, and consist of some communal goal such as preparing and eating a meal (Howe, 2002). Family *rituals* are also patterned behaviors, but these events have a stronger emotional and existential meaning for the family. Rituals define and reinforce family identity and relationship expectations and are symbolic in nature. They may mark occasions reflecting such family transitions as weddings or funerals (Howe, 2002), as well as more mundane events that harbor special meaning for the family such as Sunday dinners (Fiese et al., 2002). Both routines and rituals involve multiple family members and complex communication patterns (Denham, 2003) and may be passed down in the family across generations. Routines can involve ritual aspects and, over time, may evolve into rituals. Given these definitions, it becomes clear that the diagnosis of an illness can impinge on both routines and rituals. When routines are disrupted, the family may experience a sense of daily hassle; when rituals are disrupted or become negative, the fabric of the family may be threatened (Fiese et al., 2002).

Medically related routines have the potential to enhance medical adherence and play an important role in promoting health and managing illness. The meaning of that routine, the ritual aspect, may have a positive or potentially negative impact on the family and its individual members (Fiese, 2006). Routines may help the patient feel secure and cared for; however, if those routines are perceived as overwhelming or burdensome and these interactions come to define the family then family functioning and medical outcomes may be compromised.

EMPIRICAL EVIDENCE

Qualitative research examining family routines and rituals documents the manner in which the demands of illness and treatment greatly impact existing behavioral patterns (e.g., Buchbinder, Longhofer, & McCue, 2009). Furthermore, in samples ranging from the families of ill children to the elderly, this research provides examples of the ways in which the medical needs of a family member are integrated into such family routines as meals, morning routines, exercise, and medical appointments (e.g., Gallant, Spitze, & Prohaska, 2007; Gregory, 2005; Segal, 2004). Because of developmental shifts in responsibilities for medical management during the adolescent and young adult years, many reports focus on the challenges of creating, maintaining, and effectively adapting family routines to manage illness during this phase of family life (e.g., Newbould, Smith, & Francis, 2008; B. Williams, Mukhopadhyay, Dowell, & Coyle, 2007).

Family routines have been found to be protective in a range of illnesses and throughout the lifespan. For example, the creation of regular family routines has facilitated improved nutrition in infants diagnosed with failure-to-thrive (Yoos, Kitzman, & Cole, 1999). An early study demonstrated that fewer family routines and poorer family organization were linked to increased incidents and severity of upper respiratory infections among preschool children (Boyce et al., 1977). Families with children with asthma who reported more routines related to filling and taking asthma medications were more adherent to their prescribed regimen and forgot medications less frequently (Fiese, Wamboldt, & Anbar, 2005). Further, those families describing their asthma management strategy as reactive to symptomatology, characterized by little planning or forethought, were less adherent to treatment and three times more likely to use the emergency department for care than those with more coordinated, deliberate, and cooperative asthma management strategies (Fiese et al., 2005). Studies of adolescents with diabetes have found that inconsistencies in summer routines were associated with poorer metabolic control and higher HbA1cs when school resumed (Boland, Grey, Mezger, & Tamborlane, 1999). Ethnographic studies have uncovered that adults with diabetes whose families adapted their routines to meet nutritional recommendations (e.g., providing meals on time, including fresh fruits and vegetables) had better glycemic control than did those adults whose families failed to make such changes (Gerstle, Varenne, & Contento, 2001). Also, more routine within families has been linked to fewer pain-related episodes for adults with chronic pain (Bush & Pargament, 1997) and children with chronic headaches (Frare, Axia, & Battistella, 2002).

Family rituals, the emotionally meaningful component of family routines, may be preexisting family events maintained despite the illness, changed to incorporate the illness, or developed specifically because of the illness. Eloquent examples of such rituals are described in Buchbinder et al. (2009). Though the available research evidence is scant, the ritual aspects of family life seem most strongly related to the quality of life or emotional well-being of the family members, but there is some evidence linking such rituals to medical well-being. For example, parents' reports of greater meaning or symbolic significance in family events (e.g., dinner times, weekends, vacations, celebrations, and cultural traditions) have been linked to less anxiety for children with asthma (Markson & Fiese, 2000), whereas parents' reports of greater burden associated with medical care were related to self-reports of poorer physical and emotional health and more child-reported episodes of wheezing (Fiese, 2006).

IMPLICATIONS FOR INTERVENTION

The routines and rituals framework for understanding family influence on health and illness clearly indicates that interventions targeting the development and maintenance of family routines and the establishment of rituals with positive adaptive meanings are indicated when a family is having difficulties meeting the health care needs of its members. The authors of this model have outlined different family types based on the enactment of and engagement in routines and rituals and propose specific recommendations for intervention (Fiese, 2000, 2007; Fiese & Walmboldt, 2000). These recommendations recognize that a change in family health routines typically requires reorganization of daily behavioral patterns and possibly a change in the family belief system.

BIOBEHAVIORAL FAMILY MODEL

The biobehavioral family model (Wood, 2001; Wood, Klebba, & Miller, 2000), building on the early work of Minuchin (1974), proposes that the emotional climate of the family, the quality of the relationships and feelings of security between family members, and the biobehavioral reactivity of members influence one another and interact to either mitigate or exacerbate disease severity in stress-related illnesses such as asthma, cardiovascular incidents, and diabetes (Wood et al., 2008). Each of these factors may negatively impact disease management through decreased adherence, but each is also predicted to directly impact disease severity through physiological effects.

The *emotional climate* of the family can be characterized by its valence and intensity. A negative emotional climate includes hostility, criticism, and verbal attacks; whereas a positive emotional climate includes warmth, affection, and support. The intensity of the emotional climate can be characterized by the balance between positive and negative emotional aspects. Various factors influence the emotional climate of the family, including the extent to which family members (a) share space, information, and emotions; (b) have interactional patterns characterized by mutual support and understanding as opposed to hostility, rejection, and conflict; and (c) respond to each other appropriately emotionally, behaviorally, and physiologically. In determining the emotional climate of the family, researchers also pay attention to the quality and integrity of the parental relationship and the marital subsystem.

Biobehavioral reactivity is a pivotal construct in this model, which links psychological and emotional processes at the level of the family to disease processes in the individual family member. This reactivity is displayed in the manner with which an individual family member responds physiologically, emotionally, and behaviorally to emotional stimuli (Thayer & Lane, 2000). Emotional dysregulation, a response that does not match the requirements of the external or internal environment, can influence such physiological pathways as the hypothalamic-pituitary-adrenal axis and the autonomic nervous system that are implicated in health and illness (Wood et al., 2008). For example, sympathetic arousal in response to chronic anxiety, fear, and interpersonal stress may disrupt immune function and promote infectious disease, cardiovascular disease, or diabetes. Emotionally induced parasympathetic activation may complicate asthma or gastrointestinal disorders (Wood, 2001). Thus, any illnesses with stress reactivity, or the presence of a biobehavioral or psychophysiological pathway, may be impacted by emotional dysregulation of the individual and the emotional climate of the family (Wood & Miller, 2005).

Conceived to capture the impact of the family on child health and illness, revisions of this model have included *emotional security and attachment* within the parent-child relationship to be another important component, mediating or moderating the relationships between family emotional climate and physiological processes (Wood et al., 2000). The authors argue, however, that this model may be applicable to any type of physical or psychologically manifested disease in any family member (i.e., child or adult; Wood et al., 2000). This model is most frequently researched within the context of pediatric asthma.

EMPIRICAL EVIDENCE

Conceptualizing family interactional patterns as triggers of physiological processes within family members is not a new proposal, (e.g., Minuchin et al., 1975); evidence of this concept has been accumulating for decades (for a recent, relatively comprehensive review, see Wood & Miller, 2005). Among healthy adults, marital conflict has been found to increase blood pressure, heart rate, and stress hormones and alter immune functioning (e.g., Broadwell & Light, 1999; Mayne, O'Leary, McCrady, Contrada, & Labouvie, 1997; Nealy-Moore, Smith, Uchino, Hawkins, & Olson-Cerny, 2007; Robles & Kiecolt-Glaser, 2003). Among women with heart disease, marital stress has been linked with increased risk for reoccurring coronary problems and cardiac-related death (Orth-Gomer et al., 2000). Marital distress has also been linked to higher levels of child urinary catecholamines and cardiovascular reactivity (e.g., El-Sheikh & Harger, 2001; Gottman & Katz, 1989; see Troxel & Matthews, 2004, for a review). Furthermore, a negative emotional climate within the family characterized by cold, unsupportive, and neglectful parenting styles has been found to predict abnormal cortisol responses, suppressed immunity, and increased illness frequency for children (Flinn & England, 1997; see Repetti, Taylor, & Seeman, 2002, for a review). In addition, the emotional regulation processes of the child are empirically supported as a key pathway linking child health outcomes with marital discord or a negative emotional climate within the family (Calkins, 1994; Cummings & Davies, 2002; Cummings, Iannotti, & Zahn-Waxler, 1985).

Recent research specifically examining the biobehavioral family model has provided evidence that among families of children with asthma, a negative emotional climate contributes to depressive symptoms in the child, which in turn contribute to asthma disease severity (Wood et al., 2007; Wood et al., 2008; Wood et al., 2006). For example, in their most recently published study, Wood and colleagues report that families with greater observed conflict and less warmth had children who self-reported more symptoms of depression, and greater child depression was related to objective indices of their asthma severity (Wood et al., 2008). Other studies of this model have found similar patterns using parental reports of emotional climate and parent and observer reports of child depression. Child-reported depression was associated with objective measures of disease severity even after controlling for medical adherence (Wood et al., 2006). Findings regarding the specific role of attachment or relationship security in the model are inconsistent across studies.

IMPLICATIONS FOR INTERVENTION

Stemming from a family systems perspective, the biobehavioral family model calls for family therapy approaches to improve the physiological functioning of individual family members. This approach to intervention holds that careful assessment of family patterns and their specific outcomes needs to occur for each and every family because no particular family pattern or configuration is necessarily maladaptive for all families (Wood, 1994). Special attention should, however, be paid to aspects of the family structure (e.g., patterns of alliance between family members, strength of the marital subsystem) and the emotional climate of the family, the individual physiological reactivity of the family members, and the cyclical patterns of interpersonal behaviors, emotional reactions, and physical symptoms. Therapy that realigns the structure of the family, promotes a more positive emotional climate, fosters security within familial relationships, and helps the family develop skills for modulating emotion (as needed) is proposed to break the cyclical maladaptive patterns the family has developed. For case studies, see Wood (1994, 2001).

SUMMARY

Two specific pathways have been identified as possible mechanisms for the influence of the family on health and illness: behavioral pathways and physiological pathways. Empirical evidence exists to support both of these models, and it is quite likely that these mechanisms of effect coexist and collaboratively determine the influence of the family on health maintenance and disease management. The empirical evidence supporting these models suggests that interventions focusing on skills for establishing family routines and rituals and/or on remediating the emotional climate of the family (e.g., cohesion, warmth, conflict) are pathways through which an individual's health can be improved.

FAMILY-BASED INTERVENTION RESEARCH

Acknowledgment of the importance of the family's role in health and illness shifts the focus of behavioral medicine interventions from the individual patient to the family. Family-based interventions may take various forms ranging from simply educating a patient about the importance of enlisting family support, to inviting a spouse, adult child, or parent into the patient's medical appointment to increase knowledge and understanding of a disease or treatment regimen, to therapy involving multiple family members aimed at improving communication and family functioning and reducing distress in an effort to improve management of health and illness. Family-based intervention studies are more common with families of children with illness, but important examples of family-based interventions for adults with illness are emerging. Evidence for the superiority of family-based interventions relative to patient-only interventions is not overwhelming (Lewandowski, Morris, Draucker, & Risko, 2007; Martire, 2005), and there are many challenges in conducting family-based intervention research with illness populations (Lutz Stehl et al., 2009); therefore, high-quality studies are rare (Campbell, 2003; Martire & Schulz, 2007). To illustrate this clinical approach and area of investigation, next are provided examples of interventions involving multiple family members and targeting aspects of family functioning with the express purpose of improving illness course and medical or psychosocial outcomes.

CHILDHOOD ILLNESSES

Various family-based interventions have been examined for families of children with a range of disorders, including diabetes, asthma, cystic fibrosis, obesity, cancer, sickle cell disease, HIV, and recurrent abdominal pain (see Alderfer & Rourke, 2009, for an overview), and are emerging as part of medical care for obesity (e.g., Kitzmann & Beech, 2006), traumatic brain injury (e.g., Wade, Carey, & Wolfe, 2006a, 2006b), and sickle cell disease (e.g., Kaslow, 2000). Interventions to improve psychological distress among families of children with cancer have also been tested with some success (i.e., Hoekstra-Weebers, Heuvel, Jaspers, Kamps, & Klip, 1998; Kazak, Alderfer, Streisand, et al., 2004; Kazak et al., 2005). The majority of these interventions target multiple aspects of the family, including emotional and organizational components, as well as such relationship skills as collaborative problem solving and communication. Many interventions also include psychoeducational components and disease training; and some emphasize building skills, clarifying expectations and roles, setting goals, and establishing disease-management routines (e.g., Bartholomew et al., 1997; Barlett, Lukk, Butz, Lampros-Klein, & Rand, 2002; Bruzzese, Unikel, Gallagher, Evans, & Colland, 2008; Ellis, Naar-King, Cunningham, & Secord, 2006; Ellis et al., 2005; Georgiou et al., 2003; Goldbeck & Babka, 2001; Naar-King, Ellis, Kolmodin, Cunnigham, & Secord, 2009; Ng et al., 2008; von Schlippe, Theiling, Lob-Corzilius, & Szczepanski, 2001; Weinstein, Chenkin, & Faust, 1997). A few examples of well-researched family-based interventions for children include Behavioral Family Systems Therapy (BFST; Wysocki et al., 2006) and the Family Teamwork Intervention (Anderson, Brackett, Ho, & Laffel, 2000).

Although adapted for use with various childhood diseases (e.g., Quittner et al., 2000), BFST has been examined most closely when used with families of children with diabetes (Harris, Harris, & Mertlich, 2005; Wysocki, Greco, Harris, Bubb, & White, 2001; Wysocki et al., 2000). The intervention involves (a) training in communication and problem-solving skills; (b) cognitive restructuring to address counterproductive beliefs, attributions, and assumption held by family members regarding one another's behaviors; and (c) systemic family therapy techniques to strengthen appropriate boundaries, roles, and relationships. A recent revision of the intervention includes rigorous diabetes-management-training components—for example, behavioral contracting around adherence, clinical algorithms for modifying insulin injections based on blood glucose readings, and parents' simulatations of living with diabetes for one week—in part patterned after a successful trial by Satin, La Greca, Zigo, and Skyler (1989). Randomized clinical trials of BFST have found greater improvements in parent–teen relations, reductions in diabetes-specific conflict, and improved treatment adherence when compared to standard care and an educational support group (Wysocki et al., 2001; Wysocki et al., 2000). The most recent version has also been found to improve metabolic control (Wysocki et al., 2006).

A brief Family Teamwork Intervention has also been developed and evaluated for families of children with diabetes (Anderson et al., 2000). This intervention focuses on the importance of sharing diabetes management tasks among parents and teens and establishing ways to avoid conflicts that undermine teamwork. The intervention includes written educational materials about diabetes and ways parents and teens can work together effectively (i.e., without blaming or shaming). A plan of shared responsibility is tailored to each family, and the plan is reviewed, reinforced, and/or renegotiated as part of routine medical visits. When compared to treatment as usual and an attention control group in a randomized controlled trial, the Family Teamwork Intervention group demonstrated maintenance of or increases in parental involvement in diabetes care without increases in parent–child conflict or decreases in adolescent quality of life (Anderson, Brackett, Ho, & Laffel, 1999; Laffel et al., 2003).

ADULT ILLNESSES

Although impacting many more families than do childhood illnesses, adult illnesses are less commonly managed with the help of family-based interventions that involve multiple family members and are focused on improving family functioning as a means of improving medical outcomes. Many empirically based, theory-driven family interventions have been suggested in the literature (e.g., Fisher et al., 1998; Kayser & Scott, 2008; Lewandowski et al., 2007; Power & Dell Orto, 2004; Stiell, Naaman, & Lee, 2007; Watson & McDaniel, 2005), but few have been scientifically evaluated. This lack of empirical evaluation is even true for Medical Family Therapy (Linville, Hertlein, & Lyness, 2007; Ruddy & McDaniel, 2003; Sholevar & Sahar, 2003), first appearing in the literature over 15 years ago.

Because a thorough review of this literature is beyond the scope of this chapter, just a few examples will be provided here. Two examples of larger-scale randomized clinical trials of family-based interventions with adults experiencing chronic illness include Scott, Halford, and Ward's (2004) couples intervention for women newly diagnosed with cancer and Martire, Schulz, Keefe, Rudy, and Starz's (2008) couples intervention for patients with osteoarthritis. The first of these randomly assigned women with early-stage cancer to either a couples-based coping intervention with their partners, an individual coping intervention for the patient alone, or an education control group. The second randomly assigned patients with osteoarthritis to one of three similar groups: a couples-oriented education and support intervention, a patient-oriented intervention, or standard care. In both studies, the couples-based interventions produced better outcomes than did the other groups, documenting decreased distress, decreased spousal anger and irritation, and increased empathic communication and mutual support.

Also emerging in the literature over the past five years have been small-scale pilot feasibility studies of family-based interventions spanning other adult diseases. For example, Keogh and colleagues have presented pilot data indicating that a three-session family-based intervention to improve outcomes for adults with poorly controlled Type 2 diabetes is feasible to conduct (Keogh et al., 2007). Allen (2009) found that a pilot investigation of the Legacy Project fulfilled its intended goals of increasing communication and positive emotional experiences within families of adults with chronic, life-limiting illnesses. Likewise, Baucom and colleagues (2009) found that couples-based interventions to enhance relationships and psychological functioning of women newly diagnosed with breast or gynecological cancer and their partners were successful in achieving their aims. Finally, a randomized pilot study by Dunbar and colleagues (2005) revealed that patients with heart failure displayed better health outcomes when a family intervention targeting increased family support, empathy, and communication regarding health–related matters was added to an education intervention.

Intervention research aimed at evaluating programs that include or target adjustment of children of adults with illness is scarce (see Spath, 2007, for a review), though emerging (e.g., Laroche, Davis, Forman, Palmisano, & Heisler, 2007; Rotheram-Borus et al., 2006).

CONCLUSION

Conceptualizing health and illness within the context of the family allows the researcher and clinician to begin to appreciate the influence of individuals on their social environment and the impact of the social environment on the individual. Clearly, stable, secure family environments support the behaviors needed for sustaining health and managing disease. They also help buffer distress arising from the diagnosis and treatment of illness while ensuring that normative developmental goals are accomplished for the family and its members. Illness also has a large impact on the family, however.

The diagnosis may raise negative emotions for family members, thereby disrupting their ability to adequately support and interact positively with one another. Differences in coping styles and problem-solving strategies among family members may lead to conflict. Furthermore, the demands of treatment may necessitate uncomfortable shifts in family roles, responsibilities, and routines. The exchange of negative emotions among family members may lead to physiological reactivity that may further exacerbate illness. On the other hand, the adversity of an illness may bring the family members closer together, realign their priorities, and give them a broader sense of belonging in the world, thus allowing them to become more resilient.

As illustrated in the foregoing discussion, consideration of the family context provides a rich, vibrant, dynamic perspective of health and illness. This perspective allows for the identification of potential sources of support and mechanisms for improved health while also suggesting potential barriers to effective medical care. Various models have been developed to capture the ways in which illness impacts families and families impact illness. These models agree that the diagnosis of illness in a family member will cause turmoil within the family, impacting the family's emotional climate (e.g., cohesion, affective environment) and organizational structure (e.g., adaptability, roles). In turn, theorists have proposed that the family has a direct influence on the health and illness of its members through these same channels (i.e., emotional climate and organizational structure), as evidenced in the routines and rituals of family life and in the biobehavioral processes that unfold within familial interactions. The empirical base supporting these theories is growing. Though empirical evidence of the efficacy of family-based interventions for fostering health and improving disease management is not plentiful, the existing data indicate that attending to the family—the social context of health and illness—is important.

LIMITATIONS OF CURRENT RESEARCH

Despite this progress in conceptualizing and understanding health and illness in the context of the family, there are many limitations to the current empirical base and there remain gaps in our knowledge. For example, most of the research investigating family functioning and medical outcomes is cross-sectional in nature, thereby hampering our true understanding of the ways in which families and illness reciprocally impact one another. Population-based research longitudinally assessing the family dynamics of a large pool of families prior to and then repeatedly after the occurrence of a health crisis would provide a clear window into the ways illness impacts families and families impact illness; but given the relatively low incidence and often unpredictable nature of any single type of medical event, such research would be incredibly time intensive and costly. Still, longitudinal research after a medical event has occurred would provide valuable information as to how families and illness interact over time. Such longitudinal research is rare.

Another limitation of our current research is evident in our measurement techniques. Some research attempting to focus on the family uses a single family member's self-reported perspective to operationalize such constructs. Though this approach may be time efficient, it may also produce a biased or incomplete picture of the family. Seeking the perspectives of multiple family members or observing and coding the interactions of families may be more challenging to accomplish in the context of a research study but may provide a more reliable and valid picture of the family as a whole.

A third limitation in our current research is a lack of precision in applying models or theories of family functioning and illness to our study designs. As evidenced in this chapter, detailed models outline important family and illness characteristics believed to influence their interplay; however, research studies may not specifically adopt a model on which to base their research design; that is, they may fail to measure all the factors deemed to be important. Further, the studies may be underpowered to systematically evaluate all aspects of these models. For example, many of the models presented discuss the importance of considering characteristics of the family (e.g., their configuration, their developmental stage, their past experiences and beliefs about illness) and characteristics of the illness (e.g., specific diagnosis, stage of treatment, course, prognosis) and the fit between these sets of variables. Examining such models in research would require very large or very homogeneous samples that are difficult to achieve, hampering our efforts to validate models and to understand the true complexities in the interactions between families and illness.

A final example of a limitation of the current research concerns family-based intervention research. Family-based intervention research in the context of acute or chronic medical conditions is scarce, probably because it is very challenging. To ensure the internal validity of intervention research findings, studies need to adhere to strict inclusion criteria to ensure homogeneity of the sample, collect repeated assessments, and randomize families to condition. Specific to family-based research, multiple members of the family must also be present. These research requirements may seem unreasonable to families dealing with the stress of illness. Such participant reactions, attributable to the research process itself, are often inextricably entangled with data regarding the acceptability and feasibility of the interventions (see Lutz Stehl et al., 2009). This confounding may inadvertently lead to the conclusion that family-based interventions are unacceptable to participants, unfeasible to conduct, or not worth the effort. More research regarding the efficacy and effectiveness of family-based interventions for improving medical outcomes is vital. Methodologies other than randomized clinical trials (e.g., case-series reports, patient-preference designs) can contribute to our understanding of the usefulness of family-based intervention research and should be used in concert with randomized clinical trials as we strive for ways to reduce the burden of intervention research on families (Laurenceau, Hayes, & Feldman, 2007).

FUTURE DIRECTIONS

In sum, the complexity of family-based conceptualizations of health and illness makes this domain of research inherently interesting but also uniquely difficult. Fortunately, methodological and statistical advances are allowing this field of research to move forward. Efforts are emerging to discuss and address limitations in our measurement of family-level variables within illness populations (e.g., Alderfer et al., 2008). For example, the validity of family measures needs to be considered when examining family functioning when a member has an illness. Such families may score in "unhealthy" or "dysfunctional" ranges on certain family-functioning dimensions using norms and cutoffs developed in the general population; however, these patterns of functioning may actually assist the family in managing treatment or adapting to illness (e.g., high levels of rigidity may improve adherence). Calls are being made for additional research in these realms, and new work in this area is emerging (e.g., Marsac & Alderfer, 2011).

Combining data from multiple members of a family reporting on family functioning has been a long-standing challenge in family-based research. Although no perfect answers exist, recent recommendations have been made regarding ways to integrate data from multiple family members in either research or treatment contexts (e.g., Atkins, 2005; Cook & Kenny, 2004; Dekovic & Buist, 2005). Furthermore, multilevel statistical models are allowing researchers to consider the family as the unit of analysis, recognizing dependencies inherent in data emerging from a single family, and allowing for exploration of within- and between-family variability (e.g., Kenny, Kashy, & Cook, 2006). When used with longitudinal data, information about changes within individuals and families across time can be considered in the context of changes in other family members or illness symptomatology revealing the complex, dynamic interplay that is postulated in our theoretical models. Although large-scale studies are still needed to capture the intricacies of our theoretical models, such statistical advances are allowing for more accurate evaluation of the proposed effects.

As we move forward in this research, we must also consider the broader social context of our work and the evolving nature of both family and illness. Families vary greatly in structure, and that variety abounds in our country, which is seeing a growing number of single-parent households and blended families (Teachman, Tedrow, & Crowder, 2000). In these and in other families, "extended" family members, fictive kin, or friends may actually be part of the primary family unit and should be considered for family-based research studies. Our family assessment methods are challenged by these issues, but valuable suggestions have recently been published regarding ways to ensure assessment quality, given these circumstances (see Hofferth & Casper, 2007). Likewise, the ethnic, cultural, and linguistic backgrounds of families are becoming more diverse in America; those individuals at greatest physical risk may be more likely to reside in poverty with limited educational backgrounds (Repetti et al., 2002). Again, such variation in family background may result in lower reliability, validity, and generalizability of our studies. However, item response theory is allowing researchers to more adequately address issues of measure equivalence across diverse sociocultural groups (see Bingenheimer, Raudenbush, Leventhal, & Brooks-Gunn, 2005).

Furthermore, the nature of illness is changing as medical advances continue to transform acute, life-threatening illnesses into chronic ones (e.g., cancer, cardiac conditions), and complex, time-consuming medical treatment regimens into more efficient, automated processes (e.g., insulin pumps). The evolving nature of illness and the larger social contexts in which it exists—whether national health care policy, direct-to-consumer drug advertising, or increased reliance on outpatient and home-based care—need to be considered because these cultural changes may pose new and different challenges for families.

CONCLUDING REMARKS

Despite the challenging nature of conceptualizing health and illness in the context of the family, more research is needed in this area. New heuristics, methodologies, and statistical procedures are emerging that will enable researchers to better address the complex reciprocal interplay of families and health and illness as conceptualized in our models. As mentioned earlier, larger scale, theoretically-based longitudinal research is greatly needed to move this field forward. Specific areas of emphasis in future research should include family-based intervention research with attention to theoretically-based mechanisms of effect. Although research is emerging regarding family-based interventions when a child is ill and couples-based interventions when an adult is ill, very little attention has been paid to interventions addressing the needs of children of parents with illness or exploring the role of children in the management of parental illness. Likewise, more knowledge is needed regarding the way in which different family types, defined possibly by structure (e.g., single-parent versus two-parent) or cultural background (e.g., ethnicity, race), manage illness most effectively. Finally, examination of the ways in which the family responds to and manages illness within the context of such broader social systems as friends, schools, workplaces, communities, and public policy is important. Taking a broad systemic view will further enhance our understanding of health and illness in the context of the family and also the greater social ecology.

REFERENCES

Alderfer, M. A., Fiese, B., Gold, J., Cutuli, J. J., Holmbeck, G., Goldbeck, L., … Patterson, J. (2008). Evidence based assessment in pediatric psychology: Family measures. *Journal of Pediatric Psychology*, *33*, 1046–1061.

Alderfer, M. A., & Kazak, A. E. (2006). Family issues when a child is on treatment for cancer. In R. Brown (Ed.), *Pediatric hematology/oncology: A biopsychosocial approach* (pp. 53–74). New York, NY: Oxford University Press.

Alderfer, M. A., Long, K. A., Lown, E. A., Marsland, A. L., Ostrowski, N. L., Hock, J. M., & Ewing, L. J. (2010). Psychosocial adjustment of siblings of children with cancer: A systematic review. *Psycho-oncology*, *19*, 789–805.

Alderfer, M. A., Navsaria, N., & Kazak, A. E. (2009). Family functioning and posttraumatic stress disorder in adolescent survivors of childhood cancer. *Journal of Family Psychology*, *23*, 717–725.

Alderfer, M. A., & Rourke, M. T. (2009). Family psychology in the context of pediatric medical conditions. In J. H. Bray & M. Stanton (Eds.), *Handbook of family psychology* (pp. 527–538). West Sussex, England: Wiley Blackwell.

Allen, R. S. (2009). The Legacy Project intervention to enhance meaningful family interactions: Case examples. *Clinical Gerontologist*, *32*, 164–176.

Ammerman, R. T., Kane, V. R., Slomka, G. T., Reigel, D. H., Franzen, M. D., & Gadow, K. D. (1998). Psychiatric symptomatology and family functioning in children and adolescents with spina bifida. *Journal of Clinical Psychology in Medical Settings, 5*, 449–465.

Anderson, B. J., Brackett, J., Ho, J., & Laffel, L. M. (1999). An office-based intervention to maintain parent-adolescent teamwork in diabetes management. *Diabetes Care, 22*, 713–721.

Anderson, B. J., Brackett, J., Ho, J., & Laffel, L. M. B. (2000). An intervention to promote family teamwork in diabetes management tasks. In D. Drotar (Ed.), *Promoting adherence to medical treatment in chronic childhood illness: Concepts, methods, and interventions* (pp. 347–365). Mahwah, NJ: Erlbaum.

Atkins, D. C. (2005). Using multilevel models to analyze couple and family treatment data: Basic and advanced issues. *Journal of Family Psychology, 19*, 98–110.

Barakat, L. P., Smith-Whitley, K., & Ohene-Frempong, K. (2002). Treatment adherence in children with sickle cell disease: Disease-related risk and psychosocial resistance factors. *Journal of Clinical Psychology in Medical Settings, 9*, 201–209.

Bartholomew, L. K., Czyzewski, D. I., Parcel, G. S., Swank, P. R., Sockrider, M. M., Mariotto, M. J., … Seilheimer, D. K. (1997). Self-management of cystic fibrosis: Short-term outcomes of the Cystic Fibrosis Family Education Program. *Health Education & Behavior, 24*, 652–666.

Bartlett, S. J., Lukk, P., Butz, A., Lampros-Klein, F., & Rand, C. S. (2002). Enhancing medication adherence among inner-city children with asthma: Results from pilot studies. *Journal of Asthma, 39*, 47–54.

Baucom, D., Porter, L., Kirby, J., Gremore, T. M., Wiesenthal, N., Aldridge, W., … Keefe, F. J. (2009). A couple-based intervention for female breast cancer. *Psycho-oncology, 18*, 276–283.

Beals, K. P., Wight, R. G., Aneshensel, C. S., Murphy, D. A., & Miller-Martinez, D. (2006). The role of family caregivers in HIV medication adherence. *AIDS Care, 18*, 589–596.

Bender, B., Milgrom, H., Rand, C., & Ackerson, L. (1998). Psychological factors associated with medication nonadherence in asthmatic children. *Journal of Asthma, 35*, 347–353.

Berge, J. M., & Patterson, J. M. (2004). Cystic fibrosis and the family: A review and critique of the literature. *Families, Systems & Health, 22*, 74–100.

Beverly, E. A., Miller, C. K., & Wray, L. A. (2008). Spousal support and food related behavior change in middle-aged and older adults living with type 2 diabetes. *Health Education & Behavior, 35*, 707–720.

Beverly, E. A., Penrod, J., & Wray, L. A. (2007). Living with type 2 diabetes. *Journal of Psychosocial Nursing, 45*, 25–32.

Bingenheimer, J. B., Raudenbush, S. W., Leventhal, T., & Brooks-Gunn, J. (2005). Measurement equivalence and differential item functioning in family psychology. *Journal of Family Psychology, 19*, 441–455.

Blair, C., Freeman, C., & Cull, A. (1995). The families of anorexia nervosa and cystic fibrosis patients. *Psychological Medicine, 25*(5), 985–993.

Boland, E. M., Grey, M., Mezger, J., & Tamborlane, W. V. (1999). A summer vacation from diabetes: Evidence from a clinical trial. *Diabetes Education, 25*, 31–40.

Boss, P. (1988). *Family stress management: Family studies text series* (Vol. 8). Thousand Oaks, CA: Sage.

Boyce, W., Jensen, E., Cassel, J., Collier, A., Smith, A., & Ramey, C. (1977). Influences of life events and family routines on childhood respiratory tract illness. *Pediatrics, 17*, 609–615.

Broadwell, S. D., & Light, K. C. (1999). Family support and cardiovascular responses in married couples during conflict and other interactions. *International Journal of Behavioral Medicine, 6*, 40–63.

Brody, G. H., Kogan, S. M., Murry, V. M., Chen, Y., & Brown, A. C. (2008). Psychological functioning, support for self-management, and glycemic control among rural African American adults with diabetes mellitus type 2. *Health Psychology, 27*, S83–S90.

Bronfenbrenner, U. (1977). Toward an experimental ecology of human development. *American Psychologist, 32*, 513–531.

Brown, C., Pikler, V., Lavish, L., Keune, K., & Hutto, C. (2008). Surviving childhood leukemia: Career, family, and future expectations. *Qualitative Health Research, 18*, 19–30.

Bruzzese, J. M., Unikel, L., Gallagher, R., Evans, D., & Collard, V. (2008). Feasibility and impact of a school-based intervention for families of urban adolescents with asthma: Results from a randomized pilot trial. *Family Process, 47*, 95–113.

Buchbinder, M., Longhofer, J., & McCue, K. (2009). Family routines and rituals when a parent has cancer. *Family, Systems, & Health, 27*, 213–227.

Bush, E., & Pargament, K. (1997). Family coping with chronic pain. *Families, Systems, & Health, 15*, 147–160.

Calkins, S. D. (1994). Origins and outcomes of individual differences in emotional regulation. *Monographs of the Society for Research in Child Development, 59*, 53–72.

Campbell, T. L. (2003). The effectiveness of family interventions for physical disorders. *Journal of Marital & Family Therapy*, *29*, 263–281.

Chesla, C. A. (1999). Becoming resilient: Skill development in couples living with non–insulin dependent diabetes. In H. I. McCubbin, E. A. Thompson, A. I. Thompson, & J. A. Futrell (Eds.), *The dynamics of resilient families* (pp. 99–134). Thousand Oaks, CA: Sage.

Chesla, C. A., Fisher, L., Skaff, M. M., Mullan, J. T., Gilliss, C. L., & Kanter, R. (2003). Family predictors of disease management over one year in Latino and European American patients with type 2 diabetes. *Family Process*, *42*, 375–390.

Cochrane, B. B., & Lewis, F. M. (2005). Partner's adjustment to breast cancer: A critical analysis of intervention studies. *Health Psychology*, *24* (3), 327–332.

Cohen, D. M., Lumley, M. A., Naar-King, S., Partridge, T., & Cakan, N. (2004). Child behavior problems and family functioning as predictors of adherence and glycemic control in economically disadvantaged children with type 1 diabetes. *Journal of Pediatric Psychology*, *29*, 171–184.

Compas, B. E., Worsham, N. L., Epping-Jordan, J. E., Grant, K. E., Mireault, G., Howell, D. C., & Malcarne, V. (1994). When mom or dad has cancer: Markers of psychological distress in cancer patients, spouses, and children. *Health Psychology*, *15*, 167–175.

Cook, W. L., & Kenny, D. A. (2004). Application of the social relations model to family assessment. *Journal of Family Psychology*, *18*, 361–371.

Cooper J., Bloch, S., Love, A., Macvean, M., Duchesne, G. M., & Kissane, D. (2006). Psychosocial adjustment of female partners of men with prostate cancer. *Psycho-oncology*, *15*, 937–953.

Cummings, M. E., & Davies, P. (2002). Effects of marital conflict on children: Recent advances & emerging themes in process-oriented research. *Journal of Child Psychology & Psychiatry*, *43*, 31–63.

Cummings, M. E., Iannotti, R. J., & Zahn-Waxler, C. (1985). Influence of conflict between adults on the emotions and aggression of young children. *Developmental Psychology*, *21*, 495–507.

Dashiff, C. J. (1993). Parents' perceptions of diabetes in adolescent daughters and its impact on the family. *Journal of Pediatric Nursing*, *8*, 361–369.

Dekovic, M., & Buist, K. (2005). Multiple perspectives within the family: Family relationship patterns. *Journal of Family Issues*, *26*, 467–490.

DeLambo, K. E., Ievers-Landis, C. E., Drotar, D., & Quittner, A. L. (2004). Association of observed family relationship quality and problem-solving skills with treatment adherence in older children and adolescents with cystic fibrosis. *Journal of Pediatric Psychology*, *29*, 343–353.

Denham, S. A. (2002). Family routines: A structural perspective for viewing family health. *Advanced Nursing Science*, *24*, 60–74.

Denham, S. A. (2003). Relationships between family rituals, family routines, and health. *Journal of Family Nursing*, *9*, 305–330.

Dumont, R. H., Jacobson, A. M., Cole, C., Hauser, S. T., Wolfsdorf, J. I., Willett, J. B., … Wertlieb, D. (1995). Psycho-social predictors of acute complications of diabetes in youth. *Diabetic Medicine*, *12*, 612–618.

Dunbar, S., Clark, P., Deaton, C., Smith, A., De, A., & O'Brien, M. (2005). Family education and support interventions in heart failure: A pilot study. *Nursing Research*, *54*, 158–166.

Dura, J. R., & Beck, S. J. (1988). A comparison of family functioning when mothers have chronic pain. *Pain*, *35*, 79–89.

El-Sheikh, M., & Harger, J. (2001). Appraisals of marital conflict and children's adjustment, health, and physiological reactivity. *Developmental Psychology*, *37*, 875–885.

Ellis, D. A., Naar-King, S., Cunningham, P., & Secord, E. (2006). Use of multisystemic therapy to improve antiretroviral adherence and health outcomes in HIV-infected pediatric patients: Evaluation of a pilot program. *AIDS Patient Care and STDs*, *20*, 112–121.

Ellis, D. A., Naar-King, S., Frey, M., Templin, T., Rowland, M., & Greger, N. (2005). Multisystemic treatment of poorly controlled type 1 diabetes: Effects on medical resource utilization. *Journal of Pediatric Psychology*, *30*, 656–666.

Engle, G. L. (1980). The clinical application of the biopsychosocial model. *American Journal of Psychiatry*, *137*, 535–544.

Eriksson, M., & Svedlund, M. (2006). "The intruder": Spouses' narratives about life with a chronically ill partner. *Journal of Clinical Nursing*, *15*, 324–333.

Evans, R., Bishop, D., & Haselkorn, J. (1991). Factors predicting satisfactory home care after stroke. *Archives of Physical Medicine and Rehabilitation*, *72*, 144–147.

Evans, R. L., & Northwood, L. K. (1983). Social support needs in adjustment to stroke. *Archives of Physical Medicine and Rehabilitation*, *64*, 61–64.

Fiese, B. H. (2000). Family routines, rituals, and asthma management: A proposal for family-based strategies to increase treatment adherence. *Families, Systems & Health, 18*, 405–418.

Fiese, B. H. (2006). *Family routines and rituals.* New Haven, CT: Yale University.

Fiese, B. H. (2007). Routines and rituals: Opportunities for participation in family health. *OTJR: Occupation, Participation, and Health, 27*, S41–S49.

Fiese, B. H., Tomsho, T. J., Douglas, M., Josephs, K., Poltrock, S., & Baker, T. (2002). A review of 50 years of research on naturally occurring family routines and rituals: Cause for celebration? *Journal of Family Psychology, 16*, 381–390.

Fiese, B. H., & Wamboldt, F. (2000). Family routines, rituals, and asthma management: Family-based strategies to increase treatment adherence. *Families, Systems, & Health, 18*, 405–415.

Fiese, B. H., Wamboldt, F. S., & Anbar, R. D. (2005). Family asthma management routines: Connections to medical adherence and quality of life. *Journal of Pediatrics, 146*, 171–176.

Fisher, L., Chesla, C., Bartz, R., Gilliss, C., Skaff, M. A., Sabogal, F., … Lutz, C. P. (1998). The family and type 2 diabetes: A framework for intervention. *Diabetes Educator, 24*, 599–607.

Fisher, L., & Weihs, K. L. (2000). Can addressing family relationships improve outcomes in chronic disease? *Journal of Family Practice, 49*, 561–566.

Flinn, M. V., & England, B. G. (1997). Social economics of childhood glucocorticoid stress responses and health. *American Journal of Physical Anthropology, 102*, 33–53.

Frare, M., Axia, G., & Battistella, A. (2002). Quality of life, coping strategies, and family routines in children with headache. *Headache: The Journal of Head and Face Pain, 42*, 953–962.

Gallant, M. P., Spitze, G. D., & Prohaska, T. R. (2007). Help or hindrance: How families and friends influence chronic illness self-management among older adults. *Research on Aging, 29*, 375–409.

Geffken, G. R., Lehmkuhl, H., Walker, K. N., Storch, E. A., Heidgerken, A. D., Lewin, A., … Silverstein, J. (2008). Family functioning processes and diabetic ketoacidosis in youths with type I diabetes. *Rehabilitation Psychology, 53*, 231–237.

Georgiou, A., Buchner, D. A., Ershoff, D. H., Blasko, K. M., Goodman, L. V., & Feigin, J. (2003). The impact of a large-scale population-based asthma management program on pediatric asthma patients and their caregivers. *Annals of Allergy, Asthma, & Immunology, 90*, 308–315.

Gerstle, J., Varenne, H., & Contento, I. (2001). Post-diagnosis family adaptation influences glycemic control in women with type 2 diabetes mellitus. *Journal of the American Dietetic Association, 101*, 918–922.

Glass, T. A., & Maddox, G. L. (1992). The quality and quantity of social support: Stroke recovery as a psychosocial transition. *Social Science & Medicine, 34*, 1249–1261.

Goldbeck, L., & Babka, C. (2001). Development and evaluation of a multi-family psychoeducational program for cystic fibrosis. *Patient Education and Counseling, 44*, 187–192.

Gottman, J. M., & Katz, L. F. (1989). Effects of marital discord on young children's peer interaction and health. *Developmental Psychology, 25*, 373–381.

Gowers, S. G., Jones, J. C., Kiana, S., North, C. D., & Price, D. A. (1995). Family functioning: A correlate of diabetic control? *Journal of Child Psychology and Psychiatry, 36*, 993–101.

Grabiak, B. R., Bender, C. M., & Puskar, K. R. (2007). The impact of parental cancer on the adolescent: An analysis of the literature. *Psycho-oncology, 16*, 127–137.

Gray, R. E., Fitch, M., Phillips, C., Labrecque, M., & Fergus, K. (2000). Managing the impact of illness: The experiences of men with prostate cancer and their spouses. *Journal of Health Psychology, 5*, 531–548.

Gregory, S. (2005). Living with chronic illness in the family setting. *Sociology of Health & Illness, 27*, 372–392.

Harris, M. A., Harris, B. S., & Mertlich, D. (2005). In-home family therapy for adolescents with poorly controlled diabetes: Failure to maintain benefits at 6-month follow-up. *Journal of Pediatric Psychology, 30*, 683–688.

Hill, R. (1949). *Families Under Stress.* New York, NY: Harper & Bros.

Hilton, B., Crawford, J., & Tarko, M. (2000). Men's perspectives on individual and family coping with their wives' breast cancer and chemotherapy. *Western Journal of Nursing Research, 22*, 438–459.

Hobfoll, S. E., & Spielberger, C. D. (1992). Family stress: Integrating theory and measurement. *Journal of Family Psychology, 6*, 99–112.

Hoekstra-Weebers, J. E. M., Heuvel, F., Jaspers, J. P. C., Kamps, W.A., & Klip, E. C. (1998). Brief report: An intervention program for parents of pediatric cancer patients: A randomized controlled trial. *Journal of Pediatric Psychology, 23*, 207–214.

Hofferth, S. L., & Casper, L. M. (Eds.). (2007). *Handbook of measurement issues in family research.* Mahwah, NJ: Erlbaum.

Hoffman, L. (1981). *Foundations of family therapy.* New York, NY: Basic Books.

Horwitz, W. A., & Kazak, A. E. (1990). Family adaptation to childhood cancer: Siblings and family systems variables. *Journal of Clinical Child Psychology, 19*, 221–228.

Howe, G. W. (2002). Integrating family routines and rituals with other family research paradigms: Comment on the special section. *Journal of Family Psychology, 16*, 437–440.

Jones, R., Utz, S., Williams, I., Hinton, I., Alexander, G., Moore, C., ... Oliver, N. (2008). Family interactions among African Americans diagnosed with type 2 diabetes. *Diabetes Educator, 34*, 318–326.

Kanervisto, M., Paavilainen, E., & Heikkila, J. (2007). Family dynamics in families of severe COPD patients. *Journal of Clinical Nursing, 16*, 1498–1505.

Kaslow, N. J. (2000). The efficacy of a pilot family psychoeducational intervention for pediatric sickle cell disease. *Families, Systems & Health, 18*, 381–404.

Kaugars, A. S., Klinnert, M. D., & Bender, B. G. (2004). Family influences on pediatric asthma. *Journal of Pediatric Psychology, 29*, 475–491.

Kayser, K., & Scott, J. (2008). *Helping couples cope with women's cancers: An evidence-based approach for practitioners.* New York, NY: Springer Science & Business Media.

Kazak, A. E., Alderfer, M. A., Rourke, M. T., Simms, S., Streisand, R., & Grossman, J. R. (2004). Posttraumatic stress symptoms (PTSS) and Posttraumatic Stress Disorder (PTSD) in families of adolescent cancer survivors. *Journal of Pediatric Psychology, 29*, 211–219.

Kazak, A. E., Alderfer, M. A., Streisand, R., Simms, S., Rourke, M. T., Barakat, L. P., ... Cnaan, A. (2004). Treatment of posttraumatic stress symptoms in adolescent survivors of childhood cancer and their families: A randomized clinical trial. *Journal of Family Psychology, 18*, 493–504.

Kazak, A. E., Simms, S., Alderfer, M. A., Rourke, M. T., Crump, T., McClure, K., ... Reilly, A. (2005). Feasibility and preliminary outcomes from a pilot study of a brief psychological intervention for families of children newly diagnosed with cancer. *Journal of Pediatric Psychology, 30*, 644–655.

Kenny, D. A., Kashy, D. A., & Cook, W. L. (2006). *Dyadic data analysis.* New York, NY: Guilford Press.

Keogh, K., White, P., Smith, S., McGilloway, S., O'Dowd, T., & Gibney, J. (2007). Changing illness perceptions in patients with poorly controlled type 2 diabetes, a randomized controlled trial of a family-based intervention: Protocol and pilot study. *BMC Family Practice, 8*, 36–46.

Kitzmann, K. M., & Beech, B. M. (2006). Family-based interventions for pediatric obesity. *Journal of Family Psychology, 20*, 175–189.

Laffel, L. M., Vangsness, L., Connell, A., Goebel-Fabbri, A., Butler, D., & Anderson, B. J. (2003). Impact of ambulatory, family-focused teamwork intervention on glycemic control in youth with type I diabetes. *Journal of Pediatrics, 142*, 409–416.

Laroche, H., Davis, M., Forman, J., Palmisano, G., & Heisler, M. (2007). What about the children? The experience of families involved in an adult-focused diabetes intervention. *Public Health Nutrition, 11*, 427–436.

Laurenceau, J. P., Hayes, A. M., & Feldman, G. C. (2007). Some methodological and statistical issues in the study of change processes in psychotherapy. *Clinical Psychology Review, 27*, 682–695.

Lawler, M., Volk, R., Viviani, N., & Mengel, M. (1990). Individual and family factors impacting diabetic control in the adolescent: A preliminary study. *Maternal-Child Nursing Journal, 19*, 331–345.

Leonard, B. J., Jang, Y. P., Savik, K., & Plumbo, M. A. (2005). Adolescents with type 1 diabetes: Family functioning and metabolic control. *Journal of Family Nursing, 11*, 102–121.

Lewandowski, W., Morris, R., Draucker, C. B., & Risko, J. (2007). Chronic pain and the family: Theory-driven treatment approaches. *Issues in Mental Health Nursing, 28*, 1019–1044.

Lewin, A. B., Heidgerken, A. D., Geffken, G. R., Williams, L. B., Storch, E. A., Gelfand, K. M., & Silverstein, J. H. (2006). The relation between family factors and metabolic control: The role of diabetes adherence. *Journal of Pediatric Psychology, 31*, 174–183.

Lewis, F. M., & Hammond, M. A. (1996). The father's, mother's and adolescent's functioning with breast cancer. *Family Relations, 45*, 456–465.

Liakopoulou, M., Alifieraki, T., Katideniou, A., Peppa, M., Maniati, M., Tzikas, D., ... Dacou-Voutetakis, C. (2001). Maternal expressed emotion and metabolic control of children and adolescents with diabetes mellitus. *Psychotherapy and Psychosomatics, 70*, 78–85.

Linville, D., Hertlein, K., & Lyness, A. (2007). Medical family therapy: Reflecting on the necessity of collaborative healthcare research. *Families, Systems, & Health, 25*, 85–97.

Lutz Stehl, M., Kazak, A. E., Alderfer, M. A., Rodriguez, A., Hwang, W. T., Pai, A. L. H., ... Reilly, A. (2009). The feasibility of conducting a randomized clinical trial of an intervention for parent caregivers of children newly diagnosed with cancer. *Journal of Pediatric Psychology, 34*, 803–816.

Madan-Swain, A., Brown, R., Sexson, S., Baldwin, K., Pais, R., & Ragab, A. (1994). Adolescent cancer survivors: Psychosocial and familial adaptation. *Psychosomatics, 35*, 453–459.

Malbasa, T., Kodish, E., & Santacroce, S. J. (2007). Adolescent adherence to oral therapy for leukemia: A focus group study. *Journal of Pediatric Oncology Nursing, 24*, 139–151.

Markson, S., & Fiese, B. H. (2000). Family rituals as a protective factor for children with asthma. *Journal of Pediatric Psychology, 25*, 471–479.

Marsac, M., & Alderfer, M. A. (2011). Psychometric properties of the FACES-IV in families of children with cancer. *Journal of Pediatric Psychology, 36*(5), 528–538. doi: 10.1093/jpepsy/jsq003

Marteau, T. M., Bloch, S., & Baum, J. D. (1987). Family life and diabetic control. *Journal of Child Psychology and Psychiatry, 28*, 823–833.

Martire, L. (2005). The "relative" efficacy of involving family in psychosocial interventions for chronic illness: Are there added benefits to patients and family members? *Families, Systems, & Health, 23*, 312–328.

Martire, L. M., & Schulz, R. (2007). Involving family on psychosocial interventions for chronic illness. *Current Directions in Psychological Science, 16*, 90–94.

Martire, L. M., Schulz, R., Keefe, F. J., Rudy, T. E., & Starz, T. (2008). Couple oriented education and support intervention for osteoarthritis: Effects on spouses' support and responses to patient pain. *Families, Systems, and Health, 26*, 185–195.

Mayne, T. J., O'Leary, A., McCrady, B., Contrada, R., & Labouvie, E. (1997). The differential effects of acute marital distress on emotional, physiological and immune functions in martially distressed men and women. *Psychology and Health, 12*, 277–288.

McCubbin, H. I., & Patterson, J. M. (1983). The family stress process: The double ABCX model of adjustment and adaptation. *Marriage & Family Review, 6*, 7–37.

McEwen, B. S., & Stellar, E. (1993). Stress and the individual: Mechanisms leading to disease. *Archives of Internal Medicine, 153*, 2093–2101.

Meijer, A. M., Griffioen, R. W., van Nierop, J. C., & Oppenheimer, L. (1995). Intractable or uncontrolled asthma: Psychosocial factors. *Journal of Asthma, 32*, 265–274.

Miller-Johnson, S., Emery, R. E., Marvin, R. S., Clarke, W., Lovinger, R., & Martin, M. (1994). Parent-child relationships and the management of insulin-dependent diabetes mellitus. *Journal of Consulting and Clinical Psychology, 62*, 603–610.

Minuchin, S. (1974). *Families and family therapy.* Cambridge, MA: Harvard University Press.

Minuchin, S., Baker, L., Rosman, B. L., Liebman, R., Milman, L., & Todd, T. C. (1975). A conceptual model of psychosomatic illness in children. *Archives of General Psychiatry, 32*, 1031–1038.

Mukherjee, S., Sloper, P., & Lewin, R. (2002). The meaning of parental illness to children: The case of inflammatory bowel disease. *Child: Care, Health & Development, 28*, 479–485.

Naar-King, S., Ellis, D., Kolmodin, K., Cunningham, P., & Secord, E. (2009). Feasibility of adapting multisystemic therapy to improve illness management behaviors and reduce asthma morbidity in high risk African American youth. *Journal of Child and Family Studies, 18*, 564–573.

Naar-King, S., Podolski, C. L., Ellis, D. A., Frey, M. A., & Templin, T. (2006). Social ecology model of illness management in high-risk youths with type 1 diabetes. *Journal of Consulting and Clinical Psychology, 74*, 785–789.

Nealey-Moore, J., Smith, T., Uchino, B., Hawkins, M., & Olson-Cerny, C. (2007). Cardiovascular reactivity during positive and negative marital interactions. *Journal of Behavioral Medicine, 30*, 505–519.

Newbould, J., Smith, F., & Francis, S. A. (2008). "I'm fine doing it on my own": Partnerships between young people and their parents in the management of medication for asthma and diabetes. *Journal of Child Health Care, 12*, 116–128.

Ng, S., Li, A., Lou, V., Tso, I., Wan, P., & Chan, D. (2008). Incorporating family therapy into asthma group intervention: A randomized waitlist-controlled trial. *Family Process, 47*, 115–130.

Nichols, M. P., & Schwartz, R. C. (2001). *The essentials of family therapy.* Boston, MA: Allyn & Bacon.

Northam, E., Anderson, P., Adler, R., Werther, G., & Warne, G. (1996). Psychosocial and family functioning in children with insulin-dependent diabetes at diagnosis and one year later. *Journal of Pediatric Psychology, 21*, 699–717.

Northouse, L. (1989). A longitudinal study of the adjustment of patients and husbands to breast cancer. *Oncology Nursing Forum, 16*, 511–516.

Nostlinger, C., Bartoli, G., Gordillo, M., Roberfroid, D., & Colebunders, R. (2006). Children and adolescents living with HIV positive parents: Emotional and behavioural problems. *Vulnerable Children and Youth Studies, 1*, 1–15.

Olson, D. H. (2000). Circumplex model of marital and family systems. *Journal of Family Therapy, 22*, 144–167.

Olson, D. H., & Gorall, D. M. (2003). Circumplex model of marital and family systems. In F. Walsh (Ed.), *Normal Family Processes* (3rd ed., pp. 514–548). New York, NY: Guilford Press.

Olson, D. H., Russel, C. S., & Sprenkle, D. H. (1983). Circumplex model of marital and family systems: VI. Theoretical update. *Family Process, 22,* 69–83.

Orth-Gomer. K., Wamala, S., Horsten, M., Schenck-Gustafsson, K., Schneiderman, N., & Mittleman, M. (2000). Marital stress worsens prognosis in women with coronary heart disease: The Stockholm female coronary risk study. *Journal of American Medical Association, 284,* 3008–3014.

Osborn, T. (2007). The psychosocial impact of parental cancer on children and adolescents: A systematic review. *Psycho-Oncology, 16,* 101–126.

Pai, A. L. H., Greenley, R. N., Lewandowski, A., Drotar, D., Youngstrom, R., & Peterson, C. C. (2007). A meta-analytic review of the influence of pediatric cancer on parent and family functioning. *Journal of Family Psychology, 21,* 407–415.

Paisley, J., Beanlands, H., Goldman, J., Evers, S., & Chappell, J. (2008). Dietary change: What are the responses and roles of significant others? *Journal of Nutrition Education and Behavior, 40,* 80–88.

Patiño-Fernández, A., Pai, A., Alderfer, M. A., Hwang, W., Reilly, A., & Kazak, A. E. (2008). Acute stress in parents of children newly diagnosed with cancer. *Pediatric Blood & Cancer, 50,* 289–292.

Patterson, J. M. (1988). Families experiencing stress: I. The family adjustment and adaptation response model: II. Applying the FAAR model to health-related issues for intervention and research. *Family Systems Medicine, 6,* 202–237.

Patterson, J. M., & Garwick, A. W. (1994). Levels of meaning in family stress theory. *Family Process, 33,* 287–304.

Patterson, J. M., Goetz, D., Budd, J., & Warwick, W. J. (1993). Family correlates of a 10-year pulmonary health trend in cystic fibrosis. *Pediatrics, 9,* 383–389.

Patterson, J. M., & McCubbin, H. I. (1983). The impact of family life events and changes on the health of a chronically ill child. *Family Relations: Journal of Applied Family & Child Studies, 32,* 255–264.

Piazza-Waggoner, C., Modi, A. C., Powers, S. W., Williams, L. B., Dolan, L. M., & Patton, S. R. (2008). Observational assessment of family functioning in families with children who have type 1 diabetes mellitus. *Journal of Developmental and Behavioral Pediatrics, 29,* 101–105.

Pinquart, M., & Sorensen, S. (2003). Associations of stressors and uplifts of caregiving with caregiver burden and depressive mood: A meta-analysis. *Journals of Gerontology: Psychological Sciences and Social Sciences, 58,* P112–P128.

Pollock, K. G. J., Duncan, E., & Cowden, J. M. (2009). Emotional and behavioral changes in parents of children affected by hemolytic-uremic syndrome associated with verocytotoxin-producing escherichia coli: A qualitative analysis. *Psychosomatics, 50,* 263–269.

Power, P., & Dell Orto, A. E. (2004). *Families living with chronic illness and disability: Interventions, challenges, and opportunities.* New York, NY: Springer.

Quittner, A., Drotar, D., Ievers-Landis, C., Seidner, D., Slocum, N., & Jacobsen, J. (2000). Adherence to medical treatments in adolescents with cystic fibrosis: The development and evaluation of family-based interventions. In D. Drotar (Ed.), *Promoting adherence to medical treatment in childhood chronic illness: Interventions and methods* (pp. 383–407). Hillsdale, NJ: Erlbaum.

Rapoff, M. A. (2009). Adherence issues among adolescents with chronic diseases. In S. Shumaker, J. K. Ockene, & K. A. Riekert (Eds.), *The handbook of health behavior change* (3rd ed., pp. 545–583). New York, NY: Springer.

Repetti, R. L., Taylor, S. E., & Seeman, T. E. (2002). Risky families: Family social environments and the mental and physical health of offspring. *Psychological Bulletin, 128,* 330–366.

Revenson, T. A., & DeLongis, A. (2011). Couples coping with chronic illness. In S. Folkman (Ed.), *Oxford handbook of stress, health, and coping.* New York, NY: Oxford University Press.

Robles, T. F., & Kiecolt-Glaser, J. K. (2003). The physiology of marriage: Pathways to health. *Physiology & Behavior, 79,* 409–416.

Rolland, J. S. (1984). Toward a psychosocial typology of chronic and life-threatening illness. *Family Systems Medicine, 2,* 245–262.

Rolland, J. S. (1987). Chronic illness and the life cycle. *Family Process, 26,* 203–221.

Rolland, J. S. (2003). Mastering family challenges in illness and disability. In F. Walsh (Ed.), *Normal family processes* (3rd ed., pp. 460–489). New York, NY: Guilford Press.

Rotheram-Borus, M., Lester, P., Song, J., Lin, Y. Y., Leonard, N. R., Beckwith, L., … Lord, L. (2006). Intergenerational benefits of family-based HIV intervention. *Journal of Consulting and Clinical Psychology, 74,* 622–627.

Ruddy, N., & McDaniel, S. (2003). Medical family therapy. In T. Sexton, G. Weeks, & M. Robbins (Eds.), *Handbook of family therapy,* (pp. 365–379). New York, NY: Brunner Routledge.

Sambuco, M., Brookes, N., & Lah, S. (2008). Pediatric traumatic brain injury: A review of siblings' outcome. *Brain Injury, 22,* 7–17.

Satin, W., La Greca, A. M., Zigo, M. A., & Skylar, J. S. (1989). Diabetes in adolescence: Effects of multifamily group intervention and parent simulation of diabetes. *Journal of Pediatric Psychology*, *14*, 259–275.

Schobinger, R., Florin, I., Reichbauer, M., Lindemann, H., & Zimmer, C. (1993). Childhood asthma: Mothers' affective attitude, mother-child interaction and children's compliance with medical requirements. *Journal of Psychosomatic Research*, *37*, 697–707.

Scott, J., Halford, K. W., & Ward, B. G. (2004). United we stand? The effects of a couple-coping intervention on adjustment to early stage breast or gynecological cancer. *Journal of Consulting and Clinical Psychology*, *72*, 1122–1135.

Segal, R. (2004). Family routines and rituals: A context for occupational therapy interventions. *American Journal of Occupational Therapy*, *58*, 499–508.

Shalowitz, M. U., Berry, C. A., Quinn, K. A., & Wolf, R. L. (2001). The relationship of life stressors and maternal depression to pediatric asthma morbidity in a subspecialty practice. *Ambulatory Pediatrics*, *1*, 185–193.

Sharpe, D., & Rossiter, L. (2002). Siblings of children with chronic illness: A meta-analysis. *Journal of Pediatric Psychology*, *27*, 699–710.

Sholevar, G., & Sahar, C. (2003). Medical family therapy. In G. Sholevar & L. Schwoeri (Eds.), *Textbook of family and couples therapy: Clinical applications* (pp. 747–767). Washington, DC: American Psychiatric Publishing.

Spath, M. L. (2007). Children facing a family member's acute illness: A review of intervention studies. *International Journal of Nursing Studies*, *44*, 834–844.

Stiell, K., Naaman, S., & Lee, A. (2007). Couples and chronic illness: An attachment perspective and emotionally focused therapy interventions. *Journal of Systemic Therapies*, *26*, 59–74.

Stodberg, R., Sunvisson, H., & Ahlstrom, G. (2007). Lived experience of significant others of persons with diabetes. *Journal of Clinical Nursing*, *16*, 215–222.

Streisand, R., Mackney, E., Elliot, B., Mednick, L., Slaughter, I. M., Turek, J., & Austin, A. (2008). Parental anxiety and depression associated with caring for a child newly diagnosed with type I diabetes: Opportunities for education and counseling. *Patient Education and Counseling*, *73*, 333–338.

Swift, E. E., Chen, R., Hershberger, A., & Holmes, C. S. (2006). Demographic risk factors, mediators, and moderators in youths' diabetes metabolic control. *Annals of Behavioral Medicine*, *32*, 39–49.

Teachman, J., Tedrow, L., & Crowder, K. (2000). The changing demography of American families. *Journal of Marriage and the Family*, *62*, 123–146.

Thayer, J. F., & Lane, R. D. (2000). A model of neurovisceral integration in emotion regulation and dysregulation. *Journal of Affective Disorders*, *61*, 201–216.

Thompson, H. S., & Ryan, A. (2009). The impact of stroke consequences on spousal relationships from the perspective of the person with stroke. *Journal of Clinical Nursing*, *18*, 1803–1811.

Trief, P. M., Morin, P. C., Izquierdo, R., Teresi, J., Starren, J., Shea, S., & Weinstock, R. S. (2006). Marital quality and diabetes outcomes: The IDEATel Project. *Families, Systems, & Health*, *24*, 318–331.

Trollvik, A., & Severinsson, E. (2004). Parents' experiences of asthma: Process from chaos to coping. *Nursing and Health Sciences*, *6*, 93–99.

Troxel, W. M., & Matthews, K. A. (2004). What are the costs of marital conflict and dissolution to children's physical health? *Clinical Child and Family Psychology Review*, *7*, 29–57.

Turpin, M., Leech, C., & Hackenberg, L. (2008). Living with parental multiple sclerosis: Children's experiences and clinical implications. *Canadian Journal of Occupational Therapy*, *75*, 149–156.

Van der Poel, A., & Greeff, A. P. (2003). The influence of coronary bypass graft surgery on the marital relationship and family functioning of the patient. *Journal of Sex & Marital Therapy*, *29*, 61–77.

Varni, J., Katz, E., Colegrove, R., & Dolgin, M. (1996). Family functioning predictors of adjustment in children with newly diagnosed cancer: A prospective analysis. *Journal of Child Psychology and Psychiatry and Allied Disciplines*, *37*, 321–328.

Von Bertalanffy, L. (1968). *General systems theory*. New York, NY: Braziller.

Von Schlippe, A., Theiling, S., Lob-Corzilius, T., & Szczepanski, R. (2001). The "Luftikurs": Innovative family focused training of children with asthma in Germany. *Families, Systems, & Health*, *19*, 263–284.

Wade, S. L., Carey, J., & Wolfe, C. R. (2006a). The efficacy of an online cognitive-behavioral family intervention in improving child behavior and social competence following pediatric brain injury. *Rehabilitation Psychology*, *51*, 179–189.

Wade, S. L., Carey, J., & Wolfe, C. R. (2006b). An online family intervention to reduce parental distress following pediatric brain injury. *Journal of Consulting and Clinical Psychology*, *74*, 445–454.

Walsh, F. (2002). A family resilience framework. *Family Relations*, *51*, 130–137.

Walsh, F. (2003). Family resilience: Strengths forged through adversity. In F. Walsh (Ed.), *Normal family processes: Growing diversity and complexity* (3rd ed., pp. 399–423). New York, NY: Guilford Press.

Walsh, F. (2006). *Strengthening family resilience* (2nd ed.). New York, NY: Guilford Press.

Watson, W., & McDaniel, S. (2005). Managing emotional reactivity in couples facing illness: Smoothing out the emotional roller coaster. In M. Harway (Ed.), *Handbook of couples therapy* (pp. 253–271). Hoboken, NJ: Wiley.

Weihs, K., Fisher, L., & Baird, M. (2002). Families, health, and behavior. A section of the commissioned report by the Committee on Health and Behavior. Research, Practice, and Policy Division of Neuroscience and Behavioral Health and Division of Health Promotion and Disease Prevention Institute of Medicine, National Academy of Sciences. *Families, Systems, & Health, 20,* 7–46.

Weinstein, A. G., Chenkin, C., & Faust, D. (1997). Caring for the severely asthmatic child and family: I. The rationale for psychological treatment. *Journal of Asthma, 34,* 345–352.

Wiebe, D. J., Berg, C. A., Korbel, C., Palmer, D. L., Beveridge, R. M., Upchurch, R., … Donaldson, D. L. (2005). Children's appraisals of maternal involvement in coping with diabetes: Enhancing our understanding of adherence, metabolic control, and quality of life across adolescence. *Journal of Pediatric Psychology, 30,* 167–178.

Wiener, L., Steffen-Smith, E., Battles, H., Wayne, A., Love, C., & Fry, T. (2008). Sibling stem cell donor experiences at a single institution. *Psycho-Oncology, 17,* 304–307.

Williams, B., Mukhopadhyay, S., Dowell, J., & Coyle, J. (2007). From child to adult: An exploration of shifting family roles and responsibilities in managing physiotherapy for cystic fibrosis. *Social Sciences & Medicine, 65,* 2135–2146.

Williams, P. D. (1997). Siblings and pediatric chronic illness: A review of the literature. *International Journal of Nursing Studies, 34,* 312–323.

Wood, B. L. (1994). One articulation of the structural family therapy model: A biobehavioral family model of chronic illness in children. *Journal of Family Therapy, 16,* 53–72.

Wood, B. L. (2001). Physically manifested illness in children and adolescents: A biobehavioral family approach. *Child and Adolescent Psychiatric Clinics of North America, 10,* 543–562.

Wood, B. L., Klebba, K. B., & Miller, B. D. (2000). Evolving the biobehavioral family model: The fit of attachment. *Family Process, 39,* 319–344.

Wood, B. L., Lim, J., Miller, B. D., Cheah, P. A., Simmens, S., Stern, T., … Ballow, M. (2007). Family emotional climate, depression, emotional triggering of asthma, and disease severity in pediatric asthma: Examination of pathways of effect. *Journal of Pediatric Psychology, 32,* 542–551.

Wood, B. L., Lim, J., Miller, B. D., Cheah, P., Zwetsch, T., Ramesh, S., & Simmens, S. (2008). Testing the biobehavioral family model in pediatric asthma: Pathways of effect. *Family Process, 47,* 21–40.

Wood, B. L., & Miller, B. D. (2005). Families, health and illness: The search for mechanisms within a systems paradigm. In W. M. Pinsof & J. L. Lebow (Eds.), *Family psychology: The art of the science* (pp. 493–520). New York, NY: Oxford University Press.

Wood, B. L., Miller, B. D., Lim, J., Lillis, K., Ballow, M., Stern, T., & Simmens, S. (2006). Family relational factors in pediatric depression and asthma: Pathways of effect. *Journal of the American Academy of Child and Adolescent Psychiatry, 45,* 1494–1502.

Wynne, L. C. (2003). Systems theory and the biopsychosocial approach. In R. M. Frankel, T. E. Quill, & S. H. McDaniel (Eds.), *The biopsychosocial approach: Past, present, and future* (pp. 219–230). Rochester, NY: University of Rochester Press.

Wysocki, T., Greco, P., Harris, M. A., Bubb, J., & White, N. H. (2001). Behavior therapy for families of adolescents with diabetes. *Diabetes Care, 24,* 441–446.

Wysocki, T., Harris, M. A., Greco, P., Bubb, J., Danda, C. E., Harvey, L. M., … White, N. H. (2000). Randomized, controlled trial of behavior therapy for families of adolescents with insulin-dependent diabetes mellitus. *Journal of Pediatric Psychology, 25,* 22–33.

Wysocki, T., Harris, M. A., Buckloh, L. M., Mertlich, D., Lochrie, A. S., Taylor, A., & White, N. H. (2006). Effects of behavioral family systems therapy for diabetes on adolescents' family relationships, treatment adherence, and metabolic control. *Journal of Pediatric Psychology, 31,* 928–938.

Yoos, H. L., Kitzman, H., & Cole, R.(1999). Family routines and the feeding process. In D. B. Kessler & P. Dawson (Eds.), *Failure to thrive and pediatric undernutrition: A transdisciplinary approach* (pp. 375–384). Baltimore, MD: Brookes.

Section IV

Macro-Level and Structural
Influences on Health

22 Gender and Health
A Social Psychological Perspective

Vicki S. Helgeson
Carnegie Mellon University

Sex and gender are politically charged topics. Depending on the domain, there are often two camps of people—one arguing that there are no sex differences in the domain, that any differences found are small and insignificant, and that it would be best if sex was ignored, and the other arguing that there are important sex differences in the domain that should be taken seriously and subject to further study. One reason that people feel so passionately about the study of sex differences has to do with the underlying basis of any differences found. Is the sex difference a result of biology or of socialization? If a sex difference has a biological basis, does that mean there are inherent differences in men and women that cannot be changed and thus justify the current social structure? In most cases, both biology and socialization contribute. However, I as well as others take issue with the argument that a biological basis for a difference implies that it cannot be changed.

The present chapter is devoted to the study of gender and health. Of all the controversies in the area of sex and gender, one indisputable fact is that there are a multitude of sex differences in health. The basis for those differences, however, is complex and multifactorial. In the present chapter, I first present an overview of some of the primary differences in men's and women's health. I acknowledge the role of several biological factors (e.g., genes, hormones, immune system), and use heart disease and depression as examples. I briefly discuss how such contextual factors as physician and researcher bias could influence the presentation of some sex differences in health. Then, I turn to four classes of explanations for sex differences in health: (1) health behaviors, which include smoking, alcohol, diet, and exercise; (2) social roles, which include the male social role's link to paid employment, risk-taking behavior, and physical strength and the female social role's link to the domestic sphere and caretaking in general; (3) stressful life events, distinguishing between stress exposure and stress vulnerability; and (4) gender-related traits, which include agency and communion, as well as their unmitigated counterparts. When the explanatory factor is influenced by life-span factors, I discuss the influence of age (e.g., health behaviors).

SEX DIFFERENCES IN MORTALITY AND MORBIDITY

There are sex differences in mortality throughout the lifespan. At every age, males are more likely than females to die (see Table 22.1). Today, men in the United States can expect to live an average of 75.1 years, whereas women can expect to live an average of 80.2 years (Centers for Disease Control and Prevention, 2009a). This is a difference of 5.1 years. This sex difference is not as interesting as the fact that it has changed so much over the past century. As shown in Table 22.2, the sex difference in life expectancy increased dramatically over the first half of the 20th century; in 1900, men lived to be 46.3 years and women lived to be 48.3 years, a difference of only two years. With better nutrition, better health care, and the development of vaccinations against many acute illnesses, people began living longer and dying of such chronic diseases as heart disease and cancer. Women benefited more than men. The gap in men's and women's lifespan was attributable to the reduction in women's mortality during childbirth and men's heightened rates of heart disease and lung cancer, a

TABLE 22.1
Number of Deaths per 100,000 in 2005

Age	Male	Female	Male/Female Ratio
1–4	32	28	1.14
5–14	19	14	1.36
15–24	113	43	2.63
25–34	137	63	2.17
35–44	240	142	1.69
45–54	539	311	1.73
55–64	1121	706	1.59
65–74	2647	1761	1.50
75–84	6409	4539	1.41
85 and over	15100	13355	1.13

Source: Adapted from U.S. Census Bureau, 2007.

product of men's smoking. Today, the leading causes of death are heart disease, cancer, cerebrovascular disease, chronic lower respiratory disease (e.g., emphysema), and accidents, as shown in Table 22.3. Each of these leading causes of death is multidetermined, and each involves such behavioral risk factors as smoking, alcohol, diet, and exercise. It also is the case that males are more likely than females to die of most leading causes of death. Males are more likely than females to die of 12 of the top 15 causes of death (see Table 22.3).

The sex difference in mortality peaked in 1979 with women outliving men by 7.8 years. Since that time, the gap has narrowed. There are two primary explanations for the shrinkage of the sex difference in life expectancy (Pampel, 2002; Rieker & Bird, 2005). First, the women's movement in the 1960s brought smoking to women, and women have not quit smoking at the same rate that men have. Although lung cancer is the leading cancer death for both men and women, there has been a relatively greater increase in lung cancer among women than men over the past 25 years (American Cancer Society, 2009). The rate of lung cancer has been declining among men since 1984, whereas it is just

TABLE 22.2
Life Expectancies

	Men	Women	White Men	White Women	Black Men[a]	Black Women[a]
2006	75.1	80.2	75.7	80.6	69.7	76.5
2000	74.1	79.3	74.7	79.9	68.2	75.1
1990	71.8	78.8	72.7	79.4	64.5	73.6
1980	70.0	77.5	70.7	78.1	63.8	72.5
1970	67.1	74.7	68.0	75.6	60.0	68.3
1960	66.6	73.1	67.4	74.1	61.1	66.3
1950	65.6	71.1	66.5	72.2	59.1	62.9
1940	60.8	65.2	62.1	66.6	51.5	54.9
1930	58.1	61.6	59.7	63.5	47.3	49.2
1920	53.6	54.6	54.4	55.6	45.5	45.2
1910	48.4	51.8	48.6	52.0	33.8	37.5
1900	46.3	48.3	46.6	48.7	32.5	33.5

Source: Adapted from Centers for Disease Control and Prevention, *National Vital Statistics Report*, 57, 14, 2009.
[a] The figures from 1900 to 1960 for Blacks reflect "Blacks and others."

TABLE 22.3
Age-Adjusted Death Rates (per 100,000) for the Leading Causes of Death in 2005

Cause of Death	All	M/F	B/W	H/W
Heart disease	211.0	1.5	1.3	0.7
Cancer	187.0	1.4	1.2	0.6
Cerebrovascular disease	45.8	1.0	1.5	0.8
Chronic lower respiratory disease	41.6	1.3	0.7	0.4
Accidents	40.6	2.2	0.9	0.7
Diabetes mellitus	24.2	1.4	2.1	1.5
Alzheimer's disease	24.2	0.7	0.8	0.6
Pneumonia and influenza	18.8	1.4	1.1	0.8
Kidney disease	15.1	1.4	2.3	1.0
Septicemia	11.4	1.2	2.1	0.8
Suicide	11.1	4.0	0.4	0.4
Liver disease	9.2	2.1	0.8	1.5
Hypertension and renal disease	8.0	1.0	2.7	1.0
Parkinson's disease	6.5	2.2	0.4	0.6
Homicide	6.2	3.9	5.8	2.7

Source: Adapted from Centers for Disease Control and Prevention, *National Vital Statistics Report*, 57, 14, 2009.

B/W = Black to White ratio; H/W = Hispanic to White ratio; M/F = male to female ratio.

now plateauing among women. In 1989, lung cancer surpassed breast cancer as the leading cause of cancer death among women. Thus, men's and women's patterns of smoking not only explains the widening of the sex difference in longevity during the 20th century but also the more recent narrowing of that gap. Some researchers speculate that as women increase their rates of smoking cessation, the sex gap in longevity will once again widen (Pampel, 2002). The second reason for the narrowing of the sex gap in longevity is that the medical advances in treating cardiovascular disease have been more successful for men than women. I will expand on this issue later in the chapter.

Sex differences in mortality are not limited to the United States. In 2006, for the first time, women lived longer than men in almost all countries in the world (Barford, Dorling, Smith, & Shaw, 2006). The sex difference is more variable in developing countries where the lifespan is much shorter, but women outlive men even among the poorest countries in the world. Among the richest nations of the world, mortality rates for both men and women have been on the decline, but young women's mortality rates have declined much faster compared to those of young men (J. E. Rigby & Dorling, 2007). Researchers have attributed this difference to the increase in status and societal position young women have gained in these countries.

Despite men's higher mortality rates compared to those of women, women have higher morbidity rates than men. This is often referred to as the "gender paradox." Women perceive their health as worse than men do (Case & Paxson, 2005). In a national survey of U.S. adults, 17% of women compared to 12% of men said that they had at least one physical difficulty (Pleis & Lethbridge-Cejku, 2007). Women suffer higher rates of arthritis, immune disorders, and digestive conditions compared to men. Women suffer from more painful disorders, such as migraines, musculoskeletal pain, rheumatoid arthritis, and multiple sclerosis, than do men (LeResche, 2000). Women report more psychological and physical symptoms compared to men (Gijsbers van Wijk, Huisman, & Kolk, 1999), and women are more depressed than men (Hyde, Mezulis, & Abramson, 2008). A study in the Netherlands showed that morbidity-free life expectancy (i.e., life without chronic illness) declined for both men and women between 1989 and 2000, but the decline was greater for women such that men have a longer life expectancy without chronic illness (53.9 years) than women (51.0 years; Perenboom, van Herten, Boshuizen, & van den Bos, 2005).

Many of the sex differences in morbidity first appear in adolescence. Sex differences in health perceptions arise around age 14 and persist until about age 65 (Case & Paxson, 2005). The sex difference in depression (females more than males) also first appears during adolescence and then persists across the lifespan (Hyde et al., 2008). In childhood, boys have higher rates of chronic illnesses, such as asthma and migraine headaches, than do girls; but in adolescence, girls have higher rates than boys (Sweeting, 1995). A longitudinal study of 11-year-olds showed that such physical symptoms as headaches and stomach problems increased with age for both boys and girls, but the age-related increase was larger for girls (Sweeting & West, 2003). A study of 11- to 15-year-olds across 29 European and North American countries showed that girls reported more health complaints than did boys overall, but the sex difference increased with age (Torsheim et al., 2006). Of interest is that the sex difference was smaller in more egalitarian countries where women had relatively more education and income compared to other countries.

One explanation for the morbidity/mortality paradox is that women suffer more than men do from more acute illnesses and nonfatal chronic illnesses that are debilitating but pose less of a threat to mortality, whereas men suffer from more severe chronic illnesses such as cardiovascular disease and respiratory conditions that pose a greater threat to mortality (Case & Paxson, 2005). Sex differences in morbidity are a function of not only the morbidity measure but also age (Gorman & Read, 2006). Among adults, men report better health than do women at younger ages, but this sex difference decreases with age. By contrast, women's greater functional limitations compared to men's increase with age. The smallest sex difference occurs for life-threatening conditions; with age, this difference increases in the direction of men having higher morbidity than women.

EXPLANATIONS

There are a variety of explanations for these sex differences in morbidity and mortality (also see Oksuzyan, Juel, Vaupel, & Christensen, 2008, for a review). Although biological factors undoubtedly play a role, biology alone cannot explain the changes in life expectancy over the past 20th century, as just described. Therefore, this chapter adopts more of a social-psychological perspective on gender and health, identifying both person factors and situational forces that may be implicated in sex differences in morbidity and mortality. I focus on four categories of explanations: health behaviors, social roles, stressful life events, and gender-related traits. Before turning to these broad categories of explanations, I want to briefly acknowledge the role that biology and methodological issues contribute to sex differences in health.

Please note that I use the phrase *sex differences* rather than *gender differences* in health. Sex represents the biological categories of being male and female, whereas gender connotes the more social categories to which we assign the psychological traits that are associated with being male and female. In the studies reviewed in this chapter, researchers typically note differences in health between the biological categories of being male and female without reference to their origins. Thus, *sex differences* is a more appropriate term than *gender differences*. However, here this usage does not imply anything about the origin of those differences.

NOTE ON BIOLOGY

Biology contributes to sex differences in health in a variety of ways, one of which has to do with sex-linked chromosomes. Some disorders are associated with abnormalities on the X chromosome. Because women have a second X chromosome, they can override the disorder, whereas men cannot. This ability explains why males suffer more congenital disorders than do females (e.g., hemophilia, meningitis, muscular dystrophy; Migeon, 2006).

Hormones also contribute to sex differences in health. Their role, however, is complicated. Estrogen may play a role in women's vulnerability to such autoimmune disorders as lupus (American Lupus Foundation, 2008), as well as breast cancer (American Cancer Society, 2009). On the other hand, estrogen is thought to protect women from heart disease. As I explain next, the relation of estrogen to heart disease is complicated.

Women are protected from heart disease before menopause as a result of their higher levels of estrogen. Estrogen is associated with lower levels of the "bad" cholesterol (low-density lipoproteins) and higher levels of the "good" cholesterol (high-density lipoproteins). Thus, it was logical for researchers and clinicians alike to believe that prescribing hormone replacement therapy (HRT) after menopause would protect women longer from heart disease. And, in fact, correlational studies showed that women who were on HRT had less heart disease than women who were not on HRT. Correlation does not necessarily imply causation, however. It was always a possibility that the women who were on HRT differed in some ways from the women who were not on HRT. The only definitive test of this hypothesis was a randomized trial in which some women would receive HRT and some would not. Much to many researchers' and clinicians' surprise, the experimental studies did not confirm the hypothesis that exogenously administered estrogen protected against heart disease. In 2002, the randomized HRT trial from the Women's Health Initiative was called to a halt because early findings showed that women on HRT had a significant increased risk of breast cancer and heart attacks (Writing Group for the Women's Health Initiative Investigators, 2002). Subsequent trials have confirmed the link of HRT with increased risk of heart problems (Lowe, 2004). One reason that the correlational studies linked HRT to reduced heart disease is that the women who were on HRT did differ from the women not on HRT in terms of socioeconomic status. Women on HRT were of higher socioeconomic status than the women not on HRT (Lawlor, Smith, & Ebrahim, 2004), and higher socioeconomic status is linked to better health.

One of the most recent areas of research on hormones and health focuses on oxytocin. Oxytocin is a hormone that increases during puberty and has been shown to promote affiliative behavior in women (Gonzaga, Turner, Keltner, Campos, & Altemus, 2006). In attempts to understand the role of oxytocin in affiliative behavior, experimental studies have manipulated intranasal infusions of oxytocin and observed behavior. Such manipulations have linked oxytocin to increased generosity (Zak, Stanton, & Ahmadi, 2007), increased ability to accurately identify positive facial expressions (Marsh, Yu, Pine, & Blair, 2010), and persistence of trust in the face of betrayal (Baumgartner, Heinrichs, Vonlanthen, Fischbacher, & Fehr, 2008). There is some suggestions that oxytocin's link to affiliative behavior reduces stress in women, thus promoting better health (Grewen, Girdler, Amico, & Light, 2005; Light, Grewen, & Amico, 2005). However, another possibility is that oxytocin and affiliative behavior interact with some of the events that occur during adolescence to place females at risk for depression (Cyranowski, Frank, Young, & Shear, 2000; Klein, Corwin, & Ceballos, 2006). As will be described later in the chapter, interpersonal stressors arise during adolescence, especially for females. The increase in oxytocin and subsequent affiliation during adolescence could make females more reactive to these interpersonal stressors. As with the estrogen story, the relation of oxytocin to health is likely to be complicated.

There also is some suggestion that men's and women's immune systems function differently. Owens (2002) argues that the sex difference in mortality is largely explained by men's greater vulnerability to parasitic disease or infection compared to women. It is unclear, however, if this sex difference is a result of men's greater exposure to infection because of a larger body mass or if men are more vulnerable than women to parasite-induced disease. Again, much more research is needed in this area to explicate the role of the immune system in sex differences in health.

NOTE ON CONTEXT: PHYSICIAN BIAS

At the outset of the chapter, I stated that health is one domain in which sex differences are fairly clear-cut. That is, there is much less controversy about sex differences in morbidity and mortality than there is about sex differences in cognition and social attributes. However, both the health care establishment and the patients themselves can contribute to some of the observed sex differences in health. That is, the field of gender and health is vulnerable to experimenter (or clinician) bias and subject demand characteristics. Two key examples of clinician bias, or in this case physician bias, are in the areas of heart disease and depression.

Heart Disease

Women are less likely than men to receive each of the three major treatments for heart disease: drug therapy, percutaneous transluminal coronary angioplasty, and coronary bypass surgery (Kattainen et al., 2005; Travis, 2005). Women also are less likely than men to be referred for cardiac catheterization, the primary diagnostic tool that leads to such procedures as angioplasty and bypass surgery (Stoney, 2003). There are a variety of explanations for these differences, one of which is that women do not match the profile of the "typical cardiac patient"—an older White male. To the extent that women deviate from physicians' schematic representations of a person with heart disease, that diagnosis may be less likely to be called to mind. This problem is further exacerbated by the fact that women present with more ambiguous symptoms of heart disease compared to men. Whereas men's first symptoms of heart disease are heart attacks, women's first symptoms are more likely to be chest pain and shortness of breath, both of which are more ambiguous and can be misdiagnosed as psychological distress (Stoney, 2003). The ambiguity in symptoms makes it more difficult for physicians to recognize heart problems in women. In support of this hypothesis, one study showed that physicians are equally likely to diagnosis heart disease when symptoms are clear and in the absence of stress (Chiaramonte & Friend, 2006). However, in the presence of stress, medical students and residents were less likely to diagnosis heart disease among women than men, presumably because they attributed women's symptoms to stress. Thus, to the extent physician bias exists, it seems to be influenced by situational factors.

A second reason women are less likely than men to be referred for angioplasty and bypass surgery is that women fare more poorly than men after these procedures. Women are more likely to have complications and die in the hospital following angioplasty and bypass surgery, although these differences have become smaller in recent years (Kim, Redberg, Pavlic, & Eagle, 2006; Travis, 2005). There are a variety of reasons for these differential outcomes. First, women's coronary arteries are smaller than men's, making the procedures technically more difficult on women. Second, because heart disease is not recognized in women as early as it is in men, it is often more advanced than that of men, contributing to poorer outcomes from these procedures.

Depression

Physicians also might respond to symptoms of depression differently among men than women. Here, it is men who deviate from the typical profile of the "depressed person." Physicians are well aware of the fact that women have higher rates of depression than men, which may make physicians less likely to recognize depression in men. Depression is a disease accompanied by a series of relatively vague and diffuse symptoms. For example, symptoms of fatigue and difficulty concentrating are symptoms of depression but also can be indicators of a wide variety of other illnesses. Presentation with these symptoms might be more likely to activate a depression schema when the patient is female than when the patient is male. One study of primary care physicians showed that they were less likely to detect depression in men than women when physician diagnosis was compared to an independent screening of depression (Borowsky et al., 2000). However, another study of primary care physicians showed that they correctly classified patients as depressed in 85% of the cases and equally so for men and women (Kales et al., 2005). In the latter study, mental health diagnoses might have been primed because physicians were told that the study was about mental health issues. Physicians are more likely to prescribe antidepressants for women than men (National Center for Health Statistics, 2011), even when they present with the same symptoms (Simoni-Wastila, 1998). It is not clear, however, if this rate of prescription is a result of physician behavior or patient requests.

Health Behaviors

Health behaviors are an obvious explanation for sex differences in morbidity and mortality because men and women differ on so many of them. One of the important questions in this area has to do with *differential exposure* versus *differential vulnerability*. Is one sex at risk for disease because individuals of that sex engage (or fail to engage) in a health behavior or because that health behavior is more strongly related to disease for one sex compared to the other? For many health behaviors, both apply.

Smoking

Smoking has been referred to as the single-most preventable cause of death and is responsible for nearly 20% of deaths (American Cancer Society, 2009). Smoking is associated with an increased risk of heart disease, stroke, lung disease, gastric ulcers, and at least 15 different cancers. Among those 18 years of age and older, more men smoke compared to women (23% vs. 18%; Centers for Disease Control, 2008a) in each ethnic and racial group in the United States. Among children, the sex difference is less clear. In 2007, 19% of girls and 21% of boys in high school reported smoking cigarettes at least one day in the past month (Centers for Disease Control, 2008c). The question remains as to whether the lack of a sex difference in teens is a cohort effect or an age effect. When these adolescents reach adulthood, will the sex difference in smoking reemerge?

Despite men's higher rates of smoking compared to those of women, smoking is more hazardous for women for several reasons. First, the same level of smoking is associated with more negative health consequences for women than men. Specifically, women are more susceptible to chronic obstructive pulmonary disease (COPD) and lung cancer compared to men (Ben-Zaken Cohen, Paré, Man, & Sin, 2007). The rates of COPD and lung cancer have increased more in women compared to men despite the fact that men still smoke more than women. Thus, rates of smoking alone cannot explain this differential increase. Biologic processes are thought to play a role (Ray et al. 2006). Second, men are more likely to quit than women, and men's quit attempts are more successful than those of women (Wetter et al., 1999).

There are at least four theories as to why women have more difficulty quitting smoking than men. First, smoking is associated with depression, and women are more depressed than men. Second, smoking has more of a physiological basis among men than women, making physiological-based therapies such as the nicotine patch more effective for men than women (Perkins, Donny, & Caggiula, 1999). Third, external factors that are associated with smoking, such as taste and smell, are more reinforcing for women than men (Perkins et al., 2001). Fourth, women are more concerned with gaining weight when they quit smoking compared to men, and quitting smoking is associated with a modest weight gain (Jeffery, Hennrikus, Lando, Murray, & Liu, 2000).

Alcohol

Drinking large quantities of alcohol is associated with an increased risk of heart disease, cancer, cirrhosis of the liver, accidents, suicide, and homicide (Centers for Disease Control and Prevention, 2008b). More men than women classify themselves as regular drinkers (57% vs. 39%; Pleis & Lethbridge-Cejka, 2007). Men are nearly three times as likely as women to be binge drinkers, which is defined as drinking five or more drinks on the same occasion in the past month (Centers for Disease Control and Prevention, 2009b). Among children between the ages of 12 and 17, 40% of boys and 41% of girls reported having ever used alcohol, with slightly lower figures for the past month (32% male, 34% female; U.S. Department of Health and Human Services, 2008). As with smoking, it remains to be seen whether the lack of a sex difference in teens prevails in adulthood.

Alcohol also has different implications for men's and women's health (Nolen-Hoeksema & Hilt, 2006). Women have a lower genetic risk for alcohol-use disorders, and the physiological consequences of alcohol are more damaging to women than men. That is, it takes proportionally less alcohol to affect women in the same way it affects men because men have more water available in their system to dilute alcohol and more of the alcohol is metabolized by stomach enzymes among men than women. This biology may explain why alcohol is more strongly related to cirrhosis of the liver among women than men and why women progress more rapidly from the first drink to problem drinking compared to men.

Obesity

The rate of obesity in the United States has doubled over the past 30 years among adults. In the 2007–2008 National Health and Nutrition Examination Survey, 34% of adults over 20 years of age were obese, defined as a body mass index of 30 or more (Flegal, Carroll, Ogden, & Curtin, 2010). Although men and women have similar rates of obesity (32% vs. 34%), men are more likely than women to be classified as overweight, defined as a body mass index between 25 and 29.9. Obesity rates vary by ethnicity—at least for women. Whereas men have similar rates of obesity across ethnic groups, non-Hispanic Black women and Mexican-American women have much higher rates of obesity compared to non-Hispanic White women.

The percentage of overweight children has more than tripled in the past 30 years (Ogden, Carroll, Curtin, Lamb, & Flegal, 2010). More boys than girls are overweight among Whites and Hispanics, but more girls than boys are overweight among African Americans. One unfortunate result of the increase in obesity among children is an increase in Type 2 diabetes—a disease that used to be observed almost exclusively among older adults.

Obesity is not a health behavior, but it is a health problem caused, in part, by health behaviors, most notably diet and exercise. One reason for women's higher rates of obesity compared to that of men has to do with women's lower rates of leisure time exercise and lower rates of vigorous physical activity compared to men (Pleis & Lethbridge-Cejku, 2007). Even among children, girls engage in less physical exercise than boys (Duncan, Duncan, Strycker, & Chaumeton, 2007). Rates of physical activity decline over adolescence, and equally so for boys and girls. Thus, the sex difference persists throughout adulthood. One explanation for the lack of exercise among children is heavy television viewing and video game usage (Berkey et al., 2000).

Obesity is also influenced by diet. Here, women fare better than men. Women (and girls) have better nutrition than men (and boys), eating more fruits and vegetables, less fast food, more whole grains, less red meat, and less soda (Kiefer, Rathmanner, & Kunze, 2005; Pettinato, Loud, Bristol, Feldman, & Gordon, 2006; von Bothmer & Fridlund, 2005). The one exception is calcium. Adolescent males are more likely than adolescent females to meet the recommended daily allowance for calcium (Pettinato et al., 2006). A study of college students across 23 countries found that these sex differences in nutrition prevailed across the majority of countries (Wardle et al., 2004). The authors examined whether sex differences in nutrition were attributable to women's greater likelihood of dieting or to women attaching more importance to healthy eating compared to men. Although both explanations accounted for some of the sex differences in nutrition, the importance that women attached to healthy eating was a stronger explanatory variable. Other research has shown that women have greater knowledge than men of the nutritional aspects of food (von Bothmer & Fridlund, 2005), and women are more likely than men to read the nutritional labels on food (Huang et al., 2004). Like many of the sex differences in health, the sex difference in nutrition seems to emerge during adolescence around the age of 12 (Kiefer et al., 2005).

SOCIAL ROLES

Men and women hold distinct social roles in our society. Men's primary social role is paid employment, and women's primary social role is domestic. Although roles have become more fluid over the past several decades, with more women in the workforce and some men choosing to stay at home to take care of children, it is the case that 86% of men between the ages of 25 and 54 work outside the home compared to 72% of women (U.S. Department of Labor, 2009). Among employed individuals a greater percentage of men work full time (89%) compared to women (75%). In addition, when there are children under 6 years of age, only 64% of women work compared to 95% of men. When children are between the ages of 6 and 17, the figures increase to 78% for women compared to 93% for men. In a study of college students' future work intentions, 98% of both men and women expected to work full time after they completed their education, but 84% of men compared to 20% of women planned to work full time when they had children under the age of 5 (Fillo, 2008). When they had children in elementary school, 90% of men expected to work full-time compared to 42% of women; 51% of women said they planned to work part time. These differences appeared despite the fact that men and women had the same income expectations 10 years after graduation. Thus, men and women still have some distinct expectations about their social roles.

Male Social Role

Men's primary social role is paid employment. Men's higher rate of paid employment compared to that of women has been attributed to a mental health advantage for men. However, it also is the case that men work at jobs that have greater physical health risks compared to women. Job fatalities disproportionally affect men (93%; U.S. Department of Labor, 2010). Men are more likely than women to be employed in manual labor positions that are associated with exposure to hazardous substances and the potential for injury.

In addition to being the family breadwinner, men have other social roles, including driving the family car and taking risks more generally. Men drive more than women, which partly explains why men account for 70% of traffic fatalities (U.S. Department of Transportation, 2008). Given the same amount of driving, men also are riskier drivers compared to women. Male drivers are almost three times as likely as female drivers to be involved in a fatal crash, male drivers are more likely than female drivers to speed, and men are less likely than women to wear seatbelts (U.S. Department of Transportation, 2008). Men's leisure-time activities also are riskier than women's. Men are more likely to engage in such risky activities as downhill skiing, skydiving, mountain climbing, and hunting (Waldron, 1997). Men engage in riskier sexual behavior than do women, including inconsistent condom use and sex with multiple partners (Beadnell et al., 2005). Across an array of activities, a meta-analytic review showed that men are greater risk takers compared to women, but that the size of the sex difference depends on a combination of age and specific activity (Byrnes, Miller, & Schafer, 1999). For example, sex differences in risky driving increase with age, sex differences in drinking and drug use increase with age through college but then decrease with age, and sex differences in risky sexual behaviors decrease with age.

Another aspect of the male social role that may be hazardous to men's health is the link of masculinity to physical strength. In recent years, this has been to the detriment of men's health with the increased use of anabolic steroids (Sabo, 2005). Anabolic steroids increase the risk of liver disease, cardiovascular disease, depression, and aggression. Despite the media attention given to this issue, the use of steroids is not confined to athletes. A recent Internet-based survey showed that the typical user of anabolic steroids is a 30-year-old Caucasian, well-educated male who is not an athlete (Cohen, Collins, Darkes, & Gwartney, 2007). The primary motivation for steroid use was to increase muscle mass and enhance physical appearance rather than enhance athletic performance.

Female Social Role

Despite the increase in women working outside the home in our society, it is still the female social role to take care of the home and children. One reason that women suffer from more role conflict than men when they work outside the home is that paid employment is congruent with men's social role but detracts from women's social role. There is a large literature on the effect of paid employment on women's health, largely concluding that women who work outside the home are healthier than those who do not, even controlling for the selection effect of healthier people entering the workforce (Fokkema, 2002; Klumb & Lampert, 2004; McMunn, Bartley, & Kuh, 2006). The literature also is clear that the effect of work on women's health depends on myriad factors, including the presence, age, and number of children; socioeconomic status; and the involvement of husbands in household labor (Ozer, 1995). For these reasons, there is controversy over whether married women with children have better health when they work full time or part time (Fokkema, 2002; Schnittker, 2007).

The caretaking social role of women has mixed implications for health. On the negative side, the "nurturant role hypothesis" suggests that taking care of others has costs to health in terms of exposure to more pathogens, vulnerability to illness as a result of exhaustion from tending to the needs of others, and the fact that taking care of others interferes with taking care of oneself (Gove & Hughes, 1979). Women assume nurturant roles as mothers, spouses, and also daughters. When parents get older and become ill, women are more likely than men to be the primary caretakers. In a nationwide study of caregivers (defined as providing care to someone aged 18 or older), 61% were found to be female (National Alliance for Caregiving and AARP, 2004). Women not only were more likely to be caregivers than men but also provided more care in terms of hours per week, provided more intensive care, and were more likely to say they did not have a choice in assuming the caregiver role. As caregivers, women also report more overall strain associated with caregiving compared to men and greater increases in strain over time (Lyons, Stewart, Archbold, & Carter, 2009). Women were more likely than men to report that caregiving interfered with work (e.g., reduced hours, took leave, passed up promotion), which likely contributes to women's greater dissatisfaction with retirement compared to men. Other research has shown that women are more likely than men to retire in order to take care of an ill spouse or relative (Szinovacz & Washo, 1992) and that women's retirement is more strongly affected than men's retirement by having to take care of an ill or disabled spouse (Szinovacz & Davey, 2004).

However, there are aspects of the female caretaking role that benefit women's health. Because women are traditionally responsible for the health of the entire family, women are often more knowledgeable about health and more likely to take advantage of existing health services (Oksuzyan et al., 2008). Even this role has its downside, however, because caring for the family can interfere with caring for oneself. The female role is one in which it is acceptable to ask for help and admit not feeling well in our society. According to the "sick role hypothesis" (Nathanson, 1978), women are more likely than men to adopt the sick role when ill and seek help for symptoms.

Intensification of Social Roles During Adolescence

Social-role explanations for gender differences in health may explain why many of the sex differences in health and health behaviors arise during adolescence. It is at this time in life that boys and girls become keenly aware of what the expectations are for the male and female roles—a process referred to as "gender intensification" (Hill & Lynch, 1983). Depression could increase for girls as they become aware of the limitations of the female gender role, in particular that the female gender role is inconsistent with achievement. It also is the case that pubertal hormones and the physical changes that occur during puberty interact with these societal expectations to influence health. For example, in the case of females, puberty is associated with an increase in weight just at the time that girls become more self-conscious about their bodies and aware of societal expectations for females to be thin. One study showed that the transition to puberty was associated with an increase in depression among females *not* because of an actual weight increase (i.e., body mass index) but because of self-perceptions of being overweight (Yuan, 2007). For boys, the transition to puberty might be associated with some short-term negative effects, but puberty is associated with an increase in body size and muscle mass, which is consistent with gender-role expectations for males.

STRESSFUL LIFE EVENTS

Do men or women experience more stressful life events? A meta-analysis of sex differences in traumatic events found that men experienced more trauma than women (Tolin & Foa, 2006). However, the sex difference depended on the nature of the trauma. Whereas women were six times as likely as men to report adult sexual assault and 2.5 times as likely as men to report child sexual assault, men were 3.5 times as likely as women to report combat, war, and terrorism and over 1.5 times as likely as women to experience nonsexual assault. When stressful life events were examined more generally, a meta-analysis showed that women reported more stressful events than did men, but the size of the sex difference was small (Davis, Matthews, & Twamley, 1999). When measurement issues were taken into consideration, it turned out that the sex difference was larger for measures that asked respondents to rate the impact of events than measures that asked respondents to rate whether or not an event occurred. Thus, when stressful life events occurred, women reported that the events had stronger effects on them compared to men.

When the nature of the stressful event was examined in the last meta-analysis (Davis et al., 1999), the sex difference was larger for interpersonal events than noninterpersonal events. In addition, the sex difference in stressful life events was larger among adolescents than children and adults. Interpersonal stress increases during adolescence more so for girls than boys. A study of preadolescent (ages 8 to 12) and adolescent (ages 13 to 18) boys and girls showed that there were no sex differences in the total number of events reported but that females reported more interpersonal stress and males reported more noninterpersonal stress (Rudolph & Hammen, 1999). These differences, however, were confined to the adolescent group; there were no sex differences in either category of stress for the preadolescent group. Other studies have shown that adolescent females report more interpersonal stressors and adolescent males report more noninterpersonal stressors (Murberg & Bru, 2004; Shih, Eberhart, Hammen, & Brennan, 2006).

The differential exposure versus differential vulnerability hypotheses are relevant to this area of research. Are sex differences in health a result of the fact that one sex experiences more stressors than the other sex (i.e., differential exposure to stress), or do such differences reflect the fact that one sex is more strongly affected by a category of stressors than the other sex (i.e., differential vulnerability to stress)? In the area of depression, the research has clearly come in on the side of vulnerability among adults (Maciejewski, Prigerson, & Mazure, 2001; Turner & Avison, 1989). Even studies of children have shown that interpersonal conflict or stress is more strongly related to psychological health among girls than boys (Demir & Urberg, 2004; Shih et al., 2006).

GENDER-RELATED TRAITS

One approach to understanding more about the area of gender and health is to examine some of the ways in which we socialize men and women that could have implications for their health. Differential socialization can be examined in terms of gender-related traits. That is, males are socialized to have an instrumental or agentic orientation, whereas females are socialized to have an expressive or communal orientation. To the extent that males and females adhere to societal norms, males score higher on trait measures of agency than do females, and females score higher on trait measures of communion than do males (Spence & Buckner, 2000). Although women's agentic scores have increased over the past several decades, the sex difference persists.

What are the implications of agency and communion for health? Agency is linked to high self-esteem, fewer physical symptoms, and good mental health (Ghaed & Gallo, 2006; Helgeson, 1994). Agency has also been found to buffer the effects of stressful life events on interpersonal functioning (Lam & McBride-Chang, 2007). Agency has been related to a variety of good health practices, including physical activity, healthy eating, and good dental hygiene (Danoff-Burg, Mosher, & Grant, 2006). By contrast, communion is related to good relationships but largely unrelated to mental or physical health (Ghaed & Gallo, 2006; Helgeson, 1994; Wang, Heppner, & Berry, 1997). Because measures of agency and communion reflect the socially desirable aspects of the male and female roles, in the 1990s I began to examine the more negative forms of these traits—*unmitigated agency* and *unmitigated communion*.

Unmitigated Agency

Unmitigated agency is a construct that was first defined by Bakan (1966) in his book *The Duality of Human Existence*. He argued that it was important for agency to be mitigated by communion and that unmitigated agency would be destructive to the self and society. Spence, Helmreich, and Holahan (1979) developed a measure of unmitigated agency to reflect this idea. Men score higher than women on unmitigated agency (Helgeson & Fritz, 1999). Unmitigated agency is a focus on the self to the exclusion of others and includes an overly inflated view of the self and a disregard and mistrust of others (Helgeson, 1994).

Unmitigated agency has been associated with a variety of indicators of poor health, including depressed mood among adolescents (Craighead & Green, 1989) and college students (Ghaed & Gallo, 2006; Nagurney, 2007); hostility and aggression among college students (Ghaed & Gallo, 2006) and cardiac patients (Helgeson & Fritz, 1999); and reckless driving, substance abuse, and binge eating among college students (Danoff-Burg et al., 2006). In a study of adults, unmitigated agency was related to the severity of a first heart attack (Helgeson, 1990). Among the chronically ill, unmitigated agency has been related to poor adjustment to illness (Helgeson, 1993; Helgeson & Lepore, 1997; Helgeson & Lepore, 2004; Trudeau, Danoff-Burg, Revenson, & Paget, 2003). One study did not measure unmitigated agency per se but found that men who scored high on agency and low on communion—a profile consistent with unmitigated agency—were more likely to die of coronary heart disease 17 years later (Hunt, Lewars, Emslie, & Batty, 2007).

What are some of the reasons that unmitigated agency is associated with poor health? One is that unmitigated agency is related to a reluctance to seek help (see Helgeson & Fritz, 2000, for a review), which may explain why men are less likely than women to seek help (Galdas, Cheater, & Marshall, 2005). In a study of freshmen college students, unmitigated agency was related to fewer visits to advisors during the first semester (Helgeson & Fritz, 2000). When asked by researchers trying to understand the reasons for the reluctance to ask for help, individuals characterized by unmitigated agency were more likely to say that asking for help is a sign of weakness and that others are unable to help. These reasons are consistent with the unmitigated-agency individual's perception of the self as invincible and perception of others as incapable. In the area of health, a reluctance to seek help can have more damaging consequences. In a study of people who had sustained a heart attack, unmitigated agency was associated with longer delays before seeking help for symptoms (Helgeson, 1990). Other research suggests that men delay longer than women before seeking help for symptoms. In a study of the Danish health registry, women had greater contact with general practitioners than did men, but men had more hospitalizations than did women in the study, controlling for sex-specific conditions (Juel & Christensen, 2008). The authors suggested that the results are compatible with the idea that men delay treatment until symptoms are more severe, ultimately leading to hospitalization or more serious disease.

Unmitigated agency is related to difficulties with emotional expression as well (Helgeson & Lepore, 1997). In a study of men with prostate cancer, these emotional difficulties accounted for the relation of unmitigated agency to poor functioning. Emotional expression may be necessary in order to receive needed help. Difficulties with emotional expression may also explain why unmitigated agency individuals tend to have more negative interactions with other people (Helgeson & Fritz, 1999). People have difficulty knowing how to help someone who does not reveal his or her feelings.

Finally, a third explanation for the relation of unmitigated agency to poor health is that unmitigated agency is related to poor health behavior and noncompliance with physician instructions (Helgeson, 1993; Helgeson, 1995; Helgeson & Fritz, 1999). Research with college students has shown that unmitigated agency is associated with a variety of risky behaviors, including alcohol and drug use as well as getting into fights and shoplifting (Snell, Belk, & Hawkins, 1987; Spence et al., 1979). Finally, a study of adolescents showed that unmitigated agency was related to becoming involved in more delinquent behavior (Helgeson & Fritz, 2000).

Unmitigated Communion

Although Bakan (1966) never explicitly used the term *unmitigated communion*, he talked about the destructive effects of communion not mitigated by agency—that is, a focus on others to the exclusion of the self. Unmitigated communion is characterized by an overinvolvement in others' problems and a neglect of the self (Helgeson, 1994; Fritz & Helgeson, 1998). Women score higher than men on unmitigated communion (Helgeson & Fritz, 1999).

Unmitigated communion has been related to depression and more general measures of psychological distress in a variety of populations, including college students (Bruch, 2002; Fritz & Helgeson, 1998; Nagurney, 2007), healthy adolescents (Craighead & Green, 1989; Fritz & Helgeson, 1998), healthy adults (Fritz & Helgeson, 1998), women with breast cancer (Helgeson, 2003b; Piro, Zeldow, Knight, Mytko & Gradishar, 2001), women with rheumatoid arthritis (Danoff-Burg, Revenson, Trudeau, & Paget, 2004; Trudeau et al., 2003), and adults with heart disease (Fritz, 2000; Helgeson, 1993; Helgeson & Fritz, 1999). Two longitudinal studies of adolescents with diabetes have linked unmitigated communion with psychological distress and poor metabolic control and an increase in psychological distress and a deterioration of metabolic control over time (Helgeson & Fritz, 1996; Helgeson, Escobar, Siminerio, & Becker, 2007). In one study, unmitigated communion was related to higher levels of LDL cholesterol as well (Helgeson et al., 2007).

One of the mechanisms that links unmitigated communion to distress and poor health has to do with interpersonal relationships. A study of adolescents with diabetes showed that those who scored high on unmitigated communion reported greater interpersonal stress, which then explained the link of unmitigated communion to both depressive symptoms and poor metabolic control four months later (Helgeson & Fritz, 1996). The link between relationship stressors and poor health for unmitigated communion individuals is partly related to the fact that people who score high on unmitigated communion take on other people's problems as their own; thus, involvement in relationships becomes an additional source of stress. Two studies of college students showed that individuals who score high on unmitigated communion respond to exposure to another's problems with intrusive thoughts several days later—even when the other person who discloses a problem is a stranger (Fritz & Helgeson, 1998). Because relationships are so central to the lives of those who score high on unmitigated communion, there is an oversensitivity to relationship difficulties. Two longitudinal studies of college students have shown that people who score high on unmitigated communion are more reactive to daily or weekly interpersonal stress compared to others (Nagurney, 2007; Reynolds et al., 2006).

A second mechanism linking unmitigated communion to poor health is poor health care. Individuals who score high on unmitigated communion neglect the self in favor of caring for others, as evidenced by a host of interpersonal problems that reflect self-neglect (e.g., difficulties asserting one's needs, being exploitable, inhibiting self-expression to avoid conflict with others, difficulties with self-disclosure, self-effacement, and self-subjugation; Fritz & Helgeson, 1998; Helgeson & Fritz, 1999). In studies of people with chronic illness, unmitigated communion has been directly related to a range of poor health behaviors as well as noncompliance with physician instructions (Fritz, 2000; see Helgeson & Fritz, 2000, for a review; Helgeson, 2003a).

More recently, a new mechanism has been identified that links unmitigated communion to poor psychological and physical health outcomes during adolescence—disturbed eating behavior. Individuals who score high on unmitigated communion have an externalized self-perception (Fritz & Helgeson, 1998), meaning that their view of themselves depends on others. In fact, some of the overly other-focused behavior evidenced by unmitigated communion individuals may be aimed at enhancing their self-image in the eyes of others. Being concerned about how others view oneself may be reflected in a self-consciousness about appearance. There is evidence that unmitigated communion is related to a poor body image among women with breast cancer (Helgeson, 2003b). Among adolescents, those individuals who score high on unmitigated communion may be more vulnerable to societal pressures to be thin. In a study of adolescents, unmitigated communion was related to disturbed eating behavior, a poor body image, and increased psychological distress (Helgeson et al., 2007). Disturbed eating behavior accounted for some of the link between unmitigated communion and psychological distress.

CONCLUSION

In the area of health, there is a gender paradox in that men have higher mortality rates but women have higher morbidity rates. We reviewed several explanations for these sex differences. Each explanation makes some contribution to the paradox. Experimenter or clinician bias and research methodology are not likely causes of sex differences in health but can certainly exaggerate them. Health behaviors are an important contributor to men's mortality rates because men are more likely than women to engage in many of the risky health behaviors. However, differential vulnerability to the risks associated with health behaviors (e.g., cigarettes, alcohol) also contributes to women's mortality and morbidity. Social roles, stressful life events, and gender-related traits are major factors in men's higher mortality rates and women's higher morbidity rates. Here, personality variables interact with situational variables (societal roles, stressful life events) to pose risks to health.

Future research in this area should focus not on one category of explanations but on multiple categories. We will learn more about gender and health when we examine how factors from one category interact with factors from another category—for example, how genes interact with stressful life events or how hormones interact with gender-related traits or social roles. Although some people would suggest that research will be more objective if one is blind to subject sex, the point of this chapter was to make one aware of the importance and relevance of subject sex in understanding health. Knowledge of sex as a risk factor or protective factor for health behaviors and responses to stress can only help to protect against and treat disease.

REFERENCES

American Cancer Society. (2009). *Cancer facts & figures, 2009.* Atlanta, GA: American Cancer Society.

American Lupus Foundation. (2008). *Causes of lupus.* Retrieved from http://www.lupus.org

Bakan, D. (1966). *The duality of human existence.* Chicago: Rand McNally.

Barford, A., Dorling, D., Smith, G. D., & Shaw, M. (2006). Life expectancy: Women now on top everywhere. *British Medical Journal, 332,* 808.

Baumgartner, T., Heinrichs, M., Vonlanthen, A., Fischbacher, U., & Fehr, E. (2008). Oxytocin shapes the neural circuitry of trust and trust adaptation in humans. *Neuron, 58,* 639–650.

Beadnell, B., Morrison, D. M., Wilsdon, A., Wells, E. A., Murowchick, E., Hoppe, M., ... & Nahom, D. (2005). Condom use, frequency of sex, and number of partners: Multidimensional characterization of adolescent sexual risk-taking. *Journal of Sex Research, 42,* 192–202.

Ben-Zaken Cohen, S., Paré, P. D., Man, S. F. P., & Sin, D. D. (2007). The growing burden of chronic obstructive pulmonary disease and lung cancer in women. *American Journal of Respiratory and Critical Care Medicine, 176,* 113–120.

Berkey, C. S., Rockett, H. R., Field, A. E., Gillman, M. W., Frazier, A. L., Camargo, C. A. J., & Colditz, G. A. (2000). Activity, dietary intake, and weight changes in a longitudinal study of preadolescent and adolescent boys and girls. *Pediatrics, 105,* E56.

Borowsky, S. J., Rubenstein, L. V., Meredith, L. S., Camp, P., Jackson-Triche, M., & Wells, K. B. (2000). Who is at risk of nondetection of mental health problems in primary care? *Journal of General Internal Medicine, 15,* 381–388.

Bruch, M. A. (2002). The relevance of mitigated and unmitigated agency and communion for depression vulnerabilities and dysphoria. *Journal of Counseling Psychology, 49,* 449–459.

Byrnes, J. P., Miller, D. C., & Schafer, W. D. (1999). Gender differences in risk taking: A meta-analysis. *Psychological Bulletin, 125,* 367–383.

Case, A., & Paxson, C. (2005). Sex differences in morbidity and mortality. *Demography, 42,* 189–214.

Centers for Disease Control and Prevention. (2008a). Cigarette smoking among adults & trends in smoking cessation. *Morbidity and Mortality Weekly Report, 58*(44), 1127–1232. Retrieved from http://www.cdc.gov/mmwr/preview/mmwrhtml/mm5844a2.htm

Centers for Disease Control and Prevention. (2008b). *Quick stats: General information on alcohol use and health.* Available: http://www.cdc.gov/alcohol/quickstats/general_info.htm

Centers for Disease Control and Prevention (2008c). Youth risk behavior surveillances. *Morbidity and Mortality Weekly Report, 57*(SS–4). Retrieved from http://www.cdc.gov/mmwr/PDF/ss/ss5704.pdf

Centers for Disease Control and Prevention. (2009a). Deaths: Final data for 2006. *National Vital Statistics Report*, *57*(14). Retrieved from http://www.cdc.gov/nchs/data/nvsr/nvsr57/nvsr57_14.pdf

Centers for Disease Control and Prevention. (2009b). Sociodemographic differences in binge drinking among adults—14 states, 2004. *Morbidity and Mortality Weekly Report*, *58*(12), 301–304. Retrieved from http://www.cdc.gov/mmwr/preview/mmwrhtml/mm5812a1.htm

Chiaramonte, G. R., & Friend, R. (2006). Medical students' and residents' gender bias in the diagnosis, treatment, and interpretation of coronary heart disease symptoms. *Health Psychology*, *25*, 255–266.

Cohen, J., Collins, R., Darkes, J., & Gwartney, D. (2007). A league of their own: Demographics, motivations and patterns of use of 1,955 male adult non-medical anabolic steroid users in the United States. *Journal of the International Society of Sports Nutrition*, *4*, 12.

Craighead, L. W., & Green, B. J. (1989). Relationship between depressed mood and sex-typed personality characteristics in adolescents. *Journal of Youth and Adolescence*, *18*, 467–474.

Cyranowski, J. M., Frank, E., Young, E., & Shear, K. (2000). Adolescent onset of the gender difference in lifetime rates of major depression: A theoretical model. *Archives of General Psychiatry*, *57*, 21–27.

Danoff-Burg, S., Mosher, C. E., & Grant, C. A. (2006). Relations of agentic and communal personality traits to health behavior and substance use among college students. *Personality and Individual Differences*, *40*, 353–363.

Danoff-Burg, S., Revenson, T. A., Trudeau, K. J., & Paget, S. A. (2004). Unmitigated communion, social constraints, and psychological distress among women with rheumatoid arthritis. *Journal of Personality*, *72*, 29–46.

Davis, M. C., Matthews, K. A., & Twamley, E. W. (1999). Is life more difficult on Mars or Venus? A meta-analytic review of sex differences in major and minor life events. *Annals of Behavioral Medicine*, *21*, 83–97.

Demir, M., & Urberg, K. A. (2004). Friendship and adjustment among adolescents. *Journal of Experimental Child Psychology*, *88*, 68–82.

Duncan, S. C., Duncan, T. E., Strycker, L. A., & Chaumeton, N. R. (2007). A cohort-sequential latent growth model of physical activity from ages 12 to 17 years. *Annals of Behavioral Medicine*, *33*, 80–89.

Fillo, J. (2008). *College students' intentions for the future division of labor*. Unpublished Manuscript, Carnegie Mellon University, Pittsburgh, Pennsylvania.

Flegal, K. M., Carroll, M. D., Ogden, C. L., & Curtin, L. R. (2010). Prevalence and trends in obesity among U.S. adults, 1999–2008. *Journal of the American Medical Association*, *303*, 235–241.

Fokkema, T. (2002). Combining a job and children: Contrasting the health of married and divorced women in the Netherlands. *Social Science & Medicine*, *54*, 741–752.

Fritz, H. L. (2000). Gender-linked personality traits predict mental health and functional status following a first coronary event. *Health Psychology*, *19*, 420–428.

Fritz, H. L., & Helgeson, V. S. (1998). Distinctions of unmitigated communion from communion: Self-neglect and over involvement with others. *Journal of Personality and Social Psychology*, *75*, 121–140.

Galdas, P. M., Cheater, F., & Marshall, P. (2005). Men and health help-seeking behaviour: Literature review. *Journal of Advanced Nursing*, *49*, 616–623.

Ghaed, S. G., & Gallo, L. C. (2006). Distinctions among agency, communion, and unmitigated agency and communion according to the interpersonal circumplex, five-factor model, and social-emotional correlates. *Journal of Personality Assessment*, *86*, 77–88.

Gijsbers van Wijk, E. M. T., Huisman, H., & Kolk, A. M. (1999). Gender differences in physical symptoms and illness behavior: A health diary study. *Social Science & Medicine*, *49*, 1061–1074.

Gonzaga, G. C., Turner, R. A., Keltner, D., Campos, B., & Altemus, M. (2006). Romantic love and sexual desire in close relationships. *Emotion*, *6*, 163–179.

Gorman, B. K., & Read, J. G. (2006). Gender disparities in adult health: An examination of three measures of morbidity. *Journal of Health and Social Behavior*, *47*, 95–110.

Gove, W. R., & Hughes, M. (1979). Possible causes of the apparent sex differences in physical health: An empirical investigation. *American Sociological Review*, *44*, 126–146.

Grewen, K. M., Girdler, S. S., Amico, J., & Light, K. C. (2005). Effects of partner support on resting oxytocin, cortisol, norepinephrine, and blood pressure before and after warm partner contact. *Psychosomatic Medicine*, *67*, 531–538.

Helgeson, V. S. (1990). The role of masculinity in a prognostic predictor of heart attack severity. *Sex Roles, 22*, 755–774.

Helgeson, V. S. (1993). Implications of agency and communion for patient and spouse adjustment to a first coronary event. *Journal of Personality and Social Psychology*, *64*, 807–816.

Helgeson, V. S. (1994). The relation of agency and communion to well-being: Evidence and potential explanations. *Psychological Bulletin*, *116*, 412–428.

Helgeson, V. S. (1995). Masculinity, men's roles, and coronary heart disease. In D. Sabo & D. Gordon (Eds.), *Men's health and illness: Gender, power and the body* (pp. 68–104). Thousand Oaks, CA: Sage.

Helgeson, V. S. (2003a). Gender-related traits and health. In J. Suls & K. A. Wallston (Eds.), *Social psychological foundations of health and illness* (pp. 367–394). Malden, MA: Blackwell Publishing.

Helgeson, V. S. (2003b). Unmitigated communion and adjustment to breast cancer: Associations and explanations. *Journal of Applied Social Psychology, 33*, 1643–1661.

Helgeson, V. S., Escobar, O., Siminerio, L., & Becker, D. (2007). Unmitigated communion and health among adolescents with and without diabetes: The mediating role of eating disturbances. *Personality and Social Psychology Bulletin, 33*, 519–536.

Helgeson, V. S., & Fritz, H. L. (1996). Implications of communion and unmitigated communion for adolescent adjustment to type 1 diabetes. *Women's Health: Research on Gender, Behavior and Policy, 2*, 169–194.

Helgeson, V. S., & Fritz, H. L. (1999). Unmitigated agency and unmitigated communion: Distinctions from agency and communion. *Journal of Research in Personality, 33*, 131–158.

Helgeson, V. S., & Fritz, H. L. (2000). The implications of unmitigated agency and unmitigated communion for domains of problem behavior. *Journal of Personality, 68*, 1031–1057.

Helgeson, V. S., & Lepore, S. J. (1997). Men's adjustment to prostate cancer: The role of agency and unmitigated agency. *Sex Roles, 37*(3/4), 251–267.

Helgeson, V. S., & Lepore, S. J. (2004). Quality of life following prostate cancer: The role of agency and unmitigated agency. *Journal of Applied Social Psychology, 34*, 2559–2585.

Hill, J. P., & Lynch, M. E. (1983). The intensification of gender-related role expectations during early adolescence. In J. Brooks-Gunn & A. C. Petersen (Eds.), *Girls at puberty* (pp. 201–228). New York, NY: Plenum Press.

Huang, T. T. K., Kaur, H., McCarter, K. S., Nazir, N., Choi, W. S., & Ahluwalia, J. S. (2004). Reading nutrition labels and fat consumption in adolescents. *Journal of Adolescent Health, 35*, 399–401.

Hunt, K., Lewars, H., Emslie, C., & Batty, G. D. (2007). Decreased risk of death from coronary heart disease amongst men with higher "femininity" scores: A general population cohort study. *International Journal of Epidemiology, 36*, 612–620.

Hyde, J. S., Mezulis, A. H., & Abramson, L. Y. (2008). The ABCs of depression: Integrating affective, biological, and cognitive models to explain the emergence of the gender difference in depression. *Psychological Review, 115*, 291–313.

Jeffery, R. W., Hennrikus, D. J., Lando, H. A., Murray, D. M., & Liu, J. W. (2000). Reconciling conflicting findings regarding postcessation weight concerns and success in smoking cessation. *Health Psychology, 19*, 242–246.

Juel, K., & Christensen, K. (2008). Are men seeking medical advice too late? Contacts to general practitioners and hospital admissions in Denmark 2005. *Journal of Public Health, 30*, 111–113.

Kales, H. C., Neighbors, H. W., Valenstein, M., Blow, F. C., McCarthy, J. F., Ignacio, R. V., … Mellow, A. M. (2005). Effect of race and sex on primary care physicians' diagnosis and treatment of late-life depression. *Journal of the American Geriatrics Society, 53*, 777–784.

Kattainen, A., Salomaa, V., Jula, A., Kesaniemi, Y. A., Kukkonen-Harjula, K., Kahonen, M., … Reunanen, A. (2005). Gender differences in the treatment and secondary prevention of CHD at population level. *Scandinavian Cardiovascular Journal, 39*, 327–333.

Kiefer, I., Rathmanner, T., & Kunze, M. (2005). Eating and dieting differences in men and women. *Journal of Men's Health & Gender, 2*, 194–201.

Kim, C., Redberg, R. F., Pavlic, T., & Eagle, K. A. (2006). A systematic review of gender differences in mortality after coronary artery bypass graft surgery and percutaneous coronary interventions. *Clinical Cardiology, 30*, 491–495.

Klein, L. C., Corwin, E. J., & Ceballos, R. M. (2006). The social costs of stress: How sex differences in stress responses can lead to social stress vulnerability and depression in women. In C. L. M. Keyes & S. H. Goodman (Eds.), *Women and depression: A handbook for the social, behavioral, and biomedical sciences* (pp. 199–218). New York, NY: Cambridge University Press.

Klumb, P. L., & Lampert, T. (2004). Women, work, and well-being, 1950–2000: A review and methodological critique. *Social Science & Medicine, 58*, 1007–1024.

Lam, C. B., & McBride-Chang, C. A. (2007). Resilience in young adulthood: The moderating influences of gender-related personality traits and coping flexibility. *Sex Roles, 56*, 159–172.

Lawlor, D. A., Smith, G. D., & Ebrahim, S. (2004). Socioeconomic position and hormone replacement therapy use: Explaining the discrepancy in evidence from observational and randomized controlled trials. *American Journal of Public Health, 94*, 2149–2154.

LeResche, L. (2000). Epidemiologic perspectives on sex differences in pain. In R. B. Fillingim (Ed.), *Sex, gender and pain* (pp. 233–249). Seattle, WA: IASP Press.

Light, K. C., Grewen, K. M., & Amico, J. A. (2005). More frequent partner hugs and higher oxytocin levels are linked to lower blood pressure and heart rate in premenopausal women. *Biological Psychology, 69*, 5–21.

Lowe, G. D. O. (2004). Hormone replacement therapy and cardiovascular disease: Increased risks of venous thromboembolism and stroke, and no protection from coronary heart disease. *Journal of Internal Medicine, 256*, 361–374.

Lyons, K. S., Stewart, B. J., Archbold, P. G., & Carter, J. H. (2009). Optimism, pessimism, mutuality, and gender: Predicting 10-year role strain in Parkinson's disease spouses. *The Gerontologist, 49*, 378–387.

Maciejewski, P. K., Prigerson, H. G., & Mazure, C. M. (2001). Sex differences in event-related risk for major depression. *Psychological Medicine, 31*, 593–604.

Marsh, A. A., Yu, H. H., Pine, D. S., & Blair, R. J. R. (2010). Oxytocin improves specific recognition of positive facial expressions. *Psychopharmacology, 209*, 225–232.

McMunn, A., Bartley, M., & Kuh, D. (2006). Women's health in mid-life: Life course social roles and agency as quality. *Social Science & Medicine, 63*, 1561–1572.

Migeon, B. R. (2006). The role of x inactivation and cellular mosaicism in women's health and sex-specific diseases. *Journal of the American Medical Association, 295*, 1428–1433.

Murberg, T. A., & Bru, E. (2004). Social support, negative life events and emotional problems among Norwegian adolescents. *School Psychology International, 25*, 387–403.

Nagurney, A. J. (2007). The effects of relationship stress and unmitigated communion on physical and mental health outcomes. *Stress and Health, 23*, 267–273.

Nathanson, C. A. (1978). Sex roles as variables in the interpretation of morbidity data: A methodological critique. *International Journal of Epidemiology, 7*, 253–262.

National Alliance for Caregiving and AARP. (2004). Caregiving in the U.S.: MetLife Foundation.

National Center for Health Statistics. (2011). *Health, United States, 2010: With special feature on death and dying.* Retrieved June 23, 2011, from http://www.cdc.gov/nchs/data/hus/hus10.pdf

Nolen-Hoeksema, S., & Hilt, L. (2006). Possible contributors to the gender differences in alcohol use and problems. *Journal of General Psychology, 133*, 357–374.

Ogden, C. L., Carroll, M. D., Curtin, L. R., Lamb, M. M., & Flegal, K. M. (2010). Prevalence of high body mass index in U.S. children and adolescents, 2007–2008. *Journal of the American Medical Association, 303*, 242–249.

Oksuzyan, A., Juel, K., Vaupel, J. W., & Christensen, K. (2008). Men: good health and high mortality. Sex differences in health and aging. *Aging Clinical and Experimental Research, 20*, 91–102.

Owens, I. P. F. (2002). Sex differences in mortality rate. *Science, 297*, 2008–2009.

Ozer, E. M. (1995). The impact of childcare responsibility and self-efficacy on the psychological health of professional working mothers. *Psychology of Women Quarterly, 19*, 315–335.

Pampel, F. C. (2002). Cigarette use and the narrowing sex differential in mortality. *Population and Development Review, 28*, 77–104.

Perenboom, R. J. M., van Herten, L. M., Boshuizen, H. C., & van den Bos, G. A. M. (2005). Life expectancy without chronic morbidity: Trends in gender and socioeconomic disparities. *Public Health Reports, 120*, 46–54.

Perkins, K. A., Donny, E., & Caggiula, A. R. (1999). Sex differences in nicotine effects and self-administration: Review of human and animal evidence. *Nicotine & Tobacco Research, 1*, 301–315.

Perkins, K. A., Gerlach, D., Vender, J., Grobe, J., Meeker, J., & Hutchison, S. (2001). Sex differences in the subjective and reinforcing effects of visual and olfactory cigarette smoke stimuli. *Nicotine & Tobacco Research, 3*, 141–150.

Pettinato, A. A., Loud, K. J., Bristol, S. K., Feldman, H. A., & Gordon, C. M. (2006). Effects of nutrition, puberty, and gender on bone ultrasound measurements in adolescents and young adults. *Journal of Adolescent Health, 39*, 828–834.

Piro, M., Zeldow, P. B., Knight, S. J., Mytko, J. J., & Gradishar, W. J. (2001). The relationship between agentic and communal personality traits and psychosocial adjustment to breast cancer. *Journal of Clinical Psychology in Medical Settings, 8*, 263–271.

Pleis, J. R., & Lethbridge-Cejku, M. (2007). Summary health statistics for U.S. adults: National Health Interview Survey, 2006. *Vital and health statistics: Series 10. Data from the National Health Survey, 235*, 1–153.

Ray, R., Jepson, C., Patterson, F., Strasser, A., Rukstalis, M., Perkins, K., … Lerman, C. (2006). Association of *OPRM1* A118G variant with the relative reinforcing value of nicotine. *Psychopharmacology, 188*, 355–363.

Reynolds, K. A., Helgeson, V. S., Seltman, H., Janicki, D., Page-Gould, E., & Wardle, M. (2006). Impact of interpersonal conflict on individuals high in unmitigated communion. *Journal of Applied Social Psychology, 36*, 1595–1616.

Rieker, P. P., & Bird, C. E. (2005). Rethinking gender differences in health: Why we need to integrate social and biological perspectives. *Journal of Gerontology, 60B*, 40–47.

Rigby, J. E., & Dorling, D. (2007). Mortality in relation to sex in the affluent world. *Journal of Epidemiology and Community Health, 61*, 159–164.

Rigby, K. (2000). Effects of peer victimization in schools and perceived social support on adolescent well-being. *Journal of Adolescence, 23*, 57–68.

Rudolph, K. D., & Hammen, C. (1999). Age and gender as determinants of stress exposure, generation, and reactions in youngsters: A transactional perspective. *Child Development, 70*, 660–677.

Sabo, D. (2005). The study of masculinities and men's health. In M. S. Kimmel, J. Hearn, & R. W. Connell (Eds.), *Handbook of studies on men and masculinities* (pp. 326–352). Thousand Oaks, CA: Sage.

Schnittker, J. (2007). Working more and feeling better: Women's health, employment, and family life, 1974–2004. *American Sociological Review, 72*, 221–238.

Shih, J. H., Eberhart, N. K., Hammen, C. L., & Brennan, P. A. (2006). Differential exposure and reactivity to interpersonal stress predict sex differences in adolescent depression. *Journal of Clinical Child and Adolescent Psychology, 35*, 103–115.

Simoni-Wastila, L. (1998). Gender and psychotropic drug use. *Medical Care, 36*, 88–94.

Snell, W. E., Belk, S. S., & Hawkins, R. C. (1987). Alcohol and drug use in stressful times: The influence of the masculine role and sex-related personality attributes. *Sex Roles, 16*, 359–373.

Spence, J. T., & Buckner, C. E. (2000). Instrumental and expressive traits, trait stereotypes, and sexist attitudes: What do they signify? *Psychology of Women Quarterly, 24*, 44–62.

Spence, J. T., Helmreich, R. L., & Holahan, C. K. (1979). Negative and positive components of psychological masculinity and femininity and their relationships to self-reports of neurotic and acting out behaviors. *Journal of Personality and Social Psychology, 37*, 1673–1682.

Stoney, C. M. (2003). Gender and cardiovascular disease: A psychobiological and integrative approach. *Current Directions in Psychological Science, 12*, 129–133.

Sweeting, H. (1995). Reversals of fortune? Sex differences in health in childhood and adolescence. *Social Science & Medicine, 40*, 77–90.

Sweeting, H., & West, P. (2003). Sex differences in health at ages 11, 13, and 15. *Social Science & Medicine, 56*, 31–39.

Szinovacz, M. E., & Davey, A. (2004). Retirement transitions and spouse disability: Effects on depressive symptoms. *Journal of Gerontology: Social Sciences, 59B*, S333–S342.

Szinovacz, M., & Washo, C. (1992). Gender differences in exposure to life events and adaptation to retirement. *Journal of Gerontology: Social Sciences, 47*, S191–S196.

Tolin, D. F., & Foa, E. B. (2006). Sex differences in trauma and posttraumatic stress disorder: A quantitative review of 25 years of research. *Psychological Bulletin, 132*, 959–992.

Torsheim, T., Ravens-Sieberer, U., Hetland, J., Valimaa, R., Danielson, M., & Overpeck, M. (2006). Cross-national variation of gender differences in adolescent subjective health in Europe and North America. *Social Science & Medicine, 62*, 815–827.

Travis, C. B. (2005). 2004 Carolyn Sherif Award address: Heart disease and gender inequality. *Psychology of Women Quarterly, 29*, 15–23.

Trudeau, K. J., Danoff-Burg, S., Revenson, T. A., & Paget, S. A. (2003). Agency and communion in people with rheumatoid arthritis. *Sex Roles, 49*, 303–311.

Turner, R. J., & Avison, W. R. (1989). Gender and depression: Assessing exposure and vulnerability to life events in a chronically strained population. *Journal of Nervous and Mental Disease, 177*, 443–455.

U.S. Census Bureau. (2007). Death rates by age, sex, and race: 1950 to 2005. Retrieved from http://cdc.gov/NCHS/data/nvsr/nvsr57/nvsr57_14.pdf

U.S. Department of Health and Human Services. (2008). *Tobacco product and alcohol use in lifetime, past year, and past month among persons aged 12 or older: Percentages, 2005 and 2006*. Retrieved from http://www.oas.samhsa.gov/NSDUH/2k6NSDUH/tabs/Sect2peTabs1to42.htm

U. S. Department of Labor. (2009). *Women in the labor force: A databook*. Retrieved August 17, 2010, from www.bls.gov/cps/wlf-databook2009.htm

U. S. Department of Labor. (2010). *Hours worked and fatal work injuries, by gender of worker, 2008*. Retrieved September 23, 2010, from http://www.bls.gov/iif/oshcfoi1.htm

U.S. Department of Transportation. (2008). *Traffic safety facts, 2006*. Retrieved from http://www-nrd.nhtsa.dot.gov/Pubs/810809.pdf

Von Bothmer, M. I. K., & Fridlund, B. (2005). Gender differences in health habits and in motivation for a healthy lifestyle among Swedish university students. *Nursing and Health Sciences, 7*, 107–118.

Waldron, I. (1997). Changing gender roles and gender differences in health behavior. In D. S. Gochman (Ed.), *Handbook of health behavior research: I. Personal and social determinants* (pp. 303–328). New York, NY: Plenum Press.

Wang, L., Heppner, P. P., & Berry, T. R. (1997). Role of gender-related personality traits, problem-solving appraisal, and perceived social support in developing a mediational model of psychological adjustment. *Journal of Counseling Psychology, 44*, 245–255.

Wardle, J., Haase, A. M., Steptoe, A., Nillapon, M., Jonwotiwes, K., & Bellisle, F. (2004). Gender differences in food choice: The contribution of health beliefs and dieting. *Annals of Behavioral Medicine, 27*, 107–116.

Wetter, D. W., Kenford, S. L., Smith, S. S., Fiore, M. C., Jorenby, D. E., & Baker, T. B. (1999). Gender differences and smoking cessation. *Journal of Consulting and Clinical Psychology, 67*, 555–562.

Writing Group for the Women's Health Initiative Investigators. (2002). Risks and benefits of estrogen plus progestin in healthy postmenopausal women: Principal results from the Women's Health Initiative randomized controlled trial. *Journal of the American Medical Association, 288*, 321–333.

Yuan, A. S. V. (2007). Gender differences in the relationship of puberty with adolescents' depressive symptoms: Do body perceptions matter? *Sex Roles, 57*, 69–80.

Zak, P. J., Stanton, A. A., & Ahmadi, S. (2007). Oxytocin increases generosity in humans. *Public Library of Science, 2*(11). Retrieved from http://www.plosone.org/article/info%3Adoi%2F10.1371%2Fjournal.pone.0001128

23 Socioeconomic Status and Health

John M. Ruiz and Courtney C. Prather
University of North Texas

Patrick Steffen
Brigham Young University

Forty-eight-year-old Arthur Johnson grew up poor in southeast Dallas with his mother and four younger siblings. At age 13 he dropped out of school in order to work to help provide for his family. At the age of 27 he enrolled in a trade school and became an electrician. Working 12- to 15-hour days, six days a week, he's been able to purchase a modest house in an economically challenged neighborhood. He's also begun to accumulate a small savings, relieving him of the burden of living paycheck to paycheck and with hopes of sending his two children to college one day. Arthur is a success story in his community, where he and his wife enjoy Sundays tending the front garden and conversing with their neighbors. His quick wit and eagerness to help have earned him close friends and many acquaintances, along with a loyal customer base. Despite a recent downturn in business, Arthur has remained upbeat, telling his wife that he's weathered hard times before.

Arthur's calm demeanor belies his physical health challenges. Arthur has diabetes and high blood pressure, which he manages with medication he pays for out-of-pocket. He would like health insurance but cannot afford the monthly premiums because of the variations in his income as work ebbs and flows. The long hours of work also make it difficult for him to engage in any meaningful physical exercise or eat small frequent meals as is prescribed for his diabetes. Arthur's health and economic worlds collided last month when he suffered a substantial stroke paralyzing his left side and impairing his speech. Now home from the hospital, he requires physical rehabilitation and nursing care, which further strain his economic situation. He doesn't know when or if he will be able to return to work and worries about the accumulating debt that threatens all he has worked for. "Why did this happen?" he asks.

Did poverty in early life set a trajectory for Arthur's poor health in adulthood, or are the effects of socioeconomic status (SES) more acute or time limited? Does his SES have a direct physiological effect on his health, or are such effects mediated by behavior or such psychological processes as stress? To what extent is Arthur's health a result of not only his individual SES but also the economic status of his community as reflected in availability of healthy food, quality health care, and exposure to stress in his neighborhood? Alternatively, to what extent does Arthur's health impact his SES and his ability to afford the rehabilitation and care that will affect his ability to work again in the future?

OVERVIEW

The aims of this chapter are to (a) review a model for conceptualizing SES and a framework for understanding its relationship to health, (b) examine the major approaches to measurement and discuss the associated pros and cons, (c) review the evidence regarding SES and physical disease, (d) discuss key moderating and mediating pathways, and (e) explore exceptions to the relationship as well as discuss emerging areas of inquiry.

A GRADED RELATIONSHIP

Although the idea that wealth and health are inextricably linked has been around for centuries, contemporary research on the relationship largely began with the landmark "Whitehall" studies. Initiated in 1967, Whitehall began as a 10-year prospective study of 18,000+ British civil servant men (Reid et al., 1976). The original aim was to examine social determinants of cardiorespiratory disease and mortality. A key, if surprising, finding was a relationship between employment grade and mortality: Men in the lowest employment grade (e.g., manual laborers, doormen) were at significantly greater risk of cardiovascular and all-cause mortality than were men in the higher grades (Marmot, Shipley, & Rose, 1984). A follow-up study, Whitehall II, was initiated in 1985 to further investigate these relationships in a sample of 10,308 men and women (Marmot et al., 1991). Data collection moved beyond simple epidemiological relationships to explore mediating psychological, social/environmental, and biological pathways. Since 1991, more than 400 papers have been published from the Whitehall data. Whitehall demonstrated that the relationship between social position and health was *graded* as opposed to a dichotomy between the most disadvantaged and everyone else. Over four decades after Whitehall, data continue to demonstrate this graded relationship (see Figure 23.1), making it among the most robust findings in psychosocial health research.

WHAT IS SOCIOECONOMIC STATUS AND WHAT IS IT NOT?

A sociological ranking index, SES can be applied to individuals, groups, neighborhoods, communities, or populations and is used to make relative comparisons as well as predictions for a variety of outcomes, including health. Generally, SES is conceptualized as an amalgam or mix of multiple interrelated yet unique factors, including but not limited to economics (e.g., income, wealth, resources), occupation, education, and social status (see Figure 23.2). Whereas these markers are generally correlated and trend in the same direction (e.g., better occupation status and higher income), exceptions are not uncommon (e.g., high-status position, low pay).

It is important to note that SES is not synonymous with race or ethnicity. Although these factors are generally correlated, substantial evidence demonstrates that they have unique effects on health. For example, Clarke and colleagues (2010) examined race, ethnicity, and SES differences in life

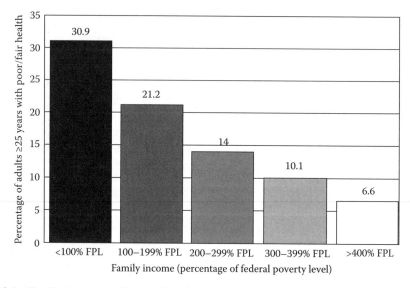

FIGURE 23.1 Family income gradient on health in the United States. In 2005 the federal poverty level (FPL) was $16,090 for a family of three. Findings from the *National Health Interview Survey, 2005* consistently show a relationship between lower family income and worse self-reported health. (Adapted from Robert Wood Johnson Foundation, 2009.)

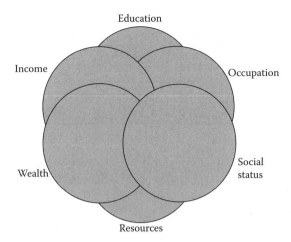

FIGURE 23.2 Socioeconomic status (SES) is conceptualized as an amalgam or mix of income or monetary wealth, education, and social status as exemplified in one's job or standing in the community.

expectancy in a study of all deaths occurring in California between 1999 and 2001. In examining race and SES main effects, the study found a nearly 20-year life expectancy gap between racial and ethnic groups living in neighborhoods with the highest SES quintile (Asian women: 84.9 years) as compared to the lowest (African American men: 65.3 years). It is also important to note that life expectancy did not vary as a function of SES among Hispanics. These and similar findings demonstrate that SES and race exert substantial independent influences on health (Baquet & Commiskey, 2000; Harper et al., 2009; D. R. Williams, 1999).

MEASUREMENT

GENERAL CONSIDERATIONS

Although SES is an amalgam of several factors, it is often assessed with a single construct such as income, education level, or occupation as in the Whitehall I study. There are several reasons for this approach. First, most SES markers are reliably correlated, suggesting that although none are perfect, all are similarly effective predictors. Second, SES is often operationalized based on available data or convenience, with psychometric standards largely ignored (Oakes & Rossi, 2003). Third, SES is often examined simply as a covariate, and as such minimal effort is put forth into rigorous assessment.

Researchers must also choose whether to use self-report or objective measures. This choice often reflects ease of consent and the measure's relevance to the specific aims of the study. In some cases, researchers may be more interested in perceptions; whereas other research questions may involve entire communities, thereby making self-report data too cumbersome to collect. It is important to note here that growing evidence suggests that objective SES indicators offer no appreciable benefit with respect to predicting health compared to subjective sources (Ostrove, Adler, Kuppermann, & Washington, 2000).

INCOME

Income refers to the flow of revenue or monetary resources. Some researchers suggest that income is the most important of the SES concepts because it either moderates or mediates the relationship of most of the other SES variables on health (cf. McDonough, Duncan, Williams, & House, 1997). Income is easy to stratify and interpret and can be assessed as a continuous variable or with categorical ranges (e.g., $25,000 to $49,999). Although income is associated with the highest response refusal rates among economic indicators (Liberatos, Link, & Kelsey, 1988), and when estimated it may be subject to more error than other indicators, measurement strategies such as the use of categories can minimize associated challenges. When measuring income, it is important to clarify the source (individual, family, business dividends, etc.) and time frame in which the income is accrued (e.g., hourly, monthly, annually). An alternative to asking several income questions is to specify the range in the question (e.g., "What is your total individual annual income?").

Several related concepts are also used as financial markers of SES. For example, *wealth* refers to the sum of such acquired resources as monetary savings, property, and investments, which have monetary value and may be crucial to overcoming disruptions in income flow or emergencies. *Benefits* are a form of compensation with monetary value and include, but are not limited to, health and life insurance, retirement pensions, paid leave, child care, credit unions, and pretax payment options for a variety of services that thereby reduce employees' taxable income. Likewise, such *indicators* as use of food stamps or Medicaid may reflect some relative economic status based on a financial demarcation (e.g., income level indicating poverty). Despite the relevance of these various indices, current income is the most commonly assessed economic indicator, and often the only economic indicator, yet it remains a significant predictor of health outcomes, including mortality (McDonough et al., 1997; Wilkinson, 1990).

EDUCATION

Education is a multidimensional SES construct reflecting status and income. A simple search of PubMed records for 2008 reveals nearly five times as many hits for "education *and* health" compared to "income *and* health" (20,904 vs. 3,426). This difference may be a result of a number of measurement strengths associated with education. Education represents an easily measured variable that is quantifiable for individuals outside the labor force. Education level is also relatively stable after young adulthood, precluding reverse-causation explanations, because most health outcomes of interest manifest after education has been established. Education also, presumably, provides or impedes access to future occupational status and income and may alternatively be conceptualized as a higher order moderator of SES. Furthermore, the relatively standard approach to quantifying education (in years) facilitates meta-analysis and cross-study comparisons (Liberatos et al., 1988). These qualities have made education one of the most popular approaches to SES measurement used in the United States (Krieger, Chen, & Ebel, 1997).

Given the simplicity of the variable, education is generally assessed with ad hoc questions rather than standardized measures. A common approach is to assess one to 12 years of education continuously and then offer categorical choices for higher education achievements (degrees, certifications). Some investigators choose entirely categorical options. For example, Molla, Madan, and Wagener (2004) used three education categories (0–8 years, 9–12 years, and 13+ years) to examine 1998 National Center for Health Statistics mortality data. Albano and colleagues (2007) used six categories (0–8 years, 9–11 years, 12 years, 13–15 years, 16 years, and 17+ years) to look at the relationship between SES and cancer mortality rates in the 2000 National Health Interview Survey. This approach emphasized specific educational milestones (12 years indicating high school graduation, 16 years indicating attainment of a bachelor's degree). Categorical approaches have the added benefit of denoting appreciable milestones in education. For example, in the American education system, the difference between junior high and high school is generally more meaningful than the difference between seventh and eighth grade.

There are a few noteworthy limitations in the use of education as a socioeconomic marker. For example, the variance in education is rather constricted, inhibiting observation of possible gradient effects. Further, higher education does not always predict earning status. For example, in the 2009

Forbes ranking of the 400 richest Americans, no one in the top ten had a doctoral-level education (Forbes.com, 2009). In addition, education is almost exclusively a predictor and rarely an outcome of health among adults.

OCCUPATION

Occupation generally reflects educational attainment and is a determinant of income and thus is an adequate, and perhaps more stable, index of the two (D. R. Williams & Collins, 1994). Moreover, occupation can be conceptualized as representing an individual's relationship to others in society, thereby determining not only access to resources that may have an impact on health (Mare, 1990) but also an individual's environment. In some cases, job characteristics appear to mediate the relationship between SES indicators and health outcomes (Karmakar & Breslin, 2008; Robert Warren, Hoonakker, Carayon, & Brand, 2004). For example, higher status occupations, or "white collar" jobs, are associated with greater control, lower stress, and lower exposure to environmental toxins (Johnson, Stewart, Hall, Fredland, & Theorell, 1996). Also, the characteristics of an occupation may influence such health behaviors as sedentary activity and risk of accidents (Wandel & Roos, 2005).

In order to capture the general social status of an occupation, ranking systems are commonly used to code occupations into a score. These scores are based on subjective hierarchical ordering of the relative status of occupations (i.e., prestige) by either investigators or survey. The Socioeconomic Index (SEI; Duncan, 1961) ranks 446 occupations and is among the most commonly used measures of SES in the United States. An advantage of the SEI is that its rankings have been updated several times to meet the needs of different populations (Blau & Duncan, 1967; Nakao, Hodge, & Treas, 1990; Nakao & Treas, 1994). Likewise, the Index of Social Position (ISP) developed by Hollingshead and Redlich (1958) is a widely used community-based scale of prestige. The ISP has the added advantage of using a two-factor measurement approach (occupation, education) yielding a composite index that is more consistent with the conceptualization of SES as a multifactoral index (Hollingshead, 1971, 1975).

It is important to note that the prestige associated with an occupation may be moderated by a number of factors, including race or ethnicity, region, gender, and time (e.g., "Disco dance instructor isn't quite what it used to be"; Berkman & Macintyre, 1997; Treiman, McKeever, & Fodor, 1996). More broadly, several caveats exist for the use of occupation as an indicator of SES, including the challenge of classifying individuals outside the workforce (Martikainen & Valkonen, 1999).

CENSUS DATA

One of the most reliable methods for objectively assessing community-based socioeconomic characteristics is through the use of census tracking. Although census tracking yields little individual-level data, it is an excellent approach for assessing broader neighborhood and community factors ranging from median family income to percentage unemployed as well as the number of hospitals and other environmental resources for a given area. The gold-standard approach begins with obtaining participants' street addresses, which are then entered into a census database. Zip or postal codes are an alternative tracking code useful for obtaining neighborhood information, particularly when specific street address information is unavailable (Geronimus & Bound, 1998). The U.S. Census Bureau has national data collected decennially, with more focused and frequent data available from many regional sources (e.g., cities, states).

Studies typically use neighborhood divisions as defined by the U.S. Census Bureau in regions of increasing specificity: *Census tracts* representing the largest grouping variable, followed by *census block-groups* and *census blocks*. Although census blocks represent the most homogenous group, with about 85 residents in each region, such blocks tend to yield less socioeconomic data (C. P. Kaplan & Van Valey, 1980). Block-groups, consisting of about 1,000 residents, tend to be more homogenous than census tracts, with about 4,000 residents, and thus they more accurately represent demarcations in the socioeconomic characteristics of a given area (Krieger, 1992). It is important to note that evidence suggests that census blocks-groups and census tracts appear to perform equally well (Diez Roux et al., 2001; Krieger et al., 2002). Census estimates of SES based on block-groups have been shown to correlate with individual-level indicators from 0.5 to 0.8, with census tracts correlating slightly higher (Diez Roux et al., 2001).

SUBJECTIVE SOCIAL STATUS

A recent advance in the measurement of SES is the use of a composite subjective rating scale. The emerging measure of choice is the MacArthur Scale of Subjective Social Status (SSS; Adler, Epel, Castellazzo, & Ickovics, 2000). The single-item measure includes a figure of a ladder. Participants are instructed to rank their perceived social status by choosing a rung on the ladder that represents their location relative to others', from low to high. Modifications in the wording of the instrument are used to reflect social status within different contexts (i.e., neighborhood, community, country). It is hypothesized that social standing at the national level may be more analogous to traditional measures of SES, whereas community standing may be an indication of resource distribution and perception of relative status in the immediate environment (MacArthur Foundation, 2009). Indeed, results appear to differ as a function of the comparative context (Ritterman et al., 2009). The MacArthur Foundation SES Research Network suggests using both a community version and a national version whenever possible in order to observe differential outcomes as function.

The MacArthur SSS scale correlates with measures of education, income, and occupation (Ghaed & Gallo, 2007; Goldman, Cornman, & Chang, 2006; Ostrove et al., 2000; Singh-Manoux, Adler, & Marmot, 2003) yet appears to explain unique variance not accounted for by these traditional measures (Thurston & Matthews, 2009). This result has led some researchers to posit that the MacArthur SSS is a "cognitive average" of objective SES indices, adding a subjective weighting element not assessed in the conventional indicators (Singh-Manoux et al., 2003). Given the scale's subjective nature, it is not surprising that the SSS is most predictive of self-rated health (de Castro, Gee, & Takeuchi, 2010; Franzini & Fernanez-Esquer, 2006; Ostrove et al., 2000). However, in limited-data lower SSS is also associated with objective health variables, including higher levels of cholesterol, C-reactive protein, elevated ambulatory blood pressure, and diabetes status (de Castro et al., 2010; Demakakos, Nazroo, Breeze, & Marmot, 2008; Ghaed & Gallo, 2007; Lemeshow et al., 2008). In spite of its simplicity, the SSS represents a potentially exciting advancement in the assessment of SES.

PHYSICAL DISEASE OUTCOMES

As illustrated in the opening vignette, the relationship between SES and health is not unidirectional. Although Arthur grew up poor, his SES had risen significantly by the time of his stroke. Still, his education, job, and income are all intertwined and contributed to his level of stress, his ability to behaviorally manage his health, and his ability to afford health insurance. Consequently, his stroke is now lowering his SES because he is unable to work and is accumulating debt. This transactional pattern where Arthur's SES influences his health, which then influences his SES, is characteristic of the relationship between SES and health (see Figure 23.3). In this section, we will review the evidence regarding SES as a determinant of health. In subsequent sections, we will discuss the impact of health on SES.

ALL-CAUSE MORTALITY

Evidence from the landmark Whitehall studies regarding the graded relationship between lower SES and greater mortality serves as the cornerstone to SES-health research (Marmot, 2003;

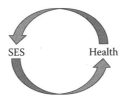

FIGURE 23.3 Transactional relationship between socioeconomic status (SES) and health. Although SES is often viewed as a determinant of future health, poor health can negatively impact financial aspects of SES, including the ability to work and accumulate wealth.

Marmot & Feeney, 1997). This incremental risk associated with socioeconomic disparities has been replicated in several population-based studies and broadened to include multiple socioeconomic indicators (Borrell, Diez Roux, Rose, Catellier, & Clark, 2004; Pickett & Pearl, 2001; Subramanian, Chen, Rehkopf, Waterman, & Krieger, 2005; Van Lenthe et al., 2005). For example, lower individual and neighborhood SES markers predicted future all-cause mortality in the Alameda County Study (Frank, Cohen, Yen, Balfour, & Smith, 2003; Haan, Kaplan, & Camacho, 1987; G. A. Kaplan, Baltrus, & Raghunathan, 2007; Turrell, Lynch, Leite, Raghunathan, & Kaplan, 2007; Yen & Kaplan, 1999).

Although the Whitehall study focused on examining incremental risk associated with occupational class, the general issue of employment versus unemployment has garnered more attention. In a study of Swedish twins, unemployment was associated with an increased risk of mortality at 10-year and 25-year follow-ups as indicated by the Swedish Causes of Death Registry (Nylen, Voss, & Floderus, 2001; Voss, Nylen, Floderus, Diderichsen, & Terry, 2004). Similarly, data from the Office of Population Censuses and Surveys longitudinal study in England (Moser, Fox, & Jones, 1984) showed an increased risk of mortality for men seeking work in the week previous to the 1971 census. Recent evidence suggests that unemployment and economic hardship are associated with lower frequency of automobile accidents but higher suicide rates (Stuckler, Basu, Suhrcke, Coutts, & McKee, 2009). It is of interest that a higher rate of mortality was also observed in the wives of unemployed males, and these effects were only partly explained by differences in SES. As part of the Coronary Artery Risk Development in Young Adults (CARDIA) Study, Janicki-Deverts, Cohen, Matthews, and Cullen (2008) found recent or current unemployment at 7-year or 10-year follow-up in males to be associated with increased levels of circulating C-reactive protein, a biomarker of inflammation and hypothesized preclinical indicator of cardiovascular disease (CVD; Danesh et al., 2000). Although this research provides insight into health disparities relative to absolute position in the workforce, it does not appreciate the more subtle, stepwise health implications of occupations.

Similar to the employment question are issues related to poverty status. Several studies have examined the relative risk associated with individual versus neighborhood poverty. In the Alameda County Study, individuals residing in a federally designated poverty area had a 71% greater relative risk of mortality compared to those in nonpoverty areas after controlling for baseline health, race, marital status, body mass index, and individual-level socioeconomic indicators (Haan et al., 1987). Similarly, a recent study of 293,138 middle-aged men screened in 14 states for participation in the Multiple Risk Factor Intervention Trial (MRFIT) found that neighborhood poverty was predictive of mortality over a 25-year-follow-up (Thomas, Eberly, Davey Smith, & Neaton, 2006). At the individual level, the graduated relationship between income and mortality risk appears nonlinear, with substantially greater risk associated with gradients near and below poverty status (Backlund, Sorlie, & Johnson, 1996; Frank et al., 2003). For example, data from the National Health and Nutrition Examination Survey (NHANES) demonstrated that in contrast to a steep slope reflecting increasing mortality risk with lower income, there is little decreasing mortality benefit associated with incomes above the median level (Rehkopf, Berkman, Coull, & Krieger, 2008).

The effects of economic disparities are not limited to adults. National and international population-based studies have documented a strong inverse association between parental income, education, poverty status, and neighborhood economic factors and greater risk of neonatal, post-natal, and infant mortality (Jahan, 2008; Jorgensen, Mortensen, & Andersen, 2008; Pena, Wall, & Persson, 2000; Singh & Kogan, 2007). Thus, the accumulated evidence strongly supports a robust relationship between SES and mortality across the lifespan.

INFECTIOUS DISEASES

Infectious diseases refer to conditions caused by bacteria, viruses, parasites, or fungi and can be spread directly or indirectly from one person to another. Substantial evidence links lower SES to higher incidence rates of a range of infectious conditions, including tuberculosis (Cantwell, McKenna, McCray, & Onorato, 1998; Lopez De Fede, Stewart, Harris, & Mayfield-Smith, 2008), sexually transmitted infections (Aral, Adimora, & Fenton, 2008; Krieger, Waterman, Chen, Soobader, & Subramanian, 2003), and various forms of hepatitis (Nguyen & Thuluvath, 2008; Stuver, Boschi-Pinto, & Trichopoulos, 1997), as well as the common cold (Cohen et al., 2008). Such findings are important, given that infectious diseases may influence mortality directly, enable secondary infections, or exacerbate preexisting conditions leading to worse outcomes.

Among the most studied infectious disease conditions is HIV. The Centers for Disease Control (CDC, 2009) estimates that there are over one million cases of HIV in the United States with nearly one-half million living with AIDS. Approximately 56,000 people are newly infected annually, though there are significant variations in the infection rate over time, including an estimated peak of 130,000 in 1984–1985 and low of 49,000 in the early 1990s (CDC, 2009). Several studies have demonstrated an inverse relationship between SES and HIV incidence (Diaz et al., 1994; Hankins et al., 1998; Murrain & Barker, 1997; Zierler et al., 2000). In addition to having a link with greater risk, lower SES is associated with worse survival outcomes. For example, Cunningham and colleagues (2005) examined individual-level SES effects on survival in a national probability sample of 2,864 adults receiving care for HIV. Socioeconomic indices included wealth (accumulated financial assets), annual income, education, employment status, and insurance status. Participants were followed from 1996 to 2000. Individuals with no accumulated wealth and those with less than a high school education were significantly more likely than their counterparts to have died over the follow-up (RR = 1.89 and RR = 1.53, respectively).

Community-level SES indicators also appear to modulate survival. McDavid Harrison, Ling, Song, and Hall (2008) examined survival in data from the national HIV/AIDS Reporting System. Five-year survival rates were significantly lower for patients living in counties with higher poverty rates and higher unemployment ($RR_{men} = 1.3$, $RR_{women} = 1.8$). Moreover, the effect of neighborhood SES appears to be stronger in the era of highly active antiretroviral therapy (HAART; McFarland, Chen, Hsu, Schwarcz, & Katz, 2003). It is mportant to note that neighborhood SES may provide a positive buffer. Joy and colleagues (2008) found that neighborhoods with higher levels of postsecondary education conferred a relative survival benefit (HR = 0.80, 95% CI: 0.71–0.91).

CARDIOVASCULAR DISEASE

A large and relatively consistent body of research has documented substantial socioeconomic disparities in heart disease risk, particularly coronary heart disease (CHD; G. A. Kaplan & Keil, 1993; Marmot, 1996; Pollitt, Rose, & Kaufman, 2005; Skodova et al., 2008; Smith & Ruiz, 2002). This relationship is among the most reliable in psychosocial health research. Lower SES individuals are at greater risk of experiencing a myocardial infarction (MI; Foraker et al., 2008; Rose et al., 2009; Rosengren et al., 2009) and experiencing complications following coronary artery bypass surgery (Gibson et al., 2009; F. C. Taylor, Ascione, Rees, Narayan, & Angelini, 2003). For example, Kelly and Weitzen (2010) found that individuals with less than a high school education were 1.5 to 3.0

times more likely to experience an MI compared to those with a college degree. It is important to note that SES markers may work synergistically to increase risk (Gerber, Goldbourt, & Frory, 2008). Finally, lower SES is predictive of lower post-MI survival, with substantial evidence documenting a relationship not only between individual-level factors but also with area deprivation as well (Goldberg, Yarzebski, Lessard, & Gore, 1999; Singh & Siahpush, 2002; Tonne et al., 2005; Tyden, Hansen, Engstrom, Hedblad, & Janzon, 2002).

More tentative are the data demonstrating a relationship between SES and preclinical markers of CHD. Limited cross-sectional studies show associations between lower individual-level SES factors and atherosclerotic development in the carotid arteries (Diez-Roux, Nieto, Tyroler, Crum, & Szklo, 1995; Lynch, Kaplan, Salonen, Cohen, & Salonen, 1995; Lynch, Kaplan, Salonen, & Salonen, 1997; Rosvall et al., 2000, 2006). In a study examining coronary artery calcification (CAC), Yan and colleagues (2006) estimated the relative risk for the presence of significant plaque in the coronary arteries was 4.14 (95% CI: 2.33–7.35) for individuals with less than a high school education compared to those with more than a college education. Building upon this finding, Dragano and colleagues (2007) found that the rate of increase in CAC, reflecting atherosclerotic progression, was 70% greater in men and 80% greater in women with less than 10 years of education compared to their more educated counterparts. Although more work is needed, these findings contribute to an emerging picture wherein SES influences CHD at multiple stages of the disease from development to its clinical endpoints.

CANCER

Cancer accounts for nearly one quarter (23.1%) of all deaths in the United States, exceeded only by diseases of the heart (ACS, 2009). The American Cancer Society predicts that over 1.5 million new cancer diagnoses will be made in 2009, adding to the 11 million people currently living with cancer. To put this number in perspective, one in two men and one in three women in the United States will develop cancer in their lifetime (ACS, 2009). However, there are significant disparities in cancer burden, including well-documented associations by race and ethnicity (Chu, Miller, & Springfield, 2007; Haynes & Smedley, 1999).

Gory and Vena (1994) examined the relationship between SES, race, and cancer incidence in 10 epidemiological studies drawing data from six national samples and four state and regional samples. They determined SES by dichotomizing income and education data and examining associations with mean estimates for a variety of cancers. Results revealed a relative risk of 1.19 for all cancers with the strongest associations observed for stomach, lung, cervix, and rectal sites. Although Blacks were four times more likely to be low in SES compared to Whites (52.8% vs. 12.3%, respectively), the aggregate effect of low SES on cancer incidence was similar across race (e.g., stomach cancer: $RR_{Black} = 2.14$, $RR_{White} = 2.12$). These findings suggest that the effect of low SES on cancer risk may be independent of race.

Similar data come from the National Cancer Institute's Surveillance, Epidemiology, and End Results (SEER) program. SEER is a population-based cancer registry covering approximately 26% of the U.S. population and serving as a significant database for U.S. cancer statistics. In a recent SEER-based study, lower education and income were independently associated with greater risk of lung cancer relative to higher levels of each (Clegg et al., 2009). Similar findings have been reported for cervical cancer (Singh, Miller, Hankey, & Edwards, 2004), suggesting an overall trend in the relationship between lower SES and higher cancer incidence across numerous sites.

Incidence reflects new diagnoses of cancer, which may be influenced by the frequency and quality of screening. Thus, the relationship between SES and cancer incidence is more complicated. Higher incidence rates for cancers identified through routine screening procedures (e.g., mammograms, prostrate-specific antigen/prostate exams) are typically associated with higher as opposed to lower SES, particularly as indexed by area or neighborhood SES (Hemminki & Li, 2003; Liu, Cozen, Bernstein, Ross, & Deapen, 2001; Lund Nilsen, Johnsen, & Vatten, 2000). Moreover, poverty is associated with not only a lower frequency of diagnosis but also diagnoses of more advanced cancers at numerous sites, including breast (Clegg et al., 2009; Echeverria, Borrell, Brown, & Rhoads, 2009; Harper et al., 2009), prostate (Clegg et al., 2009; Rapiti et al., 2009), cervix (Singh et al., 2004), and head and neck (Molina et al., 2008), with these stage differences contributing to differential mortality rates (Brookfield, Cheung, Lucci, Fleming, & Koniaris, 2009; Harper et al., 2009; Molina et al., 2008; Rapiti et al., 2009; Shackley & Clarke, 2005). Thus, area SES appears to moderate the stage of diagnosis, particularly for routinely screened cancers, with implications for survival.

Regardless of the mechanism, lower SES is broadly associated with reduced survival time following diagnosis and treatment for a range of cancer types. Schrijvers and Mackenbach (1994) examined the relationship between SES and cancer survival in 19 studies representing seven countries, most published in the 1970s and 1980s. The authors focused on cancers with a minimum of three studies of significant size (i.e., > 200 deaths reported). Patients were divided into four SES groupings and survival times between them were compared with survival risk reported by comparing the lowest and highest quartiles. Lower SES was associated with shorter survival times for cancers of the colon, rectum, breast, and cervix. Similar survival differences have been documented elsewhere for these cancer sites (Wrigley et al., 2003) as well as for cancer of the breast (Du, Fang, & Meyer, 2008; Pollock & Vickers, 1997; Yu, 2009), bladder (Shackley & Clarke, 2005), lung (Chang, Shema, Wakelee, Clarke, & Gomez, 2009; Ou, Ziogas, & Zell, 2009), prostate (Gilligan, 2005), and malignant melanoma (MacKie & Hole, 1996).

In summary, the literature supports the association between lower SES and higher cancer risk, reduced chance of early detection, and lower survival. Individual-level factors (e.g., income, education) are most often documented as determinants of incidence and mortality, whereas infrastructure disparities appear to be key to early detection and associated survival.

Summary

The accumulated evidence supports a significant and reliable inverse relationship between SES and a broad range of diseases. Although the relationship is generally characterized as graded, emerging evidence suggests the slope of effect is nonlinear with stronger effects at the lower relative to the higher end of the SES continuum. In addition, the accumulated literature has not coalesced into meaningful index-risk clusters. Rather, many of the measures appear interchangeable, though some relationships, such as the effect of area deprivation on diagnosis and survival, appear stronger than others.

MEDIATING PATHWAYS

In the first part of this chapter, we discussed how SES is conceptualized and measured and the existing evidence on the relationship between SES and health. We now address the potential mechanisms and pathways through which SES may affect health. In this section, we address health care and health behavior, physical and social environments, and psychological and physiological functioning as potential factors in the relationship between SES and health. Each of these constructs has been related to both SES and health and may potentially mediate that relationship.

Health Behaviors

Health risk behaviors are one of the more studied pathways in the relationship between SES and health. Decades of research document the relationship between lower SES and higher rates of smoking (Schaap & Kunst, 2009; Schaap, van Agt, & Kunst, 2008), poor dietary habits (Darmon & Drewnowski, 2008; Shimakawa et al., 1994; Turrell & Kavanagh, 2006), and obesity (Drewnowski, 2009; Roskam & Kunst, 2008). In addition to being linked with these negative health behaviors, lower individual and community SES indicators are associated with less engagement in such potentially health-promoting behaviors as physical activity (Burton & Turrell, 2000; Kaleta & Jegier, 2005; Makinen et al., 2010). Lower SES individuals also appear to have more difficulty changing negative health behaviors (Winkelby, Flora, & Kraemer, 1994). Although research psychologists rarely "conclude" anything, the magnitude, reliability, and strength of the evidence lead these authors to conclude that SES is a significant determinant of health behaviors.

ACCESS

A major barrier to better health and disease management is access to health resources, including healthy food choices and quality health care. Lower SES neighborhoods generally have fewer larger grocery stores and health food options and higher numbers of fast-food restaurants, convenience stores, and liquor stores (Larson, Story, & Nelson, 2009; Pearce, Hiscock, Blakely, & Witten, 2008; Zenk et al., 2009). For example, Cummins, McKay, and MacIntyre (2005) examined the distribution of McDonald's Restaurants across England and Scotland by community SES. Communities in the highest economic quartile had a total of 76 McDonald's for a mean of 0.007 per 1,000 persons. In contrast, communities in the lowest economic quartile had over four times the number of McDonald's (321), or a mean of 0.03 per 1,000 persons, a statistically significant difference ($p < .0001$). Numerous studies have shown that proximity is an important determinant of intake, including healthy and unhealthy foods, tobacco, and other consumable resources (Dubowitz et al., 2008; Truong & Sturm, 2009; Zenk et al., 2009).

Socioeconomic factors influence not only risk and resilience factors but also access to the health care mechanisms associated with identification and treatment (Kirby & Kaneda, 2005). Lower SES individuals are less likely to have insurance or have a regular source of care (Andersen et al., 2002; Institute of Medicine, 1993). Substantial evidence suggests that they are less likely to receive preventive care or receive health screening (Blackwell, Martinez, Gentleman, Sanmartin, & Berthelot, 2009; Lasser, Himmelstein, & Woolhandler, 2006). As a result, lower SES individuals are more likely to be diagnosed at later stages of disease, which impacts prognosis and survival. Lower SES is also associated with significant treatment-seeking delays. For example, patients reporting significant delay in treatment seeking following the onset of chest pain are significantly more likely to be of low SES or live in low-SES communities (Ghali, Cooper, Kowatly, & Liao, 1993; Harralson, 2007; Henderson, Magana, Korn, Genna, & Bretsky, 2002). Finally, lower SES is associated with greater use of emergency rooms for emergent and nonemergent issues (Padgett & Brodsky, 1992; R. S. Stern, Weissman, & Epstein, 1991). Such use may be moderated by lack of a usual care provider, lack of health insurance, and greater treatment-seeking delay.

PHYSICAL AND SOCIAL ENVIRONMENTAL EXPOSURE

Exposure to unhealthy environments appears to play an important role in the relationship between SES and health (Evans & Kantrowtiz, 2002; S. E. Taylor, Repetti, & Seeman, 1997). Lower SES individuals are more likely to be exposed to hazardous waste, air and water pollution, and high levels of noise in their neighborhoods and work environments and to live in crowded neighborhoods with higher levels of violence. Because people spend the majority of their time at home and at work, exposure to unhealthy environments is a chronic, constantly present condition. Unfortunately, there is evidence that even during recreation, lower income individuals are more likely to be exposed to unhealthy conditions, such as swimming in contaminated waters (Cabelli & Dafour, 1983).

Likelihood of exposure to hazardous waste is directly related to SES. Lower income individuals are more likely to be exposed to hazardous waste in or near their neighborhoods as compared to those people higher in income (Mohai & Saha, 2006; White 1998). Blood levels of lead (Pb) have been of particular note: Low-income children have significantly higher levels of lead in their blood (Gump et al., 2007) and are more likely to be classified in the unhealthy range of blood levels (CDC, 2005).

Exposure to air and water pollution is another important pathway through which SES may be related to health. Low income is related to increased exposure to air pollution, particularly with poorer neighborhoods having poorer air quality than that found in wealthier neighborhoods (Brajer & Hall, 1992; Crouse, Ross, & Goldberg, 2009; Stuart, Mudhasakul, & Sriwatanapongse, 2009). Air pollution can occur both outdoors and indoors. Lower income individuals are more likely to be exposed to secondhand smoke, and children in lower income neighborhoods are more likely to have parents who smoke. Such toxic indoor pollutants as carbon monoxide are more common in low-income neighborhoods, where the probability of being exposed to radon is also higher, likely attributable to substandard housing construction (Chi & Laquatra, 1990; Goldstein, Andrews, & Hartel, 1988; Laquatra, Maxwell, & Pierce, 2005). Exposure to allergens, mold, and fungus is also higher for those people with lower income (Cho et al., 2008; Gold, 1992; Rosenstreich et al., 1997). Water pollution is also more common for lower SES individuals, who are more likely to have contaminated water (Calderon et al., 1993). Lower income individuals are also more likely to swim in contaminated water and fish from contaminated rivers (Cabelli & Dufour, 1983).

High levels of noise are common in lower SES neighborhoods. Low-income residents are twice as likely to report problems with noise (Sherman, 1994). There is a strong negative correlation between income and neighborhood noise (U.S. Environmental Protection Agency, 1977). In a study of exposure to aircraft noise and test performance, it was found that lower SES children, as measured by percentage receiving free lunch, were exposed to more aircraft noise in their neighborhoods (Haines, Stansfeld, Head, & Job, 2002). Exaggerated exposure to ambient environmental noise may lead to a variety of negative outcomes, including impaired learning, hearing difficulties, increased mental stress, and heightened risk of mood disorders or exacerbation of psychopathology (Satterwaite, 1993; Stansfeld et al., 2005; Warr, Feldman, Tacticos, & Kelaher, 2009).

In addition to having direct effects on individuals, environmental exposure may indirectly affect their health through increases in psychological stress. In this respect, such environmental factors as noise may be particularly problematic because they influence health through direct and indirect stress pathways. Other sources of SES-related stress include job stress and urbanization. For example, lower SES individuals are more likely to have higher job strain, defined as the combination of high demands with low control, than do higher SES individuals (Brand, Warren, Carayon, & Hoonakker, 2007; Landbergis, Schnall, Pickering, Warren, & Schwartz, 2003). Lower SES individuals are more likely to live in crowded urban areas and be exposed to crime and violence (Evans & Kantrowitz, 2002). Crowded living conditions are related to increased stress and negative health outcomes (Baum, Garofalo, & Yali, 1999). Crowding is also associated with less satisfaction with living conditions and neighborhood quality (Nelson, 1978). Crowding appears to be particularly stressful for children, with crowding associated with higher behavioral problems and poor academic achievement as well as negative health outcomes (Evans, Lepore, Shejwal, & Palsane, 1998). Low-SES neighborhoods also have higher levels of crime and a greater likelihood that its residents will experience violence (Koshal & Koshal, 1975; Morenoff & Sampson, 1997).

PSYCHOLOGICAL AND PHYSIOLOGICAL FUNCTIONING

Compelling evidence documents a graded relationship between lower SES and risk of negative affect, mood, and psychopathology. Lower SES is associated with higher incidence of depression and anxiety (Ansseau et al., 2008; Grant et al., 2005; Himmelfarb & Murrell, 1984; Warheit et al., 1975), anger (Mittleman, Maclure, Nachnani, Sherwood, & Muller, 1997; Ranchor, Bouma, & Sanderman, 1996), and hostility (Barefoot et al., 1991; Lynch, Kaplan, & Salonen, 1997; Scherwtiz, Perkins, Chesney, & Hughes, 1991). Some of these associations appear to be stronger among ethnic minorities (Barefoot et al., 1991; Scherwitz, Perkins, Chesney, & Hughes, 1991), and some studies suggest that the relationship begins in childhood (Gump, Matthews, & Raikkonen, 1999; Lynch, Kaplan, & Shema, 1997).

It is important to note that the level of risk is not negligible. A meta-analysis examining SES and depression found that low-SES individuals are 1.81 times more likely to be depressed in general and that the relationship follows a dose-response pattern (Lorant et al., 2003). Lower SES also predicted the likelihood of a new episode of depression and the likelihood of depression persisting over time. Similarly, a seven-year longitudinal study found that declining SES predicted increased risk of depression over time (Lorant et al., 2007). In contrast, improvements in SES indices (e.g., attaining more education; wealth or an increase in income) predicted decreases in depression risk.

Gallo and Matthews (2003) call attention to the potential role of negative emotions as mediators of the relationship between SES and health. Specifically, they posit that intrapsychic and emotional resources buffer stress-related pathogenic pathways and that lower SES is associated with fewer of these resources (i.e., reserve capacity) and, thus, with less buffering capability. Although much of the current evidence is still of an indirect nature, the existing findings are supportive of the theory that negative emotions, among them depression, anxiety, and hostility, play a key role in how SES contributes to negative health outcomes (Gallo, Bogart, Vranceanu, & Matthews, 2005; Gallo, Penedo, Espinosa de los Monteros, & Arguelles, 2009; Matthews, Raikkonen, Gallo, & Kuller, 2008). These authors also emphasize the idea that low-SES neighborhoods and work environments are stressful and contribute to a high stress burden.

Psychological stress may impact health through exaggerated changes in such acute physiological parameters as blood pressure and neuroendocrine and immune functioning (Uchino, Ruiz, & Holt-Lunstad, 2009). In general, low SES appears to be related to increased cardiovascular reactivity to stressful situations (Chen & Matthews, 2001; Everson et al., 2001; Gump et al., 1999; Wilson, Kliewer, Plybon, & Sica, 2000). For example, Everson et al. (2001) found that men with excessive blood pressure reactivity to stress had a greater risk of stroke, with this effect being stronger among those men with less education: Those individuals who had high stress responses in combination with low education were three times more likely to have a stroke compared to those who were low stress responders and had more education. However, several studies have found high SES to be related to increased cardiovascular reactivity (Carroll et al., 1997; Suchday, Krantz, & Gottdiener, 2005). It is not clear if the differences in findings are attributable demographic differences, methodological differences, or some combination.

As with cardiovascular reactivity, the majority of published research studies have found low SES to be related to increased neuroendocrine reactivity to stressful situations (Cohen, Doyle, & Baum, 2006; Cohen et al., 2006; Li, Power, Kelly, Kirschbaum, & Hertzman, 2007; Steptoe, Brydon, & Kunz-Ebrecht, 2005). Lower SES is associated with higher basal cortisol levels and a flattened cortisol rhythm from day to night, which is typically associated with increased stress (Cohen et al., 2006). Cortisol is also related to low SES measured across the lifespan, which may be indicative of having to cope with adversity over long periods of time (Li et al., 2007). Changes in SES are also predictive of neuroendocrine functioning, with improved financial situation being related to decreased cortisol response upon awakening (Steptoe et al., 2005).

EMERGING ISSUES

In this last section, we focus on three emerging issues in the relationship between SES and health. First, we address the effects of SES on health over the life course, examining the relative contributions of childhood SES and adult SES to health outcomes. Second, we address exceptions to the social gradient, situations where a reversed social gradient has been observed, with those individuals with low SES actually having better health outcomes. Third, we address the concepts of social capital, income inequality, and relative deprivation, which may partially explain the reversed social gradient. These three new emerging issues in the research on SES and health provide unique perspectives from which to consider how SES and health are related.

TIME IN THE LIFE COURSE

Are the health effects of SES acute or pervasive? Research has begun to focus on the effects of childhood and adolescent SES on health over time. A number of studies have found that both childhood and adult SES have significant effects on health (Galobardes, Davey Smith, & Lynch 2006; Galobardes, Lynch, & Davey Smith, 2004, 2008). Such findings have led to the development of various life course models to explain how SES is related to health over time (Berkman, 2009). These include the latency/sensitive periods model, cumulative exposure model, and the social trajectory model (Ben-Shlomo & Kuh, 2002; Berkman, 2009; Hertzman, 1999).

The first model, latency/sensitive periods, focuses on early life conditions that become embodied and then influence adult health outcomes directly (Hertzman, 1999). Although it is assumed that early life conditions contribute to adult social conditions, adult social conditions are not considered a pathway between early conditions and adult health. Rather, it is theorized that critical early life experiences affect how the brain and body develop, creating a predisposition for negative health outcomes later on.

As an example, the Johns Hopkins Precursor Study followed medical student graduates for an average period of 40 years and found that physicians who came from lower SES families had a 2.4 times increased hazard of developing CHD before the age of 50 compared to graduates from higher SES families (Kittleson et al., 2006). This difference in CHD risk was not mediated by such traditional risk factors as obesity and was evident despite identical education levels, occupational status, and earning potential, thus suggesting that something about the early SES environment may have conferred a greater risk trajectory.

How does early childhood deprivation affect health decades later? A number of studies have found that lower childhood SES is related to poorer health care access and negative health behaviors in childhood and adolescence (Chen, Matthews, & Boyce, 2002; Starfield, Riley, Witt, & Robertson, 2002; Starfield, Roberston, & Riley, 2002). Lower SES children are less likely to receive vaccinations or receive all their vaccinations, and they are less likely to see a doctor regularly during childhood (T. Williams, Milton, Farrell, & Graham, 1995). Lower SES children are more likely to receive injuries. Lower SES children and adolescents are more sedentary and are more likely to smoke.

Second, lower childhood SES influences the calibration of hypothalamic-pituitary-adrenal (HPA) stress-response mechanisms (Hertzman, 1999; Meaney & Szyf, 2005), resulting in increased sensitivity to evocative stimuli over the life course. In a study of stress hormone and inflammatory markers, Miller and colleagues (2009) found compelling evidence that SES impacts genetic expression as well as current levels of stress hormones and inflammatory markers. Specifically, lower childhood SES defined by parental occupation during the first five years of life was associated with higher levels of stress and inflammatory responses, even though there were no significant differences in current SES. These physiologic differences represent an emerging pathway through which childhood socioeconomic deprivation may influence lifetime health trajectories.

The second model, cumulative exposure (Lynch, Kaplan, & Shema, 1997), views adult social conditions as a partial pathway through which early childhood experiences affect adult health, in addition to the early childhood direct effects on health. Instead of only early childhood experiences leading to later negative health outcomes, there is a chronic accumulation of exposure across the life course that begins to take its toll in adulthood. This model appears to account for a larger proportion of research findings compared to the other models (Galobardes et al., 2006; Galobardes et al., 2004; Galobardes et al., 2008; Lynch, Kaplan, & Shema, 1997). For example, several studies indicate that childhood and adult SES have significant independent contributions to adult health (Harper et al., 2002; Lynch, Kaplan, & Solonen, 1997).

The third model, social trajectory, assumes that all the effects of early childhood conditions are mediated by adult social conditions (Ben-Shlomo & Kuh, 2002). The case where this relationship appears to be most true is that of occupational stress. Early childhood conditions, such as lack of educational opportunities, have a negative impact on future occupational possibilities. Low SES (e.g., lack of childhood education) therefore contributes to adult conditions by the increased likelihood of dangerous work environments and high-stress employment, and it is the employment status that then contributes directly to health outcomes (Brand et al., 2007).

EXCEPTIONS TO THE SOCIAL GRADIENT

Is it always the case that more wealth equals better health? Surprisingly, the answer appears to be a resounding no. Studies conducted in Africa, Asia, Polynesia, and South America have documented an "inverse" gradient, suggesting that lower SES individuals may actually have better health outcomes (Steffen, Smith, Larsen, & Butler, 2006). One of the first studies to indicate a reversed social gradient was published by C.P. Donnison in *The Lancet* in 1929. In the 1920s, C. P. Donnison, a medical officer in the East African Medical Service, observed that heart disease was virtually nonexistent in natives of Kenya (Donnison, 1929). In a sampling of over 1,000 patients studied in a hospital setting, no patients had signs of atherosclerosis, nor did blood pressure rise with age, as seen in Western countries. Donnison concluded that the simple way of life of the Kenyans studied was related to a lower stress lifestyle, whereas the higher SES of Europeans was related to a "high pressure existence" (p. 7). Studies from various parts of Africa also reached similar conclusions; specifically, Africans are healthier than Europeans in terms of such chronic conditions as heart disease, possibly because Africans face less stress and lead a healthier lifestyle (Steffen et al., 2006).

Building on this line of research, some researchers have hypothesized that low SES in some non-Western countries is associated with better health because individuals in non-Western countries live a more traditional lifestyle (Bunker et al., 1996; Cockerham & Yamori, 2000; Waldron, Nowotarksi, et al., 1982). This lifestyle often involves an agrarian or hunter-gatherer economy with a strong sense of community and strong social networks, which may reflect the broader concepts of social support and social integration (Waldron, Nowotarksi, et al., 1982). Okinawans, for example, are one of the longest lived people in the world and yet have relatively low SES compared to Japanese in other areas of Japan (Cockerham & Yamori, 2000). Most Okinawans work in agriculture or fishing and have a strong sense of community and strong social networks. In contrast, low-SES people in Western countries are more likely to work in industrial settings and have a weaker sense of community and weaker social networks (Marmot et al., 1991).

An emerging hypothesis suggests that cultural values may moderate health outcomes (Steffen, 2006). Cultural values embodying such psychosocial resilience factors as social support may buffer against risk and thus lead to better health outcomes. For example, more collectivistic cultures emphasizing community and interpersonal interconnectedness are more likely to value social support, a well-established health moderator (House, Landis, & Umberson, 1988). Many non-Western cultures appear to be healthy in spite of low SES at least partly because of this emphasis on social support and community (Cockerham, Hattori, & Yamori, 2000). In contrast, more individualistic cultures may be health damaging through an emphasis on individual achievement and competition, which often require adoption of social dominance and aggression, factors associated with disease risk (Siegman et al., 2000; Smith et al., 2008; Spence, 1985; Triandis, 1995; Waldron, Heron et al., 1982). Achievement and competition may also erode social support and fracture community ties, leading to adverse health outcomes. Moreover, for many Westerners, identity is strongly tied to SES (Spence, 1985), whereas non-Westerners are more likely to derive identity through group membership and social ties (Carpenter, 2000; Carpenter & Radhakrishnan, 2000; Dabul, Bernal, & Knight, 1995; Triandis, 1995). This cultural difference in how identity is defined may explain why the social gradient works differently between Western and non-Western societies. That is, because SES is more important to an individual's identity in Western countries, lower SES may be stressful because it indicates less worth as a person.

Studies of immigrants allow for observation of how acculturation—that is, loss of traditional cultural values and the acquisition of the dominant cultural values—affects health. Immigrants from non-Western countries to the United States generally have lower rates of infant mortality and better overall health relative to the naturalized citizens despite significant SES disadvantages (Escobar, Nervi, & Gara, 2001; M. P. Stern & Wei, 1999; D. R. Williams, 2005).

Hispanic immigrants in particular show a significant health advantage relative to U.S. citizens. This effect has been called the "Hispanic Paradox" because Hispanic immigrants are one of the poorest groups in the United States and yet have better health than those individuals higher in SES (Turra & Goldman, 2007). The paradox, which has implications both for theories of population health and for social policy, refers to Hispanics' lower all-cause mortality rate, relative to non-Latino Whites, despite the greater proportion of Latinos in disadvantaged social classes and the robust relationship between lower SES and poorer health. The innovative work of Abraído-Lanza and colleagues has demonstrated that Latinos' lower mortality is neither an artifact of migrant selectivity nor a result of undercounting of migrant deaths because of aging migrants returning to their countries of origin (Abraido-Lanza, Dohrenwend, Ng-Mak, & Turner, 1999).

As Hispanic immigrants acculturate to life in the United States, however, the immigrant health advantage disappears, with the immigrants becoming more like native-born Americans (Vega, Sribney, Aguilar-Gaxiola, & Kolody, 2004). Vega et al. (1998) found that there was a gradient of increased depression with increased time lived in the United States. Lifetime prevalence of major depressive episodes was 3.2% for Mexican immigrants who had lived less than 13 years in the United States, 7.9% for those living more than 13 years in the United States, and 14.4% for Mexican Americans born in the United States. As the prevalence of major depressive episodes increased, so did income and education, with U.S.-born Mexican Americans having significantly higher levels of SES as compared to immigrants. Given that Mexicans and Mexican immigrants are healthier than European Americans and U.S.-born Mexican Americans and that acculturation to Western culture leads to an increase in both distress and SES, it is possible that cultural factors (e.g., socially oriented versus individualistically oriented cultural values) explain the differences in health between immigrants and U.S.-born Mexican Americans.

The effects of acculturation on health can occur in a relatively short time frame (Dixon, Sundquist, & Winkleby, 2000; Forrester, Cooper, & Weatherall, 1998; Marmot & Syme, 1976; Sundquist & Winkelby, 2000; Vega et al., 2004; Wei et al., 1996). Several studies have noted that significant changes can occur early during the acculturation process, sometimes in as little as three years. Burszytn and Raz (1995) and Green, Etzion, and Jucha (1991) found that on arriving in Israel, Ethiopian immigrants were healthier than Israelis; but after three years of acculturation, the health difference had disappeared. In a meta-analysis of 125 studies on acculturation and blood pressure, it was found that the largest effect sizes were found within the first three years of acculturation (Steffen et al., 2006). More research is needed to determine whether these effects relate to the loss of traditional cultural identity or the acquisition of more Western cultural values.

Acculturation to Western society also impacts cultural values and social orientation (Cuellar, Arnold, & Gonzalez, 1995; Marin & Gamba, 2003). In a study comparing high- and low-acculturated Mexican American immigrants with Anglo Americans, more acculturated Mexican immigrants appeared more similar to Anglo Americans on a measure of cultural values than to less acculturated Mexican immigrants (Domino & Acosta, 1987). Hispanics score significantly higher on measures of familialism as compared to European Americans, but as Hispanics acculturate to Western society, their scores on familialism tend to decrease (Sabogal, Marin, Otero-Sabogal, Marin, & Perez-Stable, 1987).

SOCIAL CAPITAL, INCOME INEQUALITY, AND RELATIVE DEPRIVATION

High levels of social support and connectedness play a key role in the reversed social gradient. Having significant social resources is also referred to as *social capital*. Social capital "refers to features of a social organization, such as trust, norms and networks that can improve the efficiency of society by facilitating coordinated actions" (Putnam, 1993, p. 167) and at the individual level consists of social trust, sense of belonging, volunteer activity, and community participation (Fujiwara & Kawachi, 2008; Islam, Merlo, Kawachi, Lindstrom, & Gerdtham, 2006; Kawachi, Kennedy, Lochner, & Prothrow-Stith, 1997). High social capital predicts better self-reported mental and physical health (Fujiwara & Kawachi, 2008; Islam et al., 2006).

Income inequality studies focus on income differences within a given country or community. A number of studies have found that increased differences in income predict negative health outcomes and increased mortality for those less fortunate (Kawachi et al., 1997; Wilkinson & Pickett, 2006). One interesting way to assess income inequality is to assess what is called the Robin Hood Index, which is calculated by estimating the amount of income that must be redistributed from those above the mean to those below the mean in order to achieve income equality for everyone in a given community. The larger the index, the greater the income disparity. The Robin Hood Index has been found to be strongly related to mortality in several studies, with correlations between .54 and .65 (Kawachi et al., 1997; Kennedy, Kawachi, & Prothrow-Smith, 1996). Perhaps not surprisingly, the Robin Hood Index is also negatively correlated with such measures of social capital as social trust and group membership.

Relative deprivation is another conceptual way to assess income inequality. Relative deprivation focuses on the emotions resulting from social comparisons involving inequality. Invidious social comparisons can lead to increased stress, maladaptive coping responses, and negative health behaviors as an attempt to deal with the negative emotions resulting from negative social comparisons (Subramanian & Kawachi, 2006; Wilkinson & Pickett, 2006). The Yitzhaki index of relative deprivation is frequently used to determine hierarchy and position relative to one's social reference groups. Studies have found that relative deprivation is related to worse self-reported mental and physical health (Kondo, Kawachi, Subramanian, Takeda, & Yamagata, 2008; Subramanyam, Kawachi, Berkman, & Subramanian, 2009).

The concepts of social capital, income inequality, and relative deprivation are frequently studied together and represent an emerging area of interest for a number of researchers interested in understanding how socioeconomic factors "get under the skin." These concepts also appear to provide a strong explanation for why some countries show a reversed social gradient. Specifically, countries where citizens are rich not in money but in social capital (and do not experience relative deprivation through comparisons to reference groups) are healthy in spite of not being financially well off.

CONCLUSION

Convincing evidence strongly supports an association between SES and health, broadly defined. This relationship tends to be graded though nonlinear, with greater risk at the low end of the SES spectrum. Moreover, the effects of SES are mediated through multiple pathways, with emerging evidence suggesting that one's SES in early life moderates subsequent health trajectories into adulthood. Further, SES can itself be modulated by the financial and physical costs of disease. Four decades after the original Whitehall study, the basic relationship between SES and health is widely regarded as fact, with efforts now concentrated on mediating processes. It will be important to see how these efforts translate into interventions that benefit all.

REFERENCES

Abraido-Lanza, A. F., Dohrenwend, B. P., Ng-Mak, D. S., & Turner, J. B. (1999). The Latino mortality paradox: A test of the "salmon bias" and healthy immigrant hypotheses. *American Journal of Public Health*, 89, 1543–1548.

Adler, N., Epel, E., Castellazzo, G., & Ickovics, J. (2000). Relationship of subjective and objective social status with psychological and physiological functioning: Preliminary data in healthy, White women. *Health Psychology*, 19, 586–592.

Albano, J. D., Ward, E., Jemal, A., Anderson, R., Cokkinides, V. E., Murray, T., ... Thun, M. J. (2007). Cancer mortality in the United States by education level and race. *Journal of the National Cancer Institute*, 99, 1384–1394.

American Cancer Society (ACS). (2009). *Cancer facts and figures 2009.* Atlanta, GA: American Cancer Society.

Andersen, R. M., Yu, H., Wyn, R., Davidson, P. L., Brown, E. R., & Teleki, S., (2002). Access to medical care for low-income persons: How do communities make a difference? *Medical Care Research and Review, 59,* 384–411.

Ansseau, M., Fischler, B., Dierick, M., Albert, A., Leyman, S., & Mignon, A. (2008). Socioeconomic correlates of generalized anxiety disorder and major depression in primary care: The GADIS II Study (Generalized Anxiety and Depression Impact Survey II). *Depression and Anxiety, 25,* 506–513.

Aral, S. O., Adimora, A. A., & Fenton, K. A. (2008). Understanding and responding to disparities in HIV and other sexually transmitted infections in African Americans. *Lancet, 372,* 337–340.

Backlund, E., Sorlie, P. D., & Johnson, N. J. (1996). The shapes of the relationship between income and mortality in the United States: Evidence from the National Longitudinal Mortality Study. *Annals of Epidemiology, 6,* 12–20.

Baquet, C. R., & Commiskey, P. (2000). Socioeconomic factors and breast carcinoma in multicultural women. *Cancer, 88,* 1256–1264.

Barefoot, J. C., Peterson, B. L., Dahlstrom, W. G., Siegler, I. C., Anderson, N. B., & Williams, R. B., Jr. (1991). Hostility patterns and health implications: Correlates of Cook-Medley Hostility Scale scores in a national survey. *Health Psychology, 10,* 18–24.

Baum, A., Garofalo, J. P., & Yali, A. M. (1999). Socioeconomic status and chronic stress: Does stress account for SES effects on health? In N. E. Adler, M. Marmot, B. S. McEwen, & J. Stewart (Eds.), *Socioeconomic status and health in industrial nations: Social, psychological, and biological pathways.* New York, NY: New York Academy of Sciences.

Ben-Shlomo, Y., & Kuh, D. (2002). A life course approach to chronic disease epidemiology: Conceptual models, empirical challenges and interdisciplinary perspectives. *International Journal of Epidemiology, 31,* 285–293.

Berkman, L. F. (2009). Social epidemiology: Social determinants of health in the United States: Are we losing ground? *Annual Review of Public Health, 30,* 27–41.

Berkman, L. F., & Macintyre, S. (1997). The measurement of social class in health studies: Old measures and new formulations. In M. Kogevinas, N. Pearce, M. Susser, & P. Boffetta (Eds.), *Social Inequalities and Cancer* (pp. 51–64). Lyon, France: International Agency for Research on Cancer.

Blackwell, D. L., Martinez, M. E., Gentleman, J. F., Sanmartin, C., & Berthelot, J. M. (2009). Socioeconomic status and utilization of health care services in Canada and the United States: Findings from the binational health survey. *Medical Care, 47,* 1136–1146.

Blau, P. M., & Duncan, O. D. (1967). *The American occupational structure.* New York, NY: Wiley.

Borrell, L. N., Diez Roux, A. V., Rose, K., Catellier, D., & Clark, B. L. (with the Atherosclerosis Risk in Communities Study). (2004). Neighbourhood characteristics and mortality in the Atherosclerosis Risk in Communities Study. *International Journal of Epidemiology, 33,* 398–407.

Brajer, V., & Hall, J. (1992). Recent evidence on the distribution of air pollution effects. *Contemporary Policy Issues, 10,* 63–71.

Brand, J. E., Warren, J. R., Carayon, P., & Hoonakker, P. (2007). Do job characteristics mediate the relationship between SES and health? Evidence from sibling models. *Social Science Research, 36,* 222–253.

Brookfield, K. F., Cheung, M. C., Lucci, J., Fleming, L. E., & Koniaris, L. G. (2009). Disparities in survival among women with invasive cervical cancer: A problem of access to care. *Cancer, 115,* 166–178.

Bunker, C. H., Ukolib, F. A., Okoroc, F. I., Olomud, A. B., Kriskaa, A. M., … Hustona, S. L. (1996). Correlates of serum lipids in a lean black population. *Atherosclerosis, 123*(2), 215–225.

Bursztyn, M., & Raz, I. (1995). Blood pressure and insulin in Ethiopian immigrants: Longitudinal study. *Journal of Human Hypertension, 9,* 245–248.

Burton, N. W., & Turrell, G. (2000). Occupation, hours worked, and leisure-time physical activity. *Preventive Medicine, 31,* 673–681.

Cabelli, V., & Dufour, A. (1983). *Health effects criteria for marine recreational waters.* Research Triangle Park, NC: U.S. EPA.

Calderon, R., Johnson, C., Craun, G., Dufour, A. P., Karlin, R. J., Sinks, T., & Valentine, J. L. (1993). Health risks from contaminated water: Do class and race matter? *Toxicology and Industrial Health, 9,* 879–900.

Cantwell, M. F., McKenna, M. T., McCray, E., & Onorato, I. M. (1998). Tuberculosis and race/ethnicity in the United States: Impact of socioeconomic status. *American Journal of Respiratory Critical Care Medicine, 157,* 1016–1020.

Carpenter, S. (2000). Effects of cultural tightness and collectivism on self-concept and causal attributions. *Cross-Cultural Research, 34,* 38–56.

Carpenter, S., & Radhakrishnan, P. (2000). Allocentrism and idiocentrism as predictors of in-group perceptions: An individual difference extension of cultural patterns. *Journal of Research in Personality, 34,* 262–268.

Carroll, D., Davey Smith, G., Sheffield, D., Shipley, M. J., & Marmot M. G. (1997). The relationship between socioeconomic status, hostility, and blood pressure reactions to mental stress in men: Data from the Whitehall II Study. *Health Psychology, 16,* 131–136.

Centers for Disease Control and Prevention (CDC). (2005). Blood lead levels—United States, 1999–2002. *Morbidity and Mortality Weekly Report, 54,* 513–516.

Centers for Disease Control and Prevention (CDC). (2009). *HIV/AIDS Surveillance Report, 2007* (Vol. 19). Atlanta, GA: U.S. Department of Health and Human Services, Centers for Disease Control and Prevention; 2009. Retrieved from http://www.cdc.gov/hiv/topics/surveillance/resources/reports/

Chang, E. T., Shema, S. J., Wakelee, H. A., Clarke, C. A., & Gomez, S. L. (2009). Uncovering disparities in survival after non-small-cell lung cancer among Asian/Pacific Islander ethnic populations in California. *Cancer Epidemiology, Biomarkers, & Prevention, 18,* 2248–2255.

Chen, E., & Matthews, K. A. (2001). Cognitive appraisal biases: An approach to understanding the relation between socioeconomic status and cardiovascular reactivity in children. *Annals of Behavioral Medicine, 23,* 101–111.

Chen, E., Matthews, K. A., & Boyce, W. T. (2002). Socioeconomic differences in children's health: How and why do these relationships change with age? *Psychological Bulletin, 128,* 295–329.

Chi, P., & Laquatra, J. (1990). Energy efficiency and radon risks in residential housing. *Energy, 15,* 81–89.

Cho, S. J., Ramachandran, G., Grengs, J., Ryan, A. D., Eberly, L. E., & Adgate, J. L. (2008). Longitudinal evaluation of allergen and culturable fungal concentrations in inner-city households. *Journal of Occupational and Environmental Hygiene, 5,* 107–118.

Chu, K. C., Miller, B. A., & Springfield, S. A. (2007). Measures of racial /ethnic health disparities in cancer mortality rates and the influence of socioeconomic status. *Journal of the National Medical Association, 99,* 1092–1104.

Clarke, C. A., Miller, T., Chang, E. T., Yin, D., Cockburn, M., & Gomez, S. L. (2010). Racial and social class gradients in life expectancy in contemporary California. *Social Science & Medicine, 70,* 1371–1380.

Clegg, L. X., Reichman, M. E., Miller, B. A., Hankey, B. F., Singh, G. K., Lin, Y. D., … Edwards, B. K. (2009). Impact of socioeconomic status on cancer incidence and stage at diagnosis: Selected findings from the surveillance, epidemiology, and end results: National Longitudinal Mortality Study. *Cancer Causes Control, 20,* 417–435.

Cockerham, W. C., Hattori, H., & Yamori, Y. (2000). The social gradient in life expectancy: The contrary case of Okinawa in Japan. *Social Science & Medicine, 51,* 115–122.

Cockerham, W. C., & Yamori, Y. (2000). Okinawa: An exception to the social gradient of life expectancy in Japan. *Asia Pacific Journal of Clinical Nutrition, 10,* 154–158.

Cohen, S., Alper, C. M., Doyle, W. J., Adler, N., Treanor, J. J., & Turner, R. B. (2008). Objective and subjective socioeconomic status and susceptibility to the common cold. *Health Psychology, 27,* 268–274.

Cohen, S., Doyle, W. J., & Baum, A. (2006). Socioeconomic status is associated with stress hormones. *Psychosomatic Medicine, 68,* 414–420.

Cohen, S., Schwartz, J. E., Epel, E., Kirschbaum, C., Sidney, S., & Seeman, T. (2006). Socioeconomic status, race, and diurnal cortisol decline in the Coronary Artery Risk Development in Young Adults (CARDIA) Study. *Psychosomatic Medicine, 68,* 41–50.

Crouse, D. L., Ross, N. A., & Goldberg, M. S. (2009). Double burden of deprivation and high concentrations of ambient air pollution at the neighbourhood scale in Montreal, Canada. *Social Science & Medicine, 69,* 971–981.

Cuellar, I., Arnold, B., & Gonzalez, G. (1995). Cognitive referents of acculturation: Assessment of cultural constructs in Mexican Americans. *Journal of Community Psychology, 23,* 339–356.

Cummins, S. C., McKay, L., & MacIntyre, S. (2005). McDonald's restaurants and neighborhood deprivation in Scotland and England. *American Journal of Preventive Medicine, 29,* 308–310.

Cunningham, W. E., Hays, R. D., Duan, N., Andersen, R., Nakazono, T. T., Bozzette, S. A., & Shapiro, M. F. (2005). The effect of socioeconomic status on the survival of people receiving care for HIV infection in the United States. *Journal of Health Care for the Poor and Underserved, 16,* 655–676.

Dabul, A. J., Bernal, M. E., & Knight, G. P. (1995). Allocentric and idiocentric self-description and academic achievement among Mexican American and Anglo adolescents. *Journal of Social Psychology, 135,* 621–630.

Darmon, N., & Drewnowski, A. (2008). Does social class predict diet quality? *American Journal of Clinical Nutrition, 87,* 1107–1117.

Danesh, J., Whincup, P., Walker, M., Lennon, L., Thomson, A., Appleby, P., … Pepys, M. B. (2000). Low grade inflammation and coronary heart disease: Prospective study and updated meta-analysis. *British Medical Journal, 321,* 199–204.

de Castro, A. B., Gee, G. C., & Takeuchi, D. T. (2010). Examining alternative measures of social disadvantage among Asian Americans: The relevance of economic opportunity, subjective social status, and financial strain for health. *Journal of Immigrant and Minority Health, 12,* 659–671.

Demakakos, P., Nazroo, J., Breeze, E., & Marmot, M. (2008). Socioeconomic status and health: The role of subjective social status. *Social Science & Medicine, 67,* 330–340.

Diaz, T., Chu, S. Y., Buehler, J. W. Boyd, D., Checko, P. J., Conti, L., … Levy, A. (1994). Socioeconomic differences among people with AIDS: Results from a Multistate Surveillance Project. *American Journal of Preventive Medicine, 10,* 217–222.

Diez Roux, A. V., Kiefe, C. I., Jacobs, D. R., Haan, M., Jackson, S. A., & Nieto, F. J. (2001). Area characteristics and individual-level socioeconomic position indicators in three population-based epidemiologic studies. *Annals of Epidemiology, 11,* 395–405.

Diez-Roux, A. V., Nieto, F. J., Tyroler, H. A., Crum, L. D., & Szklo, M. (1995). Social inequalities and arteriosclerosis: The Atherosclerosis Risk in Communities Study. *American Journal of Epidemiology, 141,* 960–972.

Dixon, L. B., Sundquist, J., & Winkelby, M. (2000). Differences in energy, nutrient, and food intakes in a US sample of Mexican-American women and men: Findings from the Third National Health and Nutrition Examination Survey, 1988–1994. *American Journal of Epidemiology, 152,* 548–557.

Domino, G., & Acosta, A. (1987). The relation of acculturation and values in Mexican Americans. *Hispanic Journal of Behavioral Sciences, 9,* 131–150.

Donnison, C. (1929). Blood pressure in the African natives: Its bearing upon aetiology of hyperpiesia and arteriosclerosis. *Lancet, 1,* 6–7.

Dragano, N., Verde, P. E., Moebus, S., Stang, A., Schmermund, A., Roggenbuck, U., … Siegrist, J., (with the Heinz, Nixdorf Recall Study). (2007). Subclinical coronary atherosclerosis is more pronounced in men and women with lower socioeconomic status: Associations in a population-based study: Coronary atherosclerosis and social status. *European Journal of Cardiovascular Prevention and Rehabilitation, 14,* 568–574.

Drewnowski, A. (2009). Obesity, diets, and social inequalities. *Nutrition Review, 67,* S36–S39.

Du, X. L, Fang, S., & Meyer, T. E. (2008). Impact of treatment and socioeconomic status on racial disparities in survival among older women with breast cancer. *American Journal of Clinical Oncology, 31,* 125–132.

Dubowitz, T., Heron, M., Bird, C. E., Lurie, N., Finch, B. K., Basurto-Davila, R., … Escarce, J. J. (2008). Neighborhood socioeconomic status and fruit and vegetable intake among Whites, Blacks, and Mexican Americans in the United States. *American Journal of Clinical Nutrition, 87,* 1883–1891.

Duncan, O. D. (1961). A socioeconomic index for all occupations. In A. Reiss Jr. (Ed.), *Occupations and social status.* New York, NY: Free Press.

Echeverria, S. E., Borrell, L. N., Brown, D., & Rhoads, G. (2009). A local area analysis of racial, ethnic, and neighborhood disparities in breast cancer staging. *Cancer Epidemiology, Biomarkers, & Prevention, 18,* 3024–3029.

Escobar, J. I., Nervi, C. H., & Gara, M. A. (2001). Immigration and mental health: Mexican Americans in the United States. *Harvard Review of Psychiatry, 8,* 64–72.

Evans, G. W., & Kantrowitz, E., (2002). Socioeconomic status and health: The potential role of environmental risk exposure. *Annual Review of Public Health, 23,* 303–331.

Evans, G. W., Lepore, S. J., Shejwal, B. R., & Palsane, M. N. (1998). Chronic residential crowding and children's well being: an ecological perspective. *Child Development, 69,* 1514–1523.

Everson, S. A., Lynch, J. W., Kaplan, G. A., Lakka, T. A., Sivenius, J., & Salonen, J. T. (2001). Stress-induced blood pressure reactivity and incident stroke in middle-aged men. *Stroke, 32,* 1263–1270.

Foraker, R. E., Rose, K. M., McGinn, A. P., Suchindran, C. M., Goff, D. C., Jr., Whitsel, E. A., … Rosamond, W. D. (2008). Neighborhood income, health insurance, and prehospital delay for myocardial infarction: The atherosclerosis risk in communities study. *Archives of Internal Medicine, 168,* 1874–1879.

Forbes.com (2009). The 400 richest Americans [Special report]. Retrieved from http://www.forbes.com/lists/2009/54/rich-list-09_The-400-Richest-Americans_Rank.html

Forrester, T., Cooper, R. S., & Weatherall, D. (1998). Emergence of Western diseases in the tropical world: The experience with chronic cardiovascular diseases. *British Medical Bulletin, 54,* 463–473.

Frank, J. W., Cohen, R., Yen, I., Balfour, J., & Smith, M. (2003). Socioeconomic gradients in health status over 29 years of follow-up after midlife: The Alameda County Study. *Social Science & Medicine, 57,* 2305–2323.

Franzini, L., & Fernandez-Esquer, M. E. (2006). The association of subjective social status and health in low-income Mexican-origin individuals in Texas. *Social Science & Medicine, 63*, 788–804.

Fujiwara, T., & Kawachi, I. (2008). Social capital and health: A study of adult twins in the U.S. *American Journal of Preventive Medicine, 35*, 139–144.

Gallo, L. C., Bogart, L. M., Vranceanu, A. M., & Matthews, K. A. (2005). Socioeconomic status, resources, psychological experiences, and emotional responses: A test of the reserve capacity model. *Journal of Personality and Social Psychology, 88*, 386–399.

Gallo, L. C., & Matthews, K. A. (2003). Understanding the association between socioeconomic status and physical health: Do negative emotions play a role? *Psychological Bulletin, 129*, 10–51.

Gallo, L. C., Penedo, F. J., Espinosa de los Monteros, K., & Arguelles, W. (2009). Resiliency in the face of disadvantage: Do Hispanic cultural characteristics protect health outcomes? *Journal of Personality, 77*, 1707–1746.

Galobardes, B., Davey Smith, G., & Lynch, J. W. (2006). Systematic review of the influence of childhood socioeconomic circumstances on risk for cardiovascular disease in adulthood. *Annals of Epidemiology, 16*, 91–104.

Galobardes, B., Lynch, J. W., & Davey Smith, G. (2004). Childhood socioeconomic circumstances and cause-specific mortality in adulthood: Systematic review and interpretation. *Epidemiologic Reviews, 26*, 7–21.

Galobardes, B., Lynch, J. W., & Davey Smith, G. (2008). Is the association between childhood socioeconomic circumstances and cause-specific mortality established? Update of a systematic review. *Journal of Epidemiology and Community Health, 62*, 387–390.

Gerber, Y., Goldbourt, U., & Frory, Y. (with the Israel Study Group on First Acute Myocardial Infarction). (2008). Interaction between income and education in predicting long-term survival after acute myocardial infarction. *European Journal of Cardiovascular Prevention and Rehabilitation, 15*, 526–532.

Geronimus, A. T., & Bound, J. (1998). Use of census-based aggregate variables to proxy for socioeconomic group: Evidence from national samples. *American Journal of Epidemiology, 148*, 475–486.

Ghaed, S. G., & Gallo, L. C. (2007). Subjective social status, objective socioeconomic status and cardiovascular risk in women. *Health Psychology, 26*, 668–674.

Ghali, J. K., Cooper, R. S., Kowatly, I., & Liao, Y. (1993). Delay between onset of chest pain and arrival to the coronary care unit among minority and disadvantaged patients. *Journal of the National Medical Association, 85*, 180–184.

Gibson, P. H., Croal, B. L., Cuthbertson, B. H., Gibson, G., Jeffrey, R. R., Buchan, K. G., … Hillis, G. S. (2009). Socioeconomic status and early outcome from coronary artery bypass grafting. *Heart, 95*, 793–798.

Gilligan, T. (2005). Social disparities and prostate cancer: Mapping the gaps in our knowledge. *Cancer Causes and Control, 16*, 45–53.

Gold, D. (1992). Indoor air pollution. *Clinics in Chest Medicine, 13*, 215–219.

Goldberg, R. J., Yarzebski, J., Lessard, D., & Gore, J. M. (1999). A two-decades (1975 to 1995) long experience in the incidence, in-hospital and long-term case-fatality rates of acute myocardial infarction: A community wide perspective. *Journal of the American College of Cardiology, 33*, 1533–1539.

Goldman, N., Cornman, J. C., & Chang, M. (2006). Measuring subjective social status: A case study of older Taiwanese. *Journal of Cross Cultural Gerontology, 21*, 71–89.

Goldstein, I., Andrews, L., & Hartel, D. (1988). Assessment of human exposure to nitrogen dioxide, carbon monoxide and respirable particulates in New York inner city residents. *Atmosphere and Environment, 22*, 2127–2139.

Gory, K. M., & Vena, J. E. (1994). Cancer differentials among US Blacks and Whites: Quantitative estimates of socioeconomic-related risks. *Journal of the National Medical Association, 86*, 209–215.

Grant, B. F., Hasin, D. S., Stinson, F. S., Dawson, D. A., June Ruan, W., Goldstein, R. B., … Huang, B. (2005). Prevalence, correlates, co-morbidity, and comparative disability of DSM-IV generalized anxiety disorder in the USA: Results from the National Epidemiological Survey on Alcohol and Related Conditions. *Psychological Medicine, 35*, 1747–1759.

Green, M. S., Etzion, T., & Jucha, E. (1991). Blood pressure and serum cholesterol among male Ethiopian immigrants compared to the other Israelis. *Journal of Epidemiology and Community Health, 45*, 281–286.

Gump, B. B., Matthews, K. A., & Raikkonen, K. (1999). Modeling relationships among socioeconomic status, hostility, cardiovascular reactivity, and left ventricular mass in African American and White children. *Health Psychology, 18*, 140–150.

Gump, B. B., Reihman, J., Stewart, P., Lonky, E., Darvill, T., & Matthews, K. A. (2007). Blood lead (Pb) levels: A potential environmental mechanism explaining the relation between socioeconomic status and cardiovascular reactivity in children. *Health Psychology, 26*, 296–304.

Haan, M., Kaplan, G. A., & Camacho, T. (1987). Poverty and health: Prospective evidence from the Alameda County Study. *American Journal of Epidemiology, 125*, 989–998.

Haines, M. M., Stansfeld, S. A., Head, J., & Job, R. F. S. (2002). Multilevel modeling of aircraft noise on performance tests in schools around Heathrow Airport London. *Journal of Epidemiology and Community Health, 56*, 139–144.

Hankins, C., Tran, T., Hum, L., Laberge, C., Lapointe, N., Lepine, D., … O'Shaughnessy, M. V. (1998). Socioeconomic geographical links to human immunodeficiency virus seroprevalence among childbearing women in Montreal, 1989–1993. *International Journal of Epidemiology, 27*, 691–697.

Harper, S., Lynch, J., Hsu, W. L., Everson, S. A., Hillemeier, M. M., Raghunathan, T. E., … Kaplan, G. A. (2002). Life course socioeconomic conditions and adult psychosocial functioning. *International Journal of Epidemiology, 31*, 395–403.

Harper, S., Lynch, J., Meersman, S. C., Breen, N., Davis, W. W., & Reichman, M. C. (2009). Trends in area-socioeconomic and race-ethnic disparities in breast cancer incidence, stage at diagnosis, screening, mortality, and survival among women ages 50 years and over (1987–2005). *Cancer Epidemiology, Biomarkers & Prevention, 18*, 121–131.

Harralson, T. L. (2007). Factors influencing delay in seeking treatment for acute ischemic symptoms among lower income, urban women. *Heart and Lung, 36*, 96–104.

Haynes, M. A., & Smedley, B. D. (1999). *The unequal burden of cancer: An assessment of NIH research and programs for ethnic minorities and the medically underserved.* Washington, DC: National Academy Press.

Hemminki, K., & Li, X. (2003). Level of education and the risk of cancer in Sweden. *Cancer Epidemiology Biomarkers Prevention, 12*, 796–802.

Henderson, S. O., Magana, R. N., Korn, C. S., Genna, T., & Bretsky, P. M. (2002). Delayed presentation for care during acute myocardial infarction in a Hispanic population of Los Angeles County. *Ethnicity and Disease, 12*, 38–44.

Hertzman, C. (1999). The biological embedding of early experience and its effects on health in adulthood. *Annals of the New York Academy of Sciences, 896*, 85–95.

Himmelfarb, S., & Murrell, S. A. (1984). The prevalence and correlates of anxiety symptoms in older adults. *Journal of Psychology, 116*, 159–167.

Hollingshead, A. B. (1971). Commentary on the indiscriminate state of social class measurement. *Social Forces, 49*, 563–567.

Hollingshead, A. B. (1975). *Four factor index of social status* (Unpublished manuscript). Yale University, New Haven, CT.

Hollingshead, A. B., & Redlich, F. C. (1958). *Social class and mental illness.* New York, NY: Wiley.

House, J. S., Landis, K. R., & Umberson, D. (1988). Social relationships and health. *Science, 241,* 540–545.

Institute of Medicine (IOM), Committee on Monitoring Access to Personal Health Care Services. (1993). M. Millman (Ed.), *Access to health care in America.* Washington, DC: National Academy Press.

Islam, M. K., Merlo, J., Kawachi, I., Lindstrom, M., & Gerdtham, U.G. (2006). Social capital and health: Does egalitarianism matter? A literature review. *International Journal for Equity in Health, 5*, 1–28. doi:10.1186/1475-9276-5-3

Jahan, S. (2008). Poverty and infant mortality in the eastern Mediterranean region: A meta-analysis. *Journal of Epidemiology and Community Health, 62*, 745–751.

Janicki-Deverts, D., Cohen, S., Matthews, K. A., & Cullen, M. R. (2008). History of unemployment predicts future elevations in C-reactive protein among male participants in the Coronary Artery Risk Development in Young Adults (CARDIA) Study. *Annals of Behavioral Medicine, 36*, 176–185.

Johnson, J. V., Stewart, W., Hall, E. M., Fredland, P., & Theorell, T. (1996). Long-term psychosocial work environment and cardiovascular mortality among Swedish men. *American Journal of Public Health, 86*, 324–331.

Jorgensen, T., Mortensen, L. H., & Andersen, A. M. (2008). Social inequality in fetal and perinatal mortality in the Nordic countries. *Scandinavian Journal of Public Health, 36*, 635–649.

Joy, R., Druyts, E. F., Brandson, E. K., Lima, V. D., Rustad, C. A., Zhang, W., … Hogg, R. S. (2008). Impact of neighborhood-level socioeconomic status on HIV disease progression in a universal health care setting. *Journal of Acquired Immune Deficiency Syndrome, 47*, 500–505.

Kaleta, D., & Jegier, A. (2005). Occupational energy expenditure and leisure-time physical activity. *International Journal of Occupational Medicine and Environmental Health, 18*, 351–356.

Kaplan, C. P., & Van Valey, T. L. (1980). *Census '80: Continuing the fact finding tradition.* Washington, DC: U.S. GPO.

Kaplan, G. A., Baltrus, P. T., & Raghunathan, T. E. (2007). The shape of health to come: Prospective study of the determinants of 30–year health trajectories in the Alameda County Study. *International Journal of Epidemiology, 36*, 542–548.

Kaplan, G. A., & Keil, J. E. (1993). Socioeconomic factors and cardiovascular disease: A systematic review of the literature. *Circulation, 88*, 1973–1998.

Karmakar, S. D., & Breslin, F. C. (2008). The role of educational level and job characteristics on the health of young adults. *Social Science & Medicine, 66*, 2011–2022.

Kawachi, I., Kennedy, B. P., Lochner, K., & Prothrow-Stith, D. (1997). Social capital, income inequality, and mortality. *American Journal of Public Health, 87*, 1491–1498.

Kelly, M. J., & Weitzen, S. (2010). The association of lifetime education with the prevalence of myocardial infarction: An analysis of the 2006 behavioral risk factor surveillance system. *Journal of Community Health, 35*, 76–80.

Kennedy, B. P., Kawachi, I., & Prothrow-Stith, D. (1996). Income distribution and mortality: Cross-sectional ecological study of the Robin Hood Index in the United States. *British Medical Journal, 312*, 1004–1007.

Kirby, J. B., & Kaneda, T. (2005). Neighborhood socioeconomic disadvantage and access to health care. *Journal of Health and Social Behavior, 46*, 15–31.

Kittleson, M. M., Meoni, L. A., Wang, N. Y., Chu, A. Y., Ford, D. E., & Klag, M. J. (2006). Association of childhood socioeconomic status with subsequent coronary heart disease in physicians. *Archives of Internal Medicine, 166*, 2356–2361.

Kondo, N., Kawachi, I., Subramanian, S. V., Takeda, Y., & Yamagata, Z. (2008). Do social comparisons explain the association between income inequality and health? Relative deprivation and perceived health among male and female Japanese individuals. *Social Science & Medicine, 67*, 982–987.

Koshal, R. K., & Koshal, M. (1975). Crimes and socio-economic environments. *Social Indicators Research, 2*, 223–227.

Krieger, N. (1992). Overcoming the absence of socioeconomic data in medical records: Validation and application of a census-based methodology. *American Journal of Public Health, 82*, 703–710.

Krieger, N., Chen, J. T., & Ebel, G. (1997) Can we monitor socioeconomic inequalities in health? A survey of US Health Departments' data collection and reporting practices. *Public Health Reporting, 112*, 481–491.

Krieger, N., Chen, J. T., Waterman, P. D., Soobader, M., Subramanian, S. V., & Carson, R. (2002). Geocoding and monitoring of US socioeconomic inequalities in mortality and cancer incidence: Does the choice of area-based measure and geographic level matter? The Public Health Disparities Geocoding Project. *American Journal of Epidemiology, 156*, 471–482.

Krieger, N., Waterman, P. D., Chen, J. T., Soobader, M. J., & Subramanian, S. V. (2003). Monitoring socioeconomic inequalities in sexually transmitted infections, tuberculosis, and violence: Geocoding and choice of area-based socioeconomic measures—The Public Health Disparities Geocoding Project (US). *Public Health Reports, 118*, 240–260.

Landbergis, P. A., Schnall, P. L., Pickering, T. G., Warren, K., & Schwartz, J. E. (2003). Lower socioeconomic status among men in relation to the association between job strain and job pressure. *Scandinavian Journal of Work, Environment, & Health, 29*, 206–215.

Laquatra, J., Maxwell, L. E., & Pierce, M. (2005). Indoor air pollutants: Limited-resource households and children care facilities. *Journal of Environmental Health, 67*, 39–43, 61.

Larson, N. I., Story, M. T., & Nelson, M. C. (2009). Neighborhood environments: Disparities in access to healthy foods in the U.S. *American Journal of Preventive Medicine, 36*, 84–81.

Lasser, K. E., Himmelstein, D. U., & Woolhandler, S. (2006). Access to care, health status, and health disparities in the United States and Canada: Results of a cross-national population-based survey. *American Journal of Public Health, 96*, 1300–1307.

Lemeshow, A. R., Fisher, L. Goodman, E., Kawachi, I., Berkey, C. S., & Colditz, G. A. (2008). Subjective social status in the school and change in adiposity in female adolescents: Findings from a prospective cohort study. *Archives of Pediatrics & Adolescent Medicine, 162*, 23–28.

Li, L., Power, C., Kelly, S., Kirschbaum, C., & Hertzman, C. (2007). Life-time socioeconomic position and cortisol patterns in mid-life. *Psychoneuroendocrinology, 32*, 824–833.

Liberatos, P., Link, B. G., & Kelsey, J. L. (1988). The measurement of social class in epidemiology. *Epidemiology Review, 10*, 87–121.

Liu, L., Cozen, W., Bernstein, L., Ross, R. K., & Deapen, D. (2001). Changing relationship between socioeconomic status and prostate cancer incidence. *Journal of the National Cancer Institute, 93*, 705–709.

Lopez De Fede, A., Stewart, J. E., Harris, M. J., & Mayfield-Smith, K. (2008). Tuberculosis in socio-economically deprived neighborhoods: Missed opportunities for prevention. *International Journal of Tuberculosis and Lung Disease, 12*, 1425–1430.

Lorant, V., Croux, C., Weich, S., Deliege, D., Mackenbach, J., & Ansseau, M. (2007). Depression and socioeconomic risk factors: 7-year longitudinal study. *British Journal of Psychiatry, 190*, 293–298.

Lorant, V., Deliege, D., Eaton, W., Robert, A., Philippot, P., & Ansseau, M. (2003). Socioeconomic inequalities in depression: A meta-analysis. *American Journal of Epidemiology, 157*, 98–112.

Lund Nilsen, T. I., Johnsen, R., & Vatten, L. J. (2000). Socioeconomic and lifestyle factors associated with the risk of prostate cancer. *British Journal of Cancer, 82*, 1358–1363.

Lynch, J. W., Kaplan, G. A., & Salonen, J. T. (1997). Why do poor people behave poorly? Variation in adult health behaviors and psychosocial characteristics by stages of the socioeconomic life course. *Social Science & Medicine, 44*, 809–819.

Lynch, J., Kaplan, G. A., Salonen, R., Cohen, R. D., & Salonen, J. T. (1995). Socioeconomic status and carotid aterosclerosis. *Circulation, 92*, 1786–1792.

Lynch, J., Kaplan, G. A., Salonen, R., & Salonen, J. T. (1997). Socioeconomic status and progression of carotid atherosclerosis: Prospective evidence from the Kuopio Ischemic Heart Disease Risk Factor Study. *Arteriosclerosis, Thrombosis, and Vascular Biology, 17*, 513–519.

Lynch, J. W., Kaplan, G. A., & Shema, S. J. (1997). Cumulative impact of sustained economic hardship on physical, cognitive, psychological, and social functioning. *New England Journal of Medicine, 337*, 1889–1895.

MacArthur Foundation. (2009). Notebook on the social and physical environment. Retrieved from http://www.macses.ucsf.edu/Research/Social%20Environment/chapters.html

MacKie, R. M., & Hole, D. J. (1996). Incidence and thickness of primary tumours and survival of patients with cutaneous malignant melanoma in relation to socioeconomic status. *British Medical Journal, 313*, 627–628.

Makinen, T., Kestila, L., Borodulin, K., Martelin, T., Rahkonen, O., Leino-Arjas, P., & Pratala, R. (2010). Occupational class differences in leisure-time physical inactivity—Contribution of past and current physical workload and other working conditions. *Scandinavian Journal of Work, Environment, and Health, 36*, 62–70.

Mare, R. D. (1990). Socio-economic careers and differential mortality among older men in the United States. In J. Vallin, S. D'Souza, & A. Palloni (Eds.), *Measurement and analysis of mortality* (pp. 362–387). Oxford, England: Clarendon Press.

Marin, G., & Gamba, R. J. (2003). Acculturation and changes in cultural values. In K. M. Chun, P. B. Organista, & G. Marin (Eds.), *Acculturation: Advances in theory, measurement, and applied research* (pp. 83–93). Washington, DC: American Psychological Association.

Marmot, M. G. (1996). Socio-economic factors in cardiovascular disease. *Journal of Hypertension, 14*, S201–S205.

Marmot, M. G. (2003). Understanding social inequalities in health. *Perspectives in Biology and Medicine, 46*, S9–S23.

Marmot, M., & Feeney, A. (1997). General explanations for social inequalities in health. *IARC Scientific Publications, 138*, 207–228.

Marmot, M. G., Shipley, M. J., & Rose, G. (1984). Inequalities in death—Specific explanations of a general pattern? *Lancet, 1*, 1003–1006.

Marmot, M. G., Smith, G. D., Stansfeld, S., Patel, C., North, F., Head, J., … Feeney, A. (1991). Health inequalities among British civil servants: The Whitehall II Study. *Lancet, 337*, 1387–1393.

Marmot, M. G., & Syme, S. L. (1976). Acculturation and coronary heart disease in Japanese-Americans. *American Journal of Epidemiology, 104*, 225–247.

Martikainen, P., & Valkonen, T. (1999). Bias related to the exclusion of the economically inactive in studies on social class differences in mortality. *International Journal of Epidemiology, 28*, 899–904.

Matthews, K. A., Raikkonen, K., Gallo, L. C., & Kuller, L. H. (2008). Association between socioeconomic status and metabolic syndrome in women: Testing the reserve capacity model. *Health Psychology, 27*, 576–583.

McDavid Harrison, K., Ling, Q., Song, R., & Hall, H. I. (2008). County-level socioeconomic status and survival after HIV diagnosis, United States. *Annals of Epidemiology, 18*, 919–927.

McDonough, P., Duncan, G. J., Williams, D., & House, J. (1997). Income dynamics and adult mortality in the United States, 1972–1989. *American Journal of Public Health, 87*, 1476–1483.

McFarland, W., Chen, S., Hsu, L., Schwarcz, S., & Katz, M. (2003). Low socioeconomic status is associated with a higher rate of death in the era of highly active antiretroviral therapy, San Francisco. *Journal of Acquired Immune Deficiency Syndrome, 33*, 96–103.

Meaney, M. J., & Szyf, M. (2005). Environmental programming of stress responses through DNA methylation: Life at the interface between a dynamic environment and a fixed genome. *Dialogues in Clinical Neuroscience, 7*, 103–123.

Miller, G. E., Chen, E., Fok, A. K., Walker, H., Lim, A., Nicholls, E. F., … Kobor, M. S. (2009). Low early-life social class leaves a biological residue manifested by decreased glucocorticoid and increased proinflammatory signaling. *Proceedings of the National Academy of Science, 106*, 14716–14721.

Mittleman, M. A., Maclure, M., Nachnani, M., Sherwood, J. B., & Muller, J. E. (1997). Educational attainment, anger, and the risk of triggering myocardial infarction onset: The determinants of Myocardial Infarction Onset Study investigators. *Archives of Internal Medicine*, *157*, 69–75.

Mohai, P., & Saha, R. (2006). Reassessing racial and socioeconomic disparities in environmental justice research. *Demography*, *43*, 383–399.

Molina, M. A., Cheung, M. C., Perez, E. A., Byrne, M. M., Franceschi, D., Moffat, F. L., … Koniaris, L. G. (2008). African American and poor patients have a dramatically worse prognosis for head and neck cancer: An examination of 20,915 patients. *Cancer*, *113*, 2797–2806.

Molla, M. T., Madan, J. H., & Wagener, D. K. (2004). Differential in adult mortality and activity limitation by years of education in the United States at the end of the 1990's. *Population and Development Review*, *30*, 625–646.

Morenoff, J. D., & Sampson, R. J. (1997). Violent crime and the spatial dynamics of neighborhood transition: Chicago, 1970–1990. *Social Forces*, *76*, 31–64.

Moser, K. A, Fox, A. J., & Jones, D. R. (1984). Unemployment and mortality in the OPCS Longitudinal Study. *Lancet*, *2*, 1324–1329.

Murrain, M., & Barker, T. (1997). Investigating the relationship between economic status and HIV risk. *Journal of Health Care for the Poor Underserved*, *8*, 416–423.

Nakao, K., Hodge, R., & Treas, J. (1990). On revising prestige scores for all occupations (GSS Methods Report No. 69). Irvine, CA: University of California, Department of Psychology.

Nakao, K., & Treas, J. (1994). Updating occupational prestige and socioeconomic scores: How the new measures measure up. *Sociological Methodology*, *24*, 1–72.

Nelson, F. (1978). Residential dissatisfaction in the crowded urban neighborhood. *International Review of Modern Sociology*, *8*, 227–238.

Nguyen, G. C., & Thuluvath, P. J. (2008). Racial disparity in liver disease: Biological, cultural, or socioeconomic factors. *Hepatology*, *47*, 1058–1066.

Nylen, L., Voss, M., & Floderus, B. (2001). Mortality among women and men relative to unemployment, part time work, overtime work, and extra work: a study based on data from the Swedish twin registry. *Occupational Environmental Medicine*, *58*, 52–57.

Oakes, J. M., & Rossi, P. H. (2003). The measurement of SES in health research: Current practice and steps toward a new approach. *Social Science & Medicine*, *56*, 769–784.

Ostrove, J. M., Adler, N. E., Kuppermann, M., & Washington, A. E. (2000). Objective and subjective assessments of socioeconomic status and their relationship to self-rated health in an ethnically diverse sample of pregnant women. *Health Psychology*, *19*, 613–618.

Ou, S. H., Ziogas, A., & Zell, J. A. (2009). Prognostic factors for survival in extensive stage small cell lung cancer (Ed-SCLC): The importance of smoking history, socioeconomic and marital statuses, and ethnicity. *Journal of Thoracic Oncology*, *4*, 37–43.

Padgett, D. K., & Brodsky, B. (1992). Psychosocial factors influencing non-urgent use of the emergency room: A review and recommendations for research and improved service delivery. *Social Science & Medicine*, *35*, 1189–1197.

Pearce, J., Hiscock, R., Blakely, T., & Witten, K. (2008). The contextual effects of neighbourhood access to supermarkets and convenience stores on individual fruit and vegetable consumption. *Journal of Epidemiology and Community Health*, *62*, 198–201.

Pena, R., Wall, S., & Persson, L. A. (2000). The effect of poverty, social inequity, and maternal education on infant mortality in Nicaragua, 1988–1993. *American Journal of Public Health*, *90*, 64–69.

Pickett, K. E., & Pearl, M. (2001). Multilevel analyses of neighbourhood socioeconomic context and health outcomes: A critical review. *Journal of Epidemiology and Community Health*, *55*, 111–122.

Pollitt, R. A., Rose, K. M., & Kaufman, J. S. (2005). Evaluating the evidence for models of life course socioeconomic factors and cardiovascular outcomes: A systematic review. *BMC Public Health*, *5*(7), 1–13. doi:10.1186/1471-2458-5-7

Pollock, A. M., & Vickers, N. (1997). Breast, lung, and colorectal cancer incidence and survival in South Thames region, 1987–1992: The effect of social deprivation. *Journal of Public Health Medicine*, *19*, 288–294.

Putnam, R. D. (1993). *Making democracy work*. Princeton, NJ: Princeton University Press.

Ranchor, A. V., Bouma, J., & Sanderman, R. (1996). Vulnerability and social class: Differential patterns of personality and social support over the social classes. *Personality and Individual Differences*, *20*, 229–237.

Rapiti, E., Fioretta, G., Schaffar, R., Neyroud-Caspar, I., Verkooijen, H. M., Schmidlin, F., … Bouchardy, C. (2009). Impact of socioeconomic status on prostate cancer diagnosis, treatment, and prognosis. *Cancer*, *115*, 5556–5565.

Rehkopf, D. H., Berkman, L. F., Coull, B., & Krieger, N. (2008). The non-linear risk of mortality by income level in a healthy population: US National Health and Nutrition Examination Survey mortality follow-up cohort, 1988–2001. *BMC Public Health, 10*, 383. Retrieved from http://www.biomedcentral.com/1471-2458/8/383

Reid, D. D., Hamilton, P. J. S., McCartney, P., Rose, G., Jarrett, R. J., & Keen, H. (1976). Smoking and other risk factors for coronary heart disease in British civil servants. *Lancet, 2*, 979–984.

Ritterman, M. L., Fernald, L. C., Ozer, E. J., Adler, N. E., Gutierrez, J. P., & Syme, S. L. (2009). Objective and subjective social class gradients for substance use among Mexican adolescents. *Social Science and Medicine, 68*, 1843–1851.

Robert Warren, J., Hoonakker, P., Carayon, P., & Brand, J. (2004). Job characteristics as mediators in SES-health relationships. *Social Science & Medicine, 59*, 1367–1378.

Robert Wood Johnson Foundation. (2009). Race and socioeconomic factors affect opportunities for better health. *Issue brief 5: Race and socioeconomic factors*. Retrieved from http//www.rwjf.org/files/research/commission2009issuebrief5.pdf

Rose, K. M., Suchindran, C. M., Foraker, R. E., Whitsel, E. A., Rosamond, W. D., Heiss, G., & Wood, J. L. (2009). Neighborhood disparities in incident hospitalized myocardial infarction in four U.S. communities: The ARIC surveillance study. *Annals of Epidemiology, 19*, 867–874.

Rosengren, A., Subramanian, S. V., Islam, S., Chow, C. K., Avezum, A., Kazmi, K., … Uysuf, S. (with INTERHEART Investigators). (2009). Education and risk for acute myocardial infarction in 52 high, middle, and low-income countries: INTERHEART case-control study. *Heart, 95*, 2014–2022.

Rosenstreich, D., Eggleson, P., Kattan, M., Baker, D., Slavin, R., Gergen, P., … Malveaux, F. (1997). The role of cockroach allergy and exposure to cockroach allergens in causing morbidity among inner-city children with asthma. *New England Journal of Medicine, 336*, 1356–1363.

Roskam, A. J., & Kunst, A. E. (2008). The predictive value of different socioeconomic indicators for overweight in nine European countries. *Public Health and Nutrition, 11*, 1256–1266.

Rosvall, M., Ostergren, P. O., Hedblad, B., Isacsson, S. O., Janzon, L., & Berglund, G. (2000). Occupational status, educational level, and the prevalence of carotid atherosclerosis in a general population sample of middle-aged Swedish men and women: Results from the Malmo Diet and Cancer Study. *American Journal of Epidemiology, 152*, 334–346.

Rosvall, M., Ostergren, P. O., Hedblad, B., Isacsson, S. O., Janzon, L., & Berglund, G. (2006). Socioeconomic differences in the progression of carotid atherosclerosis in middle-aged men and women with subclinical atherosclerosis in Sweden. *Social Science and Medicine, 62*, 1785–1798.

Sabogal, F., Marin, G., Otero-Sabogal, R., Marin, B. V., & Perez-Stable, E. J. (1987). Hispanic familism and acculturation: What changes and what doesn't? *Hispanic Journal of Behavioral Sciences, 9*, 397–412.

Satterwaite, D. (1993). The impact on health of urban environments. *Environment and Urbanization, 5*, 87–111.

Schaap, M. M., & Kunst, A. E. (2009). Monitoring of socioeconomic inequalities in smoking: Learning from the experiences of recent scientific studies. *Public Health, 123*, 103–109.

Schaap, M. M., van Agt, H. M., & Kunst, A. E. (2008). Identification of socioeconomic groups at increased risk for smoking in European countries: Looking beyond educational level. *Nicotine and Tobacco Research, 10*, 359–369.

Scherwitz, L., Perkins, L., Chesney, M., & Hughes, G. (1991). Cook-Medley Hostility Scale and subsets: Relationship to demographic and psychosocial characteristics in young adults in the CARDIA Study. *Psychosomatic Medicine, 53*, 36–49.

Schrijvers, C. T., & Mackenbach, J. P. (1994). Cancer patient survival by socioeconomic status in the Netherlands: A review for six common cancer sites. *Journal of Epidemiology and Community Health, 48*, 441–446.

Shackley, D. C., & Clarke, N. W. (2005). Impact of socioeconomic status on bladder cancer outcome. *Current Opinion in Urology, 15*, 328–381.

Sherman, A. (1994). *Wasting America's future*. Boston, MA: Beacon Press.

Shimakawa, T., Sorlie, P., Carpenter, M. A., Dennis, B., Tell, G. S., Watson, R., & Williams, O. D. (1994). Dietary intake patterns and socioeconomic factors in the Atherosclerosis Risk in Communities Study. *Preventive Medicine, 23*, 769–780.

Siegman, A. W., Kubzansky, L. D., Kawachi, I., Boyle, S., Vokonas, P. S., & Sparrow, D. (2000). A prospective study of dominance and coronary heart disease in the Normative Aging Study. *American Journal of Cardiology, 86*, 145–149.

Singh, G. K., & Kogan, M. D. (2007). Persistent socioeconomic disparities in infant, neonatal, and postneonatal mortality rates in the United States, 1969–2001. *Pediatrics, 119*, e928–e939.

Singh, G. K., Miller, B. A., Hankey, B. F., & Edwards, B. K. (2004). Persistent area socioeconomic disparities in U.S. incidence of cervical cancer, mortality, stage, and survival, 1975–2000. *Cancer, 101*, 1051–1057.

Singh, G. K., & Siahpush, M. (2002). Increasing inequalities in all-cause and cardiovascular mortality among US adults aged 25–64 years by area socioeconomic status, 1969–1998. *International Journal of Epidemiology, 31*, 600–613.

Singh-Manoux, A., Adler, N. E., & Marmot, M. G. (2003). Subjective social status: Its determinants and its association with measure of ill-health in the Whitehall II Study. *Social Science & Medicine, 56*, 1321–1333.

Skodova, Z., Nagyova, I., van Dijk, J. P., Sudzinova, A., Vargova, H., Studencan, M., & Reijneveld, S. A. (2008). Socioeconomic differences in psychosocial factors contributing to coronary heart disease: A review. *Journal of Clinical Psychology in Medical Settings, 15*, 204–213.

Smith, T. W., & Ruiz, J. M. (2002). Psychosocial influences on the development and course of coronary heart disease: Current status and implications for research and practice. *Journal of Consulting and Clinical Psychology, 70*, 548–568.

Smith, T. W., Uchino, B. N., Berg, C. A., Florsheim, P., Pearce, G., Hawkins, M., … Yoon, H. C. (2008). Associations of self-reports versus spouse ratings of negative affectivity, dominance, and affiliation with coronary artery disease: Where should we look and who should we ask when studying personality and health? *Health Psychology, 27*, 676–684.

Spence, J. T. (1985). Achievement American style: The rewards and costs of individualism. *American Psychologist, 40*, 1285–1295.

Stansfeld, S. A., Berglund, B., Clark, C., Lopez-Barrio, I., Fischer, P., Ohrstrom, E., … Berry, B. F. (with the RANCH Study Team). (2005). Aircraft and road traffic noise and children's cognition and health: A cross-national study. *Lancet, 365*, 1942–1949.

Starfield, B., Riley, A. W., Witt, W. P., & Robertson, J. (2002). Social class gradients in health during adolescence. *Journal of Epidemiology and Community Health, 56*, 354–361.

Starfield, B., Robertson, J., & Wiley, A. W. (2002). Social class gradients and health in childhood. *Ambulatory Pediatrics, 2*, 238–246.

Steffen, P. R. (2006). The cultural gradient: Culture moderates the relationship between socioeconomic status (SES) and ambulatory blood pressure. *Journal of Behavioral Medicine, 29*, 501–510.

Steffen, P. R., Smith, T. B., Larson, M., & Butler, L. (2006). Acculturation to Western society as a risk factor for high blood pressure: A meta-analytic review. *Psychosomatic Medicine, 68*, 386–397.

Steptoe, A., Brydon, L., & Kunz-Ebrecht, S. (2005). Changes in financial strain over three years, ambulatory blood pressure, and cortisol responses to awakening. *Psychosomatic Medicine, 67*, 281–287.

Stern, M. P., & Wei, M. (1999). Do Mexican Americans really have low rates of cardiovascular disease? *Preventive Medicine, 29*, S90–S95.

Stern, R. S., Weissman, J. S., & Epstein, A. M. (1991). The emergency department as a pathway to admission for poor and high-cost patients. *Journal of the American Medical Association, 266*, 2238–2243.

Stuart, A. L., Mudhasakul, S., & Sriwatanapongse, W. (2009). The social distribution of neighborhood-scale air pollution and monitoring protection. *Journal of Waste Management Association, 59*, 591–602.

Stuckler, D., Basu, S., Suhrcke, M., Coutts, A., & McKee, M. (2009). The public health effect of economic crises and alternative policy responses in Europe: An empirical analysis. *Lancet, 374*, 315–323.

Stuver, S. O., Boschi-Pinto, C., & Trichopoulos, D. (1997). Infection with hepatitis B and C viruses, social class, and cancer. *IARC Scientific Publications, 138*, 319–324.

Subramanian, S. V., Chen, J. T., Rehkopf, D. H., Waterman, P. D., & Krieger, N. (2005). Racial disparities in context: A multilevel analysis of neighborhood variations in poverty and excess mortality among Black populations in Massachusetts. *American Journal of Public Health, 95*, 260–265.

Subramanian, S. V., & Kawachi, I. (2006). Whose health is affected by income inequality? A multilevel interaction analysis of contemporaneous and lagged effects of state income inequality on individual self-rated health in the United States. *Health Place, 12*, 141–156.

Subramanyam, M., Kawachi, I., Berkman, L., & Subramanian, S. V. (2009). Relative deprivation in income and self-rated health in the United States. *Social Science & Medicine, 69*, 327–334.

Suchday, S., Krantz, D. S., & Gottdiener, J. S. (2005). Relationship of socioeconomic markers to daily life ischemia and blood pressure reactivity in coronary artery disease patients. *Annals of Behavioral Medicine, 30*, 74–84.

Sundquist, J., & Winkleby, M. (2000). Country of birth, acculturation status and abdominal obesity in a national sample of Mexican-American women and men. *International Journal of Epidemiology, 29*, 470–477.

Taylor, F. C., Ascione, R., Rees, K., Narayan, P., & Angelini, G. D. (2003). Socioeconomic deprivation is a predictor of poor postoperative cardiovascular outcomes in patients undergoing coronary artery bypass grafting. *Heart, 89*, 1062–1066.

Taylor, S. E., Repetti, R., & Seeman, T. E. (1997). Health psychology: What is an unhealthy environment and how does it get under the skin? *Annual Review of Psychology, 48*, 411–447.

Thomas, A. J., Eberly, L. E., Davey Smith, G., & Neaton, J. D. (with the Multiple Risk Factor Intervention Trial [MRFIT] Research Group). (2006). Zip-code-based versus tract-based income measures as long-term risk-adjusted mortality predictors. *American Journal of Epidemiology, 164*, 586–590.

Thurston, R. C., & Matthews, K. A. (2009). Racial and socioeconomic disparities in arterial stiffness and intima media thickness among adolescents. *Social Science & Medicine, 68*, 807–813.

Tonne, C., Schwartz, J., Mittleman, M., Melly, S., Suh, H., & Goldberg, R. (2005). Long-term survival after acute myocardial infarction is lower in more deprived neighborhoods. *Circulation, 111*, 3063–3070.

Treiman, D. J., McKeever, M., & Fodor, E. (1996). Racial differences in occupational status and income in South Africa, 1980 and 1991. *Demography, 33*, 111–132.

Triandis, H. C. (1995). *Individualism and collectivism*. Boulder, CO: Westview Press.

Truong, K. D., & Sturm, R. (2009). Alcohol environments and disparities in exposure associated with adolescent drinking in California. *American Journal of Public Health, 99*, 264–270.

Turra, C. M., & Goldman, N. (2007). Socioeconomic differences in mortality among U.S. adults: Insights into the Hispanic Paradox. *Journal of Gerontology: Social Sciences, 62B*, S184–S192.

Turrell, G., & Kavanagh, A. M. (2006). Socio-economic pathways to diet: Modeling the association between socio-economic position and food purchasing behavior. *Public Health and Nutrition, 9*, 375–383.

Turrell, G., Lynch, J. W., Leite, C., Raghunathan, T., & Kaplan, G. A. (2007). Socioeconomic disadvantage in childhood and across the life course and all-cause mortality and physical function in adulthood: Evidence from the Alameda County Study. *Journal of Epidemiology and Community Health, 61*, 723–730.

Tyden, P., Hansen, O., Engstrom, G., Hedblad, B., & Janzon, L. (2002). Myocardial infarction in an urban population: Worse long term prognosis for patients from less affluent residential areas. *Journal of Epidemiology and Community Health, 56*, 785–790.

Uchino, B. N., Ruiz, J. M., & Holt-Lunstad, J. (2009). Stress. In D. Sanders & K. R. Scherer (Eds.), *Oxford companion to emotion and affective sciences*. New York, NY: New York University Press.

U.S. Environmental Protection Agency. (1977). *The urban noise survey*. EPA 550/9-77. Washington, DC: EPA.

Van Lenthe, F. J., Borrell, L. N., Costa, G., Diez Roux, A. V., Kauppinen, T. M., Marinacci, C., … Valkonen, T. (2005). Neighbourhood unemployment and all-cause mortality: A comparison of six countries. *Journal of Epidemiology and Community Health, 59*, 231–237.

Vega, W. A., Kolody, B., Aguilar-Gaxiola, S., Alderete, E., Catalano, R., & Caraveo-Anduaga, J. (1998). Lifetime prevalence of DSM-III-R psychiatric disorders among urban and rural Mexican Americans in California. *Archives of General Psychiatry, 55*, 771–778.

Vega, W. A., Sribney, W. M., Aguilar-Gaxiola, S., & Kolody, B. (2004). 12-month prevalence of DSM-III-R psychiatric disorders among Mexican Americans: Nativity, social assimilation, and age determinants. *Journal of Nervous and Mental Disease, 192*, 532–541.

Voss, M., Nylen, L., Floderus, B., Diderichsen, F., & Terry, P. D. (2004). Unemployment and early cause-specific mortality: A study based on the Swedish twin registry. *American Journal of Public Health, 94*, 2155–2161.

Waldron, I., Herold, J., Dunn, D., & Staum, R. (1982). Reciprocal effects of health and labor force participation among women: Evidence from two longitudinal studies. *Journal of Occupational Medicine, 24*, 126–132.

Waldron, I., Nowotarski, M., Freimer, M., Henry, J. P., Post, N., & Witten, C. (1982). Cross-cultural variation in blood pressure: A quantitative analysis of the relationships of blood pressure to cultural characteristics, salt consumption, and body weight. *Social Science and Medicine, 16*, 419–430.

Wandel, M., & Roos, G. (2005). Work, food and physical activity: A qualitative study of coping strategies among men in three occupations. *Appetite, 44*, 93–102.

Warheit, G. J., Holzer, C. E., III, & Arey, S. A. (1975). Race and mental illness: An epidemiologic update. *Journal of Health and Social Behavior, 16*, 243–256.

Warr, D., Feldman, P., Tacticos, T., & Kelaher, M. (2009). Sources of stress in impoverished neighbourhoods: Insights into links between neighbourhood environments and health. *Australian and New Zealand Journal of Public Health, 33*, 25–33.

Wei, M., Valdez, R. A., Mitchell, B. D., Haffner, S. M., Stern, M. P., & Hazuda, H. P. (1996). Migration status, socioeconomic status, and mortality rates in Mexican Americans and non-Hispanic whites: The San Antonio Heart Study. *Annals of Epidemiology, 6*, 307–313.

White, H. L. (1998). Race, class, and environmental hazards. In D. E. Camacho (Ed.), *Environmental injustices, political struggles* (pp. 61–81). Durham, NC: Duke University Press.

Wilkinson, R. G. (1990). Income distribution and mortality: A "natural" experiment. *Sociology of Health & Illness, 12*, 391–412.

Wilkinson, R. G., & Pickett, E. (2006). Income inequality and population health: A review and explanation of the evidence. *Social Science and Medicine, 62*, 1768–1784.

Williams, D. R. (1999). Race, socioeconomic status, and health. The added effects of racism and discrimination. *Annals of the New York Academy of Science, 896*, 173–188.

Williams, D. R. (2005). The health of U.S. racial and ethnic populations. *Journal of Gerontology, 60B*, 53–62.

Williams, D. R., & Collins, C. (1995). U.S. socioeconomic and racial differences in health: Patterns and explanations. *Annual Review of Sociology, 21*, 349–386.

Williams, T., Milton, J. D., Farrell, J. B., & Graham, I. (1995). N. M. H., socioeconomic status and provider practices as predictors of immunization coverage in Virginia children. *Pediatrics, 96*, 439–446.

Wilson, D. K., Kliewer, W., Plybon, L., & Sica, D. A. (2000). Socioeconomic status and blood pressure reactivity in healthy Black adolescents. *Hypertension, 35*, 496–500.

Winkelby, M. A., Flora, J. A., & Kraemer, H. C. (1994). A community-based heart disease intervention program: Predictors of change. *American Journal of Public Health, 84*, 767–772.

Wrigley, H., Roderick, P., George, S., Smith, J., Mullee, M., & Goddard, J. (2003). Inequalities in survival from colorectal cancer: A comparison of the impact of deprivation, treatment, and host factors on observed and cause specific survival. *Journal of Epidemiology and Community Health, 57*, 301–309.

Yan. L. L., Liu, K., Daviglus, M. L., Colangelo, L. A., Kiefe, C. I, Sidney, S.,…Greenland, P. (2006). Education, 15 year risk factor progression, and coronary artery calcium in young adulthood and early middle age: The Coronary Artery Risk Development in Young Adults Study. *Journal of the American Medical Association, 295*, 1793–1800.

Yen, I. H., & Kaplan, G. A. (1999). Neighborhood social environment and risk of death: Multilevel evidence from the Alameda County Study. *American Journal of Epidemiology, 149*, 898–907.

Yu, X. Q. (2009). Socioeconomic disparities in breast cancer survival: Relation to state at diagnosis, treatment and race. *BMC Cancer, 9*, 364.

Zenk, S. N., Lachance, L. L., Schulz, A. J., Mentz, G., Kannan, S., & Ridella, W. (2009). Neighborhood retail food environment and fruit and vegetable intake in a multiethnic urban population. *American Journal of Health Promotion, 23*, 255–264.

Zierler, S., Krieger, N., Tang, Y., Coady, W., Siegfried, E., DeMaria, A., & Auerbach, J. (2000). Economic deprivation and AIDS incidence in Massachusetts. *American Journal of Public Health, 90*, 1064–1073.

24 Race and Health
Racial Disparities in Hypertension and Links Between Racism and Health

Elizabeth Brondolo, Shonda Lackey, and Erica Love
Department of Psychology, St. Johns University

Racial disparities in health continue to be a pressing problem in the United States. What accounts for these racial disparities? Are there race differences in both the individual-level and the community-level health risk factors and health-related behaviors? Do racism and ethnic discrimination contribute, directly or indirectly, to these disparities? To answer these questions, we examine racial disparities in high blood pressure, or hypertension, as a model for thinking about the complex issues driving health disparities in general.

We begin by documenting Black–White differences in the prevalence, awareness, treatment, and control of hypertension. This analysis clarifies the specific nature of the disparities that must be addressed. Next, we review the literature investigating Black versus White differences in the major modifiable risk factors for hypertension, including both individual- and community-level risks. Disparities in these risk factors may contribute to racial disparities in prevalence and could provide focal points for intervention. Yet, as we will demonstrate, studies investigating race differences in modifiable risk factors have significant methodological limitations. More important, without a clear understanding of the determinants of any race differences in risk exposure, simply documenting these race differences will not provide sufficient guidance for the development of risk-reducing interventions to reduce racial disparities in hypertension.

Risk-reducing interventions target the constellation of psychological experiences (e.g., affects, behaviors, and cognitions) and environmental circumstances (e.g., resources and barriers) that contribute to the development of the health-impairing conditions. However, these contributory factors are likely to vary substantially by race and ethnicity, among other factors. We will argue that a portion of the race differences in determinants of health outcomes is a function of differential exposure to racial and ethnic discrimination. In the third section of the chapter, we examine the evidence linking racism to hypertension both directly and by means of associations with each of the modifiable risk factors for hypertension. We consider different levels of racism, including cultural, institutional, interpersonal, and internalized or intrapersonal (Harrell, 2000; Krieger, 1999). Each of these levels may act independently and synergistically with racism at other levels and with associated psychosocial factors (e.g., socioeconomic status, or SES) to affect the development and course of hypertension (Myers, 2009). Understanding the multilevel mechanisms through which racism affects cardiovascular health is essential to help clinicians understand the range of barriers facing individuals from different racial or ethnic groups as they work together to improve health outcomes. This knowledge can promote the development of tailored and, consequentially, more effective integrated treatments for hypertension.

It is important to note that there is little consensus on the best terms to use to distinguish among groups based on phenotypic or cultural characteristics, and both scientific and political factors influence the debate. Some terms—for example, *Black*—have been used to refer to "racial" groups despite the lack of biological evidence for distinct races; whereas other terms, among them the designation *Latinos*, are usually considered to be labels for ethnic groups but have also been used to refer to "races." In this chapter, we have chosen to use the terms *race* and *ethnicity* and *racism* and *ethnic discrimination* interchangeably to refer to groups based on notions of race, cultural background, and/or ethnicity.

Similarly, there are differences of opinion about the most appropriate terms to use when referring to different ethnic or racial groups. Because we discuss ethnic discrimination as maltreatment based on phenotypic or cultural characteristics, we have chosen the most general categories—that is, the terms *Black* and *Latino*—rather than more specific subcategories when referring to the participants' ethnic and racial groupings.

Our review focuses on the differences between African Americans and White Americans, because this has been the primary focus of empirical research on racial disparities in hypertension (HTN). However, it is important to note that there are also significant disparities for other ethnic groups (e.g., Angell, et al., 2008; Burt, et al., 1995; Glover, Greenlund, & Ayala, 2002; H. Kramer et al., 2004; Zhao, Ford, & Mokdad, 2008). Recently, investigators have also identified variations among subgroups within larger ethnic or racial categories (e.g., subgroups of Asians or Latinos/ Latinas; Rosamond et al., 2008)

DOCUMENTING DISPARITY: VARIATIONS IN THE PREVALENCE, AWARENESS, TREATMENT, AND CONTROL OF HYPERTENSION

Estimates of the prevalence of hypertension in Blacks and Whites in the United States have been obtained through major epidemiological studies conducted using national or regional samples. At any given time, race-group variations in hypertension prevalence may be a function of differences in underlying pathology and symptoms presentation, as well as variations in access to diagnosis and treatment, in adherence to prevention and treatment strategies, and in response to treatment. Therefore, we will examine available data on each of these issues separately.

Although there have been variations in the standards used to consider individuals eligible for treatment, the major epidemiological studies have generally considered an individual to meet criteria for current hypertension if his or her clinic blood pressure (BP) is at or above 140/90 mmHg, or if he or she reports receiving antihypertensive treatment. National studies examining prevalence rates for hypertension among adults (> = 20 years of age) consistently report substantially higher rates for Blacks than Whites. Across studies, the prevalence rates for Whites range from 24.4% to 29%; whereas the prevalence rates for Blacks range from 30.6% to 40.5% (Borrell, Crawford, Barrington, & Maglo, 2008; Fiscella & Holt, 2008; Glover et al., 2002; Glover, Greenlund, Ayala, & Croft, 2005; Hajjar & Kotchen, 2003). Black–White differences in the prevalence of hypertension have actually increased over time for men. For example, comparisons of prevalence rates from NHANES III (collected between 1988 and 1994) and NHANES IV (collected between 1999 and 2004) indicate that the prevalence of hypertension increased for all groups, but the effects were significant for Black and White women and for Black but not White men (Cutler et al., 2008).

Black–White differences in BP levels emerge at an early age, prior to concerns about treatment adherence or treatment response. Studies of children and adolescents indicate race-group discrepancies as early as 8 years of age (Muntner et al., 2006). Among every age group, BP levels of Black individuals are higher than those of White individuals (Muntner et al., 2006). The effects of persistently elevated BP on overall health accumulate over time, with hypertension-related illnesses serving as a significant contributor to the gap in lifespan between Blacks and Whites in the United States (Fiscella & Holt, 2008). In addition, long-term differences in BP may contribute to changes in brain function that in turn modify response to antihypertensive treatment (Jennings & Zanstra, 2009).

Efforts to reduce BP depend on being aware of one's hypertensive status. Recent data indicate that Blacks are more likely than Whites to be aware of their hypertensive status. Rates of awareness in Blacks range from 66.7% to 85.5%, whereas rates of awareness in Whites range from 62.9% to 82.4% (Angell et al., 2008; Glover et al., 2002; Hajjar & Kotchen, 2003; Hertz, Unger, Cornell, & Saunders, 2005; Victor et al., 2008).

There are a number of effective nonpharmacological and pharmacological treatments for hypertension (Lawes, Bennett, Feigin, & Rodgers, 2004; Schwartz, Neale, Marco, Shiffman, & Stone, 1999). Many current studies indicate that Blacks are more likely than Whites to be prescribed treatment for hypertension. Rates of treatment for hypertension in Blacks range from 53.6% to 68.2%; whereas rates of treatment for hypertension in Whites range from 48.6% to 60.4% (Glover et al., 2002; Hertz et al., 2005; Victor et al., 2008). However, at least one study in New York City (Angell et al., 2008) reported that Black adults were less likely to receive treatment than were Whites, in part because the Black individuals were less likely than Whites to receive routine primary care.

Even when treated, the majority of patients do not consistently achieve BP control (i.e., achieving levels below 140/90 with treatment). Nationally, across ethnic or racial groups, only about 31% of those diagnosed with hypertension meet criteria for good BP control (Wang & Vasan, 2005). There is some evidence that difficulties in achieving BP control are particularly problematic for Blacks in comparison to Whites, even when both groups receive treatment. Across a number of studies, the control rates among treated hypertensive Whites ranged from 55.6% to 86.3%; whereas rates for Blacks ranged from 44.1% to 65.2% (Angell et al., 2008; Hajjar & Kotchen, 2003; Hertz et al., 2005; Victor et al., 2008). However, other studies have revealed no significant race differences in BP control (Cutler et al., 2008; Wyatt et al., 2008).

There is some evidence that Black–White differences in BP control are partly a function of disparities in adherence. Several studies, including large-scale investigations emerging from samples of Veterans Administration patients, have reported that Blacks are less adherent to antihypertensive medication than are Whites, and that these differences in adherence largely account for Black–White differences in BP control (Bosworth et al., 2006; Krousel-Wood et al., 2009). In contrast, other population-based studies emerging from NHANES have indicated that Blacks are as adherent or more adherent than Whites and that Blacks continued to have poorer BP control despite adherence to treatment (Natarajan, Santa Ana, Liao, Lipsitz, & McGee, 2009). Still other studies have reported no race differences in adherence (Kressin & Peterson, 2001).

In sum, Black Americans are more likely to be aware of their hypertension and may be more likely to receive treatment for hypertension. Despite these gains, Black Americans are still more likely than White Americans to develop hypertension, and they may be less likely to achieve effective BP control. These findings suggest that influencing access to care and treatment may not be sufficient to reduce the excess burden of hypertension among Blacks. A greater understanding of the biopsychosocial determinants of hypertension may be necessary to address the racial disparities in the prevalence and course of hypertension and to modify the type and intensity of treatments offered.

RISK FACTORS FOR HYPERTENSION

Racial disparities in the prevalence and course of hypertension may be partly a function of disparities in exposure to risk factors for hypertension. Some of the risk factors are measured at an individual level (e.g., obesity), whereas others are measured at a community level (e.g., neighborhood crime). If race differences in exposure to particular risk factors account for race differences in BP, then interventions designed to reduce these risk factors should reduce racial disparities in hypertension. But the situation is not that simple or clear. As we will review, there are difficulties with the available evidence that make it difficult to evaluate the role of race differences in risk factors to the development of hypertension. Overall, the findings highlight the need for more complex models to explain racial disparities in the prevalence of hypertension (Dressler, Oths, & Gravlee, 2005).

The major *individual-level* and potentially modifiable risk factors associated with hypertension include dietary factors and obesity and exercise participation and fitness (Cossrow & Falkner, 2004; Dickson, Blackledge, & Hajjar, 2006; Hajjar & Kotchen, 2003; Halpert et al., 1997; Narkiewicz,

2006; Okosun, Choi, Dent, Jobin, & Dever, 2001; Wexler et al., 2008), as well as psychosocial stressors and stress-related personal characteristics (e.g., stressful events, negative affect–related traits; Jonas & Lando, 2000; Matthews et al., 2004). *Community-level* risk factors include neighborhood SES and neighborhood stressors (e.g., crime, marital instability; see Dressler et al., 2005, for review; Harburg, Gleiberman, Roeper, Schork, & Schull, 1978; Nguyen, Evans, & Zonderman, 2008; D. K. Wilson, Kliewer, & Domenic, 2004).

We briefly review evidence supporting the link between each individual-level and community-level risk factor and hypertension. Next, we examine the evidence documenting racial disparities in the level of exposure to the risk factor and/or suggesting racial differences in the relationship of this risk factor to BP levels. Finally, we evaluate the evidence investigating the degree to which these risk factors can explain racial disparities in hypertension.

HEALTH BEHAVIORS AND RELATED OUTCOMES

OBESITY

Obesity as defined by body mass index (BMI) is a potent risk factor for hypertension (Cossrow & Falkner, 2004; Okosun et al., 2001). There are well-documented racial disparities in the prevalence of obesity, though there are variations depending on gender. The NHANES 1999–2000 survey revealed no race differences in the prevalence of obesity (i.e., BMI ≥ 30) for adult men, but substantial differences between Black and White women (White, 30.1%; Black, 49.7%; Flegal, Carroll, Ogden, & Johnson, 2002). Although BMI is associated with increased risk for hypertension in all groups, as obesity increases, the risks for hypertension grow more pronounced for Whites than Blacks (Oberg et al., 2007; Paeratakul, Lovejoy, Ryan, & Bray, 2002).

Abdominal obesity or visceral adipose tissue is a specific risk factor for hypertension (Fox et al., 2007). Studies of Black–White differences in abdominal obesity yield mixed findings (Cossrow & Falkner, 2004; Okosun et al., 2001; Perry et al., 2000). The limited available data suggest that the relationship of abdominal obesity to hypertension is stronger for Blacks than for Whites (Okosun et al., 2001).

HEALTHY DIETS

Hypertension prevalence has been associated with several dietary factors, including low levels of consumption of fruits and vegetables, low levels of consumption of potassium, and high levels of consumption of sodium, among other factors (Beitz, Mensink, & Fischer, 2003; Dickson et al., 2006; John, Ziebland, Yudkin, Roe, & Neil, 2002; Kotchen & McCarron, 1998). There are racial disparities in patterns of consumption. In comparison with White Americans, African Americans consume significantly fewer fruits and vegetables (Dickson et al., 2006) and more dietary sodium (Ervin, 2008).

There are very limited direct data on race differences in the relationship of patterns of consumption to hypertension. There is indirect evidence that the ability to purchase a healthier diet (e.g., when individuals have access to supermarkets) is associated with better improvements in BP for Black individuals rather than for Whites individuals (Morland, Wing, & Diez-Roux, 2002). There are some data suggesting that Black individuals are more affected by high sodium intake than are Whites, and Blacks respond with larger reductions in BP when exposed to a low-sodium diet (Sacks et al., 2001). However, there is also evidence that ethnicity does not influence the relationship between sodium intake and BP (Madhavan & Alderman, 1994).

ALCOHOL CONSUMPTION

The evidence concerning the relationship of alcohol consumption to hypertension has been mixed, with some studies reporting that the number of alcoholic drinks per day is associated with hypertension (Marmot et al., 1994; Russell, Cooper, & Frone, 1990; Sesso, Cook, Buring, Manson, & Gaziano, 2008; York & Hirsch, 1997). Other studies have not found a relationship of alcohol intake to hypertension (Koppes, Twisk, Van Mechelen, Snel, & Kemper, 2005). Daily alcohol consumption is higher among White adults than Black adults, but the association of alcohol intake to hypertension risk is greater for Black men. Race differences in the relationship of alcohol to hypertension are not seen in women (Svetkey et al., 2005).

Fitness and Exercise

Higher levels of fitness are associated with lower risk for hypertension (Fagard, 2005; Halpert et al., 1997). Data from national studies suggest that Whites are more likely than Blacks (33.7% vs. 25.3%) to report regular leisure-time physical activity (Rosamond et al., 2008). Black Americans are also more likely than their White counterparts to be "thinking about exercising" as opposed to actually exercising, according to one large-scale survey (Wexler et al., 2008). There is some evidence that although higher levels of fitness are associated with lower levels of hypertension for both Blacks and Whites, the relationship of fitness to hypertension was significant for Whites and not for Blacks (Bassett, Fitzhugh, Crespo, King, & McLaughlin, 2002).

Psychosocial Stressors

Individual-level psychosocial stressors include a wide variety of variables including life events and job strain. Psychosocial stressors also include personal characteristics, including negative affect and anger-related traits (i.e., trait anger, hostility, and anger expression) that may increase the frequency and intensity of stress exposure and distress responses. Community-level stressors can include neighborhood violence, marital instability, or housing instability.

Psychosocial stressors may affect risk for hypertension through both psychophysiological and behavioral pathways. Depression, anxiety, and anger-related traits all have been associated with disruptions in the autonomic and neuroendocrine systems that subserve BP regulation, though the pattern of effects differs depending on the characteristic under study (e.g., Jorgensen, Johnson, Kolodziej, & Schreer, 1996; Sloan et al., 2001). For example, there is substantial evidence that hostility and other anger-related traits are associated with increased BP or heart rate reactivity to stress, one index of altered autonomic function. Hostility and other psychosocial stressors also may contribute to poor health behaviors and may influence the relationship of particular health behaviors to hypertension (Matthews, 2005).

Many psychosocial stressors have been linked to hypertension prevalence in the general population, though the evidence is not completely consistent (Friedman et al., 2001). Work-related stressors are a significant correlate of hypertension (Levenstein, Smith, & Kaplan, 2001). There is also evidence linking chronic perceived stress (Sparrenberger et al., 2009), depression (Bosworth, Bartash, Olsen, & Steffens, 2003), anxiety (Jonas & Lando, 2000), hostility (Yan et al., 2003), and anger suppression (Schum et al., 2003) to either BP level or hypertension, (Friedman et al., 2001; Levenstein et al., 2001; Sparrenberger et al., 2009). Effects for job strain (Ohlin, Berglund, Rosvall, & Nilsson, 2007), anger, anxiety, and depression (Rutledge & Hogan, 2002) have been seen cross-sectionally as well as prospectively (i.e., in studies of changes from normotensive to hypertensive status).

There is evidence of Black–White differences in the levels of exposure to psychosocial stressors associated with hypertension, though the findings depend on the type and severity of the stressor (Jonas & Lando, 2000; Julius, 1988). For example, Black adults are more likely to suffer from unemployment and to face discrimination at work than are Whites (Mays, Coleman, & Jackson, 1996). Assessments of negative mood and overall psychological distress occur disproportionately among African Americans in comparison to Whites (Jonas & Lando, 2000); however, data on the prevalence of diagnosable depressive disorders do not yield consistent evidence of higher levels of diagnosable depression among African Americans (C. I. Cohen, Magai, Yaffee, & Walcott-Brown,

2005; Riolo, Nguyen, Greden, & King, 2005). There is also evidence of racial disparities in anger-related traits, with several studies indicating that Blacks have higher self-reported levels of trait hostility than do Whites (D. C. Cooper & Waldstein, 2004; R. B. Williams, Barefoot, & Schneiderman, 2009). There is some limited evidence that Blacks may be more likely than Whites to suppress rather than express anger (Harburg, Gleiberman, Russell, & Cooper, 1991).

The effects of stressor exposure on distress also appear to be greater for Blacks. Initial evidence cited by Williams (D. R. Williams & Collins, 1995) suggested that Blacks reported more distress from negative life events than did Whites. Prospective studies suggest that smaller changes in stress exposure are associated with greater changes in depressive symptoms for Blacks versus Whites (George & Lynch, 2003).

Stress and negative affect–related characteristics may also be more closely related to hypertension for Black adults than White adults, though the findings are not always consistent. Unemployment has been associated with greater rates of hypertension among Black men than among Whites (Levenstein et al., 2001). Prospective studies indicate that depression scores are more closely related to hypertension incidence in Blacks than Whites (Jonas & Lando, 2000; Krieger & Sidney, 1996); however, other studies have reported reverse effects (Yan et al., 2003). Some investigators have reported stronger relationships of hostility to BP for Black adults (R. S. Cooper, 2003); but Yan et al. (2003) reported that although hostility was a significant predictor of the development of hypertension, the effects were seen for both Black and White adults. Similarly, anger suppression has been associated with hypertension. Some studies suggest that these effects are more likely to emerge in studies of Blacks (Jorgensen et al., 1996), though other studies report no race differences (Schum et al., 2003).

Cardiovascular reactivity (CVR), one measure of physiological response to stress, has been prospectively associated with hypertension risk (Matthews et al., 2004). Many, though not all, studies of CVR suggest that Blacks show greater BP reactivity than do Whites across a range of stressors (Anderson, 1989; Duey et al., 1997; Light, Turner, Hinderliter, & Sherwood, 1993; Murphy, Stoney, Alpert, & Walker, 1995; Thomas, Nelesen, Malcarne, Ziegler, & Dimsdale, 2006; Treiber et al., 1993; Wilcox, Bopp, Wilson, Fulk, & Hand, 2005).

In sum, there are racial disparities in key health behaviors and related outcomes associated with hypertension risk. White individuals consume greater amounts of alcohol than do Black individuals; but Black individuals are more likely to be obese and to consume diets high in sodium but low in fruits and vegetables and are less likely to engage in physical activity than are Whites. However, the effects of these health behaviors and associated outcomes are not consistent across race and ethnic groups. The association of obesity and fitness may be slightly stronger for Whites than Blacks, whereas some evidence suggests that the association of sodium and alcohol consumption and abdominal obesity to hypertension is stronger for Blacks than Whites.

Black individuals are more likely to experience psychosocial stress, to experience distress as a function of stress exposure, and to display heightened physiological responses to these acute stressors; they may also be more likely to show slower recovery to certain stressors (Lepore et al., 2006). It is not clear if psychosocial stressors are more closely related to hypertension diagnosis in Black versus White adults.

COMMUNITY-LEVEL RISK FACTORS

In the next section, we examine contextual or community-level factors, including neighborhood SES and neighborhood measures of stress that have been identified as risk factors for hypertension. The bulk of studies of community-level factors have examined effects on coronary heart disease or mental health outcomes (Diez-Roux, Merkin, Hannan, Jacobs, & Kiefe, 2003; Leventhal & Brooks-Gunn, 2000), but there is a growing literature on the effects of neighborhood stress or economic resources on risk for hypertension or hypertension prevalence. These community-level risk factors may differentially influence the health behaviors and psychosocial stress exposure in Black versus White individuals. These community-level variables may also moderate the relationship of individual-level risk factors to BP.

NEIGHBORHOOD SES, NEIGHBORHOOD STRESS, AND HYPERTENSION

Neighborhood levels of SES are generally assessed with census-derived indices of income, education, and occupation level of the residents or the costs and types of housing. The findings from correlational studies examining neighborhood levels of SES and hypertension prevalence are clear. In general, indices associated with lower levels of SES are associated with higher levels of hypertension. Specifically, median housing values, controlling for individual-level measures of SES, have been negatively associated with hypertension prevalence in a national sample of Black women (Cozier et al., 2007). Similarly, rental costs have been inversely associated with hypertension in a regional study in the southern United States (Schlundt, Hargreaves, & McClellan, 2006). Block-group-level measures of income, education, and occupational status were associated with hypertension in a study of four different communities, though not all effects were significant and there were some variations by race (Diez-Roux et al., 1997). Neighborhood affluence (i.e., presence of educated individuals, proportion of individuals in professional or managerial occupations) was associated with decreased risk for hypertension in a national sample (Morenoff et al., 2007).

Low levels of neighborhood SES are associated with fewer nutritional and recreational resources. Specifically, in comparison to more affluent areas, low-SES neighborhoods have fewer stores selling low-cost and high-quality fruits and vegetables, more stores selling alcohol and fast food, and fewer facilities for recreation and fitness (Kwate, 2008; Schlundt et al., 2006). The lack of resources increases the barriers to positive health behavior and increases the likelihood that individuals will have one or more individual-level risk factors.

Data on the effects of community-level stress exposure are beginning to emerge and suggest that perceptions of social stress in the community, including experiences of violence, may increase risk for hypertension (see D. Wilson et al., 2004, for review). The studies of neighborhood stressors have evaluated the relationship of both objective and subjective ratings of different characteristics associated with stress to either BP level or self-reported hypertension. Neighborhood characteristics that have been assessed include residential or marital stability, cleanliness, crime, perceived safety, and violence. Crime- and violence-related stressors are likely to serve as chronic stressors, because fear of crime and behavioral preparations to prevent crime may be ongoing, even if actual personal or property damage occurs infrequently.

In a seminal set of studies, Harburg and colleagues (1978) reported that neighborhood stress (a composite of marital and residential instability and crime rates) was associated with higher levels of BP for younger, but not older, Black men and for younger Black women, but only for those who were underweight. The effects of neighborhood stress were not seen for Whites (Harburg et al., 1978). However, criteria for determining that an area was "high stress" were set separately for Blacks and Whites, and they lived in distinct neighborhoods. Consequently, it is difficult to determine if Whites would also display similar levels of BP if they were living in neighborhoods with the absolute stress levels seen in Black communities.

More recent work supports the notion that neighborhood stressors are associated with BP levels or hypertension. In adolescents, evidence suggests that reports of neighborhood levels of violence are associated with nocturnal blood pressure (D. K. Wilson, Kliewer, Teasley, Plybon, & Sica, 2002). In a study of managed-care patients with diabetes (Gary et al., 2008), perceived neighborhood problems (i.e., a combination of perceptions of crime, litter, trash, lighting, and access to transportation, exercise and supermarkets) were associated with poorer BP control. It is important to note that this was the case even when making comparisons controlling for individual-level indices of objective SES. Similarly, in the MESA Study, low levels of perceived safety and social cohesion, walkability, and access to healthy foods were associated with higher rates of hypertension (Mujahid et al., 2008).

There is substantial evidence that Blacks are more likely than Whites to live in areas with higher levels of perceived stress, lower levels of SES, and fewer health-promoting resources (Mujahid et al., 2008). This situation is particularly problematic because low-income Black individuals tend to live in more segregated neighborhoods with fewer resources than do low-income White individuals (Massey & Eggers, 1990). As D. R. Williams and Jackson (2005) have pointed out, the living conditions in impoverished Black neighborhoods are substantially worse than those in even the poorest neighborhoods in which the majority of residents are White.

The limited available evidence suggests minimal race difference in the deleterious effects of stressed or impoverished neighborhoods. In the MESA Study, low levels of key neighborhood characteristics (i.e., safety, social cohesion, walkability, and access to healthy foods) were associated with hypertension, but there were no race differences in these effects (Mujahid et al., 2008). Similarly, other researchers report that the risks of relative neighborhood disadvantage on hypertension hold for Whites as well as Black adults (Grady & Ramirez, 2008; Morenoff et al., 2007).

In sum, there is clear evidence that neighborhood SES is associated with higher levels of hypertension. There is also growing evidence of an association between neighborhood stressors and hypertension prevalence. Neighborhood-level variables (e.g., deficiencies in access to healthy food or recreational facilities or excess exposure to stress) appear to contribute to hypertension prevalence for both Blacks and Whites. However, Black individuals are more likely than White individuals to live in neighborhoods characterized by high levels of environmental stress and low levels of resources, increasing their exposure to both acute and persistent stressors and decreasing their ability to recover from stress exposure.

It is of note that there may also be other important pathways through which race affects hypertension risk, pathways not addressed here. For example, there may also be effects through the quality of medical care or through the patterns of distribution of physicians throughout poor communities (Bach, Hoangmai, Schrag, Tate, & Hargraves, 2004; Benkert, Peters, Clark, & Keves-Foster, 2006; Klonoff, 2009). There may also be other individual-level factors that serve as mediators of the relationship of racism to hypertension, including potential epigenetic influences or low birth weight (Oberg et al., 2007).

DO RACIAL DIFFERENCES IN RISK FACTORS ACCOUNT FOR RACIAL DISPARITIES IN THE PREVALENCE OF HYPERTENSION?

There is simply insufficient evidence to determine if racial differences in risk factors account for racial disparities in the prevalence of hypertension. There is, however, some evidence suggesting that racial disparities in hypertension persist despite controlling for individual-level health behaviors and even SES (see Dressler et al., 2005, for review). For example, in a population-based sample, racial disparities in untreated HTN persist when controlling for individual-level risk factors, including health behaviors (e.g., smoking, obesity, fitness), as well as individual-level education and income (Bell, Adair, & Popkin, 2004). Racial disparities in hypertension risk emerge at every education level (Mensah, Mokdad, Ford, Greenlund, & Croft, 2005; Pickering, 1999). However, the limited number of studies that have included measures of perceived stress as well as health behavior and SES find more significant reductions in racial disparities (Jones-Webb, Jacobs, Flack, & Liu, 1996).

Nonetheless, there are limits to the interpretation of data on the degree to which individual-level risk factors account for racial disparities in hypertension, because the methods of analysis may not be adequate to test the hypothesis. In most studies, unweighted scores for each of the risk factors are entered into the analyses (e.g., Bell et al., 2004). This type of modeling assumes that the impact of each individual risk factor is the same for Blacks and Whites. Yet as we have presented, there is evidence that there are Black–White differences in the association of most risk factors with hypertension. Consequently, the assumption of equivalence is likely to be incorrect, and different quantitative models may be needed to fully evaluate these effects.

There may also be moderator effects in which one risk factor influences the expression of another. Many moderator effects involve individual-level stress exposure. Stress appears to change the relationships between sympathetic nervous system activity and BP regulation (Joyner, Charkoudian, & Wallin, 2008); stress affects sodium excretion by means of the renin-angiotensin-aldosterone systems, altering BP through changes in blood volume (Harshfield, Pulliam, & Alpert, 1994); and stress influences the expression of genes involved in BP control (Esler et al., 2008). Black adults are more likely than Whites to be exposed to certain psychosocial stressors and, consequently, may be more likely to be subject to these moderator effects. Variations in stress exposure may partly account for race-related differences in the association of certain risk factors (e.g., abdominal obesity) to hypertension. Therefore, an analysis of the contribution of individual-level risk factors to racial disparities in hypertension that fails to include tests for interactions among these factors may underestimate their effects in explaining Black–White differences in hypertension.

There may also be "third variable" problems, given that race and social class are closely but not uniformly linked. Social class, and in particular education level, is associated with hypertension prevalence (see review by Colhoun, Hemingway, & Poulter, 1998). There are documented Black–White disparities in educational attainment, though the effects vary by educational subject as well as by individual age and generational cohort (U.S. Census Bureau, 2008; Jacobson, Olsen, Rice, Sweetland, & Ralph, 2001).

Education may affect hypertension through its association with health behaviors, including alcohol use and obesity (Colhoun et al., 1998) and exposure to psychosocial stressors (Diez-Roux, Northridge, Morabia, Bassett, & Shea, 1999). There is a need for further research on the prospective effects of changes in education or income on BP. This evidence could provide a clearer understanding of the causal nature of this relationship and help identify aspects of education that confer health benefits or contribute to racial disparities in risk.

The "third variable" problem is linked to a more problematic issue: The antecedents of any particular health behavior may vary by race, and these variations may also confound estimates of the relationship of each risk factor to hypertension. We can examine these issues in more detail by considering the factors that motivate individuals to exercise and by noting the effect of these factors on estimates of the relationship of exercise to hypertension.

When exercise facilities are easily accessible and the barriers to regular participation are low, then individuals may exercise even if they have only moderate levels of motivation or support. In contrast, when barriers to participation are high (e.g., limited access to child care, no peer support, insufficient leisure time, restricted ability to access safe exercise facilities), then any participation may reflect very high levels of motivation. In turn, on an individual basis, the level of motivation may be a function of the individual's level of conscientiousness, social support, and/or negative affect. Each of these antecedent variables—that is, variables that influence motivation and predict exercise participation—may have independent effects on hypertension risk.

More concretely, any given score on a measure of exercise participation includes some variance associated with motivation to exercise. However, race differences in the relationship of exercise to hypertension may be obscured if the factors that affect motivation are not assessed as well. For example, some White individuals are less likely to face barriers to participating in exercise or consuming healthy diets because, for example, they are more likely to reside in areas with accessible opportunities for physical activity, and/or to have supports that promote exercise adherence (Mechanic, 2005). Therefore, for Whites living in environments that present few barriers to participation, low levels of exercise compliance (e.g., walking one day a week) may be a function of low levels of individual motivation. In contrast, for Blacks living in environments that present high barriers to participation, an equivalent level of participation (i.e., walking one day a week) may reflect a much higher level of motivation. If motivation is partly a function of mood, then for Whites, but not necessarily for Blacks, low absolute levels of participation may be paired with high levels of negative mood. The determinant of exercise behavior or any given health behavior is likely to vary by community depending on the actual barriers and supports for those behaviors. Consequently, it may be important to conduct sample-specific evaluations of the predictors of any given health behavior.

Although studies of community variables as predictors of health behavior and outcome represent a new area of research, there is some evidence that community variables may at least partly explain racial disparities in hypertension. To underscore the importance of neighborhood resources, a recent study reports on a comparison of risk factors for hypertension in two neighborhoods in which the levels of resources available to Blacks and Whites were roughly equivalent. In this study, racial disparities in some of the variables related to hypertension were minimized (La Veist, Sellers, & Neighbors, 2001). In contrast, the one experimental study in which very low-income individuals from high-poverty neighborhoods were randomly assigned to new, less impoverished neighborhoods indicated that moving did not affect rates of hypertension over a five-year period, though there were reductions in obesity and in perceived stress and distress (Kling, Liebman, & Katz, 2007).

However, it is difficult to fully evaluate the hypothesis that community-level variables explain race differences, given that race-related and neighborhood-level variables are so heavily confounded. For example, in the Four Neighborhoods Study, the African American community was different from the fully or mostly White communities on every socioeconomic index (Diez-Roux et al., 1997). Similarly, the effects of specific indices of neighborhood stress are difficult to identify because some investigators have combined measures of access to resources (e.g., supermarkets) with measures more explicitly tied to psychosocial stress (e.g., perceptions of safety, violence, marital instability). These variables tend to cluster together, but it will be difficult to identify targets for intervention without a more systematic evaluation of their unique effects. Studies of the ways in which neighborhood or contextual factors moderate the effects of individual-level risk factors are also crucial.

The research on the effects of neighborhood stressors is much more developed in studies of childhood academic performance and mental disorders (see Leventhal & Brooks-Gunn, 2000, for review). It will be important to extend the methodologies from these studies to investigate the specific neighborhood stressors or resources that predict the development of hypertension.

IS RACISM A RISK FACTOR?

In the next section, we consider the possibility that racism contributes to the prevalence and course of hypertension. Racism is a psychosocial stressor that is disproportionately experienced by African Americans in comparison to European Americans (Brondolo, Brady, Libby, & Pencille, 2010; Krieger, Smith, Naishadham, Hartman, & Barbeau, 2005). Because it is a complex and multilevel stressor, racism may affect risk for hypertension through multiple mechanisms (Mays, Cochran, & Barnes, 2007). Figure 24.1 illustrates ways in which racism may operate to directly and indirectly influence risk.

Specifically, there may be direct relationships of racism to hypertension. Racism may also contribute to hypertension through effects on risk factors for hypertension (e.g., obesity, stress, or fitness). If racism influences the development and course of hypertension, risk-reducing interventions must consider the role of racism if they are to be successful in changing health behavior for targeted groups.

To fully evaluate the role of racism in the development of hypertension, it is necessary to first consider the complex nature of the actions and circumstances linked to racism and ethnic discrimination. There have been a number of definitions of racism and ethnic discrimination. One widely used definition, presented by Rodney Clark and colleagues in a paper published in 1999 in *American Psychologist* is that racism consists of "the beliefs, attitudes, institutional arrangements, and acts that tend to denigrate individuals or groups because of phenotypic characteristics or ethnic group affiliation" (Clark, Anderson, Clark, & Williams, 1999, p. 805). Contrada has used the more general term *ethnic discrimination* and defined it as unfair treatment received because of one's ethnicity, where "ethnicity" refers to various groupings of individuals based on race or culture of origin (Contrada et al., 2001; Contrada et al., 2000). In line with these definitions, we consider racism or

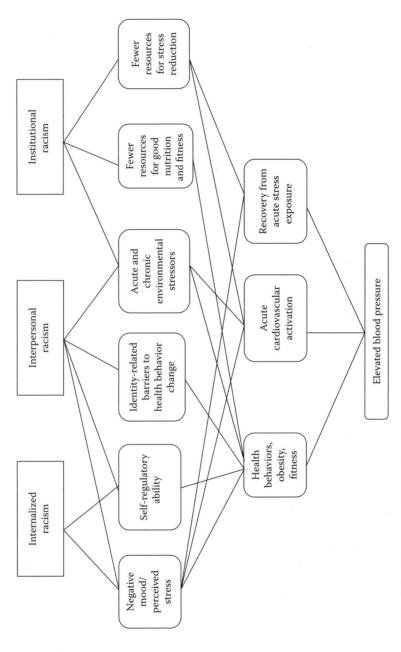

FIGURE 24.1   Possible relationships among different levels of racism, hypertension risk factors, and hypertension prevalence.

ethnic discrimination to be a form of social ostracism in which phenotypic or cultural characteristics are used to render individuals outcasts, making them targets of social exclusion, unfair treatment, and threat or harassment (Brondolo et al., 2010; Brondolo, Brady, et al., 2008).

Racism can occur on multiple levels: cultural, institutional, interpersonal, and intrapersonal or internalized (Harrell, 2000). Cultural racism occurs when the methods used to communicate cultural values (e.g., film, television, advertisements) convey negative information about a particular group. Through a variety of media, individuals are exposed to messages that influence the perceptions of a targeted group, affecting the behaviors and attitudes of all individuals both in and out of the targeted group (Major & O'Brien, 2005). The term *institutional racism* is generally used to refer to specific policies and/or procedures of institutions (i.e., government, business, schools, churches) that consistently result in unequal treatment for particular groups (Better, 2002; Griffith, Childs, Eng, & Jeffries, 2007; Lea, 2000). Jim Crow laws, forcing segregation of the races, were clear examples of institutional racism. Residential racial segregation can also be considered an outcome related to institutional racism (Williams & Mohammed, 2009).

Individual-level or interpersonal racism has been defined as "directly perceived discriminatory interactions between individuals, whether in their institutional roles or as public and private individuals" (Krieger, 1999, p. 301). Interpersonal racism may encompass different types of experiences, ranging from social exclusion, workplace discrimination, and stigmatization to physical threat, harassment, and aggression (Brondolo et al., 2005). Internalized racism has been defined as "the acceptance, by marginalized racial populations, of the negative societal beliefs and stereotypes about themselves" (D. R. Williams & Williams-Morris, 2000, p. 255). For example, individuals may come to believe themselves to be less intelligent by virtue of their group membership if they belong to a group stereotyped as inferior in intelligence.

MEASURING RACISM

Although cultural influences on the development of health attitudes and behaviors have been documented (Castro, Shaibi, & Boehm-Smith, 2009), to our knowledge there is no direct research examining the relationship of the effects of racial bias in media presentation to hypertension prevalence. Therefore, we confine our discussion of the strategies for measuring racism to assessments of institutional, interpersonal, and internalized racism.

Many studies of the health effects of institutional racism have examined outcomes of policies, rather than the policies or law themselves. Residential racial segregation (RRS) is one outcome of institutional policies and interpersonal practices that isolated African Americans and influenced patterns of housing (see M. R. Kramer & Hogue, 2009, for a review). In RRS, the types of exclusion and rejection associated with interpersonal racism are manifest in a community setting. Across all income groups, Blacks tend to live in more racially segregated areas than do Whites, but race-based residential segregation is most pronounced among low-income individuals (D. R. Williams & Mohammed, 2009). Population-based studies of attitudes toward housing confirm the degree to which race-based social ostracism drives RRS (Emerson, Yancey, & Chai, 2001).

Several different strategies used to assess RRS have been reviewed in Kramer and Hogue (2009). The indices assess the degree to which an individual is likely to encounter an individual of a different race. One of the most commonly used metrics is the proportion of Black residents in the census tract (or other defined area).

There are also investigators who have used self-reported measures of individual racism that occur in institutional settings (i.e., at work or in the criminal justice context) to serve as indices of institutional racism. However, because these scales measure directly perceived experiences, we have included them with measures of individual-level racism. Typically, interpersonal or individual-level racism is assessed with self-report questionnaires (e.g., Perceived Ethnic Discrimination Questionnaire–Community Version; Brondolo et al., 2005; Racism and Life Experiences Survey, Harrell, 1997;

Experiences of Discrimination Questionnaires, Krieger et al., 2005; Schedule of Racist Events, Landrine, Klonoff, Corral, Fernandez, & Roesch, 2006). These scales measure the frequency of exposure to either different types of race-based maltreatment or overall perceptions of exposure to discrimination in different settings. In published studies of hypertension and related risk factors, internalized racism has been assessed with the Nadolization Questionnaire, which measures agreement with common stereotypical beliefs (Taylor & Grundy, 1996).

ASSOCIATIONS OF INSTITUTIONALIZED, INTERPERSONAL AND INTERNALIZED RACISM TO HYPERTENSION AND HYPERTENSION-RELATED RISK FACTORS

INTERNALIZED RACISM

To our knowledge, there is only one study directly assessing the effects of internalized racism to resting BP, and this study did not find a relationship (S. E. Tull et al., 1999). Three studies, including one of adolescents, suggest a relationship of internalized racism to abdominal obesity, a known risk factor for HTN (Butler, Tull, Chambers, & Taylor, 2002; Chambers et al., 2004; S. E. Tull et al., 1999). However, this relationship has not been found in every study (E. S. Tull, Sheu, Butler, & Cornelious, 2005). One study also reports a relationship of internalized racism to perceived stress (E. S. Tull et al., 2005).

INTERPERSONAL RACISM

In our earlier review (Brondolo, Rieppi, Kelly, and Gerin, 2003), we reported very limited evidence of a direct relationship of interpersonal racism to blood pressure. Since that publication, new studies have emerged, and several studies have included assessments of ambulatory blood pressure as well as clinic BP. To date, there have been 13 studies examining the relationship of self-reported exposure to interpersonal racism to resting BP level or self-reported or doctor-diagnosed hypertensive status in Black adults (Barksdale, Farrug, & Harkness, 2009; Broman, 1996; J. Collins, David, Handler, Wall, & Andes, 2004; K. James, Lovato, & Khoo, 1994; S. A. James, LaCroix, Kleinbaum, & Strogatz, 1984; Krieger, 1990; Krieger & Sidney, 1996; Peters, 2004, 2006; Poston et al., 2001; Ryan, Gee, & Laflamme, 2006). There are only two studies that find a positive relationship between self-reported racism and either BP level or self-reported hypertensive status in the group overall (K. James et al., 1994) or in one subgroup (i.e., non-U.S.-born women; Cozier et al., 2006). Seven studies did not find a direct relationship of perceived racism to BP when the investigators examined the sample as a whole (Barksdale et al., 2009; Broman, 1996; Cozier et al., 2006; Din-Dzietham, Nembhard, Collins, & Davis, 2004; Dressler, 1996; Peters, 2006; Poston et al., 2001); two studies found a negative relationship either among older participants (Peters, 2004) or among the participant group as a whole (Krieger, 1990).

In contrast, the data from ambulatory blood pressure (ABP)–monitoring studies are more consistent. ABP, and in particular nocturnal ABP, is regarded as a more reliable predictor of target organ damage than are clinic measures (Pickering et al., 2005). The five studies investigating these effects in adults reported positive relationships for either daytime ABP (Steffen, McNeilly, Anderson, & Sherwood, 2003), or nighttime (Brondolo, Libby, et al., 2008; Singleton, Robertson, Robinson, Austin, & Edochie, 2008), or both (Hill, Kobayashi, & Hughes, 2007; Tomfohr, Cooper, Mills, Nelesen, & Dimsdale, 2010).

It is surprising that although evidence shows that racism is related to obesity among Asian individuals (Gee, Ro, Gavin, & Takeuchi, 2008), there has been little research on the effects among African Americans. A recent study suggests that racism may be associated with changes in weight gain over an eight-year period (Cozier, Wise, Palmer, & Rosenberg, 2009). The one study investigating the effects of racism on exercise participation did not find an association (Shelton Puleo, Bennett, McNeill, Goldman, & Emmons, 2009).

There is clear evidence that interpersonal racism is associated with negative affect, anger, depression, and anxiety, all potential risk factors for HTN (Brondolo, Brady, et al., 2008; Kessler, Mickelson, & Williams, 1999; Moghaddam, Taylor, Ditto, Jacobs, & Bianchi, 2002). Some data confirm the relationship of interpersonal racism to CVR, itself a risk factor for HTN and a potential mediator of the relationship between psychosocial stress and HTN (Clark, 2000; Guyll, Matthews, & Bromberger, 2001).

In a new area of research, investigators have consistently documented a link between interpersonal racism and low birth weight (Collins et al., 2004; Collins, et al., 2000; Dole et al., 2004; Lespinasse, David, Collins, Handler, & Wall, 2004; Mustillo et al., 2004). Low birth weight is also a risk factor for HTN, possibly through its association with heightened stress responsivity (Feldt et al., 2007). These effects may be stronger for African Americans than for European Americans (Oberg et al., 2007).

INSTITUTIONALIZED RACISM

There has been limited research specifically examining the degree to which HTN prevalence is increased as a function of RRS, as assessed by the degree to which Black individuals live primarily with other Blacks. In two studies, the proportion of individuals who were African American was associated with increased risk for hypertension (Grady & Ramirez, 2008). However, in only one study did the investigators control for neighborhood poverty and related factors (Grady & Ramirez, 2008). Consequently, it is difficult to determine if other characteristics of the neighborhood, rather than simply the presence of Black individuals, account for the higher prevalence of HTN. In contrast, two studies, one of adults (Morenoff et al., 2007) and one of adolescents (McGrath, Matthews, & Brady, 2006), report that a higher percentage of Blacks in the neighborhood was not associated with greater prevalence of HTN, controlling for other neighborhood conditions, including affluence and disadvantage.

Data from several studies suggest that living in neighborhoods with high concentrations of Black individuals is associated with a higher prevalence of obesity, higher rates of distress, and lower levels of fitness (Diez-Roux et al., 1999; Schlundt et al., 2006). However, there have been very little data examining these effects while controlling for the concomitant presence of high levels of neighborhood stress and disadvantage. Therefore, it is difficult to determine if these effects are directly associated with the presence of Blacks in the neighborhood or if they are a function of the economic and social conditions that ensue when resources are not available.

INDIRECT EFFECTS OF INSTITUTIONAL, INTERPERSONAL, AND INTERNALIZED RACISM

Most individual-level behavior change interventions to reduce weight or improve fitness require some intrinsic motivation, self-awareness, and the ability to experience positive mood in response to progress and to anticipate positive affect when achieving goals. Exposure to racism may affect each of these intrapersonal motivation-related factors. Consequently, interventions may need to target these racism-related outcomes prior to considering health behavior change.

All levels of racism may indirectly affect the intrinsic motivation to engage in some activities to change health behavior through their effects on stigma sensitivity and racial identity. Cultural racism may influence the development and maintenance of stereotypes of African Americans and may engender the development of concerns about *stereotype threat*. Stereotype threat is experienced when individuals are anxious that their performance in a particular arena will confirm the potentially biased and overgeneralized beliefs other people hold about their group (Speight, 2007; Steele, 1997). Direct exposure to racism may intensify awareness of the dangers associated with racial-group membership and strengthen concerns about stereotype threat (Contrada et al., 2001).

Concerns about stereotype threat may influence health behavior when individuals may be concerned that they are not capable of changing these health-related behaviors for fear of confirming a weakness associated with the group as a whole (G. L. Cohen & Garcia, 2005). Similarly, if individuals have internalized stereotypes about their group's ability to engage in health behavior change, self-stereotyping may undermine individuals' beliefs in their self-efficacy or ability to engage in health behavior change.

Racism may also influence motivation through processes related to identity. Adhering to behaviors that are associated with one's own racial or ethnic group and rejecting behaviors associated with other groups can be seen as a strategy for promoting in-group identification and esteem (Fordham & Ogbu, 1986). There is evidence suggesting that experiences of discrimination serve to shift internal schemas about the self, increasing the investment in and attention paid to racial or ethnic aspects of identity (Quintana, 2007). This shift can limit the motivation to participate in activities that do not conform to the individual's ethnic or racial identity. For example, investigators have reported that some urban African Americans view efforts to control weight and to exercise as characteristics that are associated with middle-class and White individuals (Oyserman & Harrison, 1998). The more participants viewed these behaviors as inconsistent with their racial or ethnic identity, the less likely they were to engage in healthy eating habits.

Studies of RRS, a form of institutional racism, suggest that neighborhoods with higher percentages of African Americans are also associated with higher prevalence of obese individuals and with lower rates of exercise participation. These concentrations of obesity or inactivity can change group norms about health eating and fitness and alter the motivation or perceived need to change health behaviors (Kwate, 2008).

Racism may also influence risk through its effects on self-regulation and self-awareness. For example, we and others have underscored the importance of considering racism to be a form of race-based social ostracism (Brondolo et al., 2010; Brondolo, Gallo, Myers, & Hector, 2009). Ostracism of any kind, even potential ostracism, has been demonstrated to be associated with impairments in self-awareness as individuals seek to avoid the pain of social exclusion and rejection. This lack of self-awareness contributes to ostracism-related deficits in behavioral self-regulation (see Baumeister, DeWall, Ciarocco, & Twenge, 2005). Inzlicht and others have demonstrated specific effects of race-based ostracism on behavioral self-regulation, including eating behavior (Inzlicht, McKay, & Aronson, 2006). The impairments in self-awareness that are a function of ostracism may be particularly problematic when they are combined with high levels of negative mood. Negative mood can make self-evaluation more painful and consequently increase the level of effort required to initiate behavioral self-control.

Negative mood and subjective experiences of stress can diminish the experience of positive affect that can fuel efforts at health behavior change. Research from our laboratory (Brondolo et al., 2005) as well as others suggests that racism changes perceptions of new events, making a broader range of experiences capable of evoking distress. Specifically, the degree to which individuals have been exposed to racism in their past influences the ways in which they view new episodes of race-based maltreatment and other ongoing interpersonal exchanges. Ambulatory monitoring studies indicate that the more individuals had been exposed to racism over the course of their lifetime, the more likely they were to view ongoing interpersonal interactions as harassing and unfair (Brondolo, Brady, et al., 2008) and to view new episodes of ethnicity-related maltreatment as threatening and harmful (Brondolo et al., 2005). This reaction increases the type and intensity of events that can evoke acute stress responses and may contribute to higher levels of ongoing stress exposure.

Racism may exhaust the available coping resources required to promote health behavior change (Brondolo, ver Halen, Pencille, Beatty, & Contrada, 2009). Targeted individuals must address the specific threats presented by actual or anticipated episodes of ethnicity-related maltreatment, such as interpersonal conflict, blocked opportunities, and social exclusion. They must also manage the emotional consequences, including painful feelings of anger, nervousness, sadness, and hopelessness, and their physiological correlates, as well as potential damage to self-concept and self-esteem (Mellor, 2004). Targeted individuals must manage their concerns about the effects of racism on other individuals who share their phenotypic or cultural characteristics, including their friends and family members. The effects of RRS, including greater exposure to neighborhood poverty and stress, may require additional coping efforts.

Consequently, individuals who are targeted for racism must develop a broad range of racism-related coping responses to permit them to respond to different types of situations and to adjust the response depending on factors that might influence the effectiveness of any particular coping strategy. This level of coping flexibility is beneficial, but it is difficult to achieve (Cheng, 2003). The effort to develop and deploy all the coping strategies necessary to manage responses to different situations is an obvious burden and may limit the cognitive, affective, and self-control resources that are available to tackle additional challenges (Baumeister et al., 2005).

Finally, if race-based ostracism results in the creation of communities in which Black individuals are relatively isolated, fewer social, education, and economic resources will be available to support health and positive health behaviors. This lack of resources will make the barriers to health promotion efforts much higher. Relative isolation can lead to disenfranchisement from mainstream political and economic processes (Emerson et al., 2001; Feldt et al., 2007). Withdrawal from these processes may limit the ability of residents to attract additional health-promoting resources into the area, contributing to restricted access to a broader range of care (Bach et al., 2004).

Summary

In sum, the evidence directly linking internalized, interpersonal, and institutionalized racism directly to hypertension is limited, though there are variations in findings depending on the ways in which these variables are operationalized and assessed (see D. R. Williams & Mohammed, 2009). The data suggest that interpersonal racism is associated with ABP, a measure that is sensitive to stress-related variations in BP. There are some studies that suggest that RRS is associated with elevated BP, but further research is needed to understand the degree to which the findings are a function of racial segregation specifically versus a function of the lack of resources and high levels of stress commonly associated with highly racially segregated communities. This is an important issue to understand, because there are some data suggesting that when individuals gain access to neighborhoods with more resources, they show a decrease in risk factors for hypertension (i.e., distress and obesity), though not in hypertension incidence itself. In addition, when comparisons are made between predominantly Black versus predominantly White neighborhoods with roughly equivalent resources, racial differences in the rates of some risk factors decrease. This finding suggests that examining resources and stress may be more critical than considering racial composition.

The clearest evidence suggests that racism may affect risk for hypertension through two primary pathways: (1) by increasing stress exposure and decreasing opportunities for recovery, and (2) by both directly and indirectly compromising the ability to engage in health-promoting behaviors.

All types of racism appear to increase stress exposure. Internalized racism has been directly associated with higher levels of perceived stress (E. S. Tull et al., 2005). Interpersonal racism has been directly, consistently, and uniformly associated with depressive symptoms and anger. Both stereotype threat and interpersonal racism also affect perceptions of new situations, such that a broader range of events become capable of eliciting a stress response. The physiological correlates of stress also appear to be influenced by exposure to racism, as evidence suggests that interpersonal racism is associated with greater cardiovascular reactivity to both race- and non-race-related stressors. This may partly explain the evidence linking racism to ABP, which captures daily stress reactivity.

As a consequence of institutionalized racism, Black individuals, even those with relatively high levels of income or education, are more likely to reside in segregated neighborhoods (D. R. Williams & Jackson, 2005). In comparison to neighborhoods in which White individuals predominate, neighborhoods in which Black individuals comprise a majority of the population are more likely to be deprived of social and economic resources. In part, this deprivation is a function of the withdrawal of the economic and social resources of Whites and other races unwilling to live in areas with substantial proportions of Black residents. These effects are compounded by the relative economic disadvantage of Black households. Disadvantaged, or low-resource, neighborhoods increase exposure to acute and persistent stressors, including greater violence, crime, and noise.

Equally important, high-stress, low-income communities also present many fewer opportunities for stress reduction and recovery. The aesthetics of the environment do not provide respite, there are fewer recreational or cultural facilities that provide opportunities for casual relaxation, and there is often less social cohesion to promote social support among residents. This combination of greater stress exposure and fewer opportunities or supports for recovery is likely to create an overall stress burden that is much higher and more sustained for Black Americans than that experienced by members of other, less stigmatized ethnic groups.

There is also substantial evidence that racism influences health behaviors that increase the risk for hypertension. Internalized racism has been directly associated with abdominal obesity. Institutionalized racism indirectly affects health behavior through its effects on neighborhood SES. Low levels of community resources make the barriers to effective health promotion high. Consequently, very high levels of motivation and initiative are necessary for individuals to surmount these barriers and pursue beneficial health behaviors.

However, interpersonal and internalized racism raise the internal barriers to health promotion. Racism may indirectly influence the motivation to participate in health-promoting behaviors that either engender concerns about stereotype threat (i.e., because Blacks have been portrayed as incapable of succeeding in these arenas) or are seen as irrelevant to Black identity (i.e., because they are overly identified with White individuals or individuals of other races). Continued ostracism limits the type of self-awareness and self-regulation required to make consistent efforts at behavior change. The depressed and angry moods that are a persistent effect of interpersonal racism can sap the will to change.

CONCLUSION

Despite improvements in awareness and treatment, Black individuals remain at higher risk for the development of hypertension than do White individuals. At least a portion of this disparity is likely to be a function of racial disparities in individual- and community-level risk factors. However, some of the determinants of risk exposure appear to differ for Blacks and Whites, and racism may play a substantial role in fostering conditions that increase the likelihood that individuals will develop hypertension.

The risk factors for hypertension are interrelated. For example, variations in individual SES are linked to exposure to neighborhood stressors, as well as to individual psychosocial stressors and health behaviors. When individuals face multiple risk factors, a single-focus intervention (e.g., exercise training) may be inadequate. Multiple-risk-factor interventions (e.g., simultaneously addressing diet, exercise, and stress) may be needed. In addition, race-based variations in the relationship of each risk factor to HTN may affect the intensity of intervention required. The duration and level of support offered to individuals facing high environmental and intrapersonal barriers should be greater than those offered to individuals with more resources (Castro et al., 2009).

The effect of each risk factor may be moderated by other, co-occurring variables (e.g., stress may moderate the effect of diet on insulin levels). Stress reduction interventions, on an individual as well as community level, may be needed before other types of health promotion interventions can be successful. However, the sources of stress may vary by race or ethnic group, affecting the types of interventions needed. For example, risk reduction interventions for highly stigmatized groups may need to consider the broad range of interpersonal stressors that emerge as a function of exposure to racism. Interventions may need to address interpersonal relations, conflict management, and generalized depressive symptoms before they address health behavior.

In addition, the presence of some stressors may be a function of environmental or personal circumstances that are disproportionately associated with one group versus the other. Black

Americans are more likely than White Americans to live in high-density neighborhoods characterized by the presence of environmental-social stressors. Individual-level interventions to decrease stress responses may not be sufficient to manage persistent and high-intensity neighborhood-level stressors (e.g., crime or crowding). It may not be sufficient or appropriate to encourage relaxation in the face of some unjust environmental exposures if the intervention does not also provide an opportunity to advocate for changes in the social environment.

Individual-level interventions to change motivation depend on the ability to increase self-awareness and generate enthusiasm. These interventions may fail if they do not first consider the role race-based social ostracism plays in self-awareness and negative mood. Self-awareness can increase negative affect, and this may be intolerable for individuals who are already experiencing high levels of negative affect as a function of exposure to racism.

It may be necessary to first develop and implement individual-level interventions to identify and ameliorate the effects of racism on mood and self-regulation. In highly ostracized groups, interventions designed to change health behaviors may also need to consider the degree to which hypertension-related health behaviors are portrayed in the media and incorporated into notions of Black identity. Preliminary assessments of the degree to which individuals associate certain health behaviors with particular types of identity may need to be evaluated and addressed before motivational interventions can be implemented.

Individual-level motivational interventions may be irrelevant without community level interventions to increases access to health-promoting resources and to challenge race-related stereotypes about health behavior. Increasing access to improved neighborhood conditions appears to be associated with reductions in obesity and improvements in mental health (Kling et al., 2007; Morland et al., 2002). Targeted efforts to address identity-based or stereotype threat–based concerns about health promotion on a community-wide level may reduce intrapersonal barriers to motivation (Oyserman & Harrison, 1998; Steele, 1997).

In sum, data on ethnic and racial or class differences in the determinants of health behaviors have clear implications for interventions. For individuals facing low environmental barriers to making health-related changes, individual-level interventions focused on motivation and adherence may be appropriate. In contrast, for individuals facing high environmental barriers to health-related change, individual-level motivational interventions may fail or potentially lead to further distress or self-hatred. Environmental interventions aimed at barrier reduction may be both more appropriate and effective.

Careful research can guide the development and implementation of effective risk reduction efforts. More consistent methods and use of assessment tools will help clarify the causes for the mixed findings in much of the literature on race and hypertension. Research that examines effects both across groups and within specific groups is needed. Multidisciplinary approaches considering intrapersonal, interpersonal, and community-level risk factors are needed to achieve the goal of reducing hypertension across all groups.

ACKNOWLEDGMENTS

Preparation of this manuscript was supported by NHLBI R01 HL58690 to E. Brondolo. A portion of the ideas and information included in this chapter have previously been presented in Brondolo, Love, Pencille, Schoenthaler, and Ogedegbe (2011).

REFERENCES

Anderson, N. B. (1989). Racial differences in stress-induced cardiovascular reactivity and hypertension: Current status and substantive issues. *Psychological Bulletin, 105*(1), 89–105.

Angell, S. Y., Garg, R. K., Gwynn, R. C., Bash, L., Thorpe, L. E., & Frieden, T. R. (2008). Prevalence, awareness, treatment, and predictors of control of hypertension in New York City. *Circulation: Cardiovascular Quality and Outcomes, 1*, 46–53.

Bach, P. B., Hoangmai, H., Schrag, D., Tate, R. C., & Hargraves, J. L. (2004). Primary care physicians who treat Blacks and Whites. *New England Journal of Medicine, 351,* 575–584.

Barksdale, D. J., Farrug, E. R., & Harkness, K. (2009). Racial discrimination and blood pressure: Perceptions, emotions, and behaviors of Black American adults. *Issues in Mental Health Nursing, 30,* 104–111.

Bassett, D. R., Fitzhugh, E. C., Crespo, C. J., King, G. A., & McLaughlin, J. E. (2002). Physical activity and ethnic differences in hypertension prevalence in the United States. *Preventive Medicine, 34,* 179–186.

Baumeister, R. F., DeWall, C. N., Ciarocco, N. J., & Twenge, J. M. (2005). Social exclusion impairs self-regulation. *Journal of Personality and Social Psychology, 88*(4), 589–604.

Beitz, R., Mensink, G. B., & Fischer, B. (2003). Blood pressure and vitamin C and fruit and vegetable intake. *Annals of Nutrition and Metabolism, 47,* 214–220.

Bell, A. C., Adair, L. S., & Popkin, B. M. (2004). Understanding the role of mediating risk factors and proxy effects in the association between socio-economic status and untreated hypertension. *Social Science & Medicine, 59*(2), 275–283.

Benkert, R., Peters, R. M., Clark, R., & Keves-Foster, K. (2006). Effects of perceived racism, cultural mistrust and trust in providers on satisfaction with care. *Journal of the National Medical Association, 98*(9), 1532–1540.

Better, S. (2002). *Institutional racism: A primer on theory and strategies for social change.* Chicago, IL: Rowman & Littlefield.

Borrell, L. N., Crawford, N. D., Barrington, D. S., & Maglo, K. N. (2008). Black/White disparity in self-reported hypertension: The role of nativity status. *Journal of Health Care for the Poor and Underserved, 19,* 1148–1162.

Bosworth, H. B., Bartash, R. M., Olsen, M. K., & Steffens, D. C. (2003). The association of psychosocial factors and depression with hypertension among older adults. *International Journal of Geriatric Psychiatry, 18,* 1142–1148.

Bosworth, H. B., Dudley, T., Olsen, M. K., Voils, C. I., Powers, B., Goldstein, M. K., & Oddone, E. Z. (2006). Racial differences in blood pressure control: Potential explanatory factors. *The American Journal of Medicine, 119*(1), 70.e9–70.e15.

Broman, C. L. (1996). The health consequences of racial discrimination: A study of African Americans. *Ethnicity & Disease, 6,* 148–153.

Brondolo, E., Brady, N., Libby, D. J., & Pencille, M. (2010). Racism as a psychosocial stressor. In R. J. Contrada & A. Baum (Eds.), *The handbook of stress science: Biology, psychology, and health* (pp. 167–184). New York, NY: Springer.

Brondolo, E., Brady, N., Thompson, S., Tobin, J. N., Cassells, A., Sweeney, M., … Contrada, R. (2008). Perceived racism and negative affect: Analyses of trait and state measures of affect in a community sample. *Journal of Social & Clinical Psychology, 27*(2), 150–173.

Brondolo, E., Gallo, L. C., Myers, H. F., & Hector, F. (2009). Race, racism and health: Disparities, mechanisms, and interventions. *Journal of Behavioral Medicine, 32*(1), 1–8.

Brondolo, E., Kelly, K. P., Coakley, V., Gordon, T., Thompson, S., Levy, E., … Contrada, R. (2005). The perceived ethnic discrimination questionnaire: Development and preliminary validation of a community version. *Journal of Applied Social Psychology, 35*(2), 335–365.

Brondolo, E., Libby, D. J., Denton, E., Thompson, S., Beatty, D. L., Schwartz, J. E., … Gerin, W. (2008). Racism and ambulatory blood pressure in a community sample. *Psychosomatic Medicine, 70*(1), 49–56.

Brondolo, E., Love, E., Pencille, M., Schoenthaler, A., & Ogedegbe, G. (2011). Racism and hypertension: A review of the empirical evidence and implications for clinical practice. *American Journal of Hypertension.* Advance online publication. doi:10.1038/ajh.2011.9

Brondolo, E., Rieppi, R., Erickson, S. A., Bagiella, E., Shapiro, P. A., McKinley, P., & Sloan, R. (2003). Hostility, interpersonal interactions, and ambulatory blood pressure. *Psychosomatic Medicine, 65,* 1003–1011.

Brondolo, E., Rieppi, R., Kelly, K.P., & Gerin, W. (2003). Perceived racism and blood pressure: A review of the literature and conceptual and methodological critique. *Annals of Behavioral Medicine, 25,* 55–65.

Brondolo, E., ver Halen, N. B., Pencille, M., Beatty, D., & Contrada, R. J. (2009). Coping with racism: A selective review of the literature and a theoretical and methodological critique. *Journal of Behavioral Medicine, 32,* 64–88.

Burt, V. L., Whelton, P., Roccella, E. J., Brown, C., Cutler, J. A., Higgins, M., … Labarthe, D. (1995). Prevalence of hypertension in the US adult population. results from the third national health and nutrition examination survey, 1988–1991. *Hypertension, 25*(3), 305–313.

Butler, C., Tull, E. S., Chambers, E. C., & Taylor, J. (2002). Internalized racism, body fat distribution, and abnormal fasting glucose among African-Carribean women in Dominica, West Indies. *Journal of the National Medical Association, 94*(3), 143–148.

Castro, F. G., Shaibi, G. Q., & Boehm-Smith, E. (2009). Ecodevelopmental contexts for preventing type 2 diabetes in Latino and other racial/ethnic minority populations. *Journal of Behavioral Medicine, 32*(2), 89–105.

Chambers, E. C., Tull, E. S., Fraser, H. S., Mutunhu, N. R., Sobers, N., & Niles, E. (2004). The relationship of internalized racism to body fat distribution and insulin resistance among African adolescent youth. *Journal of the National Medical Association, 96*(12), 1594–1598.

Cheng, C. (2003). Cognitive and motivational processes underlying coping flexibility: A dual-process model. *Journal of Personality and Social Psychology, 84*(2), 425–438.

Clark, R. (2000). Perceptions of interethnic group racism predict increased vascular reactivity to a laboratory challenge in college women. *Annals of Behavioral Medicine, 22*(3), 214–222.

Clark, R., Anderson, N. B., Clark, V. R., & Williams, D. R. (1999). Racism as a stressor for African Americans. *American Psychologist, 54*(10), 805–816.

Cohen, C. I., Magai, C., Yaffee, R., & Walcott-Brown, L. (2005). Racial differences in syndromal and subsyndromal depression in an older urban population. *Psychiatric Services, 56*, 1556–1563.

Cohen, G. L., & Garcia, J. (2005). "I am us": Negative stereotypes as collective threats. *Journal of Personality and Social Psychology, 89*(4), 566–582.

Colhoun, H. M., Hemingway, H., & Poulter, N. R. (1998). Socio-economic status and blood pressure: An overview analysis. *Journal of Human Hypertension, 12*, 91–110.

Collins, J., David, R., Handler, A., Wall, S., & Andes, S. (2004). Very low birthweight in African American infants: The role of maternal exposure to interpersonal racial discrimination. *American Journal of Public Health, 94*, 2132–2138.

Collins, J. W., David, R. J., Symons, R., Handler, A., Wall, S., & Dwyer, L. (2000). Low income African American mothers' perception of exposure to racial discrimination and infant birth weight. *Epidemiology and Community Health, 11*, 337–339.

Contrada, R. J., Ashmore, R. D., Gary, M. L., Coups, E., Egeth, J. D., Sewell, A., ... Chasse, V. (2000). Ethnicity-related sources of stress and their effects on well-being. *Current Directions in Psychological Science, 9*(4), 136–139.

Contrada, R. J., Ashmore, R. D., Gary, M. L., Coups, E., Egeth, J. D., Sewell, A., ... Chasse, V. (2001). Measures of ethnicity-related stress: Psychometric properties, ethnic group differences, and associations with well-being. *Journal of Applied Social Psychology, 31*, 1775–1820.

Cooper, D. C., & Waldstein, S. R. (2004). Hostility differentially predicts cardiovascular risk factors in African American and White young adults. *Journal of Psychosomatic Research, 57*(5), 491–499.

Cooper, R. S. (2003). Gene–environment interactions and the etiology of common complex disease. *Annals of Internal Medicine, 139*, 437–440.

Cossrow, N., & Falkner, B. (2004). Race/ethnic issues in obesity and obesity-related comorbidities. *Journal of Clinical Endocrinology & Metabolism, 89*(6), 2590–2594.

Cozier, Y. C., Palmer, J. R., Horton, N. J., Fredman, L., Wise, L. A., & Rosenberg, L. (2006). Racial discrimination and the incidence of hypertension in US Black women. *Annals of Epidemiology, 16*(9), 681–687.

Cozier, Y. C., Palmer, J. R., Horton, N. J., Fredman, L., Wise, L. A., & Rosenberg, L. (2007). Relation between neighborhood median housing value and hypertension risk among Black women in the United States. *American Journal of Public Health, 97*, 718–724.

Cozier, Y. C., Wise, L. A., Palmer, J. R., & Rosenberg, L. (2009). Perceived racism in relation to weight change in the Black Women's Health Study. *Annals of Epidemiology, 19*(6), 379–387.

Cutler, J. A., Sorlie, P. D., Wolz, M., Thom, T., Fields, L. E., & Roccella, E. J. (2008). Trends in hypertension prevalence, awareness, treatment, and control rates in United States adults between 1988–1994 and 1999–2004. *Hypertension: Journal of the American Heart Association, 52*, 818–827.

Dickson, B. K., Blackledge, J., & Hajjar, I. M. (2006). The impact of lifestyle behavior on hypertension awareness, treatment, and control in a southeastern population. *American Journal of the Medical Sciences, 332*(4), 211–215.

Diez-Roux, A. V., Merkin, S. S., Hannan, P., Jacobs, D. R., & Kiefe, C. I. (2003). Area characteristics, individual-level socioeconomic indicators, and smoking in young adults: The Coronary Artery Disease Risk Development in Young Adults Study. *American Journal of Epidemiology, 157*, 315.

Diez-Roux, A. V., Nieto, F. J., Muntaner, C., Tyroler, H. A., Comstock, G. W., Shahar, E., ... Szklo, M. (1997). Neighborhood environments and coronary heart disease: A multilevel analysis. *American Journal of Epidemiology, 146*, 48–63.

Diez-Roux, A. V., Northridge, M. E., Morabia, A., Bassett, M. T., & Shea, S. (1999). Prevalence and social correlates of cardiovascular disease risk factors in Harlem. *American Journal of Public Health, 89*(3), 302–307.

Din-Dzietham, R., Nembhard, W. N., Collins, R., & Davis, S. K. (2004). Perceived stress following race-based discrimination at work is associated with hypertension in African–Americans: The Metro Atlanta Heart Disease Study, 1999–2001. *Social Science & Medicine, 58*(3), 449–461.

Dole, N., Savitz, D. A., Siega-Riz, A. M., Hertz-Picciotto, I., McMahon, M. J., & Buekens, P. (2004). Psychosocial factors and preterm birth among African American and White women in central North Carolina. *American Journal of Public Health, 94*(8), 1358–1365.

Dressler, W. W. (1996). Social identity and arterial blood pressure in the African-American community. *Ethnicity & Disease, 6*(1–2), 176–189.

Dressler, W. W., Oths, K. S., & Gravlee, C. C. (2005). Race and ethnicity in public health research: Models to explain health disparities. *Annual Review of Anthropology, 34*, 231–252.

Duey, W. J., Bassett, D. R., Jr, Walker, A. J., Torok, D. J., Howley, E. T., Ely, D., & Pease, M. O. (1997). Cardiovascular and plasma catecholamine response to static exercise in normotensive blacks and whites. *Ethnicity & Health, 2*(1–2), 127–136.

Emerson, M. O., Yancey, G., & Chai, K. J. (2001). Does race matter in residential segregation? Exploring the preferences of White Americans. *American Social Review, 66*(6), 922–935.

Ervin, R. B. (2008). Healthy eating index scores among adults, 60 years of age and over, by sociodemographic and health characteristics: United States, 1999–2002. *Advance Data, 395*, 1–20.

Esler, M., Eikelis, N., Schlaich, M., Lambert, G., Alvarenga, M., Kaye, D., … Lambert, E. (2008). Human sympathetic nerve biology: Parallel influences of stress and epigenetics in essential hypertension and panic disorder. *Annals of the New York Academy of Sciences, 1148*, 338–348.

Fagard, R. H. (2005). Effects of exercise, diet and their combination on blood pressure. *Journal of Human Hypertension, 19*(Suppl. 3), S20–S24.

Feldt, K., Raikkonen, K., Eriksson, J. G., Andersson, S., Osmond, C., Barker, D. J. P., … Kajantie, E. (2007). Cardiovascular reactivity to psychological stressors in late adulthood is predicted by gestational age at birth. *Journal of Human Hypertension, 21*, 401–410.

Fiscella, K., & Holt, K. (2008). Racial disparity ion hypertension control: Tallying the death toll. *Annals of Family Medicine, 6*(6), 497–502.

Flegal, K. M., Carroll, M. D., Ogden, C. O., & Johnson, C. L. (2002). Prevalence and trends in obesity among US adults, 1999–2000. *Journal of the American Medical Association, 288*(14), 1723–1727.

Fordham, S., & Ogbu, J. U. (1986). Black students' school success: Coping with the "burden of acting White." *Urban Review, 18*, 176–206.

Fox, C., Massaro, J., Hoffman, U., Pou, K., Maurovich-Horvat, P., Liu, C., & … O'Donnell, C. (2007). Abdominal visceral and subcutaneous adipose tissue compartments: Association with metabolic risk factors in the Framingham Heart Study. *Circultion, 116*(1), 39-48.

Friedman, R., Schwartz, J. E., Schnall, P. L., Landsbergis, P. A., Pieper, C., Gerin, W., & Pickering, T. G. (2001). Psychological variables in hypertension: Relationship to causal or ambulatory blood pressure in men. *Psychosomatic Medicine, 63*, 19–31.

Gary, T. L., Safford, M. M., Gerzoff, R. B., Ettner, S. L., Karter, A. J., Beckles, G. L., & Brown, A. F. (2008). Perception of neighborhood problems, health behaviors, and diabetes outcomes among adults with diabetes in managed care: The translating research into action for diabetes (TRIAD) study. *Diabetes Care, 31*(2), 273–278.

Gee, G. C., Ro, A., Gavin, A., & Takeuchi, D. T. (2008). Disentangling the effects of racial and weight discrimination on body mass index and obesity among Asian Americans. *American Journal of Public Health, 98*, 493–500.

George, L. K., & Lynch, S. M. (2003). Race differences in depressive symptoms: a dynamic perspective on stress exposure and vulnerability. *Journal of Health And Social Behavior, 44*(3), 353–369.

Glover, M. J., Greenlund, K. J., & Ayala, C. (2002). Racial/ethnic disparities in prevalence, treatment, and control of hypertension—United States, 1999–2002. *MMWR, 53*(1), 7–9.

Glover, M. J., Greenlund, K. J., Ayala, C., & Croft, J. B. (2005). Racial/ethnic disparities in prevalence, treatment, and control of hypertension—United States, 1999–2002. *MMWR, 54*(1), 7–9.

Grady, S. C., & Ramirez, I. J. (2008). Mediating medical risk factors in the residential segregation and low birthweight relationship by race in New York City. *Health & Place, 14*, 661–667.

Griffith, D. M., Childs, E. L., Eng, E., & Jeffries, V. (2007). Racism in organizations: The case of a county public health department. *Journal of Community Psychology, 35*(3), 287–302.

Guyll, M., Matthews, K. A., & Bromberger, J. T. (2001). Discrimination and unfair treatment: Relationship to cardiovascular reactivity among African American and European American women. [Print Electronic; Print]. *Health Psychology, 20*(5), 315–325.

Hajjar, I. M., & Kotchen, T. A. (2003). Trends in prevalence, awareness, treatment and control of hypertension in the United States, 1988–2000. *JAMA: Journal of the American Medical Association, 290*(2), 199–206.

Halpert, J. A., Silagy, C. A., Finucane, P., Withers, R. T., Hamdorf, P. A., & Andrews, G. R. (1997). The effectiveness of exercise training in lowering blood pressure: A meta-analysis of randomized controlled trials of 4 weeks or longer. *Journal of Human Hypertension, 11*, 641–649.

Harburg, E., Gleiberman, L., Roeper, P., Schork, M. A., & Schull, W. J. (1978). Skin color, ethnicity and blood pressure in Detroit Blacks. *American Journal of Public Health, 68*, 1177–1183.

Harburg, E., Gleiberman, L., Russell, M., & Cooper, M. L. (1991). Anger-coping styles and blood pressure in Black and White males: Buffalo, New York. [Print]. *Psychosomatic Medicine, 53*(2), 153–164.

Harrell, S. P. (1997). *The racism and life experiences scales.* Unpublished manuscript.

Harrell, S. P. (2000). A multidimensional conceptualization of racism-related stress: Implications for the well-being of people of color. [Print]. *American Journal of Orthopsychiatry, 70*(1), 42–57.

Harshfield, G. A., Pulliam, D. A., & Alpert, B. S. (1994). Ambulatory blood pressure and renal function in healthy children and adolescents. *American Journal of Public Health, 7*, 282–285.

Hertz, R. P., Unger, A. N., Cornell, J. A., & Saunders, E. (2005). Racial disparities in hypertension prevalence, awareness and management. *Archives of Internal Medicine, 165*, 2098–2104.

Hill, L. K., Kobayashi, I., & Hughes, J. W. (2007). Perceived racism and ambulatory blood pressure in African American college students. *Journal of Black Psychology, 33*(4), 404–421.

Inzlicht, M., McKay, L., & Aronson, J. (2006). Stigma as ego depletion: How being the target of prejudice affects self-control. [Electronic Electronic; Print]. *Psychological Science, 17*(3), 262–269.

Jacobson, J., Olsen, C., Rice, J. K., Sweetland, S., & Ralph, J. (2001). *Education achievement and Black–White inequality. Statistical Analysis Report.* Washington, DC: Mathematica Policy Research.

James, K., Lovato, C., & Khoo, G. (1994). Social identity correlates of minority workers' health. *Academy of Management Journal, 37*(2), 383–396.

James, S. A., LaCroix, A. Z., Kleinbaum, D. G., & Strogatz, D. S. (1984). John Henryism and blood pressure differences among Black men: II. The role of occupational stressors. *Journal of Behavioral Medicine, 7*, 259–275.

Jennings, J. R., & Zanstra, Y. (2009). Is the brain the essential in hypertension? *NeuroImage, 47*, 914–921.

John, J. H., Ziebland, S., Yudkin, P., Roe, L. S., & Neil, H. A. W. (2002). Effects of fruit and vegetable consumption on plasma antioxidant concentrations and blood pressure: A randomized controlled trial. *Lancet, 359*, 1969–1974.

Jonas, B. S., & Lando, J. F. (2000). Negative affect as a prospective risk factor for hypertension. *Psychosomatic Medicine, 62*, 188–196.

Jones-Webb, R., Jacobs, D. R., Flack, J. M., & Liu, K. (1996). Relationships between depressive symptoms, anxiety, alcohol consumption, and blood pressure: Results from the CARDIA Study. *Alcoholism: Clinical and Experimental Research, 20*, 420–427.

Jorgensen, R. S., Johnson, B. T., Kolodziej, M. E., & Schreer, G. E. (1996). Elevated blood pressure and personality: A meta-analytic review. *Psychological Bulletin, 120*, 293–320.

Joyner, M. J., Charkoudian, N., & Wallin, B. G. (2008). A sympathetic view of the sympathetic nervous system and human blood pressure regulation. *Experimental Physiology, 93*(6), 715–724.

Julius, S. (1988). Transition from high cardiac output to elevated vascular resistance in hypertension. *American Heart Journal, 116*(2 Pt 2), 600–606.

Kessler, R. C., Mickelson, K. D., & Williams, D. R. (1999). The prevalence, distribution, and mental health correlates of perceived discrimination in the United States. *Journal of Health and Social Behavior, 40*(3), 208–230.

Kling, J. R., Liebman, J. B., & Katz, L. F. (2007). Experimental analysis of neighborhood effects. *Econometrica, 75*, 83–119.

Klonoff, E. A. (2009). Disparities in the provision of medical care: An outcome in search of an explanation. *Journal of Behavioral Medicine, 32*, 48–63.

Koppes, L. L., Twisk, J. W., Van Mechelen, W., Snel, J., & Kemper, H. C. (2005). Cross-sectional and longitudinal relationships between alcohol consumption and lipids, blood pressure and body weight indices. *Journal of Studies on Alcohol, 66*(6), 713–721.

Kotchen, T. A., & McCarron, D. (1998). Dietary electrolytes and blood pressure: A statement for healthcare professionals from the American Heart Association Nutrition Committee. *Circulation, 98*, 613–617.

Kramer, H., Han, C., Post, W., Goff, D., Diez-Roux, A., Cooper, R., … Shea, S. (2004). Racial/ethnic differences in hypertension and hypertension treatment and control in the multi-ethnic study of atherosclerosis (MESA). *American Journal of Hypertension, 17*, 963–970.

Kramer, M. R., & Hogue, C. R. (2009). Is segregation bad for your health? *Epidemiology Review, 31*(1), 178–194.

Kressin, N. R., & Peterson, L. A. (2001). Racial differences in the use of invasive cardiovascular procedures: Review of the literature and prescription for the future research. *Annals of Internal Medicine, 135*(5), 352–366.

Krieger, N. (1990). Racial and gender discrimination: Risk factors for high blood pressure? *Social Science & Medicine, 30*(12), 1273–1281.

Krieger, N. (1999). Embodying inequality: A review of concepts, measures, and methods for studying health consequences of discrimination. *International Journal of Health Services, 29,* 295–352.

Krieger, N., & Sidney, S. (1996). Racial discrimination and blood pressure: The CARDIA Study of young Black and White adults. *American Journal of Public Health, 86*(10), 1370–1378.

Krieger, N., Smith, K., Naishadham, D., Hartman, C., & Barbeau, E. M. (2005). Experiences of discrimination: Validity and reliability of a self-report measure for population health research on racism and health. *Social Science & Medicine, 61*(7), 1576–1596.

Krousel-Wood, M., Islam, T., Webber, L. S., Re, R. N., Morisky, D. E., & Mutner, P. (2009). New medication adherence scale versus pharmacy fill rates in seniors with hypertension. *American Journal of Managed Care, 15*(1), 59–66.

Kwate, N. O. A. (2008). Fried chicken and fresh apples: Racial segregation as a fundamental cause of fast food density in Black neighborhoods. *Health & Place, 14*(1), 32–44.

La Veist, T. A., Sellers, R. M., & Neighbors, H. W. (2001). Perceived racism and self and system blame attribution: Consequences for longevity. *Ethnicity & Disease, 11,* 711–721.

Landrine, H., Klonoff, E. A., Corral, I., Fernandez, S., & Roesch, S. (2006). Conceptualizing and measuring ethnic discrimination in health research. *Journal of Behavioral Medicine, 29*(1), 79–94.

Lawes, C. M. M., Bennett, D. A., Feigin, V. L., & Rodgers, A. (2004). Blood pressure and stroke: An overview of published reviews. *Stroke, 35,* 776–785.

Lea, J. (2000). The Macpherson Report and question of institutional racism. *Howard Journal of Criminal Justice, 39*(3), 219–233.

Lepore, S. J., Revenson, T. A., Weinberger, S. L., Weston, P., Frisina, P. G., Robertson, R. M., … Cross, W. (2006). Effects of social stressors on cardiovascular reactivity in black and white women. *Annals of Behavioral Medicine, 31*(2), 120–127.

Lespinasse, A. A., David, R. J., Collins, W. J., Handler, A. S., & Wall, S. N. (2004). Maternal support in the delivery room and birthweight among African-American women. *Journal of the National Medical Association, 96*(2), 187–195.

Levenstein, S., Smith, M. W., & Kaplan, G. A. (2001). Psychosocial predictors of hypertension in men and women. *Archives of Internal Medicine, 161,* 1341–1346.

Leventhal, T., & Brooks-Gunn, J. (2000). The neighborhoods they live in: The effects of neighborhood residence on child and adolescent outcomes. *Psychological Bulletin, 126*(2), 309–337.

Light, K. C., Turner, J. R., Hinderliter, A. L., & Sherwood, A. (1993). Race and gender comparisons: I. Hemodynamic responses to a series of stressors. *Health Psychology, 12,* 354–365.

Madhavan, S., & Alderman, H. M. (1994). Ethnicity and the relationship of sodium intake to blood pressure. *Journal of Hypertension, 12*(1), 97–103.

Major, B., & O'Brien, L. T. (2005). The social psychology of stigma. *Annual Review of Psychology, 56*(1), 393–421.

Marmot, M. G., Elliott, P., Shipley, M. J., Dyer, A. R., Ueshima, H., Beevers, D. G., … Rose, G. (1994). Alcohol and blood pressure: The INTERSALT study. *British Medical Journal, 308,* 1263–1267.

Massey, D. S., & Eggers, M. L. (1990). The ecology of inequality: Minorities and the concentration of poverty, 1970–1980. *American Journal of Sociology, 95,* 1153–1188.

Matthews, K. A. (2005). Psychological perspectives on the development of coronary heart disease. *American Psychologist, 60*(8), 783–796.

Matthews, K. A., Katholi, C. R., McCreath, H., Whooley, M. A., Williams, D. R., Zhu, S., & Markovitz, J. H. (2004). Blood pressure reactivity to psychological stress predicts hypertension in the CARDIA study. *Circulation, 110,* 74–78.

Mays, V. M., Cochran, S. D., & Barnes, N.W. (2007). Race, race-based discrimination and health outcomes among African Americans. *Annual Review of Psychology, 58,* 201–225.

Mays, V. M., Coleman, L. M., & Jackson, J. S. (1996). Perceived race-based discrimination, employment status, and job stress in a national sample of Black women: Implications for health outcomes. *Journal of Occupational Health Psychology, 1,* 319–329.

McGrath, J. J., Matthews, K. A., & Brady, S. S. (2006). Individual versus neighborhood socioeconomic status and race as predictors of adolescent ambulatory blood pressure and heart rate. *Social Science & Medicine, 63,* 1442–1453.

Mechanic, D. (2005). Policy challenges in addressing racial disparities and improving population health. *Health Affairs (Project Hope), 24*(2), 335–338.

Mellor, D. (2004). Responses to racism: A taxonomy of coping styles used by aboriginal Australians. *American Journal of Orthopsychiatry, 74*(1), 56–71.

Mensah, G. A., Mokdad, A. H., Ford, E. S., Greenlund, K. J., & Croft, J. B. (2005). State of disparities in cardiovascular health in the United States. *Circulation, 111,* 1233–1241.

Moghaddam, F. M., Taylor, D. M., Ditto, B., Jacobs, K., & Bianchi, E. (2002). Psychological distress and perceived discrimination: A study of women from India. *International Journal of Intercultural Relations, 26,* 381–390.

Morenoff, J. D., House, J. S., Hansen, B. B., Williams, D. R., Kaplan, G. A., & Hunte, H. E. (2007). Understanding social disparities in hypertension prevalence, awareness, treatment, and control: The role of neighborhood context. *Social Science & Medicine, 65*(9), 1853–1866.

Morland, K., Wing, S., & Diez-Roux, A. V. (2002). The contextual effect of the local food environment on residents' diets: The Atherosclerosis Risk in Communities Study. *American Journal of Public Health, 92,* 1761–1768.

Mujahid, M. S., Diez-Roux, A. V., Shen, M., Gowda, D., Sanchez, B., Shea, S., … Jackson, S. A. (2008). Relation between neighborhood environments and obesity in the multi-ethnic study of atherosclerosis. American Journal of Epidemiology, 167, 1349–1357.

Muntner, P., De Salvo, K., Wildman, R., Raggi, P., He, J., & Whelton, P. (2006). Trends in the prevalence, awareness, treatment, and control of cardiovascular disease risk factors among noninstitutionalized patients with a history of myocardial infarction and stroke. *American Journal of Epidemiology, 163*(10), 913–920.

Murphy, J. K., Stoney, C. M., Alpert, B. S., & Walker, S. S. (1995). Gender and ethnicity in children's cardiovascular reactivity: 7 years of study. *Health Psychology, 14*(1), 48–55.

Mustillo, S., Krieger, N., Gunderson, E., Sidney, S., McCreath, H., & Kiefe, C. (2004). Self-reported experiences of racial discrimination and Black–White differences in preterm and low-birthweight deliveries: The CARDIA Study. *American Journal of Public Health, 94,* 2125–2131.

Myers, H. F. (2009). Ethnicity- and socio-economic status–related stresses in context: An integrative review and conceptual model. *Journal of Behavioral Medicine, 32,* 9181–9184.

Narkiewicz, K. (2006). Obesity and hypertension—The issue is more complex than we thought. *Nephrology Dialysis Transplantation, 21*(2), 264–267.

Natarajan, S., Santa Ana, E. J., Liao, Y., Lipsitz, S. R., & McGee, D. L. (2009). Effect of treatment and adherence on ethnic diffewrences in blood pressure amung adults with hypertension. *Annals of Epidemiology, 9*(3), 172–179.

Nguyen, H. T., Evans, D. A., & Zonderman, A. B. (2008). Neighborhood disorganization and blood pressure: Findings from the Healthy Aging in Neighborhoods of Diversity Across the Life Span Study (HANDLS). *Annals of Epidemiology, 18*(9), 708–741.

Oberg, S., Ge, D., Cnattingius, S., Svensson, A., Treiber, F. A., Snieder, H., & Iliadou, A. (2007). Ethnic differences in the association of birth weight and blood pressure: The Georgia cardiovascular twin study. *American Journal of Hypertension, 20*(12), 1235–1241.

Ohlin, B., Berglund, G., Rosvall, M., & Nilsson, P. M. (2007). Job strain in men, but not in women, predicts a significant rise in blood pressure after 6.5 years of follow-up. *Journal of Hypertension, 25*(3), 525–531.

Okosun, I. S., Choi, S., Dent, M. M., Jobin, T., & Dever, G. E. A. (2001). Abdominal obesity defined as a larger than expected waist girth is associated with racial/ethnic differences in risk of hypertension. *Journal of Human Hypertension, 15,* 307–312.

Oyserman, D., & Harrison, K. (1998). Implications of cultural context: African American identity and possible selves. In J. K. Swim & C. Stangor (Eds.), *Prejudice: The target's perspective* (pp. 281–300). San Diego, CA: Academic Press.

Paeratakul, S., Lovejoy, J. C., Ryan, D. H., & Bray, G. A. (2002). The relation of gender, race and socioeconomic status to obesity and obesity comorbidities in a sample of US adults. *International Journal of Obesity, 26*(9), 1205–1210.

Perry, A. C., Applegate, E. B., Jackson, M. L., Deprima, S., Goldberg, R. B., Kempner, L., & Feldman, B. B. (2000). Racial differences in visceral adipose tissue but not anthropometric markers of health-related variables. *Journal of Applied Physiology, 89,* 636–643.

Peters, R. M. (2004). Racism and hypertension among African Americans. [Print Electronic; Print]. *Western Journal of Nursing Research, 26*(6), 612–631.

Peters, R. M. (2006). The relationship of racism, chronic stress emotions, and blood pressure. *Journal of Nursing Scholarship, 38*(3), 234–240.

Pickering, T. G. (1999). Cardiovascular pathways: Socioeconomic status and stress effects on hypertension and cardiovascular function. *Annals of the New York Academy of Sciences, 896,* 262–277.

Pickering, T. G., Hall, J. E., Appel, L. J., Falkner, B. E., Graves, J., Hill, M. N., … Roccella, E. J. (2005). Recommendations for blood pressure measurement in humans and experimental animals: Part 1: Blood pressure measurement in humans: A statement for professionals from the subcommittee of professional and public education of the American Heart Association Council on high blood pressure research. *Hypertension, 45*(1), 142–161.

Poston, W. S. C., Pavlik, V. N., Hyman, D. J., Ogbonnaya, K., Hanis, C. L., Haddock, C. K., … Foreyt, J. P. (2001). Genetic bottlenecks, perceived racism, and hypertension risk among African Americans and first-generation African immigrants. *Journal of Human Hypertension, 15*, 341–351.

Quintana, S. M. (2007). Racial and ethnic identity: Developmental perspectives and research. *Journal of Counseling Psychology, 54*(3), 259–270.

Riolo, S. A., Nguyen, T. A., Greden, J. F., & King, C. A. (2005). Prevalence of depression by race/ethnicity: Findings from the National Health and Nutrition Examination Survey III. *American Journal of Public Health, 95*(6), 998–1000.

Rosamond, W. D., Flegal, K., Furie, K., Go, A., Greenlund, K., Haase, N., … Hong, Y. (2008). Heart disease and stroke statistics—2008 update: A report from the American Heart Association Statistics Committee and Stroke Statistics Subcommittee. *Circulation, 117*(4), e25–146. doi:10.1161/circulationaha.107.187998

Russell, M., Cooper, L. M., & Frone, M. R. (1990). The influence of sociodemographic characteristics on familial alcohol problems: Data from a community sample. *Alcoholism: Clinical and Experimental Research, 14*(2), 221–226.

Rutledge, T., & Hogan, B. (2002). A quantitative review of prospective evidence linking psychological factors with hypertension development. *Psychosomatic Medicine, 64*, 758–766.

Ryan, A. M., Gee, G. C., & Laflamme, D. F. (2006). The association between self-reported discrimination, physical health and blood pressure: Findings from African Americans, Black immigrants, and Latino immigrants in New Hampshire. *Journal of Health Care for the Poor and Underserved, 17*, 116–132.

Sacks, F. M., Svetkey, L. P., Vollmer, W. M., Appel, L. J., Bray, G. A., Harsha, D., … Lin, P. H. (2001). Effects on blood pressure of reduced dietary sodium and the dietary approaches to stop hypertension (DASH) diet. *The New England Journal of Medicine, 344*(1), 3–10.

Schlundt, D. G., Hargreaves, M. K., & McClellan, L. (2006). Geographic clustering of obesity, diabetes, and hypertension in Nashville, Tennessee. *Journal of Ambulatory Care Management, 29*(2), 125–152.

Schum, J. L., Jorgensen, R. S., Verhaeghen, P., Sauro, M., Thibodeau, R., & Schum, J. L. (2003). Trait anger, anger expression, and ambulatory blood pressure: A meta-analytic review. *Journal of Behavioral Medicine, 26*, 395.

Schwartz, J. E., Neale, J., Marco, C., Shiffman, S. S., & Stone, A. A. (1999). Does trait coping exist? A momentary assessment approach to the evaluation of traits. *Journal of Personality and Social Psychology, 77*, 360–369.

Sesso, H. D., Cook, N. R., Buring, J. E., Manson, J. E., & Gaziano, J. M. (2008). Alcohol consumption and the risk of hypertension in women and men. *Hypertension, 51*, 1080–1087.

Shelton, R. C., Puleo, E., Bennett, G. G., McNeill, L. H., Goldman, R. E., Emmons, K. M. (2009). Racial discrimination and physical activity among low-income–housing residents. *American Journal of Preventative Medicine, 37*, 541–545.

Singleton, J. G., Robertson, J., Robinson, J. C., Austin, C., & Edochie, V. (2008). Perceived racism and coping: Joint predictors of blood pressure in Black Americans. *Negro Educational Review, 59*(1–2), 93–113.

Sloan, R. P., Bagiella, E., Shapiro, P. A., Kuhl, J. P., Chernikhova, D., Berg, J., & Myers, M. M. (2001). Hostility, gender, and cardiac autonomic control. *Psychosomatic Medicine, 63*(3), 434–440.

Sparrenberger, F., Cichelero, F. T., Ascoli, A. M., Fonseca, F. P., Weiss, G., Berwanger, O., … Sparrenberger, F. (2009). Does psychosocial stress cause hypertension? A systematic review of observational studies. *Journal of Human Hypertension, 23*, 12–19.

Speight, S. L. (2007). Internalized racism: One more piece of the puzzle. [Electronic Electronic; Print]. *Counseling Psychologist, 35*(1), 126–134.

Steele, C. M. (1997). A threat in the air: How stereotypes shape intellectual identity and performance. *American Psychologist, 52*(6), 613–629.

Steffen, P. R., McNeilly, M. D., Anderson, N., & Sherwood, A. (2003). Effects of perceived racism and anger inhibition on ambulatory blood pressure in African Americans. [Print Electronic; Print]. *Psychosomatic Medicine, 65*(5), 746–750.

Svetkey, L. P., Erlinger, T. P., Vollmer, W. M., Feldstein, A., Cooper, L. S., Appel, L. J., … Stevens, V. J. (2005). Effect of lifestyle modifications on blood pressure by race, sex, hypertension status, and age. *Journal of Human Hypertension, 19*(1), 21–31.

Taylor, J., & Grundy, C. (1996). Measuring Black internalization of White stereotypes about African Americans: The Nadanolitization Scale. In R. L. Jones (Ed.), *The handbook of tests and measurements for Black populations* (pp. 217–226). Hampton, VA: Cobb & Henry.

Thomas, K. S., Nelesen, R. A., Malcarne, V. L., Ziegler, M. G., & Dimsdale, J. E. (2006). Ethnicity, perceived discrimination, and vascular reactivity to phenylephrine. [Print Electronic; Print]. *Psychosomatic Medicine*, *68*(5), 692–697.

Tomfohr, L., Cooper, D. C., Mills, P. J., Nelesen, R. A., & Dimsdale, J. E. (2010). Everyday discrimination and nocturnal blood pressure dipping in Black and White Americans. *Psychosomatic Medicine*, *72*, 1–7.

Treiber, F. A., Davis, H., Musante, L., Raunikar, R. A., Strong, W. B., McCaffrey, F., ... Vandernoord, R. (1993). Ethnicity, gender, family history of myocardial infarction, and hemodynamic responses to laboratory stressors in children. *Health Psychology, 12*(1), 6–15.

Tull, E. S., Sheu, Y. T., Butler, C., & Cornelious, K. (2005). Relationships between perceived stress, coping behavior and cortisol secretion in women with high and low levels of internalized racism. *Journal of the National Medical Association*, *97*(2), 206–212.

Tull, S. E., Wickramasuriya, T., Taylor, J., Smith-Burns, V., Brown, M., Champagnie, G., ... Jordan, O. W. (1999). Relationship of internalized racism to abdominal obesity and blood pressure in Afro-Caribbean women. *Journal of the National Medical Association, 91*(8), 447–452.

U.S. Census Bureau. (2008). *Census 2000 gateway.* http://www.census.gov/main/www/cen2000.html

Victor, R. G., Leonard, D., Hess, P., Bhat, D. G., Jones, J. M., Vaeth, P. A. C., ... Haley, R. W. (2008). Factors associated with hypertension awareness, treatment, and control in Dallas County, Texas. *Archives of Internal Medicine*, *168*(12), 1285–1292.

Wang, T. J., & Vasan, R. S. (2005). Epidemiology of uncontrolled hypertension in the United States. *Circulation*, *112*, 1651–1662.

Wexler, R., Feldman, D., Larson, D., Sinnott, L. T., Jones, L. A., & Miner, J. (2008). Adoption of exercise and readiness to change differ between Whites and African-Americans with hypertension: A report from The Ohio State University Primary Care Practice-Based Research Network (OSU-PCPBRN). *Journal of Behavioral Family Medicine, 21*(4), 358–360.

Wilcox, S., Bopp, M., Wilson, D. K., Fulk, L. J., & Hand, G. A. (2005). Race differences in cardiovascular and cortisol responses to an interpersonal challenge in women who are family caregivers. *Ethnicity & Disease*, *15*(1), 17–24.

Williams, D. R., & Collins, C. (1995). US socioeconomic and racial differences in health: Patterns and explanations. *Annual Review of Sociology*, *21*, 349–386.

Williams, D. R., & Jackson, P. B. (2005). Social sources of racial disparities in health. *Health Affairs*, *24*, 325–334.

Williams, D. R., & Mohammed, S. A. (2009). Discrimination and racial disparities in health: Evidence and needed research. *Journal of Behavioral Medicine*, *32*, 20–47.

Williams, D. R., & Williams-Morris, R. (2000). Racism and mental health: The African American experience. *Ethnicity & Health*, *5*, 243–268.

Williams, R. B., Barefoot, J. C., & Schneiderman, N. (2009). Psychosocial risk factors for cardiovascular disease: More than one culprit at work. *JAMA: Journal of the American Medical Association*, *290*(16), 2190–2192.

Wilson, D. K., Kliewer, W., & Domenic, A. S. (2004). The relationship between exposure to violence and blood pressure mechanisms. *Current Hypertension Reports*, *6*, 321–326.

Wilson, D. K., Kliewer, W., Teasley, N., Plybon, L., & Sica, D. A. (2002). Violence exposure, catecholamine excretion, and blood pressure nondipping status in African American male versus female adolescents. *Psychosomatic Medicine*, *64*(6), 906–915.

Wyatt, S. B., Akylbekova, E. L., Wofford, M. R., Coady, S. A., Walker, E. R., Andrew, M. E., ... Jones, D. W. (2008). Prevalence, awareness, treatment, and control of hypertension in the jackson heart study. *Hypertension, 51*(3), 650–656.

Yan, L. L., Liu, K., Matthews, K. A., Daviglus, M. L., Ferguson, T. F., & Kiefe, C. I. (2003). Psychosocial factors and risk of hypertension: The Coronary Artery Risk Development in Young Adults (CARDIA) Study. *JAMA: Journal of the American Medical Association*, *290*(16), 2138–2148.

York, J. L., & Hirsch, J. A. (1997). Association between blood pressure and lifetime drinking patterns in moderate drinkers. *Journal of Studies of Alcohol*, *58*(5), 480–485.

Zhao, G., Ford, E. S., & Mokdad, A. H. (2008). Racial/ethnic variation in hypertension-related lifestyle behaviors among US women with self-reported hypertension. *Journal of Human Hypertension*, *22*, 608–616.

25 The Health of Sexual Minorities

Ilan H. Meyer
University of California, Los Angeles

Carl Joseph Walker-Hoover of Massachusetts and Jaheem Herrera of Georgia, two unrelated Black youths, killed themselves by suicide just 10 days apart in April 2009. Both youths hanged themselves in their homes—one with an extension cord, the other with a belt. Both were only 11 years old. Both were victims of bullying at school because they were seen as gay (even though, as far as we know, neither boy defined himself as gay). From their childhood perspectives, relentless homophobic taunts made life intolerable (Blow, 2009).

Although the immediate cause of these deaths was suicide, the real cause can be identified in the social rejection and ridicule these children had experienced at the hand of peers at their schools (Friedman, Silvestre, Korr, & Sites, 2006). But it is more accurate to place the blame even far beyond the bullying peers—themselves also children—responsible for the homophobic taunts and for otherwise making the lives of Carl Joseph Walker-Hoover and Jaheem Herrera so intolerable. Why? Because these children expressed a message that they have learned through *normal* socialization— that to be gay is wrong and deserving of public condemnation and ridicule. In social-psychological terms, these children enacted a socially sanctioned stigma (Herek, 2009a). Such stigma of homosexuality has roots in Western religious thought and a footing in social structures (Katz, 1983).

In this chapter, I describe *minority stress theory* as an explanatory model that describes such social structures, including stigma, as causes of health outcomes. Minority stress theory describes how social conditions and arrangements impact the lives of lesbians, gay men, and bisexual men and women (LGBs). The minority stress theory suggests that sexual minorities, that is, LGBs, experience excess stress related to stigma and prejudice related to their disadvantaged social position. Further, the theory states that this stress is chronic because it is tied to enduring social structures and that it leads to adverse health outcomes, including suicide (Meyer, 2003). Minority stress theory originated from social and psychological theories that seek to understand the person in the context of his or her social environment (Allport, 1954; Durkheim, 1951; Merton, 1957) and from stress theories that describe how a noxious social environment can be harmful to health (Dohrenwend, 1998; Pearlin, 1999).

WHO ARE LGB PEOPLE?

Before discussing how minority stress processes affect the health of LGB people, we need to understand who LGB people are. More broadly, we need to answer, what is sexual orientation?

Most researchers agree that there are three aspects of sexual orientation that should be considered when defining LGB populations: attraction, behavior, and identity (Laumann, Gagnon, Michael, & Michaels, 1994; Sell, 2007). That is, when we consider sexual orientation, we may classify people according to the gender of the person they are attracted to, the gender of the person they have or had sex with, and how they define themselves. In each of these aspects of sexual orientation, we can also think about degrees. For example, is a person attracted to persons of the opposite or same gender a lot or a little?

Furthermore, we must consider the entire lifespan, as sexual orientation can shift over the lifetime (Diamond, 2009). Many LGB people may have thought of themselves as heterosexual at some point early on in life, only later realizing that they are not heterosexual and embarking on a process of coming out as they define their sexuality and connect with LGB communities (Eliason & Schope, 2007). Others who have been sexually involved with a person of the same gender—maybe even labeled themselves as lesbian or gay—may later marry a person of the opposite gender and continue to live as heterosexuals (Diamond, 2009). To account for lifespan variability, when asking questions about sexual orientation (whether attraction, behavior, or identity), researchers usually specify which time period of the respondent's life they refer to. For example, they may ask whether a person has been attracted to persons of the same sex, opposite sex, or both during the past year, during the past five years, or since the person was 18 years old (other periods may be selected depending on the purpose of the study). Researchers have also differentiated between sexual attraction and romantic attraction. For example, National Longitudinal Study of Adolescent Health researchers believed that their teenage research participants may have not been mature enough to respond to a question about sexual attraction; instead, they asked, "Have you ever had a romantic attraction to a male?" and "Have you ever had a romantic attraction to a female?" (Udry & Chantala, 2005).

We can consider each of these aspects of sexual orientation independently but also may consider how they align together. This scope makes definition even more complicated for researchers because the three aspects of sexual orientation—attraction, behavior, and identity—do not necessarily coincide. Many people who are attracted to a person of the same gender have sexual relationships with persons of the same gender and identify themselves as lesbian, gay, bisexual, or many other terms that refer to nonheterosexual identity (such as *queer*). But for many other people, these three aspects of sexual orientation do not overlap. Some people may be attracted to a person of the same gender but never act on this attraction and do not identify as LGBs; some may engage in sexual behavior with people of the same gender but still identify as heterosexual; others identify as LGBs but abstain from sexual behavior altogether.

Clearly, with diversity in the definition of sexual orientation, different populations of sexual minorities could be defined. Therefore, in studying or otherwise addressing the health of LGB populations, professionals first need to clarify which group exactly they mean to study. Their definition could vary depending on their purpose (Meyer & Wilson, 2009). For example, when studying male sexual risk-taking related to HIV/AIDS, health professionals may define participants based on sexual behavior because they want to study men at risk for contracting HIV/AIDS through sexual behavior regardless of sexual identity. In contrast, when studying the salutogenic role of identification and affiliation with the gay community, health professionals may use identity definitions (e.g., gay, lesbian) because it would be impossible to assess identification with the gay community for someone who does not identify as LGB even if he or she has engaged in same-sex sexual behavior. Finally, Zietsch, Verweij, Bailey, Wright, and Martin (2009) argued that in their genetic study of sexual orientation, *sexual attraction* was the most relevant measure "because … attraction is less affected by mate availability and social/cultural constraints and is, in this sense, more fundamental" (p. 135).

It is important to remember, however, that regardless of the definition a researcher focuses on all aspects of sexual orientation may be important to consider. For example, even when focusing on sexual behavior in studying men who have sex with men (MSM) to assess HIV-related sexual risk taking, researchers should be cognizant that the men's identity can play an important role in determining their community affiliation, norms, and values—all of which may also impact risk-taking behaviors (Young & Meyer, 2005). That is, a profile of an MSM who identifies as gay is different from that of an MSM who identifies as straight; such a distinction has important implications for the study and prevention of HIV/AIDS.

In addition to diversity in aspects of sexual orientation, LGB populations are diverse in many other ways. LGB people differ in socioeconomic class, education, wealth, gender, age, race and ethnicity, geographic residence, nationality, religion, immigration status, political ideologies, and so on. That is, they are diverse in all the important characteristics that population health researchers are interested in. So the designation *LGB* alone cannot tell us all that is important to know about a person or group.

In this chapter, I refer to *sexual minorities* as a broad term that is inclusive of nonheterosexual orientations, and LGBs are individuals who have a nonheterosexual identity. But the diversity of LGB people is reflected also in a multitude of identity terms that they use, including *queer*, *women-loving-women*, *two-spirit people*, and many other terms.

With all this diversity, one may ask, why talk about "LGB populations" at all? Is such a term meaningful? This question can come up when studying any population or group. When studying a population, researchers confront a dilemma about the population's definition: Should we aim for generalizability or specificity and precision? On the one hand, health researchers, as well as such consumers of research as policymakers, clinicians, and other health professionals, want knowledge that is generalizable to as large a population as possible. After all, it makes little sense to conduct research that can tell us something that is so specific as to be unique to a small subgroup of individuals. Researchers seek knowledge that is useful so that interventions or treatments can be designed that affect large populations. On the other hand, this quest for generalizability conflicts with striving for precision and specificity. Most principles we arrive at regarding a population or group as a whole can be criticized for not fully reflecting some members or even a subgroup of the population. To define a population is therefore to compromise: We focus on commonalities at the expense of some important distinctions among the individuals who compose the population. For example, to understand the continuing growth of the HIV/AIDS epidemic among Black MSM (Millett, Peterson, Wolitski, & Stall, 2006), knowledge is needed that is applicable to as large a group of Black MSM as possible while being specific enough to be relevant and meaningful to this population.

In summary, despite their diversity, research on sexual minorities as a population is important because LGBs share characteristics that transcend the many distinctions among the subgroups that compose the LGB population. Foremost among these commonalities are social forces that shape the experience of LGB people; these social forces, in particular prejudice and stigma, have important health ramifications.

HEALTH DISPARITIES IN THE UNITED STATES

Because the U.S. Department of Health and Human Services (DHHS, 2000) identified reducing health disparities as one of the main goals for the nation, reducing health disparities related to sexual orientation has been a focus for health researchers. Researchers concerned with reducing health disparities ask, why does one population, such as a racial/ethnic group or sexual minorities, have higher prevalence of a disorder than another population? Although population health is not typically a framework used in health psychology, it is a useful framework for health psychologists to consider. It is a perspective that is necessary to understand this chapter because this chapter concerns differences between LGB and heterosexual populations.

Population health has been defined as a "conceptual framework for thinking about why some populations are healthier than others as well as the policy development, research agenda, and resource allocation that flow from this framework" (Kindig & Stoddart, 2003). The main distinction between population health and health psychology investigations is that population health focuses on populations, not individuals.

Population health challenges health psychologists to address public health priorities by utilizing a health psychology orientation. It also provides a framework for investigation where both determinants of health and health outcomes are considered from a population perspective. In that sense, a real test of the veracity of health psychological models, such as the stress model presented here, is that they can explain disparities between populations (Schwartz & Meyer, 2010). An implicit aspect of a population health framework is the goal of reducing health disparities. In that, the task of researchers and public health professionals does not end in describing risk factors for disease but includes thinking about intervention approaches for health promotion (Kindig & Stoddart, 2003).

THEORIES OF HEALTH DISPARITIES

Researchers have developed several general theoretical orientations to understand health disparities. Much of the work in health psychology has focused on racial and ethnic health disparities (Clark, Anderson, Clark, & Williams, 1999; Dressler, Oths, & Gravlee, 2005). These include, most prominently, explanations that focus on *biological* and genetic causes; *socioeconomic* or class theories, which explain health disparities in terms of deprivation of resources and access; and *stress* theory, which explains health disparities as a result of the excess stressors that people in disadvantaged social position experience (Dressler et al., 2005). Minority stress (also referred to as *social stress*) theory has been most prominent in examinations of health disparities related to sexual orientation (Herek & Garnets, 2007; Meyer, 1995, 2003). It is also the model that is most reliant on psychological theory. Before turning to it, I will briefly describe the two other models.

The biological perspective on health disparities suggests that observed health disparities are a result of mostly innate biological differences such as genetic differences in the makeup of social groups. This proposition is controversial because it suggests that social groups—Black versus White, LGB versus heterosexual—are different in basic genetic makeup and biological processes. This view contradicts research in genetics that has shown, for example, that race groups cannot be biologically or genetically differentiated other than by their phenotypes (e.g., darker skin pigment). Most scientists believe that race categorization is a social phenomenon—a social construct—rather than a reflection of biological or genetic entities. That is, what makes a racial or ethnic group is the social perception that it is distinct as a group. In the case of race, social processes dating back centuries led us to place great importance on skin pigmentation as a way of classifying people. But there is no significant biological or genetic differences, other than pigmentation, that distinguish darker-skinned people from lighter-skinned people (Smedley & Smedley, 2005). In the area of sexual orientation, most people agree that there are no biological or genetic markers that define sexual minority groups—hence, the multitude of ways of defining sexual orientation described earlier (Eliason & Schope, 2007). But some researchers claim that sexual orientation does have a strong genetic basis (Zietsch et al., 2009).

Proponents of socioeconomic theories of health disparities argue that income inequality, poverty, and access to resources are the most fundamental causes of health disparities (Karwachi, 2000; Link & Phelan, 1995). Although these proponents do not deny the importance of stress related to stigma and prejudice, they claim that it is more important to study (and redress) socioeconomic factors than to examine stress related to prejudice and discrimination because socioeconomic factors underlie all health problems (Farmer, 2003). This view has, however, been challenged by other researchers, who point out that there are significant health disparities that may only be accounted for by social stress theory (Williams, 1999). For example, Black women have worse birth outcomes than do White women, but these disparities are seen even among women of the same socioeconomic class, suggesting that other factors, related to racism directed at Black women, are at play (Giscombe & Lobel, 2005).

Although the impact of socioeconomic factors on LGB health has not received significant research attention, it is important to note that socioeconomic differences may be relevant to explaining disparities in sexual orientation as well. As are other minority populations, LGB people tend to be economically disadvantaged. Research has shown that compared with their heterosexual counterparts matched on education, race, and gender, LGB people have lower income (Badgett, 2006). These findings are contrary to popular portrayals of LGBs, especially urban gay men, as a high-spending consumer group with much disposable income (Badgett, 2001). In addition to the effect of income is the effect of socioeconomic status, which can have an indirect impact on LGBs, for example, through the impact of health insurance coverage. In the United States, health insurance is most often provided through employment to employees and their spouses. Because unemployed partners of LGB workers often do not qualify for employee health insurance, LGBs are, as a group, at a disadvantage, which could explain their lower health insurance coverage (Frazer, 2009).

MINORITY STRESS IN LGB POPULATIONS[1]

The minority stress model suggests that because of stigma, prejudice, and discrimination, LGBs experience more stress than do heterosexuals and that this stress can lead to mental and physical disorders. The minority stress model is based on general stress theory. Dohrenwend (2000) has described the general stress process in terms of strengths and vulnerabilities in the individual and his or her environment. I have included here only those elements of the general stress process unique to or necessary for the description of minority stress. It is important to note, however, that the omitted elements—including advantages and disadvantages in the environment, personal predispositions, biological background, ongoing situations, and appraisal and coping—are integral parts of the stress model and are essential for a comprehensive understanding of the stress process (Dohrenwend, 2000).

Figure 25.1 depicts stress and coping and their impact on mental health outcomes. Minority stress is situated within general environmental circumstances (a), which may include advantages and disadvantages related to such factors as socioeconomic status. An important aspect of these circumstances in the environment is the person's minority statuses, for example, being gay or lesbian (b). These are depicted as overlapping boxes in the figure to indicate close relationship to other circumstances in the person's environment. For example, minority stressors for a gay man who is poor would undoubtedly be related to his poverty; these characteristics would together determine his exposure to stress and coping resources (Diaz, Ayala, Bein, Jenne, & Marin, 2001). Circumstances in the environment lead to exposure to stressors, including such general stressors as job loss or death of an intimate (c); and such minority stressors unique to minority group members as discrimination in employment (d). Similar to their source circumstances, the stressors are depicted as overlapping, representing their interdependency (Pearlin, 1999). For example, an experience of antigay violence (d) is likely to increase vigilance and expectations of rejection (f). Often minority status leads to personal identification with one's minority status (e). In turn, such minority identity leads to additional stressors related to the individual's perception of the self as a stigmatized and devalued individual (Miller & Major, 2000), including expectations of rejection, concealment, and internalized homophobia (f).

Of course, minority identity not only is a source of stress but also has important positive effects in the stress process. First, characteristics of minority identity can augment or weaken the impact of stress (g). For example, minority stressors may have a greater impact on health outcomes when the LGB identity is prominent than when it is secondary to the person's self-definition (Thoits, 1999). Second, LGB identity may also be a source of strength (h) when it is associated with opportunities for affiliation, social support, and coping that can ameliorate the impact of stress (Crocker & Major, 1989; Miller & Major, 2000). I describe the main minority stress processes briefly here.

PREJUDICE EVENTS

Prejudice events include the *structural* exclusion of LGB individuals from resources and advantages available to heterosexuals, including, for example, their exclusion from the institution of marriage and from protection against employment discrimination. Prejudice events also include *interpersonal* events, perpetrated by individuals either in violation of the law (e.g., perpetration of hate crimes) or within the law (e.g., lawful but discriminatory employment practices). There are numerous accounts of the excess exposure of LGB people to such prejudice events (see Herek, 2009a, 2009b; Meyer, 2003). Studies have also shown that unlike other minority groups, LBG groups may face prejudice events in private settings. Antigay events can, for example, occur at home and be perpetrated by family members, as when a Latino man was, at age 13, raped and brutally beaten to unconsciousness by a family member who, in the respondent's words, "raped me because I was gay and to teach

---

[1] Portions of this section, including Figure 25.1, are reproduced with permission from Meyer (2003). © American Psychological Association.

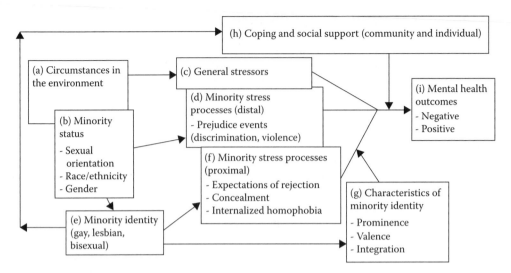

FIGURE 25.1 Minority stress process in lesbian, gay, and bisexual populations. (From Meyer, I. H., *Psychological Bulletin*, 129, 5, 674–697, 2003. With permission.)

me what a faggot goes through" (Gordon & Meyer, 2008, p. 62); or when boys and girls were kicked out of their homes to become homeless because their families rejected their homosexuality (Gordon & Meyer, 2008).

Events that are motivated by hate toward a community, such as hate crimes, are a particularly painful type of prejudice events because they inflict not only the pain of the assault itself but also the pain associated with the social disapproval of the victim's stigmatized social group. The added pain is associated with a symbolic message to the victim that he or she and his or her kind are devalued, debased, and dehumanized in society. Such victimization affects the victim's mental health, in part, because it damages his or her sense of justice and order (Garnets, Herek, & Levy, 1990; Herek, Gillis, & Cogan, 1999). Garnets and colleagues (1990) described psychological mechanisms that could explain the association between victimization and psychological distress. The authors noted that victimization interferes with perception of the world as meaningful and orderly. In an attempt to restore order to their perception of the world, survivors ask, "Why me?" To this question, they often respond with self-recrimination and self-devaluation. More generally, experiences of victimization take away the victim's sense of security and invulnerability. Health symptoms of victimization include "sleep disturbances and nightmares, headaches, diarrhea, uncontrollable crying, agitation and restlessness, increased use of drugs, and deterioration in personal relationship" (Garnett et al., 1990, p. 367). Antigay bias crimes have greater mental health impact on LGB persons than do similar crimes unrelated to bias. Such bias-crime victimization may have short- or long-term consequences, including such severe reactions as posttraumatic stress disorder (Herek et al., 1999; McDevitt, Balboni, Garcia, & Gu, 2001).

Surveys show that lesbians and gay men are disproportionately exposed to prejudice events, including discrimination and violence. For example, in a probability study of U.S. adults, LGB people were twice as likely as heterosexuals to have experienced a life event related to prejudice, such as being fired from a job (Mays & Cochran, 2001; Herek, 2009b; Herek et al., 1999). Some research has suggested variation by ethnic background. For example, Meyer, Schwartz, and Frost (2008) showed that as predicted by minority stress theory, because of their dual minority status, Black and Latino LGBs had significantly greater exposure to stressors and less access to resources than did White LGBs and White heterosexuals.

Research has suggested that LGB youths are even more likely than adults to be victimized by antigay prejudice events, and the psychological consequences of their victimization may be more severe. Surveys of schools in several regions of the United States showed that LGB youths are exposed to more discrimination and violence events than their heterosexual peers. Several such studies, conducted on population samples of high school students, converge in their findings and show that the social environment of sexual minority youths is characterized by discrimination, rejection, and violence. Compared with heterosexual youths, LGB youths are at increased risk for being threatened and assaulted, are more fearful for their safety at school, and miss more school days because of this fear (GLSEN, 2007; Ryan, Huebner, Diaz, & Sanchez, 2009). Gay men and lesbians are also discriminated against in the workplace (Huffman, Watrous-Rodriguez, & King, 2008). Waldo (1999) showed a relationship between employers' organizational climate and the experience of heterosexism in the workplace, which was subsequently related to adverse psychological, health, and job-related outcomes in gay, lesbian, and bisexual employees.

In addition to acute large events, more minor incidents and chronic conditions can be considered prejudice-related stressors. Harassment (such as being called derogative names) and other instances of rejection and disrespect—sometimes called *everyday discrimination* or *heterosexist daily hassles*—are stressful even if when they are not acute large events (Swim, Johnston, & Pearson, 2009). Such incidents do not qualify as a life event because they are minor by any objective measure; in stress language, in fact, they appear to bring about little objective change and, therefore, require little adaptation. Nonetheless, such minor instances can be damaging because of the symbolic message of rejection that they convey. Indeed, even *nonevents* can be stressful. Stressful nonevents are expected events or instances that do not happen. Examples of nonevents include expected life course milestones that were frustrated, for example, a job promotion not received when expected (Neugarten, Moore, & Lowe, 1965). Family relationship milestones, such as getting married, having children, or having grandchildren, are among the most widely expected events. Lesbian and gay persons share these expectations for life course milestones, as do their families, friends, colleagues, and acquaintances; not achieving such aims can be a significant stressor and on its own stigmatizing.

In summary, prejudice events or even everyday instances of prejudice (everyday discrimination) can have a powerful impact "more because of the deep cultural meaning they activate than because of the ramifications of the events themselves ... [; thus] a seemingly minor event, such as a slur directed at a gay man, may evoke deep feelings of rejection and fears of violence [seemingly] disproportionate to the event that precipitated them" (Meyer, 1995, pp. 41–42). Therefore, stress related to prejudice is assessed not solely by its tangible characteristics but also by its symbolic meaning within the social context; even a minor event or instance can have symbolic meaning and thus create pain and indignity beyond its seemingly low magnitude.

STIGMA: EXPECTATIONS OF REJECTION AND DISCRIMINATION

A distinct feature of prejudice-related stress is that several stress processes can be activated by the social environment through its internalization by the LGB person. Expectations of rejection and discrimination, concealment, and internalized homophobia are such processes. Even in the absence of any apparent explicit event, prejudice and the potential rejection of the LGB person and even violence are always implicit. As do other minority-group members, gay men, lesbians, and bisexuals learn to anticipate—indeed, expect—negative regard from members of the dominant culture. To ward off potential negative regard, discrimination, and violence, they must maintain vigilance. The greater one's perceived stigma, the greater the need for vigilance in interactions with dominant-group members. By definition, such vigilance is chronic in that it is repeatedly and continually evoked in the everyday life of the minority person.

Experimental social psychology research has shown that expectations of stigma can impair social and academic functioning of stigmatized persons by affecting their performance (Crocker, Major, & Steele, 1998; Farina, Allen, & Saul, 1968; Pinel, 2002; Steele, 1997; Steele & Aronson, 1995). For example, Steele (1997, p. 614) described stereotype threat as the "social-psychological threat that arises when one is in a situation or doing something for which negative stereotype about one's group applies" and showed that the emotional reaction to this threat can interfere with intellectual performance. When situations of stereotype threat are prolonged, they can lead to "disidentification," whereby a member of a stigmatized group removes from his or her self-definition a domain that is negatively stereotyped (e.g., academic success). Such disidentification with a goal undermines the person's motivation, and therefore effort, to achieve in this domain. Unlike the concept of life events, where stress stems from some concrete offense (e.g., antigay violence), here it is not necessary that any prejudice event has actually occurred.

CONCEALMENT VERSUS DISCLOSURE

Concealing LGB sexual identity is a way in which some LGB people cope with stigma and related prejudice, discrimination, and violence. School, workplace, and even family are areas where concealment occurs. For example, studies of the workplace experience of LGBs found that fear of discrimination and concealment of sexual orientation are prevalent (Huffman, Watrous-Rodriguez, & King, 2008) and have adverse psychological, health, and job-related outcomes (Waldo, 1999). These studies showed that gay men, lesbians, and bisexuals engage in identity disclosure and concealment strategies that address fear of discrimination, on the one hand, and a need for self-integrity, on the other. By concealing their LGB sexual identity, some LGB individuals hope to protect themselves from the effects of stigma. Despite offering some protections—for example, people who do not conceal their LGB identity are more likely to be victims of antigay violence than are people who conceal their LGB identity (Rosario, Hunter, Maguen, Gwadz, & Smith, 2001)—concealing one's LGB identity is itself a significant stressor for at least three reasons, described next.

First, people must devote significant psychological resources to successfully conceal their LGB identity. Writing about LGB youths, Hetrick and Martin (1987) noted that youths who conceal their sexual identity

> must constantly monitor their behavior in all circumstances: how one dresses, speaks, walks, and talks become constant sources of possible discovery. One must limit one's friends, one's interests, and one's expression, for fear that one might be found guilty by association … The individual who must hide of necessity learns to interact on the basis of deceit governed by fear of discovery … Each successive act of deception, each moment of monitoring which is unconscious and automatic for others, serves to reinforce the belief in one's difference and inferiority. (pp. 35–36)

Concealing requires constant monitoring of one's interactions and of what one reveals about one's life to others. Keeping track of what one has said and to whom is very demanding and stressful. Among the effects of concealing are preoccupation, increased vigilance of stigma discovery, and suspiciousness (Pachankis, 2007). For example, researchers studying the cognitive efforts required to conceal stigmatizing conditions described the person who attempts to conceal his or her stigma as living in a "private hell" (Smart & Wegner, 2000). The concealing effort and the required cognitive efforts can lead to significant distress, shame, anxiety, depression, and low self-esteem (Frable, Platt, & Hoey, 1998).

Second, concealing has harmful health effects by denying the person who conceals his or her LGB identity the psychological and health benefits that come from free and honest expression of emotions and sharing important aspects of one's life with others. Health psychology research has shown that expressing and sharing emotions and experiences can have a significant therapeutic effect by reducing anxiety and enhancing coping abilities (Meyer, 2003; Pachankis, 2007). In contrast, repression and inhibition can induce health problems. For example, Cole, Kemeny, Taylor, Visscher, and Fahey (1996) found that HIV-related disease advanced more rapidly in a group of gay men who concealed their sexual identity than in a group of gay men with similar HIV infection who did not conceal their sexual identity. In another study, the authors showed a similar pattern among HIV-negative men regarding health outcomes unrelated to HIV (Cole, Kemeny, Taylor, & Visscher, 1996).

More generally, concealing prevents the person from living an authentic life (Wood, Linley, Maltby, Baliousis, & Joseph, 2008). A related process has been related by the legal scholar Yoshino (2006), who described *covering* as a phenomenon where members of minority populations are censured in self-expression; that is, they are accepted as long as they do not flaunt their difference. Yoshino gives examples from such legal cases as that of an African American flight attendant fired for having a hairstyle that was inconsistent with the airline's standards or that of a lesbian who was fired because her marriage to a woman was publicized. Such instances and others are examples of modern expressions of stigma and prejudice; although overt expressions of prejudice are less common now than they were in the past, full participation and full acceptance of the minority person is still lagging (Dovidio & Gaertner, 2008).

Third, concealment prevents LGB individuals from connecting with and benefiting from social support networks and specialized services for LGB individuals. Protective coping processes can counter the stressful experience of stigma (Meyer, 2003). Access to and use of such community resources is beneficial to stigmatized minority-group members whose experiences and concerns are not typically affirmed in the larger community. For example, LGB communities have provided role models of successful same-sex intimate couples, have provided alternative values that support LGB families, and, in general, counter homophobic messages and values (Weston, 1991). However, LGB people who conceal their sexual identity would, in an effort to maintain secrecy, avoid such organizations or venues (e.g., gay or lesbian media, a gay community center, and such other gay or lesbian community events as a Gay Pride Day celebration). In addition, LGBs who need such supportive services as competent mental health services may receive better care from sources in the LGB community (e.g., a specialized gay clinic; Potter, Goldhammer, & Makadon, 2008). But individuals who conceal their LGB identity are likely to fear that their sexual identity would be exposed if they approached such sources. More generally, concealing can lead to social isolation because persons who conceal their sexual identity may avoid contact with other LGBs but also feel blocked from having meaningful, honest social relationships with non-LGB individuals.

INTERNALIZED HOMOPHOBIA

Both heterosexual and LGB individuals internalize negative social attitudes toward homosexuality as part of their socialization process, but the effects of this internalization is quite severe for LGB persons (Herek, 2009b). *Internalized homophobia* (also called *internalized heterosexism*, *homonegativity*, *internalized stigma*, and *self-stigma*) refers to an LGB person's internalization of negative societal attitudes and application of these negative attitudes toward him- or herself. Internalized homophobia is an insidious stressor because LGBs unleash it on themselves through years of socialization in a stigmatizing society even when no external stimulus is present (Meyer, 2003). Indeed, one of the developmental tasks LGB persons face on identifying as an LGB is to learn to dissociate their sense of self from what they have learned about homosexuality. In what psychologists call the coming-out process, as LGB persons unlearn negative learned values and prejudicial attitudes, they adopt new, healthier attitudes and self-perceptions (Eliason & Schope, 2007).

I demonstrate the workings of internalized homophobia in the area of intimacy. In most states of the United States and in most other nations, gay people are barred from marrying a person of the same sex. Yet, getting married is an especially important status and goal for most people in our society. One of the core stigmas about homosexuality has been the denial of intimacy for LGB couples. Recognizing intimacy as a basic human goal, society has built social structures to support the achievement of intimacy goals for heterosexual couples. Because of stigma, society has erected barriers for achievement of similar intimacy goals for LGB individuals. The denial of marriage—a structural prejudice mechanism—is the most fundamental of such barriers. The significance of denial of marriage is two pronged: It impedes the development of lasting intimate relationships by gay men and lesbians and propagates the stigma that they are undeserving or incapable of attaining satisfying intimate family relationships.

The concept of possible self (Markus & Nurius, 1986) can help in understanding another aspect of internalized homophobia. *Possible self* refers to a view of the self not only as it is but as it can become in the future. Possible selves relate to an important aspects of one's aspiration; they not only determine future success but also present hopes. These possible selves are formed from one's perception of current social norms, values, and expectations for the future. Among the important sources of possible selves are social conventions, social institutions, role models, and expectations and aspirations of others. Stigma makes it difficult for gay and lesbian youths to invoke images of getting married, having children, and other such family goals when thinking about their future because such images are typically portrayed in heterosexist form. Therefore, on realizing and accepting a gay sexual identify, an LGB person must chart a possible life course that is different from the possible life course of heterosexuals. Indeed, through socialization, gay youths often learn to

> recognize that they will not have the same course of life as their parents and heterosexual peers. They will not have a heterosexual marriage; they may not have children or grandchildren. … In a society such as ours, where much store is placed in competing and keeping up with one's friends and neighbors, such an identity crisis can unhinge not only sexuality but belief in all future life success. (Herdt & Boxer, 1996, p. 205)

In the coming-out process, LGB individuals revise these heterosexist perceptions and adopt norms and values that support an alternative notion of family and intimacy. For example, they turn to gay role models who have succeeded in establishing families. Yet, to the extent that gay persons are unsuccessful in doing so, they may believe that intimacy and family life—at least the socially sanctioned sort—are unattainable. Such internalized stigma has grave consequences for the health and well-being of LGBs. Because internalized homophobia disturbs the gay person's ability to overcome stigmatized notions of the self and envision a future life course, it is associated with mental health problems and impedes success in achieving intimate relationships. Empirical evidence has demonstrated that LGBs who have higher levels of internalized homophobia are less likely than LGBs with lower levels of or no internalized homophobia to sustain intimate relationships; even if in a relationship, the LGBs with higher internalized homophobia have poorer quality of relationships (e.g., Balsam & Szymanski, 2005; Frost & Meyer, 2009; Meyer, 1995; Meyer & Dean, 1998; Mohr, & Daly, 2008; Otis, Rotosky, Riggle, & Hamrin, 2006).

STRESS-AMELIORATING FACTORS

As early as 1954, Allport suggested that minority members respond to prejudice with coping and resilience. Modern writers agree that positive coping is common and beneficial to members of minority groups (Clark et al., 1999). Therefore, minority status is associated with not only stress but also such important resources as group solidarity and cohesiveness that protect minority members from the adverse mental health effects of minority stress (Meyer, 2003). To counteract minority stress, LGBs establish alternative structures and values that enhance their group (Crocker & Major, 1989; D'Emilio, 1983). Through coming out, LGB people learn to cope with and overcome some of the adverse effects of stress (Morris, Waldo, & Rothblum, 2001; Riggle, Rostosky, & Danner 2009).

A distinction between personal and group resources is often not addressed in the coping literature. It is important to distinguish between resources that operate on the individual level (e.g., mastery) and resources that operate on a group level. As do other individuals who cope with general stress, LGBs utilize a range of personal coping mechanisms and resources to withstand stressful experiences (Masten, 2001). In addition to such personal coping supports are social-structural factors that can have mental health benefits (Peterson, Folkman, & Bakeman, 1996). Jones and colleagues (1984) described two functions of coping achieved through minority group affiliations: (1) to allow stigmatized persons to experience social environments in which they are not stigmatized by others, and (2) to provide support for negative evaluation of the stigmatized minority group. Social evaluation theory suggests another plausible mechanism for minority coping (Pettigrew, 1967): Members of stigmatized groups who have a strong sense of community cohesiveness will evaluate themselves in comparison with others who are like them rather than with members of the dominant culture. The group may provide a reappraisal of the stressful condition, yielding it less injurious to psychological well-being. Through reappraisal, the group validates experiences and feelings of minority persons (Thoits, 1985). Indeed, reappraisal is at the core of gay-affirmative, black-affirmative, and feminist psychotherapies that aim to empower the minority person (Garnets & Kimmel, 1991; Hooks, 1993; Shade, 1990; Smith & Siegel, 1985).

The distinction between personal coping and group-level coping may be somewhat complicated because even group-level resources (e.g., services of a gay-affirmative church) need to be accessed and utilized by individuals. Whether individuals can access and use group-level resources depends on many factors, including personal strengths and resources. Nevertheless, it is important to distinguish between group-level and personal resources because when group-level resources are absent, even otherwise-resourceful individuals will have deficient coping. Group-level resources may therefore define the boundaries of individual coping efforts. Thus, *minority coping* may be conceptualized as a group-level resource, related to the group's ability to mount self-enhancing structures to counteract stigma. This formulation highlights the degree to which minority members may be able to adopt some of the group's self-enhancing attitudes, values, and structures rather than the degree to which individuals vary in their personal coping abilities. Using this distinction is important because it allows us to understand both aspects of coping. It is conceivable that an individual will have sufficient minority coping resources to overcome personal coping shortcomings. Indeed, it is a focus of affirmative therapies and interventions to provide external support, role models, and affirming experiences to counter an individual's own lack of coping resources expressed, for example, in heightened internalized homophobia. It is also conceivable that an individual with strong personal coping resources will lack minority coping resources. For example, under the U.S. *don't ask, don't tell* law, overturned by Congress in 2010, an LGB soldier was forbidden from disclosing that he or she is gay, which made affiliation and attachments with other LGB persons all but impossible. A high school student at a school that does not allow gay supportive clubs is in a similar situation. In such cases, regardless of the person's personal resources, he or she would be unable to access and utilize group-level resources. Attending to the difference between personal and group-level coping is important also because each of these scenarios calls for a different type of intervention. In a situation where personal coping is deficient, personal support, such as therapy, is called for; but in a situation where the social environmental places barriers on a person, structural interventions, aimed at reducing barriers, are called for.

HEALTH OUTCOMES RELATED TO MINORITY STRESS IN THE LGB POPULATION

MENTAL HEALTH

As depicted in Figure 25.1, the stress and stress-ameliorating processes described in the foregoing sections are damaging to the health of LGB people. Minority stress causes serious injury in the form of psychological distress, mental health problems, suicide, and lowered well-being. Studies have concluded that minority stress processes are related to an array of mental health problems, including depressive symptoms, substance use, and suicide ideation. Studies examined mental disorders, as defined by the *Diagnostic and Statistical Manual of Mental Disorders* (DSM-IV; APA, 2000) of the American Psychiatric Association and have consistently shown an increase in prevalence of disorders among LGB populations (see summaries of many published studies in Cochran & Mays, 2007; Herek & Garnets, 2007; Meyer, 2003).

Diagnosed mental disorders are not the only measure of psychological distress; such subthreshold mental health problems as mood, anxiety, or substance use problems that do not meet criteria for a formal psychiatric disorder are indicative of distress. Studies have shown that LGB populations score higher than heterosexuals on such distress measures because of minority stress resulting from stigma (Cochran, Sullivan, & Mays, 2003; Mays, & Cochran, 2001). Also, though less often studied, LGB individuals have lower levels of well-being than do heterosexuals because of exposure to such minority stress as stigma and experiences of discrimination (Frable, Wortman, & Joseph, 1997; Kertzner, Meyer, & Dolezal, 2003; Riggle et al., 2009). This is not surprising because well-being, especially *social well-being*, reflects the person's relationship with his or her social environment; it is "the fit between the individuals and their social worlds" (Kertzner, Meyer, Frost, & Stirratt, 2009, p. 500). Other studies have shown, for example, that stigma leads LGBs to experience alienation, lack of integration with the community, and problems with self-acceptance (Frable et al., 1997). Peplau and Fingerhut (2007), in their review of the literature on lesbian and gay men's intimate relationships, also note that minority stress negatively impact self-esteem, mental health, and therefore the relationship itself (e.g., Rostosky, Riggle, Gray, & Hatton, 2007).

Minority stress is also associated with a higher incidence of suicide attempts among LGBs compared with heterosexual individuals (e.g., Cochran & Mays, 2000; Gilman et al., 2001; Herrell et al., 1999; Meyer, Dietrich, & Schwartz, 2008; Russell & Joyner, 2001; Safren & Heimberg, 1999). This result is mostly related to minority stress encountered by youths in response to coming-out conflicts with family and community (Ryan et al., 2009). Youth is a time that can be particularly stressful to young LGB people; it is a time when they realize they are gay and often disclose their minority LGB identity to parents, siblings, and other family members, as well as teachers, friends, and colleagues (Flowers & Buston, 2001).

Physical Health

A number of studies have also demonstrated links between minority stress factors and such physical health outcomes as immune function, AIDS progression, and perceived physical well-being (Cole, Kemeny, Taylor, & Visscher, 1996; Cole, Kemeny, Taylor, Visscher, et al., 1996; Ullrich, Lutgendorf, & Stapleton, 2003). Unfortunately, most of these studies concerned HIV/AIDS and focused on men only, so there is less evidence regarding lesbians and bisexual women. For example, studies examined the impact of concealing one's sexual orientation as a stressor. Thus, HIV-positive but healthy gay men were followed up for nine years to assess factors that contribute to progression of HIV (e.g., moving from asymptomatic HIV infection to a diagnosis with an AIDS-defining disease such as pneumonia). The researchers showed that HIV progressed more rapidly among men who concealed their gay identity than it did among those who disclosed it. This was true even after the investigators controlled for the effects of such other potentially confounding factors as health practices, sexual behaviors, and medication use (Cole, Kemeny, Taylor, Visscher, et al., 1996). More recent studies, conducted in the context of availability of more effective HIV medications than were available to the men in the 1996 study, found, similarly, that concealment of gay identity was associated with lower CD4 count, a measure of HIV progression (Strachan, Murray Bennett, Russo, & Roy-Byrne, 2007; Ullrich et al., 2003).

The effects of concealment can be injurious in less medically vulnerable individuals too. In a study of HIV-negative gay men, Cole, Kemeny, Taylor, and Visscher (1996) showed that men who concealed their gay identity experienced a higher incidence of disease, including infectious diseases and cancer, than men who did not conceal their gay identity. As in the research in HIV-positive men, concealment was found to have a significant effect even after controlling for the effect of such other potentially confounding factors as coping styles, health behaviors, and mental health problems. Other studies examined other aspects of the minority stress model. For example, Huebner and Davis (2007) studied the impact of experiences of discrimination in gay and bisexual men. They found that exposure to discrimination was related to such outcomes as number of sick days and number of physicians visits.

Many other studies assessed the role of minority stressors in promoting risky behavior, especially HIV-related risk. For example, Hatzenbuehler, Nolen-Hoeksema, and Erickson (2008) assessed minority stress processes in a sample of bereaved gay men. They found that minority stressors, including internalized homophobia, discrimination experiences, and expectations of rejection, were associated with HIV risk behavior. Similar findings, assessing various aspects of minority stress processes and sexual risk outcome, were reported in other populations, including Latino gay and bisexual men and transgendered persons (Bruce, Ramirez-Valles, & Campbell, 2008); White and Latino lesbian, gay, and bisexual young adults (Ryan et al., 2009); gay, bisexual, and two-spirit American Indian men (Simoni, Walters, Balsam, & Meyers, 2006); rural men who have sex with men (Preston, D'Augelli, Kassab, & Starks, 2007); and transgendered women of color (Sugano, Nemoto, & Operario, 2006). One possible mechanism that explains how minority stressors are related to high-risk sexual behaviors may be that they lead to use of drugs and alcohol in sex, which reduces condom use (Kashubeck-West & Szymanski, 2008). For example, it is possible that substances are used during sex to reduce the self-reproach associated with internalized homophobia (Meyer & Dean, 1995).

DISCUSSION

WHY STUDY LGB HEALTH PSYCHOLOGY?

There are at least two important reasons for health psychologists to study LGB populations: (1) LGBs present unique health problems that must be addressed by health professionals and the public health system, and (2) studying LGB populations can help advance psychological science. First, regarding the health needs of the population, LGBs have distinct health problems that require distinct approaches for treatment and prevention. Better understanding of their special strengths and liabilities and of the psychological processes that affect their health would allow psychologists, health workers, and policy makers to design better interventions and treatments. Some areas of health disparities, where LGBs have increased risk as compared with heterosexuals, include mental health and suicide among men and women, HIV and AIDS, eating disorders, and anal cancer among men (Dean et al., 2000; U.S. DHHS, 2000). Health disparities are also suspected or recorded in behaviors that place people at risk for disease, including smoking, which is a risk factor for many diseases, in both gay men and lesbians (Gruskin, Greenwood, Matevia, Pollack, & Bye, 2007), and high body mass index in women (Aaron et al., 2001). In addition, LGBs are at increased risk for such health-related social conditions as prejudice, stigma, discrimination, hate crimes, and domestic violence (Herek, 2009b; Wolitsky, Stall, & Valdiserri, 2007). In terms of health services, compared with heterosexuals, LGB people have poorer access to care and lower rates of insurance coverage and also lack access to competent, culturally sensitive treatment (Frazer, 2009). At the same time, just as do members of other minority groups, LGBs have unique strengths that can protect them. These include affiliation with an LGB community that can provide support and challenge negative public attitudes (Crocker & Major, 1989). But community resources require that LGB people access them through participation in the LGB community. Those individuals who cannot or do not participate—for example, people who for fear of retribution cannot disclose their LGB sexual orientation, people in rural areas, and some older adults—are at risk for loneliness and social isolation (Frazer, 2009; Grossman, 2006).

Second, regarding the opportunity for scientific contribution to health psychology, studying LGB populations, in addition and in comparison to heterosexual populations, could enhance psychologists' understanding of health psychology theory and processes (Goldfried, 2001). One advantage of the inclusion of LGB respondents in health psychology studies is that it can introduce elements that cannot be observed by studying heterosexuals alone. By studying differences between LGB and heterosexual populations, researchers can examine the impact of variables that are invariant in one population or the other. For example, in studies of the effects of prejudice and stigma on mental health, we expect processes that lead to disease to be similar across groups that face prejudice and stigma in our society (Schwartz & Meyer, 2010). Although both LGBs and people of color are members of populations that are subject to prejudice in our society, the populations themselves differ in significant ways that can be capitalized on in research design. One important distinction is that racial and ethnic minorities are socialized within their minority communities. Racial and ethnic minority children typically grow up in families that share their race and ethnicity and are around people who have experienced prejudice similar to what they may experience. This shared familial minority status provides racial and ethnic minorities an opportunity for coping by learning about racism early on; acquiring alternative, self-affirming norms and values; and gaining access to communities that can provide them with support (Crocker & Major, 1989). These coping opportunities can help members of racial and ethnic minority groups and may have a protective effect, ameliorating the negative health effects of prejudice on health (Ryff, Keyes, & Hughes, 2003).

Unlike members of racial and ethnic minority groups, LGBs learn about and must cope with prejudice that they do not share with their families of origin. In fact, for many LGBs, families and communities of origin are sources of prejudice, discrimination, and stress, rather than sources of support (Flowers & Buston, 2001; Gordon & Meyer, 2008; Riggle et al., 2009). To connect with a supportive community, LGBs must step out of their community of origin and reach out to the LGB community. Doing so is no easy task because it requires disclosure of one's LGB identity, which can, in turn, expose the person to antigay violence and discrimination. By comparing patterns of prejudice, coping, and health outcomes in LGB versus racial or ethnic minorities, a researcher may be able to learn about how early socialization within one's minority community impacts health. Indeed, studies suggest that coping processes have a differential impact on African Americans and LGBs, with African Americans having higher well-being when compared with Whites but LGBs have lower well-being when compared with heterosexuals (Riggle et al., 2009).

CRITIQUES OF MINORITY STRESS THEORY

Minority stress theory is the most prominent in the literature on LGB populations (Herek & Garnets, 2007), but there are some critiques of the theory that should be considered. Prominent among these critques is the view that there has been so much positive change in the social environment of sexual minorities that LGBs, at least LGB youths, are no longer exposed to minority stress. Because of social changes over the past few decades in Western societies, as social attitudes are becoming more accepting and tolerant of homosexuality, this critique suggests that LGBs do not encounter the minority stressors described earlier in the chapter. Therefore, the critique goes, the minority stress model is not a viable psychological model. As Savin-Williams, one proponent of this view, wrote in his 2005 book *The New Gay Teenage*, "The culture of contemporary teenagers easily incorporates its homoerotic members. It's more than being gay-friendly. It's being gay-blind" (p. 197). Furthermore, "What if young people with same-sex desires are basically content with modern culture …? Maybe real changes in society's politics, laws and consciousness toward gay people have raised the possibility that sexual orientation is or will soon be irrelevant in all important respects" (p. 194).

This critique is valid because as a social theory, minority stress assumes certain stigmatizing social conditions. If these have truly changed, then the theory would, indeed, be out of date and would require revisiting and possibly discarding. But a theory and its critique should be assessed based on empirical evidence that supports or refutes the theory. New evidence would provide a good direction for future research and for elaboration and growth of theory. For example, if this critique is correct, then investigators should find no differences between LGB and heterosexual youths in level of stress and related mental health outcomes.

Currently, however, empirical findings do not support this view. Neither condition outlined in the foregoing critique—namely, that LGB have no more stress than heterosexuals and that they do not have more disorders—is satisfied to allow the conclusion that we live in a gay-blind (some say *postgay*) society that is as accepting of LGB people as it is accepting of heterosexual people (Herek, 2009a). Even with the many advances in gay rights over the past few decades, we continue to see such news stories as the one related in the opening of this chapter, about the negative and sometimes tragic results of bullying school children because they are perceived to be gay (Blow, 2009; Tharinger, 2008). Another indication of the continued disadvantage of LGBs is that many states and localities, as well as the U.S. Congress, have passed "defense of marriage" acts, which bar LGB people from marriage (though at the same time, as a sign of progress, a few states and localities have passed laws allowing LGB people to marry).

As did their predecessors, LGB adults and youths continue to mobilize a social movement against these and other expressions of prejudice and stigma. They do so both in schools throughout the United States, with such organizations as Gay Lesbian Straight Education Network and Gay Straight Alliance Network, and in the general political arena, as with the National Equality March in Washington, DC in 2009 (von Metzke, 2009).

CONCLUSIONS AND IMPLICATIONS

In summary, the minority stress model has been the most prominent model explaining observed disparities in health outcomes between LGB and heterosexual populations. The model points to social stress processes related to prejudice and stigma, as experienced through hate crimes, for example, and to the internalization of negative social attitudes. The model also points to the importance of considering such resiliency factors as social support and coping resources, among others, in exploring causes of health outcomes. Ultimately, according to the model, health outcomes are determined by the balance of positive (coping and social support) and negative (stressors) effects.

As described, population health is concerned with understanding not only causes of health outcomes but also implications for interventions. The minority stress model serves as a good guide to remind us about potential intervention points (Ouellette, 1998). The minority stress model is particularly well suited to community-based health interventions because it assesses causes that include the individual but go beyond to the community and, like such interventions, draws on existing individual and community strengths. Community-based health intervention aims to "[teach] individuals healthy behaviors within their natural environments" but also "creating environments that are conductive to health" (Revenson & Schiaffino, 2000, p. 474). Most important in the context of minority health, community-based interventions utilizes community organizing to bring about environmental and policy changes.

Using the community-based health interventions perspective of the minority stress model, psychologists would be directed to various intervention points. On the personal level, psychologist provide clinical services to affected individuals who suffer from mental health problems (Division 44, 2000). They can also help ensure that such clinical services are provided in a culturally competent and sensitive way (Potter et al., 2008). But following this perspective, psychologists also help design interventions and provide services that enhance community coping resources (Revenson & Schiaffino, 2000). Such interventions would include services targeting LGB youths, through a community center or school, or services to aged LGB individuals who may otherwise be isolated and unaffiliated (e.g., http://www.sageusa.org). Psychologists can also contribute to improving the health of LGB individuals by addressing the more distal parts of the processes that lead to health problems, for example, by attempting to reduce stigma and prejudice (Sears & Williams, 1997; Tharinger, 2008). Indeed, the American Psychological Association has called for the diverse and culturally relevant prevention of bullying in schools and communities (APA, 2004). Such efforts, if effective, could have saved the lives of Carl Joseph Walker-Hoover and Jaheem Herrera.

REFERENCES

Aaron, D. J., Markovic, N., Danielson, M. E., Honnold, J. A., Janosky, J. E., & Schmidt, N. J. (2001). Behavioral risk factors for disease and preventive health practices in a community sample of self-identified lesbian women. *American Journal of Public Health, 91*(6), 972–875.

Allport, G. W. (1954). *The nature of prejudice.* Reading, MA: Addison-Wesley.

American Psychiatric Association (APA). (2000). *Diagnostic and statistical manual of mental disorders* (DSM-IV-TR, 4th ed.). Washington, DC: American Psychiatric Press.

American Psychological Association (APA). (2004). APA resolution on bullying among children and youth. Retrieved from http://www.apa.org/pi/families/resources/bully_resolution.pdf

Badgett, L. M. V. (2001). *Money, myths, and change: The economic lives of lesbians and gay men.* Chicago, IL: University of Chicago Press.

Badgett, L. M. V. (2006). Discrimination based on sexual orientation: A review of the literature in economics and beyond. In W. M. Rodgers III (Ed.), *Handbook on the economics of discrimination.* Northampton, MA: Edward Elgar.

Balsam, K. F., & Szymanski, D. M. (2005). Relationship quality and domestic violence in women's same-sex relationships: The role of minority stress. *Psychology of Women Quarterly, 29*(3), 258–269.

Blow, C. M. (2009, April 24). Two little boys. *New York Times.* Retrieved from http://blow.blogs.nytimes.com/2009/04/24/two-little boys/

Bruce, R., Ramirez-Valles, J., Campbell, R. (2008). Stigmatization, substance use, and sexual risk behavior among Latino gay and bisexual men and transgender persons. *Journal of Drug Issues, 22,* 235–260.

Clark, R., Anderson, N. B., Clark, V. R., & Williams, D. R. (1999). Racism as a stressor for African Americans: A biopsychosocial model. *American Psychologist, 54*(10), 805–816.

Cochran, S. D., & Mays, V. M. (2000). Lifetime prevalence of suicide symptoms and affective disorders among men reporting same-sex sexual partners: Results from NHANES III. *American Journal of Public Health, 90*(4), 573–578.

Cochran, S. D., & Mays, V. M. (2007). Prevalence of primary mental health morbidity and suicide symptoms among gay and bisexual men. In R. J. Wolitski, R. Stall, & R. O. Valdiserri (Eds.), Unequal opportunity: Health disparities affecting gay and bisexual men in the United States (pp. 97–120). New York, NY: Oxford University Press.

Cochran, S. D., Sullivan, J. G., & Mays, V. M. (2003). Prevalence of mental disorders, psychological distress, and mental health services use among lesbian, gay, and bisexual adults in the United States. *Journal of Consulting and Clinical Psychology, 71*(1), 53–61.

Cole, S. W., Kemeny, M. E., Taylor, S. E., Visscher, B. R., & Fahey, J. L. (1996a). Accelerated course of human immunodeficiency virus infection in gay men who conceal their homosexual identity. *Psychosomatic Medicine, 58*(3), 219–231.

Cole, S. W., Kemeny, M. E., Taylor, S. E., & Visscher, B. R. (1996b). Elevated physical health risk among gay men who conceal their homosexual identity. *Health Psychology, 15*(4), 243–251.

Crocker, J., & Major, B. (1989). Social stigma and self-esteem: The self-protective properties of stigma. *Psychological Review, 96*(4), 608–630.

Crocker, J., Major, B., & Steele, C. (1998). Social stigma. In D. Gilbert, S. T. Fiske, & G. Lindzey (Eds.), *The handbook of social psychology* (Vol. 4, pp. 504–553). Boston, MA: McGraw-Hill.

Dean, L., Meyer, I. H., Sell, R. L., Sember, R., Silenzio, V., Bowen, D. J., ... White, J. (2000). Lesbian, gay, bisexual, and transgender health: Findings and concerns. *Journal of the Gay and Lesbian Medical Association, 4*(3), 101–151.

D'Emilio, J. (1983). *Sexual politics, sexual communities: The making of a homosexual minority in the United States, 1940–1970.* Chicago, IL: University of Chicago Press.

Diamond, L. (2009). Sexual fluidity: Understanding women's love and desire. Cambridge, MA: Harvard University Press.

Diaz, R. M., Ayala, G., Bein, E., Jenne, J., & Marin, B. V. (2001). The impact of homophobia, poverty and racism on the mental health of Latino gay men. *American Journal of Public Health, 91*(6), 927–932.

Division 44, Committee on Lesbian, Gay, and Bisexual Concerns Joint Task Force on Guidelines for Psychotherapy With Lesbian, Gay, and Bisexual Clients. (2000). Guidelines for psychotherapy with lesbian, gay, and bisexual clients. *American Psychologist, 55,* 1440–1451.

Dohrenwend, B. P. (1998). *Adversity, stress and psychopathology.* New York, NY: Oxford University Press.

Dohrenwend, B. P. (2000). The role of adversity and stress in psychopathology: Some evidence and its implications for theory and research. *Journal of Health and Social Behavior, 41*(March), 1–19.

Dovidio J. F., & Gaertner S. L. (2008). New directions in aversive racism research: persistence and perva-siveness. In Cynthia Willis-Esqueda (Ed.), *Motivational aspects of prejudice and racism: Nebraska Symposium on Motivation (*Vol. 53, pp. 43–67). New York, NY: Springer Science + Business Media.

Dressler, W. W., Oths, K. S., & Gravlee, C. C. (2005). Race and ethnicity in public health research: Models to explain health disparities. *Annual Review of Anthropology, 34,* 231–252.

Durkheim, E. (1951). Suicide. New York, NJ: Free Press.

Eliason, M. J., & Schope, R. (2007). Shifting sands or solid foundation? Lesbian, gay, bisexual, and transgender identity formation. In I. H. Meyer & M. E. Northridge (Eds.), The health of sexual minorities: Public health perspectives on lesbian, gay, bisexual and transgender populations (pp. 3–26). New York, NY: Springer.

Farina, A., Allen, J. G., & Saul, B. B. (1968). The role of the stigmatized person in affecting social relation-ships. *Journal of Personality,* 36(2), 169–182.

Farmer, P. (2003). *Pathologies of power: Health, human rights, and the new war on the poor.* Berkeley, CA: University of California Press.

Flowers, P., & Buston, J. (2001). "I was terrified of being different": Exploring gay men's accounts of grow-ing-up in a heterosexist society. *Journal of Adolescence,* 24, 52–65.

Frable, D. E., Platt, L., & Hoey, S. (1998). Concealable stigmas and positive self-perceptions: Feeling better around similar others. *Journal of Personality and Social Psychology,* 74(4), 909–922

Frable, D. E., Wortman, C., & Joseph, J. (1997). Predicting self-esteem, well-being, and distress in a cohort of gay men: The importance of cultural stigma, personal visibility, community networks, and positive identity. *Journal of Personality,* 65(3), 599–624.

Frazer. S. (2009). LGBT health and human Services needs in New York state. Report of the Empire State Pride Agenda Foundation and the New York State Lesbian, Gay, Bisexual and Transgender Health and Human Services Network. Retrieved from http://prideagenda.org/Portals/0/pdfs/LGBT%20Health%20and%20 Human%20Services%20Needs%20in%20New%20York%20State.pdf

Friedman, M. S., Silvestre, A. J., Korr, W. S., & Sites, E. W. (2006). The impact of gender-role nonconform-ing behavior, bullying, and social support on suicidality among gay male youth. *Journal of Adolescent Health,* 38, 621–623.

Frost, D. M., & Meyer, I. H. (2009). Internalized homophobia and relationship quality among lesbians, gay men, and bisexuals. *Journal of Counseling Psychology,* 59, 97–109.

Garnets, L. D., Herek, G. M., & Levy, B. (1990). Violence and victimization of lesbians and gay men: Mental health consequences. *Journal of Interpersonal Violence,* 5(3), 366–383.

Garnets, L. D., & Kimmel, D. C. (1991). Lesbian and gay male dimensions in the psychological study of human diversity. In J. D. Goodchilds (Ed.), *Psychological perspectives on human diversity in America.* Washington, DC: American Psychological Association.

Gilman, S. E., Cochran, S. D., Mays, V. M., Hughes, M., Ostrow, D., & Kessler, R. C. (2001). Risk of psychiat-ric disorders among individuals reporting same-sex sexual partners in the National Comorbidity Survey. *American Journal of Public Health,* 91(6), 933–939.

Giscombe, C. L., & Lobel, M. (2005). Explaining disproportionately high rates of adverse birth outcomes among African Americans: The impact of stress, racism, and related factors in pregnancy. *Psychological Bulletin,* 131, 662–683.

GLSEN. (2007). *GLSEN's national school climate survey: Lesbian, gay, bisexual and transgender students and their experiences in school.* New York, NY: GLSEN.

Goldfried, M.R. (2001). Integrating gay, lesbian, and bisexual issues into mainstream psychology. *American Psychologist, 56,* 977–988.

Gordon, A. R., & Meyer, I. H. (2008). Gender nonconformity as a target of prejudice, discrimination, and vio-lence against LGB individuals. *Journal of LGBT Health Research, 3*(3), 55–71.

Grossman, A. H. (2006). Physical and mental health of older lesbian, gay, and bisexual adults. In D. Kimmel, T. Rose, & S. David (Eds.), *Lesbian, gay, bisexual, and transgender aging: Research and clinical per-spectives* (pp. 53–69). New York, NY: Columbia University Press.

Gruskin, E. P., Greenwood, G. L., Matevia, M., Pollack, L. M., & Bye, L. L. (2007). Disparities in smoking between the lesbian, gay, and bisexual population and the general population in California. *American Journal of Public Health, 97*(8), 1496–1502.

Hatzenbuehler, M. L., Nolen-Hoeksema, S., & Erickson, S. J. (2008). Minority stress predictors of HIV risk behavior, substance use, and depressive symptoms: Results from a prospective study of bereaved gay men. *Health Psychology, 27,* 455–462.

Herdt, G., & Boxer, A. (1996). *Children of horizons.* Boston, MA: Beacon Press.

Herek, G. M. (2009a). Sexual stigma and sexual prejudice in the United States: A conceptual framework. In D. A. Hope (Ed.), *Contemporary perspectives on lesbian, gay, and bisexual identities* (pp. 65–111). New York, NY: Springer.

Herek, G. M. (2009b). Hate crimes and stigma-related experiences among sexual minority adults in the United States: Prevalence estimates from a national probability sample. *Journal of Interpersonal Violence, 24*(1), 54–74.

Herek, G. M., & Garnets, L. D. (2007). Sexual orientation and mental health. *Annual Review of Clinical Psychology, 3,* 353–375.

Herek, G. M., Gillis, J. R., & Cogan, J. C. (1999). Psychological sequelae of hate-crime victimization among lesbian, gay, and bisexual adults. *Journal of Consulting and Clinical Psychology, 67*(6), 945–951.

Herrell, R., Goldberg, J., True, W. R., Ramakrishnam, V., Lyons, M., Eisen, S., & Tsuang, M. T. (1999). Sexual orientation and suicidality: A co-twin control study in adult men. *Archives of General Psychiatry, 56*(10), 867–874.

Hetrick, E. S., & Martin, A. D. (1987). Developmental issues and their resolution for gay and lesbian adolescents. *Journal of Homosexuality, 14*(1/2), 25–43.

Hooks, B. (1993). *Sisters of the yam: Black woman and self-recovery.* Boston, MA: South End Press.

Huebner, D. M., & Davis, M. C. (2007). Perceived antigay discrimination and physical health outcomes. *Health Psychology, 26*(5), 627–634.

Huffman, A. H., Watrous-Rodriguez, K. M., & King, E. B. (2008). Supporting a diverse workforce: What type of support is most meaningful for lesbian and gay employees? Human *Resource Management, 47*(2), 237–253.

Jones, E. E., Farina, A., Hestrof, A. H., Markus, H., Miller, D. T., & Scott, R. A. (1984). *Social stigma: The psychology of marked relationships.* New York, NY: Freeman.

Karwachi, I. (2000). Income inequality and health. In L. F. Berkman & I. Kawachi (Eds.), *Social epidemiology* (pp. 76–94). New York, NY: Oxford University Press.

Kashubeck-West, S., & Szymanski, D. M. (2008). Risky sexual behavior in gay and bisexual men: Internalized heterosexism, sensation seeking, and substance use [Major contribution]. *Counseling Psychologist, 36,* 595–614.

Katz, J. N. (1983). *Gay/Lesbian almanac: A new documentary.* New York, NY: Harper & Row.

Kertzner, R. M., Meyer, I. H., & Dolezal, C. (2003). Psychological well-being in midlife older gay men. In G. Herdt & B. de Vries (Eds.), *Gay and lesbian aging research and future directions* (pp. 97–115). New York, NY: Springer.

Kertzner, R. M., Meyer, I. H., Frost, D. M., & Stirratt, M. J. (2009). Social and psychological well-being in lesbians, gay men, and bisexuals: The effects of race, gender, age, and sexual identity. *American Journal of Orthopsychiatry, 79*(4), 500–510.

Kindig, D., & Stoddart, G. (2003). What is population health? *American Journal of Public Health, 93*(3), 380–383.

Laumann, E. O., Gagnon, J. H., Michael, R. T., & Michaels, S. (1994). *The social organization of sexuality: Sexual practices in the United States.* Chicago, IL: University of Chicago Press.

Link, B. G., & Phelan, J. (1995). Social conditions as a fundamental cause of disease. *Journal of Health and Social Behavior: Vol. 35. Extra Issue: Forty Years of Medical Sociology: The State of the Art and Directions for the Future,* pp. 80–94.

Markus, H., & Nurius, P. (1986). Possible selves. *American Psychologist, 41*(9), 954–969.

Masten, A. S. (2001). Ordinary magic: Resilience processes in development. *American Psychologist, 56*(3), 227–238.

Mays, V. M., & Cochran, S. D. (2001). Mental health correlates of perceived discrimination among lesbian, gay, and bisexual adults in the United States. *American Journal of Public Health, 91*(11), 1869–1876.

McDevitt, J., Balboni, J., Garcia, L., & Gu, J. (2001). Consequences for victims—A comparison of bias- and non-bias-motivated assaults. *American Behavioral Scientist, 45*(4), 697–713.

Merton, R. K. (1957). *Social theory and social structure, revised and enlarged edition.* New York, NY: Free Press of Glencoe.

Meyer, I. H. (1995). Minority stress and mental health in gay men. *Journal of Health and Social Behavior, 36*(1), 38–56.

Meyer, I. H. (2003). Prejudice, social stress and mental health in lesbian, gay, and bisexual populations: Conceptual issues and research evidence. *Psychological Bulletin, 129*(5), 674–697.

Meyer, I. H., & Dean, L. (1995). Patterns of sexual behavior and risk taking among young New York City gay men. *AIDS Education and Prevention, 7*(Suppl.), 13–23.

Meyer, I. H., & Dean, L. (1998). Internalized homophobia, intimacy, and sexual behavior among gay and bisexual men. In B. Greene & G. M. Herek (Eds.), *Stigma and sexual orientation: Understanding prejudice against lesbians, gay men, and bisexuals* (pp. 160–186). Thousand Oaks, CA: Sage.

Meyer, I. H., Dietrich, J., & Schwartz, S. (2008). Lifetime prevalence of mental disorders and suicide attempts in diverse lesbian, gay, and bisexual populations. *American Journal of Public Health*, 98, 1004–1006.

Meyer, I. H., Schwartz, S., & Frost, D. M. (2008). Social patterning of stress and coping: Does disadvantaged social statuses confer more stress and fewer coping resources? *Social Science & Medicine*, 67(3), 368–379.

Meyer, I. H., & Wilson, P. A. (2009). Sampling lesbian, gay, and bisexual populations. *Journal of Counseling Psychology*, 56(1), 23–31.

Miller, C. T., & Major, B. (2000). Coping with stigma and prejudice. In T. F. Heatherton, R. E. Kleck, M. R. Hebl, & J. G. Hull (Eds.), *The social psychology of stigma* (pp. 243–272). New York, NY: Guilford Press.

Millett, G. A., Peterson, J. L., Wolitski, R. J., & Stall, R. (2006). Greater risk for HIV infection of Black men who have sex with men: A critical literature review. *American Journal of Public Health*, 96(6), 1007–1019.

Mohr, J. J., & Daly, C. (2008). Sexual minority stress and changes in relationship quality in same-sex couples. *Journal of Social and Personal Relationships*, 25, 989–1008.

Morris, J. F., Waldo, C. R., & Rothblum, E. D. (2001). A model of predictors and outcomes of outness among lesbian and bisexual women. *American Journal of Orthopsychiatry*, 71(1), 61–71.

Neugarten, B. L., Moore, J. W., & Lowe, J. C. (1965). Age norms, age constraints, and adult socialization. *American Journal of Sociology*, 70(6), 710–717.

Otis, M. D., Rostosky, S. S., Riggle, E. D. B., & Hamrin, R. (2006). Stress and relationship quality in same-sex couples. *Journal of Social and Personal Relationships*, 23(1), 81–99.

Ouellette, S. C. (1998). The value and limitations of stress models in HIV/AIDS. In B. P. Dohrenwend (Ed.), *Adversity, stress, and psychopathology* (pp. 142–160). New York, NY: Oxford University Press.

Pachankis, J. E. (2007). The psychological implications of concealing a stigma: A cognitive-affective-behavioral model. *Psychological Bulletin*, 133(2), 328–345.

Pearlin, L. I. (1999). The stress process revisited: Reflections on concepts and their interrelationships. In C. S. Aneshensel & J. C. Phelan (Eds.), *Handbook of the sociology of mental health* (pp. 395–415). New York, NY: Kluwer Academic/Plenum.

Peplau, L. A., & Fingerhut, A. W. (2007). The close relationships of lesbians and gay men. *Annual Review of Psychology*, 58, 405–424

Peterson, J. L., Folkman, S., & Bakeman, R. (1996). Stress, coping, HIV status, psychosocial resources, and depressive mood in African American gay, bisexual, and heterosexual men. *American Journal of Community Psychology*, 24(4), 461–487.

Pettigrew, T. F. (1967). Social evaluation theory: Convergencies and applications. In D. Levine (Ed.), *Nebraska Symposium on Motivation* (Vol. 15, pp. 241–304). Lincoln, NE: University of Nebraska Press.

Pinel, E. C. (2002). Stigma consciousness in intergroup contexts: The power of conviction. *Journal of Experimental Social Psychology*, 38(2), 178–185.

Potter, J., Goldhammer, H., & Makadon, H. J. (2008). Clinicians and the care of sexual minorities. In H. J. Makadon, K. H. Mayer, J. Potter, & H. Goldhammer (Eds.), *The Fenway guide to lesbian, gay, bisexual, and transgender health* (pp. 3–24). Philadelphia, PA: American College of Physicians.

Preston, D. B., D'Augelli, A. R., Kassab, C. D., & Starks, M. T. (2007). The relationship of stigma to the sexual risk behavior of rural men who have sex with men. *AIDS Education and Prevention*, 19(3), 218–230.

Revenson, T. A., & Schiaffino, K. M. (2000). Community-based health interventions. In J. Rappaport & E. Seidman (Eds.), *Handbook of community psychology* (pp. 471–493). New York, NY: Kleuwer Academic/Plenum.

Riggle, E. D. B., Rostosky, S. S., & Danner, F. (2009). LGB identity and eudaimonic well being in midlife. *Journal of Homosexuality*, 56(6), 786–798.

Rosario, M., Hunter, J., Maguen, S., Gwadz, M., & Smith, R. (2001). The coming-out process and its adaptational and health-related associations among gay, lesbian, and bisexual youths: Stipulation and exploration of a model. *American Journal of Community Psychology*, 29(1), 133–160.

Rostosky, S. S., Riggle, E. D. B., Gray, B. E., & Hatton, R. L. (2007). Minority stress experiences in committed same-sex couple relationships. *Professional Psychology Research and Practice*, 38(4), 392–400.

Russell, S. T., & Joyner, K. (2001). Adolescent sexual orientation and suicide risk: Evidence from a national study. *American Journal of Public Health*, 91(8), 1276–1281.

Ryan, C., Huebner, D., Diaz, R. M., & Sanchez, J. (2009). Family rejection as a predictor of negative health outcomes in White and Latino lesbian, gay, and bisexual young adults. *Pediatrics*, 129(1), 346–352.

Ryff, C. D., Keyes, C. L. M., & Hughes, D. L. (2003). Status inequalities, perceived discrimination, and eudaimonic well-being: Do the challenges of minority life hone purpose and growth? *Journal of Health and Social Behavior*, 44(September), 275–291.

Safren, S. A., & Heimberg, R. G. (1999). Depression, hopelessness, suicidality, and related factors in sexual minority and heterosexual adolescents. *Journal of Consulting and Clinical Psychology*, *67*, 859–866.

Savin-Williams, R. C. (2005). *The new gay teenager: Adolescent lives*. Cambridge, MA: Harvard University Press.

Schwartz, S., & Meyer, I. H. (2010). Mental health disparities research: The impact of within and between group analyses on tests of social stress hypotheses. *Social Science and Medicine*, *70*(8), 1111–1118.

Sears, J. T., & Williams W. L. (1997). Overcoming heterosexism and homophobia: Strategies that work. New York, NY: Columbia University Press.

Sell, R. L. (2007). Defining and measuring sexual orientation for research. In I. H. Meyer & M. E. Northridge (Eds.), *The health of sexual minorities: Public health perspectives on lesbian, gay, bisexual and transgender populations* (pp. 355–374). New York, NY: Springer.

Shade, B. J. (1990). Coping with color: The anatomy of positive mental health. In D. S. Ruiz (Ed.), *Handbook of mental health and mental disorder among Black Americans* (pp. 273–289). New York, NY: Greenwood Press.

Simoni, J. M., Walters, K. L., Balsam, K. F., & Meyers, S. (2006). Victimization, substance use, and HIV risk among gay/bisexual/two-spirit and heterosexual American Indian men in New York City. *American Journal of Public Health*, *96*(12), 2240–2245.

Smart, L., & Wegner, D. M. (2000). The hidden costs of hidden stigma. In T. F. Heatherton, R. E. Kleck, M. R. Hebl, & J. G. Hull (Eds.), *The social psychology of stigma* (pp. 220–242). New York, NY: Guilford Press.

Smedley, A., & Smedley, B. D. (2005). Race as biology is fiction, racism as a social problem is real. *American Psychologist*, *60*, 16–26.

Smith, A. J., & Siegel, R. F. (1985). Feminist therapy: Redefining power for the powerless. In L. R. Rosewater & L. E. A. Walker (Eds.), *Handbook of feminist therapy: Women's issues in psychotherapy*. New York, NY: Springer.

Steele, C. M. (1997). A threat in the air: How stereotypes shape intellectual identity and performance. *American Psychologist*, *52*(6), 613–629.

Steele, C. M., & Aronson, J. (1995). Stereotype threat and the intellectual test performance of African Americans. *Journal of Personality and Social Psychology*, *69*(5), 797–811.

Strachan, E. D., Murray Bennett, W. R., Russo, J., & Roy-Byrne, P. P. (2007). Disclosure of HIV status and sexual orientation independently predicts increased absolute CD4 cell counts over time for psychiatric patients. *Psychosomatic Medicine*, *69*, 74–80.

Sugano, E., Nemoto, T., & Operario, D. (2006). The impact of exposure to transphobia on HIV risk behavior in a sample of transgendered women in San Francisco. *AIDS and Behavior*, *10*, 217–225.

Swim, J. K., Johnston, K., & Pearson, N. B. (2009). Daily experiences with heterosexism: Relations between heterosexist hassles and psychological well-being. *Journal of Social and Clinical Psychology, 28*(5), 597–629.

Tharinger, D. (2008). Maintaining the hegemonic masculinity through selective attachment, homophobia, and gay-bashing in schools: challenges to intervention. *Social Psychology Review 37*(2), 221–227.

Thoits, P. (1985). Self-labeling processes in mental illness: The role of emotional deviance. *American Journal of Sociology*, *91*, 221–249.

Thoits, P. (1999). Self, identity, stress, and mental health. In C. S. Aneshensel & J. C. Phelan (Eds.), *Handbook of the sociology of mental health* (pp. 345–368). New York, NY: Kluwer Academic/Plenum.

Udry, J. R., & Chantala, K. (2005). Risk factors differ according to same-sex and opposite-sex interest. *Journal of Biosocial Science*, *37*(4), 481–497.

Ullrich, P. M., Lutgendorf, S. K., & Stapleton, J. T. (2003). Concealment of homosexual identity, social support and CD4 cell count among HIV-seropositive gay men. *Journal of Psychosomatic Research, 54*(3), 205–212.

U.S. Department of Health and Human Services (DHHS). (2000). *Healthy People, 2010: Understanding and improving health* [LGBT companion document] (2nd ed.). Washington, DC: U.S. Government Printing Office.

Von Metzke, R. (2009). People power. *The Advocate* (December 2009–January 2010), 94–101.

Waldo, C. R. (1999). Working in a majority context: A structural model of heterosexism as minority stress in the workplace. *Journal of Counseling Psychology*, *46*(2), 218–232.

Weston, K. (1991). *Families we choose: Lesbians, gays, kinship*. New York, NY: Columbia University Press.

Williams, D. R. (1999). Race, socioeconomic status, and health: The added effects of racism and discrimination, *Annals of the New York Academy of Sciences*, *896*, 173–188.

Wolitski, R. J., Stall, R., & Valdiserri, R. O. (2007). *Unequal opportunity: Health disparities affecting gay and bisexual men in the United States*. New York, NY: Oxford University Press.

Wood, A. M., Linley, P. A., Maltby, J., Baliousis, M., & Joseph, S. (2008). The authentic personality: A theoretical and empirical conceptualization, and the development of the Authenticity Scale. *Journal of Counseling Psychology*, *55*, 385–399.

Yoshino, K. (2006). *Covering the hidden assault in our human rights*. New York, NY: Random House.

Young, R. M., & Meyer, I. H. (2005). The trouble with "MSM" and "WSW": Erasure of the sexual-minority person in public health discourse. *American Journal of Public Health*, *95*(7), 1144–1149.

Zietsch, B. P., Verweij K. J., Bailey J. M., Wright M. J., & Martin N. G. (2009). Sexual orientation and psychiatric vulnerability: A twin study of neuroticism and psychoticism. *Archives of Sexual Behavior* [Published online July 9, 2009, Springer].

26 Aging and Health

Ilene C. Siegler
Duke University School of Medicine
and University of North Carolina School of Public Health

Merrill F. Elias
University of Maine and Maine Institute of Genetics and Health

Hayden B. Bosworth
Duke University Medical Center
and Durham Veteran's Administration Medical Center

Age has long played a central role in health psychology because age has potential interactions with all the important causal and mediating variables of interest in health psychology. Age is also a major risk factor for most chronic diseases (Siegler, Bosworth, & Elias, 2003). In the previous edition of this chapter, women's health and the menopausal transition was of major concern (Siegler, Bastian, & Bosworth, 2001). In the past seven years, the literature in health psychology that deals with aging has exploded, as is evidenced by other chapters in this volume that have aging content: age and definitions of illness (Leventhal et al., Chapter 1, this volume), caregiving (Martire & Schulz, Chapter 13, this volume), religion and spirituality (Park, Chapter 18, this volume), gender and age (Helgeson, Chapter 22, this volume), coping processes in social context (Revenson & Lepore, Chapter 9, this volume), and personality and coronary heart disease (CHD; T. W. Smith, Gallo, Shivpuri, & Brewer, Chapter 17, this volume). In addition, physical and mental health disparities are linked to age and culture in morbidity and mortality in the United States (Jackson, Antonucci, & Brown, 2004) and the global community (NIA, 2007). Development of the *Diagnostic and Statistical Manual*–5 (DSM-5) is also leading to an interest in understanding age considerations in psychiatric diagnoses (Jeste, Blazer, & First, 2007), with additional complications in medically ill elderly psychiatric patients (Katz & Ganzini, 2007). Other volumes present important reviews that readers of this chapter may want to consult: *Handbook of Health Psychology and Aging* (Aldwin, Park, & Spiro, 2007); *Recent Advances in Psychology and Aging* (Costa & Siegler, 2004), *Neuropsychology of Cardiovascular Disease* (Waldstein & Elias, 2001), *Annual Review of Gerontology and Geriatrics* focused on centenarian studies (Poon & Perls, 2007) and the epidemiology of aging (Fried, 2000). There has also been a methodological revolution in the application of sophisticated latent-variable-modeling techniques (Bosworth & Hertzog, 2009; Hertzog & Nesselroade, 2003).

In an ongoing update of psychology of normal aging for geriatric psychiatrists, our review suggests the following: (a) Individual decline in cognitive performance before age 60 is generally not normal aging. By the mid-70s, average decrement is observed for all abilities; and by the 80s, this decrement is severe except for verbal ability; (b) Empirical data from centenarian studies suggest that dementia is not inevitable; (c) Cognitive abilities that depend on perceptual speed and contextual memory tend to decline with age, even for healthy adults, whereas abilities that rely on semantic knowledge and highly overlearned patterns decline less or may even improve; (d) Continuity of personality and social preferences is expected across the adult lifespan; thus changes have potential diagnostic significance; and (e) Effects of Alzheimer's disease (AD) and care giving for relatives with AD varies in diverse populations (Siegler et al., 2009). With these findings as a generalized background, in this chapter we will focus on three broad areas of current research. First, there has been an explosion of work using personality, cognition, and other psychological predictors of survival. A variant of these concerns is the terminal-drop literature that assesses changes in psychological functioning at the end of life. The review is not exhaustive, given that this chapter does not present a meta-analysis but is meant to illustrate the exciting findings. Second, there is a new emphasis on understanding the role of cardiovascular risk factors and disease on cognitive decline and dementia, which should expand the research in health psychology. Third, in later life, eventually diseases accumulate, and thus coping with multiple comorbid conditions and having the capacity to use health services become a major focus of research interest. We end with some comments on the role health psychology of aging should play in the future.

PERSONALITY, PERSONALITY CHANGE, AND COGNITIVE CHANGE

Why is it important to understand if, how, and why personality factors are associated with mortality? In studies of all-cause or total mortality (vs. cause-specific mortality), we are not studying a particular disease process but are, rather, examining the age at death. Thus, the extent to which personality factors predict survival generally implies a longer period of healthy aging, suggests possible intervention strategies, and lead us to search for explanatory mechanisms that take into account behavior, such as risky and protective health behaviors (cf. Bogg & Roberts, 2004). The role of cognitive changes as predictors of mortality picks up on a very old terminal-drop literature (Riegel & Riegel, 1972; Siegler, 1975), which looked at intellectual development at a time when treatment for coronary heart disease (CHD) was quite different (Bosworth & Siegler, 2002). Then, cognitive decline was a proxy for CHD; now, cognitive decline may be a proxy for AD. The newer literature is moving toward a consideration of mild cognitive impairment at midlife as an early precursor of cognitive decline that may provide time for treatments to work and clues as to what types of drugs need to be developed to reduce impairment (Albert, 2008; Peterson & O'Brien, 2007).

Personality

Two recent meta-analyses organized around constructs in the positive psychology domain (but also included studies that could have been considered negative or bimodal) are good representatives of this work. Chida and Steptoe (2008) studied positive well-being and prospective observational studies through January 2008, splitting the review into studies of healthy populations and diseased populations. Effects were stronger in the initially healthy groups, with a hazard ratio (HR) of .82 versus .98; but significant reductions were seen in all groups. The positive nature of the predictors and thus the reduction in mortality may not be that different from that documented in the traditional literature on negative constructs and increased mortality (hostility, anger, depression; e.g., Suls & Bunde, 2005). However, the consistency of the personality factors that are predictive in well-controlled studies is impressive. Length of follow-up ranged from 2 to 64 years in healthy populations and 2 to 19.4 years in diseased populations. The studies include a full range of subjects from young adulthood (college students) to midlife as well as those starting with elderly cohorts. Age was controlled in the analyses, but it was not discussed in the report. Although Chida and Steptoe's (2008) findings appear to generalize across the full lifespan, it would have been useful to know age at measurement of the psychosocial predictor and average age of the survivors. The researchers proposed behavioral pathways accounting for part of the effect of positive emotions on survival, with stress-related physiological indicators also involved in the pathways. Kern and Friedman (2008) present a meta-analytic synthesis with a very broad definition of conscientiousness: Someone with conscientiousness is responsible; self-controlled, and not impulsive; orderly, organized, efficient, and disciplined; and achievement oriented, persistent, and industrious. These constructs are similar to facets from the Revised NEO Personality Inventory (NEO PI-R; Costa & McCrae, 1992), which has been one of the main instruments used to operationalize the five-factor model of personality (FFM; Goldberg, 1993; McCrae & Costa, 2003). The analyses also included studies with psychoticism from Eysenck Personality Questionnaire (EPQ) and psychopathic deviance (Pd) from Minnesotat Multiphasic Personality Inventory (MMPI). The researchers found 19 studies with an overall association of $r =$ .11 (.05-.17) that generalized across lifespan such that higher conscientiousness and lower impulsiveness were associated with greater survival.

Using data from the Baltimore Longitudinal Study of Aging (BLSA), which started measuring data in 1958, Terracciano, Lockenhoff, Zonderman, Ferrucci, and Costa (2008) reported on personality assessed on 2,359 participants aged 17–98 with a mean age of 50. In the subsequent 40 years, 943 study members had died an average of 18 years after personality was measured with the Guilford-Zimmerman Temperament Survey. Their results indicated that in general, differences in longevity for four factors—general activity (~E4), emotional stability (~N3), personal relations (~A1), and conscientiousness (~C4)—resulted in three years' longer survival. Then they tested with proportional hazard models and found that three constructs were significant: (1) general activity (~E4), (2) emotional stability (~N3), and (3) conscientiousness (~C4). These relationships were generally independent of cigarette smoking and obesity—an important finding, given that personality has often been related to health outcomes only through risky behaviors. This research report shows clever use of existing data and mapping the traits from the Guilford-Zimmerman Temperament Survey onto NEO PI-R to help increase comparability across studies. It is also impressive that the actual ages of survivors are featured showing the action is comparing a three-year difference in age at death (80 vs. 83). Smoking and obesity were not mediators in these analyses, perhaps because their impact occurs earlier in the life cycle.

Weiss and Costa (2005) studied personality and mortality in 1,444 individuals, of whom 1,076 had valid NEO Five-Factor Inventory (FFI) scores. The sample consisted of Medicare patients aged 65–100 with baseline 12- and 24-month follow-ups. Enrollment was staggered so that mortality was determined between three and five years after enrollment when 652 individuals were alive and 424 were dead. With a full set of covariates, proportionality was assumed, and results indicated that increased *neuroticism* (N) and *agreeableness* (A) were both related to survival. In a second set of analyses, proportionality was not assumed; only higher *conscientiousness* (C) was related to survival. Proportionality refers to whether hazard is equal from low to middle to high levels of the predictor. Additional analyses with continuous N and A and trichotomized C found replication for the N and C findings; that is, the A disappeared, and the C finding was robust over a 12-point range of cut-points. Then, three years later, a subset of individuals (597 of 1,082) completed the full NEO PI-R in order to look at facet-level analyses. Attrition in the three-year interval was a result of death ($n = 324$) or a subject's failing the cognitive screen ($n = 67$). Of 597 subjects who completed the NEO PI-R, there were 108 deaths. Results indicated that the facets N5 (*impulsiveness*), A2 (*straightforwardness*), and C4 (*self-discipline*) were shown to be associated with longevity in the three-year follow-up. Most interesting is that high N was associated with survival as well as high A and higher C compared to average and low A and C, respectively. This group was a much older sample that is typically studied, but it confirms reports of personality in centenarians in traits reflective of high N as measured on the 16 personality factors (PF; Martin, Long, & Poon, 2002).

Wilson et al. (2005) used very short N and E scales of four items each from NEO FFI tested at a mean age of 75 with six years of follow-up in 6,158 persons sampled from the Chicago Health and Aging Project. After 6.2 years, 39.5% of the sample had died. Those who died were more likely to be male, less educated, and White. Mortality increased with N (*neuroticism*) and decreased with E (*extraversion*), comparing top and bottom 10th percentiles; both effects remained when both N and E were simultaneously included in the models. These associations were reduced with covariates but not eliminated. This study is one of the few with a predominantly Black sample (62%) showing replication for personality constructs across race and socioeconomic status.

Shipley, Weiss, Der, Taylor, and Deary (2007) analyzed data from the UK Health and Lifestyle Survey (HALS), a representative sample aged 18–99 with 21-year follow-up completed in 2005, where they examined the relationships of *neuroticism* (N) and *extraversion* (E) to all-cause and cause-specific mortality. Results for N and E varied by the covariates in the model: For baseline models only (and with researchers controlling for age and gender), N predicted all-cause mortality of 1.09, or a 9% increase in mortality. This finding was attenuated by adding controls. There were no significant effects for E. These findings did not replicate for specific causes of death; this limitation, however, may have reflected limited statistical power.

PERSONALITY CHANGE

Turning to studies of personality change, Mroczek and Spiro (2007) studied *neuroticism* (N) and *extraversion* (E) from the EPQ for 18 years from 1988 to 2005 in the age range 43–91 ($m = 63$, $SD = 8$) at baseline personality measurement with up to six repeated measures over a 12-year interval in men from the Normative Aging Study. There were no significant findings for E; but for N, the researchers found a significant level by slope interaction, indicating that those who are higher on N become more neurotic (at the range of change of .5 SD/decade), which was associated with a 40% increase in mortality. Those individuals who were initially high-average and had increasing N were at the greatest risk (compared to low-average at any change and high average with decreasing). Such modeling holds great promise for the future. These analyses require very long-term studies to be able to model sufficient change and then observe sufficient outcomes; they also require methods that allow personality indicators from various systems to be seen as comparable.

These requirements are illustrated in a report by Martin, Friedman, and Schwartz (2007) from their continued work on the Terman Study with an additional 14 years of follow-up added onto their childhood indicators of *conscientiousness, cheerfulness,* and *sociability*. They developed indicators from the database to estimate the five-factor model of personality in 1940 and 1950 and were able to evaluate test and retest coefficients. As of 2000, median age at death was in the early 70s for men and women. Childhood and midlife personality measures were predictive across the life cycle. Consistently high conscientiousness was protective, consistently low was risky, and the change patterns did not matter.

COGNITIVE CHANGE

Wilson, Beck, Bienias, and Bennett (2007) provide an excellent update on the state of research on terminal drop with eight years of follow-up from the Rush Memory and Aging Study. Data analyses are based on 853 persons, with at least one wave of follow-up with a mean age at baseline of 80.4 years. Individuals with dementia at baseline and no follow-up were excluded. There was a large cognitive battery. Because on enrollment members of the cohort agreed to an autopsy, mortality follow-up was excellent. The researchers ran a series of mixed-effects models to assess rates of cognitive change from 6 to 60 months prior to death. The best fitting model had linear decline over 42 months (~ 3.5 years). Terminal decline was not seen in those study participants with vascular conditions (heart attack, congestive heart failure, stroke, or claudication) and varied by the presence of an e4 allele, suggesting a role for AD.

Shipley, Der, Taylor, and Deary (2007) from the UK HALS sample looked at 3,082 individuals, with complete data at both measurement points and 13 years' follow-up and five of six measures of cognition were predictive of increased mortality. Weatherbee and Allaire (2008) reported on 10-year mortality from the everyday cognitive battery in 171 persons initially aged 60–92. Baseline differences were seen for almost all of the measures, and only a few baseline factors predicted mortality in the Cox model analyses. Overall, high performers on the battery survived better than the average-high, average-low, and low performers. These findings may suggest that measures of mild cognitive impairment (MCI) are useful for assessing mortality as well as dementia.

MacDonald, Hultsch, and Dixon (2008) evaluated predictors of mortality in the Victoria Longitudinal Study from 1,014 baseline participants over 12 years with five times of measurement. There were 447 survivors and 265 deaths, an average of 5.2 years, after final measurement. By testing indicators of basic neurocognitive resources defined as level and inconsistency of speeded performance on cognitive tasks versus typical accuracy measures, they developed indicators of variation in cognition. Their results indicated that this index of variation may be a particularly sensitive measure of mortality that can be noted earlier than cognitive changes.

Gerstof, Smith, and Baltes (2006) studied personality and cognition together with four times of measurement (1990–1998) over six years from the Berlin Aging Study (BASE). They investigated four-year survival through 2002. The sample had a mean age of 78 at Time 1 and 84 at Time 4. None of the 109 study participants with dementia survived past Time 4. Data from the study battery included measures of cognition, personality from a shortened NEO FFI, and items reflecting health, well-being, and sensory functioning that were clustered into three groups: overall positive, overall average, and high cognition but low social functioning. Clusters were related to differences in length of survival for the three clusters; subgroup changers were worse off than those who were stable; and compared to the overall positive profile, relative risk of death was doubled for the other two groups—that is, the timing of death shown in the survival curves during the four-year follow-up indicated differences until the fourth year of follow-up.

Age at time of measurement and survival time are critical in understanding the personality and survivorship literature. This is the first time that we have sufficient psychological data on personality and cognition that can evaluate the impact on survival to age 60, from 60 to 80, and from 80 to 100. Having these data is important because the relationship between personality and cognitive functioning may well involve different mechanisms and disease associations over the ages. Understanding selective survival and who remains in the population at advanced ages will become increasingly important as treatment strategies need to be developed for aging persons and their caregivers.

There is growing support for relationships between measures of personality, cognition, and change in psychological function as predictors of mortality. This growth is the direct result of the continuation of a number of longitudinal studies and improvements in our statistical analyses (e.g., linear mixed models) improving our knowledge base.

CARDIOVASCULAR RISK AND COGNITION

The literature on cardiovascular risk factors and cognition has also grown significantly since the last edition of this book. A comprehensive review by A. D. Smith (2008) lists 23 nongenetic risk factors for the dementias: age, including myocardial infarction, midlife hypertension, hypertension, low blood pressure, atherosclerosis, atrial fibrillation, diabetes mellitus, obesity, smoking, low alcohol consumption, low physical activity at midlife, low fish diet, rate of decline in body mass index (BMI), low level of social and mental activities, low education, low intake of antioxidants, raised markers of inflammation, raised plasma total homocysteine, low plasma concentrations of folate and vitamin B_{12}, low testosterone in men, hormone replacement therapy in women after age 65, nonuse of nonsteroidal anti-inflammatory drugs, low thyroid-stimulating hormone (TSH), head injury in men, depression, and poor perceived health. Many of the variables in the foregoing list are also risk factors for modest cognitive deficit (Waldstein & Elias, 2001); and, as important, a lower level of cognitive functioning is a risk factor for dementia (M. F. Elias et al., 2000). Given the impossibly large literature to review, we review new developments in hypertension and touch on highlights of several areas of research with implications for aging. More in-depth reviews may be found in M. F. Elias, Robbins, et al. (2004), Purnell, Gao, Callahan, and Hendrie (2009), A. D. Smith (2008), and Waldstein and Elias (2001), for the findings and implications of the Maine–Syracuse studies of hypertension.

HYPERTENSION

Arterial hypertension is related to cognitive performance and is a risk factor for dementia (Birns & Kalra, 2008; Waldstein & Katzel, 2001), and it is clear that these relationships cannot be accounted for by use of antihypertensive medications (M. F. Elias, Wolf, D'Agostino, Cobb, & White, 1993). There has been a call for early treatment and diagnosis of hypertension (Staessen & Birkenhäger, 2004) in relation to three major sets of findings: (1) Higher levels of systolic and diastolic blood pressure in middle age or earlier are related to lowered cognitive performance in old age and are a risk factor for dementia (M. F. Elias et al., 1993; Robbins, Elias, Elias, & Budge, 2005; A. D. Smith, 2008; Waldstein & Katzel, 2001); and (2) Whereas hypertension results in accelerated longitudinal decline at all ages (e.g., M. F. Elias, Robbins, Elias, & Streeten, 1998), the rate of decline for fluid-type abilities is similar for young and older persons (P. K. Elias, Elias, Robbins, & Budge 2004). However, U- and L-shaped relations between blood pressure and cognition (Birns & Kalra, 2008; Waldstein, Giggey, Thayer, & Zonderman, 2005) indicate that overtreating elderly hypertensive individuals is not prudent. The fact that younger individuals are not significantly less vulnerable to hypertension appears to be related to the fact that the mechanisms underlying hypertension are different at different ages (Waldstein, 1995; Waldstein & Katzel, 2001). There is still more work needed to establish which regions of the brain are vulnerable or more vulnerable to hypertension and how this influences performance in specific domains of cognitive ability. There is some evidence that the frontal regions may be more vulnerable (Raz, Rodrigue, & Acker, 2003). A paper by Raz et al. (2003) and a recent review by Birns and Kalra (2008) cover this topic in more depth. Problems of purity of measurement with respect to clinical measures commonly used in studies make this a difficult issue to resolve. More studies using factor-analytic methods and information-processing paradigms would help resolve these issues. Innovative new trends in research include the following: (a) use of pulse wave velocity technology, the gold standard for measuring arterial stiffness, to obtain pressures measured closer to the heart and brain than peripheral blood pressure (brachial artery) measurements allow (Waldstein et al., 2008); (b) using left ventricular mass as an index of duration of hypertension rather than such less accurate methods as when hypertension was first diagnosed (M. F. Elias et al., 2007); and (c) increasing use of MRI and PET scan methods combined with cognitive performance (Birns & Kalra, 2008; M. F. Elias & Dore, 2008; Jennings et al., 2005).

Clinical trials featuring lowering of blood pressure will be necessary to further establish the likelihood of a causal link between blood pressure and cognition. A recent review (Birns & Kalra, 2008) indicates that only eight randomized clinical trials with a placebo arm have been completed and the results are inconclusive. More trials are needed in persons with mild cognitive deficits associated with shorter duration of hypertension, because it is possible that changes in cognition and hypertension sustained over many years, as evidenced by left ventricular hypertrophy, cannot be reversed by existing antihypertensive medications. Currently available antihypertensive medications (e.g., some types of calcium-channel-blocking agents and angiotensin-converting enzyme inhibitors or blockers) do have the potential for restoration of cognitive functioning either through prevention of undesirable hypertension-related cardiovascular remodeling or by their direct effects on neurons (see M. F. Elias & Dore, 2008; Staessen & Birkenhäger, 2004).

HOMOCYSTEINE AND B VITAMINS

Homocysteine (tHcy) is an amino acid produced during 1-carbon metabolism. In the 1990s, several studies indicated higher levels of tHcy in patients with cognitive deficits or dementia (A. D. Smith, 2008). Early in 2008 there were 77 cross-sectional studies and 33 prospective studies indicating relations between higher levels of tHcy (or lower folate, B_6 and B_{12} status) and lowered cognitive performance and dementia. Aside from homocysteineuria, high homocysteine levels have not been defined clinically, but many studies use the mediation of the distribution as a cut-point or relate homocysteine concentrations to performance. A number of mechanisms have been proposed as mediators of this association between homocysteine and cognition observed. The most direct hypothesis is that higher blood levels of tHcy have an adverse influence on cognition because they are neurotoxic (see M. F. Elias, Robbins, et al., 2006, and Smith, 2008, for reviews). However, inverse associations between homocysteine and cognition are seen at less than toxic levels (e.g., M. F. Elias, Robbins, et al., 2006; M. F. Elias, Sullivan, et al., 2005), and there is evidence that higher homocysteine levels serve as a marker for cardiovascular disease and as a marker for folic acid, vitamin B_{12} and vitamin B_6 (see A. D. Smith, 2008). Deficits in B vitamins result in lower cognitive performance (A. D. Smith, 2008). In this regard, elderly individuals are very likely to experience subclinical deficits in these B vitamins, and these deficits affect cognition negatively (A. D. Smith, 2008). Several large community-based studies indicate that B vitamin deficits and cardiovascular disease do not account for negative relations between homocysteine and lower cognitive performance (e.g., M. F. Elias, Robbins, et al., 2006; M. F. Elias, Sullivan, et al., 2005), but longitudinal data and clinical trials are necessary to resolve this issue.

See A. D. Smith (2008) for a summary and commentary of the few trials in which homocysteine has been lowered by administration of B vitamins. A. D. Smith (2008) argues that these trials have not been done in the correct study populations, that is, persons who are declining in cognitive ability. However, he describes ongoing trials in the correct study populations, including his own clinical trial at Oxford University, England, where restoration of cognitive functioning and/or slowing of the progression of decline and cerebral atrophy are the outcome measures and where homocysteine is lowered by B vitamin administration. His summary on this topic is an excellent introduction to this area of investigation.

APOE-ε4

ApoE is a lipoprotein involved in lipid transport, neuronal repair, and synaptogenesis after injury (Nathan et al., 1994). The protein has three isoforms, ApoE-ε2, ApoE-ε3, and ApoE-ε4. A recent summary of the literature (Bracco et al., 2007) and meta-analyses (Small, Rosnick, Fratiglioni, & Backman, 2004) indicate that the ApoE genotype is a risk factor for AD and is associated with lowered global, executive, episodic memory, and attentional capacity, as well as decreased hippocampal and amygdale volume. Recently, Bracco et al. (2007) reported that the ε4 allele was related to memory deficit at baseline but did not influence rate of decline in patients with mild AD. There have been a great many studies in this area; results have been mixed after initial positive findings. As discussed later, another feature of importance to the ApoE-ε4 genotype may be its role as an effect modifier with respect to other risk factors.

DIABETES MELLITUS

A review of the many studies of diabetes mellitus and cognition is not possible in this chapter. Recent reviews indicate that individuals with diabetes have a greater risk of cognitive decline and a greater risk of developing dementia than do nondiabetic individuals. Possible mechanisms for this association include oxidative stress, accelerated ischemic brain damage, and impaired glucose utilization during cognitive tasks (Jagust, Harvey, Mungas, & Haan, 2005; Taylor & MacQueen, 2007).

OBESITY AND CENTRAL ADIPOSITY

Interest in relations between obesity and cognition is relatively recent compared to such other risk factors as hypertension and diabetes. This interest may be related to the fact that it has been assumed that obesity is not a primary cause of lowered cognition but relates to cognition through its association with such other risk factors as hypertension and diabetes. The Framingham Heart Study was one of the first to examine relations between obesity and cognitive performance, adjusting for cardiovascular risk factors and disease (M. F. Elias, Elias, Sullivan, Wolf, & D'Agostino, 2003). Obesity in men, but not women, was associated with poorer cognitive performance. One explanation was that central adiposity, the lethal aspect of obesity with respect to cardiovascular disease, may have been higher in men than women, but no measures of central adiposity were available in the subset of studies employing a cognitive battery. Central adiposity has been linked to an increase in prevalence of white matter hyperintensities in the brain (Jagust et al., 2005) and to emerging risk factors for such cardiovascular disease as elevated systemic inflammation (Kershaw & Flier, 2004). At least one study, however, has reported relations between central adiposity and lowered cognitive performance with adjustment for a marker of inflammation, C-reactive protein (Dore, Elias, Robbins, Budge, & Elias, 2008). More recent studies have related central adiposity to cognitive performance. Interactions between central adiposity and high blood pressure has been reported (Waldstein & Katzel, 2006; Wolf et al., 2007), such that an inverse relationship between waist circumference, or waist-to-hip ratio, and cognitive function was observed in hypertensive but not normotensive individuals. Wolf et al. (2007) adjusted only for age, education, and gender; whereas Waldstein and Katzel (2006) adjusted for age, education, gender, multiple demographic and CVD risk factors, and components of the metabolic syndrome. Physical activity level and cardiorespiratory fitness have received relatively little attention as possible confounders of the relationship between central adiposity measures and cognitive performance. Recently, Dore et al. (2008) reported relations between central adiposity and multiple domains of cognitive functioning, with adjustment for CVD risk factors. However, with further adjustment for level of physical activity, only one association remained, namely, that between central adiposity and abstract reasoning ability. It is possible that this finding nearly reflected the high association between physical activity and cognition in this cross-sectional study.

It has been known for some time that physical activity is associated with higher levels of cognitive performance (Hillman, Erickson, & Kramer, 2008). The following mechanisms have been suggested: (a) physical activity increases serotonin and dopamine levels, as well as increasing insulin sensitivity, variables that have been shown to be positively correlated with cognition; and (b) physical activity also has beneficial effects on the vascular system, including reduction of atherosclerotic plaque accumulation, decreased blood coagulation, and subsequent reduction of cardiovascular disease risk (Hillman et al., 2008). An excellent review of metabolic syndrome, including obesity, hypertension, and diabetes, in relation to cognitive performance may be found in Taylor and MacQueen (2007).

ATRIAL FIBRILLATION

Elias, Sullivan, et al. (2006) and Vingerhoets (2001), among others, have summarized the literature on atrial fibrillation (AF). It is the most common form of sustained cardiac arrhythmia seen in clinical practice and is a major risk factor for blood coagulation, stroke, and all-cause mortality; further, its prevalence and incidence increase dramatically with aging. It is associated with cerebral hypoperfusion, systemic arterial embolism, and periventricular white matter lesions. Consequently, it is not surprising that AF is associated with lower cognitive performance and dementia despite adjustment for cerebral atrophy, history of transient ischemic attack, and brain atrophy (Tang et al., 2004). In a community-based study of 1,506 stroke- and dementia-free men participating in the Framingham Heart Study, AF was related to measures indexing global performance, abstract reasoning, visual–spatial memory, episodic memory, attention, and executive functioning. This was true despite adjustment for age, education, systolic blood pressure, smoking, alcohol consumption, BMI, total cholesterol, depressed mood, left ventricular hypertrophy, diabetes, CVD, and treatment with antihypertensive drugs (M. F. Elias, Sullivan, et al., 2006). Results were the same with women in the sample, but there were too few women with cognitive measures and AF for a separate analysis. More recently, Knecht et al. (2008) compared 122 stroke-free individuals with AF with 563 individuals free from AF. Three T (3-T) magnetic resonance imaging was employed to assess regional brain infarction, white matter lesions, and brain volume measures. Measures of learning and memory, attention and executive functions, working memory, and visuospatial skills were obtained. Compared to participants free from AF, patients with AF performed significantly worse on tests of learning and memory as well as attention and executive functioning. There was also a trend ($p < .06$) toward poorer performance in learning and memory tasks in patients with chronic as compared with paroxysmal AF. Hippocampal volume was reduced in patients with AF. Other radiographic measures did not differ between groups. Thus, in the absence of manifest stroke and dementia, AF is a risk factor for cognitive impairment and hippocampal atrophy. Because a person in late middle age and elderly individuals are at particularly high risk for AF, this area deserves much more in the way of active investigation. More longitudinal studies are needed as well as trials of cognitive functioning in relation to treatments designed to control or eliminate arrhythmias (e.g., beta-blocking agents and ablation).

CHRONIC KIDNEY DISEASE

The prevalence and incidence of kidney disease increases with advancing age (Madero, Gul, & Sarnak, 2008). There are clear parallels between kidney and brain in terms of their pulsatile response to cardiac output and vulnerability to cardiovascular risk factors (Seliger & Longstreth, 2008). End-stage renal disease, as well as less advanced stages of chronic kidney disease, are risk factors for cognitive impairment and dementia (e.g., Madero et al., 2008; Seliger et al., 2004). Only a handful of studies dealing with mild renal dysfunction in nondemented individuals have been published, generally with crude, or only a few, measures of cognitive performance thus far. Better studies are in progress, but much more work needs to be done in this area, particularly large community-based studies in which the progression of cognitive deficit from mild renal disease through end-stage renal disease is not only described but also related to functional and structural changes in the brain. Moreover, more work is needed to separate the effects of hemodialysis from the effects of kidney failure per se (Murray et al., 2006). This is a very important area of research in aging, especially since working memory and executive functioning are very important characteristics in adherence to the complex treatment regimens necessary in patients with more severe renal disease, especially those undergoing dialysis.

MULTIPLE RISK FACTORS: INTERACTIVE AND COMBINED

A review of literature from 2001 to 2007 (Purnell et al., 2009) is particularly instructive regarding interactions of risk factors in relation to Alzheimer's disease. Risk factors considered include hypertension, diabetes, exercise, alcohol intake, smoking, B complex vitamins, homocysteine, stroke, AF, apolipoprotein E (ApoE), lipids, and diet. Reports of studies with incident AD as an outcome and longitudinal studies with cohorts of 500 or more were included in the review. Interactions among one or more risk factors affecting AD were also found for exercise and physical function, APOE-ε4, diabetes, hypertension, and cholesterol. For example, in a recent study (M. F. Elias et al., 2008), ApoE-ε4 genotype interacted with homocysteine such that the lowest levels of performance in nondemented individuals were seen in the presence of high levels of tHcy and one or two ApoE-ε4. M. F. Elias et al. (2008) hypothesized that the reduced regenerative ability of neurons for persons with an ApoE-ε4 genotype may further promote the symptomatic manifestation of functional deficits resulting from the neurotoxic effects of homocysteine. Inverse associations between homocysteine and cognition are exacerbated by age (M. F. Elias et al., 2005). Robbins, Elias, Budge, Brennan, and Elias (2005) have reported that diabetes and high levels of homocysteine interacted such that the lowest level of performance was seen in the combined presence of these risk factors.

Much more work is needed on the combined impact of multiple risk factors on cognitive performance. As an example of such work, M. F. Elias, Sullivan, et al. (2004) report that the Framingham stroke risk profile (consisting of multiple cardiovascular risk variables weighted to predict future stroke) was associated with lower cognitive performance in nondemented individuals, as were almost all the cardiovascular risk factors making up the profile.

DEALING WITH COMPLEX CHRONIC DISEASES BY THE ELDERLY

The aging of the population and the increasing prevalence of chronic diseases pose challenges to the U.S health care system. Medicare data show that 65% of beneficiaries have multiple chronic conditions (Wolff, Starfield, & Anderson, 2002). Health care costs for individuals with at least three chronic conditions accounted for 89% of Medicare's annual budget (Anderson & Horvath, 2002). Multiple chronic conditions (multimorbidity) is associated with poor quality of life, increased physical disability, high health care use, use of multiple medications, and increased risk for adverse drug events and mortality (Bayliss et al., 2007). Individuals with multiple chronic conditions have complex needs. Care is provided by the patients and their caregivers away from medical supervision. Only 20% of patients' health care occurs in the office; the other 80% is performed at home and is based on the patients' knowledge, beliefs, and attitudes (Sobel, 1995). Thus, despite improvement in life expectancy, individuals are living longer with increased disability and are expected to take care of themselves for longer period of times (Rice & Fineman, 2004).

In a national survey, 17% of persons with chronic conditions report receiving conflicting information from providers—not surprising because the average Medicare beneficiary sees seven different physicians in one year (Anderson & Knickman, 2001). In addition, symptomatic depression (Foster, Taylor, Eldridge, Ramsey, & Griffiths, 2007; Jerant, Kravitz, Moore-Hill, & Franks, 2008), cognitive challenges, long-term attention, financial constraints, and being overwhelmed by one dominant condition, compound effects of multiple conditions and medications, low self-efficacy for self-management tasks, and low health literacy may impede self-management. Adherence to treatment regimens requires a high level of cognitive function. Cognitive factors are related to all the components, or "stages," of treatment adherence, including comprehension, formulating plans, and actually engaging in the behavior (Bosworth & Ayotte, 2009).

Information management in patient decision making is likely to be a significant problem among individuals with chronic diseases not only because of the complexity of regimens but also because many chronic diseases are also associated with deficits in cognitive function. Studies reviewed in this volume have identified associations between certain chronic illnesses, among them hypertension and diabetes. Although these cognitive declines are debilitating in their own right, people with complex chronic diseases are often older, and thus normal age-related declines in cognitive function may also interfere with chronic-disease self-management (Schaie, 2005).

Two meta-analyses suggest that information burden may play a role in self-management—a problem potentially exacerbated with age. In a systematic review of adherence to diabetes medications, Cramer (2004) showed medication adherence to be inversely related to the number of doses prescribed per day. In meta-analyses of regimen adherence in several patient populations, DiMatteo (2004) showed that patients are more adherent to circumscribed regimens (e.g., medication taking) than to regimens requiring pervasive behavior change that impose greater information-processing demands on the patient (e.g., diet). Thus, given challenges of self-management with chronic diseases, it is not surprising that despite the enormous impact of chronic diseases in the world and in spite of the availability of effective therapy for many chronic diseases such as diabetes, hypertension, and hypercholesterolemia, relatively few individuals achieve recommended goals of therapy for all multiple conditions (Johnson, Pietz, Battleman, & Beyth, 2006; Saydah, Fradkin, & Cowie, 2004).

SUGGESTIONS TO SUPPORT SELF-MANAGEMENT OF COMPLEX CHRONIC DISEASE

Patients with multiple chronic illnesses may best be served by a comprehensive, stepped-care menu of self-management support that varies in content, intensity, and delivery modality. Tailored interventions are a way to address the spectrum of individuals' needs by placing emphasis on participants' individual preferences. Tailored feedback has been demonstrated to be effective in multiple health behaviors (Stretcher et al., 1994). Although a generic health care intervention may improve adherence through reminders, a tailored intervention can address issues that are specifically relevant to a particular patient (Woolf, 1992). Self-management factors targeted in a tailored behavioral intervention might include education to increase knowledge base, skills to handle impairments in memory and cognition, medical and social support, relationships with health care providers, adverse affects of medications, and weight management, exercise, diet, stress, smoking, and alcohol use. Such interventions can be delivered efficiently by targeting more patients than can be targeted by a one-size-fits-all paradigm and making optimal use of technology and human capital. The ability to tailor self-management support is no less important than tailoring such other aspects of medical care as medication regimen.

An example of a self-management intervention for older adults is provided by some of our ongoing work with the Veteran–Study To Improve The Control of Hypertension (V-STITCH). The study was a randomized controlled trial that tested whether a patient intervention, a provider intervention, or combination of the two is more effective in improving blood pressure control. The mean age of the sample was 63 years, and 41% of participants were African American. Most individuals taking part in the study were of low socioeconomic status and 23% reported having inadequate income. Of the 294 patients randomized to the nurse intervention, 84% of the sample received all 12 intervention telephone calls. The average length of time to administer the intervention call was 3.7 minutes (SD = 2.5 min). After 24 months of follow-up, blood pressure control increased from 44% to 65% in the nurse intervention group compared to the control group, which increased from 44% to 53% ($p = .03$; an absolute difference of 12.6%). The mean annual cost of implementing the intervention was estimated to be $112 per patient (range $61–$259; Bosworth et al., 2009). The intervention did not lead to significant increases in overall observed inpatient or outpatient costs. There was no difference in the number of primary care visits over the two years (Bosworth et al., 2009).

In V-STITCH, the tailored behavioral intervention had its greatest impact among patients with diabetes. Among individuals with hypertension who had diabetes, those receiving the intervention had an increase in blood pressure control of 18.5% over the 24 months of the study, whereas patients receiving usual care had a decrease in blood pressure control of 6.6% (an absolute difference of 25.1%; $p = 0.038$). Patients without diabetes in both groups had a similar increase in blood pressure control. Despite the fact that the V-STITCH intervention was designed only to manage hypertension and has no diabetes-specific information, the intervention had a modest effect on A1c levels. Among the 150 patients with diabetes, those receiving the hypertension intervention had a mean absolute reduction in HbA_1c of 0.4% (95% CI: 0.8% reduction to 0.06% increase; $p = 0.09$) relative to a control group (Powers, Olsen, Oddone, & Bosworth, 2008). Thus, a focus on such self-management behaviors as exercise, medication adherence, and diet can lead to improvements in other outcomes.

IMPLICATIONS FOR HEALTH PSYCHOLOGISTS FOR PRACTICE AND RESEARCH

Self-management support for persons with chronic care needs requires an individualized approach and must acknowledge and address existing challenges patients may have. With the increasing introduction of psychologists into the primary care setting, health psychologists have a potential to play a significant role in the way health care is provided to our older and potentially vulnerable subpopulation of the United States. Areas where health psychologists may be able to provide support for individuals with chronic-care needs may include helping patients and providers prioritize multiple competing demands, educating providers to value and solicit patient preferences in developing individualized care plans including appropriate goal-setting and psychosocial support, implementing new and existing technologies to optimize such self-management as telemedicine, and proactively addressing and treating depression and other clear psychosocial barriers to effective patient self-management.

In terms of research, further investigation is needed to clarify complex chronic-care self-management needs and tasks and to develop the organizational infrastructure required to support its delivery in large populations. The development of relevant outcomes that capture the attainment of health goals and acknowledge the priorities of individuals with chronic-care needs is critical. Such measures might include achieving maximal function and independence, gaining confidence in managing diseases, minimizing preventable hospitalizations, and developing the ability to adapt to new health challenges in the face of ongoing self-management tasks. Additional areas of research require not only a focus on how to initiate behavior change but also, and perhaps just as important, how to ensure maintenance of these behaviors. As in the case of weight loss and smoking cessation, there are abundant data suggesting short-term improvements in behavior, but rates of success greater than 12 months are abysmal. Perhaps most important, it is critical that future work in this area consider the costs of implementing interventions and the ability to translate and disseminate successful models into real-world settings.

In the decades to come, the population of older adults living with chronic conditions and remaining in the community as they age will grow significantly. Individuals' ability to understand their choices, to make informed decisions about their care and actively participate in managing their chronic conditions, will be critical to maintaining their quality of life and preventing avoidable exacerbations of their illness. The traditional model of care in which patients are "fixed" by their doctor or nurse has proven too costly and ineffective. The challenge for the future will be to engage the chronically ill in collaborative care management and to prepare the health care system to provide not only the necessary medical expertise but also the requisite self-care management support.

WHAT ROLE SHOULD HEALTH PSYCHOLOGY OF AGING PLAY IN THE FUTURE?

As a research as well as a practice discipline, the health psychology of aging has many potential directions for the future. In 2006, the National Academy of Sciences Committee on the Future of Social Psychology and Aging evaluated where future contributions would make the most sense and devoted considerable time to developing models of behavior change (Carstensen & Hartel, 2006). Clinically, how can we best promote healthy aging for individuals as long as possible while providing behavioral treatments to individuals who suffer from age-related conditions and support for their families who must help them? What proportion of our effort should be aimed at basic developmental work that seeks to understand how psychosocial factors affect longevity and incident disease versus how psychosocial factors determine the coping processes required? Do we do this within the context of each disease-related specialty? Or is there some shared knowledge from taking an aging perspective? These are questions of strategy and tactics that will need to respond to the future climate for funding our research. Nonetheless, it has been extremely encouraging in a careful rereading of our key journals (*Health Psychology*, *Psychology and Aging*, and *Psychosomatic Medicine*) for the past 10 years that the number of research papers that treat aging in *Health Psychology*, health in *Psychology and Aging*, and their intersection in *Psychosomatic Medicine* are increasing in quantity, quality, and normalcy, such that the papers join maturing, exciting, and growing literatures.

CONCLUSION

The study of aging is now mainstream in health psychology. Research from a variety of sources on normal aging suggests that decrements in cognitive functioning are not generally to be expected to start until the decade of the 70s or to be severe until the decade of the 80s, whereas personality is generally stable until the end of life. Thus, changes before those times in the life cycle may have diagnostic significance. Cardiovascular risk factors also predict declines in cognition. Among the elderly, multiple chronic conditions that require management are the norm. These trends suggest an important role for health psychology as both a research and a practice discipline.

ACKNOWLEDGMENTS

This research was supported by National Institutes of Health grants R01 HL55356 from the National Heart Lung and Blood Institute (NHLBI) and cofunded by the National Institute on Aging (NIA); P01 HL36587 from NHLBI and the Duke Behavioral Medicine Research Center (BMRC) (Siegler).

We wish to acknowledge the editorial work by Danielle Briggeman, University of Maine. This chapter was supported by research grants 1RO1-HL67358 and 1R01-HL081290 from the NHLBI, The National Institutes of Health of the University of Maine. The content is solely the responsibility of the authors and does not represent the official views of the NHLBI.

This research was also supported by a NHLBI grant (R01 HL070713), a Veterans Affairs Health Services Research and Development grant (20-034), an Established Investigator Award from the American Heart Association, and a VA Career Scientist Award to Hayden B. Bosworth. The views expressed in this manuscript are those of the authors and do not necessarily represent the views of the Department of Veterans Affairs.

REFERENCES

Albert, M. (2008). Annual Busse Lecture. Duke University Department of Psychiatry and Behavioral Sciences. Durham, NC.

Aldwin, C. M., Park, C. L., & Spiro, A. (Eds.). (2007). *Handbook of health psychology and aging.* New York, NY: Guilford Press.

Anderson, G., & Horvath, J. (2002). *Chronic conditions: Making the case for ongoing care.* Princeton, NJ: Robert Wood Johnson Foundation's Partnership for Solutions.

Anderson, G., & Knickman, J. R. (2001). Changing the chronic care system to meet people's needs. *Health Affairs (Millwood)* 20(6): 146–160.

Bayliss, E. A., Bosworth, H. B., Noel, P.H., Wolff, J. L., Damush, T. M., & McIver, L. (2007). Supporting self-management for patients with complex medical needs: Recommendations of a working group. *Chronic Illness, 3*(2), 167–175.

Birns, J., & Kalra, L. (2008). Cognitive function and hypertension. *Journal of Human Hypertension, 23*(2), e86–e96.

Bogg, T., & Roberts, B. W. (2004). Conscientiousness and health-related behaviors: A meta-analysis of the leading behavioral contributors to mortality. *Psychological Bulletin, 130,* 887–919.

Bosworth, H., & Ayotte, B. J. (2009). The role of cognitive function in an applied setting: Medication adherence as an example. In H. B. Bosworth & C. Hertzog (Eds.), *Aging and cognition: Research methodologies and empirical advances* (pp. 219–240). Washington, DC: American Psychological Association.

Bosworth, H. B., & Hertzog, C. (Eds.). (2009). *Aging and cognition: Research methodologies and empirical advances.* Washington, DC: American Psychological Association.

Bosworth, H. B., Olsen, M. K., Dudley, T., Orr, M., Goldstein, M. K., Datta, S. K., … Oddone, E. Z. (2009). Patient education and provider decision support to control blood pressure in primary care: A cluster randomized trial. *American Heart Journal, 157*(3), 450–456.

Bosworth, H. B., & Siegler, I. C. (2002). Terminal change in cognitive function: An updated review of longitudinal studies. *Experimental Aging Research, 28,* 299–315.

Bracco, L., Piccini, C., Baccin, M., Bessi, V., Biancucci, F., Nacmias, B., … Sorbi, S. (2007). Pattern and progression of cognitive decline in Alzheimer's disease: Role of premorbid intelligence and ApoE genotype. *Dementia and Geriatric Cognitive Disorders, 24,* 483–491.

Carstensen, L. L., & Hartel, C. R. (Eds.). (2006). *When I'm 64.* Washington, DC: National Academies Press.

Chida, Y., & Steptoe, A. (2008). Positive psychological well-being and mortality: A quantitative review of prospective observational studies. *Psychosomatic Medicine, 70,* 741–756.

Costa, P. T., & McCrae, R. R. (1992). *Manual for the NEO PI-R.* Odessa, FL: Psychological Assessment Resources.

Costa, P. T., Jr., & Siegler, I. C. (Eds.). (2004). *Recent advances in psychology and aging. Advances in Cell Aging in Gerontology* (Vol. 15). Amsterdam, The Netherlands: Elsevier.

Cramer, J. A. (2004). A systematic review of adherence with medications for diabetes. *Diabetes Care, 27*(5), 1218–1224.

DiMatteo, M. R. (2004). Variations in patients' adherence to medical recommendations: A quantitative review of 50 years of research. *Medical Care, 42*(3), 200–209.

Dore, G. A., Elias, M. F., Robbins, M. A., Budge, M. M., & Elias, P. K. (2008). Relation between central adiposity and cognitive function in the Maine–Syracuse Study: Attenuation by physical activity. *Annals of Behavioral Medicine, 35*(3), 341–350.

Elias, M. F., Beiser, A., Wolf, P. A., Au, R., White, R. F., & D'Agostino, R. B. (2000). The preclinical phase of Alzheimer disease: A 22-year prospective study of the Framingham cohort. *Archives of Neurology, 57*, 808–813.

Elias, M. F., & Dore, G. A. (2008). Brain indices predict blood pressure control: Aging brains and new predictions. *Hypertension, 52*(6), e1014–e1015.

Elias, M. F., Elias, P. K., Sullivan, L. M., Wolf, P. A., & D'Agostino, R. B. (2003). Lower cognitive function in the presence of obesity and hypertension: The Framingham Heart Study. *International Journal of Obesity, 27*, 260–268.

Elias, M. F., Robbins, M. A., Budge, M. M., Elias, P. K., Brennan, S. L., Johnston, C., … Bates, C. J. (2006). Homocysteine, folate, and vitamins B_6 and B_{12} blood levels in relation to cognitive performance: The Maine–Syracuse Study. *Psychosomatic Medicine, 68*, 547–554.

Elias, M. F., Robbins, M. A., Budge, M. M., Elias, P. K., Dore, G. A., Brennan, S. L., … Nagy, Z. (2008). Homocysteine and cognitive performance: Modification by the ApoE genotype. *Neuroscience Letters 430*, 64–69.

Elias, M. F., Robbins, M. A., Budge, M. M., Elias, P. K., Hermann, B. A., & Dore, G. A. (2004). Studies of aging, hypertension and cognitive functioning: With contributions from the Maine–Syracuse Study, In P. T. Costa & I. C. Siegle (Eds.), *Recent advances in psychology and aging. Advances in Cell Aging in Gerontology* (Vol. 15, pp. 89–132). Amsterdam, The Netherlands: Elsevier.

Elias, M. F., Robbins, M. A., Elias, P. K., & Streeten, D. H. P. (1998). A longitudinal study of blood pressure in relation to performance on the Wechsler Adult Intelligence Scale. *Health Psychology, 17*, 486–493.

Elias, M. F., Sullivan, L. M., D'Agostino, R. B., Elias, P. K., Beiser, A., Au, R., … Wolf, P. A. (2004). The Framingham stroke risk profile and lowered cognitive performance. *Stroke, 35*, 404–409.

Elias, M. F., Sullivan, L. M., D'Agostino, R. B., Elias, P. K., Jacques, P. F., Selhub, J., … Wolf, P. A. (2005). Homocysteine and cognitive performance in the Framingham Offspring Study: Age is important. *American Journal of Epidemiology, 162*, 644–653.

Elias, M. F., Sullivan, L. M., Elias, P. K., D'Agostino, R. B., Sr., Wolf, P. A., Seshadri, S., … Vasan, R. S. (2007). Left ventricular mass, blood pressure, and lowered cognitive performance in the Framingham Offspring. *Hypertension, 49*, 439–445.

Elias, M. F., Sullivan, L. M., Elias, P. K., Vasan, R. S., D'Agostino, R. B., Seshadri, S., … Benjamin, E. J. (2006). Atrial fibrillation is associated with lower cognitive performance in the Framingham Offspring men. *Journal of Stroke and Cerebrovascular Disease, 15*, 214–222.

Elias, M. F., Wolf, P. A., D'Agostino, R. B., Cobb, J., & White, L. R. (1993). Untreated blood pressure level is inversely related to cognitive functioning: The Framingham Study. *American Journal of Epidemiology, 138*, 353–364.

Elias, P. K., Elias, M. F., Robbins, M. A., & Budge, M. M. (2004). Blood pressure-related cognitive decline: Does age make a difference? *Hypertension, 44*, 631–636.

Foster, G., Taylor, S. J., Eldridge, S. E., Ramsay, J., & Griffiths, C. J. (2007). Self-management education programmes by lay leaders for people with chronic conditions. *Cochrane Database System Review, 4*, CD005108.

Fried, L. P. (2000). Epidemiology of aging. *Epidemiologic Reviews, 22*, 95–106.

Gerstof, D., Smith, J., & Baltes, P. B. (2006). A systematic-wholistic approach to differential aging: Longitudinal findings from the Berlin Aging Study. *Psychology and Aging, 21*, 645–663.

Goldberg, L. (1993). The structure of phenotypic personality traits. *The American Psychologist, 48*, 26–34.

Hertzog, C., & Nesselroade, J. (2003). Assessing psychological change in adulthood: An overview of methodological issues. *Psychology and Aging, 18*, 639–657.

Hillman, C. H., Erickson, K. I., & Kramer, A. F. (2008). Be smart, exercise your heart: Exercise effects on brain and cognition. *Nature Reviews Neuroscience, 9*, 58–65.

Jackson, J. S., Antonucci, T. C., & Brown, E. (2004). A cultural lens on biopsychosocial models of aging, In P. T. Costa & I. C. Siegler (Eds.), *Recent advances in psychology and aging. Advances in Cell Aging in Gerontology* (Vol. 15, 221–241). Amsterdam, The Netherlands: Elsevier.

Jagust, W., Harvey, D., Mungas, D., & Haan, M. (2005). Central obesity and the aging brain. *Archives of Neurology, 62*, 1545–1548.

Jennings, J. R., Muldoon, M. F., Ryan, C., Price, J. C., Greeg, P., Sutton-Tyrell, K., … Meltzer, C. C. (2005). Reduced cerebral blood flow response and compensation among patients with untreated hypertension. *Neurology, 64*, 1358–1365.

Jerant, A., Kravitz, R., Moore-Hill, M., & Franks, P. (2008). Depressive symptoms moderated the effect of chronic illness self-management training on self-efficacy. *Medical Care, 46*(5), 523–531.

Jeste, D., Blazer, D. G., & First, M. B. (2007). Aging-related diagnostic variations. In W. E. Narrow, M. B. First, P. J. Sirovatka, & D. A. Regier (Eds.), *Age and gender considerations in psychiatric diagnoses: A research agenda for DSM-V* (pp. 273–288). Arlington, VA: American Psychiatric Association.

Johnson, M. L., Pietz, K., Battleman, D. S., & Beyth, R. J. (2006). Therapeutic goal attainment in patients with hypertension and dyslipidemia. *Medical Care, 44*(1), 39–46.

Katz, I., & Ganzini, L. (2007). Challenges of diagnosing psychiatric disorders in medically ill patients. In W. E. Narrow, M. B. First, P. J. Sirovatka, & D. A. Regier (Eds.), *Age and gender considerations in psychiatric diagnoses: A research agenda for DSM-V* (pp. 305–315). Arlington, VA: American Psychiatric Association.

Kern, M. L., & Friedman, H. S. (2008). Do conscientiousness individuals live longer? A quantitative review. *Health Psychology, 27*, 505–512.

Kershaw, E. E., & Flier, J. S. (2004). Adipose tissue as an endocrine organ. *Journal of Clinical Endocrinology and Metabolism, 89*, 2548–2556.

Knecht, S., Oelschläger, C., Duning, T., Lohmann, H., Albers, J., Stehling C, … Wersching, H. (2008). Atrial fibrillation in stroke-free patients is associated with memory impairment and hippocampal atrophy. *European Heart Journal, 29*, 2125–2132.

MacDonald, S. W. S., Hultsch, D. F., & Dixon, R. A. (2008). Predicting impending death: Inconsistency in speed is an selective and early marker. *Psychology and Aging, 23*, 595–607.

Madero, M., Gul, A., & Sarnak, M. J. (2008). Cognitive function in chronic kidney disease. *Seminars in Dialysis, 21*, 29–37.

Martin, L. R., Friedman, H. S., & Schwartz, J. E. (2007). Personality and mortality risk across the lifespan: The importance of conscientiousness as a biopsychosocial attribute. *Health Psychology, 26*(4), 428–436.

Martin, P., Long, M. V., & Poon, L. W. (2002). Age changes and differences in personality traits and states of the old and very old. *Journal of Gerontology. Series B: Psychological Sciences and Social Sciences, 57B*, 144–152.

McCrae, R. R., & Costa, P. T. (2003). *Personality in adulthood: A five-factor theory perspective* (2nd ed.). New York, NY: Guilford Press.

Mroczek, D. K., & Spiro, A. (2007). Personality change influences mortality in older men. *Psychological Science, 18*, 371–376.

Murray, A. M., Tupper, D. E., Knopman, D. S., Gilbertson, D. T., Pederson, S. L., Li, S., … Kane, R. L. (2006). Cognitive impairment in hemodialysis patients is common. *Neurology, 67*, 216–223.

Nathan, B. P., Bellosta, S., Sanan, D. A., Weisgraber, K. H., Mahley, R. W., & Pitas, R. E. (1994). Differential effects of apolipoproteins E3 and E4 on neuronal growth in vitro. *Science, 264*, 850–852.

National Institute on Aging (NIA). (2007). *Why population aging matters?* (NIA, NIH, Pub No, 07-6134). Retrieved from http://www.nia.nih.gov

Peterson, R. C., & O'Brien, J. (2007). Mild cognitive impairment should be considered for DSM-V. In T. Sunderland, D. V. Jeste, O. Baiyewu, P. J. Sirovatka, & D. A. Regier (Eds.), *Diagnostic issues in dementia: Advancing the research agenda for DSM-V* (pp. 52–65). Arlington, VA: American Psychiatric Association.

Poon, L. W., & Perls, T. T. (2007). *Biopsychosocial approaches to longevity: Annual review of gerontology and geriatrics*. New York, NY: Springer.

Powers, B., Olsen, M., Oddone, E., & Bosworth, H. (2008, April). *The effect of a hypertension self-management intervention on the unintended targets of diabetes and cholesterol.* Paper presented at the Society of General Internal Medicine 31st Annual Meeting, Pittsburgh, PA.

Purnell, C., Gao, S., Callahan, C. M., & Hendrie, H. C. (2009). Cardiovascular risk factors and incident Alzheimer disease: A systematic review of the literature. *Alzheimer Disease and Associated Disorders, 23*(1), 1–10.

Raz, N., Rodrigue, K. M., & Acker, J. D. (2003). Hypertension and the brain: Vulnerability of the prefrontal regions and executive functions. *Behavioral Neuroscience, 117*, 1169–1180.

Rice, D. P., & Fineman, N. (2004). Economic implications of increased longevity in the United States. *Annual Review of Public Health, 25*, 457–473.

Riegel, K. F., & Riegel, R. M. (1972). Development, drop and death. *Developmental Psychology, 6,* 306–319.

Robbins, M. A., Elias, M. F., Budge, M. M., Brennan, S. L., & Elias, P. K. (2005). Homocysteine, type 2 diabetes mellitus, and cognitive performance: The Maine–Syracuse Study. *Clinical Chemistry and Laboratory Medicine, 43,* 1101–1106.

Robbins, M. A., Elias, M. F., Elias, P. K., & Budge, M. M. (2005). Blood pressure and cognitive function in an African-American and a Caucasian-American sample: The Maine–Syracuse Study. *Psychosomatic Medicine, 67,* 707–714.

Saydah, S. H., Fradkin, J., & Cowie, C. C. (2004). Poor control of risk factors for vascular disease among adults with previously diagnosed diabetes. *JAMA, 291*(3), 335–342.

Schaie, K. W. (2005). *Developmental influences on adult intelligence: The Seattle Longitudinal Study.* New York, NY: Oxford University Press.

Seliger, S. L., & Longstreth, W. T., Jr. (2008). Lessons about brain vascular disease from another pulsating organ, the kidney. *Stroke, 39,* 5–6.

Seliger, S. L., Siscovick, D. S., Stehman-Breen, C. O., Gillen, D. L., Fitzpatrick, A., Bleyer, A., & Kuller, L. H. (2004). Moderate renal impairment and risk of dementia among older adults: The Cardiovascular Health Cognition Study. *Journal of the American Society of Nephrology, 15,* 1904–1911.

Shipley, B. A., Der, G., Taylor, M. D., & Deary, I. J. (2007). Associations between mortality and cognitive change over 7 years in a large representative sample of UK residents. *Psychosomatic Medicine, 69,* 640–650.

Shipley, B. A., Weiss, A., Der, G., Taylor, M. D., & Deary, I. J. (2007). Neuroticism, extraversion, and mortality in the UK Health and Lifestyles survey: A 21 year prospective cohort study. *Psychosomatic Medicine, 69,* 923–931.

Siegler, I. C. (1975). The terminal drop hypothesis: Fact or artifact? *Experimental Aging Research, 1,* 169–185.

Siegler, I. C., Bastian, L. A., & Bosworth, H. B. (2001). Health, behavior and aging. In A. Baum, T. A. Revenson, & J. E. Singer (Eds.), *Handbook of health psychology* (pp. 469–476). Mahwah, NJ: Erlbaum.

Siegler, I. C., Bosworth, H. B., & Elias, M. F. (2003). Adult development and aging. In A. M. Nezu, C. M., Nezu, & P. A. Geller (Eds.), *Handbook of psychology: Vol. 9, Health psychology* (pp. 487–510). New York, NY: Wiley.

Siegler, I. C., Poon, L. W., Madden, D. J., Dilworth-Anderson, P., Schaie, K. W., Willis, S. L., & Martin, P. (2009). Psychological aspects of normal aging. In D. G. Blazer & D. C. Steffens (Eds.), *Textbook of geriatric psychiatry* (4th ed., pp. 137–155). Washington, DC: American Psychiatric Press.

Small, B. J., Rosnick, C. B., Fratiglioni, L., & Backman, L. (2004). Apolipoprotein E and cognitive performance: A meta-analysis. *Psychology and Aging, 19,* 592–600.

Smith, A. D. (2008). The worldwide challenge of the dementias: A role for B vitamins and homocysteine? *Food and Nutrition Bulletin, 29,* S143–S172.

Sobel, D. S. (1995). *Partners with our patients: Empowering the hidden healthcare systems.* Seattle, WA: Dare Lecture Series.

Staessen, J. A., & Birkenhäger, W. H. (2004). Cognitive impairment and blood pressure: Que usque tandem abutere patientia nostra? *Hypertension, 44,* 612–613.

Stretcher, V., Kreuter, M. W., DenBoer, D. J., Kobrin, S., Hospers, H. J., & Skinner, C. S. (1994). The effects of tailored smoking cessation messages in family practice setting. *Journal of Family Practice, 39*(3), 262–270.

Suls, J., & Bunde, J. (2005). Anger, anxiety and depression as risk factors for cardiovascular disease: The problem and implications of overlapping affective dispositions. *Psychological Bulletin, 313,* 260–300.

Tang, W. K., Chan, S. S., Chiu, H. F., Ungvari, G. S., Wong, K. S., Kwok, T. C., … Ahuja, A.T. (2004). Frequency and determinants of pre-stroke dementia in a Chinese cohort. *Journal of Neurology, 251,* 604–608.

Taylor, V. H., & MacQueen, G. M. (2007). Cognitive dysfunction associated with metabolic syndrome. *Obesity Reviews, 8,* 409–418.

Terracciano, A., Lockenhoff, C. E., Zonderman, A. B., Ferrucci, L., & Costa, P. T. (2008). Personality predictors of longevity: Activity, emotional stability and conscientiousness. *Psychosomatic Medicine, 70,* 621–627.

Vingerhoets, G. (2001). Cognitive consequences of myocardial infarction, cardiac arrhythmias and cardiac arrest. In S. R. Waldstein & M. F. Elias (Eds.), *Neuropsychology of Cardiovascular Disease* (pp. 143–163). Mahwah, NJ: Erlbaum.

Waldstein, S. R. (1995). Hypertension and neuropsychological function: A lifespan perspective. *Experimental Aging Research, 21,* 321–352.

Waldstein, S. R., & Elias, M. F. (Eds.). (2001). *Neuropsychology of cardiovascular disease*. Mahwah, NJ: Erlbaum.

Waldstein, S. R., Giggey, P. P., Thayer, J. F., & Zonderman, A. B. (2005). Nonlinear relations of blood pressure to cognitive function: The Baltimore Longitudinal Study of Aging. *Hypertension, 45*, 374–379.

Waldstein, S. R., & Katzel, L. I. (2001). Hypertension and cognitive function. In S. R. Waldstein & M. F. Elias (Eds.), *Neuropsychology of cardiovascular disease* (pp. 15–36). Mahwah, NJ: Erlbaum.

Waldstein, S. R., & Katzel, L. I. (2006). Interactive relations of central versus total obesity and blood pressure to cognitive function. *International Journal of Obesity, 30*, 201–207.

Waldstein, S. R., Rice, S. C., Thayer, J. F., Najjar, S. S., Scuteri, A., & Zonderman, A. B. (2008). Pulse pressure and pulse wave velocity are related to cognitive decline in the Baltimore Longitudinal Study of Aging. *Hypertension, 51*, 99–104.

Weatherbee, S. R., & Allaire, J. C. (2008). Everyday cognition and mortality: Performance differences and predictive utility of the everyday cognition battery. *Psychology and Aging, 23*, 216–221.

Weiss, A., & Costa, P. T. (2005). Domain and facet personality predictors of all-cause mortality among Medicare patients aged 65 to1000. *Psychosomatic Medicine, 67*, 724–733.

Wilson, R. S., Beck, T. L., Bienias, J. L., & Bennett, D. A. (2007). Terminal cognitive decline: Accelerated loss of cognition in the last years of life. *Psychosomatic Medicine, 69*, 131–137.

Wilson, R. S., Krueger, K. R., Gu, L., Bienias, J. L., Mendes de Leon, C., & Evans, D. A. (2005). Neuroticism, extraversion and mortality in a defined population of older persons. *Psychosomatic Medicine, 67*, 841–845.

Wolf, P. A., Beiser, A., Elias, M. F., Au, R., Vasan, R. S., & Seshadri, S. (2007). Relation of obesity to cognitive function: Importance of central obesity and synergistic influence of concomitant hypertension: The Framingham Heart Study. *Current Alzheimer Research, 4*, 111–116.

Wolff, J. L., Starfield, B., & Anderson, G. (2002). Prevalence, expenditures, and complications of multiple chronic conditions in the elderly. *Arch Intern Med, 162*(20), 2269–2276.

Woolf, B. (1992). *Customer specific marketing*. New York, NY: Rand McNally.

Section V

Applications of Health Psychology

27 Psychosocial Factors in Cardiovascular Disease
Emotional States, Conditions, and Attributes

Julia D. Betensky and Richard J. Contrada
Rutgers, The State University of New Jersey

David C. Glass
Stony Brook University

Diseases of the heart and blood vessels are major sources of mortality, morbidity, loss of function, poor quality of life, and costs resulting from health care expenditures and reduced productivity. The burden of cardiovascular diseases is widely distributed around the world. The World Health Organization (WHO) estimates that it is responsible for 10% of disability-adjusted life years lost in low- and middle-income countries, and 18% in high-income countries. Once considered primarily a problem in industrialized nations, heart disease is on the rise in developing and transitional countries, partly as a result of increasing longevity, urbanization, and lifestyle changes (WHO, 2010).

For centuries, prescientific observations pointed to social and psychological antecedents of cardiovascular diseases. Potential psychosocial risk and protective factors have now been implicated by systematic research and include psychological stress, emotional states and conditions, social integration, socioeconomic status, and anger-related personality traits. Cardiovascular health psychology and behavioral cardiology are now highly active and productive areas of research and application. Their emergence was an important part of the development of the larger fields of health psychology and behavioral medicine. Moreover, in retrospect, the so-called traditional or biomedical risk factors for heart disease identified decades before the birth of health psychology and behavioral medicine—cholesterol levels, resting blood pressure, cigarette smoking, and blood sugar problems—themselves have major psychosocial determinants and ramifications. Cardiovascular diseases can now be seen as a largely psychologically and behaviorally induced set of conditions.

The goal of this chapter is to provide a selective overview of key concepts, findings, and issues in the field of cardiovascular health psychology. We begin by briefly outlining the major forms of cardiovascular disease, the traditional/biomedical risk factors, and the chief medical and surgical treatment modalities. We then describe psychosocial factors that appear related to cardiovascular risk and outline potential mechanisms for explaining their effects. In this regard, although we do touch briefly upon social and environmental factors, our emphasis is on emotional states, conditions, and personality constructs. In the final section we discuss some conceptual issues that confront researchers seeking to build upon existing knowledge in this area.

MAJOR FORMS OF CARDIOVASCULAR DISEASE

Cardiovascular disease and *heart disease* refer to a set of specific conditions that affect the heart and circulation. In the United States, cardiovascular diseases are responsible for approximately 26%–37% of all deaths, which exceeds the mortality rates for cancer (19%–24%), accidents (3%–6%), assault (5%), diabetes mellitus (4%–5%), and kidney diseases (3%; NCHS, 2005). The ascendance of cardiovascular disease (CVD) as a global health problem has stimulated a considerable amount of research on its diagnosis, epidemiology, etiology, prevention, and treatment. Major forms of CVD are described in the following sections.

CORONARY ATHEROSCLEROSIS

Coronary atherosclerosis, or *coronary artery disease* (CAD), is the buildup of fat and other substances that form plaque on the inner lining of the coronary arteries, the vessels that supply oxygenated blood to heart muscle. A number of processes are involved, including metabolic, hemodynamic, inflammatory, and hematologic activity (Hansson, 2005). As blood vessels become narrower, blood flow to the heart muscle becomes obstructed and is diminished. This process may begin early in life and progress asymptomatically for decades. When the narrowing becomes severe or when plaque ruptures, a platelet-clotting cascade may culminate in thrombosis that causes a sudden increase in the restriction of blood flow, in some cases closing off the blood vessel completely. Coronary atherosclerosis is a substrate for several conditions, including major forms of coronary heart disease, which are responsible for much of the burden associated with cardiovascular disorders. Coronary atherosclerosis and its sequelae will therefore be the focus of this chapter.

CORONARY HEART DISEASE

Coronary heart disease (CHD) occurs when the heart is inadequately supplied with oxygenated blood. Because the generic term for such a state is *ischemia*, CHD is sometimes referred to as *ischemic heart disease*. It has several clinical manifestations, as will be outlined here. Diagnosis is based on symptom presentation and results of tests that may include a resting electrocardiogram, cardiac stress testing, assays for certain enzymes in the blood, and coronary angiography.

Myocardial infarction (MI), or "heart attack," is death of a portion of the heart muscle caused by prolonged and/or severe ischemia. An MI is often precipitated by a rupture of plaque in a coronary artery that leads to complete blockage of blood flow through that vessel. Symptoms of MI include chest pain, shortness of breath, nausea, vomiting, palpitations, sweating, and anxiety.

Angina pectoris refers to pain in the center of the chest that may radiate along the left arm to the jaw or to the back. Angina has long been considered the cardinal symptom of myocardial ischemia. *Stable* angina pectoris is a syndrome of chest pain and other symptoms that are precipitated by physical activity and then cease when the activity is discontinued. *Unstable* angina is characterized by worsening ("crescendo") angina attacks, sudden-onset angina at rest, or angina lasting more than 15 minutes.

Silent myocardial ischemia is myocardial ischemia that is not associated with angina or other symptoms. It is thought to involve dysfunction of a network of nerves surrounding the heart that normally can produce pain. Painless ischemic episodes can be precipitated by effortful physical or mental activities. Their occurrence can lead to MI and sudden death.

Sudden cardiac death refers to cardiac death without warning. Although it typically follows within minutes after symptom onset, it can be asymptomatic. Sudden cardiac death may involve *cardiac arrest* (i.e., the sudden loss of heart function), which occurs when the electrical impulses in the diseased heart become rapid, chaotic, or extremely slow.

Heart failure is a condition in which a damaged heart is unable to pump adequately to meet the demands of the body for oxygen and nutrition. It may be associated with reduced blood supply to organs, pulmonary congestion, shortness of breath, congestion of peripheral tissues, and swelling in the lower extremities. Heart failure resulting from *systolic dysfunction*, which usually develops because the heart cannot contract normally, may lead to reduced blood supply to the body and lungs as well as myocardial enlargement. Heart failure resulting from *diastolic dysfunction*, which usually develops because the heart muscle (particularly the left ventricle) stiffens, often leads to congestion in the left atrium and lung blood vessels.

Hypertension is chronically elevated blood pressure, often resulting from reduced vascular elasticity. Hypertension is a major risk factor for coronary heart disease, stroke, heart failure, and kidney problems because it puts enormous strain on the heart and circulatory system. *Primary* or *essential hypertension* refers to high blood pressure that has no identifiable medical cause. *Secondary hypertension* refers to high blood pressure that is caused by another condition, such as kidney disease.

TRADITIONAL RISK FACTORS

The traditional risk factors for atherosclerotic CVD are older age, male gender, high total cholesterol levels, hypertension, family history, cigarette smoking, and diabetes. Also implicated are obesity, a sedentary lifestyle, a high-fat and -carbohydrate diet, low levels of high-density lipoprotein cholesterol, high levels of triglycerides, and high levels of C-reactive protein and other inflammatory markers. Many of these risk factors can be modified or controlled by lifestyle behaviors (i.e., physical activity, healthy diet) or medication. Some reports suggest that traditional risk factors account for approximately 50% of the variability in the risk for developing heart disease and that unexplained variance may be partially attributable to genetics (Allen, 2000). Although it is unclear how accurate this estimate is, formulae that combine these factors using the Framingham calculation provide a projection of the 10-year risk for CHD that can be used to guide therapy (Framingham Heart Study, 2007).

MAJOR TREATMENT MODALITIES

Many different classes of medications are used to manage CVD, including ACE inhibitors, angiotensin II receptor blockers, antiarrhythmics, antiplatelet agents, aspirin, beta blockers, calcium-channel blockers, digoxin, diuretics, inotropic drugs, statins and other lipid-lowering agents, vasodilators, and warfarin. Among other effects, these drugs may help control blood pressure, reduce cholesterol levels, lower the risk of thrombosis, or help rid the body of excess fluids. Cardiovascular patients often require more than one of these medications (AHA, 2010).

Balloon angioplasty is a commonly used procedure for opening blocked arteries. A small balloon is guided toward the blockage and is inflated to stretch the artery open and increase blood flow to the heart. Following angioplasty, a small metal mesh tube, a *stent*, usually coated with an agent that reduces risk of restenosis, is inserted to maintain the enlarged arterial opening. Rates of balloon angioplasty with stenting have increased because they are minimally invasive, highly effective, and require a relatively brief recovery time (AHA, 2006).

Coronary artery bypass graft surgery (CABG) is a common treatment for severe or multivessel CAD (AHA, 2004). It is a major surgical procedure that usually requires a three- to seven-day hospital stay. A blood vessel is removed or redirected from one area of the body and grafted to points in the coronary circulation near areas of narrowing to "bypass" the blockages and restore blood flow to the heart muscle. Depending on presurgical testing, CABG may be performed with traditional open-heart surgery or with less invasive procedures.

Pacemakers and implanted cardioverter-defibrillators (ICDs) are electronic devices for maintaining heart rhythm and for reversing rhythm disturbances, respectively. They can be implanted just under the skin of the chest during a minor surgical procedure. Several clinical trials have demonstrated that ICDs reliably terminate ventricular tachycardia and improve survival compared with conventional antiarrhythmic medical therapy alone (Connolly et al., 2000; Moss, Prosser, & Goldberg, 1996). Because recent technologic advances have led to reduced device size and improved firing specificity (Glikson & Friedman, 2001), the number of implantations performed continues to rise (Mond & Whitlock, 2008).

PSYCHOSOCIAL RESEARCH ON CORONARY DISEASE: CONCEPTUAL AND EMPIRICAL FOUNDATIONS

A very large body of research has been devoted to understanding the relationships between social and psychological factors and CVD. These efforts were prompted by limitations in the predictive power of more traditional risk factors, theory and research linking stress- and emotion-related biological activity to cardiovascular dysfunction, and suggestive informal observations by clinicians and researchers. They were also stimulated by increases in the prevalence of CVD during the first part of the 20th century and the expansion of its costs to society. Much work in the broad field of research on psychosocial contributors to health outcomes, reviewed in Sections III and IV of this volume, has involved cardiovascular endpoints. Similarly, the general theoretical frameworks, paradigms, and issues discussed in Sections I and II of this volume also have been informed by research on CVD. In this section, we will take a more disease-specific focus in discussing some of these topics.

DISEASE-PROMOTING MECHANISMS IN THE NATURAL HISTORY OF CAD

As noted earlier in this chapter, CAD underlies many forms of cardiovascular disease and therefore provides a useful focus of research on psychosocial influences on these conditions. However, the natural history of CAD affords more than one specific target for psychosocial research. As represented schematically in Figure 27.1, the possibilities include: (a) initiation of CAD in the context of genetic factors and early environmental exposures, (b) progression of CAD over many decades, (c) precipitation of clinical CHD, (d) the course of CHD, and (e) case-mortality in CHD patients. Psychosocial factors also may influence the patient's adjustment to the diagnosis and experience of CHD and its treatment. The importance and even the direction of the effect of a given psychosocial risk or vulnerability factor cannot be assumed to be the same across all these time points and outcomes.

It has proved useful to distinguish among the types of mechanisms that may define pathways linking psychosocial factors to the natural history of CAD and other disease outcomes (Krantz, Glass, Contrada, & Miller, 1981; see Figure 27.1). Direct, *pathophysiological* mechanisms involve biological processes, typically identified with stress or emotion, through which psychosocial factors may initiate or contribute to the etiology, pathogenesis, and clinical manifestation and outcome of CAD. Indirect, *behavioral* mechanisms involve actions or inactions that influence CAD risk or exacerbate its course, including cigarette smoking, dietary practices, and physical inactivity. *Reactions to illness* involve cognitive and behavioral responses to the symptoms and signs of disease, as well as to its treatment, and may contribute favorably or unfavorably to CAD outcomes through effects on health care utilization, adherence to medication regimens, and adoption of recommended lifestyle behaviors. Psychosocial factors have been implicated in CAD outcomes through effects on all three types of mechanisms. For the remainder of this chapter, we will focus on direct, pathophysiological pathways to CAD that reflect the effects of stress and emotion; the reader is referred to Chapters 1, 10, 12, and 14, this volume, for discussions of indirect and behavioral mechanisms and reactions to illness.

PATHOPHYSIOLOGIC PROCESSES LINKING STRESS AND EMOTION TO CAD

Stress encompasses (a) stressors, that is, environmental events and conditions that place demands and constraints on adaptive resources; (b) psychological responses to stressors, that is, perceptual-

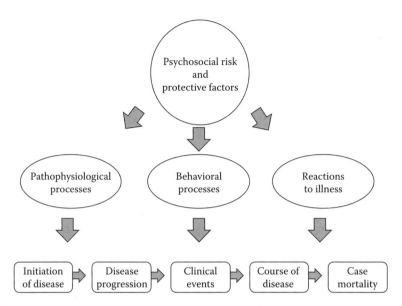

FIGURE 27.1 A general framework for research on psychosocial influences on coronary disease. Personal attributes and social-contextual factors may increase or reduce risk at multiple points in the natural history of coronary atherosclerosis and clinical heart disease. These influences may be mediated by separable though potentially overlapping and interacting pathways involving biological and behavioral processes and psychological reactions to disease and its treatment.

evaluative (appraisal) processes, emotions, and cognitive and behavioral responses, including coping activity, that may counteract or exacerbate stressors and their impact; and (c) biological responses, including potentially health-damaging activity of neuroendocrine, autonomic, cardiovascular, and immunological systems. Many stressors have been found to alter psychological and biological processes. Among those stressors linked empirically to CVD outcomes are major life events, occupational stress, and marital conflict.

There is a rich tradition of research concerning the effects of stress and emotion on the body (see Dougall & Baum, Chapter 3, this volume). Foundational contributions in this area include Cannon's (1929) characterization of the fight-or-flight response, which emphasized sympathetic-adrenomedullary (SAM) activity, and Selye's (1976) notion of a general adaptation syndrome, which emphasized hypothalamic-pituitary-adrenocortical (HPAC) activity. Considerable interest in the psychophysiology of stress and emotion was generated by the initial studies that examined cardiovascular and neuroendocrine measures as possible markers for mechanisms whereby the Type A coronary-prone behavior pattern might promote CHD independently of traditional risk factors (Dembroski, MacDougall, Shields, Petitto, & Lushene, 1978; Friedman, Byers, Diamant, & Rosenman, 1975; Glass et al., 1980).

Increasingly more sophisticated models have been developed to describe physiological processes that may explain how stress and related psychosocial factors may promote CHD (e.g., Harris & Matthews, 2004; Kamarck & Jennings, 1991; Kop & Gottdiener, 2005; Rozanski, Blumenthal, Davidson, Saab, & Kubzansky, 2005). As noted earlier and discussed at length by Kop (1999), a comprehensive framework must take into account the manner and point in the natural history of heart disease in which particular pathophysiologic processes are involved, which depends in part on whether stress and related antecedent factors operate chronically (over many years), episodically (from several months to a year or two), or acutely (in a matter of minutes or hours). Much of the physiologic activity promoted by stress is initiated and regulated by the SAM and HPAC systems. It involves multiple responses, including endocrine, autonomic, cardiovascular, hematologic, and immune and inflammatory activity.

Certain stress- and emotion-related responses have received particular emphasis in research concerning psychosocial influences on cardiac pathophysiology. These include abrupt hemodynamic changes, such as elevations in blood pressure, which may be involved in the initiation of CAD and in the precipitation of plaque rupture and coronary thrombosis. They also include elevations in myocardial oxygen demand, which may result in acute episodes of myocardial ischemia in CAD patients. In addition, stress can promote a state of hypercoagulation, permitting small thrombi to trigger blood clotting, acute coronary occlusion, and such acute cardiac episodes as MI or sudden cardiac death. Detailed reviews of these and other stress-related cardiovascular and hematologic processes thought to promote CAD and its clinical manifestations may be found elsewhere (e.g., Holmes, Krantz, Rogers, Gottdiener, & Contrada, 2006).

Many other biological processes have been studied as possible pathways through which stress and related factors may contribute to CHD. Examples include *heart rate variability* and concomitant patterns of autonomic activity, which have been linked to CHD outcomes (Carney, Freedland, Carney, & Freedland, 2009); *cardiometabolic syndrome*, a set of correlated risk factors that include an atherogenic lipid profile, elevations in resting blood pressure and plasma glucose, and insulin resistance, among others (Schneiderman, 2010); and *endothelial dysfunction*, in which changes in the inner lining of the coronary arteries cause those vessels to constrict under conditions that normally promote dilation, thereby reducing rather than increasing blood supply to the heart and potentially triggering myocardial ischemia and acute cardiac episodes (Harris & Matthews, 2004).

Perhaps the most active area of pathophysiologic mechanism–focused research in CHD since publication of the first edition of this handbook concerns immune and inflammatory activity (see Kop & Gottdiener, 2005, for a review). Although it is well beyond the scope of this chapter to detail the complexities of these systems and their potential role in accounting for the effects of stress-related psychosocial factors on CAD and its clinical manifestations, a few key points are worth highlighting. One is that immune and inflammatory processes involved in CHD may, in part, reflect responses to germs (Kop & Gottdiener, 2005). That is, chronic viral and bacterial infections appear to be involved in the initiation and progression of CAD (Epstein et al., 2000). Another is that immune and inflammatory activity appears to be associated with many specific physiologic pathways that culminate in CHD, including interactions with lipids that promote the progression of CAD, as well as processes of plaque activation, rupture, and thrombosis that may trigger acute CHD (Ross, 1999).

A third observation concerns various forms of feedback and bidirectional influence that involve immune and inflammatory systems (Kop & Gottdiener, 2005). Some of these operate within a single, biological level of analysis. These include cyclic processes through which inflammation and pathogenic lipid transformations promote one another and thereby contribute to atherogenesis, through which damage to heart tissue promotes inflammation, which, in turn, promotes further disease progression, and through which inflammation and blood coagulation are mutually reinforcing (Tracey, 2002). Other possible cyclic processes operate at multiple levels of analysis and involve biopsychological feedback in which such emotional factors as depression, which are potential causes of CAD and CHD (see below), are also promoted by CAD and CHD, through effects of proinflammatory factors on brain mechanisms that, in turn, alter mood states (Maier & Watkins, 1998). Although these complexities challenge simplistic notions about pathways linking psychosocial factors to CHD, they also present exciting opportunities in which contributions to the understanding of CHD pathophysiology may both inform and be informed by basic biobehavioral research.

Life Stress and CHD

Widely varying life stressors have been studied as potential risk factors for CHD. These include major life events such as bereavement (e.g., Kaprio, Koskenvuo, & Rita, 1987; Rozanski, Blumenthal, & Kaplan, 1999), as well as traumatic events such as earthquakes and terrorist incidents (Leor & Kloner, 1996; Steptoe & Brydon, 2009), all of which have been examined as precipitants of cardiac episodes. In addition, also receiving attention have been such chronic stressors as occupational stress (Bunker et al., 2003; Kuper, Marmot, & Hemingway, 2002; Yusuf et al., 2004), marital stress (Matthews & Gump, 2002; Orth-Gomer et al., 2000), and caregiver stress (Dimsdale, 2008; Lee, Colditz, Berkman, & Kawachi, 2003; Schulz & Beach, 1999). Ethnic discrimination has been identified as a source of both chronic and acute episodic stress for minority-group members (e.g., Brondolo, Gallo, & Myers, 2009; Thomas, Bardwell, Ancoli-Israel, & Dimsdale, 2006), and the study of daily hassles is emerging as a focus of research on chronic stress and CHD (see Bekkouche, Holmes, Whittaker, & Krantz, 2011), in part because of their purported association with increased inflammatory and procoagulant markers (Jain, Mills, von Känel, Hong, & Dimsdale, 2007). At least three studies found that risk of myocardial ischemia was elevated during periods of daily life stress (Barry et al., 1988; Bekkouche et al., 2011; Gabbay et al., 1996; Gullette et al., 1997).

Bekkouche et al. (2011) recently provided a useful framework for organizing research on the effects of stress and related psychosocial factors on pathophysiologic processes culminating in CHD. They proposed that these processes may operate at four stages, such that psychosocial factors influence (1) traditional CHD risk factors, (2) intermediate markers for CAD, (3) nonfatal clinical events, and/or (4) cardiac mortality. Bekkouche et al. then evaluated the evidence that stress-related physiological activity plays a role at each of these stages. Available findings indicate that stress may influence behavioral risk factors for CHD (e.g., smoking and poor diet), as well as biological risk factors (e.g., cholesterol and resting blood pressure levels). Stress also appears linked to changes in intermediate markers reflecting the progression of CAD, including endothelial function, inflammation, and platelet aggregation, as well as to processes that trigger nonfatal and fatal cardiac events, including myocardial ischemia, MI, and arrhythmias.

Interplay of Stress With Psychosocial Risk and Protective Factors

In the first edition of this handbook, Contrada and Guyll (2001) described a general framework for conceptualizing the ways in which personality factors might operate as stress moderators by interacting with stress processes in promoting or protecting against the development of CHD and other physical diseases. Here, we extend that framework to incorporate psychosocial factors other than personality that also may promote CHD through their interactions with stress (see Figure 27.2). Elements of this framework are based on a number of theoretical models, including those described by Leventhal et al. (Chapter 1, this volume), Scheier, Carver, and Armstrong (Chapter 4, this volume), and Smith, Gallo, Shivpuri, and Brewer (Chapter 17, this volume).

Stressor Exposure

The frequency and duration with which the individual confronts potentially stressful environmental demands and constraints may be influenced by three general processes whereby individuals determine their extent of contact with particular types of environments, referred to by Buss (1987) as selection, evocation, and manipulation. Stressor selection involves choosing whether or not to enter into potentially demanding environments, whereas evocation and manipulation refer to the person's impact on the environment once entered. In stressor evocation, the person passively elicits or provokes stressful responses from the social environment (e.g., because of a hostile demeanor or reputation), whereas stressor manipulation involves intentionally creating or modifying an environment in ways that increase its potential to initiate stress processes (e.g., through overtly aggressive behavior). A fourth way a person can influence stressor exposure is to prolong or minimize the duration of such exposures (e.g., failure to turn a task over to a more capable coworker). All four of these processes represent pathways whereby psychosocial risk and protective factors may initiate, promote, avoid, or reduce episodes of stress-related pathophysiologic activity.

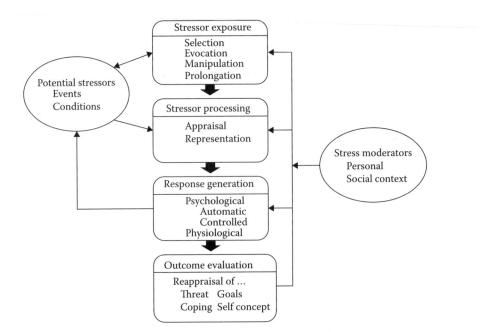

FIGURE 27.2 A model of interactions between stress processes and psychosocial moderators of stress. Personal attributes and social-contextual factors may operate as risk or protective factors in the development of coronary disease by influencing processes that determine the frequency and duration of exposure to stressors, cognitive and affective responses to stressors, physiological and behavioral activity, and feedback processes that alter the appraisal and interpretation of stressors, goals for the stressful encounter, coping activity, and self-concept and social identity.

Cognitive Appraisal

The process of cognitive appraisal is central to the influential theory of psychological stress formulated by Richard Lazarus (1966; Lazarus & Folkman, 1984). In this process, events and conditions that are recalled, ongoing, anticipated, or imagined are judged with respect to their relevance to physical and psychological well-being. Stress appraisals arise when the individual perceives that such circumstances tax or exceed his or her adaptive resources (Lazarus & Folkman, 1984). Whereas primary appraisal involves an evaluation of harm or loss that has already been sustained or is threatened, secondary appraisal involves an evaluation of available strategies and resources for managing the problem and its effects on the person. Stressful appraisals include harm or loss (damage already sustained), threat (possible damage), and challenge (threat accompanied by possible gain). Although often discussed in terms of conscious thought, appraisal is probably best defined as an automatic, effortless, cognitive–evaluative process. Given exposure to a particular environmental demand or constraint, psychological structures associated with risk-enhancing or risk-reducing psychosocial factors may act to increase or decrease the probability of a stress appraisal, thereby influencing the initiation, intensity, and/or duration of bouts of health-damaging biological activity.

Cognitive Representations

In their commonsense model of illness cognition, Leventhal and associates (Chapter 1, this volume) use the term *problem representation* to describe an interpretive process that is activated by the perception of health threats, a process that presumably is initiated by non-health-related threats as well. Problem representation refers to the formation of a mental structure that characterizes the stressor, reflecting both its specific attributes and the influence of preexisting schemas for particular kinds of stressors. Mental representations of stressors initiate and guide cognitive, affective, and behavioral responses and therefore play a role in the elicitation and regulation of physiologic responses that accompany stressful encounters. As with stressor exposure and cognitive appraisal, psychosocial factors associated with disease risk may influence the stress process by shaping problem representation.

Coping

Contrada and Guyll (2001) used the term *response generation* to encompass all the affected individual's psychological reactions following the initiation of cognitive appraisal and problem representation processes. Of chief interest in health psychology are *coping responses*, that is, cognitive and behavioral activities that are aimed at managing either the stressor or its effects on the person (Lazarus & Folkman, 1984). If the coping construct is to be useful, however, it cannot refer to all cognitive and behavioral responses to stressors. Lazarus and Folkman (1984) therefore restrict "coping" to activity that is conscious, deliberate, and effortful.

Many forms of coping have been identified in stress research and are often divided into two or more categories, with the most common distinction between *problem-focused* responses and *emotion-focused* responses. Problem-focused coping involves responses aimed at altering the situation that gave rise to the stress appraisal—for example, planning, seeking information, and attempting to master the situation. Emotion-focused coping involves responses aimed at managing subjective responses to stressors—for example, suppression of negative affect or fatigue, self-distraction, and denial. Several alternative coping classifications have been suggested in the coping literature (see Carver, 2011). Coping activity presumably plays a major role in determining how psychosocial risk and protective factors influence both the intensity and duration of health-damaging, physiological responses to stressors, as well as processes of stress modulation, including recovery and restoration (P. G. Williams, Smith, Gunn, & Uchino, 2011). In particular, effortful cognitive and behavioral responses to stressors, sometimes referred to as *active coping*, appear to be associated with potentially health-damaging elevations in sympathetic adrenomedullary activity and concomitant increases in blood pressure and heart rate (Krantz & Manuck, 1984).

Uncontrolled Psychological Responses to Stress

Exposure to stressors may elicit other, more automatic psychological responses that, like coping, may reflect the effects of psychosocial risk and vulnerability factors and may play a role in determining the course and outcome of the stressful encounter. Examples include motor patterns involved in the expression of emotion though facial movements (Tomkins, 1962) or vocal tone (Scherer, 1986), processes involved in the inhibition of communication between brain centers involved in emotion and language (Davidson, 1984), and implicit, nonconscious cognitive processes traditionally referred to in terms of such ego-defense mechanisms as repression (Haan, 1977). Rather than being conceived as a categorical distinction, the difference between coping and what might be referred to as automatic self-regulation may be conceptualized in terms of a continuum involving differences in the degree to which the activity is mediated by verbal-propositional cognition as opposed to schematic cognitive processing or, at a more rudimentary level, reflex circuits (Leventhal, 1979, 1980). Recently, Carver, Johnson, and Joormann (2008) made use of this distinction in an analysis of two potential CHD risk factors discussed later in this chapter, impulsive aggression and depression.

Outcome Evaluation

Self-regulation theories assign a key role to cognitive feedback processes whereby the person engages in information acquisition and interpretation on an ongoing basis, potentially altering cognitive appraisal and modifying problem representation (see Leventhal et al., Chapter 1, this volume; Scheier, Carver, & Armstrong, Chapter 4, this volume). Possible changes include perceived increases or decreases in the severity of the stressor or in the effectiveness of initial coping activity. Feedback may also lead to the addition, deletion, and reprioritization of specific coping goals and to broader psychological changes that affect self-perception (e.g., giving up and becoming helpless, or experiencing growth and a sense meaning from the experience). By influencing the evaluation

of coping activity, psychosocial risk and vulnerability factors form part of a dynamic conception of psychological stress and coping as ever-changing, transactional processes (Lazarus &
Folkman, 1984).

TYPE A BEHAVIOR: THE PROTOTYPICAL PSYCHOSOCIAL RISK FACTOR

A significant portion of the work that supports the observations outlined in the preceding section
involved or was stimulated by the Type A construct. The Type A behavior pattern (TABP) is a set of
behaviors that include competitive achievement striving, impatience and time urgency, hostility and
anger, and vigorous speech stylistics (Friedman & Rosenman, 1974). Measures of dominance and
self-confidence correlate with Type A behavior (e.g., Glass, 1977; Swan, Carmelli, & Rosenman,
1990); at the same time, however, feelings of self-worth and self-esteem in Type A individuals are
contingent on achieving success and recognition from others (R. A. Martin, Kuiper, & Westra,
1989; Sturman, 1999). The TABP construct initially attracted considerable attention as a psychosocial risk factor for CHD. Subsequently, research findings led to diminished interest in Type A in
favor of alternative constructs.

The prospective Western Collaborative Group Study (WCGS; Rosenman et al., 1975) first documented a predictive association between TABP and CHD endpoints. Over 3,000 healthy men were
recruited in 1960 and reexamined periodically over the next decade. After 8.5 years, 257 had been
diagnosed with CHD, reflecting an incidence that is almost two times higher in Type A than Type B
men, the latter group being more relaxed, less impatient, and less irritable. This result was obtained
after controlling for traditional risk factors such as cholesterol and cigarette smoking.

Subsequent prospective studies did not fully confirm the WCGS results (Booth-Kewley &
Friedman, 1987; Matthews, 1988). The association between global TABP and CHD was confined
largely to population-based studies with participants free of CHD at initiation of the study period.
Later reviews of TAPB and CHD research reached more negative conclusions (Myrtek, 1995), and
some researchers argued for abandoning Type A research altogether (Conduit, 1992). A 2002 review
paper on psychosocial factors and CHD devoted scant attention to global TABP, although it did
review evidence for a relationship between a TABP component—hostility—and CHD (Krantz &
McCeney, 2002).

TABP AND HOSTILITY

It was at about the time of waning interest in Type A that investigators began to minimize the role
of achievement striving and impatience in precipitating CHD and argued that hostility and anger
form the "toxic" components of the TABP (e.g., Siegman, 1994). Subsequent prospective studies
examined a variety of hostility and anger constructs, including cynical hostility (as measured by the
Ho Scale; Cook & Medley, 1954) and different forms of anger expression. The bulk of the research
relied on the Ho Scale (e.g., Dembroski & Costa, 1987; R. B. Williams, 1987), though studies using
other measures also yielded promising findings (e.g., Glass & Contrada, 1984; Kent & Shapiro,
2009).

It appears that hostility, characterized by general cynicism and interpersonal mistrust, may be
related to CAD outcomes and premature cardiovascular mortality (Miller, Smith, Turner, Guijarro, &
Hallet, 1996). Significant, albeit modest, effects of hostility on CHD morbidity (e.g., severity of atherosclerosis) and all-cause mortality have also been reported (e.g., J. E. Williams et al., 2000; see
also Kent & Shapiro, 2009, and Miller et al., 1996), but there have been negative findings as well
(e.g., Booth-Kewley & Friedman, 1987; Schulman & Stromberg, 2007). The risk ratio in studies
reporting an association ranges from 1.40 to 9.60 (Suls & Bunde, 2005). Suls and Bunde (2005)
observed that 7 of the 11 studies concerning hostility in healthy individuals showed that cynical hostility was statistically associated with subsequent development of documented CHD at either conventional or marginally significant levels. In patients with a history of CVD, higher hostility levels

have been associated with an increased risk for cardiac death, MI, and angina (Hecker, Chensney, Black, & Frautschi, 1988), as well as with more ischemia during stress testing (Helmers et al., 1993), more rapid progression of carotid atherosclerosis (Julkunen, Salonen, Kaplan, Chesney, & Salonen, 1994), and platelet activation (Markovitz, 1998). Anger may also interact with mental stress to contribute to the onset of malignant arrhythmias and elevation in markers of arrhythmic vulnerability (Lampert, Jain, Burg, Batsford, & McPherson, 2000; Strike & Steptoe, 2005).

A growing body of research suggests that hostility might alter several physiological processes relevant to the pathophysiology of CHD (Smith & Ruiz, 2002; see Kop, 1999; Rozanski, Blumenthal, & Kaplan, 1999, for reviews). For example, in healthy individuals, hostility is associated with exaggerated cardiovascular reactivity (Smith, Ruiz, & Uchino, 2004) and delayed recovery of cardiovascular responses to stressful situations, especially those that relate to interpersonal stress (Suls & Wan, 1993). It is also thought that hostility may contribute to CAD and CHD through behavioral pathways (Smith & Gallo, 2001), among them health habits (e.g., smoking, inactivity) and behavioral components of standard care (e.g., adherence to medication regimens, diet restrictions). Moreover, the purported role of hostility in social isolation, inadequate social support (Siegler et al., 2003), and marital conflict (Baron et al., 2007) may also partially explain its cardiotoxic effects. That is, in an example of stressor exposure processes described earlier, hostile individuals may interact with others in a quarrelsome manner that may both increase the frequency of exposure to stressful circumstances and reduce access to stress-buffering social support (Smith et al., 2004).

Anger has also been identified as an independent cardiotoxic factor. Where hostility is primarily an attitudinal construct, anger is characterized by affective experience and expression. In healthy individuals, some evidence indicates a positive relationship between anger and fatal and nonfatal MI (J. E. Williams et al., 2000), whereas other evidence is mixed. One longitudinal study reported that physically healthy older men with high levels of anger have a twofold to threefold increase in the risk of total CHD and angina pectoris compared with men reporting lower levels of anger, even after adjusting for potential medical confounds (Kawachi, Sparrow, Spiro, Vokonas, & Weiss, 1996). In another study, it was only when high levels of expressed anger were combined with low perceived social support that CAD patients were at significant risk for accelerated progression of atherosclerosis (Angerer et al., 2000; but cf. Matthews, Owens, Kuller, Sutton-Tyrrell, & Jansen-McWilliams, 1998). Among individuals with known CHD, investigations have variously reported a relationship between trait anger and CHD that was significant (Denollet & Brutsaert, 1998), marginally significant (Mendes de Leon, Kop, de Stuart, Bar, & Appels, 1996), or nonsignificant (Welin, Lappas, & Wilhelmsen, 2000). This work also has examined anger expression—that is, the tendency to be verbally or physically antagonistic—with several studies in healthy individuals reporting null findings, but others reporting that anger expression is associated with significantly greater CHD risk, especially among women (Haynes, Levine, Scotch, Feinlieb, & Kannel, 1978) and 48–59-year-olds (Carmelli et al., 1991). Findings are also mixed among populations with known CHD (see Suls & Bunde, 2005).

On balance, it appears that hostility, anger, and anger expression may increase CHD risk. Inconsistency in the findings precludes drawing firm conclusions in all populations (Krantz & McCeney, 2002). Nonetheless, it remains a plausible hypothesis that warrants continued examination (see Smith et al., Chapter 17, this volume).

TABP AND TIME URGENCY OR IMPATIENCE

Despite the current focus on hostility and anger, researchers must consider that other aspects of TABP may also be health-damaging. Support for this hypothesis comes from older research on Type A showing that irritation at time delay and competitive achievement striving predicted CHD incidence (Del Pino Perez, Gaos Meizoso, & Dorta Gonzalez, 1999; Matthews, Glass, Rosenman, & Bortner, 1977). The impatience or irritability factor has been related to general ill health and negative health-risk profiles (Hart, 1997). Exemplars of this line of research include a study by Spence, Helmreich, and Pred (1987) showing that impatience or irritability was significantly related to poorer health. Similar results have been reported for the relationship between time urgency and self-reported sleep problems (Conte, Schwenneker, Dew, & Romano, 2001). Moreover, Suls and Marco (1990) report that impatience was uniquely predictive of both illness incidence and severity. The cited studies assessed general somatic complaints, however, and their implications for CHD have yet to be determined.

Further support for the role of impatience or irritability in CHD risk comes from research examining sympathetic nervous system activation in stressful situations. A recent meta-analysis concluded that among TABP characteristics, impatience, not only hostility, is associated with cardiovascular hyper-reactivity to laboratory stressors (Chida & Hamer, 2008). Similarly, a review of studies of ambulatory blood pressure (ABP)—another index of SAM activation—concluded that impatience or irritability was associated with higher ABP levels in nonlaboratory settings, although the effect depended on the environmental circumstances in which measurements were made (Carels, Sherwood, & Blumenthal, 1998).

OTHER EMOTIONAL STATES AND CONDITIONS

As interest in Type A behavior gave over to a focus on its anger-related components, investigators began to examine other negative emotions as well. Research on depression has dominated in this work, but anxiety and neuroticism have also been examined. An overview of the main findings is presented next.

DEPRESSION AND CHD

Depression has emerged as one of the most promising predictors of CHD both in healthy populations and among coronary patients. In other words, depression may contribute to both the manifestation and worsening of CHD (Frasure-Smith & Lespérance, 2005). Research in this domain has encompassed various forms of depression along a continuum of severity and, occasionally, in terms of its components and such variable forms as hopelessness and vital exhaustion. Although prevalence rates of depression in patients with CAD range from 16% to 23% (Musselman, Evans, & Nemeroff, 1998), it is possible that depression is underdiagnosed in primary care environments (Freedland, Lustman, Carney, & Hong, 1992). Findings suggest that depressive symptoms and major depression are associated with increased cardiovascular morbidity and mortality even after controlling for other risk factors (Musselman et al., 1998).

Cardiac outcomes reported more than once include all-cause mortality, fatal and nonfatal MI, angina, cardiovascular death, and heart failure (Frasure-Smith & Lespérance, 2005). In one longitudinal study lasting 19.4 years, patients with moderate to severe depression at baseline were at 69% greater risk for cardiac death and 78% greater risk for all-cause death (Barefoot et al., 1996). A four-year longitudinal study revealed that individuals with major depressive disorder (MDD) were 3.9 times more likely to die of cardiac causes compared with nondepressed individuals at baseline, controlling for coronary risk factors and disease severity (Penninx et al., 2001). Recent meta-analyses continue to support an association between depression and CHD, though the consistency of the findings varies across prospective versus prognostic studies and they remain open to alternative causal interpretations (e.g., Nicholson, Kuper, & Hemingway, 2006; Suls & Bunde, 2005). Heterogeneity of samples and proper control of coronary risk factors across studies require greater scrutiny. Nonetheless, the sheer volume of findings provides a strong case for viewing depression as a likely CHD risk factor (Goldston & Baillie, 2007; Kent & Shapiro, 2009).

ANXIETY

Like hostility and anger, anxiety has been linked to the development of CVD in physically healthy populations (Kubzansky, Kawachi, Weiss, & Sparrow, 1998; Rozanski et al., 1999). As discussed by Suls and Bunde (2005), evidence for an association between anxiety and CVD is mixed. In healthy populations, studies report either a significant association (e.g., Kubzansky et al., 1997), a marginally significant association (e.g., Kawachi et al., 1994), mixed results (Coryell, Noyesm, & Housem, 1986), or no significant risk (Allgulander & Lavori, 1992; Hippisley-Cox, Fielding, & Pringle, 1998; R. L. Martin, Cloninger, Guze, & Clayton, 1985) associated with anxiety after adjusting for other CHD risk factors. There is a growing emphasis on research examining the effects of anxiety on prognosis in patients already diagnosed with CAD. For example, some research supports an association between anxiety and ischemic and arrhythmic events following MI (Frasure-Smith, Lespérance, & Talajic, 1995; Moser & Dracup, 1996). Likewise, in anxiety disorder patients, there is an increased incidence of MI, CHD, and other CVD conditions (Csaba, 2006). Similar to studies in healthy populations, however, several studies in populations with known CHD report null effects (see Suls & Bunde, 2005) or an inverse relationship (Ketterer et al., 1998).

NEUROTICISM

Neuroticism refers to individual differences in negative emotional responses (i.e., irritability, anger, sadness, anxiety, worry, hostility, self-consciousness, and vulnerability) to threat, frustration, or loss (Costa & McCrae, 1992; Goldberg, 1993). There is growing evidence that neuroticism is a correlate of multiple mental and physical disorders (Lahey, 2009). Individuals with high scores on neuroticism scales are more likely to express medically unexplained somatic complaints (Chaturvedi, 1986; Costa & McCrae, 1987), interpret their symptoms catastrophically, and seek medical care (Goubert, Crombez, & Van Damme, 2004). Neuroticism may be linked to CAD through its strong association with depression and anxiety disorders (Currie & Wang, 2005; Robles, Glaser, & Kiecolt-Glaser, 2005; Sareen, Cox, Clara, & Asmundson, 2005; Watkins et al., 2006), which are associated with abnormalities in cardiac (Barger & Sydeman, 2005) and immune (Maier & Watkins, 1998; Pace et al., 2006; Robles et al., 2005) functioning. Alternatively, some work also suggests that neuroticism itself is associated with CVD (Suls & Bunde, 2005) and a statistically significant 10% greater mortality from CVD, after controlling for many other risk factors (Shipley, Weiss, Der, Taylor, & Deary, 2007). More prospective studies that adequately control for potential confounds are necessary to elucidate potential direct and/or indirect effects of neuroticism on various cardiac endpoints.

STRESS REACTIVITY

Stress reactivity refers to physiologic changes provoked by stressors, usually in comparison with resting or baseline levels of the same variables (Holmes et al., 2006). Most often, reactivity is assessed with measures of heart rate or blood pressure, with fewer studies using methods for assessing underlying myocardial and vascular activity or for directly detecting alterations in neuroendocrine and autonomic systems. Initially examined primarily as a single-occasion response to stressors and a correlate of the TABP, evidence began to accumulate to suggest that stress reactivity is a stable characteristic, demonstrating temporal and cross-situational consistency (Krantz & Manuck, 1984).

Prospective studies have provided evidence to suggest that individuals who display excessive physiologic reactivity to stress may show heightened risk for carotid atherosclerosis CHD (Jennings et al., 2004; Kamarck, Everson, Kaplan, Manuck, & Salonen, 1997), coronary calcification (Matthews, Zhu, Tucker, & Whooley, 2006), and clinical CHD (Keys et al., 1971; but cf. Coresh, Klag, Mead, Liang, & Whelton, 1992). A program of research on cynomolgus monkeys fed a high-cholesterol diet demonstrated an association between heart rate reactivity to a laboratory maneuver (threatened capture) and extent of CAD (Kaplan & Manuck, 1999).

Studies in cardiac patients have implicated stress reactivity in the course and outcome of CHD. More reactive patients are more likely to show stress-induced myocardial ischemia (Blumenthal et al., 1995; Krantz et al., 1991) and more negative clinical outcomes over time (Krantz et al., 1999; Manuck, Olsson, Hjemdahl, & Rehnqvist, 1992). Several studies have shown that CAD patients in whom myocardial ischemia can be provoked by mental stress are at greater risk of subsequent clinical events (for a review, see Holmes et al., 2006).

MODIFICATION OF EMOTIONAL RISK FACTORS FOR CHD

Given evidence to support a possible role for emotion as a CHD risk factor, there has been a great deal of interest in determining whether interventions designed to modify emotional states, conditions, and personality attributes can have a positive impact on cardiovascular health outcomes. The goal has been to adapt typically effective psychotherapeutic interventions by making them compatible with the medication regimen, older age, and functional status of CHD patients (Lett, Davidson, & Blumenthal, 2005). The primary research questions in this intervention work include these: (a) Do pharmacologic and/or nonpharmacologic treatments aimed at reducing psychosocial factors linked with CHD (e.g., depression, Type A characteristics, stress) reduce psychological distress in CHD populations? (b) Do these treatments also affect CHD outcomes? (c) Do existing treatments need to be modified for a CHD population, and if so, how should they be modified?

EFFORTS TO REDUCE TYPE A BEHAVIORS AND EMOTIONAL DISTRESS

Early research suggested that modification of Type A behaviors was associated with better short-term outcomes (e.g., less incapacitation by disease when walking, higher maximal workload in an exercise test) as well as better long-term outcomes (e.g., lowered risk of recurrent MI compared with standard cardiologic counseling; Burell, Ohman, & Sundin, 1994; Friedman et al., 1986). Several studies that have examined the effects of empirically validated psychosocial interventions on depressive symptoms in CHD patients without documented MDD appear mixed in terms of their psychological and cardiovascular outcomes (Blumenthal et al., 1997; Frasure-Smith et al., 1997; Jones & West, 1996; Stern, Gorman, & Kaslow, 1983).

For example, among 106 post-MI patients, group counseling substantially reduced depression and improved other psychological variables but had no effect on mortality; patients in the exercise group, however, reported fewer major cardiovascular sequelae (Stern et al., 1983). In the Ischemic Heart Disease Life Stress Monitoring Program, psychological interventions that in part were designed to reduce stress initially appeared to reduce rates of cardiac mortality in nondepressed men with CHD (Frasure-Smith & Prince, 1985). However, in a follow-up trial, positive effects in men were not replicated, and there was a greater risk of cardiac mortality among women (Frasure-Smith et al., 1997).

A third study reported no reduction in anxiety, depression, or 12-month mortality among 2,328 post-MI patients participating in rehabilitation programs (e.g., psychotherapy, counseling, relaxation training, and stress management), although it reported a lower frequency of angina and medication use (Jones & West, 1996). In the Myocardial Ischemia Intervention Trial (Blumenthal et al., 1997), patients who took part in a cognitive-behavioral stress management intervention showed reduced ischemia and were less likely to suffer a cardiac event over a five-year period. More recent studies also indicated that exercise training, including formal cardiac rehabilitation, is associated with reductions in mortality, an effect that seems to be mediated in part by the effects of exercise in reducing psychosocial stress (Lavie, Thomas, Squires, Allison, & Milani, 2009; Milani & Lavie, 2007, 2009).

INTERVENTIONS FOR MAJOR DEPRESSION

One of the largest studies to date—the Enhancing Recovery in Coronary Heart Disease (ENRICHD) Trial—tested the efficacy of cognitive-behavioral therapy (CBT) versus usual care among postmyocardial infarction patients with major depression, minor depression, or dysthymia with a history of major depression (Carney et al., 2004). Although there was a statistically significant albeit small effect of treatment on depression at a six-month follow-up, there was no effect on recurrent MI or survival over the 3.5 year follow-up. However, patients whose depression persisted despite treatment had worse long-term survival than those whose depression remitted, suggesting that treatment-refractory patients may require more aggressive cardiologic care (Carney et al., 2004).

Given the efficacy of antidepressants among noncardiac patients with depression, several large randomized controlled trials have studied newer antidepressants (e.g., fluoxetine, sertraline, citalopram, and mirtazapine) to determine their safety and effect on both psychiatric and medical outcomes in CHD patients (see Kent & Shapiro, 2009; O'Keefe, Carter, & Lavie, 2009). In general, the findings suggest that these antidepressants are superior to placebo in reducing depression and psychosocial stress, but they typically fail to affect markers for pathophysiological mechanisms (e.g., inflammatory activity) thought to contribute to cardiac events and have not been shown to favorably alter the prognosis of patients with CVD. However, in line with some behavioral interventions described previously, a recent study suggests that compared to standard care, a CBT stress intervention is associated with a 41% reduction of fatal and nonfatal CVD and a 45% reduced acute MI rate at eight-year follow-up (Burell, Svardsudd, & Gulliksson, 2010).

CURRENT ISSUES AND FUTURE DIRECTIONS

The foregoing overview suggests many issues that might profitably be addressed in future work on stress- and emotion-related psychosocial factors in CHD. In epidemiological research, there is a need for more long-term, prospective research, better coverage of the more established risk factors, and greater attention to rigorous measurement of objective disease endpoints. Other issues concern pathophysiological mechanisms. Studies of blood pressure and heart rate reactivity should more often include assessments of underlying hemodynamic and autonomic events, and cardiovascular work could be better integrated with the use of neuroendocrine, immunological or inflammatory, and central nervous system assessments.

In addition to these kinds of epidemiologic and mechanism-related concerns, there are issues that arise from a distinctly psychological perspective. They are derived from a larger set of principles concerned with the generation and assessment of evidence regarding the validity of psychological measures and the relationships among constructs (Messick, 1981, 1995): (a) construct overlap and distinctiveness, (b) the genotype-phenotype distinction, (c) the nomological network, and (d) person–situation interactionism. Following is a brief discussion of these considerations.

OVERLAP AND DISTINCTIVENESS OF EMOTION-RELATED RISK AND PROTECTIVE FACTORS

Clear interpretation of psychological measurements depends on evidence of both *convergent* and *discriminant* validity. Convergent validity emphasizes commonality and concerns evidence that an instrument shows the expected associations with other measures of the same construct. Discriminant validity emphasizes distinctiveness and concerns evidence that an instrument shows the expected lack of association with measures of different constructs. It is often the case in health psychology that an instrument is prematurely considered to have validity based solely on convergence with other measures of the same attribute. As discussed next, neglect of discriminant validity considerations is involved in two sets of questions regarding the role of emotion constructs in promoting CHD.

Relationships Among Anger, Hostility, Anxiety, and Depression

Suls and Bunde (2005) have discussed the ambiguity created by conceptual and measurement-level overlap among health-related emotion constructs. The implicit model in much research on anger, hostility, anxiety, and depression appears to assume that their effects are independent and therefore does not address their intercorrelations, which are substantial. The few epidemiologic studies that have measured two or three of these constructs (e.g., Frasure-Smith & Lespérance, 2003; Mendes de Leon et al., 1996) have generated inconsistent findings. Suls and Bunde (2005) encouraged systematic research based on more sophisticated models that specify both the unique effects of anger, hostility, anxiety, and depression, including possible interactions among these constructs, and the role of their shared components.

Depression, Bipolar Disorder, and CHD: Type A Redux?

In addition to overlap across anger, anxiety, and depression, measures of each of these constructs may reflect characteristics from other conceptual domains. A case in point is the relationship between depressive and manic or hypomanic tendencies. Although depression has received considerable attention as a possible CHD risk factor, there has been less research on two bipolar subtypes of depressive disorder—Bipolar I and Bipolar II. According to the *Diagnostic and Statistical Manual of Mental Disorders* (American Psychiatric Association, 2000), their shared characteristics, in addition to periods of depression, include elevated, expansive, and/or irritable mood, inflated self-esteem or grandiosity, reduced need for sleep, pressured speech, flight of ideas, distractibility, increased goal-directed activity or psychomotor agitation, and greater involvement in pleasurable activities with potential negative consequences. Bipolar I is more severe and, unlike Bipolar II, also entails delusions and/or hallucinations accompanying manic episodes.

Limited available evidence has shown that individuals with bipolar illness are at greater risk for CVD than are normal individuals (e.g., Baune, Adrian, Avolt, & Berger, 2006; Sharma & Markar, 1994), have a higher prevalence of such CHD risk factors as diabetes mellitus and hypertension compared with general population estimates (Birkenaes et al., 2007; Cassidy, Ahearn, & Carroll, 1999; Johannessen, Strudsholm, Foldager, & Munk-Jorgensen, 2006), and show greater risk of cardiovascular mortality than do those individuals with other mental illnesses, including unipolar depression (e.g., Angst, Stassen, Clayton, & Angst, 2002; Osby, Brandt, Correia, Ekbom, & Sparen, 2001; Weeke, Juel, & Vaeth, 1987). Angst et al. (2002) documented greater risk of death from both cardiovascular and cerebrovascular disease in Bipolar I compared with Bipolar II. Fiedorowicz and colleagues (2009) found that a symptom burden index reflecting the proportion of weeks with manic or hypomanic symptoms was a significant predictor of cardiovascular death controlling for age, gender, bipolar subtype, antidepressive medications, and a depressive symptom burden index.

It therefore appears possible that manic or hypomanic symptoms play a role in the onset and progression of CHD. Use of self-report instruments for assessing severity of depressive symptoms may fail to identify individuals with milder forms of bipolar illness. Thus, as discussed by Barrick (1999) and Glass and Contrada (in press), there is a possibility that past research on unipolar depression and CHD has obscured important associations between cardiovascular disease and mania or hypomania. This suggestion takes on added significance in light of the overlap between features of bipolar mania or hypomania and of TABP, which appear to include irritability and anger, enthusiastic goal-striving, impatience and time-urgency, psychomotor agitation, less need for sleep, and energetic speech stylistics (Glass & Contrada, in press). Although there are also differences in the descriptors for bipolar mania or hypomania and TABP, the shared features appear extensive enough to warrant systematic attention.

GENOTYPE VERSUS PHENOTYPE

Greater understanding of a psychological construct is achieved when research goes beyond a descriptive level of analysis and begins to characterize factors that underlie its observable manifestations. In the case of emotion constructs implicated as CHD risk factors, the state–trait distinction may be a useful starting point (Suls & Bunde, 2005). Measures of time-limited states of anger, anxiety, and depression may, in part, reflect corresponding dispositions, in addition to other influences. Advanced multivariate statistical methods make it possible to model the effects of both trait and state forms of these constructs in relation to markers for pathophysiological mechanisms and disease outcomes.

Other ways to conceptualize the underpinning of health-related emotion constructs include cognitive, genetic, and neurobiological approaches. In most theories, cognitive processes are viewed as the initiating event in stress (Lazarus & Folkman, 1984) and emotion (Lazarus, 1991). Cognitive factors are also thought to play a key role in emotional disorders (Mathews & MacLeod, 2005) and emotional personality factors (e.g., Wilkowski & Robinson, 2008). The emotional symptoms represented in widely used measures of anger, anxiety, and depression may fail to capture upstream cognitive factors with potential explanatory power for models of stress, emotion, and disease. Similarly, research on psychosocial factors in cardiovascular disease is likely to benefit from consideration of the possible genetic bases of emotional conditions and traits (Lau & Eley, 2010), as well as from the utilization of conceptual models and methodological tools for understanding the neurobiology of threat-related information processing and the regulation of stress responses (Carver et al., 2008; Gianaros & O'Connor, 2011; Harmon-Jones, 2003).

The Nomological Network

Statistical control of better established predictors is essential in efforts to identify psychosocial risk and protective factors that may exert an independent influence on CHD outcomes. However, this is only a first step in causal analysis, and even at that the results can be misleading. Greater attention should be given to the potentially extensive set of causal and noncausal connections, or nomological network (Messick, 1981), through which antecedents of CHD are linked together. Kraemer, Stice, Kazdin, Offord, and Kupfer (2001) discuss several analytic problems that arise when standard approaches are applied to the study of medical conditions that reflect multiple genetic, environmental, social, and biological risk factors. They propose formal definitions and discuss statistical methods for distinguishing among five types of relationships among risk factors. Two of these are given ample attention in research on emotion and CHD: The possibility that *Risk Factor B is a proxy for Risk Factor A*, which can spuriously suggest a causal association, provides the motivation for controlling statistically for established risk factors; only then can it be determined whether *A and B are independent risk factors*, which is usually the focal hypothesis. Kraemer et al. also discuss the case in which *A and B are overlapping*, which we discussed in the preceding section. In the two remaining scenarios, *B mediates the effect of A*, and *A moderates the effect of B*. Given that mediation, moderation, and statistical methods for demonstrating their presence are becoming increasingly familiar in health research, they warrant greater attention in the analysis of epidemiological data. Moreover, as discussed by Kraemer et al., relationships among risk factors can take more complex forms that require even more sophisticated statistical modeling.

Person–Situation Interactionism

The TABP, discussed in the foregoing section as the prototypical CHD risk factor, was conceptualized as the observable outcome of a person–situation interaction in which susceptible individuals respond to certain kinds of environmental events and conditions (Friedman et al., 1975). Similarly, the concept of psychological stress emphasizes interactions involving a person's preexisting resources and vulnerabilities and situational demands and constraints (Lazarus & Folkman, 1984). From these theoretical considerations, from research linking measures of life stress to cardiovascular endpoints (e.g., Rozanski et al., 2005), and from the possibility of causal chains involving moderator effects (Kraemer et al., 2001), it follows that measures of stressful events and conditions warrant more frequent inclusion in epidemiological studies of anger, hostility, anxiety, and depression and CHD, which too often have focused solely on the main effects of either person attributes or stressors. In this sense, the study of mechanism-focused research on psychosocial risk and protective factors might provide a useful guide to its epidemiological counterpart.

CONCLUSION

Systematic research has substantially confirmed early speculation regarding the role of social and psychological factors in CVD. Although many questions remain unanswered and the field is not without its controversies and disappointing findings, it is difficult to deny that significant progress has been made since initial findings suggested that stress- and emotion-related variables may operate as independent risk factors for CHD. The study of psychosocial risk and protective factors for CHD is an inherently multidisciplinary endeavor. Nonetheless, psychologists have played a key role and should continue to do so in the future.

ACKNOWLEDGMENTS

We would like to thank David S. Krantz for his helpful comments on an earlier version of this chapter.

REFERENCES

Allen, J. K. (2000). Genetics and cardiovascular disease. *Nursing Clinics of North America, 35,* 653–662.

Allgulander, C., & Lavori, P. W. (1991). Excess mortality among 3302 patients with "pure" anxiety neurosis. *Archives of General Psychiatry, 48,* 599–602.

American Heart Association (AMA). (2004). ACC/AHA 2004 Guideline update for coronary artery bypass graft surgery. *Circulation, 110,* e340–e437.

American Heart Association (AMA). (2006). ACC/AHA/SCAI Practice guidelines, February 21, 2006. *Circulation, 113,* e166–e286.

American Heart Association (AMA). (2010). *Medications commonly used to treat heart failure.* Retrieved from http://www.americanheart.org/presenter.jhtml?identifier=118

American Psychiatric Association (APA). (2000). *Diagnostic and statistical manual of mental disorders* (DSM-IV-TR, 4th ed.). Washington, DC: American Psychiatric Press.

Angerer P., Siebert, U., Kothny, W., Mühlbauer, D., Mudra, H., & von Schacky, C. (2000). Impact of social support, cynical hostility and anger expression on progression of coronary atherosclerosis. *Journal of the American College of Cardiology, 36,* 1781–1788.

Angst, F., Stassen, H. H., Clayton, P. J., & Angst, J. (2002). Mortality of patients with mood disorders: Follow-up over 34–38 years. *Journal of Affective Disorders, 68,* 167–181.

Barefoot, J. C., Helms, M. J., Mark, D. B., Blumenthal, J. A., Califf, R. M., Haney, T. L., … Williams, R. B. (1996). Depression and long-term mortality risk in patients with coronary artery disease. *American Journal of Cardiology, 78,* 613–617.

Barger, S. D., & Sydeman, S. J. (2005). Does generalized anxiety disorder predict coronary heart disease risk factors independently of major depressive disorder? *Journal of Affective Disorders, 88,* 87–91.

Baron, K. G., Smith, T. W., Butner, J., Nealey-Moore, J., Hawkins, M. W., & Uchino, B. N. (2007). Hostility, anger, and marital adjustment: concurrent and prospective associations with psychosocial vulnerability. *Journal of Behavioral Medicine, 30,* 1–10.

Barrick, C. B. (1999). Sad, glad or mad hearts? Epidemiological evidence for a causal relationship between mood disorders and coronary artery disease. *Journal of Affective Disorders, 53,* 193–201.

Barry, J., Selwyn, A. P., Nabel, E. G., Rocco, M. B., Mead, K., Campbell, S., & Rebecca, G. (1988). Frequency of ST-segment depression produced by mental stress in stable angina pectoris from coronary artery disease. *American Journal of Cardiology. 61,* 989–993.

Baune, B. T., Adrian, I., Avolt, V., & Berger, K. (2006). Associations between major depression, bipolar disorders, dysthymia and cardiovascular diseases in the general adult population. *Psychotherapy and Psychosomatics, 75,* 319–326.

Bekkouche, N. S., Holmes, S., Whittaker, K. S., & Krantz, D. S. (2011). Stress and the heart: Psychosocial stress and coronary heart disease. In R. J. Contrada & A. Baum (Eds.), *Handbook of stress science: Psychology, biology, and health,* (pp. 385–398). New York, NY: Springer.

Birkenaes, A. B., Opjordsmoen, S., Brunborg, C., Engh, J. A., Jonsdottir, H., & Andreassen, O. A. (2007). The level of cardiovascular risk factors in bipolar disorder equals that of schizophrenia: A comparative study. *Journal of Clinical Psychiatry, 68,* 917–923.

Blumenthal, J. A., Jiang, W., Babyak, M. A., Krantz, D. S., Frid, D. J., Coleman, R. E., … Morris, J. J. (1997). Stress management and exercise training in cardiac patients with myocardial ischemia: effects on prognosis and evaluation of mechanisms. *Archives of Internal Medicine, 157*, 2213–2223.

Blumenthal, J. A., Jiang, W., Waugh, R. A., Frid, D. J., Morris, J. J., Coleman, R. E., … O'Connor, C. (1995). Mental stress–induced ischemia in the laboratory and ambulatory ischemia during daily life: Association and hemodynamic features. *Circulation, 92*, 2102–2108.

Booth-Kewley, S., & Friedman, H. S. (1987). Psychological predictors of heart disease: A quantitative review. *Psychological Bulletin, 101*, 343–362.

Brondolo, E., Gallo, L. C., & Myers, H. F. (2009). Race, racism and health: disparities, mechanisms, and interventions. *Journal of Behavioral Medicine, 32*, 1–8.

Bunker, S. J., Colquhoun, D. M., Esler, M. D., Hickie, I. B., Hunt, D., Jelinek, V. M., … Tonkin, A. M. (2003). "Stress" and coronary heart disease: psychosocial risk factors. *Medical Journal of Australia, 178*, 272–276.

Burell, G., Ohman, A., & Sundin, O. (1994). Modification of the type A behavior pattern in Post-myocardial infarction patients: A route to cardiac rehabilitation. *International Journal of Behavioral Medicine, 1*, 32–54.

Burell, G. K., Svardsudd, M. D., & Gulliksson, M. (2010, March). *Stress management prolongs life for CHD patients: A randomized clinical trial assessing the effects of group intervention on all cause mortality, recurrent cardiovascular disease and quality of life.* Abstract 1624 from Paper Session 7 at American Psychosomatic Society meeting. Abstract retrieved from http://www.psychosomatic.org/events/meeting2010/APSProgram2010.pdf

Buss, D. M. (1987). Selection, evocation, and manipulation. *Journal of Personality and Social Psychology, 53*, 1214–1221.

Cannon, W. B. (1929). *Bodily changes in pain, hunger, fear, and rage* (2nd ed.). Oxford, England: Appleton.

Carels, R. A., Sherwood, A., & Blumenthal, J. A. (1998). Psychosocial influences on blood pressure during daily life. *International Journal of Psychophysiology, 28*, 117–129.

Carmelli, D., Halpern, J., Swan, G. E., Dame, A., McElroy, M., Gelb, A. B., & Rosenman, R. H. (1991). 27-year mortality in the Western Collaborative Group Study: Construction of risk groups by recursive partitioning. *Journal of Clinical Epidemiology, 44*, 1341–1351.

Carney, R. M., Blumenthal, J. A., Freedland, K. E., Youngblood, M., Veith, R. C., Burg, M. M., … Jaffe, A. S [ENRICHD Investigators]. (2004). Depression and late mortality after myocardial infarction in the Enhancing Recovery in Coronary Heart Disease (ENRICHD) Study. *Psychosomatic Medicine, 66*, 466–474.

Carney, R. M., Freedland, K. E., Carney, R. M., & Freedland, K. E. (2009). Depression and heart rate variability in patients with coronary heart disease. *SO—Cleveland Clinic Journal of Medicine, 76*(Suppl. 2), S13–S17.

Carver, C. S. (2011). Coping. In R. J. Contrada & A. Baum (Eds.), *Handbook of stress science: Psychology, biology, and health.* (pp. 221–229). New York, NY: Springer.

Carver, C. S., & Connor-Smith, J. (2010). Personality and coping. *Annual Review of Psychology, 61*, 679–704.

Carver, C. S., Johnson, S. L., & Joormann, J. (2008). Serotonergic function, two-mode models of self-regulation, and vulnerability to depression: What depression has in common with impulsive aggression. *Psychological Bulletin, 134*, 912–943.

Cassidy, F., Ahearn, E., & Carroll, B. J. (1999). Elevated frequency of diabetes mellitus in hospitalized manic-depressive patients. *American Journal of Psychiatry, 156*, 1417–1420.

Chaturvedi, S. K. (1986). Chronic idiopathic pain disorder. *Journal of Psychosomatic Research, 30*, 199–203.

Chida, Y., & Hamer, M. (2008). Chronic psychosocial factors and acute physiological responses to laboratory-induced stress in healthy populations: A quantitative review of 30 years of investigations. *Psychological Bulletin, 134*, 829–885.

Conduit, E. H. (1992). If A-B does not predict heart disease, why bother with it? A clinician's view. *British Journal of Medical Psychology, 65*, 289–296.

Connolly, S. J., Gent, M., Roberts, R. S., Dorian, P., Roy, D., Sheldon, R. S., … O'Brien, B. (2000). Canadian implantable defibrillator study (CIDS): A randomized trial of the implantable cardioverter defibrillator against amiodarone. *Circulation, 101*, 1297–1302.

Conte, J. M., Schwenneker, H. H., Dew, A. F., & Romano, D. M. (2001). Incremental validity of time urgency and other type A subcomponents in predicting behavioral and health criteria. *Journal of Applied Social Psychology, 31*, 1727–1748.

Contrada, R. J., & Guyll, M. (2001). On who gets sick and why: The role of personality, stress, and disease (pp. 59–81). In A. Baum, T. A. Revenson, & J. E. Singer (Eds.), *Handbook of health psychology.* Hillsdale, NJ: Erlbaum.

Cook, W., & Medley, D. (1954). Proposed hostility for pharisaic-virtue skills of the MMPI. *Journal of Applied Psychology, 38*, 414–418.

Coresh, J., Klag, M. J., Mead, L. A., Liang, K. Y., & Whelton, P. K. (1992). Vascular reactivity in young adults and cardiovascular disease. A prospective study. *Hypertension, 19*, II218–II223.

Coryell, W., Noyesm, R., Jr., & Housem, J. D. (1986). Mortality among outpatients with anxiety disorders. *American Journal of Psychiatry, 143*, 508–510.

Costa, P. T., & McCrae, P. T. (1987). Neuroticism, somatic complaints, and disease: Is the bark worse than the bite? *Journal of Personality, 55*, 299–316.

Costa, P. T., Jr., & McCrae, R. R. (1992). Normal personality assessment in clinical practice: The NEO Personality Inventory. *Psychological Assessment, 4*, 5–13.

Csaba, B. M. (2006). Anxiety as an independent cardiovascular risk. *Neuropsychopharmacologia Hungarica, 8*, 5–11.

Currie, S. R., & Wang, J. (2005). More data on major depression as an antecedent risk factor for first onset of chronic back pain. *Psychological Medicine, 35*, 1275–1282.

Davidson, R. (1984). Affect, cognition, and hemispheric specialization. In C. E. Izard, J. Kagan, & R. B. Zajonc (Eds.), *Emotions, cognition, and behavior* (pp. 320–365). New York, NY: Cambridge University Press.

Del Pino Perez, A., Gaos Meizoso, M. T., & Dorta Gonzalez, R. (1999). Validity of the structured interview for the assessment of type A behavior pattern. *European Journal of Psychological Assessment, 15*, 39–48.

Dembroski, T. M., & Costa, P. (1987). Coronary-prone behavior: Components of the type A pattern and hostility. *Journal of Personality, 55*, 211–236.

Dembroski, T. M., MacDougall, J. M., Shields, J. L., Petitto, J., & Lushene, R. (1978). Components of the type A coronary-prone behavior pattern and cardiovascular responses to psychomotor performance challenge. *Journal of Behavioral Medicine, 1*, 159–176.

Denollet, J., & Brutsaert, D. L. (1998). Personality, disease severity, and the risk of long-term cardiac events in patients with a decreased ejection fraction after myocardial infarction. *Circulation, 97*, 167–173.

Dimsdale, J. E. (2008). Psychological stress and cardiovascular disease. *Journal of the American College of Cardiology, 51*, 1237–1246.

Epstein, S. E., Zhu, J., Burnett, M. S., Zhou, Y. F., Vercellotti, G., & Hajjar, D. (2000). Infection and atherosclerosis: potential roles of pathogen burden and molecular mimicry. *Arteriosclerosis, Thrombosis, and Vascular Biology, 20*, 1417–1420.

Fiedorowicz, J. G., Solomon, D. A., Endicott, J., Leon, A. C., Crunshan, Li, Rice J. P., & Coryell, W. H. (2009). Manic/hypomanic symptom burden and cardiovascular mortality in bipolar disorder. *Psychosomatic Medicine, 71*, 598–606.

Framingham Heart Study. (2007, September 20). Retrieved from National Institutes of Health National Heart, Lung, and Blood Institute website http://www.nhlbi.nih.gov/about/framingham/index.html

Frasure-Smith, N., & Lespérance, F. (2003). Depression—A cardiac risk factor in search of a treatment. *Journal of the American Medical Association, 289*, 3171–3173.

Frasure-Smith, N., & Lespérance, F. (2005). Reflections on depression as a cardiac risk factor. *Psychosomatic Medicine, 67*, S19–S25.

Frasure-Smith, N., Lespérance, F., Prince, R. H., Verrier, P., Garber, R. A., Juneau, M., … Bourassa, M. G. (1997). Randomised trial of home-based psychosocial nursing intervention for patients recovering from myocardial infarction. *Lancet, 350*, 473–479.

Frasure-Smith, N., Lespérance, F., & Talajic, M. (1995). The impact of negative emotions on prognosis following myocardial infarction: is it more than depression? *Health Psychology, 14*, 388–398.

Frasure-Smith, N., & Prince, R. (1985). The ischemic heart disease life stress monitoring program: impact on mortality. *Psychosomatic Medicine, 47*, 431–445.

Freedland, K. E., Lustman, P. J., Carney, R. M., & Hong, B. A. (1992). Underdiagnosis of depression in patients with coronary artery disease: The role of nonspecific symptoms. *International Journal of Psychiatry in Medicine, 22*, 221–229.

Friedman, M., Byers, S. O., Diamant, J., & Rosenman, R. H. (1975). Plasma catecholamine response of coronary-prone subjects (type A) to a specific challenge. *Metabolism: Clinical & Experimental, 24*, 205–210.

Friedman, M., & Rosenman, R. H. (1974). *Type A behavior and your heart.* New York, NY: Knopf.

Friedman, M., Thoresen, C., Gill, J., Ulmer, D., Powell, L. H., Price, V. A., … Bourg, E. (1986). Alteration of type A behavior and its effect on cardiac recurrences in post myocardial infarction patients: summary results of the recurrent coronary prevention project. *American Heart Journal, 112*, 653–665.

Gabbay, F. H., Krantz, D. S., Kop, W. J., Hedges, S. M., Klein, J., Gottdiener, J. S., & Rozanski, A. (1996). Triggers of myocardial ischemia during daily life in patients with coronary artery disease: physical and mental activities, anger and smoking. *Journal of the American College of Cardiology, 27*, 585–592.

Gianaros, P. J., & O'Connor, M. F. (2011). Neuroimaging methods in human stress science. In R. J. Contrada & A. Baum (Eds.), *Handbook of stress science: Psychology, biology, and health.* (pp. 543–563). New York, NY: Springer.

Glass, D. C. (1977). *Behavior patterns, stress, and coronary disease.* Hillsdale, NJ: Erlbaum.

Glass, D. C., & Contrada, R. J. (1984). Type A behavior and catecholamines: A critical review. In M. G. Ziegler & C. R. Lake (Eds.), *Norepinephrine: Frontiers in clinical neuroscience* (Vol. 2). Baltimore, MD: Williams & Wilkins.

Glass, D. C., & Contrada, R. J. (in press). Bipolar disorder, Type A behaviour, and coronary disease. *Health Psychology Review.*

Glass, D. C., Krakoff, L. R., Contrada, R., Hilton, W. F., Kehoe, K., Mannucci, E. G., … Elting, E. (1980). Effect of harassment and competition upon cardiovascular and plasma catecholamine responses in type A and type B individuals. *Psychophysiology, 17,* 453–463.

Glikson M, & Friedman, P. A. (2001). The implantable cardioverter defibrillator. *Lancet, 357,* 1107–1117.

Goldberg, L. R. (1993). The structure of phenotypic personality traits. *American Psychologist, 48,* 26–34.

Goldston, K., & Baillie, A. J. (2007). Depression and coronary heart disease: A review of the epidemiological evidence, explanatory mechanisms and management approaches. *Clinical Psychology Review, 28,* 288–306.

Goubert, L., Crombez, G., & Van Damme, S. (2004). The role of neuroticism, pain catastrophizing and pain-related fear in vigilance to pain: A structural equations approach. *Pain, 107,* 234–241.

Gullette, E. C., Blumenthal, J. A., Babyak, M., Jiang, W., Waugh, R.A., Frid, D. J., … Krantz, D. S. (1997). Effects of mental stress on myocardial ischemia during daily life. *Journal of the American Medical Association, 277,* 1521–1526.

Haan, N. (1977). *Coping and defending.* New York, NY: Academic Press.

Hansson, J. K. (2005). Inflammation, atherosclerosis, and coronary artery disease. *New England Journal of Medicine, 352,* 1685–1695.

Harmon-Jones, E. (2003). Anger and the behavioral approach system. *Personality and Individual Differences, 35,* 995–1005.

Hart, K. E. (1997). A moratorium on research using the Jenkins Activity Survey for type A behavior. *Journal of Clinical Psychology, 53,* 905–907.

Harris, K. F., & Matthews, K. A. (2004). Interactions between autonomic nervous system activity and endothelial function: A model for the development of cardiovascular disease. *Psychosomatic Medicine, 66,* 153–164.

Haynes, S. G., Levine, S., Scotch, N., Feinlieb, M., & Kannel, W. B. (1978). The relationship of psychosocial factors to coronary heart disease in the Framingham Study: I. Methods and risk factors. *American Journal of Epidemiology, 107,* 362–383.

Hecker, M. H., Chesney, M. A., Black, G. W., & Frautschi, N. (1988). Coronary-prone behaviors in the Western Collaborative Group Study. *Psychosomatic Medicine, 50,* 153–164.

Helmers, K. F., Krantz, D. S., Howell, R. H., Klein, J., Bairey, C. N., & Rozanski, A. (1993). Hostility and myocardial ischemia in coronary artery disease patients: evaluation by gender and ischemic index. *Psychosomatic Medicine, 55,* 29–36.

Hippisley-Cox, J., Fielding, K., & Pringle, M. (1998). Depression as a risk factor for ischaemic heart disease in men: Population based case-control study. *British Medical Journal, 316,* 1714–1719.

Holmes, S. D., Krantz, D. S., Rogers, H., Gottdiener, J., & Contrada, R. J. (2006). Mental stress and coronary artery disease: a multidisciplinary guide. *Progress in Cardiovascular Disease, 49,* 106–122.

Jain, S., Mills, P. J., von Känel, R., Hong, S., & Dimsdale, J. E. (2007). Effects of perceived stress and uplifts on inflammation and coagulability. *Psychophysiology, 44,* 154–160.

Jennings, J. R., Kamarck, T. W., Everson-Rose, S. A., Kaplan, G. A., Manuck, S. B., & Salonen, J. T. (2004). Exaggerated blood pressure responses during mental stress are prospectively related to enhanced carotid atherosclerosis in middle-aged Finnish men. *Circulation, 110,* 2198–2203.

Johannessen, L., Strudsholm, U., Foldager, L., & Munk-Jorgensen, P. (2006). Increased risk of hypertension in patients with bipolar disorder and patients with anxiety compared to background population and patients with schizophrenia. *Journal of Affective Disorders, 95,* 13–17.

Jones, D. A., & West, R. R. (1996). Psychological rehabilitation after myocardial infarction: multicentre randomised controlled trial. *British Medical Journal, 313,* 1517–1521.

Julkunen, J., Salonen, R., Kaplan, G. A., Chesney, M. A., & Salonen, J. T. (1994). Hostility and the progression of carotid atherosclerosis. *Psychosomatic Medicine, 56,* 519–525.

Kamarck, T. W., Everson, S. A., Kaplan, G. A., Manuck, S. B., & Salonen, J. T. (1997). Exaggerated blood pressure responses during mental stress are associated with enhanced carotid atherosclerosis in middle-aged Finnish men: Findings from the Kuopio Ischemic Heart Disease Study. *Circulation, 96,* 3842–3848.

Kamarck, T. W., & Jennings, J. (1991). Biobehavioral factors in sudden cardiac death. *Psychological Bulletin, 109*, 42–75.

Kaplan, J. R., & Manuck, S. B. (1999). Status, stress, and atherosclerosis: The role of environment and individual behavior. *Annals of the New York Academy of Science, 896*, 145–161.

Kaprio, J., Koskenvuo, M., & Rita, H. (1987). Mortality after bereavement: a prospective study of 95,647 widowed persons. *American Journal of Public Health, 77*, 283–287.

Kawachi, I., Colditz, G. A., Ascherio, A., Rimm, E. B., Giovannucci, E., Stampfer, M. J., & Willett, W. C. (1994). Prospective study of phobic anxiety and risk of coronary heart disease in men. *Circulation, 89*, 1992–1997.

Kawachi, I., Sparrow, D., Spiro, A., 3rd, Vokonas, P., & Weiss, S. T. (1996). A prospective study of anger and coronary heart disease. The Normative Aging Study. *Circulation, 94,* 2090–2095.

Kent, L. K., & Shapiro, P. A. (2009). Depression and related psychological factors in heart disease. *Harvard Review of Psychiatry, 17*, 377–388.

Ketterer, M. W., Huffman, J., Lumley, M. A., Wassef, S., Gray, L., Kenyon, L., … Goldberg, A. D. (1998). Five year follow-up for adverse outcomes in males with at least minimally positive angiograms: Importance of "denial" in assessing psychosocial risk factors. *Journal of Psychosomatic Research, 44*, 241–250.

Keys, A., Taylor, H. L., Blackburn, H., Brozek, J., Anderson, J. T., & Simonson, E. (1971). Mortality and coronary heart disease among men studied for 23 years. *Archives of Internal Medicine, 128*, 201–214.

Kop, W. J. (1999). Chronic and acute psychological risk factors for clinical manifestations of coronary artery disease. *Psychosomatic Medicine, 61*, 476–487.

Kop, W. J., & Gottdiener, J. S. (2005). The role of immune system parameters in the relationship between depression and coronary artery disease. *Psychosomatic Medicine, 67*(Suppl. 1), S37–S41.

Kraemer, H. C., Stice, E., Kazdin, A., Offord, D., & Kupfer, D. (2001). How do risk factors work together? Mediators, moderators, and independent, overlapping, and proxy risk factors. *American Journal of Psychiatry, 158*, 848–856.

Krantz, D. S., Glass, D. C., Contrada, R. J., & Miller, N. E. (1981). Behavior and health. In the National Science Foundation's five year outlook on science and technology: 1981 Source Materials (Vol. 2, pp. 561–588). Washington, DC: U.S. Government Printing Office.

Krantz, D. S., Helmers, K. F., Bairey, C. N., Nebel, L. E., Hedges, S. M., & Rozanski, A. (1991). Cardiovascular reactivity and mental stress-induced myocardial ischemia in patients with coronary artery disease. *Psychosomatic Medicine, 53*, 1–128.

Krantz, D. S., & Manuck, S. B. (1984). Acute psychophysiologic reactivity and risk of cardiovascular disease: A review and methodologic critique. *Psychological Bulletin, 96*, 435–464.

Krantz, D. S., & McCeney, M. K. (2002). Effects of psychological and social factors on organic disease: A critical assessment of research on coronary heart disease. *Annual Review of Psychology, 53*, 341–369.

Krantz, D. S., Santiago, H. T., Kop, W. J., Bairey Merz, C. N., Rozanski, A., & Gottdiener, J. S. (1999). Prognostic value of mental stress testing in coronary artery disease. *American Journal of Cardiology, 84*, 1292–1297.

Kubzansky, L. D., Kawachi, I., Spiro, A., III, Weiss, S. T., Vokonas, P. S., & Sparrow, D. (1997). Is worrying bad for your heart? A prospective study of worry and coronary heart disease in the Normative Aging Study. *Circulation, 95*, 818–824.

Kubzansky, L. D., Kawachi, I., Weiss, S. T., & Sparrow, D. (1998). Anxiety and coronary heart disease: a synthesis of epidemiological, psychological, and experimental evidence. *Annals of Behavioral Medicine, 20*, 47–58.

Kuper, H., Marmot, M., & Hemingway, H. (2002). Systematic review of prospective cohort studies of psychosocial factors in the etiology and prognosis of coronary heart disease. *Seminars in Vascular Medicine, 2*, 267–314.

Lahey, B. B. (2009). Public health significance of neuroticism. *American Psychologist, 64*, 241–256.

Lampert, R., Jain, D., Burg, M. M., Batsford, W. P., & McPherson, C. A. (2000). Destabilizing effects of mental stress on ventricular arrhythmias in patients with implantable cardioverter-defibrillators. *Circulation, 101*, 158–164.

Lau, J. Y., & Eley, T. C. (2010). The genetics of mood disorders. *Annual Review of Clinical Psychology, 6,* 313–337.

Lavie, C. J., Thomas, R. J., Squires, R. W., Allison, T. G., & Milani, R. V. (2009). Exercise training and cardiac rehabilitation in primary and secondary prevention of coronary heart disease. *Mayo Clinic Proceedings, 84*, 373–383.

Lazarus, R. S. (1966). *Psychological stress and the coping process.* New York, NY: McGraw-Hill.

Lazarus, R. S. (1991). *Emotion and adaptation.* New York, NY: Oxford University Press.

Lazarus, R. S., & Folkman, S. (1984). *Stress, appraisal and coping*. New York, NY: Springer.

Lee, S., Colditz, G. A., Berkman, L. F., & Kawachi, I. (2003). Caregiving and risk of coronary heart disease in U.S. women: A prospective study. *American Journal of Preventative Medicine, 24*, 113–119.

Leor, J., & Kloner, R. A. (1996). The Northridge earthquake as a trigger for acute myocardial infarction. *American Journal of Cardiology, 77*, 1230–1232.

Lett, H., Davidson, R., & Blumenthal, J. (2005). Nonpharmacologic treatments for depression in patients with coronary heart disease. *Psychosomatic Medicine, 67*, S58–S62.

Leventhal, H. (1979). A perceptual-motor processing model of emotion. In P. Pliner, K. Blankenstein, & I. M. Spigel (Eds.), *Perception of emotion in self and others* (Vol. 5).

Leventhal, H. (1980). Toward a comprehensive theory of emotion. *Advances in Experimental Social Psychology, 13*, 139–207.

Maier, S. F., & Watkins, L. R. (1998). Cytokines for psychologists: implications of bidirectional immune-to-brain communication for understanding behavior, mood, and cognition. *Psychological Review, 105*, 83–107.

Manuck, S. B., Olsson, G., Hjemdahl, P., & Rehnqvist N. (1992). Does cardiovascular reactivity to mental stress have prognostic value in postinfarction patients? A pilot study. *Psychosomatic Medicine, 54*, 102–108.

Markovitz, J. H. (1998). Hostility is associated with increased platelet activation in coronary heart disease. *Psychosomatic Medicine, 60*, 586–591.

Martin, R. A., Kuiper, N. A., & Westra, H. A. (1989). Cognitive and affective components of the Type A behavior pattern: Preliminary evidence for a self-worth contingency model. *Personality and Individual Differences, 10*, 771–784.

Martin, R. L., Cloninger, C. R., Guze, S. B., & Clayton, P. J. (1985). Mortality in a follow-up of 500 psychiatric outpatients. *Archives of General Psychiatry, 42*, 47–54.

Mathews, A., & MacLeod, C. (2005). Cognitive vulnerability to emotional disorders. *Annual Review of Clinical Psychology, 1*, 167–195.

Matthews, K. A. (1988). Coronary heart disease and Type A behaviors: Update on and alternative to the Booth-Kewley and Friedman (1987) quantitative review. *Psychological Bulletin, 104*, 373–380.

Matthews, K. A., Glass, D. C., Rosenman, R. H., & Bortner, R. W. (1977). Competitive drive, Pattern A, and Coronary Heart Disease: A further analysis of some data from the Western Collaborative Group Study. *Journal of Chronic Diseases, 30*, 489–498.

Matthews, K. A., & Gump, B. B. (2002). Chronic work stress and marital dissolution increase risk of posttrial mortality in men from the Multiple Risk Factor Intervention Trial. *Archives of Internal Medicine, 162*, 309–315.

Matthews, K. A., Owens, J. F., Kuller, L. H., Sutton-Tyrrell, K., & Jansen-McWilliams, L. (1998). Are hostility and anxiety associated with carotid atherosclerosis in healthy postmenopausal women? *Psychosomatic Medicine, 60*, 633–638.

Matthews, K. A., Zhu, S., Tucker, D. C., & Whooley, M. A. (2006). Blood pressure reactivity to psychological stress and coronary calcification in the Coronary Artery Risk Development in Young Adults Study. *Hypertension, 47*, 391–395.

Mendes de Leon, C. F., Kop, W. K., de Stuart, H. B., Bar, F. W., & Appels, A. P. (1996). Psychosocial characteristics and recurrent events after percutaneous transluminal coronary angioplasty. *American Journal of Cardiology, 77*, 252–255.

Messick, S. (1981). Constructs and their vicissitudes in educational and psychological measurement. *Psychological Bulletin, 89*, 575–588.

Messick, S. (1995). Validity of psychological assessment: Validation of inferences from persons' responses and performances as scientific inquiry into score meaning. *American Psychologist, 50*, 741–749.

Milani, R. V., & Lavie, C. J. (2007). Impact of cardiac rehabilitation on depression and its associated mortality. *American Journal of Medicine, 120*, 799–806.

Milani, R. V., & Lavie, C. J. (2009). Reducing psychosocial stress: a novel mechanism of improving survival from exercise training. *American Journal of Medicine, 122*, 931–938.

Miller, T. Q., Smith, T. W., Turner, C. W., Guijarro, M. L., & Hallet, A. J. (1996). A meta-analytic review of research on hostility and physical health. *Psychological Bulletin, 119*, 322–348.

Mond, H. G., & Whitlock, R. M. (2008). The Australian and New Zealand cardiac pacing and implantable cardioverter-defibrillator survey: Calendar year 2005. *Heart, Lung and Circulation, 17*, 85–89.

Moser, D. K., & Dracup, K. (1996). Is anxiety early after myocardial infarction associated with subsequent ischemic and arrhythmic events? *Psychosomatic Medicine, 58*, 395–401.

Moss, S., Prosser, H., & Goldberg, D. (1996). Validity of the schizophrenia diagnosis of the psychiatric assessment schedule for adults with developmental disability (PAS-ADD). *British Journal of Psychiatry, 168*, 359–367.

Musselman, D. L., Evans, D. L., & Nemeroff, C. B. (1998). The relationship of depression to cardiovascular disease: epidemiology, biology, and treatment. *Archives of General Psychiatry, 55,* 580–592.

Myrtek, M. (1995). Type A behavior pattern, personality factors, disease, and physiological reactivity. *Personality and Individual Differences, 18,* 491–502.

NCHS Update. (2005). NAPHSIS. Centers for Disease Control and Prevention National Center for Health Statistics. Retrieved from http://www.naphsis.org/NAPHSIS/files/ccLibraryFiles/Filename/000000000198/v-2%20 sondik.nchs%20update.naphsis.2005.ppt#478,1,Slide 1

Nicholson, A., Kuper, H., & Hemingway, H. (2006). Depression as an aetiologic and prognostic factor in coronary heart disease: a meta-analysis of 6362 events among 146 538 participants in 54 observational studies. *European Heart Journal, 27,* 2763–2774.

O'Keefe, J. H., Carter, M. D., & Lavie, C. J. (2009). Depression screening in patients with heart disease. *Journal of the American Medical Association, 301,* 1337–1337.

Orth-Gomer, K., Wamala, S. P., Horsten, M., Schenck-Gustafsson, K., Schneiderman, N., & Mittleman, M. A. (2000). Marital stress worsens prognosis in women with coronary heart disease: The Stockholm Female Coronary Risk Study. *Journal of the American Medical Association, 284,* 3008–3014.

Osby, U., Brandt, L., Correia, N., Ekbom, A., & Sparen, P. (2001). Excess mortality in bipolar and unipolar disorder in Sweden. *Archives of General Psychiatry, 58,* 844–850.

Pace, T. W., Mletzko, T. C., Alagbe, O., Musselman, D. L., Nemeroff, C. B., Miller, A. H., & Heim, C.M. (2006). Increased stress-induced inflammatory responses in male patients with major depression and increased early life stress. *American Journal of Psychiatry, 163,* 1630–1633.

Penninx, B. W., Beekman, A. T., Honig, A., Deeg, D. J., Schoevers, R. A., van Eijk, J. T., & van Tilburg, W. (2001). Depression and cardiac mortality: results from a community-based longitudinal study. *Archives of General Psychiatry, 58,* 221–227.

Robles, T. F., Glaser, R., & Kiecolt-Glaser, J. K. (2005). Out of balance: A new look at chronic stress, depression, and immunity. *Current Directions in Psychological Science, 14,* 111–115.

Rosenman, R. H., Brand, R. J., Jenkins, C. D., Friedman, M., Straus, K., & Wurm, M. (1975). Coronary heart disease in the Western Collaborative Group Study: Final follow-up experience of 8.5 years. *Journal of the American Medical Association, 22,* 872–877.

Ross, R. (1999). Atherosclerosis: an inflammatory disease. *New England Journal of Medicine, 340,* 115–126.

Rozanski, A., Blumenthal, J. A., Davidson, K. W., Saab, P. G., & Kubzansky, L. (2005). The epidemiology, pathophysiology and management of psychosocial risk factors in cardiac practice—The emerging field of behavioral cardiology. *Journal of the American College of Cardiology, 45,* 637–651.

Rozanski, A., Blumenthal, J. A., & Kaplan, J. (1999). Impact of psychological factors on the pathogenesis of cardiovascular disease and implications for therapy. *Circulation, 99,* 2192–2217.

Sareen, J., Cox, B. J., Clara, I., & Asmundson, G. J. (2005). The relationship between anxiety disorders and physical disorders in the U.S. National Comorbidity Survey. *Depression and Anxiety, 21,* 193–202.

Scherer, K. R. (1986). Vocal affect expression: A review and a model for future research. *Psychological Bulletin, 99,* 143–165.

Schneiderman, E. H. (2010). Gestational diabetes: an overview of a growing health concern for women. *Journal of Infusion Nursing, 33,* 48–54.

Schulman, J., & Stromberg, S. (2007). On the value of doing nothing. Anger and cardiovascular disease in clinical practice. *Cardiology Review, 15,* 123–132.

Schulz, R., & Beach, S. R. (1999). Caregiving as a risk factor for mortality. *Journal of the American Medical Association, 282,* 2215–2219.

Selye, H. (1976). *The stress of life* (Rev. ed.). New York, NY: McGraw-Hill.

Sharma, R., & Markar, H. R. (1994). Mortality in affective disorder. *Journal of Affective Disorders, 31,* 91–96.

Shipley, B. A., Weiss, A., Der, G., Taylor, M. D., & Deary, I. J. (2007). Neuroticism, extraversion, and mortality in the UK Health and Lifestyle Survey: a 21-year prospective cohort study. *Psychosomatic Medicine, 69,* 923–931.

Siegler, I. C., Costa, P. T., Brummett, B. H., Helms, M. J., Barefoot, J. C., Williams, R. B., … Rimer, B. K. (2003). Patterns of change in hostility from college to midlife in the UNC Alumni Heart Study predict high-risk status. *Psychosomatic Medicine, 65,* 738–745.

Siegman, A. W. (1994). From Type A to hostility to anger: Reflections on the history of coronary-prone behavior. In A. W. Siegman & T. W. Smith (Eds.), *Anger, hostility and the heart* (pp. 1–21). Hillsdale, NJ: Erlbaum.

Smith, T. W., & Gallo, L. C. (2001). Personality traits as risk factors for physical illness. In A. Baum, T. Revenson, & J. Singer (Eds.), *Handbook of health psychology* (pp. 139–174). Hillsdale, NJ: Erlbaum.

Smith, T. W., & Ruiz, J. (2002). Psychosocial influences on the development and course of coronary heart disease: Current status and implications for research and practice. *Journal of Consulting and Clinical Psychology, 70*, 548–568.

Smith, T. W., Ruiz, J. M., & Uchino, B. N. (2004). Mental activation of supportive ties, hostility, and cardiovascular reactivity to laboratory stress in young men and women. *Health Psychology, 23*, 476–485.

Spence, J. T., Helmreich, R. L., & Pred, R. S. (1987). Impatience versus achievement strivings in the Type A pattern: Differential effects on students' health and academic achievement. *Journal of Applied Psychology, 72*, 522–528.

Steptoe, A., & Brydon, L. (2009). Emotional triggering of cardiac events. *Neuroscience and Biobehavioral Reviews, 33*, 63–70.

Stern, M. J., Gorman, P. A., & Kaslow, L. (1983). The group counseling v exercise therapy study: a controlled intervention with subjects following myocardial infarction. *Archives of Internal Medicine, 143*, 1719–1725.

Strike, P., & Steptoe, A. (2004). Psychosocial factors in the development of coronary artery disease. *Progress in Cardiovascular Diseases, 46*, 337–347.

Sturman, T. S. (1999). Achievement motivation and Type A behavior as motivational orientations. *Journal of Research in Personality, 33*, 189–207.

Suls, J., & Bunde, J. (2005). Anger, anxiety, and depression as risk factors for cardiovascular disease: the problems and implications of overlapping affective dispositions. *Psychological Bulletin, 131*, 260–300.

Suls, J., & Marco, C. A. (1990). Relationship between JAS- and FTAS-Type A behavior and non-CHD illness: a prospective study controlling for negative affectivity. *Health Psychology, 9*, 479–492.

Suls, J., & Wan, C. (1993). The relationship between trait hostility and cardiovascular reactivity: A quantitative review and analysis. *Psychophysiology, 30*, 615–626.

Swan, G. E., Carmelli, D., & Rosenman, R. H. (1990). Cook and Medley hostility and the Type A behavior pattern: Psychological correlates of two coronary-prone behaviors. *Journal of Social Behavior and Personality, 5*, 89–106.

Thomas, K. S., Bardwell, W. A., Ancoli-Israel, S., & Dimsdale, J. E. (2006). The toll of ethnic discrimination on sleep architecture and fatigue. *Health Psychology, 25*, 635–642.

Tomkins, S. S. (1962). *Affect, imagery, consciousness* (Vol. 1). *The positive affects*. New York, NY: Springer.

Tracey, K. J. (2002). The inflammatory reflex. *Nature, 420*, 853–859.

Watkins, L. L., Blumenthal, J. A., Davidson, J. R., Babyak, M. A., McCants, C. B., Jr., & Sketch, M. H., Jr. (2006). Phobic anxiety, depression, and risk of ventricular arrhythmias in patients with coronary heart disease. *Psychosomatic Medicine, 68*, 651–656.

Weeke, A., Juel, K., & Vaeth, M. (1987). Cardiovascular death and manic-depressive psychosis. *Journal of Affective Disorders, 13*, 287–292.

Welin, C., Lappas, G., & Wilhelmsen, L. (2000). Independent importance of psychosocial risk factors for prognosis after myocardial infarction. *Journal of Internal Medicine, 247*, 629–639.

Wilkowski, B. M., & Robinson, M. D. (2008). The cognitive basis of trait anger and reactive aggression: An integrative analysis. *Personality and Social Psychology Review, 12*, 3–21.

Williams, J. E., Paton, C. C., Siegler, I. C., Eigenbrodt, M. L., Nieto, F. J., & Tyroler, H. A. (2000). Anger proneness predicts coronary heart disease risk: Prospective analysis from the Atherosclerosis Risk in Communities (ARIC) Study. *Circulation, 101*, 2034–2039.

Williams, P. G., Smith, T. W., Gunn, H. E., & Uchino, B. N. (2011). Personality and Stress: Individual Differences in Exposure, Reactivity, Recovery, and Restoration. In R. J. Contrada & A. Baum (Eds.), *Handbook of stress science: Psychology, biology, and health* (pp. 231–245). New York, NY: Springer.

Williams, R. B., Jr. (1987). Psychological factors in coronary artery disease: Epidemiological evidence. *Circulation, 76*(Suppl. 1), 1117–1123.

World Health Organization (WHO). (2010). *Fact sheet No. 317. September 2009*. Retrieved from http://www .who.int/mediacentre/factsheets/fs317/en/index.html

Yusuf, S., Hawken, S., Ounpuu, S., Dans, T., Avezum, A., Lanas, F., … Lisheng, L., on behalf of the INTERHEART Study Investigators. (2004). Effect of potentially modifiable risk factors associated with myocardial infarction in 52 countries (the INTERHEART study): case-control study. *Lancet, 364*, 937–952.

28 Treatment in Cardiovascular Disease

Stanton P. Newman, Shashivadan P. Hirani,
Jan Stygall, and Theodora Fteropoulli
University College London and City University London

Cardiovascular diseases (CVDs) are a group of disorders of the heart and blood vessels. The conditions that result are congenital or acquired. For example, congenital heart disease encompasses a range of conditions where the heart is poorly formed at birth. In most cases, these conditions require some form of surgical intervention. Others are acquired and range from such disorders as peripheral vascular disease (PVD), which leads to claudication of the extremities, to blockages of the coronary arteries and malfunctioning of the valves of the heart. For each of these cardiovascular disorders, there are myriad treatments, including early broad-based interventions that involve attempts to encourage general behavior change, pharmacological solutions, and different levels of invasive treatments. Which treatment is applied is often related to the severity of the condition. In some cases, such as cardiac valve disease, treatment consists of careful monitoring of the condition to determine if and when an invasive treatment is required. In others, a major event, such as a myocardial infarction (MI) is frequently followed rapidly by some form of invasive treatment, often surgery. Each treatment is designed to alleviate symptoms, reduce the risks of a major cardiac event occurring or reoccurring, and reduce mortality. In most cases, treatments are accompanied by both medication and recommendations for behavior change. In some cases, these behavioral recommendations generally involve diet and exercise. In others, such as congestive heart failure, the recommendations involve daily monitoring of signs to assess changes in severity and the need for alterations of medications or a consultation with a health care professional.

In this chapter, we have selected to focus on coronary artery disease (CAD) and its treatments. We first describe the condition and the three most common treatments in the area, pharmacological therapy, percutaneous coronary intervention (PCI), and coronary artery bypass grafting (CABG). We then look at three phases of the "journey with illness" that patients with these conditions may encounter, specifically pretreatments, during treatments, and following interventions. We focus within each stage on a single topic that is particularly relevant to that stage of a patient's journey but can have implications or be applied to other stages. For the first stage, pretreatment, we look at how people think about their illness and treatment in CAD and how these cognitions convey a patient's perspective of the condition. At the next stage, we examine the possible consequences of undergoing coronary artery bypass surgery as one of the dominant and most invasive treatments for CAD. Finally, at the postintervention stage, we examine the most general and dominant of psychosocial interventions that fall under the rubric of cardiac rehabilitation, focusing specifically on depression and its treatment after cardiac events.

Given space limitations and our focus on only this condition, a number of important aspects of research in this area being left unaddressed or not addressed in detail within the chapter. We must acknowledge that such factors as gender, culture and ethnicity, and coexisting diseases may have important implications within treatments and outcomes for CAD. We direct the reader to excellent reviews and articles to cover this limitation (Baker, Richter, & Anand, 2001; Berry, Tardif, & Bourassa, 2007a, 2007b; Correa-de-Araujo, 2006; Davidson et al., 2010; Gupta, Birnbaum, &

Uretsky, 2004; Jacobs, 2009; Kim, Redberg, Pavlic, & Eagle, 2007; Lip et al., 2007; Webinski, 2008) and the chapters in this volume (e.g., Betensky, Glass, & Contrada, Chapter 27).

MEDICAL AND SURGICAL TREATMENTS IN CORONARY ARTERY DISEASE

THE CONDITION

Coronary artery disease is a common condition involving the narrowing or total occlusion of one or more of the heart's major arteries. More than 95% of all CAD results from a buildup of plaque on the inside of the walls of the arteries (atherosclerosis). This plaque is made up of lipids, inflammatory cells, smooth muscle cells, connective tissue, thrombi, and calcium deposits. Atherosclerotic plaques can be classified as stable or unstable. Stable plaques regress, remain static, or grow slowly over decades until they may cause stenosis or occlusion. Unstable plaques are vulnerable to spontaneous erosion, fissure, or rupture, causing acute thrombosis, occlusion, and infarction long before they cause stenosis. Total occlusion can rapidly lead to ischemia and death of heart muscle or to MI. Therefore, plaque stabilization may be a way to reduce morbidity and mortality (Beers & Berkow, 2005).

The clinical presentation of CAD is extremely variable, and most often people are asymptomatic. The most distinctive symptom is pain or tightening in the chest that radiates to the arms and jaw. Symptoms emanating from stable plaque (stable angina) usually occur during exercise when the heart muscle's need for oxygenated blood exceeds the ability of the coronary arteries to deliver. However, most clinical events result from unstable plaques. Here, symptoms occur unexpectedly and when at rest (unstable angina). These symptoms may develop when unstable plaques rupture and occlude a major coronary artery.

Treatments for CAD aim to reduce the rate of mortality, improve symptoms, and prevent such further cardiac events as MI, stroke, and repeat invasive procedures (Almeda & Snell, 2005). The three major treatments are pharmacological therapy, percutaneous coronary intervention (PCI), and coronary artery bypass grafting (CABG).

PHARMACOLOGICAL THERAPY

Medications are often considered the first line of interventional treatment and principally function to reduce the workload on the heart by (a) limiting myocardial oxygen needs through slowing the heart rate both at rest and exercise; (b) relaxing the smooth muscle of the heart; (c) blocking the actions of catecholamine, which increases heart rate, blood pressure, and cardiac contractility; or (d) acting as vasodilators and venodilators on coronary and peripheral vessels to increase blood flow, enabling more oxygen and nutrients to reach the heart muscle.

REVASCULARIZATION

Both PCI and CABG aim to reestablish blood flow through the arteries to the areas of the heart supplied by sections of arteries distal of the atherosclerotic blockages, thereby relieving symptoms. PCI involves the advancing of a guided, deflated balloon-tipped catheter through an artery into the aorta, into the affected coronary artery, and on to the obstruction. The balloon is then inflated compressing the plaque and thereby enlarging the inner diameter of the coronary artery. At this point, a mesh tube (stent) that covers the balloon is opened and the balloon is deflated and removed, leaving the stent in place to support the artery wall and increase the blood flow. Originally directed at patients with single-vessel disease, PCI it has been increasingly employed for multivessel disease.

CABG is a major surgical procedure generally performed under general anaesthesia and takes on average three to four hours. The heart is reached by making a midline chest incision and dividing the sternum. Depending upon which arteries are stenosed, the internal mammary artery from inside the chest wall and/or segments of saphenous vein are taken from the patient's leg or radial arteries from the arm. These are used to make a vessel that is attached to the coronary artery above and below the stenosis, allowing the blood to flow through this conduit "bypassing" the stenosis.

Initially, CABG surgery involved the surgeon working on a beating heart. With the introduction of cardiopulmonary bypass (CPB), which is a machine that takes over the work of the heart and lungs during cardiac surgery, the surgeon is able to work on a relatively still heart in a clean field. However, because of concerns that many of the complications of cardiac surgery were secondary to the bypass machine (CPB), there has been resurgence in CABG surgery without the use of CPB, a procedure often referred to as off-pump coronary artery bypass (OPCAB). Of the estimated 300,000 CABG surgery procedures currently conducted in the United States, it has been reported that between 18% and 25% are performed off-pump (Sellke, Chu, & Cohn, 2010). However, over the last decade a number of studies have been conducted to examine the efficacy of OPCAB compared to conventional CABG, and these have produced inconsistent results. Some studies have found that OPCAB is associated with shorter length of hospital stay, reduced transfusion requirements, reduced pulmonary morbidity, and fewer postoperative neurologic events; whereas other studies have found no difference (Chu et al., 2009). Therefore, which surgical revascularization approach is better is still controversial, and uptake of OPCAB varies widely between centers and individual surgeons.

PREINTERVENTION STAGE: ILLNESS AND TREATMENT BELIEFS IN CARDIOVASCULAR DISEASE

PATIENT-CENTERED PERSPECTIVE

Given the success of invasive interventions in CAD, mortality and morbidity (in terms of subsequent nonfatal MIs) are no longer considered as the only outcomes by which to differentiate and evaluate these clinical procedures. Many researchers have gone beyond the biomedical approach to consider quality of life and psychosocial outcomes as means by which to gauge the efficacy of therapies. In addition, the variables used to predict outcomes from these interventions are now also being selected from a broader range of disciplines. Besides the biomedical, these include the psychological, interpersonal, functional, and economic domains. The result is a shift in emphasis from a biomedical to an increasingly patient-centered perspective of treatment and recovery. Furthermore, as the importance of psychological factors in the management of illness receives more attention, the emphasis placed on the role of patients in the successful management of their illness has also increased.

Central to the patient perspective of illness is the manner in which patients perceive their illness and their treatments. The ways in which ill individuals think about their illness, that is, their *illness cognitions*, have the capacity to influence their behavioral and emotional responses and, as a consequence, the outcome of an illness. Psychosocial interventions attempt to change these cognitions to improve outcomes by addressing misconceptions or damaging beliefs that lead to adoption of health-damaging behaviors or lead to the avoidance of behaviors that protect, maintain, and enhance health.

Cognitions regarding illness can be expected to change over the illness journey. At the pretreatment stage, illness cognitions are likely to represent patients' expectations of the future state of their illness and the role of their treatments and behaviors in addressing the illness state (Hirani, 2009). The extent to which expectations are met posttreatment are likely to impact upon patients' evaluations of the treatments they received and the future course of their illness- and health-related behaviors. Thus, the examination of the perspective of the patient, the pretreatment, is an important aspect of psychosocial interventions (Leventhal, Weinman, Leventhal, & Phillips, 2008).

There is a rich history of psychological models utilized to explain health-related cognitions and behaviors and how chronically ill individuals think about and manage their conditions; these models include the theory of planned behavior (Ajzen, 1991) protection motivation theory (Rogers, 1975), the health belief model (Rosenstock, 1966), and the health action process approach (Schwarzer, 1992). A theoretical model that is increasingly utilized and influential in understanding the patient's perspective in the health care context and guiding interventions is the self-regulatory model (SRM) of illness by Leventhal and colleagues (Leventhal, Meyer, & Nerenz, 1980; Leventhal, Nerenz, & Steele, 1984).

SELF-REGULATORY MODEL

The SRM postulates that when confronted with an illness or a threat to their health, individuals instigate a complex set of cognitions to conceptualize and manage the situation. In such situations people are active problems solvers; their behavioral responses to ill health are an interaction between the physical presence of a disease and the person's subjective perception and interpretation of the disease state. They generate parallel cognitive and emotional *representations* of the health threat from interpretations of somatic sensations and social stimuli (previous experiences, advice from health care professionals, vicarious learning, etc.). Then through a partially independent process, these representations inform individuals on how to *cope* with their predicament, for example, to address any illness consequences or attendant issues with problem-focused coping and to respond to the emotional reactions to the illness threat with emotion-focused strategies. The outcomes of these coping efforts are *appraised* and fed back into the representational and coping systems such that the self-regulatory process is a constantly developing and active system (Leventhal & Leventhal, 1993).

The SRM predicts that illness representations are directly related to coping and through coping to adaptive outcomes, among them disability and quality of life. Thus, coping is considered to mediate between the representations and outcomes (Heijmans, 1998). Subsequent work has demonstrated a direct link between representations and outcomes (Hagger & Orbell, 2003). The SRM can be seen as a heuristic device to assist the understanding of individuals' responses to the threat of illness (Cohen, Trippreimer, Smith, Sorofman, & Lively, 1994).

ILLNESS COGNITIONS

Integral to the SRM are the illness cognitions that specify different domains of beliefs people have regarding their illness. These cognitions have been the focus of research in coronary disease and many other chronic and acute illnesses (see Hagger & Orbell, 2003). Numerous categorizations for the manner in which people think about illnesses have been formulated, for example, illness representations within the SRM (Leventhal et al., 1984), the generic implicit illness model (Turk, Rudy, & Salovey, 1986), and personal models (Hampson, Glasgow, & Toobert, 1990). Although these models differ in their terminology, methodology, theoretical background, and focus, they have a significant degree of conceptual overlap and similar components that tend to closely follow the seminal framework of the *illness representations* (IR) portion of the SRM developed by Leventhal and colleagues.

The standard formulation of IR includes five components: (1) identity: the bodily symptoms and label associated with the illness; (2) causality: beliefs about factors contributing to the onset of the illness; (3) consequences: both long- and short-term expected outcomes and sequelae of the condition; (4) timeline: beliefs concerning the moment of onset and expectations about the illness's duration and periodicity (acute, cyclic, or chronic); and (5) cure or control: how one may mediate or recover from the disease. Studies collectively suggest that the individual components of such models form a generic knowledge *structure* that is stable and outside the influence of significant experience in individual medical history, whereas the *content* of these illness models may emerge as idiosyncratic and reflective of medical history.

The SRM's five components have come to be accepted as the main categories of illness beliefs and remain the most influential schema and the typical starting point for IR operationalization and measurement (Heijmans & de Ridder, 1998). It is acknowledged that dependent on the illness being investigated and the context of the investigation, the relative importance of each component may vary; dimensions may become redundant, merge, or emerge as divergent from the original formulation. Recent iterations of the questionnaires utilized to measure IR—for example, the Illness Perceptions Questionnaire–Revised (Moss-Morris et al., 2002) and the Brief-IPQ (Broadbent, Petrie, Main, & Weinman, 2006)—have expanded the number of dimensions investigated (e.g., treatment control, personal control, cyclical timeline), yet they remain centered on the core components.

Further, IR have been associated with or found to predict various types of outcomes in cardiac health–related behaviors, including attendance at cardiac rehabilitation, psychosocial adjustment, quality of life, depression, medication adherence, delay in reaching hospital, exercise, alcohol consumption, and return to work (e.g., Broadbent et al., 2006; Byrne, Walsh, & Murphy, 2005; French, Cooper, & Weinman, 2006; French, Lewin, Watson, & Thompson, 2005; Grace et al., 2005; Steed, Newman, & Hardman, 1999; Walsh, Lynch, Murphy, & Daly, 2004). Much of the work with IRs has, however, considered beliefs and outcomes after the treatment stage of the condition.

TREATMENT REPRESENTATIONS

In recent years, the illness cognition sector of the SRM has been extended to include a wider range of cognition. Besides the fractionation of core IR components as a result of empirical investigations (Broadbent et al., 2006; Hirani, Pugsley, & Newman, 2006), important beliefs that have been identified are related to the treatment of the condition. These treatment representations (TR) concern the beliefs patients have about the interventions that are being offered to address their illnesses.

In influential work, Horne and colleagues (Horne & Weinman, 1999, 2002; Horne, Weinman, & Hankins, 1999) have integrated treatment beliefs about medication into an extended self-regulatory model. They postulate that *medication beliefs* comprise four factors: the necessity of prescribed medication (specific-necessity); the danger of dependence, toxicity, and disruptiveness of medication (specific-concerns); the harmful, addictive, poisonous nature of medications (general-harm); and the overuse and excessive prescription of medications by health professionals (general-overuse). In CAD-related conditions, these scales have been found to be related to IR; such important health-related outcomes and processes as a strong belief in the necessity of one's medication and a lower level of concern about one's medication are associated with higher levels of adherence (Byrne et al., 2005). Medication-related treatment beliefs measured over time have been demonstrated as both remaining relatively stable (Porteous, Francis, Bond, & Hannaford, 2010) and showing changes (LaPointe et al., 2010).

However, it is clear from the beliefs addressed in studies over time that this work specifically focuses on medication rather than such other medical treatments as surgery or percutaneous procedures found in CAD. Where used in illnesses where surgical or other nonmedication treatments are the primary form of therapy, beliefs about medication have been found to have little role in predicting outcome (Llewellyn, McGurk, & Weinman, 2007). This approach is useful for investigating treatment representation with regards to medications; it is not appropriate for investigating representations for nonpharmacological treatments.

Leventhal and colleagues (Leventhal et al., 1997; Leventhal, Musumeci, & Contrada, 2007) suggest that because treatments are designed to counteract illness, they may be viewed along dimensions similar to those of IR. For instance, treatments may be perceived with respect to time for effectiveness, ability to cure or control, consequences on functioning, the symptoms and illness targets, and routes of action (causal). Thus, just as IR address many illness conditions; the TR can address many treatments. Qualitative work on treatments has focused on psychiatric illnesses, the doctor–patient relationship, and the psychotherapeutic process (e.g., Kampman et al., 2000). Other work has concentrated on treatment efficacy and expectations (e.g., Whittle, 1996). The conglomeration of research has highlighted the important role of treatment representations and their relationship to such health-related behaviors as functioning and adherence and has indicated a number of dimensions that need to be considered. These dimensions include:

- Expected improvements (e.g., relief of symptoms, return to normal life)
- Treatment decisions (e.g., decision satisfaction, level of information provided)
- Necessity of treatment (e.g., life impossible or be very ill without it)
- Possible side effects
- Concerns regarding the treatment (e.g., anxiety, worry)
- Time scales for improvements
- Changes required in personal behavior and lifestyle (e.g., dietary changes, increase in exercise)

An empirical investigation of treatment beliefs addressing these domains, within a group of CAD patients prior to undergoing treatments of CABG, PCI, or continuing medication, revealed that in this cardiac population, patients' TR were centered around four dimensions: (1) treatment value: representing patients' beliefs regarding the positive benefits of their treatment in controlling and arresting their CAD; (2) treatment concerns: reflecting trepidation, mainly anxiety and worry at undergoing treatment, and concerns with regards to the nature of the treatment; (3) decision satisfaction: an assessment of the decision process in choosing the course of treatment, including informational needs, satisfaction with the decision-making process, and suitability of the chosen treatment; and (4) cure: examining beliefs regarding the ability of the treatment to remove the disease and return the patient to his or her normal life (Hirani, Patterson, & Newman, 2009). These dimensions somewhat overlap with the factors for medications identified by Horne and colleagues (2009) but also address additional domains relevant to the other treatments for CAD.

This study provided the opportunity to address how people about to face one of the three different treatments (CABG, PCI, and medication) available for CAD may lead to differing pretreatment expectations from their recipients. The different treatment group had treatment cognitions that reflected the nature of the treatment to be undertaken and took into account the vastly different "drama" involved in the procedures.

The CABG surgery patients expected their treatment to offer a cure for their condition, were most satisfied with the treatment decision, valued the treatment most, and had the most concerns about undergoing treatment. This profile of treatment beliefs reflected the fact that they were to receive the most invasive and dramatic treatment and what appears to be the perceived (even among those patients not receiving it) as the definitive treatment for CAD. In contrast, medication patients, though valuing their treatment, were least satisfied with the treatment decision, had the least concerns with the treatment, and were equivocal regarding cure. In general, this response appeared to reflect that the average patient was uncertain regarding the benefits of this therapy. Of interest is that the PCI group occupied a midway position between the two other therapies on the TR for concerns, satisfaction, and cure. However, the PCI group was found to value the procedure slightly less than did the medication group, possibly because the PCI is often perceived as an interim procedure before the inevitable CABG and has a relatively high failure rate (S. C. Smith et al., 2006). Despite these different profiles it is of note that all three treatment groups retained a relatively high value of their treatment and had relatively low concerns to undergo them, despite the rather daunting prospects of CABG.

The differing profiles of the three CAD intervention groups provide an insight into how the different treatments are viewed by patients. However, treatment representations can also be considered across treatment groups to examine how they relate to other illness-related cognition. Treatment beliefs have been found to have a limited degree of conceptual overlap with the five dimensions of the illness representation model as assessed by an adapted Illness Perceptions Questionnaire (Weinman, Petrie, Moss-Morris, & Horne, 1996). The treatment representations of cure and, to a limited degree, the treatment value were found to be similar to IR beliefs of illness cure and control. The treatment concerns and decision satisfaction subscales are quite distinct from the IR components and add additional dimensions to how people think about both illness and treatments. The findings suggest that although illness and treatment may be closely related, they do not share a similar structure and should therefore be considered in conjunction. When considered together, illness and treatment representations in CAD are well integrated and explain greater variance in outcomes than when each area is considered alone.

It is important to note how individuals' perceptions of their treatment influence their perceptions about their illness (e.g., greater perceived value of one's treatment increases one's belief in the ability to control the illness) and, vice versa, how people think about their illness influences their thought on their treatments (e.g., patients' beliefs about the emotional causes of their illness influence their satisfaction with the treatment decisions and the concerns they have about the treatment; Hirani, 2009). These notions support Leventhal and colleagues' (2008) assertion that TR and IR are intrinsically linked. These beliefs also reflect stages in the patient's CAD journey, which is punctuated by different treatments. As such, treatment and illness beliefs should be integrated into psychological models to account for patients' responses to CAD and, by implication, to other conditions. An understanding of a patient's cognitions when treatments or changes in treatment occur may facilitate important "windows of opportunity" (Petrie, Cameron, Ellis, Buick, & Weinman, 2002) in which to bring about change, probably because patients are likely to be in an unstable situation and uncertain state.

This section has demonstrated how including treatment beliefs along with illness beliefs provides a more elaborate portrait of the CAD patient's perspectives prior to receiving discrete interventions. Here, IR have been shown to be malleable to interventions, as in cardiac rehabilitation efforts that improved outcomes for MI patients (Petrie et al., 2002). If the same success is demonstrable in TR to ensure that patients have realistic expectations, such that IR and TR can form a cohesive pattern, self-regulation processes and psychosocial outcomes may be enhanced (Leventhal et al., 2008).

ACUTE PERIPROCEDURAL STAGE: COGNITIVE COMPLICATIONS ASSOCIATED WITH CABG TREATMENT FOR CAD

Most clinical treatments have some side effects. In some cases, the side effects may have a significant impact on psychosocial functioning. Although the most invasive CAD treatment, CABG surgery, has been found to be effective in relieving angina, it has also been associated with significant cerebral morbidity, manifesting itself in a range of disorders from lethal or incapacitating stroke to subtle neuropsychological decline. Given that the cardiac cause of death after CABG has declined since the 1970s, the proportion of deaths attributable to central nervous system (CNS) complications resulting in death have risen from 7.2% to nearly 20% in the 1980s and is still on the increase (M. F. Newman et al., 2006). The incidence of stroke in patients following CABG surgery has been reported to be approximately 3%, dependent upon the method of clinical assessment and patient characteristics. Obviously, a stroke can have devastating consequences on the patient and the patient's family. However, more subtle and less apparent effects on CNS functioning have also been found. This neuropsychological decline, involving for example problems with memory, concentration, attention, and speed of mental response, has been found to be associated with increased medical costs and decreased quality of life (M. F. Newman, Grocott, et al., 2001; Roach et al., 1996).

It has been suggested that physicians and patients alike may be unaware of these cognitive problems and that where patients have noticed decline, many hesitate to report these problems because of embarrassment (Funder, Steinmetz, & Rasmussen, 2009). However, it was because of patients' reports of cognitive decline following CABG surgery in the 1980s that researchers began investigating neuropsychological outcome following cardiac surgery. The reported incidence of cognitive decline in these studies has varied widely. Investigators assessing participants 5 to 10 days postoperatively have reported the incidence of neuropsychological morbidity to range from 12.5% to 79%. Whereas later assessments, conducted between six weeks and six months, have detected neuropsychological dysfunction in 12%–37% of participants (S. P. Newman & Stygall, 2000). Longer term consequences have shown a significant deterioration in a small number of patients up to five years postsurgery (e.g. M. F. Newman, Kirchner, et al., 2001; Selnes et al., 2001; Stygall et al., 2003). All the aforementioned studies involved CABG surgery using CPB.

For health psychology, these changes in cognition can be used to evaluate the impact of variations in surgical and anaesthetic techniques and the findings used to alter practice to improve outcomes for patients. The variation occurring in these studies has been attributed not only to differing surgical techniques (e.g., blood pressure during CPB, rewarming rate, surgeon's attention to aortic atherosclerosis) but also to such methodological issues as timings of assessments, NP tests used, patient characteristics, definitions of decline, and analysis. In an attempt to reduce this variability consensus, meetings were held and guidelines were drawn up regarding the methodology involved in the design of research investigating NP decline (Murkin, Newman, Stump, & Blumenthal, 1995; Murkin, Stump, Blumenthal, & McKhann, 1997). It has been suggested that refinements to study design and methodology have improved the reliability of findings in the recent literature (Sweet et al., 2008).

Despite the variability in the incidence of NP decline in studies, it has been generally accepted that cognitive decline does exist in a subset of patients undergoing CABG surgery (Colon, Grocott, & Macksen, 2008; Sellke et al., 2010). Several factors have been cited as accounting for this neuropsychological decline (e.g., age, genetic predisposition, blood pressure, cerebral blood flow). These factors are often presented as competing hypotheses; and although the mechanisms are likely to be multifactorial, one of the principal mechanisms is microemboli occurring as a result of aortic manipulations and the use of CPB.

Differences between men and women in neuropsychological outcome following CABG surgery have rarely been examined; where examined, however, no significant differences were found (Phillips-Bute et al., 2003; M. H. Smith et al., 2000). Phillips-Bute and colleagues (2003) found that women report more cognitive problems than do men. The relationship between patients' perceptions of cognitive difficulties and formally assessed cognitive performance is unclear. Many studies have found a stronger association between mood and subjective reports of cognitive problems than between neuropsychological tests scores and subjective reports, with those patients who are more anxious and depressed reporting more cognitive problems (e.g., Gallo Malek, Gilbertson, & Moore, 2005; Johnson et al., 2002: Khatri et al., 1999; Vingerhoets, de Soete, & Jannes, 1995). It has been argued that patients who are emotionally distressed develop a negative information bias leading to a distorted perception of their cognitive performance (Gallo et al., 2005).

Studies gradually moved on from examining the incidence of cognitive decline to exploring factors that could be associated with this decline and then to intervention studies designed to reduce cognitive decline. These studies have initiated changes in the CPB equipment and anaesthetic and surgical technique. In our own institution we have seen a decline in cognitive dysfunction since 1985, when 33% of patients demonstrated significant cognitive decline, to 11% using the same NP tests and same measurement of change. This improvement for patients has been the result of the application of neuropsychological assessment and reflects the changes in surgical and anaesthetic equipment and practice that have been introduced.

The concerns regarding the impact of CABG on the brain and the potential role of using CPB fueled the resurgence of conducting surgery on the beating heart, thereby avoiding the CPB machine (OPCAB surgery, as noted earlier). The first large randomized controlled trial ($n = 281$) conducted by van Dijk and colleagues (2002) found that avoiding CPB resulted in a trend toward a better cognitive outcome at three months after surgery (21% decline after off-pump vs. 29% decline after on-pump; $p = 0.15$); but by 12 months, this trend had diminished (31% vs. 34% respectively; $p = 0.69$). The same team found no difference in mortality, cardiac outcome, or quality of life at these time-points (Nathoe et al., 2003). At five years, though half the patients had cognitive decline, there was no difference between groups. Also, there were no differences between groups in cardiovascular events, angina, or quality of life (van Dijk et al., 2007).

Recently, more randomized controlled trials have emerged reporting no difference between groups in either short- or long-term changes in cognitive outcome (e.g. Jensen, Hughes, Rasmussen, Pedersen, & Steinbruchel, 2006; Selnes & McKhann, 2009; Takagi, Tananbashi, Kawai, & Umemoto, 2007), suggesting that the problems are no longer inherent in the CPB equipment and appear to reflect improvements of this equipment over time.

Very few studies have been conducted to examine cognitive outcome of different treatment strategies. Rosengart and colleagues compared patients undergoing PCI with CABG surgery patients and a group of healthy controls at baseline, three weeks and four months postprocedure (Rosengart et al., 2006). Using four different analytic techniques, which produced a wide variability in findings, they were unable to demonstrate a consistent finding of group differences or change in cognition when comparing PCI and CABG groups with healthy controls. They had similar results at a one-year follow-up (Sweet et al., 2008). In a more recent study, Selnes et al. (2009) conducted a longitudinal study to examine cognitive outcome in four groups: patients undergoing on-pump coronary artery bypass surgery ($n = 152$), off-pump surgery ($n = 75$), nonsurgical CAD ($n = 99$), and heart-healthy controls ($n = 69$). Although the CAD groups had a greater degree of decline over the six-year follow-up compared to the healthy controls, the researchers found no differences between the therapy groups and suggested that the type of management strategy did not impact long-term cognitive outcome. However, in common with Rosengart et al. (2006), they found that compared with healthy controls, the CAD patients had lower baseline cognitive performance and greater degrees of decline over six years. These results are consistent with other studies that have reported preexisting cognitive dysfunction in patients' pre-CABG surgery (e.g., Baird, Murkin, & Lee 1997; Millar, Asbury, & Murray, 2001; Rankin, Kochamba, Boone, Petitti, & Buckwalter, 2003). This finding suggests that the cognitive performance of CAD patients may be influenced more by their vascular disease than by treatment strategy (Selnes et al., 2009).

The findings in this section indicate that even though patients consider surgery as the most favoured and definitive form of treatment, surgery has a hidden impact that may lead to greater psychosocial difficulties for patients.

THE POSTINTERVENTION STAGE: PSYCHOSOCIAL TREATMENT AFTER CARDIAC EVENTS

CARDIAC REHABILITATION

The dominant psychosocial intervention for a wide range of cardiac conditions, normally after a cardiac event and associated treatment, is what is termed cardiac rehabilitation. *Cardiac rehabilitation* (CR) is a multidisciplinary intervention that is, in practice, very varied but always involves a variety of components around altering risk behaviors. It is common for CR to include the provision of information on the value of behavior change and consequent risk reduction (e.g., smoking, diet) and some form of structured exercise, along with pharmacological therapy. In some cases, one of a range of psychological therapy or counseling is offered. This therapy or counseling may involve psychological support, cognitive restructuring, relaxation, and stress management (see Figure 28.1). Some CR programs offer specific treatments for depression or anxiety. Evidence from systematic reviews and meta-analyses demonstrate that regardless of the diversity of the CR programs, attending them reduces mortality by approximately 25% (Brown, Taylor, Noorani, Stone, & Skidmore, 2003; Clark, Hartling, Vandermeer, & McAlister, 2005; Taylor et al., 2004).

Despite the overwhelming evidence of CR's benefit, some, but not all, patients are offered some form of cardiac rehabilitation after cardiac surgery or MI (Thomas et al., 2007). Key features that are predictive of referral by a physician include the attitudes of the physician and the physician's endorsement or support of the program (Grace et al., 2008; Jackson, Leclerc, Erskine, & Linden,

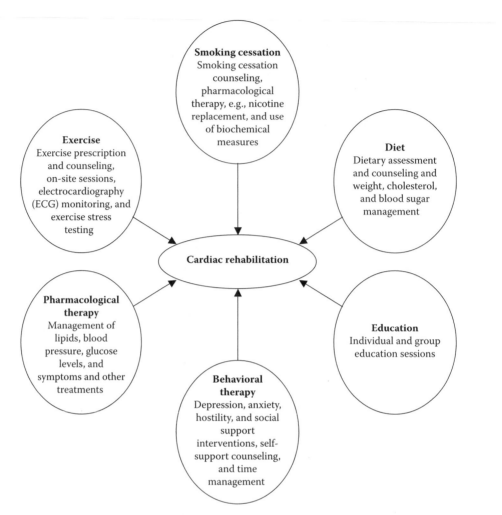

FIGURE 28.1   Modern cardiac rehabilitation program (Adapted from Lear, S. A. and Ignaszewski, A., *Current Controlled Trials in Cardiovascular Medicine*, 2, 221–232, 2001.)

2005). Even if referred, a number of patients do not attend CR programs. The result is that overall rates of attendance at CR programs is in the region of 15%–30% (Bunker & Goble, 2003; Grace et al., 2002; Sharp & Freeman, 2009; Wyer, Joseph, & Earll, 2001).

The factors that have been reported as barriers to the attendance and adherence to CR include such environmental issues as the distance from the rehabilitation center, male gender, socioeconomic status, educational level, the presence of comorbidities, medical insurance, and whether the individual is a smoker (Deskur-Smielecka et al., 2009). Other barriers include depression; anxiety; self-efficacy; social support (Grace et al., 2002); patients' motivation (Daly et al., 2002); and as with other treatments (see earlier), the patients' perception of the usefulness of CR (Dunlay et al., 2009).

Many proposals have been offered in order to facilitate and promote referral, uptake, and adherence to CR. Some procedural approaches include referring patients to CR while they are still hospitalized, which has been demonstrated to increase the likelihood of participation (Dunlay et al., 2009). Moreover, some individuals have advocated the use of telehealth interventions, where phone, Internet, and video conferencing between patients and physicians are used. Telehealth intervention is a technique to provide more convenience for patients, avoid the barrier of distance, and enable an easy and potentially cost-effective means for delivering CR. Providing individuals with a choice of the type of CR they prefer—whether home, hospital, community, or telehealth—has been argued as the technique most likely to enhance participation (Thompson & Clark, 2009).

A number of approaches have been used to address the modifiable psychological factors that influence uptake and adherence to CR. For example, for patients who lack motivation, interventions that include motivational interviewing appear to have had some success (Sharp & Freeman, 2009).

TREATMENT FOR MOOD DISORDERS IN CARDIOVASCULAR DISEASE

The psychological impact of a such a cardiac event as MI or cardiac surgery can be significant and may influence well-being (Kristofferzon, Lofmark, & Carlsson, 2005). In the short term, patients experience a range of emotions, among them feelings of sadness, shock, disbelief, and anxiety (Nemeroff, Musselman, & Evans, 1998). It is only when these feelings extend to long periods of time or are extremely severe that they may indicate a more serious psychological problem and thereby suggest the need for intervention.

Many studies have documented the high prevalence of depression among people with cardiac disease. Epidemiological studies report that figures range form 16% to 23% for post-MI and -CAD patients (Musselman, Evans, & Nemeroff, 1998). Between 15% and 20% of patients hospitalized for an MI meet the DSM (*Diagnostic and Statistical Manual of Mental Disorders*) criteria for major depression (Lichtman et al., 2008). In addition, according to Frasure-Smith, Lespérance, and Talajic (1993), significant depressive symptomatology is evident in 65% of post-MI patients. Women appear to experience more depressive symptomatology after an MI than do men (Grace et al., 2002). This high prevalence rate of depression is also apparent in patients hospitalized for unstable angina, PCI, CABG surgery, valve surgery, and congestive heart failure (Rutledge, Reis, Linke, Greenberg, & Mills, 2006).

Anxiety disorders have been reported to range between 10% and 29% (Serber, Todaro, Tilkemeier, & Niaua, 2009). Bankier, Januzzi, and Littman (2004) found that high rates of such other psychiatric disorders as dysthymic disorder, generalized anxiety disorder, and posttraumatic stress disorder are also observable in patients with CAD.

Some earlier studies suggested that depression was not associated with mortality in cardiac disease (Kaufman et al., 1999; Ladwig, Kieser, Konig, Breithardt, & Borggrefe, 1991). However, recent studies have documented that across many cardiac disease groups, the likelihood of mortality is increased for both men and women when depression is present (Frasure-Smith, Lespérance, Juneau, Talajic, & Bourassa, 1999). For instance, CABG patients have been found to have a greater risk for further nonfatal cardiac events when depressed (Burg, Benedetto, Rosenberg, & Soufer, 2001). Depressed post-MI patients have three to four times more chance of dying in the subsequent six months compared to nondepressed patients after adjusting for medical and demographic risk factors (Frasure-Smith et al., 1993). Similarly, depressed patients with unstable angina were also more likely than their nondepressed counterparts to die or have a further nonfatal MI (Lespérance & Frasure-Smith, 2000). Recent meta-analyses reported that the risk of mortality is twice as high for depressed as opposed to nondepressed MI and CAD patients (Barth, Schumacher, & Herrmann-Lingen, 2004; Van Melle et al., 2004).

Findings in relation to anxiety are less consistent. Denollet, Sys, and Brutsaert (1995) found a correlation between anxiety symptoms and mortality post-MI. Other studies have indicated that anxiety predicts further cardiac events but not mortality, and some studies report no association between anxiety and prognosis (Ahern et al., 1990; Lane, Douglas, Ring, Beevers, & Lip, 2001).

Besides having a link to mortality and further cardiac events, depression and anxiety have detrimental effects on patients' well-being and quality of life. The Heart and Soul Study (Ruo et al., 2003) showed that the presence of depressive symptoms predicted greater physical limitations and a diminished overall quality of life. Mayou et al. (2000) reported that anxiety and depression predict poor outcomes in terms of life quality, use of primary care resources, and lifestyle changes.

Similarly, depression scores accounted for 49% of the variance in quality of life scores in the study by Conn, Taylor, and Wiman (1991).

One proposed route for the poor outcomes of people with cardiac disease and depression or anxiety is through their adherence to treatments. Ziegelstein et al. (2000) found that MI patients who exhibit mild, moderate, and major depression are less adherent to such healthy behaviors as exercise and diet; whereas those patients with major depression and/or dysthymia are less likely to adhere to prescribed medication than are nondepressed patients. Depression and anxiety are associated with inconsistent attendance, higher drop-out rates, and higher chances of noncompletion of CR (McGrady, McGinnia, Badenhop, Bentle, & Rajput, 2009). The evidence of the widespread impact of mood disorders in this group has important implications for the identification of patients with depression and the need to identify effective treatments for this group.

Several interventions have been conducted targeting cardiac patients with depression. These include pharmacological, exercise-based, and psychological interventions. Patients with severe depressive symptoms usually receive pharmacological therapy. Recent trials support the usefulness and efficacy of Selective Serotonin Reuptake Inhibitors (SSRI) in treating depression. The Sertraline Antidepressant Heart Attack (SADHART) Trial showed that Sertraline is effective in treating depression, particularly for recurrent and severe forms of depression in post-MI patients. The patients treated with the specific SSRI had a decreased risk of death and reinfarction compared to untreated patients (Glassman et al., 2002). In addition to this, treatment with SSRIs was found to have positive effects on heart rate variability, a significant prognostic factor in CAD. For a comprehensive review of antidepressant medication interventions for clinical depression in cardiac patients, see Davies, Jackson, Potokar, and Nutt (2004).

In addition, exercise has been found to reduce depression in cardiac patients (Lawlor & Hopker, 2001). Stern, Gorman, and Kaslow (1983) conducted a randomized controlled trial of 106 MI patients with depression, anxiety, or low fitness levels. They randomized participants into those who received the usual care (control group), those who received group therapy, and those who received 12 weeks of exercise training. Their findings indicated that participants who received either group therapy or exercise training showed improvement in depression in relation to controls after one year. Moreover, a meta-analysis by Kugler, Seelbach, and Kruskemper (1994) supported the beneficial effect of exercise on depression and anxiety in the CR settings. An extensive review of exercise-based interventions in CAD has been conducted by Taylor et al. (2004). This review included 48 studies in which 67% of the population were MI patients. It is of interest that although more than half the studies included women, the latter accounted for only 20% of all recruited participants. The review provided support for the usefulness of exercise interventions in CAD patients. Specifically, exercise intervention had positive effects in terms of physical outcomes (blood pressure, cholesterol, and triglyceride levels), health-related quality of life, and mortality.

Psychological interventions have been widely used to treat depression in cardiac patients. Interventions of a psychological nature include stress management (e.g., learning relaxation, use of cognitive techniques and cognitive challenge, coping strategies to deal with stress); counseling; and psychodynamic, educational, and self-management interventions. Stress management is the most commonly used psychological intervention in cardiac populations and appears to be successful in reducing anxiety and depression but not mortality (see Rees, Bennett, West, Davey, & Ebrahim, 2004, for a full review). The American Psychological Association (APA) task force report defined three categories of interventions based on the support that these have received from previous research. Category I includes such treatments as behavioral therapy, behavioral marital therapy, cognitive behaviorial therapy, and interpersonal therapy; these treatments are supported by at least two control studies. Category II includes such treatments as dynamic therapy, self-control therapy, and social problem-solving therapy; these treatments are supported by at least one control study. Finally, Category III includes either innovative treatments, treatments with no support from trials, or treatments that have not been adequately tested (Chamless & Ollendick, 2001). There are several distinctive trials that use psychological approaches to treating depression, and these are discussed next.

Probably the most well-known trial in the treatment of depression is the ENRICHD (Enhancing Recovery in Coronary Heart Disease) Study (Carney et al., 2004). In this trial, acute MI patients with depression, dysthymia, or low social support were randomized to usual care or psychological intervention. The latter consisted of 6 to 12 sessions of cognitive-behavioral therapy and antidepressant medication when required. The cognitive-behavioral therapy sessions involved active problem-solving, behavioral activation, and the challenging of depressing thoughts. The results of the trial indicated that there was a modest reduction of depression for both groups (mean decrease in the Beck Depression Inventory score of 49% in the intervention group vs. 33% in the usual care group), but there were no effects of the treatment on mortality.

The CREATE (Canadian Cardiac Randomized Evaluation of Antidepressant and Psychotherapy Efficacy) Trial used interpersonal therapy for treating depression in CAD patients, but the findings did not support the usefulness of interpersonal therapy in the treatment of depression (Lespérance et al., 2007). In the Montreal Heart Attack Readjustment Trial (MHART), patients were randomized to monthly telephone monitoring with or without support for psychological distress. The treatment was not successful in improving mortality rates and psychological outcomes, and it even increased mortality in women who received it (Frasure-Smith et al., 1997). These findings do not concur with those of other trials that were successful in reducing recurrent MI (Ischemic Heart Disease Life Stress Monitoring Study [IHDLSM]; Frasure-Smith & Prince, 1989) and distress (Blumenthal et al., 1997).

These studies have important implications for the way researchers approach the treatment of depression. Some authors have argued that the results of the SADHART, ENRICHD, and MHART studies may be attributed to the fact that treatments were initiated shortly after diagnosis. In such cases, symptoms of depression may be situational, and therefore treatment will be less effective in reducing them (Whooley, 2006). This argument has been supported by the meta-analysis of Linden, Phillips, and Leclerc (2007). They found that when psychological treatment was initiated within two months of the cardiac event, it failed to produce any beneficial effects; whereas if it was initiated at a later stage, it tended to be more successful. This finding has important implications in terms of both the diagnosis and the treatment of mood disorders. It emphasizes the need to evaluate patients on multiple occasions and to refer patients for treatment when symptoms persist over time.

Moreover, there have been indications that previous history of depression is of great importance and therefore should be taken into consideration. Goodman, Shimbo, Haas, Davidson, and Rieckmann (2008) conducted a study in order to explore whether there is a difference in CAD severity in first-time incident versus recurrent depression. The findings suggested that patients with incident depression had more severe CAD than those with recurrent depression. This finding is supported by the results of the CREATE Trial, which showed that patients with incident depression were more responsive to the treatment in relation to the placebo group than were patients with previous history of depression (Lespérance et al., 2007). The foregoing finding raises questions about whether incident and recurrent depression should be treated separately.

Another assumption about the failure of these studies to reduce mortality is attributed to the lack of understanding of the processes that link depression to mortality. One potential mechanism is adherence to medication. Depression is known to be associated with poor medication adherence across many patient groups, including cardiac patients (DiMatteo, Lepper, & Croghan, 2000; Kronish et al., 2006). As mentioned earlier, Ziegelstein et al. (2000) found that MI patients who exhibit depression (mild, moderate, and major) are less adherent to such healthy behaviors as exercise and diet, and those with major depression and/or dysthymia are less likely to adhere to prescribed medication than are nondepressed patients. Depression is also associated with inconsistent attendance, higher drop-out rates, and higher chances of noncompletion of cardiac rehabilitation (McGrady et al., 2009). Rieckmann et al. (2006) explored whether improvements in depression over time had an effect on adherence to aspirin medication. They reported that there is a gradient relationship between the two, indicating that when depressive symptoms improve, the improvement leads to subsequent improvements in medication adherence one to three months after discharge.

Project COPES, a randomized controlled trial by Burg et al. (2008) was designed to examine the effect of treatment on two key pathophysiological pathways between depression and event-free survival; namely, medication adherence and inflammation. The treatment included sessions based on problem-solving therapy, a form of CBT that teaches patients how to solve psychosocial problems that promote depression, and a "stepped-care" approach. The latter entailed that symptom severity was reviewed regularly and treatment was adapted accordingly. The results of this trial are yet to be known but it is hoped they will shed some light upon the areas that previous studies have ignored.

Some authors have argued that the reason why interventions appear to be unsuccessful in reducing depression and mortality may be the duration of the treatment (Shimbo, Davidson, Haas, Fuster, & Badimon, 2004). Although it is still not clear what the ideal length for the treatment is, the ENRICHD and SADHART trials showed that a six-month duration is not sufficient to generate significant changes in depression.

Overall, although depression is a significant obstacle to survival after cardiac disease, psychological interventions have been fairly unsuccessful in reducing depression and mortality. This failure has been attributed to such various factors as initiation timing, duration, history of previous depressive episodes, and the mechanisms linking depression to mortality. All these factors should be taken into consideration when designing future interventions. If depression also affects CR uptake, then the issue is whether depression should be treated before initiating CR, to increase success chances, or after as part of CR. Future studies and interventions, should take into consideration all the mentioned limitations for both depression treatment and CR in general so that the key role of depression is clarified and appropriate policy steps are taken.

It is apparent, though, that some psychological treatments have a positive effect for some patients (Rees et al., 2004), and so the challenge for researchers is to determine which intervention works for which patient. Future trials should adapt their content in relation to the outcomes that these studies are designed to change over time. For example, it has been extensively argued that not only mortality but depression and anxiety could serve as endpoints in clinical trials (Linden, 2000). This approach is especially important when there is evidence indicating that patients' overall quality of life is diminished by high levels of anxiety and depression (Ruo et al., 2003). Treatment should not only aim at reducing mortality but also focus on "adding life to years" by improving the patients' overall quality of life (Linden, 2000).

CONCLUSION

In this chapter, we have attempted to indicate the central role of treatments in the patients' journey in CAD. We have considered progress in this journey within three stages: pre-, peri-, and postintervention. Integral to understanding how individuals respond to CAD disease in the preintervention stage is their thoughts regarding the different treatments available. The perceptions people hold regarding the range of treatments appear to shape their understanding of their disease; these, in turn, have an impact on emotions and behavior. To understand the CAD patients' journey necessitates an examination of the treatments they receive or are about to receive because these are integral to their understanding of where they are in their journey with their condition. An important issue is that an understanding of the interventions that address patients' false perceptions about their condition and its treatment are scarce, and thus there is an increasing need to examine the role and usefulness of these perceptions in the adaptation to chronic illness.

Cardiovascular disease and its treatments in the peri-intervention stage have some unintended consequences. We have illustrated this reality by examining the effects of surgery for occlusion of the arteries that provide blood to the heart. The impact on the brain and on cognitive abilities is important for a number of reasons. The cognitive abilities are important for patients and their family as they appear to influence their life course and its quality. They may also influence the capacity to deal with their chronic disease although these relationships are currently not well integrated into our understanding of coping with the demands of CAD. The assessment of brain function through neuropsychological testing has provided an extremely valuable tool through which to judge the impact of different forms of surgery and anaesthesia in this area. It is through using neuropsychological assessment in the systematic examination of how this form of surgery affects the brain that both surgical procedures and anaesthesia have been improved.

Finally, in the postintervention stage, the role of emotions, and in particular depression and its treatment, constitutes a central problem in long-term CAD rehabilitation. More well-designed and -structured interventions that aim to treat depression in these patients will help to shed light on the ideal approach to treating mood disorders in CR settings. The integration of patient's beliefs into their condition and the systematic integration of these into models of behavior change may lead to more success than presently experienced in dealing with the behavior change and mood difficulties that some CAD patients experience.

REFERENCES

Ahern, D. K., Gorkin, L., Anderson, J. L., Tierney, C., Hallstrom, A., Ewart, C., ... and The CAPS Investigators. (1990). Biobehavioral variables and mortality or cardiac arrest in the Cardiac Arrhythmia Pilot Study (CAPS). *American Journal of Cardiology, 66*, 59–62.

Ajzen, I. (1991). The theory of planned behavior. *Organizational Behavior and Human Decision Processes, 50*, 179–211.

Almeda, F. Q., & Snell, R. J. (2005). Coronary revascularization in multivessel disease: Which is better, stents or surgery? *Postgraduate Medicine, 118*, 1–17.

Baird, D. L., Murkin, J. M., & Lee, D. L. (1997). Neurologic findings in coronary artery bypass patients: Perioperative or preexisting? *Journal of Cardiothoracic amd Vascular Anesthesia, 11*(6), 694–698.

Baker, B., Richter, A., & Anand, S. S. (2001). From the heartland: Culture, psychological factors, and coronary heart disease. In S. S. Kazarian & D. R. Evans (Eds), *Handbook of cultural health psychology* (pp. 141–162). London, England: Academic Press.

Bankier, B., Januzzi, J. L., & Littman, A. B. (2004). The high prevalence of multiple psychiatric disorders in stable outpatients with coronary heart disease. *Psychosomatic Medicine, 66*, 645–650.

Barth, J., Schumacher, M., & Herrmann-Lingen, C. (2004). Depression as a risk factor for mortality in patients with coronary heart disease: A meta-analysis. *Psychosomatic Medicine, 66*, 802–813.

Beers, M. H., & Berkow, R. (2005). *The Merk manual of diagnosis and therapy* (17th ed.) Whitehouse Station, NJ: Merk Research Laboratories.

Berry, C., Tardif, J. C., & Bourassa, M. G. (2007a). Coronary heart disease in patients with diabetes: Part I. Recent advances in prevention and noninvasive management. *Journal of the American College of Cardiology, 49*(6), 631–642.

Berry, C., Tardif, J. C., & Bourassa, M. G. (2007b). Coronary heart disease in patients with diabetes: Part II. Recent advances in coronary revascularization. *Journal of the American College of Cardiology, 49*(6), 643–656.

Blumenthal, J. A., Jiang, W., Babyak, M. A., Krantz, D. S., Frid, D. J., Coleman, R. E., ... Morris, J. J. (1997). Stress management and exercise training in cardiac patients with myocardial ischemia: Effects on prognosis and evaluation of mechanisms. *Archives of Internal Medicine, 157*(19), 2213–2223.

Broadbent, E., Petrie, K. J., Main, J., & Weinman, J. (2006). The Brief Illness Perception Questionnaire. *Journal of Psychosomatic Research, 60*, 631–637.

Brown, A., Taylor, R., Noorani, H., Stone, J., & Skidmore, B. (2003). Exercise-based cardiac rehabilitation programs for coronary artery disease: a systematic clinical and economic review. *Technology Report*, No. 34.

Bunker, S. J., & Goble, A. J. (2003). Cardiac rehabilitation: under-referral and underutilisation. *Medical Journal of Australia, 179*, 332–333.

Burg M. M., Benedetto, C. M., Rosenberg, R., & Soufer, R. (2001). Depression prior to CABG predicts 6-month and 2-year morbidity and mortality. *Psychosomatic Medicine, 63*, 103.

Burg, M. M., Lespérance, F., Rieckmann, N., Clemow, L., Skotzko, C., & Davidson, K. W. (2008). Treating persistent depressive symptoms in post-ACS patients: The project COPES phase-I randomized controlled trial. *Contemporary Clinical Trials, 29*, 231–240.

Byrne, M., Walsh, J., & Murphy, A. (2005). Secondary prevention of coronary heart disease: patient beliefs and health-related behavior. *Journal of Psychosomatic Research, 58*, 403–415.

Carney, R. M., Blumenthal, J. A., Freedland, K. E., Youngblood, M., Veith, R. C., Burg, M. M., ... Jaffe, A. S. (for the ENRICHD Investigators). (2004). Depression and late mortality after myocardial infarction in the Enhancing Recovery in Coronary Heart Disease (ENRICHD) Study. *Psychosomatic Medicine, 66,* 466–474.

Chambless, D. L., & Ollendick, T. H. (2001). Empirically supported psychological interventions: controversies and evidence. *Annual Review of Psychology, 52,* 685–716.

Chu, D., Bakaeen, F. G., Dao, T. K., LeMaire, S. A., Coselli, J. S., & Huh, J. (2009). On-pump versus off-pump coronary artery bypass grafting in a cohort of 63,000 patients. *Annals of Thoracic Surgery, 87,* 1820–1827.

Clark, A. M., Hartling, L., Vandermeer, B., & McAlister, F. A. (2005). Meta-analysis: Secondary prevention programs for patients with coronary artery disease. *Annals of Internal Medicine, 143,* 659–672.

Cohen, M. Z., Trippreimer, T., Smith, C., Sorofman, B., & Lively, S. (1994). Explanatory models of diabetes: Patient practitioner variation. *Social Science & Medicine, 38,* 59–66.

Colon, N., Grocott, H. P., & Macksen, G. B. (2008). Neuroprotection during cardiac surgery. *Expert Review of Cardiovascular Therapy, 6,* 503–520.

Conn, W. S., Taylor, S. G., & Wiman, P. (1991). Anxiety, depression, quality of life, and self-care among survivors of myocardial infarction. *Issues in Mental Health Nursing, 12*(4), 321–331.

Correa-de-Araujo, R. (2006). Serious gaps: How the lack of sex/gender-based research impairs health. *Journal of Women's Health, 15,* 1116–1122.

Daly J., Sindone, A. P., Thompson, D. R., Hancock, K., Chang, E., & Davidson, P. (2002). Barriers to participation in and adherence to cardiac rehabilitation programs: A critical literature review. *Progress in Cardiovascular Nursing, 17,* 8–17.

Davidson, P. M., Gholizadeh, L., Haghshenas, A., Rotem, A., DiGiacomo, M., Eisenbruch, M., & Salamonson, Y. (2010). A review of the cultural competence view of cardiac rehabilitation. *Journal of Clinical Nursing, 19,* 1335–1342.

Davies, S. J. C., Jackson, P. R., Potokar, J., & Nutt, D. J. (2004). Treatment of anxiety and depressive disorders in patients with cardiovascular disease. *BMJ, 328,* 939–943.

Denollet, J., Sys, S. U., & Brutsaert, D. L. (1995). Personality and mortality after myocardial infarction. *Psychosomatic Medicine, 57*(6), 582–591.

Deskur-Smielecka, E., Borowicz-Bienkowska, S., Brychcy, A., Wilk, M., Przywarska, I., & Dylewicz P. (2009). Why patients after acute coronary syndromes do not participate in an early outpatient rehabilitation programme? *Kardiologia Polska, 67,* 632–638.

DiMatteo, R. M., Lepper, H. S., & Croghan, T. W. (2000). Depression is a risk factor fornoncompliance with medical treatment. Meta-analysis of the effects of anxiety and depression on patient adherence. *Archives of Internal Medicine, 160,* 2101–2107.

Dunlay, S. M., Witt, B. J., Allison, T. G., Hayes, S. N., Weston, S. A., Koepsell, E., & Roger, V. L. (2009). Barriers to participation in cardiac rehabilitation. *American Heart Journal, 158,* 852–857.

Frasure-Smith, N., Lespérance, F., Juneau, M., Talajic, M., & Bourassa, M. G. (1999). Gender, depression, and one-year prognosis after myocardial infarction. *Psychosomatic Medicine, 61,* 26–37.

Frasure-Smith, N., Lespérance, F., Prince, R. H., Verrier, P., Garber, R. A., Juneau, M., ... Bourassa, M. G. (1997). Randomised trial of home-based psychosocial nursing intervention for patients recovering from myocardial infarction. *Lancet, 350,* 473–479.

Frasure-Smith, N., Lespérance, F., & Talajic, M. (1993). Depression following myocardial infarction: impact on 6-month survival. *Journal of the American Medical Association, 270*(15), 1819–1825.

Frasure-Smith, N., & Prince, R. (1989). Long-term follow-up of the Ischemic Heart Disease Life Stress Monitoring Program. *Psychosomatic Medicine, 51,* 485–513.

French, D., Cooper, A., & Weinman, J. (2006). Illness perceptions predict attendance at cardiac rehabilitation following acute myocardial infarction: a systematic review with meta-analysis. *Journal of Psychosomatic Research, 61*(6), 757–767.

French, D. P., Lewin, R. J. P., Watson, N., & Thompson, D. R. (2005). Do illness perceptions predict attendance at cardiac rehabilitation and quality of life following myocardial infarction? *Journal of Psychosomatic Research, 59,* 315–322.

Funder, K. S., Steinmetz, J., & Rasmussen, L. S. (2009). Cognitive dysfunction after cardiovascular surgery. *Minerva Anestesiologica, 75,* 329–332.

Gallo, L. C., Malek, M. J., Gilbertson, A. D., & Moore, J. L. (2005). Perceived cognitive function and emotional distress following coronary artery bypass surgery. *Journal of Behavioral Medicine, 28,* 433–442.

Glassman, A. H., O'Connor, C. M., Califf, R. M., Swedberg, C., Schwartz, P., Bigger, T. Jr., ... Harrison, W. M. (for the Sertraline Antidepressant Heart Attack Randomized Trial [SADHART] Group). (2002). Sertraline treatment of major depression in patients with acute MI or unstable angina. *Journal of the American Medical Association, 288,* 701–709.

Goodman, J., Shimbo, D., Haas, D. C., Davidson, K. W., & Rieckmann, N. (2008). Incident and recurrent major depressive disorder and coronary artery disease severity in acute coronary syndrome patients. *Journal of Psychiatric Research, 42*, 670–675.

Grace, S. L., Abbey, S. E., Shnek, Z. M., Irvine, J., Franche, R.-L., & Stewart, D. E. (2002). Cardiac rehabilitation II: Referral and participation. *General Hospital Psychiatry, 24*(3), 127–134.

Grace, S. L., Gravely-Witte, S., Brual, J., Suskin, N., Higginson, L., Alter, D., & Stewart, D. E. (2008). Contribution of patient and physician factors to cardiac rehabilitation enrolment: a prospective multilevel study. *European Journal of Cardiovascular Prevention & Rehabilitation, 15*(5), 548–556.

Grace, S. L., Krepostman, S., Brooks, D., Arthur, H., Scholey, P., Suskin, N., ... Steward, D. E. (2005). Illness perceptions among cardiac patients: Relation to depressive symptomatology and sex. *Journal of Psychosomatic Research, 59*, 153–160.

Gupta, R., Birnbaum, Y., & Uretsky, B. F. (2004). The renal patient with coronary artery disease: Current concepts and dilemmas. *Journal of the American College of Cardiology, 44*, 1343–1353.

Hagger, M. S., & Orbell, S. (2003). A meta-analytic review of the common-sense model of illness representations. *Psychology and Health, 18*, 141–184.

Hampson, S. E., Glasgow, R. E., & Toobert, D. J. (1990). Personal models of diabetes and their relations to self-care activities. *Health Psychology, 9*, 632–646.

Heijmans, M. (1998). Coping and adaptive outcome in chronic fatigue syndrome: importance of illness cognitions. *Journal of Psychosomatic Research, 45*, 39–51.

Heijmans, M., & de Ridder, D. (1998). Assessing illness representations of chronic illness: Explorations of their disease-specific nature. *Journal of Behavioral Medicine, 21*, 485–503.

Hirani, S. P. (2009). *An exploration of the relationships within and between illness and treatment beliefs in coronary artery disease patients undergoing coronary artery bypass, percutaneous coronary interventions and medical therapy interventions* [Doctoral thesis]. University College London (UCL), London, England.

Hirani, S. P., Patterson, D. L. H., & Newman, S. (2009). What do coronary artery disease patients think about their treatments? An assessment of patients' treatment representations. *Journal of Health Psychology, 13*, 311–322.

Hirani, S. P., Pugsley, W. B., & Newman, S. P. (2006). Illness representations of coronary artery disease: An empirical examination of the illness perceptions questionnaire (IPQ) in patients undergoing surgery, angioplasty and medication. *British Journal of Health Psychology, 11*, 199–220.

Horne, R., & Weinman, J. (1999). Patients' beliefs about prescribed medicines and their role in adherence to treatment in chronic physical illness. *Journal of Psychosomatic Research, 47*, 555–567.

Horne, R., & Weinman, J. (2002). Self-regulation and self-management in asthma: exploring the role of illness perceptions and treatment beliefs in explaining non-adherence to preventer medication. *Psychology & Health, 17*, 17–32.

Horne, R., Weinman, J., & Hankins, M. (1999). The Beliefs about Medicines Questionnaire: The development and evaluation of a new method for assessing the cognitive representation of medication. *Psychology & Health, 14*, 1–24.

Jackson, L., Leclerc, J., Erskine, Y., & Linden, W. (2005). Getting the most out of cardiac rehabilitation: A review of referral and adherence predictors. *Heart, 91*(1), 10–14.

Jacobs, A. K. (2009). Coronary interventions in 2009: Are women no different than men? *Circulation: Cardiovascular Interventions, 2*, 69–78.

Jensen, B. O., Hughes, P., Rasmussen, L. S., Pedersen, P. U., & Steinbruchel, D. A. (2006). Cognitive outcomes in elderly high-risk patients after off-pump versus conventional coronary artery bypass grafting: a randomized trial. *Circulation, 113*, 2790–2795.

Johnson, T., Monk, T., Rasmussen, L. S., Abildstrom, H., Houx, P., Korttila, K., ... Jakob, M. (for the ISPOCD2 investigators). (2002). Postoperative cognitive dysfunction in middle-aged patients. *Anesthesiology, 96*, 1351–1357.

Kampman, O., Lehtinen, K., Lassila, V., Leinonen, E., Poutanen, O., & Koivisto, A.-M. (2000). Attitudes towards neuroleptic treatment: Reliability and validity of the Attitudes Towards Neuroleptic Treatment (ANT) Questionnaire. *Schizophrenia Research, 45*, 223–234.

Kaufman, M. W., Fitzgibbons, J. P., Sussman, E. J., Reed, J. F. III, Einfalt, J. M., Rodgers, J. K., & Fricchione, G. L. (1999). Relation between myocardial infarction, depression, hostility, and death. *American Heart Journal, 138*(3), 549–554.

Khatri, P., Babyak, M., Clancy, C., Davis, R., Croughwell, N., Newman, M., ... Blumenthal, J. A. (1999). Perception of cognitive function in older adults following coronary artery bypass surgery. *Health Psychology, 18*, 301–306.

Kim, C., Redberg, R. F., Pavlic, T., & Eagle, K. A. (2007). A systematic review of gender differences in mortality after coronary artery bypass graft surgery & percutaneous coronary interventions. *Clinical Cardiology*, *30*(10), 491–495.

Kristofferzon, M. L., Löfmark, R., & Carlsson, M. (2005). Perceived coping, social support, and quality of life 1 month after myocardial infarction: A comparison between Swedish women and men. *Heart & Lung*, *34*(1), 39–50.

Kronish, I. M., Rieckmann, N., Halm, E. A., Shimbo, D., Vorchheimer, D., Haas, D. C., ... Davidson, K. W. (2006). Persistent depression affects adherence to secondary prevention behaviors after acute coronary syndromes. *Journal of General Internal Medicine*, *21*, 1178–1183.

Kugler, J., Seelbach, H., & Kruskemper, G. M. (1994). Effects of rehabilitation exercise programmes on anxiety and depression in coronary patients: A meta-analysis. *British Journal of Clinical Psychology*, *33*, 401–410.

Ladwig, K. H., Kieser, M., Konig, J., Breithardt, G., & Borggrefe, M. (1991). Affective disorders and survival after acute myocardial infarction. *European Heart Journal*, *12*, 959–964.

Lane, D., Douglas, C., Ring, C., Beevers, D. G., & Lip, G. Y. H. (2001). Mortality and quality of life 12 months after myocardial infarction: Effects of depression and anxiety. *Psychosomatic Medicine*, *63*, 221–230.

LaPointe, N. M. A., Ou, F. S., Calvert, S. B., Melloni, C., Stafford, J. A., Harding, T., ... Peterson, E. D. (2010). Changes in beliefs about medications during long-term care for ischemic heart disease *American Heart Journal*, *159*, 561–569.

Lawlor, D. A., & Hopker, S. W. (2001). The effectiveness of exercise as an intervention in themanagement of depression: systematic review and meta-regression analysis of randomised controlled trials. *BMJ*, *322*(7289), 763–767.

Lear, S. A., & Ignaszewski, A. (2001). Cardiac rehabilitation: a comprehensive review. *Current Controlled Trials in Cardiovascular Medicine*, *2*, 221–232.

Lespérance, F., & Frasure-Smith, N. (2000) . Depression in patients with cardiac disease: A practical review. *Journal of Psychosomatic Research*, *48*(4–5), 379–391.

Lespérance, F., Frasure-Smith, N., Koszycki, D., Laliberte, M.-A., van Zyl, L. T., Baker, B., ... Guertin, M.-C. (for the CREATE Investigators). (2007). Effects of citalopram and interpersonal psychotherapy on depression in patients with coronary artery disease: The Canadian Cardiac Randomized Evaluation of Antidepressant and Psychotherapy Efficacy (CREATE) Trial. *Journal of the American Medical Association*, *297*, 367–379.

Leventhal, H., Benyamini, Y., Brownlee, S., Diefenbach, M., Leventhal, E., Patrick-Miller, L. & Robitaille, C. (1997). Illness representations: Theoretical foundations. In K. J. Petrie & J. A. Weinman (Eds.), *Perceptions of health and illness: Current research and applications* (pp. 19–46). Amsterdam, Netherlands: Harwood Academic.

Leventhal, H., & Leventhal, E. A. (1993). Affect, cognition, and symptom perception. In K. M. Foley & C. R. Chapman (Eds.), *Current and emerging issues in cancer pain: Research and practice* (pp. 153–173). New York, NY: Raven Press.

Leventhal, H., Meyer, D., & Nerenz, D. (1980). The common sense model of illness danger. *Medical Psychology*, *2*, 7–30.

Leventhal, H., Musumeci, T. J., & Contrada, R. J. (2007). Current issues and new directions in psychology and health: Theory, translation, and evidence-based practice. *Psychology & Health*, *22*, 381–386.

Leventhal, H., Nerenz, D., & Steele, D. J. (1984). Illness representation and coping with health threats. In A. S. Baum, S. E. Taylor, & J. E. Singer (Eds.), *Handbook of psychology and health: Social psychological aspects of health* (Vol. 4, pp. 219–252). Hillsdale, NJ: Erlbaum.

Leventhal, H., Weinman, J., Leventhal, E., & Phillips, L. A. (2008). Health psychology: The search for pathways between behavior and health. *Annual Review of Psychology*, *59*, 477–505.

Lichtman, J. H., Bigger, J. T., Jr., Blumenthal, J. A., Frasure-Smith, N., Kaufmann, P. G., Lesperance, F., ... Sivarajan Froelicher, E. (2008). Depression and coronary heart disease: Recommendations for screening, referral, and treatment: A science advisory from the American Heart Association Prevention Committee of the Council on Cardiovascular Nursing, Council on Clinical Cardiology, Council on Epidemiology and Prevention, and Interdisciplinary Council on Quality of Care and Outcomes Research: Endorsed by the American Psychiatric Association. *American Psychiatric Association*, *7*, 406–413.

Linden, W. (2000). Psychological treatments in cardiac rehabilitation: review of rationales and outcomes. *Journal of Psychosomatic Research*, *48*(4–5), 443–454.

Linden, W., Phillips, M. J., & Leclerc, J. (2007). Psychological treatment of cardiac patients: A meta-analysis. *European Heart Journal*, *28*(24), 2972–3984.

Lip, G. Y. H., Barnett, A. H., Bradbury, A., Cappuccio, F. P., Gill, P. S., Hughes, E., ... Patel, K. (2007). Ethnicity and cardiovascular disease prevention in the United Kingdom: A practical approach to management. *Journal of Human Hypertension, 21*, 183–211.

Llewellyn, C. D., McGurk, M., & Weinman, J. (2007). Illness and treatment beliefs in head and neck cancer: Is Leventhal's common sense model a useful framework for determining changes in outcomes over time? *Journal of Psychosomatic Research, 63*, 17–26.

Mayou, R. A., Gill, D., Thompson, D. R., Day, A., Hicks, N., Volmink, J., & Neil., A. (2000). Depression and anxiety as predictors of outcome after myocardial infarction. *Psychosomatic Medicine, 62*, 212–219.

McGrady, A., McGinnis, R., Badenhop, D., Bentle, M., & Rajput, M. (2009). Effects of depression and anxiety on adherence to cardiac rehabilitation. *Journal of Cardiopulmonary Rehabilitation and Prevention, 29*, 358–364.

Millar, K., Asbury, A. J., & Murray, J. D. (2001). Pre-excognitive impairment as a factor influencing outcome after cardiac surgery. *British Journal of Anesthesia, 86*(1), 63–67.

Moss-Morris, R., Weinman, J., Petrie, K. J., Horne, R., Cameron, L. D., & Buick, D. (2002). The Revised Illness Perception Questionnaire (IPQ-R). *Psychology & Health, 17*, 1–16.

Murkin, J. M., Newman, S. P., Stump, D. A., & Blumenthal, J. A. (1995). Statement of consensus on assessment of neurobehavioral outcomes after cardiac surgery. *Annals of Thoracic Surgery, 59*, 1289–1295.

Murkin, J. M., Stump, D. A., Blumenthal, J. A., & McKhann, G. (1997). Defining dysfunction: Group means versus incidence analysis—A statement of consensus. *Annals of Thoracic Surgery, 64*, 904–905.

Musselman, D. L., Evans, D. L., & Nemeroff, C. B. (1998). The relationship of depression to cardiovascular disease: Epidemiology, biology, and treatment. *Archives of General Psychiatry, 55*, 580–592.

Nathoe, H. M., van Dijk, D., Jansen, E. W. L., Suyker, W. J. L., Diephuis, J. C., van Boven, W.-J., ... de Jaegere, P. P. T. (2003). A comparison of on-pump and off-pump coronary bypass surgery in low-risk patients. *New England Journal of Medicine, 348*, 394–402.

Nemeroff, C. B., Musselman, D. L., & Evans, D. L. (1998). Depression and cardiac disease. *Depression and Anxiety, 8*(Suppl. 1), 71–79.

Newman, M. F., Grocott, H. P., Mathew, J. P., White, W. D., Landolfo, K., Reves, J. G., ... Blumenthal, J. A. (for the Neurologic Outcome Research Group and the Cardiothoracic Anesthesia Research Endeavors [CARE] Investigators of the Duke Heart Center). (2001). Report of the substudy assessing the impact of neurocognitive function on quality of life 5 years after cardiac surgery. *Stroke, 32*, 2874–2881.

Newman, M. F., Kirchner, J. L., Phillips–Bute, B., Gaver, V., Grocott, H., Jones, R. H., ... Blumenthal, J. A. (for the Neurological Outcome Research Group and the Cardiothoracic Anesthesiology Research Endeavors Investigators). (2001). Longitudinal assessment of neurocognitive function after coronary artery bypass surgery. *New England Journal of Medicine, 344*, 395–402.

Newman, M. F., Mathew, J. P., Grocott, H. P., Mackensen, B. G., Monk, T., Welsh-Bohmer, K. A., ... Mark, D. B. (2006). Central nervous system injury associated with cardiac surgery. *Lancet, 368*, 694–703.

Newman, S. P., & Stygall, J. (2000). Neuropsychological outcome following cardiac surgery. In S. P. Newman & M. J. G. Harrison (Eds.), *The brain and cardiac surgery* (pp. 21–50). London, England: Harwood Academic.

Petrie, K. J., Cameron, L. D., Ellis, C. J., Buick, D., & Weinman, J. (2002). Changing illness perceptions after myocardial infarction: An early intervention randomized controlled trial. *Psychosomatic Medicine, 64*, 580–586.

Phillips-Bute, B., Mathew, J., Blumenthal, J. A., Welsh-Bohmer, K., White, W. D., Mark, D., Landolfo, K., & Newman, M. F. (for the Neurological Outcome Research Group and C.A.R.E. Investigators of the Duke Heart Center). (2003). Female gender is associated with impaired quality of life 1 year after coronary artery bypass surgery. *Psychosomatic Medicine, 65*, 944–951.

Porteous, T., Francis, J., Bond, C., & Hannaford, P. (2010). Temporal stability of beliefs about medicines: Implications for optimising adherence. *Patient Education & Counselling, 79*, 225–230.

Rankin, K. P., Kochamba, G., S., Boone, K. B., Petitti, D. B., & Buckwalter, J. G. (2003). Presurgical deficits in patients receiving coronary artery bypass graft surgery. *Journal of the International Neuropsychological Society, 9*, 913–924.

Rees, K., Bennett, P., West, R., Davey, S. G., & Ebrahim, S. (2004). Psychological interventions for coronary heart disease. *Cochrane Database of Systematic Reviews*, No. 2., Art. No. CD002902. doi:10.1002/14651858. CD002902.pub2

Rieckmann, N., Kronish, I. M., Haas, D., Gerin, W., Chaplin, W. F., Burg, M. M., ... & Davidson, K. W. (2006). Persistent depressive symptoms lower aspirin adherence after acute coronary syndromes. *American Heart Journal, 152*, 922–927.

Roach, G. W., Kanchuger, M., Mangano, C. M., Newman, M., Nussmeier, N., Wolamn, R., … Mangano, D. T. (for the Multicenter Study of Perioperative Ischemia Research Group and the Ischemia Research and Education Foundation Investigators). (1996). Adverse cerebral outcomes after coronary bypass surgery. *New England Journal of Medicine, 335*, 1857–1863.

Rogers, R. W. (1975). A protection motivation theory of fear appeals and attitude change. *Journal of Psychology, 91*, 93–114.

Rosengart, T. K., Sweet, J. J., Finnin, E., Wolfe, P., Cashy, J., Hahn, E., … Sanborn, T. (2006). Stable cognition after coronary artery bypass grafting: comparisons with percutaneous intervention and normal controls. *Annals of Thoracic Surgery, 82*, 597–607.

Rosenstock, I. M. (1966). Why people use health services. *Milbank Memorial Fund Quarterly, 44*, 94–127.

Ruo, B., Rumsfeld, J. S., Hlatky, M. A., Liu, H., Browner, W. S., & Whooley, M. A. (2003). Depressive symptoms and health-related quality of life: The Heart and Soul Study. *Journal of the American Medical Association, 290*, 215–221.

Rutledge, T., Reis, V. A., Linke, S. E., Greenberg, B. H., & Mills, P. J. (2006). Depression in heart failure: A meta-analytic review of prevalence, intervention effects, and associations with clinical outcomes. *Journal of the American College of Cardiology, 48*(8), 1527–1537.

Schwarzer, R. (1992). Self-efficacy in the adoption and maintenance of health behaviors: Theoretical approaches and a new model. In R. Schwarzer (Ed.), *Self-efficacy: Thought control of action* (pp. 217–242). Washington, DC: Hemisphere.

Sellke, F .W., Chu, L. M., & Cohn, W. E. (2010). Current state of surgical myocardial revascularization. *Circulation, 74*, 1031–1037.

Selnes, O. A., Grega, M. A., Bailey, M. M., Pham, L. D., Zeger, S. L., Baumgartner, W. A., & McKhann, G. M. (2009). Do management strategies for coronary artery disease influence 6-year cognitive outcomes? *The Annals of Thoracic Surgery, 88*(2), 445–454.

Selnes, O. A., & McKhann, G. M. (2009). Neurocognitive complications after coronary artery bypass surgery. *Annals of Neurology, 57*(5), 615–21.

Selnes, O. A., Royall, R. M., Grega, M. A., Borowicz, L. M., Quaskey, S., & McKhann, G. M. (2001). Cognitive changes 5 years after coronary artery bypass grafting: Is there evidence of late decline? *Archives of Neurology, 58*, 598–604.

Serber, E. R., Todaro, J. F., Tilkemeier, P. L., & Niaura, R. (2009). Prevalence and characteristics of multiple psychiatric disorders in cardiac rehabilitation patients. *Journal of Cardiopulmonary Rehabilitation and Prevention, 29*(3), 161–168.

Sharp, J., & Freeman, C. (2009). Patterns and predictors of uptake and adherence to cardiac rehabilitation. *Journal of Cardiopulmonary Rehabilitation and Prevention, 29*, 241–247.

Shimbo, D., Davidson, K. W., Haas, D. C., Fuster, V., & Badimon, J. J. (2004). Negative impact of depression on outcomes in patients with coronary artery disease: mechanisms, treatment, considerations, and future directions. *Journal of Thrombosis and Haemostasis, 3*, 897–908.

Smith, M. H., Wagenknecht, L. E., Legault, C., Goff, D. C., Stump, D. A., Todd Troost, B., & Rogers, A. T. (2000). Age and other risk factors for neuropsychological decline in patients undergoing coronary artery bypass graft surgery. *Journal of Cardiothoracic and Vascular Anesthesia, 14*, 428–432.

Smith, S. C., Jr., Feldman, T. E., Hirshfeld, J. W., Jr., Jacobs, A. K., Kern, M. J., King, S. B., III, … Riegel, B. (2006). ACC/AHA/SCAI 2005 Guideline update for percutaneous coronary intervention—Summary article: A report of the American College of Cardiology/American Heart Association Task Force on Practice Guidelines [ACC/AHA/SCAI writing committee to update the 2001 guidelines for percutaneous coronary intervention]. *Circulation, 113*, 156–175.

Steed, E., Newman, S. P., & Hardman, S. M. C. (1999). An examination of the self-regulation model in atrial fibrillation. *British Journal of Health Psychology, 4*, 337–347.

Stern, M. J., Gorman, P. A., & Kaslow, P. (1983). The Group Counseling v Exercise Therapy [Study]: A controlled intervention with subjects following myocardial infarction. *Archives of Internal Medicine, 143*, 1719–1725.

Stygall, J., Newman, S. P., Fitzgerald, G., Steed, L., Mulligan, K., Arrowsmith, J. E., … Harrison, M. J. (2003). Cognitive change five years after coronary artery bypass surgery. *Health Psychology, 22*, 579–586.

Sweet, J. J., Finnin, E., Wolfe, P. L., Beaumont, J. L., Hahn, E., Marymont, J., … Rosengart, T. K. (2008). Absence of cognitive decline one year after coronary bypass surgery: Comparison to nonsurgical and healthy controls. *Annals of Thoracic Surgery, 85*, 1571–1578.

Takagi, H., Tananbashi, T., Kawai, N., & Umemoto, T. (2007). Cognitive decline after off-pump versus on-pump coronary artery bypass graft surgery: Meta-analysis of randomized controlled trials. *Journal of Thoracic and Cardiovascular Surgery, 134*, 512–513.

Taylor, R. S., Brown, A., Ebrahim, S., Jolliffe, J., Noorani, H., Rees, K., … Oldridge, N. (2004). Exercise-based rehabilitation for patients with coronary heart disease: Systematic review and meta-analysis of randomized controlled trials. *American Journal of Medicine, 116,* 682–692.

Thomas, R. J., King, M., Lui, K., Oldridge, N., Pina, I. L., Spertus, J., … Whitman, G. R. (2007). AACVPR/ACC/AHA 2007 Performance measures on cardiac rehabilitation for referral to and delivery of cardiac rehabilitation/secondary prevention services. *Journal of American College of Cardiology, 50,* 1400–1433.

Thompson, D. R., & Clark, A. M. (2009). Cardiac rehabilitation—Into the future. *Heart.* Retrieved from http://heart.bmj.com/content/early/2009/10/08/hrt.2009. 173732.full.pdf

Turk, D. C., Rudy, T. E., & Salovey, P. (1986). Implicit models of illness. *Journal of Behavioral Medicine, 9,* 453–474.

Van Dijk, D., Jansen, E. W., Hijman, R., Nierich, A. P., Diephuis, J. C., Moons, K. G. M., … Kalkman, C. J. (for the Octopus Study Group). (2002). Cognitive outcome after off-pump and on-pump coronary artery bypass graft surgery: A randomized trial. *Journal of the American Medical Association, 287,* 1405–1412.

Van Dijk, D., Spoor, M., Hijman, R., Nathoe, H. M., Borst, C., Jansen, E. W. L., … Kalkman, C. J. (for the Octopus Study Group). (2007). Cognitive and cardiac outcomes 5 years after off-pump vs on-pump coronary artery bypass graft surgery. *Journal of the American Medical Association, 297,* 701–708.

Van Melle, J. P., de Jonge, P., Spijkerman, T. A., Tijssen, I. G. P., Ormel, J., van Veldhuisen, D. J., … van den Berg, M. P. (2004). Prognostic association of depression following myocardial infarction with mortality and cardiovascular events: A meta-analysis. *Psychosomatic Medicine, 66,* 814–822.

Vingerhoets, G., de Soete, G., & Jannes, C. (1995). Subjective complaints versus neuropsychological test performance after cardiopulmonary bypass. *Journal of Psychosomatic Research, 39,* 843–853.

Walsh, J. C., Lynch, M., Murphy, A. W., & Daly, K. (2004). Factors influencing the decision to seek treatment for symptoms of acute myocardial infarction—An evaluation of the self-regulatory model of illness behaviour. *Journal of Psychosomatic Research, 56,* 67–73.

Webinski, J. (2008). American Medical Women's Association position paper on sex- and gender-specific medicine. *Journal of Women's Health, 10,* 1557.

Weinman, J., Petrie, K. J., Moss-Morris, R., & Horne, R. (1996). The Illness Perception Questionnaire: A new method for assessing the cognitive representation of illness. *Psychology & Health, 11,* 431–445.

Whittle, P. (1996). Causal beliefs and acute psychiatric admission. *British Journal of Medical Psychology, 69,* 355–370.

Whooley, M. A. (2006). Depression and cardiovascular disease: Healing the broken-hearted. *Journal of the American Medical Association, 295,* 2874–2881.

Wyer S., Joseph, S., & Earll, L. (2001). Predicting attendance at cardiac rehabilitation: A review and recommendations. *Coronary Health Care, 5,* 171–177.

Ziegelstein, R. C., Fauerbach, J. A., Stevens, S. S., Romanelli, J., Richter, D. P., & Bush, D. E. (2000). Patients with depression are less likely to follow recommendations to reduce cardiac risk during recovery from a myocardial infarction. *Archives of Internal Medicine, 160,* 1818–1823.

29 Randomized Clinical Trials
Psychosocial-Behavioral Interventions for Cardiovascular Disease

Neil Schneiderman
University of Miami

Kristina Orth-Gomér
Karolinska Institute

Cardiovascular disease, including coronary artery disease (CAD) and stroke, is the leading cause of death worldwide (WHO, 2011). Over 80% of cardiovascular disease deaths take place in low- and middle-income countries and occur almost equally in men and women. According to INTERHEART, modifiable risk factors are implicated in almost all CAD mortality (Yusuf et al., 2004). INTERHEART was a standardized case-control study of acute myocardial infarction (MI) carried out in 52 countries and including every inhabited continent. The study compared 15,152 post-MI cases with 14,820 age- and sex-matched control participants in terms of self-reported smoking, hypertension, diabetes, psychosocial factors, physical activity, dietary patterns, and consumption of alcohol as well as measurements of adiposity and apolipoproteins. The investigators found that the above nine potentially modifiable risk factors accounted for more than 90% of the population attributable risk for an acute initial MI. These risks held for men and women, across geographic regions and for all racial and ethnic groups. It is important to note that daily consumption of fruits or vegetables, moderate or strenuous exercise, and moderate consumption of alcohol were found to be protective.

INTERHEART provided a broad listing of risk factors that need to be addressed for the primary and secondary prevention of CAD. This listing included the importance of attending to psychosocial risk (Rosengren et al., 2004). Although the population attributable risk for severe global stress was less than for smoking, it was comparable to that posed by abnormal lipids, hypertension, diabetes, and abdominal obesity. Psychosocial factors including depression and financial, marital, and work stress, as well as recent adverse life events, accounted for 32.5% of the population attributable risk for MI in the INTERHEART study. The findings from this major investigation suggest that behavioral intervention trials designed to decrease CAD risk and improve health outcomes should attend to relevant psychosocial variables as well as other modifiable risk factors.

At present only a few psychosocial and behaviorally based randomized clinical trials have provided reasonable evidence that when behavior change techniques are applied by trained interventionists, the interventions either reduced cardiovascular risk in participants at high risk (Knowler et al., 2002; Tuomilehto et al., 2001; Wing et al., 2010) or decreased CAD morbidity (Friedman et al., 1986; Gulliksson et al., 2011) or mortality (Orth-Gomér et al., 2009) in post-MI patients. In contrast, other clinical trials using psychosocial-behavioral intervention procedures have reported null results (Berkman et al., 2003; Frasure-Smith et al., 1997; Jones & West, 1996). The purpose of the present chapter is therefore to examine the current state of research in this area and attempt to clarify some of the issues that may have contributed to discrepancies in outcome among randomized clinical trials.

LIFESTYLE INTERVENTIONS IN PERSONS AT HIGH RISK

Type 2 diabetes mellitus is a major risk factor for CAD in both men and women (AHA, 2010). Diabetics have two to four times higher risk of developing CAD than do nondiabetics (Eckel, Kahn, Robertson, & Rizza, 2006). In fact, the risk of MI in diabetics is equal to that of persons who have had a previous MI (Haffner, Lehto, Rönnemaa, Pyörälä, & Laakso, 1998). Therefore, two major randomized clinical trials were conducted to assess whether lifestyle interventions targeting weight loss and an increase in physical activity could reduce the incidence of diabetes in persons at high risk for developing Type 2 diabetes (Knowler et al., 2002; Tuomilehto et al., 2001).

The Finnish Diabetes Prevention Study (Tuomilehto et al., 2001) randomly assigned 522 middle-aged overweight men and women to either an intervention or a control group. Participants in the intervention group received individual counseling aimed at reducing weight, total intake of fat, and intake of saturated fat. Those individuals in the intervention group had seven sessions with a nutritionist during the first year of the study and one session every three months thereafter. The participants also were given individual guidance on increasing physical activity, improving endurance, and undertaking resistance-training sessions. After four years, the cumulative incidence of diabetes was 23% in the control group but only 11% in the intervention group. Thus, the risk of Type 2 diabetes was significantly reduced by 58% in the intervention group, and the reduced incidence of diabetes was found to be directly related to changes in lifestyle.

In the United States, the Diabetes Prevention Program Research Group (Knowler et al., 2002) randomly assigned 3,234 nondiabetic persons with elevated fasting and post-glucose-load plasma glucose concentrations to either placebo ($n = 1,082$); metformin ($n = 1,073$), which is an antihyperglycemic agent that increases peripheral glucose uptake and utilization; or to lifestyle modification ($n = 1,079$) aiming at a 7% reduction in weight and at least 150 minutes of physical activity per week. The lifestyle intervention began with a 16-lesson curriculum covering diet, exercise, and behavior modification taught by case managers on a one-to-one basis during the first 24 weeks after enrollment. The program was designed to be flexible, culturally sensitive, and individualized. Subsequent individual monthly sessions as well as group sessions with the case managers were designed to reinforce the behavioral changes. After an average of 2.8 years, the mean incidence of diabetes was 11.0, 7.8, and 4.8 cases in the placebo, metformin, and lifestyle groups, respectively. Thus, the lifestyle intervention reduced the incidence of diabetes by 58% and metformin reduced the incidence by 31% compared to the placebo condition. These differences were both statistically significant.

Based on the success of the Diabetes Prevention Research Program and the Finnish Diabetes Prevention Trial, the Look AHEAD (Action for Health in Diabetes) randomized clinical trial is comparing the effects of an intensive lifestyle intervention versus a diabetes support and education control group on the major CAD events in 5,145 overweight or obese participants with Type 2 diabetes (Wing et al., 2010; see also Wing & Phelan, 2011). The lifestyle intervention included diet modification and physical activity designed to induce at least a 7% weight loss at Year 1 and to maintain this weight loss in subsequent years. To increase dietary adherence, a portion controlled diet was used, with liquid-meal replacements provided free. The exercise goal was at least 175 minutes of physical activity per week, using activities similar in intensity to brisk walking. Behavioral strategies, including self-monitoring, goal setting, and problem solving, were stressed. Intervention participants were seen weekly for the first six months and three times per week for the next six months, with a combination of individual and group contacts. During Years 2 through 4, participants were seen individually at least once a month, contacted another time each month by telephone or e-mail, and offered a variety of ancillary group choices. At each session, participants were weighed, self-monitoring records were reviewed, and a new lesson was presented. Participants in the control condition were invited to three group sessions per year and received educational instruction on diet, physical activity, or social support. At four years, intervention participants showed greater improvement than control participants in terms of weight loss, fitness, hemoglobin A1c, systolic blood pressure, and high-density lipoprotein cholesterol. Not totally unexpected, reduction in low-density cholesterol was greater in the control than in the intervention participants owing to greater use of lipid-lowering medication. The trial is scheduled to last for a total of 11.5 years, which should permit assessment of CAD event data.

The Finnish Diabetes Prevention Study (Tuomilehto et al., 2001), Diabetes Prevention Program (Knowler et al., 2002), and the ongoing Look AHEAD Trial (Wing et al., 2010) have all proven to be efficacious. They clearly indicate that under rigorously controlled conditions, behavioral interventions using behavioral-change techniques administered by trained interventionists can produce lifestyle changes leading to improvements in health outcomes in individuals at high risk for diabetes and/or CAD. The extent to which these interventions can be shown to be effective in clinical practice is still to be determined. Given the explosive growth in Type 2 diabetes that is occurring worldwide, it is noteworthy that the techniques developed by the Finnish Prevention Study, the Diabetes Prevention Program, and Look AHEAD have become available. At the same time, it should be recognized that a large proportion of those at high risk for CAD, including obese Type 2 diabetes patients suffering from major comorbidities, currently lack access to treatment and the motivation to adhere to rigorous lifestyle interventions. Nevertheless, aspects of the skill sets developed in the lifestyle intervention studies most certainly will prove to be useful in a variety of settings.

PSYCHOSOCIAL INTERVENTIONS AFTER MAJOR ADVERSE CORONARY EVENTS

Although there has been considerable consistency in results among the three large-scale randomized clinical trials concentrating on lifestyle interventions, the few randomized clinical trials reporting on psychosocial-behavioral interventions among patients who have previously suffered major adverse coronary events have provided both null and positive outcomes. The three major studies that reported positive results are the Recurrent Coronary Prevention Project (RCPP) conducted by Friedman et al. (1986), the Secondary Prevention in Uppsala Primary Health Care Project (SUPRIM) conducted by Gulliksson et al. (2011), and the Stockholm Women's Intervention Trial for Coronary Heart Disease (SWITCHD) conducted by Orth-Gomér et al. (2009). Conversely, three large-scale trials that obtained null results include a study by Jones and West (1996), the Montreal Heart Attack Readjustment Trial (M-HART) led by Frasure-Smith et al. (1997), and the Enhancing Recovery in Coronary Heart Disease (ENRICHD) Trial conducted by Berkman et al. (2003).

The RCPP was the first major randomized clinical trial using a psychosocial-behavioral intervention on post-MI patients (Friedman et al., 1986). This trial randomized 862 post-MI patients in a ratio of 2:1, so that there were 592 participants in the psychosocial-behavioral condition and 270 participants in the control condition. The trial included 90% men of whom 98% were white. Those individuals in the control condition, administered by cardiologists, received advice and information concerning diet, exercise, medications, possible surgical regimens, medication adherence, and cardiovascular pathophysiology. Participants enrolled in the psychosocial intervention condition received the same information as those in the control condition, but they also had relaxation training to decrease behavioral arousal as well as group-based cognitive behavior therapy designed to decrease Type A behaviors, specifically hostility, impatience, and time urgency. Group process was used to examine these behaviors and to explore healthier, more productive alternatives. This intervention, carried out by trained psychologists and psychiatrists, emphasized behavioral self-management techniques, group support, and therapist support. Intervention participants, who attended both the cardiac counseling (control) sessions as well as the psychosocial-behavioral sessions, participated in a mean of 38 sessions (61%) over 4.5 years, whereas control participants attended a mean of 25 sessions (76%) during the same period of time. Rate of nonfatal infarctions was significantly lower in the intervention (6.6%) than in the control (17.2%) condition. Compared to the control condition, the intervention participants also revealed significant reductions in hostility, impatience, time urgency, and depressed mood as well as significant gains in perceived self-efficacy (Mendes de Leon, Powell, & Kaplan, 1991).

The second major randomized clinical trial using a psychosocial-behavioral intervention that reported a positive outcome was SWITCHD, which was conducted on women in Sweden who had suffered a major adverse coronary event, primarily MI (Orth-Gomér et al., 2009). This trial randomized 237 women into either a group-based cognitive behavior therapy program or into usual care and followed the women for a mean duration of 7.1 years. The intervention methods followed basic principles of cognitive behavior therapy and included communication of cardiovascular health knowledge, applying methods for self-monitoring, recognizing cognitive distortions, cognitive restructuring, skills training, and role playing. Contents of the intervention focused on women's specific psychosocial risk factor profile and on controlling behavioral risk factors, attenuating negative emotions, developing coping skills, reducing stress, and improving social support. The intervention was carried out by nurses with extensive experience in coronary care, who subsequently received extensive training in cognitive behavior therapy training from an expert clinical psychologist. This intervention was provided during 20 sessions carried out during the course of a year. Groups of four to eight women met weekly with a therapist for 10 weeks and thereafter monthly. Some 75% of the women attended 15–20 sessions that included skills training and practice in relaxation to decrease arousal as well as provide education about cardiovascular pathophysiology, risk factors, self-care and adherence to medical advice, and coping with stress exposure from family and work. The program, which used detailed therapist manuals, covered specific topics. Opportunities were offered for smoking cessation, physical exercise, and weight change. Therapists also made sure that every patient was engaged and talked during each session. From randomization until the end of follow-up (mean duration 7.1 years), the intervention compared with the control group showed an almost threefold protective effect on mortality rate (OR = 0.33; 95% CI = 0.1–.74). The third major randomized clinical trial that used a psychosocial-behavioral outcome and reported a positive outcome was SUPRIM, which was conducted on women and men in Sweden who had suffered a major adverse coronary event (Gulliksson et al., 2011). Patients were randomized to receive traditional care (usual care, 170 patients) or traditional care plus cognitive behavior therapy (intervention group, 192 patients). The cognitive behavior therapy program focused upon stress management and other topics similar to those covered by Orth-Gomér et al. (2009) and featured 20 two-hour group sessions during one year. Median attendance at each group session was 85%. Women and men were enrolled in separate groups. During a mean 94 month follow-up period, the intervention group had a 41% lower rate of fatal and non-fatal first recurrent CAD event (OR = 0.59; 95% CI = 0.42–0.83), 45% fewer recurrent acute MI (OR = 0.55; 95% CI = 0.36–0.85), and a nonsignificant 28% lower all-cause mortality (OR = 0.72; 95% CI = 0.40–1.30) than the usual care group after adjustment for other outcome-affecting variables. During the first two years of follow-up, there were no significant group differences in traditional risk factors.

Previously, Jones and West (1996) randomized 2,328 post-MI patients into either an intervention condition receiving seven weekly, two-hour psychological counseling and therapy, relaxation, and stress-management sessions or into a usual care condition. The intervention program was initiated soon after hospital discharge and was led by clinical psychologists and health care visitors. Spouses (or partners) were invited to attend the first two sessions. Intervention sessions included group and individual counseling. Principal objectives of the intervention were to (a) provide information about the cardiovascular system, heart disease, MI, treatment and management; (b) increase awareness of stress and stressful situations; (c) teach relaxation skills; (d) improve responses to stressful situations and develop coping skills; (e) promote positive adjustment to illness; and (f) rebuild confidence in patients and spouses. Sessions included teaching practical exercises with patient participation, group discussion, and individual counseling. The importance of practice between sessions was emphasized. Also, patients were asked to keep records of progress with diaries of activity, stress, and relaxation. However, such other components of comprehensive rehabilitation as consideration of diet, weight control, and exercise were explicitly omitted. Data on the age, sex distribution, and racial, ethnic, and other demographic information about participants were not described in the published article.

According to Jones and West (1996), 25% of the randomized participants did not attend any sessions. From the write-up of the publication, it appears that many of these no-shows may never have agreed to participate in the trial but were included in the "intent-to-treat" analysis. Data were also not provided on how many sessions were attended by the other participants. The investigators found no significant differences within or between groups in reported anxiety and depression between baseline and six months, suggesting that although attempts to elicit changes in these variables were at least secondary objectives of the trial, the psychosocial intervention was ineffective. Finally, the investigators found no differences between conditions in clinical complications, clinical sequela, or mortality after one year. In this respect, it is worth noting that the Friedman et al. (1986), Orth-Gomér et al., (2009) and Gulliksson et al. (2011) trials, which reported positive results, followed patients for a mean of 4.5, 7.1 and 7.8 years, respectively. An examination of the published figure showing cumulative all-cause mortality rates in the SWITCH Trial, conducted by Orth-Gomér and colleagues, indicates that mortality differences between groups did not really begin to diverge until after two years. It would thus appear that after comparing the studies conducted by Jones and West on the one hand with those of Friedman and colleagues, Orth-Gomér and colleagues, and Gulliksson and collaborators on the other, the differences in outcomes were likely attributable to differences in the extensiveness, adequacy, and comprehensiveness of the methods used.

In another psychosocial-behavioral intervention study, Frasure-Smith et al. (1997) randomized 1,376 post-MI patients (903 men, 473 women) into an intervention program ($n = 692$) or a usual care condition ($n = 684$) for one year in the Montreal Heart Attack Readjustment Trial (M-HART). Intervention participants were telephoned by a research assistant beginning one week after hospital discharge for acute MI and then monthly for a year. This research assistant administered a 20-item General Health Questionnaire that assesses psychological distress from symptoms of anxiety, depression, and impairment in activities (Goldberg, 1972). If a patient scored 5 or more out of 20 on this scale or was readmitted to the hospital, the research assistant contacted the project nurse responsible for that patient. The nurse then arranged to visit the patient as soon as possible at home or at another convenient location. During the initial one-hour visit, the nurse evaluated extensively the patient's psychosocial difficulties, needs, and cardiac status. Immediate difficulties were addressed; and if the patient agreed, the nurse scheduled a second visit within a month. Thereafter, intervention visits continued as required until the nurse and project team decided that further contact was not needed. Intervention visits were individually adjusted, but they typically involved the combination of emotional support, reassurance, education, practical advice, and referral to family physicians, cardiologists, and other health resources as needed. The nurses were experienced in cardiology nursing, but they received no special professional training concerning the implementation of the research protocol. All patients completed a baseline interview that included assessment of depression and anxiety. Survivors were also interviewed after one year.

Approximately 75% of intervention condition participants in M-HART received about 5–6 one-hour nursing visits. The program had no influence on psychological outcomes (e.g., depressive symptoms, anxiety, anger, or perceived social support) between conditions nor upon cardiac or all-cause mortality over the year. Treated women, however, showed marginally greater all-cause mortality (10.3% intervention vs. 5.4% usual care, $p = 0.051$), suggesting that the intervention may have been harmful to women. The reasons for this marginal finding remain speculative.

The Enhancing Recovery in Coronary Heart Disease (ENRICHD) Trial randomized 2,481 post-MI patients (44% women; 34% racial- or ethnic-minority participants) into a cognitive-behavioral intervention condition or into usual care (Berkman et al., 2003). Post-MI patients were selected because they were depressed and/or had low perceived social support. Among those individuals who were randomized, 39% were depressed, 26% had low perceived social support, and 34% met both criteria. Cognitive behavior therapy was used as the basis for the ENRICHD intervention. For depressed patients, cognitive behavior therapy was given as described by Beck (1995). For patients with low perceived social support, cognitive behavior therapy techniques were used to address the cognitions, behaviors, and emotions that accompany low perceived social support, supplemented with techniques based on social learning theory. Intervention-group patients with very high depression scores or failure to lower such scores after five weeks of psychosocial-behavioral intervention were referred to study psychiatrists for consideration of pharmacotherapy. In instances where group-based psychosocial-behavioral intervention was available, intervention participants were allowed to begin the group treatment provided they first completed at least three sessions of individual cognitive-behavioral therapy. The maximum duration of the psychosocial-behavioral intervention was six months. Group therapy could extend an additional 12 weeks, and adjunctive pharmacotherapy for up to 12 months. Approximately 30% of intervention participants received group-based psychotherapy, whereas 70% did not. Cognitive behavior therapy was initiated at a median of 17 days after the index MI for a median of 11 individual sessions throughout six months.

The major finding in ENRICHD was that after an average follow-up of 29 months, there was no significant difference in event-free survival between usual care (75.9%) and the psychosocial intervention (75.8%). There was also no difference in survival between the psychosocial intervention and usual-care arms in any of the three psychosocial risk groups (i.e., depression, low perceived social support, and both). In contrast, there was some improvement in psychosocial outcomes at six months that favored treatment in terms of decreased depression and increased social support scores. The decline in depression scores in the intervention group was significant and comparable to the reduction in depression observed in other clinical trials of depression in post-MI patients (e.g., Veith et al., 1982). However, patients in the usual-care group also improved substantially, resulting in very modest, although significant, differences between groups. This result raises the issue of how much the depression seen immediately after MI is attributable to psychological factors and how much may be related to the role of proinflammatory cytokines. The cytokines associated with MI influence the central nervous system to produce behaviors that may be described in terms of depression symptoms (for a full discussion of this issue, see Siegel & Schneiderman, 2005). In any event, the findings from ENRICHD were that the psychosocial intervention did not decrease the combined endpoint of all-cause mortality and recurrent MI, but it did produce a modest decrease in depression and low perceived social support.

Because ENRICHD was designed to enroll large numbers of women and minority participants, it was possible to conduct a post hoc secondary analysis examining the outcome of sex by race/ethnicity subgroups (Schneiderman et al., 2004). The 2,481 patients with MI (973 White men, 424 minority men, 674 White women, and 410 minority women) in ENRICHD were examined in a 2×2 factorial design. Analyses indicated that among White men, those in the intervention group had significantly lower cardiac mortality (OR = 0.63; 95% CI = 0.40–0.99, p = <.05) and nonfatal MI (OR = 0.61; 95% CI = 0.40–0.92, p < .05). The difference between the intervention and the control condition was not significant among either minority men or White or minority women. Although these results are exploratory, they raise the issue of the extent to which interventions are culturally appropriate. Recall that in M-HART (Frasure-Smith et al., 1997), women, but not men, may actually have been harmed by the intervention. Based on such concerns, SWITCHD (Orth-Gomér et al., 2009) and SUPRIM (Gulliksson, 2011) conducted on same-sex groups and specifically attempted to address issues relevant to women or men. It cannot be said with certainty that attention to gender issues accounted for the differences in biomedical outcomes between ENRICHD versus SWITCHD and SUPRIM, but the differences in results suggest that attention to gender and other cultural factors needs to be considered in future clinical trials.

There are, of course, many other differences in procedure between ENRICHD (Berkman et al., 2003), which produced a null result, and the studies that reported positive outcomes (Friedman et al., 1986; Gulliksson et al., 2011; Orth-Gomér et al., 2009). For example, ENRICHD specifically focused on patients who have traditionally been difficult to work with in terms of behavior change (i.e., individuals who are clinically depressed or socially isolated). Putting such people into group settings in which cooperative behavior is important can be extremely challenging. It should also be noted that SUPRIM, SWITCHD, and the RCPP exposed all intervention participants to relaxation training and gave attention to lifestyle problems during treatment, whereas only the 30% of participants who were exposed to the group-based intervention received such treatment in ENRICHD. Furthermore, SUPRIM, SWITCHD, and the RCPP used a longer intervention period than did ENRICHD (an average of 38 sessions over 4.5 years in RCPP; up to 20 sessions over a year in SWITCHD and SUPRIM) and followed up patients for a longer time (at least 4.5 years in RCPP, and a mean of 7.1 years in SWITCHD and 7.4 years in SUPRIM), in contrast to participants in ENRICHD, who were followed up for an average of 29 months. Finally, it is worth mentioning that both intervention and control participants received extensive traditional risk factor counseling (i.e., diet, exercise, and medication adherence) in the RCPP and that knowledge of the heart, medication adherence, healthy lifestyle, and training skills were covered to a greater extent in SWITCHD and SUPRIM than they were in ENRICHD.

THE GREAT DEBATE

Thus far we have stressed the commonalities between lifestyle intervention and psychosocial treatments. Not everyone accepts this view (Relman & Angell, 2002). In an editorial in the *New England Journal of Medicine*, Angell (1985) wrote, "It is time to acknowledge that our belief in disease as a direct reflection of mental state is largely folklore" (p. 1571). Whereas most people trained in health psychology and behavioral medicine might translate "mental state" into the concepts of cognitive and affective processes that influence our brain and autonomic nervous, endocrine, and immune systems, to some folks in the biomedical community the terms *mental state* and *psychosocial intervention* apparently conjure up the concept of power of mind to change the course of disease independent of biological processes. This difference in viewpoint led to what became known as "The Great Debate" on the contribution of behavioral interventions to organic outcomes (Kaplan & Davidson, 2010; Markovitz, 2002). The debate as to whether "psychosocial interventions can improve clinical outcomes in organic disease" was held in 1991 and pitted Neil Schneiderman and Redford Williams, representing the American Psychosomatic Society, versus Marcia Angell and Arnold Relman, both former editors of the *New England Journal of Medicine*. Prior to the debate, the participants and others took part in a conference call to establish the ground rules. At the outset, Angell and Relman argued strongly against the use of meta-analyses in the debate because they felt meta-analysis is a flawed methodology and not scientific (Williams, Schneiderman, Relman, & Angell, 2002). Although Williams and Schneiderman indicated that they were strong proponents of the position that psychosocial interventions improve clinical outcomes in organic disease through lifestyle changes as well as changes involving stress autonomic, endocrine, and immune system changes (Williams et al., 2002), Relman and Angell insisted that they would only debate the proposition that psychological and social variable per se can directly change the course of serious organic disease. At this point, Williams and Schneiderman considered dropping out of the debate, but they decided against it. In a previous debate with Andrew Weil, Relman had contended, "Practitioners of alternative medicine believe in the power of mind and thought to change physical matter and heal organic disease, a concept which basically contradicts the laws of physics in the modern scientific view of nature" (Dalen, 1999, p. 2123). Relman then insisted on introducing into the debate a research paper by Kabat-Zinn (Kabat-Zinn et al., 1998). He then criticized this paper for being unscientific even though it had never been mentioned by the affirmative side.

Hippocrates, the father of medicine argued as long ago as 400 BC that disturbances in temperament were associated with disease (Asimov, 1982; Porter, 1994). Although Hippocrates was a keen observer of both human behavior and disease and was therefore moved to comment on relationships between temperament and disease, the science of his day precluded his being able to identify the biological pathways mediating these relationships. The rapprochement of biological reductionism and a modern biopsychosocial model was subsequently dependent upon scientists establishing (a) statistically significant associations in well-controlled epidemiological studies between cognitive, emotional, and psychosocial processes and disease outcomes (Anda et al., 1993; Mayne, Vittinghoff, Chesney, Barrett, & Coates, 1996); (b) discovery of plausible biological pathways that can mediate these associations (Gonzales et al., 2005; Kaplan, Manuck, Adams, Weingand, & Clarkson, 1987; see also the review by Miller, Chen, & Cole, 2009); and (c) describing randomized clinical trials. These psychosocial-behavioral intervention trials have since attempted to capitalize on intervention-induced reductions in physiological arousal (e.g., relaxation training), changes in psychosocial, autonomic-endocrine-immune interactions, and improvements in health behaviors (Friedman et al., 1986; Gullikesson et al., 2011; Orth-Gomér et al., 2009). This three-pronged strategy of (1) describing associations between psychosocial variables and disease outcome in well-controlled clinical investigations (Cohen, Tyrrell, & Smith, 1991) and large-scale epidemiological studies (Anda et al., 1993); (2) identifying plausible biological pathways in laboratory experiments (e.g., Kaplan et al., 1987); and (3) describing randomized clinical trials was adopted by Williams and Schneiderman for The Great Debate. Although Williams and Schneiderman described such studies as the trial by Friedman et al. (1986), Angell and Relman discounted that trial because they felt the outcome could have been influenced by changes in lifestyle, including diet and exercise. Thus the debaters were talking past one another because the assumptions about scientific evidence held by each side differed. For Williams and Schneiderman, the fact that participants in each condition had about the same number of lifestyle sessions, whereas intervention participants also received training that significantly decreased hostility, time urgency, impatience, and depressed mood, indicated that the differences were a result of the psychosocial aspects of the intervention. For Relman and Angell, the fact that Friedman et al. did not adjust statistically for potential differences in diet, exercise, weight gain or loss, and medication adherence weakened the case for a purely psychosocial relationship to disease outcome. Relman and Angell also hammered home the point that there are still very few large-scale randomized clinical trials that have attempted to show that psychosocial interventions can favorably influence organic outcome. The Great Debate turned out to be important for the fields of health psychology and behavioral medicine because it emphasized the high value that the biomedical community places on large-scale randomized clinical trials.

Because of the framework imposed by The Great Debate, important interactions between psychosocial variables and lifestyle factors were not considered. For example, such variables as depression can influence the course of disease through autonomic-endocrine-immune processes as well as through motivational factors that may lead to such risky behaviors as increased cigarette smoking, poor diet, accentuated sedentary behavior, and failure to take medications as prescribed. Conversely, psychosocial-behavioral therapeutic interventions in depressed patients may lead to decreased smoking, better control of diet, increased physical activity, and increased conscientiousness in taking medications as well as decreased sympathetic nervous system arousal and improved endocrine and immune function. Such well-designed randomized clinical trials as the RCPP (Friedman et al., 1986), SWITCHD (Orth-Gomér et al., 2009) and SUPRIM (Gullikesson et al., 2011) of course, positioned themselves to influence stress-related autonomic-endocrine-immune variables as well as lifestyle factors in their intervention conditions.

Although the present chapter has primarily focused on psychosocial-behavioral interventions for cardiovascular disease and risk, it is worth noting that a group-based cognitive-behavioral intervention for breast cancer has also shown positive mortality results (Andersen et al., 2008). Andersen and colleagues randomized 227 women who had been surgically treated for regional breast cancer into a group-based cognitive-behavioral intervention condition or into usual care. The intervention consisted of 26 sessions conducted over a one-year period and included strategies to reduce stress (i.e., progressive muscle relaxation), improve mood, alter health behaviors (i.e., diet, exercise, and smoking cessation), and maintain adherence to cancer treatment and care. After a median of 11 years of follow-up, intervention patients as compared to control patients showed a reduced risk of death from breast cancer (OR = 0.44; 95% CI = 0.22–0.86) or breast cancer recurrence (OR = 0.55; 95% CI = 0.32–0.96). Previously, in the same cohort, Andersen et al. (2004) found that compared to the control condition, participants in the intervention condition showed significant decreases in smoking and anxiety as well as improvement in perceived social support, dietary habits, and T-cell proliferative response to plant mitogens.

The important findings by Andersen et al. (2008) in breast cancer patients add confirmation and generality to the findings in coronary patients reported by Friedman et al. (1986), Orth-Gomér et al. (2009), and Gullikesson et al. (2011). It is important to note that these randomized clinical trials had a number of features in common. The trials all used group-based cognitive-behavior therapy and also included relaxation training, encouragement of specific lifestyle changes (e.g., diet and exercise), and medication adherence training. All three interventions were designed to last at least a year (20 sessions during a year in SWITCHD and SUPRIM; an average of 38 sessions over 4.5 years in RCPP; and 26 sessions during a year in the study by Andersen and collaborators). The follow-up of patients was long term in each study, being at least 4.5 years in the RCPP, a median of 7.1 years in SWITCHD, 7.4 years in SUPRIM, and a median of 11 years in the Andersen et al. trial. It is interesting that all four trials included only members of one sex within intervention groups. In contrast to the trials by Berkman et al. (2003), Frasure-Smith et al. (1997), and Jones and West (1996), which began intervention soon after hospital discharge, the interventions by Orth-Gomér et al., Gullikesson et al., and Friedman et al. did not commence until at least several months after discharge. Whereas interventions beginning soon after a major adverse event might be expected to focus on acute management of a crisis situation, psychosocial-behavioral interventions beginning at least several months after hospital discharge would more likely focus on long-term lifestyle adjustments that might occur over a relatively long period of time.

CONCLUSION

The robust findings reported by Andersen et al. (2008), Friedman et al. (1986), Orth-Gomér et al. (2009), and Gullikesson et al. (2011) suggest that the time is appropriate to initiate large-scale, multicenter psychosocial-behavioral randomized clinical trials in breast cancer and post-MI patients. The consistency of positive results in these four trials makes a persuasive case for using group-based cognitive behavior therapy but also including relaxation training and attention to medication adherence, as well as attention to lifestyle factors, including diet and exercise. However, the comments made by Relman and Angell (2002) during The Great Debate also speak to the desirability of attempting to partial out the relative contribution of intervention components as well as studying their interactions. It is important to note that all the successful trials described in this chapter, including the ones by Knowler et al. (2002), Tuomilehto et al. (2001), and Wing et al. (2010), relied upon treatment manuals and skilled interventionists. They also built on a strong foundation of well-established behavior change and coping strategies as well as on a literature that has identified modifiable risk factors (Rosengren et al., 2004; Yusuf et al., 2004). The trials all employed 16 or more sessions conducted over at least a year and had reasonable long-term follow-up.

It is important to note that one can often learn as much from well-conducted randomized clinical trials that have a null result as from trials that report a positive one. Thus, the study by Frasure-Smith et al. (1997) suggests that the intervention may have been harmful to women, but not men. Similarly, the secondary analysis conducted on ENRICHD by Schneiderman et al. (2004) suggests that the ENRICHD intervention may have actually benefited men, whereas it clearly did not benefit women or minorities. Such findings emphasize the need to tailor psychosocial-behavioral randomized clinical trials to various demographic groups differing in gender, racial and ethnic background, socioeconomic status, and age. To the extent possible, randomized clinical trials also need to partial out psychosocial (e.g., temperament, marital and work stressors, social support) and lifestyle (e.g., medication adherence, diet, physical activity) factors, as well as examine the interactions between intervention components and these factors.

Because the randomized clinical trials by Andersen et al. (2008), Friedman et al. (1986), Gullikesson et al. (2011), and Orth-Gomér et al. (2009) addressed the multiple, modifiable risk factors identified in INTERHEART (Yusuf et al., 2004), it is reasonable to ask whether subsequent trials should have a narrower focus. To the extent that the aforementioned four trials used a relatively small number of participants, did not completely adjust for all the relevant treatment components, and did not allow for studying intervention impact on different demographic groups, there is need for replicating these results in comprehensive, large-scale multicenter trials. Randomized clinical trials investigating psychosocial-behavioral interventions are very costly, and positive results clearly need to be replicated. The disaggregation of treatment components will inevitably become important but should follow the replication of the smaller scale trials. Small-scale trials are more nimble than large randomized clinical trials, but they cannot substitute for them. In the social and behavioral sciences tradition, dissecting complexity is often a major goal. However, when designing large-scale randomized clinical trials, such a virtue has to be balanced against the potentially high cost to science of a null result in a highly visible trial.

Although the cited randomized clinical trials that had positive results demonstrated treatment efficacy, the methods used need to be proven effective in clinical practice. One important issue is cost-benefit. Here, it is interesting to note that the trials by Andersen et al. (2008), Friedman et al. (1986), Orth-Gomér et al. (2009), and Gullikesson et al. (2011) showed health benefits over the course of quite a few years. Thus, if the cost of the behavioral intervention is prorated across several years, the group-based treatments of 20–25 sessions would be cheaper than some individual medications (e.g., statins), quite possibly with equivalent results. An added value of the psychosocial-behavioral interventions is that they benefit not only physical clinical outcomes but also quality-of-life variables.

As previously mentioned, issues of effectiveness need to be examined carefully in patients enrolled in demanding lifestyle interventions involving weight loss and exercise. This can be a major issue in patients with serious comorbidities, including diabetes mellitus, morbid obesity, and motor impairment. Lack of community health resources and poor access to appropriate health care in many countries, including the United States, pose major problems for implementing lifestyle and other psychosocial-behavioral interventions. These problems notwithstanding, the psychosocial-behavioral randomized clinical trials that are now underway or have been completed clearly demonstrate that psychosocial-behavioral treatments can improve clinical outcomes in organic disease. In order for psychosocial-behavioral interventions to become a significant part of evidence-based medicine, the number of comprehensive, large-scale randomized clinical trials in this area will have to be increased.

REFERENCES

American Heart Association (AMA). (2010). Heart disease and stroke statistics—2010 update [Glance version]. Retrieved from http://www.americanheart.org/downloadable/heart_1265665152970DS-3241%20HeartStrokeUpdate_2010.pdf

Anda, R., Williamson, D., Jones, D., Macera, C., Eaker, E., Glassman, A., … Marks, J. (1993). Depressed affect, hopelessness, and the risk of ischemic heart disease in a cohort of U.S. adults. *Epidemiology, 4,* 285–294.

Andersen, B. L., Yang, H. C., Farrar, W. B., Golden-Kreutz, D. M., Emery, C. F., Thornton, L. M., … Carson, W. E., 3rd. (2008). Psychologic intervention improves survival for breast cancer patients: a randomized clinical trial. *Cancer, 113*(12), 3450–3458.

Angell, M. (1985). Disease as a reflection of the psyche. *New England Journal of Medicine, 312,* 1570–1572.

Asimov, I. (1982). *Asimov's biographical encyclopedia of science and technology* (2nd rev. ed.). Garden City, NY: Doubleday.

Beck, J. (1995). *Cognitive therapy: Basics and beyond.* New York, NY: Guilford Press.

Berkman, L. F., Blumenthal, J., Burg, M., Carney, R. M., Catellier, D., Cowan, M. J., … Schneiderman, N. (Enhancing Recovery in Coronary Heart Disease Patients Investigators [ENRICHD]). (2003). Effects of treating depression and low perceived social support on clinical events after myocardial infarction: The Enhancing Recovery in Coronary Heart Disease Patients (ENRICHD) Randomized Trial. *Journal of the American Medical Association, 289*, 3106–3116.

Cohen, S., Tyrrell, D. A., & Smith, A. P. (1991). Psychological stress in humans and susceptibility to the common cold. *New England Journal of Medicine, 325*, 606–612.

Dalen, J. E. (1999). Is integrative medicine the medicine of the future: A debate between Arnold S. Relman, MD, and Andrew Weil, MD. *Archives of Internal Medicine, 159*, 2122–2126.

Eckel, R., Kahn, R., Robertson, R., & Rizza, R. (2006). Preventing cardiovascular disease and diabetes: A call to action from the American Diabetes Association and the American Heart Association. *Circulation, 113*(25), 2943–2946. Retrieved from MEDLINE database.

Frasure-Smith, N., Lespérance, F., Prince, R. H., Verrier, P., Garber, R. A., Juneau, M., … Bourassa, M. G. (1997). Randomised trial of home–based psychosocial nursing intervention for patients recovering from myocardial infarction. *Lancet, 350*, 473–479.

Friedman, M., Thoresen, C. E., Gill, J. J., Ulmer, D., Powell, L. H., Price, V. A., … Dixon, T. (1986). Alteration of type A behavior and its effect on cardiac recurrences in post myocardial infarction patients: Summary results of the Recurrent Coronary Prevention Project. *American Heart Journal, 112*, 653–665.

Goldberg, D. P. (1972). *The assessment of psychiatric illness by questionnaire.* London, England: Oxford University Press.

Gonzales, J. A., Szeto, A., Mendez, A. J., Goldberg, R. B., Caperton, C. V., Paredes, J., … McCabe, P. M. (2005). Effect of behavioral interventions on insulin sensitivity and atherosclerosis in the Watanabe Heritable Hyperlipidemic Rabbit. *Psychosomatic Medicine, 67*, 172–178.

Gullikesson, M., Burell, G., Vessby, B., Lundin, L., Toss, H., & Svärdsudd, K. (2011). Randomized controlled trial of cognitive behavioral therapy vs. standard treatment to prevent recurrent cardiovascular events in patients with coronary heart disease. *Archives of Internal Medicine, 171*, 134–140.

Haffner, S., Lehto, S., Rönnemaa, T., Pyörälä, K., & Laakso, M. (1998). Mortality from coronary heart disease in subjects with type 2 diabetes and in nondiabetic subjects with and without prior myocardial infarction. *New England Journal of Medicine, 339*(4), 229–234.

Jones, D. A., & West, R. R. (1996). Psychological rehabilitation after myocardial infarction: Multicentre randomized controlled trial. *BMJ, 313*, 1517–21.

Kabat-Zinn, J., Wheeler, E., Light, T., Skillings, A., Schart, M. J., Cropley, T. G., … Bernhard, J. D. (1998). Influence of a mindfulness mediation-based stress reduction intervention on rates of skin clearing in patients with moderate to severe psoriasis undergoing phototherapy (UVB) and photochemotherapy (PUVA). *Psychosomatic Medicine, 60*, 625–632.

Kaplan, J. R. Manuck. S. B., Adams, M. R., Weingand, K. W., & Clarkson, T. B. (1987). Inhibition of coronary atherosclerosis by propranolol in behaviorally predisposed monkeys fed an atherogenic diet. *Circulation, 76*, 1364–1372.

Kaplan, R. M., & Davidson, K. W. (2010). The great debate on the contribution of behavioral interventions. In J. M. Suls, K. W. Davison, & R. M. Kaplan (Eds.), *Handbook of health psychology and behavioral medicine* (pp. 3–14). New York, NY: Guilford Press.

Knowler, W. C., Barrett-Connor, E., Fowler, S. E., Hamman, R. F., Lachin, J. M., Walker, E. A., & Nathan, D. M. (Diabetes Prevention Program Research Group). (2002). Reduction in the incidence of type 2 diabetes with lifestyle intervention or metformin. *New England Journal Medicine, 346*(6), 393–403.

Markovitz, J. H. (2002). Resolved: psychosocial interventions can improve clinical outcomes in organic disease—Moderator introduction. *Psychosomatic Medicine, 64*(4), 549–551.

Mayne, T. J., Vittinghoff, E., Chesney, M. A., Barrett, D. C., & Coates, T. J. (1996). Depressive affect and survival among gay and bisexual men infected with HIV. *Archives of Internal Medicine, 156*, 2233–2238.

Mendes de Leon, C. F., Powell, L. H., & Kaplan, B. (1991). Change in coronary-prone behaviors in the recurrent coronary prevention project. *Psychosomatic Medicine, 53*, 407–419.

Miller, G., Chen, E., & Cole, S. W. (2009). Health psychology: Developing biologically plausible mechanisms linking the social world and physical health. *Annual Review of Psychology, 60*, 501–524.

Orth-Gomér, K., Schneiderman, N., Wang, H., Walldin, C., Bloom, M., & Jernberg, T. (2009). Stress reduction prolongs life in women with coronary disease: The Stockholm Women's Intervention Trial for Coronary Heart Disease (SWITCHD). *Circulation: Cardiovascular Quality and Outcomes, 2*, 25–32.

Porter, R. (1994). *The biographical dictionary of scientists* (2nd ed.). New York, NY: Oxford University Press.

Rosengren, A., Hawken, S., Ounpuu, S., Silwa, K., Zubaid, M., Almahmeed, W. A., ... Yusuf, S. (INTERHEART investigators). (2004). Association of psychosocial risk factors with risk of acute myocardial infarction in 11119 cases and 13648 controls from 52 countries (the INTERHEART Study): Case-control study. *Lancet, 11-17*; 364, 953–62.

Relman, A. S., & Angell, M. (2002). Resolved: Psychosocial interventions can improve clinical outcomes in organic disease (con). *Psychosomatic Medicine, 64*(4), 558–563.

Schneiderman, N., Saab, P. G., Catellier, D. J., Powell, L. H., DeBusk, R. F., Williams, R. B., ... Kaufmann, P. G. (2004). Psychosocial treatment within gender by ethnicity subgroups in the Enhancing Recovery in Coronary Heart Disease (ENRICHD) Clinical Trial. *Psychosomatic Medicine, 66*, 475–483.

Siegel, S., & Schneiderman, N. (2005). Heart disease, cardiovascular functioning, and fatigue. In J. DeLuca (Ed.), *Fatigue as a window to the brain* (pp. 229–242). Boston, MA: MIT Press.

Tuomilehto, J., Lindstrom, J., Eriksson, J. G., Valle, T. T., Hamalainen, H., Ilanne-Parikka, P., ... Uusitupa, M. (Finnish Diabetes Prevention Study Group). (2001). Prevention of type 2 diabetes mellitus by changes in lifestyle among subjects with impaired glucose tolerance. *New England Journal of Medicine, 344*(18), 1343–1350.

Veith, R. C., Raskind, M. A., Caldwell, J. H., Barnes, R. F., Gumbrecht, G., & Ritchie, J. L. (1982). Cardiovascular effects of tricyclic antidepressants in depressed patients with chronic heart disease. *New England Journal of Medicine, 306*, 954–959.

Williams, R., Schneiderman, N., Relman, A., & Angell, M. (2002). Resolved: Psychosocial interventions can improve clinical outcomes in organic disease—Rebuttals and closing arguments. *Psychosomatic Medicine, 64*(4), 564–567.

Wing, R. R., Bahnson, J. L., Bray, G. A., Clark, J. M., Coday, M., Egan, C., ... Yanovski, S. Z. (2010). Long-term effects of a lifestyle intervention on weight and cardiovascular risk factors in individuals with type 2 diabetes mellitus [Look AHEAD Trial]. *Archives of Internal Medicine, 170*, 1566–1575.

World Health Organization (WHO). (2011). Cardiovascular diseases (CVDs). (Fact sheet No. 317). Retrieved from http://www.who.int/mediacentre/factsheets/fs317/en/#

Yusuf, S., Hawken, S., Ounpuu, S., Dans, T., Avezum, A., Lanas, F., ... Lisheng, L. (INTERHEART Study Investigators). (2004). Effect of potentially modifiable risk factors associated with myocardial infarction in 52 countries (the INTERHEART Study): Case-control study. *Lancet, 11–17*, 364, 937–52.

30 Psychosocial Interventions for People With Cancer

Leigh Anne Faul
Georgetown University

Paul B. Jacobsen
University of South Florida

Approximately one out of every two American men and one out of every three American women will develop cancer at some point during their lifetime (American Cancer Society, 2010). The chances for these individuals to survive cancer vary considerably depending on the specific type diagnosed, the extent of disease at the time of initial diagnosis, and the responsiveness of the disease to treatment. Much of the early effort to combat cancer focused exclusively on testing new therapies to improve the quantity of patients' lives (i.e., survival). These efforts, combined with improvements in early detection, have yielded impressive gains for certain forms of the disease.

More recently, there has been growing recognition that comprehensive cancer care should also seek to preserve or restore the quality of patients' lives (Institute of Medicine, 2007). This recognition is, in part, a result of the large body of evidence documenting the adverse psychological impact for many individuals of a cancer diagnosis and the adverse psychological and physical impact of many forms of cancer treatment (e.g., surgery, chemotherapy, and radiotherapy). These problems do not appear to be confined to the period of active cancer treatment. The burgeoning field of cancer survivorship research has shown that many problems, which first arise during treatment, can persist for months or years following treatment completion. In addition, research has shown that new problems can arise even after treatment has been completed.

Research on the quality of life of cancer patients has not been confined to describing the characteristics, course, and correlates of the problems that patients experience. Considerable effort has been devoted to developing and testing interventions to prevent or relieve these problems. Rather than attempt to review the vast body of research on this topic, the current chapter will focus on interventions to address depression, pain, and fatigue, three of the most common problems experienced by cancer patients. The importance of these problems and the extent of scientific interest in them is underscored by the fact they were the topic of the first State-of the-Science Conference on Symptom Management in Cancer conducted by the National Institutes of Health (Patrick et al., 2004).

In the sections that follow, each of these problems is described in terms of its common presentations and prevalence. We then review current clinical practice guidelines for the management of each problem, with a focus on the role of psychosocial interventions. Next, the existing evidence base on the efficacy of psychosocial interventions in addressing each problem is discussed. Our approach to this topic involves summarizing the findings of existing systematic reviews and meta-analyses of the effects of psychosocial interventions on depression, fatigue, and pain in adults with cancer. To help bridge the gap between research and practice, we then provide examples of interventions found to be effective for each problem that we believe have good potential for dissemination and implementation. Finally, we identify promising future directions for research on psychosocial interventions to improve quality of life in people with cancer.

DEPRESSION

Depressive symptoms worsen quality of life (Capuron, Ravaud, & Dantzer, 2000; Grassi et al., 1996). In adults with cancer, depression may also reduce compliance with cancer treatment (Grassi et al., 1996) and prolong hospitalization (Prieto et al., 2002). Possible sources of depression include preexisting psychological problems (predating cancer diagnosis), reactions to the diagnosis of a severe and potentially life-threatening illness, and the presence of unpleasant symptoms (e.g., pain, nausea, and fatigue). Concerns about disruptions in life plans, diminished quality of life, and disease recurrence or progression can also elicit depressive symptoms. In addition, the physiologic effects of certain treatments (e.g., high-dose interferon therapy) on the central nervous system may directly produce depression (Capuron et al., 2000). Studies indicate that heightened depression is not limited to the active treatment period but may persist for months or even years following successful treatment (Kim et al., 2008).

Depression has also been identified as a factor that may affect survival after cancer diagnosis through biological or behavioral pathways (Spiegel & Giese-Davis, 2003). Evidence for its impact includes the finding, based on a meta-analysis of 68 prospective studies, of a pooled relative risk ratio of 1.18 ($p < .001$) for the relationship of depression with cancer mortality (Pinquart & Duberstein, 2010). Drawing conclusions about the prognostic importance of depression from observational studies is complicated, however, by the difficulty of controlling for relevant confounding variables. Randomized controlled trials of interventions to address depression and related psychological symptoms have the potential to address this methodological challenge and provide more definitive evidence. Positive findings for the impact on mortality from at least two such trials (Andersen et al., 2008; Speigel, Bloom, Kramer, & Gottheil, 1989) have been used to argue that psychological interventions can enhance the survival of cancer patients. This conclusion has been disputed by others (Coyne, Stefanek, & Palmer, 2007; Stefanek, Palmer, Thombs, & Coyne, 2009), who cite numerous studies that found no significant effects for psychological interventions on cancer survival and can identify important methodological limitations in those studies that have reported effects on survival. Accordingly, the question of whether depression affects cancer survival cannot be answered conclusively at this time.

PREVALENCE OF DEPRESSION

Depression among adult cancer patients is well documented (Fallowfield, Ratcliffe, Jenkins, & Saul, 2001). However, estimates vary as to the prevalence of depression in cancer patients, ranging from 1.5% to 50% (Pirl, 2004). Broadly speaking, this variability can be attributed to sample characteristics and methodology. With regard to sample characteristics, variability in prevalence rates reflects differences across studies in such patient factors as age and disease severity. Evidence suggests depression is greater in younger patients and patients with more advanced disease (Fallowfield et al., 2001). With regard to the methods used, differences in prevalence may reflect whether depression was assessed using a multisymptom approach or a clinical syndrome approach. Studies of the prevalence of depression in other populations have typically relied on a clinical syndrome approach using mood disorder criteria from the American Psychiatric Association's *Diagnostic and Statistical Manual of Mental Disorders* (DSM-IV) (APA, 1994). However, the multisymptom approach is the most commonly used method in psychosocial oncology research. The multisymptom approach refers to assessment methods that focus on measuring constellations of depressive symptoms. Common multisymptom approaches to measuring depression in cancer patients include such self-report scales as the Center for Epidemiologic Studies Depression Scale (CES-D) (Radloff, 1977). The chief advantages of these methods are their established reliability and validity, their ability to detect change over time, and the availability of reference values for a variety of medical and nonmedical populations. The chief disadvantage is the presence on some measures of item content that might reflect disease symptoms or treatment side effects (e.g., loss of appetite) rather

than emotional difficulties. Cutoff scores indicative of clinically significant depressive symptomatology have been developed for such multisymptom measures as the CES-D (Radloff, 1977) and the
Hospital Anxiety and Depression Scale (Zigmond & Snaith, 1983). Although prevalence estimates
vary considerably, depression is among the most common symptoms experienced by cancer patients
and survivors (Chang, Hwang, Feuerman, Kasimis, & Thaler, 2000; Cleeland et al., 2000).

CLINICAL PRACTICE GUIDELINES FOR MANAGEMENT OF DEPRESSION IN CANCER PATIENTS

Clinical practice guidelines for the management of depression in cancer patients have been proposed from two sources. The National Comprehensive Cancer Network (NCCN) has developed
several clinical practice guidelines for the supportive care of cancer patients. The *NCCN Guidelines
for Distress Management*, first issued in 1999 and updated annually, proffers recommendations
for evaluation, treatment, and follow-up care (NCCN, 2010c). Recommendations for the management of depression appear primarily in sections of the guidelines focusing on mood disorders.
These recommendations are based on consensus among members of an expert panel and generally
rely on lower level research evidence. In 2003, the National Breast Cancer Centre (NBCC) and
the National Cancer Control Initiative (NCCI) in Australia published the first edition of *Clinical
Practice Guidelines for the Psychosocial Care of Adults With Cancer* (NBCC & NCCI, 2003).
The guidelines are presented mostly in the form of specific recommendations for the psychosocial
care of people with cancer. These recommendations are based on available research evidence and
are accompanied by identification of the levels and sources of research support (e.g., Level I or II
evidence). Some of the evidence cited in support of these guidelines includes systematic reviews
and randomized trials conducted on populations other than cancer patients. More recently, Dy,
Lorenz, et al. (2008) published evidence-based recommendations for the management of depression in adults with cancer. Their review of the literature indicated empirical support for depression
screening and identified risk factors for depression and psychosocial distress (e.g., advanced disease
and worsening physical symptoms). Recommendations for screening include screening new at-risk
patients (e.g., newly diagnosed patients), advanced-stage patients, and patients receiving chemotherapy or radiotherapy (Dy, Lorenz, et al., 2008). Evidence also indicated support for the creation
of a treatment plan (for patients subsequently diagnosed with depression after screening), and monitoring of treatment response throughout follow-up (Dy, Lorenz, et al., 2008).

SYSTEMATIC REVIEWS AND META-ANALYSES OF PSYCHOSOCIAL
INTERVENTIONS FOR DEPRESSION IN ADULTS WITH CANCER

To determine the effects of psychosocial interventions on depression in adults with cancer, Jacobsen
and Jim (2008) compiled and compared existing systematic reviews and meta-analyses on this topic
(see Table 30.1). The researchers identified 13 publications that reached conclusions regarding intervention efficacy for depression (Barsevick, Sweeney, Haney, & Chung, 2002; Bottomley, 1998;
Devine & Westlake, 1995; Jacobsen, Donovan, Swaine, & Watson, 2006; Lovejoy & Matteis, 1997;
Luebbert, Dahme, & Hasenbring, 2001; Newell, Sanson-Fisher, & Savolainen, 2002; Osborn,
Demoncada, & Feuerstein, 2006; Rodin et al., 2007; Sellick & Crooks, 1999; Sheard & Maguire,
1999; Uitterhoeve et al., 2004; Williams & Dale, 2006). Nine of the 13 publications reached positive conclusions about the efficacy of psychosocial interventions for depression in cancer patients
(Barsevick et al., 2002; Bottomley, 1998; Devine & Westlake, 1995; Jacobsen et al., 2006; Lovejoy &
Matteis, 1997; Luebbert et al., 2001; Osborn et al., 2006; Sellick & Crooks, 1999; Uitterhoeve et al.,
2004). Differences in the scope of the reviews, the methods used to summarize findings across studies, and the manner in which recommendations were reached seriously limit the conclusions that
can be drawn from these publications. Indeed, two recent reviews of many of the same publications
reached very different conclusions about the overall effectiveness of psychosocial interventions.
Whereas one review (Andrykowski & Manne, 2006) concluded that the preponderance of evidence

TABLE 30.1

Systematic Reviews and Meta-Analyses of Psychosocial Interventions for Depression in Adults With Cancer

Reference	Intervention Focus	Psychosocial Intervention Studies Reviewed	Findings for Psychosocial Studies	Conclusions
Devine & Westlake (1995)	Psychoeducational care	Randomized and nonrandomized studies of cancer patients	Positive results in 92% of studies; $d = 0.54$, 95% CI = 0.43–0.65	Many types of psychoeducational care show beneficial effects.
Lovejoy & Matteis (1997)	Cognitive-behavioral interventions	Randomized and nonrandomized studies of cancer patients	In the beginning phases of development, knowledge base for management of cancer-related depression with cognitive-behavioral therapy	Several studies suggest that simple, brief therapy (six sessions or less) provides effective relief in milder cases of cancer-related depression.
Bottomley (1998)	Pharmacological and psychosocial interventions	Randomized and nonrandomized studies	Positive results with individual and group interventions	A number of psychosocial approaches demonstrate positive effects.
Sellick & Crooks (1999)	Individual psychosocial counseling interventions	Randomized studies of cancer patients	10 studies reviewed; magnitude of treatment effects classified as large (5), moderate (2), low (2), and none (1)	Positive effect of statistical and clinical significance shown.
Sheard & Maguire (1999)	Psychosocial interventions	Randomized studies of cancer patients	Depression: $d = 0.36$, 95% CI = 0.06–0.66; $d = 0.19$ with positive outliers removed	No effect of preventative psychosocial interventions shown.
Luebbert et al. (2001)	Relaxation training	Randomized studies of nonsurgical cancer patients	Depression: $d = 0.54$, 95% CI = 0.30–0.78	Relaxation training has a significant (medium) effect.
Barsevick et al. (2002)	Psychoeducational interventions	Randomized and nonrandomized studies of cancer patients	Positive results reported in 63% of studies reviewed	Positive effect of psychoeducational interventions shown. In particular, behavioral therapy, psychotherapy, and either of these combined with education had positive outcomes.
Newell et al. (2002)	Psychosocial interventions	Randomized studies of cancer patients of fair or better quality	Recommendations tentatively against 7 strategies and neither for or against 6 strategies	Several intervention strategies warrant further exploration.
Uitterhoeve et al. (2004)	Psychosocial interventions for advanced cancer	Randomized studies of cancer patients	Significant intervention effect in 6 of 10 reviewed studies	The main benefit of psychosocial interventions is an improvement of depression and feelings of sadness.

TABLE 30.1 (Continued)
Systematic Reviews and Meta-Analyses of Psychosocial Interventions for Depression in Adults With Cancer

Reference	Intervention Focus	Psychosocial Intervention Studies Reviewed	Findings for Psychosocial Studies	Conclusions
Jacobsen et al. (2006)	Psychosocial and pharmacological interventions	Randomized studies of cancer patients	Significant results in 41% of analyses favoring the intervention condition	Numerous evidence-based recommendations can be made for the use of psychosocial interventions in the management of depression.
Osborn et al. (2006)	Psychosocial interventions	Randomized studies of cancer patients with posttreatment follow-up evaluations	Depression; $g = 1.21$, 95% CI = 0.22–2.19 (cognitive-behavioral therapy); $g = -0.06$, 95% CI = −0.24–0.13 (psychoeducation)	Cognitive-behavioral therapy is effective for the short-term (<8 months) management of depression in cancer survivors.
Williams & Dale (2006)	Psychosocial and pharmacological interventions	Randomized studies of cancer patients	Benefit of psychosocial intervention in 3 of 4 studies; CBT benefit in reducing depression in 7 of 10 trials	Cognitive-behavioral therapy appears effective in reducing depressive symptoms, but limited trial data.
Rodin et al. (2007)	Psychosocial and pharmacological interventions	Randomized and nonrandomized studies of cancer patients	Benefit of psychosocial intervention in 2 of 4 studies	Evidence for nonpharmacological treatment of depression is mixed.

furnished by these systematic reviews, particularly that gleaned from meta-analyses, suggests that psychological interventions are effective in managing distress, the other review (Lepore & Coyne, 2006) concluded that "our review of reviews, particularly the more systematic reviews, provides no compelling evidence of broadly effective psychological interventions for reducing a wide range of distress outcomes in cancer patients" (p. 90).

Rather than attempt to reach an overall conclusion about the efficacy of psychosocial interventions, we believe it is more valuable to examine how previous systematic reviews and meta-analyses can be used to derive specific evidence-based recommendations for the management of depression in adults with cancer. An approach we developed previously that may be useful is to summarize the literature in terms of the number of randomized controlled trials (RCTs) that demonstrated efficacy in managing depression based on intervention type and patient disease or treatment status (Jacobsen & Jim, 2008). Providing this information to practitioners can serve several useful purposes. First, it readily identifies when in the disease course or at what point in the treatment process a specific intervention strategy has been shown to be effective. Second, the number of unique citations next to each listing indicates the strength of the evidence for that application of an intervention strategy. Finally, the citations themselves identify publications that provide information about the content and delivery of an intervention and the methodology that was used to evaluate it.

EXAMPLES OF EVIDENCE-SUPPORTED INTERVENTIONS FOR DEPRESSION

In this section, we provide examples of psychological interventions found to be effective in managing depression in people with cancer. Two considerations were foremost in our selection of intervention examples: evidence of efficacy in a published RCT and reasonable potential for dissemination based on the time and resources required for implementation.

Project Genesis

Nezu, Nezu, McClure, Felgoise, and Houts (2003) developed a professionally administered problem-solving intervention for cancer patients experiencing significant distress. The intervention is comprised of problem-solving training for major depression tailored for adults with cancer. Training in problem orientation and problem solving is delivered by trained staff once per week over 10 weeks in 90-minute individual sessions. To evaluate the intervention, participants were randomly assigned to one of three conditions: problem-solving therapy with the patient alone, problem-solving therapy that also included a significant other, or wait-list control. Findings indicated that patients receiving problem-solving therapy demonstrated less distress, less depressive symptomatology, and improved quality of life compared to wait-list controls. As expected, problem-solving therapy enhanced problem-solving coping, which was, in turn, associated with improved quality of life and attenuated depression. In addition, involvement of a significant other appeared to enhance the positive effects of problem-solving therapy on depressive symptoms.

Stress Management Training for Chemotherapy Patients

Jacobsen et al. (2002) developed a self-administered form of stress management training designed specifically for patients undergoing chemotherapy. The intervention uses print and audiovisual materials to instruct patients in three common stress-management techniques: paced abdominal breathing, progressive muscle-relaxation training with guided imagery, and use of coping self-statements. As part of the intervention, patients scheduled for outpatient chemotherapy meet for approximately 10 minutes with a clinician who provides the packet of instructional resources (booklet, audiotape, and videotape) and explains their use in managing common physical and mental stressors encountered during chemotherapy treatment. Patients receive instructions on how to practice the techniques before the start of chemotherapy and when to use the techniques after the start of chemotherapy. The clinician who provides the materials subsequently meets with the patient in the chemotherapy clinic for approximately five minutes just before the start of the first treatment cycle to answer any questions and encourage use of the techniques after the start of chemotherapy. Using an RCT design, the investigators compared the efficacy of this intervention to usual care only and professionally administered training in the same three techniques. Patient-reported outcomes were assessed before the start of chemotherapy (prior to randomization) and at the start of the second, third, and fourth treatment cycles. Findings indicated that patients who received self-administered training reported significantly less depression than did patients who received only usual care. Differences between the professionally administered intervention and usual-care-only conditions were in the same direction but were not statistically significant. As part of the same study, the investigators also calculated the costs of delivering the two stress-management interventions. The average per-patient cost of the self-administered intervention was found to be 57% less than that of the professionally administered intervention ($47 versus $110).

Collaborative Depression Care for People With Cancer

Strong et al. (2008) evaluated the use of a collaborative care model to identify and treat depressed cancer patients. In this study of cancer patients being treated at a regional center, patients found to have major depressive disorder through screening were randomly assigned to usual care or usual care plus a collaborative care intervention (Strong et al., 2008). The intervention consists of up to 10 sessions with a cancer nurse who provides education about depression and its treatment (including antidepressant medication) and engages in problem-solving therapy to overcome feelings of helplessness. In addition, the nurse consults with each patient's oncologist and primary care physician about management of depression. Findings showed significantly lower scores on a measure of depressive symptomatology three months postrandomization for patients who received the collaborative care intervention relative to usual care controls. These differences are reflected in the percentages of usual care patients (45%) versus collaborative care patients (68%) whose major depressive disorder had remitted in the three-month period. The beneficial effects of collaborative care observed at three months were still evident at 6-month and 12-month follow-up assessments. As part of the same study, the investigators also calculated the costs of delivering the depression-management intervention versus provision of usual care only. Incremental cost of the intervention was $668 over six months.

FATIGUE

Cancer-related fatigue has been described as "a persistent subjective sense of tiredness related to cancer or cancer treatment that interferes with usual functioning" (Mock et al., 1994, p. 889). Research suggests that the fatigue experienced by cancer patients is both quantitatively and qualitatively different from that of healthy individuals. As Poulson (2001) notes, "The deadening fatigue which invades the very bones of cancer patients is totally unlike even the most profound fatigue of an otherwise well person" (p. 4180). Normal fatigue is usually described as physical exhaustion or sleepiness that is alleviated by rest (Glaus, Crow, & Hammond, 1996). In contrast, cancer-related fatigue endures; energy is not replenished even after long periods of sleep or rest (Cella, Davis, Breitbart, & Curt, 2001; Rhodes, Watson, & Hanson, 1988). Patients often describe fatigue as one of the most difficult and disruptive aspects of the cancer experience (Baker, Denniston, Smith, & West, 2005; Rhodes et al., 1988). In one survey, more than one third of patients treated with chemotherapy or radiotherapy reported that fatigue has negatively affected their ability to work, their social relationships, and/or their mental and physical well-being (Vogelzang et al., 1997). Finally, cancer-related fatigue is pervasive; it saps the energy to function effectively in cognitive, physical, and psychological domains. Patients often report problems with short-term memory and concentration, generalized weakness, reduced ability to carry out normal activities, decreased motivation, and heightened frustration and depression (Geinitz et al., 2004; Glaus et al., 1996; Jacobsen, Donovan, & Weitzner, 2003). Many cancer patients with no clinical evidence of disease continue to experience fatigue for months or even years following treatment completion (Jacobsen, Donovan, Vadaparampil, & Small, 2007). The etiology of cancer-related fatigue presents a complex picture for which the mechanisms are only partially understood. Fatigue can occur as a result of direct biological or metabolic changes associated with the tumor itself (Groopman & Itri, 1999) or cancer treatment (anemia, hypothyroidism) (Groopman & Itri, 1999; NCCN, 2010b), as well as occur as secondary to such side effects and symptoms as nausea and pain (Cella, 1998). In addition, cognitive and behavioral factors (e.g., catastrophizing and physical inactivity) may contribute to the exacerbation and persistence of fatigue (Jacobsen, Andrykowski, & Thors, 2004; Jacobsen et al., 1999). Once treatment is completed, persistent immune changes and late effects may also contribute to fatigue among long-term survivors (Bower, Ganz, Aziz, & Fahey, 2002). In sum, the factors that precipitate and perpetuate fatigue are multifaceted and present multiple targets for assessment and intervention.

PREVALENCE OF FATIGUE

Fatigue is one of the most common symptoms experienced by cancer patients with advanced disease and those undergoing radiotherapy and chemotherapy (Mitchell & Berger, 2006; NCCN, 2010b). Depending on the patient sample and methodology, an estimated 75% to 100% of cancer patients experience fatigue (Curt et al., 2000; NCCN, 2010b). Demographic variables (e.g., age, ethnicity, marital status, education) do not appear to be strongly correlated with fatigue severity (Jacobsen et al., 2004). Instead, type of treatment appears to be the most important contributor. Chemotherapy (Broeckel, Jacobsen, Horton, Balducci, & Lyman, 1998; Jacobsen et al., 1999) and bone marrow transplantation (Hann et al., 1997) are both reliably associated with increases in fatigue. With radiotherapy, fatigue levels tend to peak during treatment (Greenberg, Sawicka, Eisenthal, & Ross,

1992), then decrease to rates comparable to healthy controls (Hann, Jacobsen, Martin, Azzarello, & Greenberg, 1998). Fatigue also tends to be high in palliative care settings (Stone, Richards, Ahern, & Hardy, 2000). For example, in a study comparing palliative care inpatients to age- and sex-matched healthy controls, 75% of patients reported a fatigue score in excess of the 95th percentile of controls (Stone et al., 1999).

CLINICAL PRACTICE GUIDELINES FOR MANAGEMENT OF FATIGUE IN CANCER PATIENTS

NCCN's cancer-related fatigue management guidelines recommend that patients reporting fatigue in the moderate or severe range receive further evaluation and treatment (NCCN, 2010b). Management of fatigue should occur in two stages: (1) Health care professionals should identify and treat contributing factors to fatigue, and (2) residual fatigue should be treated. The guidelines identify seven contributing factors: pain, emotional distress, sleep disturbance, anemia, nutrition, activity level, and comorbidities. The guidelines also suggest the provision of methods for dealing with stress, depression, and anxiety, which co-occur with fatigue, especially during active treatment (Stark et al., 2002). The complexity of the mechanisms underlying fatigue is reflected in these guidelines, as well as in current management strategies. Interventions target a broad array of possible causes. As a result, to reduce fatigue, multiple interventions may be required ranging from concurrent treatment of anemia and/or hypothyroidism to recommendations for dietary intake (e.g., to avoid dehydration and imbalance of sodium, potassium, or magnesium).

Dy, Lorenz, et al. (2008) recently published evidence-based recommendations for the management of cancer-related fatigue. Advanced stage and receipt of chemotherapy as treatment were identified as risk factors for fatigue. Their review indicated support for the screening for fatigue at the initial visit with an oncologist and ongoing screening for fatigue at all chemotherapy visits. They also recommended assessing depression and insomnia in patients with newly identified fatigue and conducting ongoing follow-ups with patients treated for fatigue.

SYSTEMATIC REVIEWS OF PSYCHOSOCIAL INTERVENTIONS FOR FATIGUE

Our examination of the literature identified one systematic reviews and two meta-analyses that encompassed psychosocial interventions for fatigue in adults with cancer (Jacobsen et al., 2007; Kangas, Bovbjerg, & Montgomery, 2008; Lawrence, Kupelnick, Miller, Devine, & Lau, 2004) (see Table 30.2). It should be noted that several systematic reviews and meta-analyses solely of exercise interventions for cancer-related fatigue have also been published (Conn, Hafdahl, Porock, McDaniel, & Nielsen, 2007; Cramp & Daniel, 2008; Kirshbaum, 2006; Luctkar-Flude, Groll, Tranmer, & Woodend, 2007; Markes, Brockaw, & Resch, 2006; McNeely et al., 2006; Schmitz et al., 2005; Speck, Courneya, Masse, Duval, & Schmitz, 2010; Stevinson, Lawlor, & Fox, 2004)

Lawrence et al. (2004) performed a systematic review of research on interventions for fatigue in cancer patients that included studies published through 2001. The search identified 10 RCTs that assessed the efficacy of interventions for cancer-related fatigue. For nonpharmacological interventions, the authors concluded from the results of two trials that exercise might be helpful in reducing or preventing cancer-related fatigue (Lawrence et al., 2004).

Jacobsen et al. (2007) performed a meta-analysis of RCTs of psychological and activity-based interventions with cancer patients in which fatigue was measured as an outcome. the researchers identified 41 studies, of which 24 evaluated psychological interventions and 17 evaluated activity-based interventions. Overall, 50% of psychological intervention trials and 44% of activity-based intervention trials rated fair or better in quality yielded significant findings favoring the intervention condition. Meta-analysis of 30 studies yielded an overall effect size of 0.09 (95% CI = 0.02–0.16) favoring nonpharmacological conditions. Further analysis indicated that effect sizes were significant for psychological interventions ($d_w = 0.10$, 95% CI = 0.02–0.18), but not activity-based interventions ($d_w = 0.05$, 95% CI = −0.08–0.19). The authors concluded that the findings provide limited

TABLE 30.2

Systematic Reviews and Meta-Analyses of Psychosocial Interventions for Fatigue in Adults With Cancer

Reference	Intervention Focus	Psychosocial Intervention Studies Reviewed	Findings for Psychosocial Studies	Conclusions
Lawrence et al. (2004)	Pharmacological and nonpharmacological interventions	Randomized studies of cancer patients	Four studies reviewed; results described	Psychosocial interventions are among several promising approaches requiring further study.
Jacobsen et al. (2007)	Psychosocial and exercise interventions	Randomized studies of cancer patients	Fatigue: $d = 0.09$, 95% CI $= 0.02$–0.18	Results provide limited support for the use of psychosocial interventions to prevent or relieve fatigue.
Kangas et al. (2008)	Nonpharmacological interventions	Randomized and nonrandomized studies of cancer patients	Fatigue: $d = 0.31$, 95% CI $= -0.38$ to -0.25	Overall effect of psychosocial interventions on fatigue was in the small to moderate range and clinically meaningful.

support for the use of nonpharmacological interventions to manage cancer-related fatigue. The lack of studies with heightened fatigue as an eligibility criterion was identified as a notable weakness of the existing evidence base.

More recently, Kangas et al. (2008) performed a meta-analysis of studies published through 2006 of nonpharmacological interventions in which fatigue and related constructs (e.g., vitality and vigor) were measured as outcomes. Their work identified 67 RCTs, of which 50 were studies of psychosocial interventions and 17 were studies of exercise interventions. A meta-analysis that included 41 psychosocial intervention studies and 16 exercise intervention studies yielded significant results favoring the intervention condition for both psychosocial interventions ($d_w = -0.31$, 95% CI $= -0.37$ to -0.25) and exercise interventions ($d_w = -0.42$, 95% CI $= -0.60$ to -0.23). When psychosocial and exercise interventions as a whole were compared, there were no significant differences between them. Based on these and additional findings reported, the authors conclude that exercise and walking programs, restorative approaches, supportive-expressive therapy, and cognitive-behavioral interventions show promising potential for ameliorating cancer-related fatigue.

EXAMPLES OF EVIDENCE-SUPPORTED PSYCHOLOGICAL AND EXERCISE INTERVENTIONS FOR FATIGUE

Given that cancer-related fatigue is influenced by multiple factors, both pharmacological and non-pharmacological approaches have been examined to manage fatigue. A review of pharmacologic therapies is beyond the scope of this chapter, though their use has been reviewed elsewhere (Jim & Jacobsen, 2008). In this section, we provide examples of psychological and exercise interventions found to be effective in managing fatigue in people with cancer. As with interventions for depression, two considerations were foremost in our selection of examples: superiority of the intervention to a control condition in a published RCT and relative ease of dissemination.

Energy Conservation and Activity Management

Barsevick et al. (2004) developed an energy conservation and activity management (ECAM) intervention designed to reduce fatigue in adults receiving cancer treatment (i.e., chemotherapy, radiotherapy, or both). The intervention is delivered by nurses by means of telephone in three sessions that are conducted during the first five weeks of treatment. In the first session, participants receive information on cancer-related fatigue and learn energy conservation skills (e.g., activity pacing and priority setting). They are also given a homework assignment that includes keeping a journal in which they monitor their fatigue and other symptoms and make a list that prioritizes their usual activities. In the second session, the journal and priority list are used to develop an energy conservation plan that seeks to maintain valued activities and minimize interference from fatigue. In the final session, the energy conservation plan is evaluated and revised as needed. Using an RCT design, the investigators compared the efficacy of the ECAM intervention to a control condition in which participants received nutritional education. Fatigue was assessed at baseline and at two later time-points that varied depending on type of cancer treatment participants were receiving. Findings indicated that patients receiving the ECAM intervention experienced less fatigue over time compared with controls (Barsevick et al., 2004)

Exercise Training

Courneya et al. (2003) evaluated an exercise-training program with postmenopausal women with breast cancer who had completed surgery, radiotherapy, and/or chemotherapy. The exercise intervention consists of supervised training on cycle ergometers conducted three times per week for 15 weeks. Each training session lasts 15 minutes during the first three weeks. Sessions increase in five-minute intervals every three weeks, up to a maximum of 35 minutes during the final three weeks. The intervention was evaluated using an RCT design in which control participants received no exercise training. Adherence to the exercise intervention was excellent, with 98.4% of the exercise sessions completed as prescribed. Findings indicated that the exercise group reported significant improvement in fatigue relative to the control group. Additional findings suggested that the beneficial effects of exercise training on fatigue were mediated by improvements in cardiopulmonary function.

Cognitive Behavior Therapy

Gielissen, Verhagen, Witjes, and Bleijenberg (2006) examined the efficacy of cognitive behavior therapy in disease-free cancer survivors experiencing heightened fatigue. The intervention centers on seven factors thought to perpetuate fatigue in the posttreatment period: insufficient coping with the experience of cancer, fear of disease recurrence, dysfunctional cognitions regarding fatigue, dysregulation of sleep, dysregulation of activity, low social support, and negative social interactions. The intervention consists of separate modules for each of these seven factors, with participants receiving only those modules considered relevant to them based on an initial evaluation. The intervention was evaluated using an RCT design that featured a wait-list control condition. On average, the intervention was delivered in 12.5 one-hour sessions over a six-month period, followed by a maximum of two additional sessions over a subsequent six months. Study outcomes were assessed at baseline and six months later. Findings indicated that participants receiving the intervention experienced significantly less fatigue, less psychological distress, and less functional impairment compared to wait-list controls. The magnitude of these intervention effects was considered to be clinically significant based on additional analyses that used a reliable change index approach. A pooled follow-up assessment was conducted an average of 1.9 years later with participants who were randomized to receive the intervention or who eventually received the intervention following the waiting period (Gielissen, Verhagen, & Bleijenberg, 2007). Findings suggested that the initial beneficial effects of the intervention were largely maintained over the follow-up period.

PAIN

Pain is one of the most feared and burdensome symptoms experienced by cancer patients (van den Beuken van Everdingen et al., 2007). Unrelieved cancer pain is likely to adversely affect an individual's quality of life in numerous domains, including physical, social, psychological, and spiritual functioning (Allard, Maunsell, Labbe, & Dorval, 2001). Moderate or severe pain in cancer patients is often associated with interference with sleep, daily life activities, enjoyment of life, work ability, and social involvement (Allard et al., 2001). The causes of cancer pain and the mechanisms underlying its pathophysiology are numerous and complex. In general, cancer pain can be divided into three broad etiologic categories (McGuire, 2004). The first category consists of pain caused by direct tumor involvement. Examples include pain caused by injury to the central nervous system (e.g., spinal cord compression) and by activation of pain receptors in cutaneous and deep tissues (e.g., metastasis to bone and organs). The second category consists of pain that results from diagnostic or therapeutic procedures. Examples include surgery-related pain as well as pain resulting from biopsies, venipuncture, and lumbar punctures. The third category consists of pain that occurs as a side effect or toxicity of cancer treatment. Examples include peripheral neuropathy and oral mucositis pain attributable to chemotherapeutic agents and skin burns attributable to radiation therapy. Compounding the complexity of cancer pain is the possibility that patients may have more than one type of cancer-related pain at any given time.

PREVALENCE OF PAIN

A recent meta-analysis identified 160 studies published over the past 40 years that had examined the prevalence of pain in patients with cancer (van den Beuken van Everdingen et al., 2007). Among these studies, the prevalence of pain was measured using a variety of self-report formats that included visual analog scales, numerical rating scales, verbal rating scales, and "yes/no" questions. Moreover, there were differences in the recall periods (e.g., right now, today, and past week) on which ratings were based. The studies also vary considerably in terms of the demographic, disease, and treatment characteristics of the samples for which results are reported. Drawing from 52 studies that met a criterion for quality, the authors calculated pooled pain prevalence rates for four subgroups of studies. Among studies that included patients assessed after curative treatment, pain prevalence was 33%. Among studies that included patients undergoing cancer treatment, pain prevalence was 59%. Among studies that included patients characterized as having advanced, metastatic, or terminal disease, pain prevalence was 64%. Finally, among studies that included patients at all disease stages, pain prevalence was 53%. These findings suggest that pain is common among cancer patients at all stages of disease and phases of treatment, but that patients with worse disease are more likely to experience pain. The clinical significance of these findings is underscored by results showing that among patients experiencing pain, more than one third rated it as moderate or severe.

CLINICAL PRACTICE GUIDELINES FOR MANAGEMENT OF PAIN IN CANCER PATIENTS

Both evidence-based and consensus-based guidelines have been issued for the management of pain in cancer patients. The American Pain Society has supported the development of evidence-based guidelines for management of pain in adults with cancer (Miakowski, Cleary, et al., 2004). These guidelines are offered in the form of a series of evidence-based recommendations accompanied by information identifying the level and source of evidence supporting each recommendation. Many of the recommendations that concern the assessment and pharmacological management of cancer pain are beyond the scope of this chapter. Of particular relevance are guidelines that identify the central role of education in cancer pain management and identify specific content to be included in educational efforts. Among the recommended educational content is information on when and how to use nonpharmacological approaches for pain management. The guidelines also identify specific nonpharmacological approaches found to be effective in controlled studies. These include several psychological approaches such as hypnosis, relaxation training, cognitive-behaviorial therapy, and supportive therapy.

NCCN has developed consensus-based guidelines for the management of pain in adults with cancer (NCCN, 2010a). Similar to other NCCN guidelines, these are presented largely in the form of clinical pathways that identify recommendations at key treatment decision points. Although much of the focus is on pharmacological approaches, the guidelines stress the role of patient education and psychosocial support in management of cancer pain. In addition, the guidelines identify several nonpharmacological approaches that may serve as beneficial adjuncts to pharmacologic interventions. These approaches are subcategorized as physical or cognitive modalities. The latter includes such techniques as imagery and hypnosis, distraction training, relaxation training, active coping training, graded task assignments, and cognitive-behavioral training. In contrast to the American Pain Society's guidelines, recommendations regarding the use of nonpharmacological interventions in the NCCN guidelines are not linked to research that provides empirical support.

More recently, Dy, Asch, et al. (2008) published evidence-based standards for cancer pain management. Their recommendations include routine screening for pain, routine pain education, and routine follow-up to evaluate the adequacy of pain management.

Systematic Reviews and Meta-Analyses of Psychosocial Interventions for Pain in Adults With Cancer

Our examination of the literature identified one systematic review and one meta-analysis that focused specifically on the effects of psychosocial intervention on pain in adults with cancer (see Table 30.3). The systematic review that was identified (Allard et al., 2001) encompassed studies published through 1999 of educational interventions designed to improve pain control in adult cancer patients. Of the 33 studies retained for final analysis, 25 evaluated interventions directed at health professionals, seven evaluated interventions directed at patients, and one evaluated an intervention directed at family caregivers. Of the eight studies directed at patients and family caregivers, only two used randomized designs. The pain education interventions studied with patients and caregivers are quite diverse and range from a brief 15-minute counseling session to three educational home visits. Improvements in knowledge or attitudes regarding cancer pain management relative to baseline were reported in all six studies in which these variables were assessed. Improvements in pain relief were reported in three of the four studies in which this variable was assessed. Given the limited number of published RCTs identified, the authors conclude that their systematic review cannot be used to define what constitutes an evidence-based educational approach to cancer pain control.

TABLE 30.3

Systematic Reviews and Meta-Analyses of Psychosocial Interventions for Pain in Adults With Cancer

Reference	Intervention Focus	Psychosocial Intervention Studies Reviewed	Findings for Psychosocial Studies	Conclusions
Devine (2003)	Psychosocial interventions	Randomized and nonrandomized studies of cancer patients	Pain: $d = 0.41$, 95% CI $= 0.15–0.58$	Reasonably strong evidence exists for relaxation-based cognitive-behavioral interventions, education about analgesic usage, and supportive counseling.
Allard et al. (2001)	Educational interventions	Randomized and nonrandomized studies of cancer patients	Randomized designs in only 2 of 7 studies directed at patients	Systematic review findings cannot be used to define evidence-based approach to cancer pain control.

The meta-analysis that was identified (Devine, 2003) encompassed studies of psychoeducational interventions published through 2001 that included a pain outcome measure and for which an effect size could be calculated. Among the interventions that met the criteria for being psychoeducational in nature were studies of hypnosis, education, supportive-expressive therapy, relaxation training, and self-selected music. Twenty-five studies were included in the meta-analysis, and 20 of these used randomized designs. Across all studies, a moderate-sized statistically significant effect of intervention on self-reported pain was found ($d = .41, p < .05$). When the analysis was restricted to nine higher quality studies that featured random assignment and other methodological strengths, the effect was somewhat smaller but still statistically significant ($d = .36, p < .05$). Additional analyses based on type of intervention indicated that there were significant positive effects for educational interventions ($d = .65, p < .05$), cognitive-behavioral interventions that included relaxation training ($d = .36, p < .05$), and supportive counseling that may or may not have included other intervention components ($d = .44, p < .05$). These findings lead the author to conclude that despite variable methodological quality, reasonably strong evidence exists for the efficacy of the three types of psychoeducational interventions just described.

EXAMPLES OF EVIDENCE-SUPPORTED PSYCHOLOGICAL INTERVENTIONS FOR PAIN

In this section, we provide examples of three psychosocial interventions found to be effective in managing pain in people with cancer. Two considerations, similar to those described for depression and fatigue, were foremost in our selection of intervention examples: superiority to a control condition in a published RCT and relative ease of dissemination.

Patient Training in Cancer Pain Management

Syrjala et al. (2008) developed a cancer pain management intervention based primarily on print and audiovisual materials in an effort to reduce the amount of professional time and resources required to provide patients with relevant information and advice. Similar to professionally administered interventions, this intervention was expected to reduce pain management and improve pain outcomes. This single-session intervention consists of a patient watching a 15-minute video that provided basic information about pain management and then reviewing with a nurse a handbook intended to serve as a resource for pain and related symptom questions and needs that might arise over the course of cancer care. After this, the nurse assists the patient in completing a checklist of "Things to Tell Your Doctor" and encourages the patient to take the checklist to the next doctor's appointment and to take in a new checklist if a new pain occurred, pain was not well controlled, or other symptoms occurred. A telephone follow-up is conducted 72 hours later to reinforce learning from the training. Using an RCT design and a multisite sampling strategy, the investigators compared the efficacy of this intervention to a time- and attention-equivalent nutritional-counseling intervention in patients with disease-related persistent pain. Ratings of pain and barriers to pain management and information about opioid-analgesic use were collected at baseline and at one, three, and six months later. Findings indicated that patients who received the pain-management intervention reported significantly fewer barriers to pain management and less pain relative to patients in the control group. In addition, they used significantly more opioid analgesics than did the controls. Whereas the differences between intervention conditions in barriers and pain ratings tended to narrow over time, the difference in opioid use tended to increase over time.

Representational Intervention to Decrease Cancer Pain

Ward et al. (2008) developed a representational approach to cancer pain education based on theories regarding cognitive representations of illness (Leventhal & Diefenbach, 1991). The intervention is described as having five steps during which an interventionist (1) asks patients to describe their beliefs about the cause, timeline, consequences, cure, and control of cancer pain; (2) identifies and discusses misconceptions about reporting pain and using analgesics; (3) discusses limitations and losses that are a consequence of these misconceptions; (4) provides credible evidence to replace the identified misconceptions; and (5) summarizes and discusses the benefits of adopting this new information. These steps occur during a single session that may last from 20 to 60 minutes depending on the number of identified misconceptions. Using an RCT design, the investigators compared this intervention to a standard education information condition in which patients received a booklet that described common misconceptions about cancer pain management and the management of opioid side effects. The participants were ambulatory patients with pain and a diagnosis of metastatic cancer. They completed measures assessing pain, well-being, and beliefs about analgesic use and had their analgesic use recorded at baseline and one and two months later. Findings indicated that patients who received the representational intervention reported fewer barriers at both follow-up assessments and less severe usual pain at the second follow-up assessment than did patients who received the standard education intervention. There were no differences in the adequacy of analgesic regimens based on intervention assignment. Additional analyses confirmed that reductions in barriers mediated the beneficial effects of the representational intervention on patients' pain reports.

Brief Hypnosis Intervention for Breast Surgery Patients

Montgomery et al. (2007) developed a hypnosis intervention designed to decrease pain and other side effects commonly associated with breast cancer surgery. The intervention consists of a brief (15-minute) meeting with a psychologist on the morning of surgery that includes a standardized hypnotic induction, suggestions to visualize pleasant imagery and experiencing feelings of relaxation, and instruction on how to use hypnosis on one's own. Using an RCT design, the investigators compared the efficacy of this intervention to an attention control condition comprised of nondirective empathic listening. Pain and other symptoms were assessed by self-report once patients reached standardized criteria for hospital discharge and medical records were reviewed to measure use of intraoperative analgesics and sedatives and postoperative analgesics. Findings indicated that relative to the control condition, patients who received the hypnotic intervention reported less pain, nausea, fatigue, discomfort, and emotional upset postoperatively and required lesser amounts of lidocaine (an analgesic) and propfol (a sedative) intraoperatively. There were no group differences, however, in postoperative analgesic use.

CONCLUSIONS

As reviewed in this chapter, numerous psychosocial interventions have been tested and found to be efficacious in preventing or relieving depression, fatigue, and pain in cancer patients. Nevertheless, important gaps exist in the research literature. Many of the studies conducted were limited to women with breast cancer who were recruited at major cancer treatment centers. Consequently, there has been a dearth of research on men with cancer, on women with other forms of cancer, and on patients who are from racial and ethnic minority groups. In addition, few studies have focused on patients with advanced disease and on patients who have completed treatment. Perhaps the most glaring gap in the research reviewed is the very limited number of studies of patients experiencing clinically significant levels of depression or fatigue at the time of recruitment. Although not the focus of this chapter, it is also worth noting that the development of psychosocial interventions for other common problems (e.g., sexual, sleep, and cognitive difficulties) lags behind progress in treating depression, fatigue, and pain. Conducting research that addresses these gaps should be a priority for future research.

Three additional recommendations are offered that go beyond addressing existing gaps to reconsidering how studies of psychosocial interventions are conducted. All three recommendations reflect the need for research that is more relevant to clinical practice. First, studies of psychosocial interventions should be informed by the growing body of research demonstrating that cancer patients tend to experience symptoms in clusters rather than in isolation (Miakowski, Dodd, &

Lee, 2004). Depression, for example, frequently co-occurs with pain and fatigue in cancer patients (Gaston-Johansson, Fall-Dickson, Bakos, & Kennedy, 1999). Recognizing this pattern, interventions are now being designed specifically to treat symptom clusters of this type (Williams, 2007).

Second, psychosocial interventions need to be evaluated in combination with other approaches used to manage depression, fatigue, and pain. Clinical practice guidelines typically recommend that these symptoms be treated using a combination of pharmacological and nonpharmacological approaches. For example, the NCCN's consensus-based clinical practice guidelines for distress management recommend the use of psychotherapy in combination with antidepressant and/or anxiolytic medication for patients with mood disorders (NCCN, 2010c). RCTs are needed that explicitly test whether the combination of pharmacotherapy and psychotherapy is better than either approach alone. RCTs should also be conducted to test whether certain demographic, disease, or treatment characteristics predict whether a patient is more likely to benefit from psychotherapy or medication. Third, research is needed that evaluates the entire process through which patients might receive a psychosocial intervention in clinical practice. For example, NCCN's clinical practice guidelines recommend that patients be screened routinely for distress, pain, and fatigue with psychosocial interventions provided based on further evaluation of patients experiencing moderate to severe levels of these symptoms (NCCN, 2010a, 2010b, 2010c). Whether or not this strategy (i.e., routine screening followed by referral for psychosocial interventions) results in better symptom management than do other strategies (e.g., preventive interventions offered to all patients) has yet to be evaluated.

The final recommendations reflect the need to increase patient access to evidence-supported interventions. First, more research is needed on interventions that have the potential for widespread dissemination based on their being relatively inexpensive and requiring few professional resources to deliver. One approach would be to evaluate whether psychosocial interventions typically provided through face-to-face meetings with a clinician can be adapted for delivery over the Internet. Second, mechanisms need to be developed that facilitate the dissemination of evidence-supported interventions to clinicians caring for cancer patients. The National Cancer Institute (NCI) and several partners recently developed a Web site that supplies information about research-tested intervention programs (http://rtips.cancer.gov/rtips/index.do; NCI, 2010). Among the interventions described are several psychosocial interventions found to be effective in improving quality of life in cancer patients. In addition to describing research-tested interventions, the Web site provides information about how to obtain the training manuals and other materials needed to deliver these interventions. This effort has the potential to become a very valuable resource for promoting evidence-based psychosocial care for cancer patients.

REFERENCES

Allard, P., Maunsell, E., Labbe, J., & Dorval, M. (2001). Educational interventions to improve cancer pain control: A systematic review. *Journal of Palliative Medicine, 4*, 191–203.

American Cancer Society. (2010). *Cancer facts & figures*. Atlanta, GA: American Cancer Society.

American Psychiatric Association (APA). (1994). *Diagnostic and statistical manual of mental disorders* (4th ed.). Washington, DC: American Psychiatric Association.

Andersen, B. L., Yang, H.-C., Farrar, W. B., Golden-Kreutz, D. M., Emery, C., Thornton, L. M., … Carson, W. E. (2008). Psychologic intervention improves survival for breast cancer patients. *Cancer, 113*, 3450–3458.

Andrykowski, M., & Manne, S. (2006). Are psychological interventions effective and accepted by cancer patients? *Annals of Behavioral Medicine, 32*, 93–97.

Baker, F., Denniston, M., Smith, T., & West, M. (2005). Adult cancer survivors: How are they faring? *Cancer, 104*, 2565–2576.

Barsevick, A., Dudley, W., Beck, S., Sweeney, C., Whitmer, K., & Nail, L. (2004). A randomized trial of energy conservation for patients with cancer-related fatigue. *Cancer, 100*, 1302–1310.

Barsevick, A., Sweeney, C., Haney, E., & Chung, E. (2002). A systematic qualitative analysis of psychoeducational interventions for depression in patients with cancer. *Oncology Nursing Forum, 29*, 73–84.

Bottomley, A. (1998). Depression in cancer patients: A literature review. *European Journal of Cancer Care, 7*, 181–191.

Bower, J., Ganz, P., Aziz, N., & Fahey, J. (2002). Fatigue and proinflammatory cytokine activity in breast cancer survivors. *Psychosomatic Medicine, 64*, 604–611.

Broeckel, J. A., Jacobsen, P., Horton, J., Balducci, L., & Lyman, G. H. (1998). Characteristics and correlates of fatigue after adjuvant chemotherapy for breast cancer. *Journal of Clinical Oncology, 16*, 1689–1696.

Capuron, L., Ravaud, A., & Dantzer, R. (2000). Early depressive symptoms in cancer patients receiving interleukin 2, and or interferon alpha-2b therapy. *Journal of Clinical Oncology, 18*, 2143–2151.

Cella, D. (1998). Factors influencing quality of life in cancer patients: Anemia and fatigue. *Seminars in Oncology, 25*, 43–46.

Cella, D., Davis, K., Breitbart, W., & Curt, G. (2001). Cancer-related fatigue: Prevalence of proposed diagnostic criteria in a US sample of cancer survivors. *Journal of Clinical Oncology, 19*, 3385–3391.

Chang, V., Hwang, S., Feuerman, M., Kasimis, B., & Thaler, H. (2000). The Memorial Symptom Assessment Scale Short Form (MSAS-SF). *Cancer, 89*, 1162–1171.

Cleeland, C., Mendoza, T., Wang, X., Chou, C., Harle, M., & Morrissey, M. (2000). Assessing symptom distress in cancer patients: The MD Anderson Symptom Inventory. *Cancer, 89*, 1634–1646.

Conn, V., Hafdahl, A., Porock, D., McDaniel, R., & Nielsen, P. (2007). A meta-analysis of exercise interventions among people treated for cancer. *Supportive Care in Cancer, 14*, 699–712.

Courneya, K., Mackey, J., Gordon, J., Jones, L., Field, C., & Fairey, A. (2003). Randomized controlled trial of exercise training in post menopausal breast cancer survivors: Cardiopulmonary and quality of life outcomes. *Journal of Clinical Oncology, 21*, 1660–1668.

Coyne, J. C., Stefanek, M., & Palmer, S. C. (2007). Psychotherapy and survival in cancer: The conflict between hope and evidence. *Psychological Bulletin, 133*, 367–394.

Cramp, J., & Daniel, J. (2008). Exercise for management of cancer-related fatigue in adults [Review]. *Cochrane Database of Systematic Reviews*, No. 2. Art No. CD006145. doi:10.1002/14651858.CD006145.pub 2

Curt, G. A., Breitbart, W., Cella, D., Groopman, J., Horning, S., & Itri, L. (2000). Impact of cancer-related fatigue on the lives of patients: New findings from the Fatigue Coalition. *Oncologist, 5*, 353–360.

Devine, E. (2003). Meta-analysis of the effect of psychoeducational interventions on pain in adults with cancer. *Oncology Nursing Forum, 30*, 75–89.

Devine, E., & Westlake, S. K. (1995). The effects of psychoeducational care provided to adults with cancer: Meta-analysis of 116 studies. *Oncology Nursing Forum, 22*, 1369–1381.

Dy, S., Asch, S., Naeim, A., Sanati, H., Walling, A., & Lorenz, K. (2008). Evidence-based standards for cancer pain management. *Journal of Clinical Oncology, 26*, 3879–3885.

Dy, S., Lorenz, K., Naeim, A., Sanati, H., Walling, A., & Asch, S. (2008). Evidence-based recommendations for cancer fatigue, anorexia, depression, and dyspnea. *Journal of Clinical Oncology, 26*, 3886–3895.

Fallowfield, L., Ratcliffe, D., Jenkins, V., & Saul, J. (2001). Psychiatric morbidity and its recognition by doctors in patients with cancer. *British Journal of Cancer, 84*, 1011–1015.

Gaston-Johansson, F., Fall-Dickson, J., Bakos, A., & Kennedy, M. (1999). Fatigue, pain, and depression in pre-autotransplant breast cancer patients. *Cancer Practice, 7*, 240–247.

Geinitz, H., Zimmerman, F., Thamm, R., Keller, M., Busch, R., & Molls, M. (2004). Fatigue in patients with adjuvant radiation therapy for breast cancer: Long-term follow-up. *Journal of Cancer Research and Clinical Oncology, 130*, 327–333.

Gielissen, M., Verhagen, S., & Bleijenberg, G. (2007). Cognitive behaviour therapy for fatigued cancer survivors: Long-term follow-up. *British Journal of Cancer, 97*, 612–618.

Gielissen, M., Verhagen, S., Witjes, F., & Bleijenberg, G. (2006). Effects of cognitive behavior therapy (CBT) in severely fatigued disease-free cancer patients compared to patients waiting for CBT: A randomized controlled trial. *Journal of Clinical Oncology, 24*, 4882–4887.

Glaus, A., Crow, R., & Hammond, S. (1996). A qualitative study to explore the concept of fatigue/tiredness in cancer patients and in healthy individuals. *European Journal of Cancer Care, 5*, 8–23.

Grassi, L., Indelli, M., Marzola, M., Maestri, A., Santini, A., & Piva, E. (1996). Depressive symptoms and quality of life in home-care assisted cancer patients. *Journal of Pain and Symptom Management, 12*, 300–307.

Greenberg, D., Sawicka, J., Eisenthal, S., & Ross, D. (1992). Fatigue syndrome due to localized radiation *Journal of Pain and Symptom Management, 7*, 38–45.

Groopman, J., & Itri, L. (1999). Chemotherapy-induced anemia in adults: Incidence and treatment. *Journal of the National Cancer Institute, 91*, 1616–1634.

Hann, D., Jacobsen, P., Martin, S., Azzarello, L., & Greenberg, H. (1998). Fatigue and quality of life following radiotherapy for breast cancer: A comparative study. *Journal of Clinical Psychology in Medical Settings, 5*, 19–33.

Hann, D., Jacobsen, P., Martin, S., Kronish, L., Azzarello, L., & Fields, K. (1997). Fatigue in women treated with bone marrow transplantation for breast cancer: A comparison with women with no history of cancer. *Supportive Cancer Care*, *5*, 44–52.

Institute of Medicine (2007). *Cancer care for the whole patient: M eeting psychosocial health needs.* Washington, DC: National Academies Press.

Jacobsen, P., Andrykowski, M., & Thors, C. (2004). Relationship of catastrophizing to fatigue among women receiving treatment for breast cancer. *Journal of Consulting and Clinical Psychology*, *72*, 355–361.

Jacobsen, P., Donovan, K., Swaine, Z., & Watson, I. (2006). Management of anxiety and depression in adult cancer patients: Toward an evidence-based approach. In G. Chang, P. Ganz, D. Hayes, T. Kinsell, H. Pass, J. Schiller, … V. Strecher (Eds), *Oncology: An evidence-based approach* (pp. 1552–1579). New York, NY: Springer-Verlag.

Jacobsen, P., Donovan, K., Vadaparampil, S., & Small, B. (2007). Systematic review and meta-analysis of psychological and activity-based interventions for cancer-related fatigue. *Health Psychology*, *26*, 660–667.

Jacobsen, P., Donovan, K., & Weitzner, M. (2003). Distinguishing fatigue and depression in patients with cancer. *Seminars in Clinical Neuropsychiatry*, *8*, 229–240.

Jacobsen, P., Hann, D., Azzarello, L., Horton, J., Balducci, L., & Lyman, G. H. (1999). Fatigue in women receiving adjuvant chemotherapy for breast cancer: Characteristics, course, and correlates. *Journal of Pain and Symptom Management*, *18*, 233–242.

Jacobsen, P., & Jim, H. S. (2008). Psychosocial interventions for anxiety and depression in cancer patients: Achievements and challenges. *Cancer*, *58*, 214–230.

Jacobsen, P., Meade, C., Stein, K., Chirikos, T., Small, B., & Ruckdeschel, J. (2002). Efficacy and costs of two forms of stress management training for cancer patients undergoing chemotherapy. *Journal of Clinical Oncology*, *20*, 2851–2862.

Jim, H., & Jacobsen, P. (2008). Assessment and management of cancer-related fatigue. In G. Lyman & J. Crawford (Eds.), *Cancer supportive care: Advances in therapeutic strategies*. New York, NY: Informa Health.

Kangas, M., Bovbjerg, D., & Montgomery, G. (2008). Cancer-related fatigue: A systematic and meta-analytic review of non-pharmacological therapies for cancer patients. *Psychological Bulletin*, *134*, 700–741.

Kim, S. H., Son, B. H., Hwang, S. Y., Han, W., Young, J. H., & Lee, S. (2008). Fatigue and depression in disease-free breast cancer survivors: Prevalence, correlates, and association with quality of life. *Journal of Pain and Symptom Management*, *35*, 644–655.

Kirshbaum, M. (2006). A review of the benefits of whole body exercise during and after treatment for breast cancer. *Journal of Clinical Nursing*, *16*, 104–121.

Lawrence, D., Kupelnick, B., Miller, K., Devine, D., & Lau, J. (2004). Evidence report on the occurrence, assessment, and treatment of fatigue in cancer patients [Systematic review]. *Journal of the National Cancer Institute Monographs*, *32*, 40–50.

Lepore, S., & Coyne, J. (2006). Psychological interventions for distress in cancer patients: A review of reviews. *Annals of Behavioral Medicine*, *32*, 85–92.

Leventhal, H., & Diefenbach, M. (1991). The active side of illness cognition. In J. Skelton & R. Croyle (Eds.), *Mental representation of health and illness* (pp. 247–272). New York, NY: Springer.

Lovejoy, N., & Matteis, M. (1997). Cognitive-behavioral interventions to manage depression in patients with cancer: Research and theoretical initiatives. *Cancer Nursing*, *20*, 155–167.

Luctkar-Flude, M., Groll, D., Tranmer, J., & Woodend, K. (2007). Fatigue and physical activity in older adults with cancer: A systematic review of the literature. *Cancer Nursing*, *30*, E35–E45.

Luebbert, K., Dahme, B., & Hasenbring, M. (2001). The effectiveness of relaxation training in reducing treatment-related symptoms and improving emotional adjustment in acute nonsurgical cancer treatment: A meta-analytic review. *Psycho-Oncology*, *10*, 490–502.

Markes, M., Brockaw, T., & Resch, K. (2006). Exercise for women receiving adjuvant therapy for breast cancer (Publication No. CD005001). *Cochrane Database System Review.* Retrieved from http://www.ncbi.nlm.nih.gov/pubmed/17054230

McGuire, D. (2004). Occurrence of cancer pain. *Journal of the National Cancer Institute Monographs*, *32*, 51–56.

McNeely, M., Campbell, K., Rowe, B., Klaussen, T., Mackey, J., & Courneya, K. (2006). Effects of exercise on breast cancer patients and survivors: A systematic review and meta-analysis. *Canadian Medical Association Journal*, *175*, 34–41.

Miakowski, C., Cleary, J., Burney, R., Coyne, P., Finley, R., & Foster, R. (2004). *Guidelines for the management of cancer pain in adults and children.* Glenview, IL: American Pain Society.

Miakowski, C., Dodd, M., & Lee, K. (2004). Symptom clusters: The new frontier in symptom managment research. *Journal of the National Cancer Institute Monographs*, *32*, 17–21.

Mitchell, S., & Berger, A. (2006). Cancer-related fatigue: The evidence base for assessment and management. *Cancer, 12*, 374–387.

Mock, V., Burke, M., Sheehan, P., Creaton, E., Winningham, M., & McKenney-Tedder, S. (1994). A nursing rehabilitation program for women with breast cancer receiving adjuvant chemotherapy. *Oncology Nursing Forum, 21*, 899–907.

Montgomery, G., Bovberg, D., Schnur, J., David, D., Goldfarb, A., Weltz, C., … Silverstein, J. H. (2007). A randomized clinical trial of a brief hypnosis intervention to control side effects in breast surgery patients. *Journal of the National Cancer Institute, 99*, 1304–1312.

National Breast Cancer Centre and National Cancer Control Initiative. (2003). *Clinical practice guidelines for the psychosocial care of adults with cancer*. Camperdown, Australia: National Breast Cancer Centre. Retrieved from http://www.nhmrc.gov.au/publications/synopses/cp90syn.htm

National Cancer Institute (NCI). (2010). Research-tested intervention programs (RTIIPS). *Cancer Control P.L.A.N.E.T*. Retrieved from http://rtips.cancer.gov/rtips/index.do

National Comprehensive Cancer Network (NCCN). (2010a). NCCN clinical practice guidelines in oncology: Adult cancer pain. Retrieved October 11, 2010, from http:/www.nccn.org/professionals/physician_gls/PDF/pain.pdf

National Comprehensive Cancer Network (NCCN). (2010b). NCCN clinical practice guidelines in oncology: Cancer-related fatigue. Retrieved October 11, 2010, from http://www.nccn.org/professionals/physician_gls/PDF/fatigue.pdf

National Comprehensive Cancer Network (NCCN). (2010c). NCCN clinical practice guidelines in oncology: Distress management. Retrieved October 11, 2010, from http://www.nccn.org/professionals/physician_gls/PDF/distress.pdf

Newell, S., Sanson-Fisher, R., & Savolainen, N. (2002). Systematic review of psychological therapies for cancer patients: Overview and recommendations for future research. *Journal of the National Cancer Institute, 94*, 558–584.

Nezu, A., Nezu, C., McClure, K., Felgoise, S., & Houts, P. (2003). Project Genesis: Assessing the efficacy of problem-solving therapy for distressed adult cancer patients. *Journal of Consulting and Clinical Psychology, 71*, 1036–1048.

Osborn, R., Demoncada, A., & Feuerstein, M. (2006). Psychosocial interventions for depression, anxiety, and quality of life in cancer survivors: Meta-analyses. *Psychosomatic Medicine, 36*, 13–34.

Patrick, D., Ferketich, S., Frame, P., Harris, J., Hendircks, C., & Levin, B. (2004). National Institutes of Health State-of-the-Science Conference statement: Symptom management in cancer: Pain, depression and fatigue. *Journal of the National Cancer Institute Monographs, 32*, 9–16.

Pinquart, M., & Duberstein, P. R. (2010). Depression and cancer morality: A meta-analysis. *Psychological Medicine, 40*, 1797–1810.

Pirl, W. (2004). Evidence report on the occurrence, assessment, and treatment of depression in cancer patients. *Journal of the National Cancer Institute Monographs, 32*, 32–39.

Poulson, M. (2001). Not just tired. *Journal of Clinical Oncology, 19*, 4180–4181.

Prieto, J., Blanch, J., Atala, J., Carreras, E., Rovira, M., & Cirera, E. (2002). Psychiatric morbidity and impact on hospital length of stay among hematologic cancer patients receiving stem cell transplantation. *Journal of Clinical Oncology, 20*, 1907–1917.

Radloff, S. (1977). The CES-D: A self-report depression scale for research in the general population. *Applied Psychological Measurement, 1*, 385–401.

Rhodes, V., Watson, P., & Hanson, B. (1988). Patients' descriptions of the influence of tiredness and weakness on self-care abilities. *Cancer Nursing, 11*, 186–194.

Rodin, G., Lloyd, N., Katz, M., Green, E., MacKay, J. A., & Wong, R. (2007). The treatment of depression in cancer patients: A systematic review. *Supportive Care in Cancer, 15*, 123–136.

Schmitz, K., Holtzman, J., Courneya, K., Masse, L., Duval, S., & Kane, R. (2005). Controlled physical activity trials in cancer survivors: A systematic review and meta-analysis. *Cancer Epidemiology, Biomarkers, and Prevention, 14*, 1588–1595.

Sellick, S., & Crooks, D. (1999). Depression and cancer: An appraisal of the literature for prevalence, detection, and practice guideline development for psychological interventions. *Psycho-Oncology, 8*, 315–333.

Sheard, T., & Maguire, P. (1999). The effects of psychological interventions on anxiety and depression in cancer patients: Results of two meta-analyses. *British Journal of Cancer, 80*, 1770–1780.

Speck, R., Courneya, K. S., Masse, L. C., Duval, S., & Schmitz, K. H. (2010). An update of controlled physical activity trials in cancer survivors: A systematic review and meta-analysis. *Journal of Cancer Survivorship, 4*, 87–100.

Spiegel, D., Bloom, J. R., Kramer, H. C., & Gottheil, E. (1989). Effect of psychosocial treatment on survival of patients with metastatic breast cancer. *Lancet, 2,* 888–891.

Spiegel, D., & Giese-Davis, J. (2003). Depression and cancer: Mechanisms and disease progression. *Biological Psychiatry, 54,* 269–282.

Stark, D., Kiely, M., Smith, A., Velikova, G., House, A., & Selby, P. (2002). Anxiety disorders in cancer patients: Their nature, associations, and relation to quality of life. *Journal of Clinical Oncology, 20,* 3137–3148.

Stefanek, M., Palmer, S. C., Thombs, B. D., & Coyne, J. C. (2009). Finding what is not there. *Cancer, 115,* 5612–5616.

Stevinson, C., Lawlor, D., & Fox, K. (2004). Exercise interventions for cancer patients: systematic review of controlled trials. *Cancer Causes and Control, 15,* 1035–1056.

Stone, P., Hardy, J., Broadley, K., Tookman, A. J., Kurowska, A., & Ahern, R. (1999). Fatigue in advanced cancer: A prospective controlled cross-sectional study. *British Journal of Cancer, 79,* 1479–1486.

Stone, P., Richards, M., Ahern, R., & Hardy, J. (2000). A study to investigate prevalence, severity, and correlates of fatigue among patients with cancer in comparison with a control group of volunteers without cancer. *Annals of Oncology, 11,* 561–567.

Strong, V., Waters, R., Hibberd, C., Murray, G., Wall, L., Walker, J., … Sharpe, M. E. (2008). Management of depression for people with cancer (SMaRt oncology 1): A randomised trial. *Lancet, 372,* 40–48.

Syrjala, K., Abrams, J., Polissar, N., Hansbury, J., Robison, J., DuPen, S., … DuPen, A. (2008). Patient training in cancer pain management using integrated printed video materials: A multi-site randomized controlled trial. *Pain, 135,* 175–186.

Uitterhoeve, R., Vernooy, M., Litjens, M., Potting, K., Bensing, J., & DeMulder, P. (2004). Psychosocial interventions for patients with advanced cancer: A systematic review of the literature. *British Journal of Cancer, 91,* 1050–1062.

Van den Beuken van Everdingen, M., de Rijke, J., Kessels, A., Schouten, H., van Kleef, M., & Patijn, J. (2007). Prevalence of pain in patients with cancer: A systematic review of the past 40 years. *Annals of Oncology, 18,* 1437–1449.

Vogelzang, N., Breitbart, W., Cella, D., Curt, G., Groopman, J., Horning, S., … Portenoy, R. K. (1997). Patient, caregiver, and oncologist perceptions of cancer-related fatigue: Results of a tripart assessment survey. *Seminars in Hematology, 34,* 4–12.

Ward, S., Donovan, H., Gunnarsdottir, S., Serlin, R., Shapiro, G., & Hughes, S. (2008). A randomized trial of representational intervention to decrease cancer pain (RIDcancerPain). *Health Psychology, 27,* 59–67.

Williams L. (2007). Clinical management of symptom clusters. *Seminars in Oncology Nursing 23,* 113–120.

Williams, L., & Dale, J. (2006). The effectiveness of treatment for depression/depressive symptoms in adults with cancer: A systematic review. *British Journal of Cancer, 94,* 372–390.

Zigmond, A., & Snaith, R. (1983). The Hospital and Anxiety Depression Scale. *Acta Psychiatria Scandiniavica, 67,* 361–370.

31 Stress, Immunity, and Susceptibility to Upper Respiratory Infectious Disease

Anna L. Marsland
University of Pittsburgh

Elizabeth A. Bachen
Mills College

Sheldon Cohen
Carnegie Mellon University

Psychoneuroimmunology is the study of relations between psychosocial factors, the central nervous system, the immune system, and health. To date, the human literature within this field has focused on a working model that stressful life events impact immune function, which in turn modifies host resistance to immune-related disease (Cohen & Herbert, 1996). Upper respiratory infections (URIs) have served as one of the primary disease models in this literature, and early prospective studies supported popular belief and provided compelling evidence that stressful life events and psychological distress predict biologically verified infectious illness (Cohen et al., 1998; Cohen, Tyrrell, & Smith, 1991, 1993; Stone et al., 1992). More recent attention has focused on possible mechanisms of this effect. In this regard, there is substantial evidence that stress is associated with changes in immune function (Segerstrom & Miller, 2004); however, the implications of stress-induced immune changes for susceptibility to disease largely remain to be established. This chapter provides an overview of the human literature in psychoneuroimmunology, exploring evidence linking stress to immune function and susceptibility to infectious disease. Particular attention is given to individual differences in the magnitude of stress-related changes in immunity as one plausible explanation for variability in susceptibility to infectious pathogens.

STRESS AND SUSCEPTIBILITY TO INFECTIOUS DISEASE

Stress is a generalized set of diverse host responses to external or internal stimuli (stressors) that are harmful or are perceived to be harmful (Lazarus & Folkman, 1984). There is consistent evidence that persons under stress report more symptoms of infectious disease and that stress results in greater health care utilization for these infections (Cohen & Williamson, 1991). Indeed, results from numerous prospective cohort studies document a direct relationship between negative life events and/or perceived stress and increased risk for symptoms of URI (Graham, Douglas, & Ryan, 1986; Stone, Reed, & Neale, 1987; Takkouche, Regueira, & Gestal-Otero, 2001; Turner Cobb & Steptoe, 1998). For example, Takkouche and colleagues (2001) found that among 1,149 adults followed for one year, greater stressful life events, trait negative affectivity, and perceived stress predicted greater self-reported symptoms of URI. Similarly, recent findings from a prospective epidemiologic study of 5,404 adults showed that psychological stress and trait negative mood predicted the onset of self-reported symptoms of influenza, with perceived stress and trait negative affect contributing independently to symptom report (Smolderen, Vingerhoets, Croon, & Denollet, 2007). However, whereas self-reported symptoms of infectious disease may tap underlying pathology, it is also possible that they reflect a biased interpretation of physical sensations without underlying illness. The latter interpretation is supported by studies in which effects of stress on symptoms, but not verified disease, are observed, and by evidence that stress is associated with increased symptom reporting in general, not only with symptoms directly associated with infectious pathology (Cohen & Williamson, 1991).

In support of a relationship between stress and increased susceptibility to infectious disease, epidemiological studies in which the presence of pathology was verified by physician diagnosis or biological methods have found that major stressful life events, chronic family conflict, and disruptive daily events increase risk for upper respiratory disease (Graham et al., 1986; Meyer & Haggerty, 1962; Turner Cobb & Steptoe, 1996). For example, Meyer and Haggerty (1962) followed 100 members of 16 families for a 12-month period. Daily life events that disrupted family and personal life were four times more likely to precede than to follow new streptococcal and nonstreptococcal infections (as diagnosed by throat cultures and blood antibody levels) and associated symptomatology. Similar results were reported in a study of viral URIs in 235 members of 94 families (Graham et al., 1986). Here, number of major stressful and minor daily life events and ratings of psychological stress were positively associated with verified episodes and symptom days of respiratory illness. Turner Cobb and Steptoe (1996) also found that higher levels of life event stress were associated with increased clinically verified URI among 107 adults followed for 15 weeks. In sum, studies verifying infectious episodes suggest that stress increases risk for upper respiratory disease. However, community studies, such as these, do not control for the possible effects of stressful events on exposure to infectious agents. Indeed, increased incidence of infection in these studies may be attributable to stress-induced increases in exposure to infectious agents rather than to stress-induced immune modulation.

Several prospective studies have eliminated the possible role of psychological effects on exposure by experimentally inoculating healthy individuals with common cold viruses (viral challenge studies). Here, volunteers are assessed for degree of stress and then experimentally exposed to a cold virus or placebo. They are then kept in quarantine and monitored for the development of infection and illness. Early viral challenge studies were limited by a range of methodological weaknesses (Cohen & Williamson, 1991), including insufficient samples sizes and lack of control for factors known to influence susceptibility to viral infection (including preexisting antibodies to the infectious agent and age). Furthermore, the possible role of stress-elicited changes in such health practices as smoking and alcohol consumption was not considered. These limitations may account for initial failures to find consistent relations between stress and susceptibility to URI. In contrast, later viral challenge studies included multiple controls for factors known to be independently associated with susceptibility to viral infection (e.g., Cohen, Tyrell, & Smith, 1991, 1993; Cohen et al., 1998; Stone et al., 1992). These studies consistently found an association between stress and susceptibility to URI. For example, Cohen, Miller, and Rabin (1991) exposed 394 adult subjects to one of five upper respiratory viruses and assessed rates of infection and illness. Measures of negative life events in the past year, perceived stress, and negative affect were combined to form a stress index for each subject. After adjusting for control variables, the rates of verified infections and symptomatic illness increased with increasing values of the stress index for all five viruses. In a subsequent analysis of the data, Cohen, Tyrrell, and Smith (1993) reported that perceived stress and negative affect were significant predictors of becoming infected (replicating virus), whereas negative life events increased the probability of infected people developing clinical symptoms. This pattern was independently reproduced in a smaller study of 17 subjects experimentally infected with rhinovirus that found a significant positive correlation of major negative life events, but not perceived stress or negative affect, with the development of clinical colds (Stone et al., 1992). Subsequent studies showed that severe chronic negative life events (primarily underemployment or unemployment and enduring interpersonal difficulties with family and/or friends), but not severe acute negative life events, predicted increased risk for the development of a clinical cold (Cohen et al., 1998) and that negative mood prior to viral exposure predicted colds and influenza of greater severity, as determined by the amount of mucus produced over the course of illness (Cohen et al, 1995). A large group of control factors have not been able to explain increased risk for colds among persons reporting greater stress in these studies, including age, sex, allergic status, body weight, season, and virus-specific antibody status before challenge. Smoking, alcohol consumption, diet, exercise, and sleep quality also have failed to account for the relationship between stress and illness.

More recent attention has turned to an examination of psychosocial factors that may decrease susceptibility to URI by regulating emotion-sensitive biological systems and/or encouraging health-enhancing behaviors. These factors include dispositional positive affect and social dispositions and networks. Initial findings from viral challenge studies suggest that susceptibility to URI decreases in a dose-response manner with increased diversity of social network and with trait sociability (Cohen, Doyle, Skoner, Rabin, & Gwaltney, 1997; Cohen, Doyle, Turner, Alper, & Skoner, 2003b). Furthermore, higher positive affect has been associated with decreased incidence of objective symptoms of upper respiratory disease among infected people (Cohen, Alper, Doyle, Treanor, & Turner, 2006; Cohen, Doyle, Turner, Alper, & Skoner, 2003a). These relationships appear to be independent of negative emotional styles, baseline immunity, demographics, and health practices.

In sum, well-controlled studies corroborate prospective studies of community samples in indicating that psychological stress is associated with increased susceptibility to infectious disease. In addition, there is consistent evidence for increased symptom reporting under stress. More recent evidence also shows that positive emotional styles, sociability, and more diverse social networks are protective, being related to greater resistance to infection and the expression of fewer objective clinical symptoms.

MECHANISMS THAT MAY LINK STRESS TO DISEASE

A number of potential pathways exist through which stress may contribute to infectious pathology, including behavioral and immune mechanisms. In the first case, psychosocial factors could directly or indirectly influence health through changes in health-related behaviors. For example, poor nutritional status, smoking, drug and alcohol intake, lack of exercise, and poor sleep have all been shown to compromise immune status and health (e.g., Brolinson & Elliott, 2007; Diaz et al., 2002; Gleeson, 2007; Irwin et al., 1996; Kiecolt-Glaser & Glaser, 1988; McAllister-Sistilli et al., 1998; Romeo et al., 2007), with smoking (Cohen, Tyrrell, & Smith, 1993; Cohen et al., 1997), lack of regular exercise (Cohen et al., 1997), poorer diet and poorer sleep efficiency (Cohen et al., 2003b; Cohen, Doyle, Alper, Janicki-Deverts, & Turner, 2009) being associated with increased susceptibility to infectious disease. However, as noted earlier, these behavioral factors do not account for much of the stress-related variability among individuals in URI risk. Thus, other mechanisms must also be operating.

The influence of stress on the immune system is considered the primary biological pathway through which stress can influence infectious pathology. Numerous neurochemicals released during stress are associated with modulation of immune function, including catecholamines (epinephrine and norepinephrine) and corticosteroids (Rabin, 1999). In addition, direct anatomical links exist between the central nervous and immune systems, as evidenced by sympathetic and parasympathetic innervation of lymphoid organs (Felten & Olschowka, 1987; Livnat, Felten, Carlson, Bellinger, & Felten, 1985). Moreover, immune cells, which migrate between lymphoid organs and the peripheral blood stream, have receptors for a variety of hormones and neurotransmitters that are released during stress, including catecholamines, corticosteroids, and various neuropeptides (Stevens-Felten & Bellinger, 1997). Activation of these receptors has immunomodulatory effects, altering leukocyte function and providing a biological pathway for the influences of stress on susceptibility to infectious disease. Pathways connecting the central nervous and immune systems are bidirectional, with peripheral immune activation signaling the brain to effect behavioral, affective, and cognitive changes that typically accompany infectious disease (Maier & Watkins, 1998). Indeed, it is now understood that alterations in cytokine secretion that result from innate immune responses to infection mediate many of these effects (Blalock & Smith, 2007; Maier & Watkins, 1998), penetrating the blood–brain barrier directly through active transport mechanisms (Banks & Kastin, 1991) or indirectly through activation of the afferent vagus nerve (Tracey, 2002) to stimulate the production of central proinflammatory cytokines that modulate brain function. Thus, empirical evidence supports a communication network linking the nervous, endocrine, and immune systems. It is likely that psychological stress modulates immune function through direct activation of this network, by means of neural pathways that innervate lymphoid tissue and the activation of neuroendocrine systems that result in the release of hormones (e.g., cortisol) that bind to receptors on immune cells.

Conversely, activation of the immune system in response to infection results in the secretion of cytokines that affect the central nervous system, resulting in symptoms of sickness, central activation of the hypothalamic-pituitary-adrenal axis, and peripheral release of corticosteroids, which, function to shut off the immune response (Blalock & Smith, 2007). Thus, these pathways create a systemic feedback loop that fine-tunes the magnitude of the immune response.

A few studies have begun to examine whether the immune system mediates the association of chronic stressors with susceptibility to URI. However, this literature is in its infancy. Cohen and colleagues (1997) reported that higher urinary levels of epinephrine, but not norepinephrine or cortisol, measured prior to viral challenge predicted risk for developing a clinical cold; however, this effect was independent of the positive association of chronic negative life events with URI risk. In another study by the same group (Cohen et al., 2002), negative life events and physiologic responses to an acute stressor were assessed among 115 adults who were then followed for 12 weeks for the development of a URI. The results showed that individuals who produced high levels of cortisol to the acute stressor (cortisol reactors) and had high levels of negative life events were at greater risk for URI than were low reactors or those with low levels of negative life events. Immune responses to acute stress also interacted with weekly perceived stress levels to predict self-reported colds. Here, low immune reactors were more likely to report cold symptoms during weeks of high perceived stress when compared to low-stress weeks, whereas high immune reactors did not exhibit differences in colds as a function of weekly stress level (Cohen et al., 2002). Thus, initial evidence suggests that physiologic responses to acute stress may contribute to susceptibility to infectious disease in the face of life event stress; however, further research is necessary to fully understand the nature of these associations.

Other studies suggest that the magnitude of the local inflammatory response to infection may mediate positive associations of stress with symptom severity. For example, Cohen, Doyle, and Skoner (1999) showed that nasal levels of the proinflammatory cytokine interleukin (IL)-6 contributed to the relationship between perceived stress and greater symptoms of URI among 55 adults experimentally infected with influenza A virus. Similarly, nasal levels of IL-6 have been shown to partially account for the inverse association of objective and subjective symptoms of illness with positive emotional style following exposure to a rhinovirus (Doyle, Gentile, & Cohen, 2006). Together, these results are consistent with the hypothesis that IL-6 acts as a biological mediator linking psychological stress to the expression of infectious illness.

Other studies have failed to provide support for neuroendocrine or immune mediators of the association between psychosocial factors and susceptibility to infectious disease (Cohen et al., 1998). In this regard, it should be noted that the immune response to viral pathogens involves a complex cascade of events. Researchers measuring immune function in humans are limited to a few basic markers that provide a poor overall estimate of the body's ability to resist disease. Hence, it remains likely that multiple immune components operate as pathways in the link between stress and susceptibility to disease. The remainder of this chapter focuses on evidence that stress is accompanied by changes in immune function, which may in turn render individuals more susceptible to infectious disease. First, however, a brief overview of measures of immune function is offered.

MEASUREMENTS OF IMMUNOCOMPETENCE

The immune system is a highly complex, interactive network, and there is no single, adequate measure of its status (Cunnick, Lysle, Armfield, & Rabin, 1988). Human studies are limited to quantitative and functional assessments of immune parameters sampled from peripheral blood, nasal lavage, and saliva. These tests include assessment of the numbers and functional abilities of various subgroups of immune cells. In enumerative assays, the various populations of leukocytes are identified and counted by staining the unique surface molecules of each cell type with fluorescent reagents. Using this technique, the percentages or absolute numbers of circulating T-lymphocytes (and their subsets), B lymphocytes, macrophages, and NK cells can be determined. It should be noted that the normal range for circulating numbers of these cell subtypes is quite large, so that small changes in circulating levels are unlikely to have any clinical significance in healthy individuals.

In addition to quantitative measures are a number of functional assessments that provide an in vitro measure of the ability of immune cells to perform specific activities. For example, lymphocyte proliferation assays are commonly used in human research. In this assay, leukocytes are incubated with experimental antigens called mitogens that nonspecifically stimulate T or B lymphocytes to divide. The rate of resultant proliferation is taken as a measure of immunocompetence, with greater cell division reflecting a more effective immune response. Commonly used mitogens include phytohemagglutinin (PHA) and concanavalin A (Con A), which stimulate the proliferation of T lymphocytes, and pokeweed mitogen (PWM), which activates T and B lymphocytes. NK cell cytotoxicity is another frequently assessed measure of immune function. NK cells are a subset of lymphoid cells with the ability to spontaneously kill some human tumor and virally infected cells. NK cell cytotoxicity is a measure of the ability of NK cells to destroy tumor cells in vitro. Enhanced NK cell activity may also be measured by incubating NK cells with such stimulatory cytokines as IL-2 or interferon-gamma. The ability of these cytokines to increase NK cell activity is then compared to cytotoxicity levels found in unstimulated samples. Finally, in vitro assays are also used to measure cytokine concentrations in peripheral circulation, a measure of current immune activation, or the production of cytokines by lymphocytes and monocytes following stimulation with endotoxin (e.g., lipopolysaccharide) or mitogens, a measure of immune competence.

In contrast to these laboratory measures, other indices of immunocompetence are performed in vivo, assessing immune function in the living organism. One such measure is antibody production in response to inoculation with an antigen. Here, individuals ingest or are inoculated with an antigen, for example, influenza vaccine or rabbit albumin, and the amount of antibody produced in response to that specific antigen is quantified in serum. Certain antibody responses (e.g., salivary immunoglobulin A) can also be measured in saliva. In general, greater antibody response is thought to reflect better immunocompetence; however, elevated antibody levels to latent herpes virus may reflect a reactivation of virus resulting from the weakened ability of the immune system to keep such viruses in check. Therefore, high antibody levels to herpes viruses (e.g., Epstein-Barr virus, or EBV) are often interpreted as indicating poorer immunocompetence (Kiecolt-Glaser & Glaser, 1987).

CHRONIC STRESSORS AND IMMUNITY

It is now widely accepted that chronic naturalistic stress (as measured by both self-report and objective life events) is reliably associated with modulation of functional aspects of the immune system. Indeed, a comprehensive meta-analysis of more than 300 empirical articles examining associations of stress with the immune system revealed 23 studies that examined the impact of chronic stress (Segerstrom & Miller, 2004). Although there were no consistent associations between chronic stress and enumerative measures of immunity, stress was inversely related to functional measures of the immune system, including NK cell activity, lymphocyte proliferation to PHA and Con A, IL-2 cytokine production, and antibody response to influenza vaccination. Many studies also show that chronic stress is associated with increased antibody levels to latent herpes viruses, suggesting decreases in the competence of the immune system to control latent virus activity (for a review, see Herbert & Cohen, 1993a; Pierson, Mehta, & Stowe, 2007). Stress has also been associated with decreases in total serum immunoglobulin (Ig)-M (Herbert & Cohen, 1993a) and in the concentration of total salivary IgA (Evans, Bristow, Hucklebridge, Clow, & Walters, 1993). Finally, more recent evidence shows a positive association of chronic stress with circulating levels of markers of inflammation, such as C-reactive protein (CRP) and IL-6 (Kiecolt-Glaser et al., 2003; Miller, Rohleder, & Cole, 2008; von Kanel et al., 2006).

To date, the majority of studies in this literature have examined the influence of naturally occurring stressors on immune function. Numerous life event stressors and environmental demands have been associated with a down-regulation of immune function, including job stress (Arnetz et al., 1987), long-term unemployment (Arnetz et al., 1987; Dorian et al., 1985), loss of an intimate relationship because of death (Kemeny et al., 1995; Schleifer, Keller, Camerino, Thornton, & Stein, 1983) or separation and divorce (Kennedy, Kiecolt-Glaser & Glaser, 1988), caring for a relative with dementia (Kiecolt-Glaser, Glaser, et al., 1987), marital discord (Kiecolt-Glaser et al., 1997), forced displacement from home by war (Sabioncello et al., 2000), space flight (Pierson et al., 2007), natural disasters such as earthquakes (Soloman, Segerstrom, Grohr, Kemeny, & Fahey, 1997) and hurricanes (Ironson et al., 1997), missile attacks in the 1991 Persian Gulf War (Weiss et al., 1996), and residing near a damaged nuclear power plant (McKinnon, Weisse, Reynolds, Bowles, & Baum, 1989). Of interest, there is also evidence that alterations in immunity may persist (i.e., fail to habituate) for months or years with prolonged stressor exposure (e.g., Baum, 1990; Glaser, Kiecolt-Glaser, Malarkey, & Sheridan, 1998; Kiecolt-Glaser, Glaser, et al., 1987).

NATURALISTIC STRESSORS

Considerable research indicates that chronic interpersonal difficulties are particularly provocative stressors, being associated reliably with the down-regulation of immune function. For example, studies show that loss of a close relationship from death or divorce is associated with a reduction in lymphocyte proliferation responses and NK cell activity when compared with prebereavement levels (Schleifer et al., 1983) or nonbereaved controls (Bartrop, Lazarus, Luckhurst, Kiloh, & Penny, 1977; Gerra et al., 2003; Goodkin et al., 1996; Kemeny et al., 1995). In these studies, immunologic alterations persisted from 2 to 14 months after the loss, with evidence showing that the degree of immune changes associated with bereavement may be related to the severity of concomitant depressed mood (Irwin, Daniels, Smith, Bloom, & Weiner, 1987; Linn, Linn, & Jenson, 1984).

Separation, divorce, and marital conflict have similarly been associated with immune alterations. For example, Kiecolt-Glaser, Fisher, et al (1987) found decreased proliferative responses to PHA, higher antibodies to EBV, and lower percentages of circulating NK and T-helper cells among 16 recently separated or divorced women than among a matched group of married women. Higher antibody levels to two latent herpes viruses—EBV and herpes simplex Type 1—were also found among separated or divorced men when compared to matched, married controls (Kiecolt-Glaser et al., 1988). In a study of newlyweds, couples who expressed greater hostility during a discussion of marital problems showed the most pronounced down-regulation of immune function, as measured by lower NK cell activity and proliferative responses to PHA and Con A over a 24-hour period and by higher antibody titers to EBV (Kiecolt-Glaser et al., 1993). Similar findings were reported in a study of 31 older couples who had been married an average of 42 years. Here, men and women who showed greater suppression of lymphocyte proliferative response and higher antibodies to EBV displayed more negative behavior during conflict and described their usual marital disagreements as more negative than did individuals who showed more protective immune responses (Kiecolt-Glaser et al., 1997).

Other studies have examined the chronic stress of caring for a sick child or a spouse with Alzheimer's disease. Here, it has been demonstrated that caregivers suffer higher levels of mortality, depression, more frequent health complaints, and decreased life satisfaction as a result of the stressfulness of the caregiving experience (Bodnar & Kiecolt-Glaser, 1994; Light & Lebowitz, 1989; Schultz & Beach, 1999). Consistent evidence also shows that caregiving is associated with immune dysregulation. When compared to well-matched controls, caregivers show poorer antibody responses to vaccinations (Glaser, Sheridan, Malarkey, MacCallum, & Kiecolt-Glaser, 2000; Vedhara et al., 1999), lower percentages of circulating lymphocytes and T-helper cells (Kiecolt-Glaser, Glaser, et al., 1987), poorer NK cell response to stimulatory cytokines (IL-2 and interferon-gamma; Esterling, Kiecolt-Glaser, & Glaser, 1996), higher antibody titers to EBV (Esterling, Kiecolt-Glaser, Bodnar, & Glaser, 1994), and greater increases in IL-6 over a six-year period (Kiecolt-Glaser et al., 2003). It is of interest that caregivers also show slower healing of a 3.5-mm punch biopsy wound (Kiecolt-Glaser, Marucha, Malarkey, Mercado, & Glaser, 1995), making it possible that decreases in immune function observed among caregivers lead to an impairment of wound healing. In summary, there is a large body of evidence demonstrating that such chronic naturalistic stressors as loss through death or divorce, marital conflict, or caring for a sick relative modulate immune function, with immune changes occurring in a direction that is consistent with increased susceptibility to immune-related disease.

EXAMINATION STRESS

Numerous studies in the PNI literature have employed a quasi-experimental design, examining immune changes from before to after a naturally occurring event. Probably best known in this literature is the series of studies by Kiecolt-Glaser, Glaser, and colleagues (e.g., Glaser et al., 1999; Kiecolt-Glaser et al., 1986; Kiecolt-Glaser et al., 1984) examining immune responses of students to examination stress. In their meta-analytic review of the literature, Segerstrom and Miller (2004) identified 63 studies examining the impact of brief naturalistic stress (95% examination stress) on immune parameters. Results of the meta-analysis provided no evidence that examination stress affected the number of cells in peripheral circulation. However, compared to measures taken at less stressful times (e.g., summer vacation), studies consistently show modulation of immune function during examinations. These stress effects include (a) a decrease in production of the cytokine interferon-gamma, which stimulates natural and cellular immune functions; (b) an increase in the production of IL-6, which stimulates inflammation, and IL-10, which inhibits T-helper 1 cytokine production; (c) a decrease in lymphocyte proliferation in response to mitogen stimulation; (d) a decrease in NK cell cytotoxicity; and (e) an increase in antibody production to latent virus, particularly EBV (Segerstrom & Miller, 2004). Taken together, these changes suggest that acute naturalistic stress is associated with a suppression of cellular immunity and an enhancement of humoral immunity, including inflammation. These immune changes may contribute to the slower healing of wounds that is observed at examination time. For example, in dental students, punch biopsy wounds placed three days before examinations healed an average of 40% slower than did wounds made in the same students during the summer vacation (Marucha, Kiecolt-Glaser, & Favagehl, 1998).

VACCINATION RESPONSES

Other investigators have explored the impact of stress on ability to produce antibodies (develop immunity) to novel antigens. This in vivo immune measure is directly related to host resistance and may provide a more proximate mechanism of stress–infectious disease associations than in vitro markers of immune competence, which provide limited information about the status of the highly integrated and complex immune system. Although not all findings are consistent, reviews of the literature examining the impact of stress on antibody response to immunization generally support an association of chronic psychological stress with suppression of secondary antibody response (Burns, Carroll, Ring, & Drayson, 2003; Cohen et al., 2001; Wetherell & Vedhara, 2007). These conclusions are consistent with a large animal literature indicating that chronic stress is associated with reduced ability to mount an antibody response on exposure to novel antigens (Moynihan, Cohen, & Ader, 1994).

The most consistent findings in the human literature come from studies that measure severe enduring stress (e.g., caring for a spouse with Alzheimer's disease) or a traitlike stress characteristic, such as trait negative affect. These enduring measures of stress have been associated with poorer antibody responses to a number of vaccinations, including influenza (e.g., Kiecolt-Glaser, Glaser, Gravenstein, Malarkey, & Sheridan, 1996; Phillips, Carroll, Burns, & Drayson, 2005; Vedhara et al., 1999), rubella (Morag, Morag, Reichenbaum, Lerer, & Yirmiya, 1999); pneumococcus polysaccharide (Glaser et al., 2000), and hepatitis B (Burns, Ring, Drayson, & Carroll, 2002; Marsland, Cohen, Rabin, & Manuck, 2001), with older adults being at particular risk for stress-related reductions in antibody response (Glaser et al., 1998). Higher levels of perceived stress around the time of vaccination have also been associated with poorer antibody responses to meningitis C (Burns et al., 2003) and influenza (Miller et al., 2004; Moynihan et al., 2004) vaccines. For example, Miller and colleagues (2004) recorded perceived stress four times a day for the 10 days following administration of the influenza vaccine among 83 healthy, young adults. Results showed that higher mean levels of stress across this 10-day period predicted lower antibody response to one of three influenza viral strains at one- and four-month follow-up. Taken together, these results suggest that an individual's psychological "state" following the antigen challenge and antibody formation may negatively influence their levels of antibody response.

A similar pattern of findings is observed when individuals are exposed to nonpathogenic antigens, to which the individual has not had prior exposure. For example, Snyder, Roghmann, and Sigal (1993) demonstrated that three weeks after inoculation with an innocuous novel antigen (keyhole limpet hemocyanin, or KLH), individuals reporting more psychological distress and "bad" life events mounted a lower lymphocyte proliferation response to KLH than did individuals who reported "good" life events and social support. Similarly, Stone, Neale, Cox, and Napoli (1994) had volunteers ingest a capsule containing an innocuous novel antigen daily for 12 weeks. During this period, volunteers also completed daily dairies, recording positive and negative daily events, and gave saliva samples to assess secretory immunoglobulin A (sIgA), an antibody to the novel antigen. Here, more undesirable daily events were associated with lower, and more desirable with higher, antibody to the novel antigen. Thus, immune dysregulation associated with psychological stress can down-regulate both virus-specific antibody responses and T-cell-proliferative responses to specific antigens.

The impact of chronic stress on vaccination response appears to influence not only the magnitude of peak antibody levels but also their maintenance over time. In this regard, several studies suggest that chronic stress has a detrimental impact on the maintenance of antibody response (Burns et al., 2003; Glaser et al., 2000). For example, among older adults administered the pneumococcal pneumonia vaccine, dementia caregivers and matched controls mounted similar antibody responses at two weeks, one month, and three months postvaccination, but caregivers had significantly lower titers at six-month follow-up (Glaser et al., 2000). These results suggest that stress may impact the rate of deterioration of protection following vaccination.

It remains to be determined at what point during the process of antibody production and maintenance stress impacts antibody levels. As noted, studies that employ stable (enduring) measures of chronic stress that likely reflect elevated distress over the entire process show an inverse association of stress with magnitude of immune response. However, findings from studies employing more acute measures of stress—for example, perceived stress, recent life events, or level of daily hassles that are annoying or unpleasant—are less consistent. If it is assumed that physiological or behavioral responses to stress are the mechanisms of stress-related changes in immune function, then the timing of the event is a critical factor in predicting immune response. Consistent with such specula-tion, Snyder et al. (1993) found that daily minor stressors were correlated more strongly (negatively) with antibody response to immunization with KLH than were major negative life events. Similarly, Miller et al. (2004) showed that daily stress across the 10 days following influenza vaccine predicted lower antibody levels at one- and four-month follow-up. However, other studies find no significant associations of psychological distress and daily hassles around the time of exposure to a novel anti-gen with magnitude of antibody response (Glaser et al., 1992; Petrie, Booth, Pennebaker, Davison, & Thomas, 1995). Furthermore, findings from two recent experimental studies show that exposure to acute laboratory stress (mental arithmetic or physical exercise) immediately prior to influenza and meningococcal A vaccination resulted in higher peak antibody responses when compared with the responses of individuals randomly assigned to a no-stress control condition (Edwards et al., 2008, 2006). Thus, it is possible that acute and chronic stress have differential and time-dependent effects on vaccination response. This is consistent with evidence that acute stress is associated with activa-tion of innate inflammatory processes that likely potentiate the initial antibody response, whereas chronic stress is associated with the down-regulation of cellular immune processes involved in antibody production and maintenance (Segerstrom & Miller, 2004).

INDIVIDUAL DIFFERENCES IN IMMUNE RESPONSES TO NATURALISTIC STRESS

Not all individuals demonstrate immune changes following stressful life events. Indeed, there is marked variability among individuals in the magnitude of their immune responses to stress. In this regard, it is suggested that negative events have an impact on immune function only when they lead to negative affect or psychological distress. It is proposed that such distress is elicited when persons perceive that demands imposed by life events exceed their ability to cope (Lazarus & Folkman, 1984). In support of this model, meta-analytic reviews of the literature conclude that depressed mood states in clinical and nonclinical samples modulate various immune components, as evi-denced by a down-regulation of NK cell activity, lowered proliferative response of lymphocytes to the mitogens PHA, Con A, and PWM, and decreases in the total numbers of circulating lympho-cytes, NK, B, and T-cells (Herbert & Cohen, 1993b; Zorilla et al., 2001). These depression-related effects suggest a down-regulation of components of natural and cellular immune function. More recent evidence also supports depression-related activation of innate inflammatory pathways, as marked by higher levels of proinflammatory cytokines (IL-6, IL-1, tumor necrosis factor [TNF]-α) and such acute-phase proteins as CRP (Irwin & Miller, 2007).

A number of studies provide further evidence that emotional reactions and personality character-istics associated with affect regulation contribute to interindividual variability in the magnitude of immune responses to life circumstances (e.g., Locke et al., 1984; Segerstrom, 2001). For example, decreased positive mood partially mediated associations of the stress of relocating with reduced NK cell cytotoxicity among healthy older adults (Lutgendorf, Vitaliano, Tripp-Reimer, Hervey, & Lubaroff, 1999). In regard to personality characteristics, dispositional optimism—that is, general-ized positive expectations for the future—often buffers the immune system from the effects of life event stress (Segerstrom, 2005). However, at times when stressors are more difficult, persistent, and uncontrollable, optimists can show greater down-regulation of cellular immune function than can pessimists (Segerstom, 2005). In support of popular belief, recent findings suggest that indi-viduals who characterize themselves by such moods as happy, pleased, relaxed, and lively show higher NK cell number and activity (Valdimarsdottir & Bovbjerg, 1997), better control of latent EBV (Lutgendorf et al., 2001), increased T-helper Type 1 (TH1) cytokine (IL-2 and interferon-gamma) responses to in vitro stimulation with live influenza virus (Costanzo et al., 2004), higher antibody responses to hepatitis B vaccination, as measured following the first two doses of the vaccine (Marsland, Cohen, Rabin, & Manuck, 2006), and decreased incidence of experimentally induced URIs (Cohen et al., 2003b, 2006) than do their less positive counterparts. Indeed, recent evidence suggests that previously reported associations of negative affective styles with decreased antibody response to vaccination and increased susceptibility to viral infection may reflect diminished positive affect, rather than the presence of negative mood traits (Cohen et al., 2006; Marsland et al., 2006). Taken together, these findings suggest that individual differences in affective style may contribute to variability in immune response, either as a main effect or by buffering the negative impact of adverse life events.

Interindividual variability in the magnitude of immune responses to stress may also be attributable to social buffers (i.e., interpersonal resources). In this regard, literature reviews document abundant evidence that higher levels of social support and more positive social relationships improve immunoregulation and are associated with decreased morbidity and mortality (House, Landis, & Umberson, 1988; Uchino, Cacioppo, & Kiecolt-Glaser, 1996). For example, perceived inadequacy of interpersonal relationships, as measured by self-report, is related to distress and diminished immune function among medical students taking examinations (e.g., Kiecolt-Glaser & Glaser, 1991) and caregivers of relatives with dementia (Kiecolt-Glaser, Glaser, et al., 1987). There is also evidence that supportive interpersonal relationships buffer the adverse impact of negative life events on immune function. For example, Baron, Cutrona, Hicklin, Russell, and Lubaroff (1990) found that social support was associated with higher NK cell activity and greater proliferative responses to PHA (but not Con A) among 23 women whose husbands were being treated for urological cancer. Similarly, Glaser et al. (1992) showed that when compared with individuals reporting low levels of social support, medical students with more support mounted greater antibody responses to hepatitis B vaccination. In sum, although few studies examine individual differences in immune response to naturalistic stressors, it is clear that dispositional factors and interpersonal resources moderate emotional responses to life circumstances, with distress (as measured by symptoms of anxiety or depression) or reductions in positive moods being associated with immune changes that are consistent with increased risk for infectious disease.

INTERVENTION STUDIES

A number of studies have investigated whether psychological interventions designed to lower emotional distress also reduce or prevent stress-related changes in immunity. These studies use a diverse array of psychological interventions. Findings are inconsistent, with some studies showing intervention-related improvements in immune function and others not. Indeed, a meta-analytic review of this literature concluded that there is only modest evidence that interventions can reliably alter immune parameters (Miller & Cohen, 2001). Miller and Cohen (2001) attributed the many null findings to theoretical and methodological limitations of existing studies, including a general failure to (a) focus on individuals with high levels of stress, (b) use interventions demonstrated to be effective at reducing stress, or (c) measure immune parameters that are typically dysregulated by stress. When limited to studies that recruited populations experiencing heightened levels of stress, results are more consistent and document intervention-related improvements in immune function (e.g., Andersen et al., 2004; Antoni et al., 1991; Antoni et al., 2009; Carlson, Speca, Faris, & Patel, 2007; Fawzy et al., 1990; Hewson-Bower & Drummond, 2001; Witek-Janusek et al., 2008). To date, the majority of effective interventions have employed stress-management techniques, including coping skills training, cognitive restructuring, relaxation training, mindfulness-based stress reduction (MBSR), and social support.

One of the most widely cited early studies in this literature evaluated the effects of a six-session group intervention for patients with malignant melanoma (Fawzy et al., 1990). When compared with patients who received routine medical care, the intervention, comprised of psychological support and training in relaxation, stress management, problem-solving and coping skills, effectively enhanced coping and reduced psychological distress and was associated with an increase in NK cell percentage and activity. Another study suggests the down-regulation of immune components known to accompany notification of positive-HIV-antibody status can be attenuated by a 10-week group cognitive-behavioral stress-management (CBSM) intervention (Antoni et al., 1991). More recent attention has focused on the psychological and immune benefit of stress-management training for women with breast cancer. For example, both CBSM and MBSR interventions have been shown to facilitate psychological adaptation and improve cellular immune function in this population (Andersen et al., 2004; Antoni et al., 2009; Carlson et al., 2007; McGregor et al., 2004; Witek-Janusek et al., 2008), with positive associations of intervention-related improvements in psychological and immune function (McGregor et al., 2004). In sum, recent findings from studies that focus on populations with chronic diseases or heightened levels of stress suggest that interventions designed to manage or reduce stress are associated with improved immune function or an amelioration of stress-related changes in immunity. Again, the health significance of these positive, but relatively small, immunologic changes remains unclear.

SUMMARY OF NATURALISTIC STRESS

It is well established that naturalistic stress modulates functional aspects of immunity. The most consistent alterations suggest that stress suppresses immune function over protracted periods during particularly intense or prolonged stressors. Despite these central tendencies, not all individuals demonstrate immune changes following stressful life events. Indeed, there is marked variability among individuals in the magnitude of immune responses to naturalistic stress. This interindividual variability has been attributed to a number of psychosocial buffers, including trait characteristics and interpersonal resources that are proposed to modulate the negative impact of adverse life events. To date, it remains unclear how stress may contribute to changes in the immune system. Potential pathways include the impact of stress on health practices (e.g., diet, exercise, or sleep) and/or stress-induced activation of physiological pathways (e.g., neuroendocrine parameters). Few naturalistic investigations have examined relations between health practices, neuroendocrine factors, and immune measures during stress. However, growing evidence suggests that sleep disturbances may play an important role in the modulation of immune function during naturalistic stress. For example, Ironson et al. (1997) showed that the onset of sleep problems following Hurricane Andrew partially mediated the relationship between posttraumatic stress symptoms and lowered NK cell activity in a community sample affected by this disaster. Furthermore, psychological stress is reliably linked to disrupted sleep (e.g., Mezick et al., 2009), and poorer sleep efficiency and shorter sleep duration predict a greater likelihood of developing a cold following experimental exposure to a rhinovirus (Cohen et al., 2009).

LABORATORY STRESSORS AND IMMUNITY

In order to examine whether psychological stress, independent of concomitant changes in health behaviors, alters immune components, investigators have examined the effects of acute laboratory stress on immune functioning in healthy individuals. These controlled, experimental studies also provide a means to explore neuroendocrine pathways associated with stress and immunity. Findings from these studies reveal significant immunologic alterations following exposure to a range of standardized, short-term laboratory stressors that are generally perceived by subjects as aversive, demanding, or interpersonally challenging. Stressors employed in these studies include mental arithmetic, unsolvable puzzles, evaluative speech tasks, electric shocks and/or loud noise, marital discussions involving conflict, and disturbing films depicting combat surgery (for a review, see Segerstrom & Miller, 2004). In contrast to some of the less common naturalistic stressors (e.g., bereavement or caring for a relative with Alzheimer's disease), some of these challenges may more accurately characterize everyday hassles and thus account for more observed interindividual variability in immune response to stress and susceptibility to disease.

The effects of short-term laboratory challenge on immune function are not consistent with longer term changes seen following chronic forms of naturalistic stress. In their meta-analytic review, Segerstrom and Miller (2004) identified 85 studies that examined the impact of acute psychological stressors on immune parameters. Consistent findings support reliable changes in immune measures from pre- to post-task. In contrast to the chronic-stress literature, these changes include a transient increase in the number of NK cells, and cytotoxic T and large granular lymphocytes (neutrophils) in peripheral circulation, and in secretory IgA in saliva (Segerstrom & Miller, 2004). As a result of increased peripheral numbers of cytotoxic T-cells, acute stressors are also associated with a reliable decline in the ratio of helper-T to cytotoxic-T lymphocytes.

With regard to functional measures, acute laboratory stress has been associated with an increase in NK cell cytotoxicity, largely resulting from the increase in circulating numbers of NK cells (Segerstrom & Miller, 2004). Recent evidence also shows that circulating levels of the proinflammatory cytokines IL-6 and IL-1beta are increased following acute challenge (Steptoe, Hamer, & Chida, 2007), with an increase in the rate of stimulated production of both IL-6 and interferon-gamma, cytokines that stimulate activation of macrophages and NK cells, respectively (Segerstrom & Miller, 2004). Taken together, the aforementioned changes suggest an up-regulation of natural immune function in response to acute stress. It has been suggested that this response may be adaptive and a component of the fight-or-flight response, preparing the organism for possible infection or injury (Dhabhar & McEwan, 1997, 2001; Segerstrom & Miller, 2004). In contrast, evidence suggests a down-regulation of acquired immune function under conditions of acute challenge. Here, findings are more consistent with the effects of chronic naturalistic stress, with acute laboratory stress resulting in a reduction in lymphocyte proliferation on exposure to PHA, Con A, and PWM. In this regard, it is suggested that it is not adaptive to invest energy in immune responses that take longer to develop (Dhabhar & McEwan, 1997, 2001; Segerstrom & Miller, 2004).

How the transient immune responses seen following discrete acute stress relate to those responses associated with chronic naturalistic stress is unknown. However, it is hypothesized that alternative physiological mechanisms may account for these differential effects (Herbert & Cohen, 1993a; Segerstrom & Miller, 2004). In the case of acute psychological stress, research findings suggest that immune responses are largely mediated by the autonomic nervous system (ANS). For example, it has been demonstrated that immune outcomes assessed after a laboratory stressor covary with the magnitude of sympathetic activation elicited under the same stimulus conditions (e.g., Manuck, Cohen, Rabin, Muldoon, & Bachen, 1991; Zakowski, McAllister, Deal, & Baum, 1992). Pharmacological studies also indicate that the administration of physiological doses of sympathetic stimulants (e.g., exogenous catecholamines or isoproterenol) invokes functional modulations of cellular immunity that are similar to those seen during acute challenge (e.g., Crary et al., 1983). More direct evidence for sympathetic mediation derives from the observation that stress-related immune responses are blocked by adrenergic receptor inhibition (Bachen et al., 1995; Benschop et al., 1994). Indeed, it has been demonstrated that administration of an adrenergic inhibitor prevents stress-induced alterations in a variety of immune parameters, including proliferative responses to PHA and Con A, NK cell number and activity, and the ratio of T-helper to T-cytotoxic cells (Bachen et al., 1995; Benschop et al., 1994).

More recent evidence has examined the role of the parasympathetic branch of the ANS, which generally acts in opposition to the sympathetic branch of the system. Here, findings suggest that activation of efferent parasympathetic (vagal) neurons leads to the suppression of proinflammatory cytokine release through activation of nicotinic acetylcholine receptors expressed on macrophages and other immune cells involved in the inflammatory response, thus decreasing local and systemic inflammation (Czura & Tracey, 2005). Indeed, low levels of cardiac vagal activity, as measured by noninvasive indicators of heart rate variability, are associated with decreased stimulated production of the proinflammatory cytokines IL-6 and TNF-alpha (Marsland et al., 2007). This raises the possibility that increases in circulating levels of IL-6 observed one to two hours following acute psychological stress result from the decreases in parasympathetic activation that accompany acute challenge.

The exact mechanism of autonomic-immune mediation remains unclear. Evidence suggests that activation of the sympathetic nervous system may influence the immune system by both active and passive processes (Marsland et al., 1997). Under conditions of acute stress, an increase in arterial blood pressure driven by activation of the sympathetic nervous system causes fluid to filter out of circulation into extravascular spaces, leading to a passive increase in the concentration of all nondiffusible constituents of blood, including blood cells and cytokines (Jern, Wadenvik, Mark, Hallgren, & Jern, 1989). It has been shown that stress-induced increases in the concentration of circulating T-cytotoxic and NK cells are partly, but not wholly, attributable to this hemoconcentration effect (Marsland et al., 1997). The observation that this passive effect only partly accounts for acute increases in cytotoxic-T and NK cell numbers suggests that more active mechanisms are also operating (Bachen, Marsland, Manuck, & Cohen, 1998). In this regard, it has been demonstrated that sympathetically mediated alterations in adhesion molecules on cell surfaces enable cytotox-ic-T and NK cells to be mobilized into circulation from the peripheral margins of blood vessels (Mills & Dimsdale, 1996). Evidence also shows that acute stress results in rapid activation of the transcription factor nuclear factor kB (NF-kB) in peripheral blood mononuclear cells, by means of norepinephrine-dependent pathways (Bierhaus et al., 2003), and that activation of NF-kB results in the expression of genes for the production of proinflammatory cytokines. Parasympathetic activation has the opposite effect, inhibiting NF-kB activation (Pavlov & Tracey, 2005). Evidence also suggests that activation of the hypothalamic-pituitary-adrenocortical (HPA) system may also modulate immune function that accompanies acute challenge (Kunz-Ebrecht, Mohamed-Ali, Feldman, Kirschbaum, & Steptoe, 2003). Indeed, individuals who exhibited high sympathetic responses to acute stress also showed a stress-induced increase in plasma cortisol levels, when compared with low sympathetic responders, who showed no change in cortisol following stress (Cacioppo et al., 1998; Cohen et al., 2000). This finding is noteworthy, given extensive evidence that cortisol is associated with longer term down-regulation of cellular immune function (Cacioppo et al., 1995).

In contrast to the rapid immune responses associated with acute stress, exposure to more chronic stress leads to relatively stable shifts in the baseline levels of immune measures (Herbert & Cohen, 1993a; Segerstrom & Miller, 2004). Here, it is widely accepted that chronic stress can regulate immune function by direct activation of the HPA and sympathetic-adrenal-medullary axes, leading to an increase in the release of glucocorticoids (cortisol in humans). In contrast to activation of the sympathetic nervous system, which stimulates inflammatory pathways (Sondergaard, Ostrowski, Ullum, Pedersen, 2000), the HPA axis generally down-regulates immune function. Glucocorticoid receptors are expressed on a variety of immune cells, including lymphocytes and monocytes; and ligand binding to these receptors has a number of inhibitory effects, including reduced production of proinflammatory cytokines, decreased expression of cell adhesion molecules necessary for the inflammatory response, and decreased mitogen-stimulated lymphocyte proliferation (e.g., Almawi, Beyhum, Rahme, & Rieder, 1996; Cato & Wade, 1996). Based on knowledge that glucocorticoids suppress the inflammatory response, one would predict that stress would be associated with suppression of inflammatory processes. However, evidence supports the opposite, with chronic stress being associated with increased systemic inflammation and greater risk for inflammatory conditions. It has been suggested that this apparent paradox is the result of a reduction in the sensitivity of glucocorticoid receptors on immune cells, likely a result of prolonged exposure to cortisol, rendering the immune system less responsive to signals that turn off the inflammatory cascade (Miller, Cohen, & Ritchey, 2002). Animal studies support this model and show that glucocorticoid resistance is restricted to macrophages and is the result of impaired nuclear translocation of glucocorticoid receptors and a decrease in transcriptional suppression of NF-kB (Quan et al., 2003; Stark, Avitsur, Hunzeker, Padgett, & Sheridan, 2002; Stark et al., 2001).

INDIVIDUAL DIFFERENCES IN IMMUNE RESPONSES TO ACUTE LABORATORY STRESS

Although it is well established that acute and chronic stress are associated with functional and enumerative aspects of immunity, an examination of response variability reveals that individuals differ substantially in the magnitude of their immunologic reactivity to stress (Kiecolt-Glaser, Cacioppo,

Malarkey, & Glaser, 1992; Marsland, Henderson, Chambers, & Baum, 2002), with many individuals exhibiting little or no response. It is suggested that these differences reflect variability among individuals in the magnitude of their autonomic and HPA hormone responsivity to stress, aspects of individual difference that have been demonstrated to be relatively stable over time (Cohen & Hamrick, 2003; Dimsdale, Young, Moore, & Strauss, 1987). Evidence suggests that interindividual variability of behaviorally evoked immune reactivity is also reproducible over time and across stressor tasks and may therefore denote a relatively stable dimension of individual differences (Cohen & Hamrick, 2003; Marsland et al., 2002; Marsland, Manuck, Fazzari, Stewart, & Rabin, 1995). The existence of such dispositional characteristics makes it conceivable that exaggerated immune responsivity to behavioral challenge may be implicated in the pathogenesis of immune-related disease, such as host resistance to infection (Cohen & Manuck, 1995). One possibility is that individuals who show exaggerated immune responses to laboratory stressors exhibit similarly exaggerated reactions to everyday hassles (e.g., work demands and time pressures), rendering them more susceptible to infectious disease.

More recent attention has focused on the possibility that individual differences in physiologic reactivity moderate associations of psychological stress with susceptibility to infectious illness (Cohen et al., 2002). As mentioned previously, Cohen and colleagues found that individuals who showed the largest increases in cortisol following acute stress (cortisol reactors) and had high negative life event scores were more likely to develop verified URIs over the course of a three-month follow-up period. In contrast, low immune responders (T-cytotoxic cell number, NK cell number, and cytotoxicity) were more likely to experience a URI during high-stress weeks than high immune responders. Boyce and colleagues (1993, 1995) also found that cardiovascular and immune responses to acute stress were associated with increased URI risk under conditions of heightened naturalistic stress in a study of young children (ages 3–5 years). However, here, it was the children who showed larger stress-induced immune reactions (increases in B-cell numbers and in lymphocyte proliferation to PWM) who were at greatest URI risk. Interpretation of these effects is unclear because these immune changes are not typically observed following acute stress in adults. Furthermore, the interaction between immune reactivity and stress, as a predictor of infection, was attributable in large part to an unexpectedly lower incidence of disease for high-reactive children not exposed to naturalistic stress (Cohen & Manuck, 1995).

Other studies have examined whether individual differences in sympathetic and immune reactions to acute stress predict antibody responses to vaccination, an in vivo measure of host resistance to infection. Marsland et al. (2001) found that graduate students who mounted lower antibody responses to hepatitis B vaccination, as measured following the first two doses of vaccine, showed greater suppression of lymphocyte proliferation to PHA following laboratory stress than did higher antibody responders. Similarly, Burns et al. (2002) found that individuals who responded to acute stress with larger cardiac sympathetic activation exhibited lower antibody titers to hepatitis B vaccination than did their less reactive counterparts. Cacioppo (1994) also found that sympathetic activation predicted response to an influenza vaccine, with larger cardiac sympathetic activation to acute challenge being associated with poorer vaccine-specific T-cell responses. Taken together, initial evidence suggests that individual differences in the magnitude of stress-induced activation of sympathetic and HPA pathways, as well as suppression of immune function, may have clinical significance, being related to an in vivo immune response relevant for protection against infection and, in the case of cortisol, increased URI risk. Further prospective studies employing measures of individual difference as predictors of susceptibility to disease are warranted.

CONCLUSION

In support of popular belief, there is now substantial evidence for the role of psychological stress in susceptibility to URI disease (e.g., Cohen et al., 1991, 1993; Cohen et al., 1998, Stone et al. 1992). One possible mediator of this relationship is the modulation of immune function, thereby influencing host susceptibility to infectious pathogens. In this regard, it is well established that both major stressful experiences (e.g., bereavement or natural disasters) and more minor stressors (e.g., arguing with a spouse or facing an acute laboratory challenge) are associated with changes in immune function. Although the clinical significance of stress-related changes in many measures of immune function remains to be determined, recent evidence suggests that stress-related increases in the production of proinflammatory cytokines may result in greater susceptibility to URI. In this regard, chronic stress has been associated with a decrease in the sensitivity of immune cells to cortisol, a hormone that down-regulates the production of proinflammatory cytokines and thus terminates the inflammatory response. This decrease in glucocorticoid receptor sensitivity, which likely results from chronically elevated levels of cortisol, may account for the increased levels of proinflammatory cytokines, such as IL-6, that accompany chronic stress. Initial findings suggest that increases in nasal secretory levels of IL-6 mediate associations of perceived stress and lower positive emotional style with subjective and objective symptom severity following viral challenge (Cohen et al., 1999; Doyle et al., 2006). Thus, chronic stress may interfere with the immune system's ability to respond to hormonal signals that turn off the inflammatory response, resulting in increased inflammation and susceptibility to symptoms of infection.

To date, it remains unclear whether associations between psychological factors and vulnerability to infection are attributable to stress-induced changes in immunity. Indeed, the clinical significance of relatively small immunologic alterations has not been established. Many associations of stress with immune function and health may be attributable to changes in health behaviors. Growing evidence shows, however, that the autonomic nervous system mediates some immunologic changes during acute challenge stress. Furthermore, it is likely that naturalistic stress modulates immune function though activation of neuroendocrine systems that result in the release of hormones, such as cortisol, that bind to receptors on immune cells. It has been demonstrated that individuals differ substantially in the magnitude of their immunologic responsivity to stress, with evidence suggesting that these response tendencies may reflect stable attributes of individuals. Recent evidence suggests that individuals who respond to acute laboratory stressors with large increases in cortisol are at greater risk for URI when exposed to stressors in the natural environment (Cohen et al., 2002; Cohen et al., 2009). Hence, it is conceivable that there is a meaningful distribution of differences in physiologic reactivity that may form a basis for differences in susceptibility to infection.

Future research in PNI needs to continue to focus on whether the type, magnitude, or pattern of stress-related immune modulation influences host resistance, for it is likely that substantial fluctuations in immune function can be tolerated without influencing susceptibility to disease. The role of the immune system in susceptibility to infectious disease needs to be addressed with prospective studies, measuring psychosocial parameters and immune mediators relevant for the disease under study, controlling for health behavior, and documenting disease outcomes.

REFERENCES

Almawi, W. Y., Beyhum, H. N., Rahme, A. A., & Rieder, M. J. (1996). Regulation of cytokine and cytokine receptor expression by glucocorticoids. *Journal of Leukocyte Biology*, *60*, 563–572.

Andersen, B. L., Farrar, W. B., Golden-Kreutz, D. M., Glaser, R., Emery, C. F., Crespin, T. R., … Carson, W.E. (2004). Psychological, behavioral, and immune changes after a psychological intervention: A clinical trial. *Journal of Clinical Oncology*, *22*, 3570–3580.

Antoni, M. H., Baggett, L., Ironson, G., LaPerriere, A., August, S., Klimas, N., … Fletcher, M. S. (1991). Cognitive–behavioral stress management intervention buffers distress responses and immunologic changes following notification of HIV-1 seropositivity. *Journal of Consulting and Clinical Psychology*, *59*, 906–915.

Antoni, M. H., Lechner, S., Diaz, A., Vargas, S., Holley, H., Phillips, K., … Blomberg, B. (2009). Cognitive behavioral stress management effects on psychosocial and physiological adaptation in women undergoing treatment for breast cancer. *Brain, Behavior, and Immunity*, *23*, 580–591.

Arnetz, B. B., Wasserman, J., Petrii, B., Brenner, S. O., Levi, L., Eneroth, P., … Patterson, I. L. (1987). Immune function in unemployed women. *Psychosomatic Medicine 49*, 3–12.

Bachen, E. A., Manuck, S. B., Cohen, S., Muldoon, M. F., Raible, R., Herbert, T. B., & Rabin, B. S. (1995). Adrenergic blockade ameliorates cellular immune responses to mental stress in humans. *Psychosomatic Medicine, 57*, 366–372.

Bachen, E. A., Marsland, A. L., Manuck, S. B., & Cohen, S. (1998). Immunomodulation: Psychological stress and immune competence. In T. F. Kresina (Ed.), *Handbook of immune modulating agents* (pp. 145–159). New York, NY: Marcel Dekker.

Banks, W. A., & Kastin, A. J. (1991). Blood to brain transport of interleukin links the immune and central nervous systems. *Life Sciences, 48*, PL117–121.

Baron, R. S., Cutrona, C. E., Hicklin, D., Russell, D. W., & Lubaroff, D. M. (1990). Social support and immune function among spouses of cancer patients. *Journal of Personality and Social Psychology, 59*, 344–352.

Bartrop, R., Lazarus, L., Luckhurst, E., Kiloh, L. G., & Penny, R. (1977). Depressed lymphocyte function after bereavement, *Lancet, i*, 834–836.

Baum, A. (1990). Stress, intrusive imagery, and chronic distress. *Health Psychology, 9*, 653–675.

Benschop, R. J., Nieuwenhuis, E. E. S., Tromp, E. A. M., Godaert, G. L. R., Ballieux, R. E., & van Doornen, L. J. P. (1994). Effects of β–adrenergic blockade on immunologic and cardiovascular changes induced by mental stress. *Circulation, 89*, 762–769.

Bierhaus, A., Wolf, J., Andrassy, M., Rohleder, N., Humpert, P. M., Petrov, D., … Nawroth, P. P. (2003). A mechanism converting psychosocial stress into mononuclear cell activation. *Proceedings of the National Academy of Sciences, 100*, 1920–1925.

Blalock, J. E., & Smith, E. M. (2007). Conceptual development of the immune system as a sixth sense. *Brain, Behavior, and Immunity, 21*, 23–33.

Bodnar, J., & Kiecolt-Glaser, J. K. (1994). Caregiver depression after bereavement: Chronic stress isn't over when it's over. *Psychology and Aging, 9*, 372–380.

Boyce, W. T., Chesney, M., Alkon, A., Tschann, J. M., Adams, S., Chesterman, B., … Wara, D. (1995). Psychobiological reactivity to stress and childhood respiratory illnesses: Results of two prospective studies. *Psychosomatic Medicine, 57*, 411–422.

Boyce, W. T., Chesterman, E. A., Martin, N., Folkman, S., Cohen, F., & Wara, D. (1993). Immunologic changes occurring at kindergarten entry predict respiratory illnesses after the Loma Prieta earthquake. *Journal of Developmental and Behavioral Pediatrics, 14*, 296–303.

Brolinson, P. G., & Elliott, D. (2007). Exercise and the immune system. *Clinical Sports Medicine, 26*, 311–319.

Burns, V. E., Carroll, D., Ring, C., & Drayson, M. (2003). Antibody response to vaccination and psychosocial stress in humans: Relationships and mechanisms. *Vaccine, 21*, 2523–2534.

Burns, V. E., Ring, C., Drayson, M., & Carroll, D. (2002). Cortisol and cardiovascular reactions to mental stress and antibody status following hepatitis B vaccination: A preliminary study. *Psychophysiology, 39*, 361–368.

Cacioppo, J. T. (1994). Social neuroscience—Autonomic, neuroendocrine, and immune-responses to stress. *Psychophysiology, 31*, 113–128.

Cacioppo, J. T., Berntson, G. G., Malarkey, W. B., Kiecolt-Glaser, J. K., Sheridan, J. F., Poehlmann, K. M., … Glaser, R. (1998). Autonomic, neuroendocrine, and immune responses to psychological stress: The reactivity hypothesis. *Annals of the New York Academy of Sciences, 840*, 664–673.

Cacioppo, J. T., Malarkey, W. B., Kiecolt-Glaser, J. K., Uchino, B. N., Sgoutas-Emch, S. A., Sheridan, J. F., … Glaser, R. (1995). Cardiac autonomic substrates as a novel approach to explore heterogeneity in neuroendocrine and immune responses to brief psychological stressors. *Psychosomatic Medicine, 57*, 154–164.

Carlson, L. E., Speca, M., Faris, P., & Patel, K. D. (2007). One year pre-post intervention follow-up of psychological, immune, endocrine and blood pressure outcomes of mindfulness-based stress reduction (MBSR) in breast and prostate cancer outpatients. *Brain, Behavior, and Immunity, 21*, 1038–1049.

Cato, A. C., & Wade, E. (1996). Molecular mechanisms of anti-inflammatory action of glucocorticoids. *Bioessays, 18*, 371–378.

Cohen, S., Alper, C. M., Doyle, W. J., Treanor, J. J., & Turner, R. B. (2006). Positive emotional style predicts resistance to illness after experimental exposure to rhinovirus or influenza A virus. *Psychosomatic Medicine, 68*, 809–815.

Cohen, S., Doyle, W. J., Alper, C. M., Janicki–Deverts, D., & Turner, R. B. (2009). Sleep habits and susceptibility to the common cold. *Archives of Internal Medicine, 169*, 62–67.

Cohen, S., Doyle, W. J., & Skoner, D. P. (1999). Psychological stress, cytokine production, and severity of upper respiratory illness. *Psychosomatic Medicine, 61*, 175–180.

Cohen, S., Doyle, W. J., Skoner, D. P., Fireman, P., Gwaltney, J. M., & Newsom, J. T. (1995). State and trait negative affect as predictors of objective and subjective symptoms of respiratory viral infections. *Journal of Personality and Social Psychology, 68*, 159–169.

Cohen, S., Doyle, W. J., Skoner, D. P., Rabin, B. S., & Gwaltney, J. M. (1997). Social ties and susceptibility to the common cold. *Journal of the American Medical Association, 24*, 1940–1944.

Cohen, S., Doyle, W. J., Turner, R. B., Alper, C. M., & Skoner, D. P. (2003a). Sociability and susceptibility to the common cold. *Psychological Science 14*, 389–395.

Cohen, S., Doyle, W. J., Turner, R. B., Alper, C. M., & Skoner, D. P. (2003b). Emotional style and susceptibility to the common cold. *Psychosomatic Medicine, 65*, 652–657.

Cohen, S., Frank, E., Doyle, W. J., Skoner, D. P., Rabin, B. S., & Gwaltney, J. M. (1998). Types of stressors that increase susceptibility to the common cold in healthy adults. *Health Psychology, 17*, 214–223.

Cohen, S., & Hamrick, N. (2003). Stable individual differences in physiological response to stressors: Implications for stress-elicited changes in immune related health. *Brain, Behavior, and Immunity, 17*, 407–414.

Cohen, S., Hamrick, N., Rodriguez, M. S., Feldman, P. J., Rabin, B. S., & Manuck, S. B. (2000). The stability of and intercorrelations among cardiovascular, immune, endocrine, and psychological reactivity. *Annals of Behavioral Medicine, 22*, 1–10.

Cohen, S., Hamrick, N., Rodriguez, M. S., Feldman, P. J., Rabin, B. S., & Manuck, S. B. (2002). Reactivity and vulnerability to stress-associated risk for upper respiratory illness. *Psychosomatic Medicine, 64*, 302–310.

Cohen, S., & Herbert, T. B. (1996). Health psychology: Psychological factors and physical disease from the perspective of human psychoneuroimmunology. *Annual Review of Psychology 47*, 113–142.

Cohen, S., & Manuck, S. B. (1995). Stress, reactivity, and disease. *Psychosomatic Medicine, 57*, 423–426.

Cohen, S., Miller, G. E., & Rabin, B. S. (2001). Psychological stress and antibody response to immunization: A critical review of the human literature. *Psychosomatic Medicine, 63*, 7–18.

Cohen, S., Tyrrell, D. A., Russell, M. A., Jarvis, M. J., & Smith, A. P. (1993). Smoking, alcohol consumption, and susceptibility to the common cold. *American Journal of Public Health, 83*, 1277–1283.

Cohen, S., Tyrrell, D. A., & Smith, A. P. (1991). Psychological stress and susceptibility to the common cold. *New England Journal of Medicine, 325*, 606–612.

Cohen, S., Tyrrell, D. A., & Smith, A. P. (1993). Negative life events, perceived stress, negative affect, and susceptibility to the common cold. *Journal of Personality and Social Psychology, 64*, 131–140.

Cohen, S., & Williamson, G. M. (1991). Stress and infectious disease in humans. *Psychological Bulletin, 109*, 5–24.

Costanzo, E. S., Lutgendorf, S. K., Kohut, M. L., Nisly, N., Roseboom, K., Spooner, S., … McElhaney, J. E. (2004). Mood and cytokine response to influenza virus in older adults. *Journal of Gerontology, 12*, 1328–1333.

Crary, B., Hauser, S. L., Borysenko, M., Kutz, I., Hoban, C., Ault, K. A., … Benson, H. (1983). Epinephrine–induced changes in the distribution of lymphocyte subsets in peripheral blood of humans. *Journal of Immunology, 131*, 1178–1181.

Cunnick, J. E., Lysle, D. T., Armfiled, A., & Rabin, B. S. (1988). Shock-induced modulation of lymphocyte responsiveness and natural killer cell activity: Differential effects of induction. *Brain, Behavior, and Immunity, 2*, 102–113.

Czura, C. J., & Tracey, K. J. (2005). Autonomic neural regulation of immunity. *Internal Medicine, 257*, 156–166.

Dharbar, F. S., & McEwan, B. S. (1997). Acute stress enhances while chronic stress suppresses cell–mediated immunity in vivio: A potential role for leukocyte trafficking. *Brain, Behavior, and Immunity, 11*, 286–306.

Dharbar, F. S., & McEwan, B. S. (2001). Bidirectional effects of stress and glucocorticoid hormones on immune function: Possible explanations for paradoxical observations. In R. Ader, D. L. Felten, & N. Cohen (Eds.), *Psychoneuroimmunology* (3rd ed., pp. 301–338). San Diego, CA: Academic Press.

Diaz, L. E., Montero, A., Gonzalez-Gross, M., Vallejo, A. I., Romeo, J., & Marcos, A. (2002). Influence of alcohol consumption on immunological status A review. *European journal of Clinical Nutrition, 56*, S50–53.

Dimsdale, J. E., Young, D., Moore, R., & Strauss, W. (1987). Do plasma norepinephrine levels reflect behavioral stress? *Psychosomatic Medicine, 49*, 375–382.

Dorian, B., Garfinkel, P., Keystone, E., Gorczyinski, R., Darby, P., & Garner, D. (1985). Occupational stress and immunity [Abstract]. *Psychosomatic Medicine, 47*, 77.

Doyle, W. J., Gentile, D. A., & Cohen, S. (2006). Emotional style, nasal cytokines, and illness expression after experimental rhinovirus exposure. *Brain, Behavior, and Immunity, 20*, 175–181.

Edwards, K. M., Burns, V. E., Adkins, A. E., Carroll, D., Drayson, M., & Ring, C. (2008). Meningococcal A vaccination response is enhanced by acute stress in men. *Psychosomatic Medicine, 70*, 147–151.

Edwards, K. M., Burns, V. E., Reynolds, T., Carroll, D., Drayson, M., & Ring, C. (2006). Acute stress exposure prior to influenza vaccination enhances antibody response in women. *Brain, Behavior, and Immunity, 20*, 159–168.

Esterling, B. A., Kiecolt-Glaser, J. K., Bodnar, J. C., & Glaser, R. (1994). Chronic stress, social support, and persistent alterations in the natural killer cell response to cytokines in older adults. *Health Psychology, 13*, 291–298.

Esterling, B. A., Kiecolt-Glaser, J. K., & Glaser, R. (1996). Psychosocial modulation of cytokine-induced natural killer cell activity in older adults. *Psychosomatic Medicine, 58*, 264–272.

Evans, P., Bristow, M., Hucklebridge, F., Clow, A., & Walters, N. (1993). The relationship between secretory immunity, mood and life-events. *British Journal of Clinical Psychology, 32*, 227–236.

Fawzy, F. I., Kemeny, M. E., Fawzy, N. W., Elashoff, R., Morton, D., Cousins, N., & Fahey, J. L. (1990). A structured psychiatric intervention for cancer patients: Changes over time in immunological measures. *Archives of General Psychiatry, 47*, 729–735.

Felten, S. Y., & Olschowka, J. (1987). Noradrenergic sympathetic innervation of the spleen: II. Tyrosine hydroxylase (TH)–positive nerve terminals for synaptic like contacts on lymphocytes in the splenic white pulp. *Journal of Neuroscience Research, 18*, 37–48.

Gerra, G., Monit, D., Panerai, A., Sacerdote, P., Anderlini, R., Avanzini, P., … Franceschi, C. (2003). Long-term immune-endocrine effects of bereavement: relationships with anxiety levels and mood. *Psychiatry Research, 121*, 145–158.

Glaser, R., Kiecolt-Glaser, J. K., Bonneau, R. H., Malarkey, W., Kennedy, S., & Hughes, J. (1992). Stress-induced modulation of the immune response to recombinant hepatitis B vaccine. *Psychosomatic Medicine, 54*, 22–29.

Glaser, R., Kiecolt-Glaser, J., Malarkey, W. B., & Sheridan, J. F. (1998). The influence of psychological stress on the immune response to vaccines. *Annals of the New York Academy of Science, 840*, 649–655.

Glaser, R., Kiecolt-Glaser, J. K., Marucha, P. T., MacCallum, R. C., Laskowski, B. F., & Malarkey, W. B. (1999). Stress-related changes in proinflammatory cytokine production in wounds. *Archives of General Psychiatry, 56*, 450–456.

Glaser, R., Kiecolt-Glaser, J. K., Stout, J. C., Tarr, K. L., Speicher, C. E., & Holliday, J. E. (1985). Stress-related impairments in cellular immunity. *Psychiatry Research, 16*, 233–239.

Glaser, R., Sheridan, J. F., Malarkey, W. B., MacCallum, R. C., & Kiecolt-Glaser, J. K. (2000). Chronic stress modulates the immune response to a pneumococcal pneumonia vaccine, *Psychosomatic Medicine, 62*, 804–807.

Gleeson, M. (2007). Immune function in sport and exercise. *Journal of Applied Physiology, 103*, 693–699.

Goodkin, K., Feaster, D. J., Tuttle, R., Blaney, N. T., Kumar, M., Baum, M. K., … Fletcher, M. (1996). Bereavement is associated with time-dependent decrements in cellular immune function in asymptomatic human immunodeficiency virus Type 1–seropositive homosexual men. *Clinical and Diagnostic Laboratory Immunology, 3*, 109–118.

Graham, N. M. H., Douglas, R. B., & Ryan, P. (1986). Stress and acute respiratory infection. *American Journal of Epidemiology, 124*, 389–401.

Herbert, T. B., & Cohen, S. (1993a). Stress and immunity in humans: A meta-analytic review. *Psychosomatic Medicine, 55*, 364–379.

Herbert, T. B., & Cohen, S. (1993b). Depression and immunity: A meta-analytic review. *Psychological Bulletin, 113*, 472–486.

Hewson–Bower, B., & Drummond, P. D. (2001). Psychological treatment for recurrent symptoms of colds and flu in children. *Journal of Psychosomatic Research, 51*, 369–377.

House, J. S., Landis, K. R., & Umberson, D. (1988). Social relationships and health. *Science, 241*, 540–545.

Ironson, G., Wyningo, C., Schneiderman, N., Baum, A., Rodriguez, M., Greenwood, D., … Fletcher, M. A. (1997). Posttraumatic stress symptoms, intrusive thoughts, loss, and immune function after Hurricane Andrew. *Psychosomatic Medicine, 59*, 128–141.

Irwin, M., Daniels, M., Smith, T. L., Bloom, E., & Weiner, H. (1987). Impaired natural killer cell activity during bereavement. *Brain Behavior, and Immunity, 1*, 98–104.

Irwin, M., McClintick, J., Costlow, C., Fortner, M., White, J., & Gillin, J. C. (1996). Partial night sleep deprivation reduced natural killer and cellular immune responses in humans. *Journal of the Federation of American Societies for Experimental Biology, 10*, 643–653.

Irwin, M. R., & Miller, A. H. (2007). Depressive disorders and immunity: 20 years of progress and discovery. *Brain, Behavior, and Immunity, 21*, 374–383.

Jern, C., Wadenvik, H., Mark, H., Hallgren, J., & Jern, S. (1989). Haematological changes during acute mental stress. *British Journal of Haematology, 71*, 153–156.

Kemeny, M. E., Weiner, H., Duran, R., Taylor, S. E., Visscher, B., & Fahey, J. L. (1995). Immune system changes after the death of a partner in HIV-positive gay men. *Psychosomatic Medicine, 57,* 547–554.

Kennedy, S., Kiecolt-Glaser, J. K., & Glaser, R. (1988). Immunological consequences of acute and chronic stressors: Mediating role of interpersonal relationships. *British Journal of Medical Psychology, 61,* 77–85.

Kiecolt-Glaser, J. K., Cacioppo, J. T., Malarkey, W. B., & Glaser, R. (1992). Acute psychological stressors and short-term immune changes: What, why, for whom, and what extent? *Psychosomatic Medicine, 54,* 680–685.

Kiecolt-Glaser, J. K., Fisher, L. D., Ogrocki, P., Stout, J. C., Speicher, C. E., & Glaser, R. (1987). Marital quality, marital disruption, and immune function. *Psychosomatic Medicine, 49,* 13–34.

Kiecolt-Glaser, J. K., Garner, W., Speicher, C., Penn, G. M., Holliday, J., & Glaser, R. (1984). Psychosocial modifiers of immunocompetence in medical students. *Psychosomatic Medicine, 46,* 7–14.

Kiecolt-Glaser, J. K., & Glaser, R. (1987). Psychosocial moderators of immune function. *Annals of Behavioral Medicine, 9,* 16–20.

Kiecolt-Glaser, J. K., & Glaser, R. (1988). Methodological issues in behavioral immunology research with humans. *Brain, Behavior and Immunity, 2,* 67–78.

Kiecolt-Glaser, J. K., & Glaser, R. (1991). Stress and immune function in humans. In R. Ader, D. L. Felten, & N. Cohen (Eds.), *Psychoneuroimmunology* (pp. 849–867). Orlando, FL: Academic Press.

Kiecolt-Glaser, J. K., Glaser, R., Cacioppo, J. T., MacCallum, R. C., Snydersmith, M., Kim, C., & Malarkey, W. B. (1997). Marital conflict in older adults: endocrinological and immunological correlates. *Psychosomatic Medicine, 59,* 339–349.

Kiecolt-Glaser, J. K, Glaser, R., Gravenstein, S., Malarkey, W. B., & Sheridan, J. (1996). Chronic stress alters the immune response to influenza virus vaccine in older adults. *Proceedings of the National Academy of Sciences* [United States], *93,* 3043–3047.

Kiecolt-Glaser, J. K., Glaser, R., Shuttleworth, E., Dyer, C., Ogrocki, P., & Speicher, C. E. (1987). Chronic stress and immunity in family caregivers of Alzheimer's disease victims. *Psychosomatic Medicine, 49,* 523–535.

Kiecolt-Glaser, J. K., Glaser, R., Strain, E. C., Stout, J. C., Tarr, K. L., Holliday, J. E., & Speicher, C. E. (1986). Modulation of cellular immunity in medical students. *Journal of Behavioral Medicine, 9,* 5–21.

Kiecolt-Glaser, J. K., Kennedy, S., Malkoff, S., Fisher, L., Speicher, C. E., & Glaser, R. (1988). Marital discord and immunity in males. *Psychosomatic Medicine, 50,* 213–229.

Kiecolt-Glaser, J. K., Malarkey, W. B., Chee, M., Newton, T., Cacioppo, J. T., Mao, H., & Glaser, R. (1993). Negative behavior during marital conflict is associated with immunological down-regulation. *Psychosomatic Medicine, 55,* 395–409.

Kiecolt-Glaser, J. K., Marucha, P. T., Malarkey, W. B., Mercado, A. M., & Glaser, R. (1995). Slowing of wound healing by psychological stress. *Lancet, 346,* 1194–1196.

Kiecolt-Glaser, J. K., Preacher, K. J., MacCallum, R. C., Atkinson, C., Malarkey, W. B., & Glaser, R. (2003). Chronic stress and age-related increases in the proinflammatory cytokine IL-6. *Proceedings of the National Academy of Sciences, 100,* 9090–9095.

Kunz-Ebrecht, S. R., Mohamed-Ali, V., Feldman, P. J., Kirschbaum, C., & Steptoe, A. (2003). Cortisol responses to mild psychological stress are inversely associated with proinflammatory cytokines. *Brain, Behavior, and Immunity, 17,* 373–383.

Lazarus, R. S., & Folkman, S. (1984). *Stress, appraisal, and coping.* New York, NY: Springer.

Lemieux, A., Coe, C. L., & Carnes, M. (2008). Symptom severity predicts degree of T cell activation in adult women following childhood maltreatment. *Brain, Behavior, and Immunity, 22,* 994–1003.

Light, E., & Lebowitz, B. D. (1989). *Alzheimer's disease treatment and family stress: Directions for research.* Rockville, MD: National Institute of Mental Health.

Linn, M. W., Linn, B. S., & Jenson, J. (1984). Stressful events, dysphoric mood, and immune responsiveness. *Psychology Reports, 54,* 219–222.

Livnat, S., Felten, S. Y., Carlson, S. L., Bellinger, D. L., & Felten, D. L. (1985). Involvement of peripheral and central catecholamine systems in neural-immune interactions. *Journal of Neuroimmunology, 10,* 5–30.

Locke, S. E., Kraus, L., Leserman, J., Hurst, M. W., Heisel, J. S., & Williams, R. M. (1984). Life changes stress, psychiatric symptoms, and natural killer cell activity. *Psychosomatic Medicine, 46,* 411–452.

Lutgendorf, S. K., Tripp Reimer, T., Harvey, J. H., Marks, G., Hong, S-Y., Hillis, S. L., & Lubaroff, D. M. (2001). Effects of housing relocation on immunocompetence and psychosocial functioning in older adults. *Journal of Gerontology, 56A,* M97–105.

Lutgendorf, S. K., Vitaliano, P. P., Tripp-Reimer, T., Harvey, J. H., & Lubaroff, D. M. (1999). Sense of coherence moderated the relationship between life stress and natural killer cell activity in healthy older adults. *Psychology and Aging, 14,* 552–563.

Maier, S. F., & Watkins, L. R. (1998). Cytokines for psychologists: Implications of bidirectional immune-to-brain communication for understanding behavior, mood, and cognition. *Psychological Review, 105,* 83–107.

Manuck, S. B., Cohen, S., Rabin, B. S., Muldoon, M. F., & Bachen, E. A. (1991). Individual differences in cellular immune response to stress. *Psychological Science, 2,* 111–115.

Marsland, A. L., Cohen, S., Rabin, B. S., & Manuck, S. B. (2001). Associations between stress, trait negative affect, acute immune reactivity, and antibody response to hepatitis B injection in healthy young adults. *Health Psychology, 20,* 4–11.

Marsland, A. L., Cohen, S., Rabin, B. S., & Manuck, S. B. (2006). Trait positive affect and antibody response to hepatitis B vaccination. *Brain, Behavior, and Immunity, 20,* 261–269.

Marsland, A. L., Gianaros, P. J., Prather, A. A., Jennings, J. R., Neumann, S. A., & Manuck, S. B. (2007). Stimulated production of proinflammatory cytokines covaries inversely with heart rate variability. *Psychosomatic Medicine, 69,* 709–716.

Marsland, A. L., Henderson, B. N., Chambers, W. H., & Baum, A. (2002). Stability of individual differences in cellular immune responses to two different laboratory tasks. *Psychophysiology, 39,* 865–868.

Marsland, A. L., Herbert, T. B., Muldoon, M. F., Bachen, E. A., Patterson, S., Cohen, S., … Manuck, S. B. (1997). Lymphocyte subset redistribution during acute laboratory stress in young adults: Mediating effects of hemoconcentration. *Health Psychology, 16,* 1–8.

Marsland, A. L., Manuck, S. B., Fazzari, T. V., Stewart, C. J., & Rabin, B. S. (1995). Stability of individual differences in cellular immune responses to acute psychological stress. *Psychosomatic Medicine, 57,* 295–298.

Marucha, P. T., Kiecolt-Glaser, J. K., & Favagehl, M. (1998). Mucosal wound healing is impaired by examination stress. *Psychosomatic Medicine, 60,* 362–365.

McAllister–Sistilli, C. G., Caggiula, A. R., Knopf, S., Rose, C. A., Miller, A. L., & Donny, E. C. (1998). The effects of nicotine on the immune system. *Psychoneuroendocrinology, 23,* 175–187.

McGregor, B. A., Antoni, M. H., Boyers, A., Alferi, S. M., Blomberg, B. B., & Carver, C. S. (2004). Cognitive-behavioral stress management increases benefit finding and immune function among women with early-stage breast cancer. *Journal of Psychosomatic Research, 56,* 1–8.

McKinnon, W., Weisse, C. S., Reynolds, C. P., Bowles, C. A., & Baum, A. (1989). Chronic stress, leukocyte subpopulations, and humoral response to latent viruses. *Health Psychology, 8,* 389–402.

Meyer, R. J., & Haggerty, R. J (1962). Streptoccocal infections in families. *Pediatrics, 29,* 539–49.

Mezick, E. J., Matthews, K. A., Hall, M., Kamarck, T. W., Buysse, D. J., Owens, J. F., & Reis, S. E. (2009). Intra-individual variability in sleep duration and fragmentation associations with stress. *Psychoneuroendocrinology, 34,* 1346–1354.

Miller, G. E., & Cohen, S. (2001). Psychological interventions and the immune system: A meta-analytic review and critique. *Health Psychology, 20,* 47–63.

Miller, G. E., Cohen, S., Pressman, S., Barkin, A., Rabin, B. S., & Traenor, J. J. (2004). Psychological stress and antibody response to influenza vaccination: When is the critical period for stress, and how does it get inside the body? *Psychosomatic Medicine, 66,* 215–223.

Miller, G. E., Cohen, S., & Ritchey, A. K. (2002). Chronic psychological stress and the regulation of pro-inflammatory cytokines: A glucocorticoid-resistance model. *Health Psychology, 21,* 531–541.

Miller, G. E., Rohleder, N., & Cole, S. W. (2008). Chronic interpersonal stress predicts activation of pro- and anti-inflammatory signaling pathways 6 months later. *Psychosomatic Medicine, 71,* 57–62.

Mills, P. J., & Dimsdale, J. E. (1996). The effects of acute psychologic stress on cellular adhesion molecules. *Journal of Psychosomatic Research, 41,* 49–53.

Morag, M., Morag, A., Reichenberg, A., Lerer, B., & Yirmiya, R. (1999). Psychological variables as predictors of rubella antibody titers and fatigue—A prospective, double blind study. *Journal of Psychiatry Research, 33,* 389–395.

Moynihan, J. A., Cohen, N., & Ader, R. (1994). Stress and immunity. In B. Scharrer, E. M. Smith, & G. B. Stefano (Eds.), Neuropeptides and Immunoregulation (pp. 12–138). New York, NY: Springer-Verlag.

Moynihan, J. A., Larson, M. R., Treanor, J., Duberstein, P. R., Power, A., Shore, B., & Ader, R. (2004). Psychosocial factors and the response to influenza vaccination in older adults. *Psychosomatic Medicine, 66,* 950–953.

Pavlov, V. A., & Tracey, K. J. (2005). The cholinergic anti-inflammatory pathway. *Brain, Behavior, and Immunity, 19,* 493–499.

Petrie, K. J., Booth, R. J., Pennebaker, J. W., Davison, K. P., & Thomas, M. G. (1995). Disclosure of trauma and immune response to a hepatitis B vaccination program. *Journal of Consulting and Clinical Psychology, 63,* 787–792.

Phillips, A. C., Carroll, D., Burns, V. E., & Drayson, M. (2005). Neuroticism, cortisol reactivity, and antibody response to vaccination. *Psychophysiology, 42*, 232–238.

Pierson, D. L., Mehta, S. K., & Stowe, R. P. (2007). Reactivation of latent herpes viruses in astronauts. In R. Ader (Ed.), *Psychoneuroimmunology* (4th ed., pp. 851–868). Burlington, MA: Elsevier Academic Press.

Quan, N., Avitsur, R., Stark, J. L., He, L., Lai, W., Dhabhar, F., & Sheridan, J. F. (2003). Molecular mechanisms of glucocorticoid resistance in splenocytes of socially stressed male mice. *Journal of Neuroimmunology, 137*, 51–58.

Rabin, B. S. (1999). *Stress, immune function and health: The connection.* New York, NY: Wiley-Liss.

Romeo, J., Warnberg, J., Nova, E., Diez, L. E., Gomez–Martinez, S., & Marcos, A. (2007). Moderate alcohol consumption and the immune system: A review. *British Journal of Nutrition, 98*, S111–115.

Sabioncello, A., Kocijan–Hercigonja, D., Rabatic, S., Tomasic, J., Jeren, T., Matijevic, L., ... Dekaris, D. (2000). Immune, endocrine, and psychological responses to civilians displaced by war. *Psychosomatic Medicine, 62*, 502–508.

Schleifer, S. J., Keller, S. E., Camerino, M., Thornton, J. C., & Stein, M. (1983). Suppression of lymphocyte stimulation following bereavement. *Journal of American Medical Association, 250*, 374–377.

Schulz, R., & Beach, S. R. (1999). Caregiving as a risk factor for mortality: The Caregiver Health Effects Study. *Journal of the American Medical Association, 282*, 2215–2219.

Segerstrom, S. C. (2001). Optimism, goal conflict, and stressor-related immune change. *Journal of Behavioral Medicine, 24*, 441–467.

Segerstrom, S. C. (2005). Optimism and immunity: do positive thoughts always lead to positive effects? *Brain, Behavior, and Immunity, 19*, 195–200.

Segerstrom, S. C., & Miller, G. E. (2004). Psychological stress and the human immune system: A meta–analytic study of 30 years of inquiry. *Psychological Bulletin, 130*, 601–630.

Smolderen, K. G., Vingerhoets, A. J., Croon, M. A., & Denollet, J. (2007). Personality, psychological stress, and self–reported influenza symptomatology. *BMC Public Health, 7*, 339.

Snyder, B. K., Roghmann, K. J., & Sigal, L. H. (1993). Stress and psychosocial factors: Effects on primary cellular immune response. *Journal of Behavioral Medicine, 16*, 143–161.

Soloman, G. F., Segerstrom, S. C., Grohr, P., Kemeny, M., & Fahey, J. (1997). Shaking up immunity: Psychological and immunologic changes after a natural disaster. *Psychosomatic Medicine, 59*, 114–127.

Sondergaard, S. R., Ostrowski, K., Ullum, H., & Pederson, B. K. (2000). Changes in plasma concentrations of interleukin-6 and interleukin-1 receptor antagonists in response to adrenaline infusion in humans. *European Journal of Applied Physiology, 83*, 95–98.

Stark, J. L., Avitsur, R., Hunzeker, J., Padgett, D. A., & Sheridan, J. F. (2002). Interleukin-6 and the development of social disruption–induced glucocorticoid resistance. *Journal of Neuroimmunology, 124*, 9–15.

Stark, J. L., Avitsur, R., Padgett, D. A., Campbell, K. A., Beck, F. M., & Sheridan, J. F. (2001). Social stress induces glucocorticoid resistance in macrophages. *American Journal of Physiology—Regulatory, Integrative and Comparative Physiology, 280*, 1799–1805.

Steptoe, A., Hamer, M., & Chida, Y. (2007). The effects of acute psychological stress on circulating inflammatory factors in humans: A review and meta–analysis. *Brain, Behavior and Immunity, 21*, 901–912.

Stevens–Felten, S. Y., & Bellinger, D. L. (1997). Noradrenergic and peptidergic innervations of lymphoid organs. *Chemical Immunology, 69*, 99–131.

Stone, A. A., Bovbjerg, D. H., Neale, J. M., Napoli, A., Valdimarsdottir, H., Cox, D., ... Gwaltney, J. M. (1992). Development of common cold symptoms following experimental rhinovirus infection is related to prior stressful life events. *Behavioral Medicine, Fall*, 115–120.

Stone, A. A., Marco, C. A., Cruise, C. E., Cox, D. S., & Neal, J. M. (1996). *International Journal of Behavioral Medicine, 3*, 1–10.

Stone, A. A., Neale, J. M., Cox, D. S., & Napoli, A. (1994). Daily events are associated with a secretory immune response to an oral antigen in men. *Health Psychology, 13*, 440–446.

Stone, A. A., Reed, B. R., & Neale, J. M. (1987). Changes in daily event frequency precede episodes of physical symptoms. *Journal of Human Stress, 13*, 70–74.

Takkouche, B., Regueira, C., & Gestal–Otero, J. J. (2001). A cohort study of stress and the common cold. *Epidemiology, 11*, 345–349.

Tracey, K. J. (2002). The inflammatory reflex. *Nature, 420*, 853–859.

Turner Cobb, J. M., & Steptoe, A. (1996). Psychosocial stress and susceptibility to upper respiratory tract illness in an adult population sample. *Psychosomatic Medicine, 58*, 404–412.

Turner Cobb, J. M., & Steptoe, A. (1998). Psychosocial influences on upper respiratory infectious illness in children. *Journal of Psychosomatic Research, 45*, 319–330.

Uchino, B. N., Cacioppo, J. T., & Kiecolt–Glaser, J. K. (1996). The relationship between social support and physiological processes: A review with emphasis on underlying mechanisms and implications for health. *Psychological Bulletin, 119*, 488–531.

Valdimarsdottir, H. B., & Bovbjerg, D. H. (1997). Positive and negative mood: Association with natural killer cell activity. *Psychology and Health, 12*, 319–327.

Vedhara, K., Cox, N. K., Wilcock, G. K., Perks, P., Hunt, M., Anderson, S., … Shanks, N. M. (1999). Chronic stress in elderly carers of dementia patients and antibody response to influenza vaccination. *Lancet, 353*, 627–631.

Von Kanel, R., Dimsdale, J. E., Mills, P. J., Ancoli-Israel, S., Patterson, T., Mausbach, B. T., & Grant, I. (2006). Effect of Alzheimer caregiving stress and age on frailty markers interleukin-6, c-reactive protein, and d-dimer. *Journal of Gerontology, 61A*, 963–969.

Weiss, D. W., Hirt, R., Tarcic, N., Berzon, Y., Ben-Zur, H., Breznitz, S., … O'Dorisio, T. M. (1996). Studies in psychoneuroimmunology: Psychological, immunological, and neuroendocrinological parameters in Israeli civilians during and after a period of Scud missile attacks. *Behavioral Medicine, 22*, 5–14.

Wetherell, M. A., & Vedhara, K. (2007). Stress-associated immune dysregulation can affect antibody and T-cell responses to vaccines. In R. Ader (Ed.), *Psychoneuroimmunology* (4th ed., pp. 897–916). Burlington, MA: Elsevier Academic Press.

Witek-Janusek, L., Albuquerque, K., Chroniak, K. R., Chroniak, C., Durazo-Arvizu, R., & Mathews, H. L. (2008). Effect of mindfulness based stress reduction on immune function, quality of life and coping in women newly diagnosed with early stage breast cancer. *Brain, Behavior, and Immunity, 22*, 969–981.

Zakowski, S. G., McAllister, C. G., Deal, M., & Baum, A. (1992). Stress, reactivity, and immune function in healthy men. *Health Psychology, 11*, 223–232.

Zorrilla, E. P., Luborsky, L., McKay, J. R., Rosenthal, R., Houldin, A., Tax, A., … Schmidt, K. (2001). The relationship of depression and stressors to immunological assays: A meta-analytic review. *Brain, Behavior, and Immunity, 15*, 199–226.

32 Psychological Processes in Rheumatic Disease

Sharon Danoff-Burg
University at Albany, State University of New York

Asani H. Seawell
Grinnell College

My whole life has changed as a result of lupus. Social, personal, professional and spiritual. It was most difficult to leave my full time teaching position mid-year due to lupus. Learning how to modulate my time [and] energy is a challenge. Facing a fatal illness, not all that is known about, is most difficult. At times you don't look "sick" with lupus and this raises questions. Other times I look so terrible and feel so horrible I can't leave the house.

I think so many people (myself included) can't quite understand the vagaries of RA. I am unable to babysit my youngest grandchildren because I can't lift them or help them if they fall. I'm so afraid that I won't be able to protect them in certain situations. If there is any stress it may perhaps be my own fears or thoughts of inadequacy.

No one ever knows about living with a chronic illness until it happens to them.[1]

THE CHALLENGES OF LIVING WITH RHEUMATIC DISEASE

Living with chronic illness can be challenging; it can vastly affect individuals' physical and psychological functioning as well as the ability to fulfill important roles, maintain employment, or manage close relationships. Rheumatic disease, which includes over 100 different types of illnesses and conditions affecting the joints, the tissues that surround joints, and other connective tissue, can pose unique challenges. First, the initial onset of rheumatic symptoms most often occurs between the ages of 15 and 40 (Marshall, 2002), meaning that the disease can span many decades. Second, rheumatic disease flares can occur almost without warning, making it difficult to plan for the future. Some symptoms of rheumatic disease such as fatigue are largely unseen, meaning that patients may find themselves convincing others that they truly are ill and may fear being viewed as lazy or told that symptoms are all in their head (Fite & Kopala, 2003). Finally, rheumatic disease symptoms may influence patients' emotional and physical intimacy with their partners, including the frequency with which they engage in physically intimate behaviors and how readily they disclose details about their illness experience (Druley, Stephens, & Coyne, 1997).

The terms rheumatic disease and arthritis are usually used interchangeably. Common symptoms include joint pain, stiffness, and fatigue, and may affect nearly every activity of daily living and erode quality of life. Arthritis is the most common cause of disability in the United States, with costs from medical care and lost wages due to disability amounting to billions of dollars each year (Centers for Disease Control and Prevention [CDC], 2008). Based on data from the National Health

---

[1] Quotes are from participants in the authors' research programs.

Interview Survey, 46 million American adults (22%) report having physician-diagnosed arthritis, and this number is expected to increase as the population ages; it is estimated that one-quarter of American adults will have physician-diagnosed arthritis by the year 2030 (CDC, 2008). Examples include osteoarthritis (OA), fibromyalgia, rheumatoid arthritis (RA), juvenile idiopathic arthritis (previously called juvenile rheumatoid arthritis), systemic lupus erythematosus (SLE), gout, and ankylosing spondylitis.

This chapter will discuss psychological research focused on RA and SLE. These two rheumatic diseases are similar in that both are chronic, inflammatory, and thought to be autoimmune in origin. Both RA and SLE are more common among women than men. Both may have a variable disease course characterized by periods during which symptoms flare and remit, often unpredictably. Some patients experience symptoms that are mild in nature, whereas the symptoms experienced by other patients are severe. SLE in some cases can be life threatening, involving organs such as the kidneys, lungs, and brain (Marshall, 2002; Sperry, 2006).

AN ECOLOGICAL PERSPECTIVE ON RHEUMATIC DISEASE

For this chapter on psychological processes in rheumatic disease, we take an "illness-in-context" or ecological perspective, which emphasizes that health and psychosocial adaptation to disease are functions not only of individual characteristics but also broader interpersonal, social, and cultural contexts (Revenson, 1994). According to this perspective, health and illness are determined by a confluence of factors surrounding the individual, which interact in a reciprocal manner to influence disease (see Figure 32.1). For instance, not only do patients' perceptions of their own illness influence well-being, but the illness perceptions of patients' spouses can also influence psychosocial outcomes. Positive perceptions of illness on the part of the spouse have been associated with

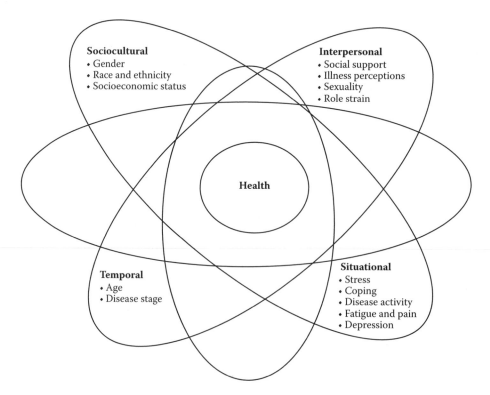

FIGURE 32.1 An ecological perspective on rheumatic disease. (Adapted from Revenson, T. A., in *Personality and Disease*, 65–94, John Wiley, New York, 1990.)

better health among medical patients, including those with RA (e.g., Figueiras & Weinman, 2003; Riemsma, Taal, & Rasker, 2000). This example illustrates that the experience of illness does not occur in isolation, but is rather the result of reciprocal relationships that exist between the individual and a particular context (Revenson, 1990). Important information about the experience of illness may be obscured if ways in which contextual variables influence health are not considered.

The research on rheumatic disease that we review here makes it apparent that illness is best understood from an ecological perspective that considers the context in which illness occurs. Hence, we review the literature on psychological processes in rheumatic disease using the four contextual domains of Revenson's (1990) ecological approach to personality and disease: interpersonal, sociocultural, situational, and temporal domains. We then discuss psychosocial interventions and conclude with directions for future research.

PSYCHOSOCIAL PROCESSES IN RHEUMATIC DISEASE

INTERPERSONAL DOMAIN

The interpersonal domain describes social and relationship variables that influence a person's illness experience. People cope with illness within the context of their relationships (Revenson, Kayser, & Bodenmann, 2005). As can be seen in the quotes from patients that opened this chapter, rheumatic disease can affect all areas of one's social network, including partners, extended family members, coworkers, and friends.

Social Support

Living with rheumatic disease can be stressful, making social support essential. Social support provides patients with valuable feedback and information, helps patients achieve new understandings of their problems, increases motivation to take positive action, and reduces emotional stress (Danoff-Burg & Revenson, 2005a; Revenson, 2003). Social support also encourages the use of adaptive coping strategies (Holtzman, Newth, & Delongis, 2004). Patients who receive helpful social support report less pain and disability (Evers, Kraaimaat, Geene, Jacobs, & Bijlsma, 2003) and fewer depressive symptoms (Druley & Townsend, 1998; Revenson, Schiaffino, Majerovitz, & Gibofsky, 1991). For example, in a study by Sutcliffe, Clarke, Levinton, and colleagues (1999), female SLE patients with higher perceived social support also had higher self-reported physical functioning, mental health, and social functioning.

As negative physical and mental health outcomes become worse, patients' needs for social support increase (Manne & Zautra, 1992). Unfortunately, patients with rheumatic disease tend to be dissatisfied with their levels of social support (Archenoltz, Burckhardt, & Segesten, 1999) and have needs that remain unmet. For instance, Moses, Wiggers, Nicholas, and Cockburn (2005) found that individuals with SLE reported unmet needs related to feelings of anxiety and stress, and Danoff-Burg and Friedberg (2009) found that SLE patients' unmet needs varied according to demographic factors. Fortunately, social support, a mechanism by which unmet needs can be addressed, is a potentially modifiable factor that may improve overall functioning (Sutcliffe, Clarke, Levinton, et al., 1999).

Social support is most beneficial when the type of support offered fits the patients' needs (Cohen & Wills, 1985). For instance, patients with rheumatic disease may expect emotional support from their partner (Fekete, Stephens, Mickelson, & Druley, 2007) and problem-focused or informational support from their healthcare providers (Revenson, 1993). As a result, patients many become distressed if the source and type of support does not meet their expectations or if the support provided is unhelpful (i.e., minimization of symptoms or pessimistic comments; Affleck, Pfeiffer, Tennen, & Fifield, 1988). Further, some research suggests that support efforts are most successful when they are undetected by the recipient, perhaps because awareness of one's need for help can negatively affect self-esteem (Bolger, Zuckerman, & Kessler, 2000). Nonetheless, relationships characterized by high levels of both support perceived as helpful and support perceived as unhelpful are better than having little or no positive support at all (Revenson, Schiaffino, Majerovitz, &

Gibofsky, 1991). Support providers must be both skillful and flexible in their provision of support because the support needs of patients may change over the course of the illness and in response to different treatment regimens.

Partners and Support

Many patients may call upon a partner as their primary source of emotional and tangible support (Revenson, 1993). Indeed, patients with SLE or RA have indicated that family and friends are the most important aspects of their lives (Archenholtz et al., 1999). In particular, committed romantic relationships are important because they provide a deeper level of intimacy and commitment compared to other types of relationships (Revenson, 1994; Revenson et al., 2005). Consequently, partners of patients with rheumatic disease are at times likely to carry much of the stress and burden related to illness (Revenson & Majerovitz, 1990). They may accompany the patient to medical appointments, assume household duties when the patient is ill, and assist the patient with activities of daily living (e.g., dressing).

Although much research focused on social support from the perspective of the patient, there is a growing body of literature examining support needs of partners. Partners are in need of their own support, given that caring for and supporting an intimate partner with chronic illness can be both rewarding and stressful. Common stressors experienced by partners of rheumatic disease patients include feelings of helplessness in response to patients' pain, frustration with the patients' physical limitations, and worries about the future (Revenson & Majerovitz, 1990). In addition to these stressors, partners may be coping with their own illnesses and may fear burdening their ill partners with their own support needs. Patients in turn may believe that they are unable to meet the needs of their partner (Bediako & Friend, 2004) or may become so focused on providing support that they neglect themselves (Danoff-Burg, Revenson, Trudeau, & Paget, 2004; Trudeau, Danoff-Burg, Revenson, & Paget, 2003), all of which may result in distress. Research suggests that partners who receive adequate support from their extended support networks are better equipped to provide support to others (Revenson & Majerovitz, 1990). For partners, receiving outside support may reduce the burden of caregiving and provide the opportunity to express emotions.

Illness Perceptions

The experience of living with rheumatic disease may lead to patients and their partners coming to view themselves and the illness in particular ways, and perceptions of illness held by one partner may influence the other partner. Shared perceptions of the illness may be beneficial in that having similar views may result in less stress and better psychosocial outcomes (Riemsma et al., 2000). In a longitudinal study of patients with RA and their partners, Sterba and colleagues (2008) found that having congruent optimistic beliefs about the ability to control illness and the belief that RA is cyclical predicted better mood and life satisfaction.

When partners' illness perceptions are incongruent, such as when there is disagreement regarding the extent of the patient's disability, then interventions aimed at modifying illness perceptions may be useful. For instance, Goodman, Morrissey, Graham, & Bossingham (2005) tested the effectiveness of a cognitive-behavioral intervention in changing the illness representations of patients with SLE. Relative to a control group, the intervention was effective in reducing stress and improving perceptions of the ability to manage treatment and emotions surrounding the illness.

Sexuality

Sexuality is a concern for many adults with rheumatic disease, and during adolescence rheumatic disease can affect evolving sexuality (Siegel & Baum, 2004). Some research suggests that sexual functioning is poorer among women with rheumatic disease relative to other women. In one study, 26% of patients with SLE abstained from sexual activities compared to only 4% of a healthy comparison sample (Curry, Levine, Jones, & Kurit, 1993). Similarly, patients with SLE have reported more gynecological problems, lower sexual functioning, greater depression, and poorer body image compared to controls (Curry, Levine, Corty, Jones, & Kurit, 1994). Druley and colleagues (1997) found that women with SLE who had recently experienced a disease flare avoided physical intimacy and had poorer well-being.

Although illness can interfere with sexual functioning, sexual dysfunction is not inevitable. Sexual problems are not uncommon in the general population, although couples with rheumatic disease often attribute such problems to the illness (Danoff-Burg & Revenson, 2005b). Whereas some aspects of sexuality may indeed be altered as a result of illness, the sexual satisfaction of couples in which one partner has rheumatic disease may not necessarily differ from that of healthy couples (Majerovitz & Revenson, 1994; Seawell & Danoff-Burg, 2005). Sexual dissatisfaction may be most likely to occur when levels of fatigue, depression (Seawell & Danoff-Burg, 2005), or pain (Curry et al., 1993; Majerovitz & Revenson, 1994) are high. It should also be noted that some women report perceiving benefits to their intimate relationships as a result of illness, such as appreciation of the support they receive from their partners (Danoff-Burg & Revenson, 2005a) or gains in self-acceptance and even self-confidence (Karlen, 2002).

Role Strain

Chronic illness can affect every aspect of family life, resulting in major lifestyle changes for patients and their loved ones (Revenson, 1994; Melamed & Brenner, 1990). Household responsibilities and activities may be altered as family members make efforts to adapt to rheumatic disease, which can be unpredictable in its symptoms and its course. Distress may occur if family members are no longer able to fulfill the roles they assumed previously, and in many families these may have aligned with traditional gender roles. For example, Karasz and Ouellette (1995) found that disease severity in female SLE patients most often resulted in psychological distress when role strain related to being a wife or mother occurred. In another study (Coty & Wallston, 2008), the ability to balance multiple roles was the sole predictor of psychological well-being in patients with RA. Some aspects of family structure may change as family members cope with illness, and families who are able to remain flexible will likely fare best (Chrisler & Parrett, 1995; Danoff-Burg & Revenson, 2000).

SOCIOCULTURAL DOMAIN

Socioeconomic status (SES) along with other variables such as gender and education comprise the sociocultural domain. These variables may exacerbate physical and mental dysfunction, or they may act as buffers against dysfunction (Revenson, 1990). For patients with rheumatic disease, sociocultural factors can have an impact on disease activity and damage, as well as on interpersonal relationships and coping.

Gender

Gender can be a key factor in understanding patients' experiences of pain and disability. Women with rheumatic disease have been shown to experience more disability than do men (e.g., lower mobility and self-care; Kraaimaat, Bakker, Jansen, & Bijlsma, 1996) and greater decline in functional capacity over time (Hommel, Wagner, Chaney, & Mullins, 1998). Interactions of gender with other variables have been identified. For example, De Roos and Callahan (1999) found that women with RA who were unable to work due to disability were more likely to have less than a high school education and higher pain scores than did employed female patients. Similar associations among disability, education, and pain were not found among male patients. Longitudinal research has indicated that women with rheumatic disease experience more depression and negative mood than do men with rheumatic disease (Dowdy, Dwyer, Smith, & Wallston, 1996).

Researchers have investigated not only whether women and men with rheumatic disease experience differences in symptoms, but also whether they cope with their experiences differently. Whereas the larger coping literature has found evidence for both the presence and absence of gender differences (for a review see Brannon, 1999), studies of patients with rheumatic disease support the idea that men and women tend to use different coping strategies. For instance, Affleck and colleagues (1999) found that, even after controlling for levels of pain, female RA patients were more likely than male patients to use emotion-focused coping. A study examining relationship-focused coping (Badr, 2004) found that women with rheumatic disease or other illnesses such as cancer or diabetes, compared to healthy husbands, were less likely to use active engagement as a form of coping when communicating with their partner. Other research (van Middendorp et al., 2005) suggests that women with RA attend more to their emotions and experience them more intensely than do male patients.

Research focused on potential gender differences among patients and their partners is particularly challenging due to the fact that diseases such as RA and SLE occur much more frequently among women than men (Petri, 1995; Theis, Helmick, & Hootman, 2007). When samples include few or no men with rheumatic disease, it can be difficult to determine the effects of gender versus the effects of patient status.

Race, Ethnicity, and Socioeconomic Status

Variables related to race, ethnicity, and SES are important to consider in the study of adaptation to rheumatic disease. Numerous studies have documented that non-Caucasian race and lower SES are associated with more serious illness (Brekke, Hjortdahl, Thelle, & Kvien, 1999), including greater disease activity and damage (Alarcon et al., 1998; Sutcliffe, Clarke, Gordon, Farwell, & Isenberg, 1999) and more serious disease at a younger age (Fernandez et al., 2007). Non-Caucasian race and higher disease activity have been associated with a lack of private health insurance, sudden disease onset, helplessness, and maladaptive illness-related behaviors among patients with SLE (Alarcon et al., 1998). The combination of personal and community poverty may result in poorer mental health outcomes such as depression (Trupin et al., 2008). In contrast, lower disease activity has been associated with higher education, higher income, and private health insurance (Karlson et al., 1995). In a longitudinal study of African Americans and Caucasians with SLE, Friedman et al. (1999) found that poorer physical functioning was associated with fatigue and pain, and in both groups self-esteem was related to mental health. In a follow-up study (Bae, Hashimoto, Karlson, Liang, & Daltroy, 2001) that reanalyzed Karlson and colleagues' (1997) data, a significant relation between social support and physical functioning was found only among Caucasian patients above poverty level who had health insurance and low pre-morbid disease activity. Among patients with RA, longitudinal research has documented that those with low SES have worse disease activity, physical and mental health, and quality of life than those with high SES (Jacobi et al., 2003).

Some studies, however, have found no link between race or ethnicity and disease outcomes (e.g., Berkanovic et al., 1996; Poole, Chiappisi, Cordova, & Sibbitt, 2007). For example, Jordan, Lumley, and Leisen (1998) found no differences in self-reported pain severity among African American and White women with RA, although African Americans were less physically active. Similarly, Lotstein and colleagues (1998) found that ethnicity was not associated with physical health outcomes in patients with SLE.

Given the mixed findings with respect to particular demographic factors and disease outcomes, additional research is needed. When studying ethnicity, researchers should consider examining the individual's level of acculturation. For example, greater disease activity has been found in Hispanic SLE patients with higher levels of acculturation (Alarcon et al., 1999), but in Hispanics with RA those with lower levels of acculturation tended to fare worse (Escalante, del Rincon, & Mulrow, 2000). Researchers should continue to examine these types of sociocultural variables and their contribution to physical and mental health outcomes rather than simply controlling for them in statistical analyses, which can obscure findings.

SITUATIONAL DOMAIN

The situational domain contains contextual variables that enhance or compromise the responses that person is able to make (Revenson, 1990). For instance, particular coping strategies in response to disease-related stress, as well as co-occurring major and minor stressors, may result in better physical and mental health outcomes. In contrast, depression, pain, and fatigue may inhibit one's ability to manage illness.

Stress

Given the immunologic basis of both RA and SLE, disease processes can be influenced by factors affecting the immune system, including stress (Keefe et al., 2002). Zautra and colleagues (Zautra, Burleson, Matt, Roth, & Burrows, 1994; Zautra, Hamilton, Potter, & Smith, 1999; Zautra & Smith, 2001) have documented relatively high levels of physiological reactivity to interpersonal stress among persons with RA compared to persons with OA, as well as relations among stress reactivity, disease activity, and depression. Similarly, daily stress among patients with SLE, particularly daily stress regarding interpersonal relationships and social duties, has been shown to predict disease activity (Pawlak et al., 2003).

Another line of research focuses on the relative contribution of major and minor life stressors to physical and psychological outcomes. One study (Da Costa et al., 1999) found that major life stress predicted functional disability at an eight-month follow-up, whereas another (Adams, Dammers, Saia, Brantley, & Gaydos, 1994) found that minor rather than major life stressors best predicted increases in symptoms. A more recent study (Nery et al., 2007) found both life stressors and hassles to be associated with major depression among patients with SLE.

Coping

The impact of stress on psychological and physical outcomes may be buffered by coping processes. Depending on the severity of the rheumatic disease, patients may need to cope on a daily basis with pain, stiffness, fatigue, and physical activity restrictions, as well as with issues related to identity, body image, and even mortality. A large body of research has examined individual-level coping among patients with RA (see Newman & Revenson, 1993; Zautra & Manne, 1992). For example, avoidant strategies and self-blame consistently have been associated with poorer functioning (Felton & Revenson, 1984; Manne & Zautra, 1989; Parker et al., 1988; Ramjeet, Smith, & Adams, 2008).

Concerned about the limitations of self-report questionnaire checklists (e.g., Coyne & Gottlieb, 1996; Danoff-Burg, Ayala, & Revenson, 2000), some stress and coping researchers have combined qualitative and quantitative approaches (e.g., Danoff-Burg & Revenson, 2005a; Dwyer, Bess, & Smith, 1996). Another alternative to the coping checklist approach is daily diary studies and ecological momentary assessment (Yoshiuchi, Yamamoto, & Akabayashi, 2008). Using daily processes analyses, investigators have been able to examine patterns of coping with RA that might not be captured using other methodologies (e.g., Holtzman et al., 2004; Keefe et al., 1997; Keefe et al., 2001; Newth & Delongis, 2004). Conner et al. (2006) noted differences in daily pain coping between patients with a history of depression and patients with no history of depression that were not revealed by examining group averages. This type of coping assessment and analysis, along with additional types of longitudinal designs, are needed to capture the complex and multidimensional nature of coping (Keefe et al., 2002).

Disease Activity

Another situational variable that has been examined by researchers interested in rheumatic disease is disease activity. Not surprisingly, patients with more active disease states, particularly those experiencing higher levels of pain and physical disability, tend to experience greater psychological distress than do patients with less active disease (Dobkin et al., 1998; Ward et al., 1999; Zautra, Hamilton, Potter, & Smith, 1999). Accordingly, those with less active disease report lower levels of distress and higher occupational and general functioning (Segui et al., 2000). Not all studies, however, have found a significant relation between disease activity and distress (Waterloo, Omdal, Husby, & Mellgren, 1998). Studies of patients with SLE have shown that disease activity and quality of life may be uncorrelated

(Abu-Shakra et al., 1999; Gladman, Urowitz, Gough, & MacKinnon, 1996; Hanly, 1997). Similarly, in a study of patients with RA, disease status predicted illness-related functioning but not emotional or social adjustment (Curtis, Groarke, Coughlan, & Gsel, 2005). With regard to the effect of psychosocial interventions on disease activity, a meta-analysis of randomized controlled trials concluded that they typically do not alter biologic markers for RA but can influence objective clinical indices of disease activity such as joint tenderness (Astin, Beckner, Soeken, Hochberg, & Berman, 2002).

Fatigue and Pain

Fatigue is part of the disease experience for many patients with chronic, systemic rheumatic disease, yet too often fatigue is not addressed as a treatment target (Hewlett et al., 2005; Repping-Wuts, Fransen, van-Achterberg, Bleijenberg, & van-Riel, 2007). This is unfortunate in light of the connection between fatigue and quality of life among patients with RA (Rupp, Boshuizen, Jacobi, Dinant, & van den Bos, 2004) and SLE (Zonana-Nacach et al., 2000). Fatigue has been shown to be related not only to outcomes such as mood and sleep, but also to contextual variables such as socioeconomic status, interpersonal events, and social support (McKinley, Ouellette, & Winkel, 1995; Parrish, Zautra, & Davis, 2008; Zonana-Nacach et al., 2000). Understanding causal pathways among these influences can be challenging for clinicians and researchers alike.

Needless to say, the research literature concerning psychological aspects of rheumatic disease includes many studies on the topic of pain. Pain is a subjective experience that is not necessarily predicted by disease activity or severity, even though it may be viewed that way by patients (Ruzicka, 1998). Not surprisingly, anxiety and depression have been shown to be related to arthritis pain (Smith & Zautra, 2008a), and psychosocial interventions can reduce arthritis pain (Dixon, Keefe, Scipio, Perri, & Abernethy, 2007). An interesting development within this large body of research is the investigation of positive affect rather than a sole focus on negative affect. For instance, positive affect has been described as a factor of resilience, in that it helps reduce the distress associated with fluctuations in pain (Strand et al., 2006).

Depression

The majority of individuals with RA and SLE do not experience clinical depression, despite the multitude of potential stressors resulting from their illness (DeVellis, 1993; Segui et al., 2000). Risk factors for depression among persons with RA include high daily stress, low perceived ability to cope with pain, physical disability, and loss of valued activities (Covic, Tyson, Spencer, & Howe, 2006; Katz & Yelin, 1995; Sharpe, Sensky, & Allard, 2001). Demographic variables are also significant, with female gender, younger age, and fewer economic and social resources predicting greater depressive symptoms (Newman, Fitzpatrick, Lamb, & Shipley, 1989; Wright et al., 1998).

Researchers and clinicians must pay careful attention to the possibility of overlap among symptoms of rheumatic disease, symptoms of depression, and side effects of medications (Blalock, DeVellis, Brown, & Wallston, 1989). Depression can worsen the pain and disability associated with rheumatic disease, in some cases leading patients and providers to interpret difficulties caused by depression as a worsening of the rheumatic disease process; this in turn can lead to unnecessary changes in the medical regimen without proper treatment of the depression. Regarding psychological interventions, the efficacy of cognitive-behavioral therapy (CBT) has been documented. For example, in a randomized controlled trial of patients with recent-onset RA, CBT was associated with decreased depressive symptoms and improved joint involvement at 6-month follow-up relative to standard medical care (Sharpe, Sensky, Timberlake, et al., 2001).

Temporal Domain

The temporal domain refers to the time at which the onset of disease occurs as well as the stage of disease. Temporal factors can influence illness perceptions as in the case when diagnosis is thought to be "off-time" due to the individual's developmental stage at the time of diagnosis (Revenson, 1990).

The stage of disease, such as whether the patient is experiencing a disease flare, can influence coping. Different coping tasks present themselves at different stages of illness, and what may be effective coping at one time will not necessarily be effective at another time (Newman & Revenson, 1993). For instance, medical treatment plans may change over time, resulting in changes in side effects and in symptoms. These changes may in turn affect interpersonal relationships and family responsibilities.

Burke, Zautra, Schultz, Reich, & Davis (2002) noted that among patients with RA, age and illness duration are diathesis factors that contribute to disease course and prognosis. Specifically, early onset is associated with more progressive disease (Harris, 1993), younger patients are at higher risk for depression (Wright et al., 1998), and the first two years of disease activity may be most amenable to treatment effects (Anderson, Wells, Verhoeven, & Felson, 2000).

Longitudinal investigations may yield results that contradict previous findings or otherwise be surprising. One study (Demange et al., 2004) found cross-sectional but not longitudinal links between RA patients' social support or social networks and their functional limitations and psychological distress. With regard to SLE, a longitudinal study by Dobkin et al. (2001) found that disease activity was more likely to improve than to worsen over time. Findings such as these, which may contradict assumptions held by some lay people or professionals, underscore the need for prospective biopsychosocial research.

PSYCHOSOCIAL INTERVENTIONS FOR RHEUMATIC DISEASE

Given the chronic course of rheumatic disease and the fact that many pharmacologic treatments produce adverse side effects, psychosocial interventions play an important role in the lives of many patients. Astin et al. (2002) conducted a meta-analytic review of studies comparing psychosocial interventions for RA to non-intervention controls (wait-list, usual care, or attention placebo). The interventions, most of which could be categorized as multimodal, included approaches such as cognitive-behavioral therapy, psychoeducation, emotional disclosure, group counseling, stress management, and biofeedback. Examining 25 randomized trials, these authors found small but significant average effect sizes at post-treatment for pain, functional disability, depression, coping, and self efficacy. At the time of treatment follow-up, which averaged 8.5 months, effect sizes for depression, coping, and tender joints were significant. Important challenges for the future include understanding which individuals are most likely to benefit from which psychosocial interventions, and identifying underlying mechanisms of action, including placebo or expectancy effects (Astin, 2004).

Randomized controlled trials of psychological interventions for SLE are less common. One such study (Dobkin et al., 2002), which compared brief supportive-expressive group psychotherapy to standard medical care for SLE, indicated that the psychological intervention was not efficacious. Another study (Greco, Rudy, & Manzi, 2004) randomized SLE patients to biofeedback-assisted cognitive-behavioral treatment (BF/CBT), symptom monitoring, or usual medical care. BF/CBT participants showed the greatest post-treatment reductions in psychological dysfunction (e.g., stress, depressive symptoms) and in pain. At a 9-month follow-up, only the effect on psychological functioning remained significant relative to usual care. A psychoeducational intervention for SLE patients and their partners (Karlson et al., 2004), compared with an attention placebo control group, resulted in better outcomes with regard to quality of life, self-efficacy, fatigue, and couples' communication. Disease activity also was measured but did not change in response to this intervention. Similarly, a recent trial comparing CBT for SLE to standard medical care (Navarrete-Navarrete et al., 2010) documented improvement in mood, quality of life, and somatic symptoms, but no change in disease activity.

The most widely disseminated psychosocial intervention for people with rheumatic disease is the Arthritis Self-Management Program (ASMP; Lorig & Fries, 2006), also known as the Arthritis Self-Help Course. ASMP is a structured group program that combines patient education with cognitive-behavioral techniques. Benefits appear to be relatively long-lasting and include increased knowledge and self-care behaviors and decreased pain (Lorig, Lubeck, Kraines, Seleznick, & Holman, 1985;

Lorig & Holman, 1989). The Systemic Lupus Erythematosus Self-Help Course (SLESH; Braden, Brodt-Weinberg, Depka, McGlone, & Tretter, 1987) also has yielded positive results (Braden, 1992; Braden, McGlone, & Pennington, 1993). Some researchers have focused on modifying these interventions to meet the needs of ethnically diverse populations, such as offering community-based programs for Spanish-speaking participants, involving family members, and addressing any negative feelings regarding health care professionals (e.g., Lorig, Gonzalez, & Ritter, 1999; Robbins, Allegrante & Paget, 1993). Needs assessment research may help guide future research in this area.

CONCLUSION

As noted above, prospective biopsychosocial research is essential, and, as emphasized throughout this chapter, researchers must attend to contextual factors. In recent years, more studies have been published examining links between patient functioning and sociocultural variables such as SES (e.g., Jacobi et al., 2003); however, many questions and challenges remain concerning the impact of SES and other contextual variables such as gender. For example, the authors of a recent multinational study (Sokka et al., 2009) concluded that RA disease activity appeared worse in women than in men, but that this gender difference may reflect the measures that were used rather than actual differences in disease.

With regard to clinically relevant research, we are pleased to see that behavioral scientists have begun to study third wave cognitive-behavioral approaches (Öst, 2008), such as mindfulness-based interventions, among patients with RA (Pradhan et al., 2007; Zautra et al., 2008). As discussed previously in this chapter, enough studies have now been conducted to produce a meta-analysis of randomized controlled trials of psychosocial interventions for RA (Astin et al., 2002), but these types of studies for SLE are relatively rare. Randomized, controlled studies of psychosocial interventions for SLE are a research priority, and investigators also should work to identify factors that predict treatment adherence, including the role of patient-provider communication (Seawell & Danoff-Burg, 2004).

Finally, we join with other health psychologists (e.g., Smith & Zautra, 2008b) in calling for the consideration of resilience—as well as other positive concomitants of illness—in psychological theory, research, and intervention. For example, Sinclair and Wallston (2004) surveyed samples of patients with RA to understand and measure resilient coping, distinguished by "the ability to promote positive adaptation despite high stress" (p. 95). Related to resilience is the ability to find benefits in adverse experiences, a process that has been associated with enhanced functioning in both SLE and RA patients (Affleck et al., 1988; Danoff-Burg, Agee, Romanoff, Kremer, & Strosberg, 2006; Danoff-Burg & Revenson, 2005a; Katz, Flasher, Cacciapaglia, & Nelson, 2001; Tennen, Affleck, Urrows, Higgins, & Mendola, 1992). Research and clinical work that is focused not only on vulnerability and pathology but also on protective factors and growth will increase positive psychological and health-related adjustment to rheumatic disease.

REFERENCES

Abu-Shakra, M., Mader, R., Langevitz, P., Friger, M., Codish, S., Neumann, L., & Buskila, D. (1999). Quality of life in systemic lupus erythematosus: A controlled study. *Journal of Rheumatology, 26*, 306–330.

Adams, S. G., Dammers, P. M., Saia, T. L., Brantley, P. J., & Gaydos, G. R. (1994). Stress, depression, and anxiety predict average symptom severity and daily symptom fluctuation is systemic lupus erythematosus. *Journal of Behavioral Medicine, 17*, 459–477.

Affleck, G., Pfeiffer, C., Tennen, H., & Fifield, J. (1988). Social support and psychosocial adjustment to rheumatoid arthritis. *Arthritis Care and Research, 1*, 71–77.

Affleck, G., Tennen, H., Keefe, F. J., Lefebvre, J. C., Kashikar-Zuck, S., Wright, K., … Caldwell, D. S. (1999). Everyday life with osteoarthritis or rheumatoid arthritis: Independent effects of disease and gender on daily pain, mood, and coping. *Pain, 83*, 601–609.

Alarcon, G. S., Rodriguez, J., Benavides, G., Brooks, K., Kurusz, H., & Reveille, J. D. (1999). Systemic lupus erythematosus in three ethnic groups: V. Acculturation, health-related attitudes and behaviors, and disease activity in Hispanic patients from the LUMINA cohort. *Arthritis Care and Research, 12*, 267–274.

Alarcon, G. S., Roseman, J. M., Bartolucci, A. A., Freidman, A. W., Moulds, J. M., Goel, N., ... Reville, J. D. (1998). Systemic lupus erythematosus in three ethnic groups: II. Features predictive of disease activity early in its course. *Arthritis & Rheumatism, 41,* 1173–1180.

Anderson, J. J., Wells, G., Verhoeven, A. C., & Felson, D. T. (2000). Factors predicting response to treatment in rheumatoid arthritis: The importance of disease duration. *Arthritis & Rheumatism, 43,* 22–29.

Archenholtz, B. C., Burckhardt, S., & Segesten, K. (1999). Quality of life of women with systemic lupus erythematosus or rheumatoid arthritis: Domains of importance and dissatisfaction. *Quality of Life Research, 8,* 411–416.

Astin, J. A. (2004). Mind–body therapies for the management of pain. *Clinical Journal of Pain, 20,* 27–32.

Astin, J. A., Beckner, W., Soeken, K., Hochberg, M. C., & Berman, B. (2002). Psychological interventions for rheumatoid arthritis: A meta-analysis of randomized controlled trials. *Arthritis & Rheumatism, 47,* 291–302.

Badr, H. (2004). Coping in marital dyads: A contextual perspective on the role of gender and health. *Personal Relationships, 11,* 197–211.

Bae, S., Hashimoto, H., Karlson, E., Liang, M., & Daltroy, L. (2001). Variable effects of social support by race, economic status, and disease activity in systemic lupus erythematosus. *Journal of Rheumatology, 28,* 1245–1251.

Bediako, S. M., & Friend, R. (2004). Illness-specific and general perceptions of social relationships in adjustment to rheumatoid arthritis: The role of interpersonal expectations. *Annals of Behavioral Medicine, 28,* 203–210.

Berkanovic, E., Oster, P., Wong, W. K., Bulpitt, K., Clements, P., Sterz, M., & Paulus, H. (1996). The relationship between socioeconomic status and recently diagnosed rheumatoid arthritis. *Arthritis Care and Research, 9,* 457–462.

Blalock, S. J., DeVellis, R. F., Brown, G. K., & Wallston, K. A. (1989). Validity of the Center for Epidemiological Studies Depression Scale in arthritis populations. *Arthritis & Rheumatism, 32,* 991–997.

Bolger, N., Zuckerman, A., & Kessler, R. (2000). Invisible support and adjustment to daily stress. *Journal of Personality and Social Psychology, 79,* 953–961.

Braden, C. J. (1992). Description of learned response to chronic illness: Depressed versus nondepressed self-help class participants. *Public Health Nursing, 9,* 103–108.

Braden, C. J., Brodt-Weinberg, R., Depka, L., McGlone, K., & Tretter, S. (1987). *Systemic lupus erythematosus (SLE) self-help course, leader's manual.* Atlanta, GA: Arthritis Foundation.

Braden, C. J., McGlone, K., & Pennington, F. (1993) Specific psychosocial and behavioral outcomes from the systemic lupus erythematosus self-help course. *Health Education Quarterly, 20,* 29–41.

Brannon, L. (1999). *Gender: Psychological perspectives* (2nd ed.). Boston, MA: Allyn and Bacon.

Brekke, M., Hjortdahl, P., Thelle, D. S., & Kvien, T. K. (1999). Disease activity and severity in patients with rheumatoid arthritis to socioeconomic inequality. *Social Science and Medicine, 48,* 1743–1750.

Burke, H. M., Zautra, A. J., Schultz, A. M., Reich, J. W., & Davis, M. C. (2002). Arthritis. In A. J. Christensen & M. H. Antoni (Eds.), *Chronic physical disorders* (pp. 268–287). Oxford, England: Blackwell.

Centers for Disease Control and Prevention (CDC). (2008, June). *Arthritis.* Retrieved from http://www.cdc.gov/arthritis

Chrisler, J. C., & Parrett, K. L. (1995). Women and autoimmune disorders. In A. L. Stanton & S. J. Gallant (Eds.), *The psychology of women's health: Progress and challenges in research and application* (pp. 171–195). Washington, DC: American Psychological Association.

Cohen, S., & Wills, T. A. (1985). Stress, social support, and the buffering hypothesis. *Psychological Bulletin, 98,* 310–357.

Conner, T., Tennen, H., Zautra, A., Affleck, G., Armeli, S., & Fifield, J. (2006). Coping with rheumatoid arthritis pain in daily life: Within-person analyses reveal hidden vulnerability for the formerly depressed. *Pain, 126,* 198–209.

Coty, M. B., & Wallston, K. (2008). Roles and well-being among healthy women and women with rheumatoid arthritis. *Journal of Advanced Nursing, 63,* 189–198.

Covic, T., Tyson, G., Spencer, D., & Howe, G. (2006). Depression in rheumatoid arthritis patients: Demographic, clinical, and psychological predictors. *Journal of Psychosomatic Research, 60,* 469–476.

Coyne, J. C., & Gottlieb, B. H. (1996). The mismeasure of coping by checklist. *Journal of Personality, 64,* 959–991.

Curry, S. L., Levine, M. N., Jones, P. K., & Kurit, D. M. (1993). Medical and psychosocial predictors of sexual outcome among women with systemic lupus erythematosus. *Arthritis Care and Research, 6,* 23–30.

Curry, S., Levine, S., Corty, E., Jones, P., Kurit, D. (1994). The impact of systemic lupus erythematosus on women's sexual functioning. *Journal of Rheumatology, 21,* 2254–2260.

Curtis, R., Groarke, A., Coughlan, R., & Gsel, A. (2005). Psychological stress as a predictor of psychological adjustment and health status in patients with rheumatoid arthritis. *Patient Education and Counseling, 59*, 192–198.

Da Costa, D., Dobkin, P. L., Pinard, L., Fortin, P. R., Danoff, D. S., Esdaile, J. M., & Clarke, A. E. (1999). The role of stress in functional disability among women with systemic lupus erythematosus: A prospective study. *Arthritis Care and Research, 2*, 112–119.

Danoff-Burg, S., Agee, J. D., Romanoff, N. R., Kremer, J. M., & Strosberg, J. M. (2006). Benefit finding and expressive writing in adults with lupus or rheumatoid arthritis. *Psychology and Health, 21*, 651–665.

Danoff-Burg, S., Ayala, J., & Revenson, T. A. (2000). Researcher knows best? Toward a closer match between the concept and measurement of coping. *Journal of Health Psychology, 5*, 183–194.

Danoff-Burg, S., & Friedberg, F. (2009). Unmet needs of patients with systemic lupus erythematosus. *Behavioral Medicine, 35*, 5–13.

Danoff-Burg, S., & Revenson, T. A. (2000). Rheumatic illness and relationships: Coping as a joint venture. In K. B. Schmaling & T. G. Sher (Eds.), *The psychology of couples and illness: Theory, research, and practice* (pp. 105–133). Washington, DC: American Psychological Association.

Danoff-Burg, S., & Revenson, T. A. (2005a). Benefit-finding among patients with rheumatoid arthritis: Positive effects on interpersonal relationships. *Journal of Behavioral Medicine, 28*, 91–103.

Danoff-Burg, S., & Revenson, T. A. (2005b). Psychosocial aspects of the rheumatic diseases. In S. A. Paget, A. Gibofsky, J. F. Beary, III, & T. Sculco (Eds.), *Manual of rheumatology and outpatient orthopedic disorders: Diagnosis and therapy* (5th ed., pp. 70–79). Philadelphia, PA: Lippincott Williams & Wilkins.

Danoff-Burg, S., Revenson, T. A., Trudeau, K. J, & Paget, S. A. (2004). Unmitigated communion, social constraints, and psychological distress among women with rheumatoid arthritis. *Journal of Personality, 72*, 29–46.

Demange, V., Guillemin, F., Baumann, M., Suurmeijer, T. P. B. M., Moum, T., Doeglas, D., … van den Heuvel, W. J. A. (2004). Are there more than cross-sectional relationships of social support and support networks with functional limitations and psychological distress in early rheumatoid arthritis? The European Research on Incapacitating Diseases and Social Support Longitudinal Study. *Arthritis & Rheumatism, 51*, 782–791.

De Roos, A. J., & Callahan, L. F. (1999). Differences by sex in correlates of work status in rheumatoid arthritis patients. *Arthritis Care and Research, 12*, 381–491.

DeVellis, B. M. (1993). Depression in rheumatologic diseases. *Balliere's Clinical Rheumatology, 7*, 241–257.

Dixon, K. E., Keefe, F. J., Scipio, C. D., Perri, L. M., & Abernethy, A. P. (2007). Psychological interventions for arthritis pain management in adults: A meta-analysis. *Health Psychology, 26*, 241–250.

Dobkin, P. L., Da Costa, D., Fortin, P. R., Edworthy, S., Barr, S., Esdaile, J. M., … Clarke, A. E. (2001). Living with lupus: A prospective pan-Canadian study. *Journal of Rheumatology, 28*, 2442–2448.

Dobkin, P. L., Da Costa, D., Joseph, L., Fortin, P. R., Edworthy, S., Barr, S., … Clarke, A. E. (2002). Counterbalancing patient demands with evidence: Results from a pan-Canadian randomized clinical trial of brief supportive-expressive group psychotherapy for women with systemic lupus erythematosus. *Annals of Behavioral Medicine, 24*(2), 88–99.

Dobkin, P. L., Fortin, P. R., Joseph, L., Esdaile, J. M., Danoff, D. S., & Clarke, A. E. (1998). Psychosocial contributors to mental and physical health in patients with systemic lupus erythematosus. *Arthritis Care and Research, 11*, 23–31.

Dowdy, S. W., Dwyer, K. A., Smith, C. A., & Wallston, K. A. (1996). Gender and psychosocial well-being of persons with rheumatoid arthritis. *Arthritis Care and Research, 9*, 449–456.

Druley, J. A., Stephens, M. A. P., & Coyne, J. C. (1997). Emotional and physical intimacy in coping with lupus: Women's dilemmas of disclosure and approach. *Health Psychology, 16*, 506–514.

Druley, J. A., & Townsend, A. L. (1998). Self-esteem as a mediator between spousal support and depressive symptoms: A comparison of healthy individuals and individuals coping with arthritis. *Health Psychology, 17*, 255–261.

Dwyer, K. A., Bess, C., & Smith, C. (1996). Active versus passive coping: An in-depth exploration of the coping profiles. *Arthritis Care and Research, 9*, S9.

Escalante, A., del Rincon, I., & Mulrow, C. D. (2000). Symptoms of depression and psychological distress among Hispanics with rheumatoid arthritis. *Arthritis Care and Research, 13*, 156–167.

Evers, A. W. M., Kraaimaat, F. W., Geene, R., Jacobs, J. W. G., & Bijlsma, J. W. J. (2003). Pain coping and social support as predictors of long-term functional disability and pain in early rheumatoid arthritis. *Behaviour Research and Therapy, 41*, 1295–1310.

Fekete, E. M., Stephens, M. A. P., Mickelson, K. M., & Druley, J. A. (2007). Couples' support provision during illness: The role of perceived emotional responsiveness. *Families, Systems and Health, 25*, 204–217.

Felton, B. J., & Revenson, T. A. (1984). Coping with chronic illness: A study of illness controllability and the influence of coping strategies on psychological adjustment. *Journal of Consulting and Clinical Psychology*, 52, 343–353.

Fernandez, M., Alarcon, G. S., Calvo-Alen, J., Andrade, R., McGwin, G., Vila, L. M., Reveille, J. D. (with the LUMINA Study Group). (2007). A multiethnic, multicenter cohort of patients with systemtic lupus erythematosus (SLE) as a model for the study of ethnic disparities in SLE. *Arthritis & Rheumatism*, 57, 576–584.

Figueiras, M. J., & Weinman, J. (2003). Do similar patient and spouse perceptions of myocardial infarction predict recovery? *Psychology and Health*, 18, 201–216.

Fite, J., & Kopala, M. (2003). Chronic fatigue syndrome, fibromyalgia, multiple sclerosis, and lupus: Meeting the challenges. In M. Kopala & M. A. Keitel (Eds.), *Handbook of Counseling Women* (pp. 392–410). Thousand Oaks, CA: Sage.

Friedman, A. W., Alarcon, G. S., McGwin, G., Straaton, K. V., Roseman, J. M., Goel, N., & Reveille, J. D. (1999). Systemic lupus erythematosus in three ethnic groups: IV. Factors associated with self-reported functional outcome in a large cohort study. *Arthritis Care and Research*, 12, 256–266.

Gladman, D. D., Urowitz, M. B., Gough, O., & MacKinnon, A. (1996). Lack of correlation among the 3 outcomes describing SLE: disease activity, damage and quality of life. *Clinical and Experimental Rheumatology*, 14, 305–308.

Goodman, D., Morrissey, S., Graham, D., & Bossingham, D. (2005). The application of cognitive-behaviour therapy in altering illness representations of systemic lupus erythematosus. *Behaviour Change*, 22, 156–171.

Greco, C. M., Rudy, T. E., & Manzi, S. (2004). Effects of a stress-reduction program on psychological function, pain, and physical function of systemic lupus erythematosus patients: A randomized controlled trial. *Arthritis & Rheumatism*, 51, 625–634.

Hanly, J. (1997). Disease activity, cumulative damage and quality of life in systemic lupus erythematosus: Results of a cross-sectional study. *Lupus*, 6, 243–247.

Harris, E. D. (1993). Clinical features of rheumatoid arthritis. In W. N. Kelley, E. D. Harris, S. Ruddy, & C. B. Sledge (Eds.), *Textbook of rheumatology* (4th ed., pp. 874–911). Philadelphia, PA: W. B. Sauders.

Hewlett, S., Cockshott, Z., Byron, M., Kitchen, K., Tipler, S., Pope, D., … Hehir, M. (2005). Patients' perceptions of fatigue in rheumatoid arthritis: Overwhelming, uncontrollable, ignored. *Arthritis & Rheumatism*, 53, 697–702.

Holtzman, S., Newth, S., & Delongis, A. (2004). The role of social support in coping with daily pain among patients with rheumatoid arthritis. *Journal of Health Psychology*, 9, 677–695.

Hommel, K. A., Wagner, J. L., Chaney, J. M., & Mullins, L. L. (1998). Gender-specific effects of depression on functional disability in rheumatoid arthritis: A prospective study. *International Journal of Rehabilitation and Health*, 4, 183–191.

Jacobi, C. E., Mol, G. D., Boshuizen, H. C., Rupp, I., Dinant, H. J., & Van Den Bos, G. A. (2003). Impact of socioeconomic status on the course of rheumatoid arthritis and on related use of health care services. *Arthritis & Rheumatism*, 49, 567–573.

Jordan, M. S., Lumley, M. A., & Leisen, J. C. C. (1998). The relationships of cognitive coping and pain control beliefs to pain and adjustment among African-American and Caucasian women with rheumatoid arthritis. *Arthritis Care and Research*, 11, 80–88.

Karasz, A., & Ouellette, S. C. (1995). Role strain and psychological well-being in women with systemic lupus erythematosus. *Women and Health*, 23, 41–57.

Karlen, A. (2002). Positive sexual effects of chronic illness: Case studies of women with lupus (SLE). *Sexuality and Disability*, 20, 191–208.

Karlson, E., Daltroy, L., Lew, R., Wright, E. A., Partridge, A. J., Fossel, A. H., … Liang, M. H. (1997). The relationship of socioeconomic status, race, and modifiable risk factors to outcomes in patients with systemic lupus erythematosus. *Arthritis & Rheumatism*, 40, 47–56.

Karlson, E., Daltroy, L., Lew, R., Wright, E. A., Partridge, A. J., Roberts, W. N., … Liang, M. H. (1995). The independence and stability of socioeconomic predictors of morbidity in systemic lupus erythematosus. *Arthritis & Rheumatism*, 38, 267–273.

Karlson, E. W., Liang, M. H., Eaton, H., Huang, J., Fitzgerald, L., Rogers, M. P., & Daltroy, L. H. (2004). A randomized clinical trial of a psychoeducational intervention to improve outcomes in systemic lupus erythematosus. *Arthritis & Rheumatism*, 50, 1832–1841.

Katz, P. P., & Yelin, E. H. (1995). The development of depressive symptoms among women with rheumatoid arthritis: The role of function. *Arthritis & Rheumatism*, 38, 49–56.

Katz, R. C., Flasher, L., Cacciapaglia, H., & Nelson, S. (2001). The psychosocial impact of cancer and lupus: A cross-validation study that extends the generality of "benefit-finding" in patients with chronic disease. *Journal of Behavioral Medicine*, 24, 561–571.

Keefe, F. J., Affleck, G., Lefebvre, J., Starr, K., Caldwell, D., S., & Tennen, H. (1997). Coping strategies and coping efficacy in rheumatoid arthritis: A daily process analysis. *Pain*, *69*, 43–48.

Keefe, F. J., Affleck, G., Lefebvre, J., Underwood, L., Caldwell, D., S., Drew, J., … Pargament, K. (2001). Living with rheumatoid arthritis: The role of daily spirituality and daily religion and spiritual coping. *Journal of Pain*, *2*, 101–110.

Keefe, F. J., Smith, S. J., Buffington, A. L. H., Gibson, J., Studts, J. L., & Caldwell, D. S. (2002). Recent advances and future directions in the biopsychosocial assessment and treatment of arthritis. *Journal of Consulting and Clinical Psychology*, *70*, 640–655.

Kraaimaatt, F. W., Bakker, A. H., Janssen, E., & Bijlsma, J. W. J. (1996). Intrusiveness of rheumatoid arthritis on sexuality in male and female patients living with a spouse. *Arthritis Care and Research*, *9*, 120–135.

Lorig, K., & Fries, J. F. (2006). *The arthritis helpbook* (6th ed.). Cambridge, MA: Da Capo Press.

Lorig, K., Gonzalez, V. M., & Ritter, P. (1999). Community-based Spanish language arthritis education program: A randomized trial. *Medical Care*, *37*, 957–963.

Lorig, K., & Holman, H. R. (1989). Long-term outcomes of an arthritis self-management study: Effects of reinforcement efforts. *Social Science and Medicine*, *29*, 221–224.

Lorig, K., Lubeck, D., Kraines, R. G., Seleznick, M., & Holman, H. R. (1985). Outcomes of self-help education for patients with arthritis. *Arthritis & Rheumatism*, *28*, 680–685.

Lotstein, D. S, Ward, M. M., Bush, T. M., Lambert, R. E., van Vollenhoven, R., & Neuwelt, C. M. (1998). Socioeconomic status and health in women with systemic lupus erythematosus. *Journal of Rheumatology*, *25*, 1720–1729.

Majerovitz, S. D., & Revenson, T. A. (1994). Sexuality and rheumatic disease: The significance of gender. *Arthritis Care and Research*, *7*, 29–34.

Manne, S. L., & Zautra, A. J. (1989). Spouse criticism and support: Their association with coping and psychological adjustment among women with rheumatoid arthritis. *Journal of Personality and Social Psychology*, *56*, 608–617.

Manne, S. L., & Zautra, A. J. (1992). Coping with arthritis: Current status and critique. *Arthritis & Rheumatism*, *35*, 1273–1280.

Marshall, E. (2002). Lupus: Mysterious disease holds its secrets tight. *Science*, *296*, 659–691.

McKinley, P., Ouellette, S., & Winkel, G. (1995). The contributions of disease activity, sleep patterns, and depression to fatigue in systemic lupus erythematosus. *Arthritis and Rheumatism*, *38*, 826–834.

Melamed, B. G., & Brenner, G. F. (1990). Social support and chronic medical stress: An interaction-based approach. *Journal of Social and Clinical Psychology*, *9*, 104–117.

Moses, N., Wiggers, J., Nicholas, C., & Cockburn, J. (2005). Prevalence and correlates of perceived unmet needs of people with systemic lupus erythematosus. *Patient Education and Counseling*, *57*, 30–38.

Navarrete-Navarrete, N., Peralta-Ramírez, M. I., Sabio-Sánchez, J. M., Coín, M. A., Robles-Ortega, H., Hidalgo-Tenorio, C., … Jiménez-Alonso, J. (2010). Efficacy of cognitive behavioural therapy for the treatment of chronic stress in patients with lupus erythematosus: A randomized controlled trial. *Psychotherapy and Psychosomatics*, *79*, 107–115.

Nery, F. G., Borba, E. F., Hatch, J. P., Soares, J. C., Bonfá, E., & Neto, F. L. (2007). Major depressive disorder and disease activity in systemic lupus erythematosus. *Comprehensive Psychiatry*, *48*, 14–19.

Newman, S. P., Fitzpatrick, R., Lamb, R., & Shipley, M. (1989). The origins of depressed mood in rheumatoid arthritis. *Journal of Rheumatology*, *16*, 740–744.

Newman, S. P., & Revenson, T. A. (1993). Coping with rheumatoid arthritis. *Balliere's Clinical Rheumatology*, *7*, 259–280.

Newth, S., & Delongis, A. (2004). Individual differences, mood, and coping with chronic pain in rheumatoid arthritis: A daily process analysis. *Psychology and Health*, *19*, 283–305.

Öst, L. (2008). Efficacy of the third wave of behavioral therapies: A systematic review and meta-analysis. *Behaviour Research and Therapy*, *46*, 296–321.

Parker, J. C., Frank, R. G., Beck, N. C., Smarr, K. L., Buescher, K. L., Phillips, L. R., … Walker, S. E. (1988). Pain management in rheumatoid arthritis patients. *Arthritis & Rheumatism*, *31*, 593–601.

Parrish, B. P., Zautra, A. J., & Davis, M. C. (2008). The role of positive and negative interpersonal events on daily fatigue in women with fibromyalgia, rheumatoid arthritis, and osteoarthritis. *Health Psychology*, *27*, 694–702.

Pawlak, L. R., Witte, T., Heiken H., Hundt, M., Schubert, J., Wiese, B., … Schedlowski, M. (2003). Flares in patients with systemic lupus erythematosus are associated with daily psychological stress. *Psychotherapy and Psychosomatics*, *72*, 159–165.

Petri, M. (1995). Clinical features of systemic lupus erythematosus. *Current Opinion in Rheumatology, 7*, 395–401.

Petri, M. (2000). Systemic lupus erythematosus: Women's health issues. *Bulletin on the Rheumatic Diseases, 49*, 1–3.

Poole, J. L., Chiappisi, H., Cordova, J. S., & Sibbitt, W., Jr. (2007). Quality of life in American Indian and White women with and without rheumatoid arthritis. *American Journal of Occupational Therapy, 61*, 280–289.

Pradhan, E. K., Baumgarten, M., Langenberg, P., Handwerger, B., Gilpin, A. K., Magyari, T., … Berman, B. M. (2007). Effect of mindfulness-based stress reduction in rheumatoid arthritis patients. *Arthritis & Rheumatism, 57*, 1134–1142.

Ramjeet, J., Smith, J., & Adams, M. (2008). The relationship between coping and psychological and physical adjustment in rheumatoid arthritis: A literature review. *Journal of Clinical Nursing. 17*, 418–428.

Repping-Wuts, H., Fransen, J., van-Achterberg, T., Bleijenberg, G., & van-Riel, O. (2007). Persistent severe fatigue in patients with rheumatoid arthritis. *Journal of Clinical Nursing, 16*, 377–383.

Revenson, T. A. (1990). Not all things are equal: An ecological approach to personality and disease. In H. S. Friedman (Ed.), *Personality and disease* (pp. 65–94). New York, NY: Wiley.

Revenson, T. A. (1993). The role of social support with rheumatic disease. *Bailliere's Clinical Rheumatology, 7*, 377–396.

Revenson, T. A. (1994). Social support and marital coping with chronic illness. *Annals of Behavioral Medicine, 16*, 122–130.

Revenson, T. A. (2003). Scenes from a marriage: Examining support, coping, and gender within the context of chronic illness. In J. Suls & K. Wallston (Eds.), *Social psychological foundations of health and illness* (pp. 530–559). Malden, MA: Blackwell.

Revenson, T. A. K., Kayser, K., & Bodenmann, G. (2005). Introduction. In T. A. Revenson, K. Kayser, & G. Bodenmann (Eds.), *Couples coping with chronic stress* (pp. 3–10). Washington, DC: American Psychological Association.

Revenson, T. A, & Majerovitz, S. D. (1990). Spouses' support provision to chronically ill patients. *Journal of Social and Personal Relationships, 7*, 575–586.

Revenson, T. A., Schiaffino, K. M., Majerovitz, S. D., & Gibofsky, A. (1991). Social support as a double-edged sword: The relation of positive and problematic support to depression among rheumatoid arthritis patients, *Social Science and Medicine, 7*, 807–813.

Riemsma, R. P, Taal, E., & Rasker, J. J. (2000). Perceptions about perceived functional disabilities and pain of people with rheumatoid arthritis: Differences between patients and their spouses and correlates with well-being. *Arthritis Care and Research, 13*, 255–261.

Robbins, L., Allegrante, J., & Paget, S. (1993). Adapting the systemic lupus erythematosus self-help (SLESH) course for Latino SLE patients. *Arthritis Care and Research, 6*, 97–103.

Rupp, I., Boshuizen, H. C., Jacobi, C. E., Dinant, H. J., & van den Bos, G. A. M. (2004). Impact of fatigue on health-related quality of life in rheumatoid arthritis. *Arthritis & Rheumatism, 51*, 578–585.

Ruzicka, S. A. (1998). Pain beliefs: What do elders believe? *Journal of Holistic Nursing, 16*, 369–383.

Seawell, A. H., & Danoff-Burg, S. (2004). Psychosocial research on systemic lupus erythematosus: A literature review. *Lupus, 13*, 891–899.

Seawell, A. H, & Danoff-Burg, S. (2005). Body image and sexuality in women with and without systemic lupus erythematosus. *Sex Roles, 53*, 865–876.

Segui, J., Ramos-Casals, M., Garcia-Carrasco, M., de Flores, T., Cervera, R., Valdes, M., … Ingelmo, M. (2000). Psychiatric and psychosocial disorders in patients with systemic lupus erythematosus: A longitudinal study of active and inactive stages of disease. *Lupus, 9*, 584–588.

Sharpe, L., Sensky, T., & Allard, S. (2001). The course of depression in recent onset rheumatoid arthritis: The predictive role of disability, illness perceptions, pain and coping. *Journal of Psychosomatic Research, 51*, 713–719.

Sharpe, L., Sensky, T., Timberlake, N., Ryan, B., Brewin, C. R., & Allard, S. (2001). A blind, randomized, controlled trial of cognitive-behavioural intervention for patients with recent onset rheumatoid arthritis: Preventing psychological and physical morbidity. *Pain, 89*, 275–283.

Siegel, D. M., & Baum, J. (2004). Rheumatic disease and sexuality. In D. Isenberg, P. Maddison, P. Woo, D. Glass, & F. Breedveld (Eds.), *Oxford textbook of rheumatology* (3rd ed., pp. 279–285). New York, NY: Oxford University Press.

Sinclair, V. G., & Wallston, K. A. (2004). The Development and Psychometric Evaluation of the Brief Resilient Coping Scale. *Assessment, 11*, 94–101.

Smith, B. W., & Zautra, A. J. (2008a). The effects of anxiety and depression on weekly pain in women with arthritis. *Pain*, *138*, 354–361.

Smith, B. W., & Zautra, A. J. (2008b). Vulnerability and resilience in women with arthritis: Test of a two-factor model. *Journal of Consulting and Clinical Psychology*, *76*, 799–810.

Sokka, T., Toloza, S., Cutolo, M., Kautiainen, H., Makinen, H., Gogus, F., … Pincus, T. (2009). Women, men, and rheumatoid arthritis: Analyses of disease activity, disease characteristics, and treatments in the QUEST-RA Study. *Arthritis Research and Therapy*, *11*, R7.

Sperry, L. (2006). Biopsychosocial aspects of some common chronic illnesses. In L. Sperry (Ed.), *Psychological treatment of chronic illness: The biopsychosocial therapy approach* (pp. 41–64). Washington, DC: American Psychological Association.

Sterba, K. R., DeVellis, R. F., Lewis, M. A., DeVellis, B. M., Jordan, J. M., & Baucom, D. H. (2008). Effect of couple illness perception congruence on psychological adjustment in women with rheumatoid arthritis. *Health Psychology*, *27*, 221–229.

Strand, E. B., Zautra, A. J., Thoresen, M., Odegård, S., Uhlig, T., & Finset, A. (2006). Positive affect as a factor of resilience in the pain–negative affect relationship in patients with rheumatoid arthritis. *Journal of Psychosomatic Research*, *60*, 477–484.

Sutcliffe, N., Clarke, A. E., Gordon, C., Farewell, V., & Isenberg, D. (1999). The association of socio-economic status, race, psychosocial factors and outcome in patients with systemic lupus erythematosus. *Rheumatology*, *38*, 1130–1137.

Sutcliffe, N., Clarke, A. E., Levinton, C., Frost, C., Gordon, C., & Isenberg, A. (1999). Associates of health status in patients with systemic lupus erythematosus. *Journal of Rheumatology*, *26*, 2352–2356.

Tennen, H., Affleck, G., Urrows, S., Higgins, P., & Mendola, R. (1992). Perceiving control, construing benefits, and daily processes in rheumatoid arthritis. *Canadian Journal of Behavioral Science*, *24*, 186–203.

Theis, K. A., Helmick, C. G., & Hootman, J. M. (2007). Arthritis burden and impact are greater among U.S. women than men: Intervention opportunities. *Journal of Women's Health*, *16*, 441–453.

Trudeau, K. J., Danoff–Burg, S., Revenson, T. A., & Paget, S. A. (2003). Agency and communion in people with rheumatoid arthritis. *Sex Roles*, *49*, 303–311.

Trupin, L., Tonner, M. C., Yazdany, J., Julian, L. J., Criswell, L. A., Katz, P. P., & Yelin, E. (2008). The role of neighborhood and individual socioeconomic status in outcomes of systemic lupus erythematosus. *Journal of Rheumatology*, *35*, 1782–1788.

Van Middendorp, H., Geenen, R., Sorbi, M. J., Hox, J. H., Vingerhoets, A. J. J. M., van Doornen, L. J. P., & Bijlsma, J. W. J. (2005). Gender differences in emotion regulation and relationships with perceived health in patients with rheumatoid arthritis. *Women and Health*, *42*, 75–97.

Ward, M., Lotstein, D., Bush, T., Lambert, E., van Vollenhoven, R., & Neuwelt, C. (1999). Psychosocial correlates of morbidity in women with systemic lupus erythematosus. *Journal of Rheumatology*, *26*, 2153–2158.

Waterloo, K., Omdal, R., Husby, G., & Mellgren, S. I. (1998). Emotional status in systemic lupus erythematosus. *Scandinavian Journal of Rheumatology*, *27*, 410–414.

Wright, G. E., Parker, J. C., Smarr, K. L., Johnson, J. C., Hewett, J. E., & Walker, S. E. (1998). Age, depressive symptoms, and rheumatoid arthritis. *Arthritis & Rheumatism*, *41*, 298–305.

Yoshiuchi, K., Yamamoto, Y., & Akabayashi, A. (2008). Application of ecological momentary assessment in stress-related diseases. *BioPsychoSocial Medicine*, *2*, 13.

Zautra, A., J., Burleson, M. H., Matt, K. S., Roth, S., & Burrows, L. (1994). Interpersonal stress, depression, and disease activity in rheumatoid arthritis and osteoarthritis patients. *Health Psychology*, *13*, 139–148.

Zautra, A. J., Davis, M. C., Reich, J. W., Nicassario, P., Tennen, H., Finan, P., … Irwin, M. R. (2008). Comparison of cognitive behavioral and mindfulness meditation interventions on adaptation to rheumatoid arthritis for patients with and without history of recurrent depression. *Journal of Consulting and Clinical Psychology*, *76*, 408–421.

Zautra, A., J., Hamilton, N. A., Potter, P., & Smith, B. (1999). Field research on the relationship between stress and disease activity in rheumatoid arthritis. *Annals of New York Academy of Sciences*, *876*, 397–412.

Zautra, A. J., & Manne, S. L. (1992). Coping with rheumatoid arthritis: A review of a decade of research. *Annals of Behavioral Medicine*, *14*, 31–39.

Zautra, A. J., & Smith, B. W. (2001). Depression and reactivity to stress in older women with rheumatoid arthritis and osteoarthritis. *Psychosomatic Medicine*, *63*, 687–696.

Zonana-Nacach, A., Roseman, J. M., McGwin, G. J., Friedman, A. W., Baethge, B. A., Reveille, J. D., & Alarcon, G. S. (2000). Systemic lupus erythematosus in three ethnic groups: VI. Factors associated with fatigue within 5 years of criteria diagnosis. *Lupus*, *9*, 101–109.

33 Psychological and Biobehavioral Processes in HIV Disease

Michael H. Antoni
University of Miami

Adam W. Carrico
University of California, San Francisco Center for AIDS Prevention Studies

This chapter will focus on the application of health psychology in the context of human immunodeficiency virus and acquired immune deficiency syndrome (HIV/AIDS). Over the past 30 years, health psychology has emerged as a mainstream area of scientific inquiry that is broadly concerned with contributing to the prevention and treatment of disease. A number of psychologists in this dynamic field draw upon basic psychobiological theory and research to develop investigations that are aimed at enhancing the capacity of individuals to manage a variety of such chronic medical conditions as coronary heart disease, different cancers, and HIV/AIDS. Although health psychology is becoming increasingly specialized as a result of dramatic advances in our understanding of the basic pathophysiology of a number of chronic diseases, the field is unified by an explicit focus on research that (a) examines the role of psychological factors in the prevention or amelioration of disease, and (b) elucidates the biobehavioral pathways that explain the effects of psychological factors on disease management and course (see Figure 33.1).

In this chapter, we build upon this basic model to summarize health psychology research that examines the biobehavioral mechanisms whereby psychological processes may modulate HIV disease outcomes. We shall demonstrate these mechanisms by summarizing longitudinal research showing that affective states, psychosocial processes, and health behaviors contribute importantly to variability in the physical course of HIV/AIDS; that numerous aspects of stress physiology and neuroendocrine regulation may mediate these associations; and that psychosocial and behavioral interventions targeting optimal stress management and health behavior changes can affect both quality of life and objective indicators of physical health (immunologic status and opportunistic disease processes) in persons dealing with the challenges of this chronic life-changing condition. As experts in understanding chronic stress, psychosocial resources, and behavior change processes in the context of disease prevention and management, health psychologists stand to make major contributions to biobehavioral research and evidence-based practice in HIV/AIDS in the coming decade.

PATHOPHYSIOLOGY OF HIV INFECTION

In the early days of what has come to be known as AIDS, there were no effective treatments for the then-fatal condition, physical symptoms were variable, and the causative agent remained undiscovered. Even after the discovery that HIV was responsible for this emerging syndrome, medical treatments would be unavailable for years. Under this set of circumstances, persons with HIV were instructed to make basic lifestyle adaptations in the hope of impacting life expectancy and

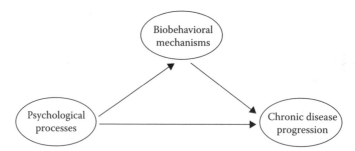

FIGURE 33.1 Associations between such psychological processes as affective states and the progression of chronic diseases may be explained by biobehavioral mechanisms studied by health psychologists.

enhancing quality of life by delaying the insidious progression to AIDS. Fortunately, since the beginning of the epidemic, scientific knowledge regarding the pathogenesis of HIV infection has grown dramatically.

HIV is a retrovirus belonging to the lentivirus subtype that displays a specific cell tropism for a subset of lymphocytes defined by the expression of a surface T4 glycoprotein (Klatzmann et al., 1984). Glycoprotein 120 (gp120) allows HIV to bind to the T4 glycoprotein and its coreceptor (CXCR4 or CCR5) at the cell surface. After binding, the virus uncoats, releasing HIV RNA into the cell cytoplasm. Utilizing the reverse transcriptase enzyme, HIV DNA is produced. Then, viral DNA migrates to the nucleus, where the integrase enzyme merges HIV with the cellular DNA to become a provirus. After integration, the viral replication mechanisms of HIV become almost entirely host dependent (Varmus, 1988). Making use of its host cell's resources, viral transcription of HIV RNA and protein synthesis ensue. Finally, the protease enzyme cleaves the HIV RNA into segments that migrate into viral capsids and bud out of the infected cell. As a result of the rapid replication rate of HIV as well as its propensity toward mutation, the arrangement of glycoproteins on its capsid is in a constant state of change, which impairs the effectiveness of both humoral and cell-mediated immune mechanisms in controlling the infection. Thus, HIV infection is characterized by the progressive decline in a subset of cells that coordinate the acquired immune response, T-helper (CD4+) cells, and the process of HIV replication is continuous (Gaines et al., 1990).

Progression to AIDS is conceptualized as occurring in three distinct stages (Rutherford, Lifson, & Hessol, 1990). Many individuals who have recently been infected with HIV develop an acute mononucleosis-like syndrome about a month after seroconversion (Tindall & Cooper, 1991). In addition, during the 4 to 12 weeks following infection, individuals display a markedly elevated HIV viral load—an index of the amount of free virus in circulation (Clerici, Berzofski, Shearer, & Tacket, 1991). Those individuals who have recently been infected with HIV appear to be at substantially elevated risk of transmitting the virus because of this elevated HIV viral load and an increased likelihood that they are not yet aware they are HIV-positive (Pinkerton, 2008). A period of clinical latency, lasting for a number of years, follows the initial sequence of acute infection, viral dissemination, development of HIV-specific immunity, and curtailment of extensive viral replication. During the clinically latent period, one observes an increasing viral load, decrements in CD4+ cell count, and an increasing proportion of HIV-infected lymphoid cells (Pantaleo, Graziosi, & Fauci, 1993). Following this period of clinical latency, most individuals develop full-blown AIDS (Kaplan, Wofsky, & Volberding, 1987). AIDS is defined as a decline in the number of CD4+ cells to critically low levels (< 200 cell/mm^3) or clinical signs consistent with the emergence of AIDS-defining opportunistic infections or neoplasias (Centers for Disease Control, 1992).

Although ongoing monitoring of the CD4+ cell count and viral load are part of the standard of care for the medical management of HIV infection, long-term follow-up is often necessary to observe clinically meaningful changes (Dybul, Fauci, Bartlett, Kaplan, & Pau, 2002). As a result, other measures may provide unique information regarding the ongoing immune status of HIV-positive persons. For example, individuals with AIDS who remain healthy despite having critically low CD4+ cell counts display a relative preservation of natural killer (NK) cells and natural killer cell cytotoxicity (NKCC), innate immune parameters that are important for the surveillance of pathogens and neoplasias (Ironson et al., 2001). Inconsistent findings have been reported regarding the clinical prognostic value of T-cytotoxic/suppressor (CD8+) cell counts. CD8+ cells are responsible for the destruction of cells that have been infected by pathogens and suppression of neoplastic cell growth. It seems that preservation of certain subsets of CD8+ cells (e.g., memory CD8+) may be associated with enhanced immunosurveillance. However, increases in activated CD8+ (CD8+38+) cells appear to predict hastened HIV disease progression, particularly in later disease stages (Giorgi et al., 1999). Furthermore, such other markers of immune activation as neopterin have been shown to independently predict more rapid HIV disease progression (Mildvan et al., 2005). Studies examining these diverse immune parameters may provide insight into the possible pathways whereby psychological factors influence HIV disease progression. It is these biological parameters that frequently constitute the outcome variables used in health psychology research in HIV/AIDS. One of the most widely studied psychological factors in this field is the affective state of individuals dealing with HIV/AIDS.

AFFECTIVE STATES AND HIV DISEASE PROGRESSION

Given the many stressors inherent in HIV infection, successful disease management involves addressing psychological as well as biomedical issues (Schneiderman et al., 1994). The anticipation and the impact of HIV antibody test notification; the emergence of the first symptoms of disease; changes in vocational plans, lifestyle behaviors, and interpersonal relationships; and the burdens of complex antiretroviral therapy (ART) regimens are all highly stressful. Although reductions in mood disturbance have been observed following the introduction of ART (Rabkin, Ferrando, Lin, Sewell, & McElhiney, 2000), recent epidemiologic investigations estimate that approximately half of a sample of 2,864 HIV-positive patients screened positive for a psychiatric disorder over a one-year period, including major depression, dysthymia, and generalized anxiety disorder (Bing et al., 2001). In fact, the risk of developing major depressive disorder is two times higher in HIV-positive samples (Ciesla & Roberts, 2001). Although effectively managing depressive symptoms and other forms of negative affect may be important, recent research informed by stress and coping theory suggests an independent role for positive affect (Folkman & Moskowitz, 2000). Positive affect can occur with relatively high frequency in the midst of a chronic stressor such as living with HIV, and investigations informed by stress and coping theory have observed that positive affect serves important adaptive functions (Folkman, 2008). The clinical relevance of distinct affective states is further supported by burgeoning research examining both negative and positive affect as predictors of HIV disease progression.

Findings across investigations provide impressive evidence that elevated depressed mood and depressive symptoms may result in decrements in immune status, hastened HIV disease progression, and mortality (Leserman, 2008). However, the directionality of this relationship has been hotly debated. Given that clinically significant reductions in HIV viral load have been observed to predict decreased distress (Kalichman, Difonzo, Austin, Luke, & Rompa, 2002), longitudinal investigations with repeated measurements of psychological and immunologic data provide the most reliable findings with regard to the temporal associations between depression and HIV disease progression. For example, previous investigations have observed that depressive symptoms were associated with reductions in CD8+ and NK cell counts over a two-year period, especially among those individuals reporting more stressful life events (Leserman et al., 1997). Although depressive symptoms have been associated with more rapid CD4+ cell count decline in cohorts of HIV-positive men (Burack et al., 1993; Vedhara et al., 1997) and women (Ickovics et al., 2001), other longitudinal investigations that utilized *only* baseline measurements of depressive symptoms have not observed similar effects (Lyketsos et al., 1993; Patterson et al., 1996). Another investigation of HIV-positive men and women who had not yet progressed to AIDS indicated that the relationship between depression and cell-mediated immunity is observed only in participants with low levels of HIV viral burden (Motivala et al., 2003). Specifically, increased distress was associated with lower total CD4+, memory CD4+, and B cell counts; but only in those subjects with viral load ≤ 1 standard deviation below the mean. These findings may partially explain discrepant results regarding the association between depressive symptoms and CD4+ cell counts, suggesting that depression may be a more potent predictor of HIV disease progression among individuals in the early stages.

Other investigations with HIV-positive women have observed that symptoms of depression are associated with more activated CD8+ cells (CD8+38+) and higher HIV viral load (Evans et al., 2002), both of which are independently associated with more rapid HIV disease progression. In this cross-sectional investigation, a diagnosis of major depression was also related to lower NKCC. More important, women whose major depression resolved over time showed concurrent increases in NKCC up to two years later (Cruess et al., 2005). The continued relevance of negative mood in the era of ART is further supported by observations that cumulative depressive symptoms, hopelessness, and avoidant-coping scores were associated with decreased CD4+ cell counts and higher HIV viral load over a two-year period in a diverse sample of HIV-positive men and women (Ironson et al., 2005). These effects of negative mood and avoidant coping on immune status held after controlling for ART adherence.

Results from one randomized controlled trial of a group-based cognitive-behavioral stress management (CBSM) intervention lend further support for the relevance of negative mood in the ART era. HIV-positive gay and bisexual men were randomized to CBSM with medication adherence training (CBSM+MAT) or MAT alone. Among those who presented with detectable HIV viral load at baseline, men in CBSM+MAT displayed a .56 $\log_{10}$ reduction in HIV viral load over the 15 months following randomization after controlling for self-reported ART adherence. This statistically significant and clinically interesting decrease in HIV viral load was mediated by reductions in depressed mood during the 10-week intervention period (Antoni, Carrico, et al., 2006). Although these findings are promising, significant methodological limitations of the randomized controlled trials conducted to date make it difficult to draw definitive conclusions about the capacity of psychological interventions to improve HIV disease markers (Carrico & Antoni, 2008).

Lending support to the clinical relevance of decrements in immune status are findings highlighting the association between depressive symptoms and disease endpoints. Specifically, depressive symptoms have been related to faster progression to AIDS (Leserman et al., 1999; Page-Shafer, Delenze, Satariano, & Winkelstein, 1996) and development of an AIDS-related clinical condition (Leserman et al., 2002). Other investigations have determined that chronically elevated depressive symptoms are associated with hastened mortality in HIV-positive men (Mayne et al., 1996) and women (Ickovics et al., 2001). Again, the majority of investigations that reported no effect of depressive symptoms on hastened mortality utilized *only* baseline measures of depression (Burack et al., 1993; Lyketsos et al., 1993; Page-Shafer et al., 1996). Interestingly, in a follow-up to one study where no effects of baseline depressive symptoms were observed on HIV disease progression, participants reported a dramatic increase in depressive symptoms 6 to 18 months before an AIDS diagnosis (Lyketsos et al., 1996). Elevated depressive symptoms in the earlier stages of infection, HIV-related symptoms, unemployment, cigarette smoking, and social isolation were all associated with greater severity of depression as AIDS developed. However, increases in depressive symptoms during this stage were not associated with mortality. Although discrepant findings have been reported, it appears that depressive symptoms may be an important predictor of HIV disease progression. In particular, investigations examining the chronic nature of depressive symptoms over time have yielded the most consistent, replicable findings that demonstrate an effect of depressive symptoms on HIV disease progression.

Although relatively few investigations have systematically examined other negative mood states, anger has been associated with faster progression to AIDS (Leserman et al., 2002). Anxiety symptoms have also been related to greater CD8+38+ cell counts and higher HIV viral load—both indicators of elevated disease activity (Evans et al., 2002). On the other side of the coin, there is some emerging evidence that "positive" psychological states may relate to slowed HIV disease progression (Ironson & Hayward, 2008). Ickovics and colleagues (2006) observed that a composite factor of positive psychological resources (including positive affect, positive HIV outcome expectancies, and benefit finding) predicted less rapid CD4+ cell decline and longevity in a cohort of HIV-positive women. These findings remained unchanged after controlling baseline depression and ART use over the five-year investigation period. Results of another recent investigation indicate that enhanced positive affect is uniquely associated with longevity in a cohort of HIV-positive men who have sex with men (Moskowitz, 2003). Taken together, it appears that both positive and negative affective states may have implications for HIV disease progression.

How do such states as depression, anxiety, and anger or such positive states as affection and joy contribute to the course of HIV infection? As shown in Figure 33.2, there are a number of biobehavioral mechanisms that could explain the effects of affective states on HIV disease progression. These include biobehavioral processes related to medication adherence, sympathetic nervous system (SNS) and hypothalamic-pituitary-adrenal (HPA) neuroendocrine regulation, and use of such controlled substances as stimulants. There is good evidence that each of these sets of variables is related to affective states on the one hand and HIV disease progression on the other. In the subsequent sections, we review evidence supporting the disease relevance of these biobehavioral processes and the role that psychological factors may play in modulating them. Together, this body of research provides a starting point for developing health psychology interventions that may ultimately serve as an adjunct to frontline biomedical therapies for HIV/AIDS. This is meant to serve not as an exhaustive list of putative biobehavioral mechanisms but, rather, as a model to guide research efforts in health psychology as applied to HIV/AIDS. Other pathways have been reviewed in depth elsewhere (Gore-Felton & Koopman, 2008).

ADHERENCE TO ANTIRETROVIRAL THERAPY

As a result of the substantial reductions in morbidity and mortality associated with the advent of ART medication regimens, HIV infection is now commonly conceptualized as a chronic illness (Bangsberg et al., 2001). By directly suppressing HIV replication, ART-treated individuals may attenuate CD4+ cell decline and delay the onset of AIDS. However, not all HIV-positive patients treated with ART display adequate viral suppression, which may in large part be a result of suboptimal levels of adherence as well as the emergence of medication-resistant strains of the virus (Bangsberg et al., 2001; Tamalet, Fantini, Tourres, & Yashi, 2003). Questions also remain regarding the appropriate time to initiate ART in HIV-positive patients because of variability in the extent of immune reconstitution, increased incidence of opportunistic infections in the months following initiation, and reports of profound drug-related toxicities (Lederman & Valdez, 2000). Bearing in mind

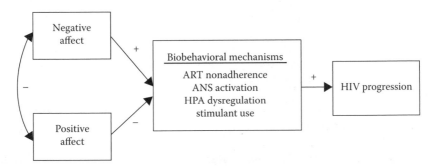

FIGURE 33.2 Both negative and positive affect states may relate to HIV disease progression through such biobehavioral processes as nonadherence to antiretroviral (ART) therapy, autonomic nervous system (ANS) activation, hypothalamic-pituitary-adrenal (HPA) axis dysregulation, and/or stimulant substance use.

these complexities involved in the medical management of HIV infection, investigators have examined barriers to initiating ART. A substantial number of individuals with advanced HIV disease in the United States experience significant structural, social, and psychological barriers to initiating treatment (Morin et al., 2002). These barriers may directly contribute to late presentation for HIV medical care and failure to initiate ART (Keruly & Moore, 2007), which can substantially increase risk for hastened AIDS-related mortality (Riley, Bangsberg, Guzman, Perry, & Moss, 2005).

A demanding, unforgiving treatment regimen, ART requires unprecedented levels of patient adherence, up to 95% to maximize the clinical benefits (Friedland & Williams, 1999). Further complicating adherence to ART are the special indications (e.g., taking medications with food) that accompany many medications in order to attenuate the severity of side effects, maximize bio-availability, and ensure a constant therapeutic dose. One key treatment-related factor that appears to be a significant obstacle to continuing ART is the side effects many patients experience. In fact, medication intolerance is the most commonly cited reason among patients for terminating ART (Park, Laura, Scalera, Tseng, & Rourke, 2002). Greater number and severity of medication side effects is also associated with poorer self-reported adherence among those individuals who continue to take ART. Such specific side effects as nausea, vomiting, skin problems, and memory impairment have been independently associated with reporting less than 90% adherence to ART (Johnson et al., 2005).

Investigations have also increasingly focused on examining psychological correlates of adherence in order to inform the development of innovative interventions designed to improve ART adherence. There is burgeoning evidence that depressive symptoms and other forms of negative affect are directly or indirectly associated with ART nonadherence (Johnson et al., 2003; Starace et al., 2002; Weaver et al., 2005). However, investigations examining whether symptoms of posttraumatic stress disorder are independently related to ART nonadherence have obtained mixed results (Delahanty, Bogart, & Figler, 2004; Sledjeski, Delahanty, & Bogart, 2005; Vranceanu et al., 2008). Delahanty and colleagues (2004) observed that HIV-specific traumatic stress was associated with poorer ART adherence, but also with higher CD4+ cell counts and lower salivary-free cortisol in the 30 to 45 minutes after awakening. In contrast to these findings, other studies have observed that HIV-specific traumatic stress as well as general symptoms of posttraumatic stress disorder from any trauma, including HIV, are not independently related to lower ART adherence after accounting for depressive symptoms (Sledjeski et al., 2005; Vranceanu et al., 2008). Further research is needed to determine whether HIV-specific traumatic stress and symptoms of posttraumatic stress impair adherence.

Relatively few investigations have examined the potential role that positive psychological resources may play in promoting ART adherence. In one of the few studies to date, Gonzalez and colleagues (2004) observed that the association between perceived social support and improved ART adherence was mediated by increased positive states of mind (sense of tranquility and other positive states). Building on these findings, another investigation with HIV-positive methamphetamine users observed that positive affect was independently associated with better self-reported ART adherence after controlling for negative affect and HIV-specific traumatic stress (Carrico, Johnson, Colfax, & Moskowitz, 2010). Taken together, findings across studies indicate that both positive and negative affective states are important correlates of ART adherence. It is possible that ART adherence is one key pathway whereby affective states influence HIV disease progression.

There is some evidence that individuals on ART regimens can be empowered to deal with treatment burdens through psychological interventions. Some of these target cognitive appraisals of ART-related side effects. For instance, Johnson, Gamarel, and Dawson-Rose (2006) observed that a time-limited psychological intervention increased adherence self-efficacy and enhanced perceptions of positive side effects among participants who were naïve to ART. Further research is needed to examine whether psychological interventions can decrease the perceived severity of side effects among ART-treated individuals as a way to improve their adherence.

Bearing in mind the association of affective states with ART adherence, enhanced affect regulation may be a key target of psychological interventions designed to improve ART adherence. Simoni, Pearson, Pantalone, Marks, and Crepaz (2006) conducted a meta-analytic review of 19 randomized controlled trials that examined the efficacy of innovative adherence interventions. The majority of these interventions employed cognitive-behavioral principles, and results indicated that participants randomized to the intervention arm were significantly more likely to achieve 95% adherence. More recent trials also lend support to cognitive-behavioral interventions that include components designed specifically to improve depressed mood. One trial examined the efficacy of a 12-week individual cognitive-behavioral intervention for adherence and depression in depressed men and women (Safren et al., 2009). Over the intervention period, individuals in the cognitive-behavioral treatment reported reductions in depressive symptoms and displayed concurrent increases in electronically monitored ART adherence compared to those who received a single-session adherence intervention. Participants in the cognitive-behavioral intervention also displayed decreases in HIV viral load through nine-month follow-up; but because of the cross-over trial design, there was no comparison condition. In the previously discussed trial of CBSM+MAT, no significant increases in ART adherence were reported, but this may have been because of the high levels of ART adherence reported by participants at baseline (Carrico et al., 2006). Despite the fact that no significant intervention effects on adherence were observed, men in CBSM+MAT displayed a significant and clinically interesting decrease in HIV viral load over the 15-month investigation period. Reductions in depressed mood during the 10-week intervention period mediated the sustained effects of CBSM+MAT on HIV viral load after controlling for adherence (Antoni, Carrico, et al., 2006). Although these trials support the efficacy of cognitive-behavioral treatments in combination with problem-focused ART adherence interventions, important questions remain. Further research is needed to identify the active element(s) of these multimodal treatments to determine whether reductions in depressed mood are necessary to improve ART adherence and reduce HIV viral load, particularly among depressed HIV-positive individuals.

NEUROENDOCRINE HORMONE REGULATION

Because HIV-positive persons endure a chronic, unpredictable disease that requires adaptation across a variety of domains, personal differences in the ways individuals adapt to these challenges may contribute not only to quality of life but also to disease processes. Research in psychoneuroimmunology has examined the potential biobehavioral mechanisms whereby such psychosocial factors as stressors, stress responses, coping, and affective states influence disease progression (Carrico, Antoni, Young, & Gorman, 2008). Psychological factors are hypothesized to relate to the immune system functioning in humans through stress- or distress-induced changes in hormonal regulatory systems (Kiecolt-Glaser, McGuire, Robles, & Glaser, 2002). Several adrenal hormones—including cortisol and catecholamines (norepinephrine and epinephrine)—are known to be altered as a function of an individual's appraisals of and coping responses to stressors (McEwen, 1998). In HIV-positive persons, elevations in these hormones have also been associated with alterations in multiple indices of immune status (Antoni & Schneiderman, 1998).

One pathway whereby stress-induced immunomodulation may occur is the HPA axis. Under conditions of stress, the parvocellular subdivision of the paraventricular nucleus of the hypothalamus releases corticotrophin-releasing factor, which subsequently triggers the pituitary to release of adrenocorticotrophic hormone (ACTH). Then, the ACTH travels through the circulatory system, where it stimulates the adrenal cortex and medulla to secrete cortisol and catecholamines (epinephrine and norepinephrine), respectively. Because the HPA axis relies on secretion of ACTH into circulation, there is an approximately 20-minute lag time between stressor onset and increased secretion of adrenal hormones (Sapolsky, Romero, & Munck, 2000). Elevated levels of cortisol inhibit cellular-immune responses through changes in DNA and RNA synthesis after binding with the receptor sites located within the cytoplasm of the lymphocyte (Cupps & Fauci, 1982). Cortisol also synergizes with gp120 to enhance rates of cell decline (Nair, Mahajan, Hou, Sweet, & Schwartz, 2000) and is associated with high rates of apoptosis (programmed cell death) in CD4+ and accessory cells in lymphoid tissue (Amendola et al., 1996). Glucocorticoids such as cortisol also influence maturational selection of CD4+ cells in these regions in addition to impacting CD4+ cell function in the periphery (Corley, 1996). Cortisol negatively impacts functioning of macrophages (Pavlidis & Chirigos, 1980) and NK cells (Herberman & Holden, 1978). Other in vitro data indicate that cortisol enhances HIV p24 antigen production in human monocyte-derived macrophages, a possible reservoir of HIV infection (Swanson, Zeller, & Spear, 1998). Finally, longitudinal investigations of HIV-positive men indicate that greater concentrations of serum cortisol were associated with progression to AIDS, development of an AIDS-related complex (ARC) symptom, and death over a nine-year period (Leserman et al., 2002).

Investigations examining the effects of stress management interventions on mood, cortisol, and immune parameters in HIV-positive persons has shed some light on the relevance of HPA axis regulation (for a review, see Carrico & Antoni, 2008). HIV-positive men assigned to a group-based 10-week CBSM intervention that combined training in relaxation, cognitive restructuring, coping skills, and interpersonal skills (Antoni, Ironson, & Schneiderman, 2007) showed decreases in 24-hour urinary cortisol output that was proportional to reductions in depressed mood (Antoni, Wagner, et al., 2000). Over a 10-week period, men assigned to CBSM showed successive improvements in their ability to reduce weekly in-session salivary cortisol levels and negative mood during relaxation induction, which were proportional to greater home practice of relaxation exercises (Cruess, Antoni, Kumar, & Schneiderman, 2000). CBSM-related decreases in cortisol and depressed mood were related to reductions in immunoglobulin G antibody titers to herpes simplex virus–Type 2 (HSV-2) over a 10-week intervention period in HIV-positive men, suggesting better immunologic control over this latent viral infection (Cruess et al., 2000; Lutgendorf et al., 1997). These reductions in cortisol were also found to comediate (along with reductions in depressed mood), increases in transitional naïve CD4+ cells at one-year follow-up in this cohort (Antoni et al. 2005), suggesting that stress management–associated improvements in HPA axis dysregulation may contribute to retarding disease progression by facilitating immune reconstitution. This multimodal cognitive-behavioral intervention may improve health outcomes in HIV-positive persons by decreasing negative affect and improving cortisol regulation.

The ANS is another plausible pathway for the effects of psychological factors on the immune system and progression of disease in HIV/AIDS. Findings from seminal neuroanatomical studies in the field of psychoneuroimmunology indicate that the sympathetic branch of the ANS innervates lymphoid tissue as well as such other important immune organs as the thymus and spleen (Nance & Sanders, 2007). In contrast to the slower acting HPA axis, an activated ANS triggers the release of norepinephrine at sympathetic nerve terminals shortly after the onset of a stressor. Because lymphoid organs are a primary site of HIV replication, sympathetic innervation of these regions may dramatically influence HIV progression. By binding with β_2 receptors on the lymphocyte membrane, norepinephrine activates the G protein–linked adenyl cyclase-cAMP-protein kinase A signaling cascade (Kobilka, 1992). Cellular changes of this nature are associated with in vitro decrements in interferon-gamma (IFN-γ) and interleukin-10 during the eight days following HIV infection of peripheral blood mononuclear cells. This suppression of IFN-γ and interleukin-10 production, in turn, predicts elevations in HIV viral load over time (Cole, Korin, Fahey, & Zack, 1998). Sympathetic innervation of both primary and secondary lymphoid tissue may provide an ideal microenvironment for ANS activation to accelerate HIV replication. This possibility is supported by data indicating that simian immunodeficiency virus replication is enhanced by 3.9-fold near-catecholaminergic varicosities (Sloan, Tarara, Capitanio, & Cole, 2006). Lending further support to the role of ANS activation, another study observed that individuals who displayed higher ANS activity at rest prior to beginning ART subsequently demonstrated poorer suppression of HIV viral load and decreased CD4+ cell reconstitution over a 3- to 11-month period (Cole et al., 2001).

Taken together, there is burgeoning evidence for the role of ANS activation in hastened HIV disease progression (Cole, 2008).

Very few studies have examined whether psychosocial interventions can modulate ANS activity in persons with HIV/AIDS. One study found that a 10-week CBSM intervention (previously described) reduced 24-hr urinary norepinephrine and anxiety levels in HIV-positive men (Antoni, Cruess, et al., 2000). It is interesting that these reductions in norepinephrine and anxiety during the 10-week intervention period mediated its effect in preserving levels of CD8+ cells at one-year follow-up. Because CD8+ T-cells are chief effector cells necessary for cell-specific cytotoxic responses, it is plausible that both psychosocial and pharmacologic interventions designed to more directly target anxiety and ANS activation may improve immune surveillance over opportunistic viral infections and neoplastic processes in HIV-infected persons (Antoni, Lutgendorf, et al., 2006).

In addition, stressors and stress management have been related to the progression and persistence of cervical neoplasia in women coinfected with HIV and such oncogenic viruses as human papilloma virus (HPV). Greater life stress predicted greater risk of developing cervical neoplasia (Pereira et al., 2003a) and HSV-2 outbreaks (Pereira et al., 2003b) over a one-year period in these HIV+HPV+ women. More recently, it was shown that HIV+HPV+ women assigned to a 10-week CBSM intervention showed decreased perceived stress and decreased odds of persistent cervical neoplasia at six-month follow-up (Antoni et al., 2008). Whether these intervention effects on neoplastic disease are mediated by some combination of health behavior changes (e.g., substance use, medication adherence) and neuroimmune pathways is currently under investigation. Health psychology research has accumulated documenting associations among stress, psychoneuroimmunologic processes, and HIV disease progression. Investigators are now seeking to identify neuroimmunologic and virologic pathways that might explain the association of psychological processes and such specific HIV-related disease endpoints as opportunistic infections and cancers. Health psychologists stand to contribute to this line of inquiry by designing prospective studies that can first identify the influence of stressors, stress responses, and stress moderators, which in turn gives rise to the development and validation of theoretically derived psychological interventions. Beyond stress physiology, it is also reasonable to examine the role of such health behaviors as substance use as a mediator of the association between affective states and HIV disease course. Another major area of health psychology research in HIV/AIDS focuses on the role of substance use in the transmission of HIV as well as on the progression of disease in infected persons.

STIMULANT USE

A national probability-based sample of adults receiving HIV care in the United States observed high rates of substance use and probable substance use disorders (Bing et al., 2001). In this investigation, approximately 38% of participants reported using substances other than marijuana during the past year, and 12.5% screened positive for a substance use disorder. In this section, we review investigations that focused on stimulant use as a predictor of HIV disease markers and more rapid HIV disease progression. We focus on stimulant use because it relates to disruptions in medication adherence as well as to ANS activation, both of which may contribute to disease progression. Health psychology studies of stimulant use among HIV-positive persons provide a unique opportunity to examine a number of biobehavioral mechanisms that are relevant to HIV disease progression.

The regular use of such stimulants as cocaine, crack, and methamphetamine has been associated with increased rates of HIV transmission risk behavior, acquisition of strains of HIV that are resistant to some classes of antiretroviral medications, impaired adherence to ART, and elevated HIV viral load (Colfax et al., 2007; Hinkin et al., 2007; Johnson, Carrico, Chesney, & Morin, 2008). Consequently, stimulant users have been identified as an important group to target for HIV prevention efforts. There is some preliminary evidence that behavioral interventions designed to enhance motivation as well as bolster self-efficacy for reducing sexual risk taking are effective in decreasing HIV transmission risk behavior in methamphetamine users (Mausbach, Semple, Strathdee,

Zians, & Patterson, 2007). However, little is known about the role of potentially modifiable psychological factors (e.g., affective states) in relation to substance use and ART adherence among HIV-positive stimulant users. One prior cross-sectional investigation observed that the ability to effectively regulate negative affect is indirectly related to elevated HIV viral load through two independent behavioral pathways—a decreased likelihood of reporting regular stimulant use and better self-reported ART adherence (Carrico et al., 2007). These findings were supported by a subsequent cross-sectional study with HIV-positive methamphetamine users where HIV-specific traumatic stress was associated with more frequent cocaine and crack use and positive affect was associated with a decreased likelihood of reporting injection drug use (Carrico et al., 2010). It is of interest that another study observed that in the three months following an HIV seropositive diagnosis, positive affect independently predicted reductions in stimulant use as well as abstinence from stimulant use (Carrico & Moskowitz, 2008). Although further research is needed to examine the potentially bidirectional relationship between substance use and affect regulation, it is plausible that stimulant use is one pathway for the effects of positive and negative affect on HIV disease progression.

Several cohort studies have examined whether substance use predicts more rapid HIV disease progression. One 11-year cohort study (1985–1996) followed HIV-positive men and women who attended a methadone maintenance clinic. In multivariate Cox proportional hazards models, crack use predicted more rapid progression to AIDS after controlling for gender, CD4+ cell count, and HIV symptoms (Webber, Schoenbaum, Gourevitch, Buono, & Klein, 1999). However, crack use did not predict more rapid CD4+ cell count decline or mortality in this cohort. In the era of ART, data from the AIDS Link to Intravenous Experience (ALIVE) cohort study indicated that active cocaine or heroin use in the past six months predicted decreased utilization of ART, ART nonadherence, and impaired immune status (Lucas, Cheever, Chaisson, & Moore, 2001). Subsequent analyses of the ALIVE cohort data lend further support to the temporal relationship between substance use and immune decrements. Participants who relapsed to heavy alcohol use or to use of any substance (i.e., cocaine or heroin) over a six-month period were substantially more likely to report impaired ART utilization and nonadherence as well as to display decreased CD4+ cell reconstitution and clinically elevated HIV viral load (Lucas, Gebo, Chaisson, & Moore, 2002). Building on these findings, further evidence from the 1,851 participants who enrolled in the ALIVE cohort since 1998 indicates that active cocaine or heroin use predicts increased risk of developing an opportunistic infection (e.g., bacterial pneumonia) and hastened mortality. It is of interest that even after adjusting for ART use and ART nonadherence, the relationship between active cocaine or heroin use and indicators of more rapid HIV disease progression was unchanged (Lucas et al., 2001). This finding indicates that there may be pathways other than ART nonadherence that explain more rapid HIV disease progression among individuals who use cocaine and/or heroin.

Concurrent support for these findings was published by the Women's Interagency HIV Study Collaborative Group. In a sample of women who initiated ART between 1995 and 2003, current use of cocaine, crack, or heroin predicted the development of an AIDS-defining illness and hastened AIDS-related mortality after adjusting for ART regimen, nadir CD4+ count, peak HIV viral load, having had an AIDS diagnosis prior to initiating ART, ART adherence, age, income, depression, and cigarette smoking (Anastos et al., 2005). Taken together, findings from these large cohort studies generally indicate that substance use predicts more rapid HIV disease progression; nonetheless, important, unanswered questions remain. It is difficult to determine whether the relationship between substance use and HIV disease progression reflects the effects of specific substances (e.g., cocaine and/or heroin), the effects of specific routes of substance administration (e.g., smoking versus injecting), or a general pattern of immune decrements among active users of any substance.

Stimulants can acutely precipitate both physical and psychological changes, including hyperthermia, elevated blood pressure, decreased appetite, insomnia, enhanced sex drive, and feelings of euphoria (Irwin et al., 20 07; Makisumi et al., 1998). Greater output of norepinephrine may partially explain observations that stimulant users on ART display a markedly elevated HIV viral load (Ellis et al., 2003). Even after accounting for higher rates of self-reported ART nonadherence, regular stimulant use several or more times per week is independently associated with 50% higher HIV viral load (Carrico et al., 2007). In the context of chronic HIV infection, elevated viral load may lead to sustained activation of the cellular immune response (Hunt et al., 2006), which could further be exacerbated by the capacity of stimulants to increase IFN-γ production in the periphery (Gan et al., 1998). As a result, stimulants may have both direct and indirect effects on immune activation. The potential direct effects of stimulants on immune activation are further supported by a recent cross-sectional study with ART-treated HIV-positive persons. In this investigation, weekly stimulant use was independently associated with higher HIV viral load, elevated neopterin, and lower tryptophan after controlling for self-reported ART adherence (Carrico, Johnson, et al., 2008). Taken together, these data provide some preliminary evidence that regular use of stimulants may independently predict more rapid HIV disease progression. This relationship should be examined in future cohort studies and if supported would justify randomized controlled trials testing the effects of psychological interventions targeting stimulant use to determine how it is related to disease progression.

CONCLUSION

Taken together, research in health psychology has yielded some compelling evidence that such psychological factors as negative and positive affect predict important health outcomes in HIV disease. Studies have also begun to map out the biobehavioral mechanisms that may explain the effects of psychological factors on HIV disease biomarkers. In particular, randomized controlled trials provide a unique opportunity to experimentally enhance psychological adjustment and examine the biobehavioral pathways whereby improved psychological adjustment is related to improvements in immune status. Although a number of randomized controlled trials have examined the efficacy of such psychological interventions as CBSM with respect to HIV disease markers, significant methodological limitations make it difficult to draw definitive conclusions. Large-scale trials with diverse groups of HIV-positive persons are needed to determine whether psychological interventions can meaningfully improve immune status and health outcomes among HIV-positive persons.

Although research reviewed in this chapter has been specific to HIV/AIDS, results of this body of work provide an excellent framework to inform health psychology research with other chronic medical conditions. Such issues as adaptation to chronic illness, adherence to medical regimens, and substance abuse are highly relevant across disease groups. Furthermore, stress-related activation of the HPA axis and ANS may also have important implications for the progression of a variety of chronic diseases, including coronary artery disease, diabetes, and various forms of cancer. By understanding the biobehavioral pathways whereby psychological factors influence chronic-disease progression, health psychologists can develop and test innovative interventions to address these specific mechanisms.

REFERENCES

Amendola, A., Gougeon, M. L., Poccia, F., Bondurand, A., Fesus, L., & Piacentini, M. (1996). Induction of tissue transglutaminase in HIV pathogenesis: Evidence for high rate of apoptosis on CD4+ T lymphocytes and accessory cells in lymphoid tissues. *Proclamation of the [U.S.] National Academy of Sciences, 93,* 11057–11062.

Anastos, K., Schneider, M. F., Gange, S. J., Minkoff, H., Greenblatt, R. M., Feldman, J., … Cohen F. (2005). The association of race, sociodemographic, and behavioral characteristics with response to highly active antiretroviral therapy in women. *Journal of Acquired Immune Deficiency Syndromes, 39,* 537–544.

Antoni, M. H., Carrico, A. W., Durán, R. E., Spitzer, S., Penedo, F., Ironson, G., … Schneiderman, N. (2006). Randomized clinical trial of cognitive behavioral stress management on human immunodeficiency virus viral load in gay men treated with highly active antiretroviral therapy. *Psychosomatic Medicine, 68,* 143–151.

Antoni, M. H., Cruess, D., Klimas, N., Carrico, A. W., Maher, K., Cruess, S., … Schneiderman, N. (2005). Increases in a marker of immune system reconstitution are predated by decreases in 24-hour urinary cortisol output and depressed mood during a 10-week stress management intervention in symptomatic HIV-infected gay men. *Journal of Psychosomatic Research, 58,* 3–13.

Antoni, M. H., Cruess, D., Wagner, S., Lutgendorf, S., Kumar, M., Ironson, G., … Schneiderman, N. (2000). Cognitive behavioral stress management effects on anxiety, 24-hour urinary catecholamine output, and T-Cytotoxic/suppressor cells over time among symptomatic HIV-infected gay men. *Journal of Consulting and Clinical Psychology*, *68*, 31–45.

Antoni, M. H., Ironson, G., & Schneiderman, N. (2007). *Stress management for persons with HIV infection.* New York, NY: Oxford University Press.

Antoni, M. H., Lutgendorf, S., Cole, S., Dhabhar, F., Sephton, S., McDonald, P., … Sood, A. K. (2006). The influence of biobehavioral factors on tumor biology, pathways and mechanisms. *Nature Reviews Cancer*, *6*, 240–248.

Antoni, M. H., Pereira, D. B., Buscher, I., Ennis, N., Peake-Andrasik, M., Rose, R., … O'Sullivan, M. J. (2008). Stress management effects on perceived stress and cervical intraepithelial neoplasia in low-income HIV infected women. *Journal of Psychosomatic Research*, *65*, 389–401.

Antoni, M. H., & Schneiderman, N. (1998). HIV/AIDS. In A. Bellack & M. Hersen (Eds.), *Comprehensive clinical psychology.* (pp. 237–275). New York, NY: Elsevier Science.

Antoni, M. H., Wagner, S., Cruess, D., Kumar, M., Lutgendorf, S., Ironson, G., … Schneiderman, N. (2000). Cognitive behavioral stress management reduces distress and 24-hour urinary free cortisol among symptomatic HIV-infected gay men. *Annals of Behavioral Medicine*, *22*, 29–37.

Bangsberg, D. R., Perry, S., Charlebois, E. D., Clark, R. A., Roberston, M., Zolopa, A. R., & Moss, A. (2001). Non-adherence to highly active antiretroviral therapy predicts progression to AIDS. *AIDS*, *15*(9), 1181–1183.

Bing, E. G., Burnam, M. A., Longshore, D., Fleishman, J. A., Sherbourne, C. D., London, A. S., … Shapiro, M. (2001). Psychiatric disorders and drug use among human immunodeficiency virus-infected adults in the United States. *Archives of General Psychiatry*, *58*, 721–728.

Burack, J. H., Barrett, D. C., Stall, R. D., Chesney, M. A., Ekstrand, M. L., & Coates, T. J. (1993). Depressive symptoms and CD4 lymphocyte decline among HIV-infected men. *Journal of the American Medical Association*, *270*, 2568–2573.

Carrico, A. W., & Antoni, M. H. (2008). The effects of psychological interventions on neuroendocrine hormone regulation and immune status in HIV-positive persons: A review of randomized controlled trials. *Psychosomatic Medicine*, *70*, 575–584.

Carrico, A. W., Antoni, M. H., Durán, R. E., Ironson, G., Penedo, F., Fletcher, M. A., … Schneiderman, N. (2006). Reductions in depressed mood and denial coping during cognitive behavioral stress management with HIV-positive gay men treated with HAART. *Annals of Behavioral Medicine*, *3*(2), 155–164.

Carrico, A. W., Antoni, M. H., Young, L., & Gorman, J. M. (2008) Psychoneuroimmunology and HIV. In M. A. Cohen & J. M. Gorman (Eds.), *Comprehensive textbook of AIDS psychiatry* (pp. 27–38). Oxford, England: Oxford University Press.

Carrico, A. W., Johnson, M. O., Colfax, G. N., & Moskowitz, J. T. (2010). Affective correlates of stimulant use and adherence to anti-retroviral therapy among HIV-positive methamphetamine users. *AIDS and Behavior, 14*(4), 769–777.

Carrico, A. W., Johnson, M. O., Morin, S. F., Remien, R. H., Riley, E. D., Hecht, F. M., & Fuchs, D. (2008). Stimulant use is associated with immune activation and depleted tryptophan among HIV-positive persons on anti-retroviral therapy. *Brain, Behavior, and Immunity*, *22*, 1257–1262.

Carrico, A. W., Johnson, M. O., Moskowitz, J. T., Neilands, T. B., Morin, S. F., Charlebois, E. D., … Chesney, M. (2007). Affect regulation, stimulant use, and viral load among HIV-positive persons on anti-retroviral therapy. *Psychosomatic Medicine*, *69*, 785–792.

Carrico, A. W., & Moskowitz, J. T. (2008). *Positive affect promotes decreases in stimulant use following a HIV seropositive diagnosis.* Poster presented at the 10th International Congress of Behavioral Medicine, Tokyo, Japan.

Centers for Disease Control. (1992). 1993 revised classification system for HIV infection and expanded surveillance case definition for AIDS among adolescents and adults. *Morbidity and Mortality Weekly Report*, *41*, 1–18.

Ciesla, J. A., & Roberts, J. E. (2001). Meta-analysis of the relationship between HIV infection and the risk for depressive disorders. *American Journal of Psychiatry*, *158*, 725–730.

Clerici, M., Berzofsky, J. A., Shearer, G. M., & Tacket, C. O. (1991). Exposure to human immunodeficiency virus type 1–specific T helper cell responses before detection of infection by polymerase chain reaction and serum antibodies. *Journal of Infectious Diseases*, *164*, 178–184.

Cole, S. W. (2008). Psychosocial influences on HIV-1 disease progression: Neural, endocrine, and virologic mechanisms. *Psychosomatic Medicine*, *70*, 562–568.

Cole, S. W., Korin, Y. D., Fahey, J. L., & Zack, J. A. (1998). Norepinephrine accelerates HIV replication via protein kinase A-dependent effects on cytokine production. *Journal of Immunology*, *161*, 610–616.

Cole, S. W., Naliboff, B. D., Kemeny, M. E., Griswold, M. P., Fahey, J. L., & Zack, J. A. (2001). Impaired response to HAART in HIV-infected individuals with high autonomic nervous system activity. *Proceedings of the [U.S.] National Academy of Sciences*, *98*, 12695–12700.

Colfax, G. N., Vittinghoff, E., Grant, R., Lum, P., Spotts, G., & Hecht, F. M. (2007). Frequent methamphetamine use is associated with primary non-nucleoside reverse transcriptase inhibitor resistance. *AIDS*, *21*(2), 239–241.

Corley, P. A. (1996). Acquired immune deficiency syndrome: The glucocorticoid solution. *Medical Hypotheses*, *47*, 49–54.

Cruess, D., Antoni, M. H., Kumar, M., & Schneiderman, N. (2000). Reductions in salivary cortisol are associated with mood improvement during relaxation training among HIV-1 seropositive men. *Journal of Behavioral Medicine*, *23*, 107–122.

Cruess, D. G., Douglas, S. D., Petitto, J. M., Have, T. T., Gettes, D., Dube, B., ... Evans, D. L. (2005). Association of resolution of major depression with increased natural killer cell activity among HIV-seropositive women. *American Journal of Psychiatry*, *162*, 2125–2130.

Cupps, T., & Fauci, A. (1982). Corticosteroid-mediated immunoregulation in man. *Immunology Review*, *65*, 694–697.

Delahanty, D. L., Bogart, L. M., & Figler, J. L. (2004). Posttraumatic stress disorder symptoms, salivary cortisol, medication adherence, and CD4 levels in HIV-positive individuals. *AIDS Care*, *16*(2), 247–260.

Dybul, M., Fauci, A. S., Bartlett, J. G., Kaplan, J. E., & Pau, A, K. (2002). Guidelines for using antiretroviral agents among HIV-infected adults and adolescents. *Annals of Internal Medicine*, *137*, 381–433.

Ellis, R. J., Childers, M. E., Cherner, M., Lazzaretto, D., Letendre, S., & Grant, I. (2003). Increased human immunodeficiency virus loads in active methamphetamine users are explained by reduced effectiveness of antiretroviral therapy. *Journal of Infectious Diseases*, *188*, 1820–1826.

Evans, D. L., Ten Have, T. R., Douglas, S. D., Gettes, D., Morrison, C. H., Chiappini, M. S., ... Petitto, J. M. (2002). Association of depression with viral load, CD8 T lymphocytes, and natural killer cells in women with HIV infection. *American Journal of Psychiatry*, *159*, 1752–1759.

Folkman, S. (2008). The case for positive emotions in the stress process. *Anxiety, Stress, and Coping*, *21*, 3–14.

Folkman, S., & Moskowitz, J. T. (2000). Positive affect and the other side of coping. *American Psychologist*, *55*, 647–654.

Friedland, G. H., & Williams, A. (1999). Attaining higher goals in HIV treatment: The central importance of adherence. *AIDS*, *13*, S61–S72.

Gaines, H., von Sydow, M. A., von Stedingk, L. V., Biberfeld, G., Bottiger, B., Hansson, L. O., ... Stranngaard, O. O. (1990). Immunological changes in primary HIV-1 infection. *AIDS*, *(4)*, 995–999.

Gan, X., Zhang, L., Newton, T., Chang, S. L., Ling, W., Kermani, V., ... Fiala, M. (1998). Cocaine infusion increases interferon-gamma and decreases interleukin-10 in cocaine-dependent subjects. *Clinical Immunology and Immunopathology*, *89*, 181–190.

Giorgi, J. V., Hultin, L. E., McKeating, J. A., Johnson, T. D., Owens, B., Jacobson, L. P., ... Detels, R. (1999). Shorter survival in advanced human immunodeficiency virus type 1 infection is more closely associated with T lymphocyte activation than with plasma virus burden or virus chemokine coreceptor usage. *Journal of Infectious Diseases*, *179*, 859–870.

Gonzalez, J. S., Penedo, F. J., Antoni, M. H., Duran, R. E., McPherson-Baker, S., Ironson, G., ... Schneiderman, N. (2004). Social support, positive states of mind, and HIV treatment adherence in men and women living with HIV/AIDS. *Health Psychology*, *23*(4), 413–418.

Gore-Felton, C., & Koopman, C. (2008). Behavioral mediation of the relationship between psychosocial factors and HIV disease progression. *Psychosomatic Medicine*, *70*, 569–574.

Herberman, R., & Holden, H. (1978). Natural cell–mediated immunity. *Advances in Cancer Research*, *27*, 305–377.

Hinkin, C. H., Barclay, T. R., Castellon, S. A., Levine, A. J., Durvasula, R. S., Marion, S. D., ... Longshore, D. (2007). Drug use and medication adherence among HIV-1 infected individuals. *AIDS and Behavior*, *11*, 185–194.

Hunt, P.,W., Deeks, S. G., Bangsberg, D. R., Moss, A., Sinclair, E., Liegler, T., ... Martin, J. N. (2006). The independent effect of drug resistance on T cell activation in HIV infection. *AIDS*, *20*, 691–699.

Ickovics, J. R., Hamburger, M. E., Vlahov, D., Schoenbaum, E. E., Schuman, P., Boland, R. J., ... Moore, J. (2001). Mortality, CD4 cell count decline, and depressive symptoms among HIV-seropositive women: Longitudinal analysis from the HIV Epidemiology Research Study. *Journal of the American Medical Association*, *285*, 1460–1465.

Ickovics, J. R., Milan, S., Boland, R., Schoenbaum, E., Schuman, P., Vlahov, D., & the HERS Group. (2006). Psychological resources protect health: 5-year survival and immune function among HIV-infected women from four U.S. cities. *AIDS*, *20*, 1851–1860.

Ironson, G., Balbin, G., Solomon, G., Fahey, J., Klimas, N., Schneiderman, N., & Fletcher, M. A. (2001). Relative preservation of natural killer cell cytotoxicity and number in healthy AIDS patients with low CD4 cell counts. *AIDS, 15*, 2065–2073.

Ironson, G., & Hayward, H. (2008). Do positive psychological factors predict disease progression in HIV-1? A review of the evidence. *Psychosomatic Medicine, 70*, 546–554.

Ironson, G., O'Cleirigh, C., Fletcher, M. A., Laurenceau, J. P., Balbin, E., Klimas, N., … Solomon, G. (2005). Psychosocial factors predict CD4 and viral load change in men and women with human immunodeficiency virus in the era of highly active antiretroviral therapy. *Psychosomatic Medicine, 67*, 1013–1021.

Irwin, M. R., Olmos, L., Wang, M., Valladares, E. M., Motivala, S. J., Fong, T., … Cole, S. W. (2007). Cocaine dependence and acute cocaine induce decreases of monocyte proinflammatory cytokine expression across the diurnal period: Autonomic mechanisms. *Journal of Pharmacology and Experimental Therapeutics, 320*, 507–515.

Johnson, M. O., Carrico, A. W., Chesney, M. A., & Morin, S. F. (2008). Internalized heterosexism among HIV-positive gay-identified men: Implicaitons for HIV prevention and care. *Journal of Consulting and Clinical Psychology, 76*, 829–839.

Johnson, M. O., Catz, S. L., Remien, R. H., Rotheram-Borus, M. J., Morin, S. F., Charlebois, E., … Chesney, M. A. (2003). Theory-guided, empirically supported avenues for intervention on HIV medication nonadherence: findings from the Healthy Living Project. *AIDS Patient Care STDS, 17*(12), 645–656.

Johnson, M. O., Charlebois, E., Morin, S. F., Catz, S. L., Goldstein, R. B., Remien, R. H., … Chesney, M. A. (2005). Perceived adverse effects of antiretroviral therapy. *Journal of Pain and Symptom Management, 29*, 193–205.

Johnson, M. O., Gamarel, K. E., & Dawson-Rose, C. (2006). Changing HIV treatment expectancies: A pilot study. *AIDS Care, 18*, 550–553.

Kalichman, S. C., Difonzo, K., Austin, J., Luke, W., & Rompa, D. (2002). Prospective study of emotional reactions to changes in HIV viral load. *AIDS Patient Care and STD's, 16*(3), 113–120.

Kaplan, L. D., Wofsky, C. B., & Volberding, P. A. (1987). Treatment of patients with acquired immunodeficiency syndrome and associated manifestations. *Journal of the American Medical Association, 257*, 1367–1376.

Keruly, J. C., & Moore, R. D. (2007). Immune status at presentation to care did not improve among antiretroviral-naïve persons from 1990 to 2006. *Clinical Infectious Diseases, 45*, 1369–1374.

Kiecolt-Glaser, J. K., McGuire, L., Robles, T. F., & Glaser, R. (2002). Psychoneuroimmunology: Psychological influences on immune function and health. *Journal of Consulting and Clinical Psychology, 70*, 537–547.

Klatzmann, D., Champagne, E., Chamaret, S., Gruest, J., Guetard, D., Hercend, T., … Montagnier, L. (1984). T-lymphocyte T4 molecule behaves as the receptor for human retrovirus LAV. *Nature, 312*, 767–768.

Kobilka, B. (1992). Adrenergic receptors as models for G-protein coupled receptors. *Annual Review of Neuroscience, 15*, 87.

Lederman, M. M., & Valdez, H. (2000). Immune restoration with antiretroviral therapies: Implications for clinical management. *JAMA, 284*(2), 223–228.

Leserman, J. (2008). Role of depression, stress, and trauma in HIV disease progression. *Psychosomatic Medicine, 70*, 539–545.

Leserman, J., Jackson, E. D., Petitto, J. M., Golden, R. N., Silva, S. G., Perkins, D. O., … Evans, D. L. (1999). Progression to AIDS: The effects of stress, depressive symptoms and social support. *Psychosomatic Medicine, 61*, 397–406.

Leserman, J., Petitto, J. M., Perkins, D. O., Folds, J. D., Golden, R. N., & Evans, D. L. (1997). Severe stress and depressive symptoms, and changes in lymphocyte subsets in human immunodeficiency virus infected men. *Archives of General Psychiatry, 54*, 279–285.

Leserman, J., Petitto, J. M., Gu, H., Gaynes, B. N., Barroso, J., Golden, R. N., … Evans, D. L. (2002). Progression to AIDS, a clinical AIDS condition and mortality: Psychosocial and physiological predictors. *Psychological Medicine, 32*, 1059–1073.

Lucas, G. M., Cheever, L. W., Chaisson, R. E., & Moore R. D. (2001). Detrimental effects of continued illicit drug use on the treatment of HIV-1 infection. *Journal of Acquired Immune Deficiency Syndromes, 27*, 251–259.

Lucas, G. M., Gebo, K. A., Chaisson, R. E., & Moore, R. D. (2002). Longitudinal assessment of the effects of drug and alcohol abuse on HIV-1 treatment outcomes in an urban clinic. *AIDS, 16*, 767–774.

Lucas, G. M., Griswold, M., Gebo, K. A., Keruly, J., Chaisson, R. E., & Moore, R. D. (2006). Illicit drug use and HIV-1 disease progression: a longitudinal study in the era of highly active antiretroviral therapy. *American Journal of Epidemiology, 163*, 412–420.

Lutgendorf, S. K., Antoni, M. H., Ironson, G., Klimas, N., Kumar, M., Starr, K., … Schneiderman, N. (1997). Cognitive behavioral stress management intervention decreases dysphoria and herpes simplex virus–type 2 titers in symptomatic HIV-seropositive gay men. *Journal of Consulting and Clinical Psychology, 65*, 23–31.

Lyketsos, C. G., Hoover, D. R., Guccione, M., Dew, M. A., Wesch, J. E., Bing, E. G., & Treisman, G. J. (1996). Changes in depressive symptoms as AIDS develops: The Multicenter AIDS Cohort Study. *American Journal of Psychiatry, 153*, 1430–1437.

Lyketsos, C. G., Hoover, D. R., Guccione, M., Senterfitt, W., Dew, M. A., Wesch, J., … Morgenstern, H. (1993). Depressive symptoms as predictors of medical outcomes in HIV infection. *Journal of the American Medical Association, 270*, 2563–2567.

Makisumi, T., Yoshida, K., Watanabe, T., Tan, N., Murakami, N., & Morimoto, A. (1998). Sympatho-adrenal involvement in methamphetamine-induced hyperthermia through skeletal muscle hypermetabolism. *European Journal of Pharmacology, 363*, 107–112.

Mausbach, B. T., Semple, S. J., Strathdee, S. A., Zians, J., & Patterson, T. L. (2007). Efficacy of a behavioral intervention for increasing safer sex behaviors in HIV-positive MSM methamphetamine users: Results from the EDGE Study. *Drug and Alcohol Dependence, 87*(2–3), 249–257.

Mayne, T. J., Vittinghoff, E., Chesney, M. A., Barrett, D. C., & Coates, T. J. (1996). Depressive affect and survival among gay and bisexual men infected with HIV. *Archives of Internal Medicine, 156*, 2233–2238.

McEwen, B. (1998). Protective and damaging effects of stress mediators. *New England Journal of Medicine, 338*, 171–179.

Mildvan, D., Spritzler, J., Grossberg, S. E., Fahey, J. L., Johnston, D. M., Schock, B. R., & Kagan, J. (2005). Serum neopterin, an immune activation marker, independently predicts disease progression in advanced HIV-1 infection. *Clinical Infectious Diseases, 40*, 853–858.

Morin, S. F., Sengupta, S., Cozen, M., Richards, T. A., Shriver, M. D., & Palacio, H. (2002). Responding to racial and ethnic disparities in the use of HIV drugs: Analysis of state policies. *Public Health Reports, 117*, 263–272.

Moskowitz, J. T. (2003). Positive affect predicts lower risk of AIDS mortality. *Psychosomatic Medicine, 65*, 620–626.

Motivala, S. J., Hurwitz, B. E., Llabre, M. M., Klimas, N., Fletcher, M. A., Antoni, M. H., … Schneiderman, N. (2003). Psychological distress is associated with decreased memory helper T-cell and B-cell counts in pre-AIDS HIV seropositive men and women but only in those with low viral load. *Psychosomatic Medicine, 65*, 627–635.

Nair, M. P. N., Mahajan, S., Hou, J., Sweet, A. M., & Schwartz, S. A. (2000). The stress hormone, cortisol, synergizes with HIV-1 gp120 to induce apoptosis of normal human peripheral blood mononuclear cells. *Cellular and Molecular Biology, 46(7)*, 122–1238.

Nance, D. W., & Sanders, V. M. (2007). Autonomic innervation and regulation of the immune system (1987–2007). *Brain, Behavior, and Immunity, 21*, 736–745.

Page-Shafer, K., Delorenze, G. N., Satariano, W., & Winkelstein, W. (1996). Comorbidity and survival in HIV-infected men in the San Francisco Men's Health Survey. *Annals of Epidemiology, 6*, 420–430.

Pantaleo, G., Graziosi, C., & Fauci, A. S. (1993). The immunopathogenesis of human immunodeficiency virus infection. *New England Journal of Medicine, 328*, 327–335.

Park, W., Laura, Y., Scalera, A., Tseng, A., & Rourke, S. (2002). High rate of discontinuations of highly active antiretroviral therapy as a result of antiretroviral intolerance in clinical practice: Missed opportunities for support? *AIDS, 16(7)*, 1084–1086.

Patterson, T. L., Williams, S. S., Semple, S. J., Cherner, M., McCutchman, A., Atkinson, J. H., … Nannis, E. (1996). Relationship of psychosocial factors to HIV disease progression. *Annals of Behavioral Medicine, 18*, 30–39.

Pavlidis, N., & Chirigos, M. (1980). Stress-induced impairment of macrophage tumoricidal function. *Psychosomatic Medicine, 42*, 47–54.

Pereira, D., Antoni, M. H., Simon, T., Efantis-Potter, J., Carver, C. S., Durán, R., … O'Sullivan, M. J. (2003a). Stress and squamous intraepithelial lesions in women with human papillomavirus and human immunodeficiency virus. *Psychosomatic Medicine, 65*, 427–434.

Pereira, D., Antoni, M. H., Simon, T., Efantis-Potter, J., Carver, C. S., Durán, R., … O'Sullivan, M. J. (2003b). Stress as a predictor of symptomatic genital herpes virus recurrence in women with human immunodeficiency virus. *Journal of Psychosomatic Research, 54*, 237–244.

Pinkerton, S. D. (2008). Probability of HIV transmission during acute infection in Rakai, Uganda. *AIDS and Behavior, 12*, 677–684.

Rabkin, J. G., Ferrando, S. J., Lin, S. H., Sewell, M., & McElihney, M. (2000). Psychological effects of HAART: A 2-year study. *Psychosomatic Medicine*, *62*, 413–422.

Riley, E. D., Bangsberg, D. R., Guzman, D., Perry, S., & Moss, A. R. (2005). Antiretroviral therapy, hepatitis C virus, and AIDS mortality among San Francisco's homeless and marginally housed. *Journal of Acquired Immune Deficiency Syndromes*, *38*, 191–195.

Rutherford, G. W., Lifson, A. R., & Hessol, N. A. (1990). Course of HIV-1 infection in a cohort of homosexual and bisexual men: An 11 year follow up study. *British Medical Journal*, *301*, 1183–1191.

Safren, S., O'Cleirigh, C., Tan, J., Raminani, S., Reilly, L., Otto, M. W., & Mayer, K. H. (2009). Cognitive behavioral therapy for adherence and depression (CBT-AD) in HIV-infected individuals. *Health Psychology*, *28*, 1–10.

Sapolsky, R. M., Romero, L. M., & Munck, A. U. (2000). How do glucocorticoids influence stress responses? Integrating permissive, suppressive, stimulatory, and preparative actions. *Endocrine Reviews*, *21*, 55–89.

Schneiderman, N., Antoni, M. H., Ironson, G., Fletcher, M. A., Klimas, N., & LaPerriere, A. (1994). HIV-1, immunity and behavior. In Glaser, R. (Ed.), *Handbook of human stress and immunity*. New York, NY: Academic Press.

Simoni, J. M., Pearson, C. R., Pantalone, D. W., Marks, G., & Crepaz, N. (2006). Efficacy of interventions in improving highly active antiretroviral therapy adherence and HIV-1 RNA viral load: A meta-analytic review of randomized controlled trials. *Journal of Acquired Immune Deficiency Syndromes*, *43*(Suppl. 1), S23–S35.

Sledjeski, E. M., Delahanty, D. L., & Bogart, L. M. (2005). Incidence and impact of posttraumatic stress disorder and comorbid depression on adherence to HAART and CD4+ counts in people living with HIV. *AIDS Patient Care STDS*, *19*(11), 728–736.

Sloan, E. K., Tarara, R. P., Capitanio, J. P., & Cole, S. W. (2006). Enhanced replication of simian immunodeficiency virus adjacent to catecholaminergic varicosities in primate lymph nodes. *Journal of Virology*, *80*, 4326–4335.

Starace, F., Ammassari, A., Trotta, M. P., Murri, R., De Longis, P., Izzo, C., … Antinori, A. (2002). Depression is a risk factor for suboptimal adherence to highly active antiretroviral therapy. *Journal of Acquired Immune Deficiency Syndromes*, *31*(Suppl. 3), S136–S139.

Swanson, B., Zeller, J. M., & Spear, G. T. (2998). Cortisol upregulates HIV p24 antigen production in cultured human monocyte-derived macrophages. *Journal of the Association of Nurses in AIDS Care*, *9*(4), 78–84.

Tamalet, C., Fantini, J., Tourres, C., & Yashi, N. (2003). Resistance of HIV-1 to Multiple antiretroviral drugs in France: A 6-year survey (1997–2002) based on an analysis of over 7000 genotypes. *AIDS*, *17*, 2383–2388.

Tindall, B., & Cooper, D. A. (1991). Primary HIV infection: Host responses and intervention strategies. *AIDS*, *5*, 1–15.

Varmus, H. (1988). Retroviruses. *Science*, *240*, 1427–1434.

Vedhara, K., Nott, K. H., Bradbeer, C. S., Davidson, E. A. F., Ong, E. L. C., Snow, M. H., … Nayagam, A. T. (1997). Greater emotional distress is associated with accelerated CD4+ cell decline in HIV infection. *Journal of Psychosomatic Research*, *42*, 379–390.

Vranceanu, A. M., Safren, S. A., Lu, M., Coady, W. M., Skolnik, P. R., Rogers, W. H., & Wilson, I. B. (2008). The relationship of post-traumatic stress disorder and depression to antiretroviral medication adherence in persons with HIV. *AIDS Patient Care STDS*, *22*, 313–321.

Weaver, K. E., Llabre, M. M., Duran, R. E., Antoni, M. H., Ironson, G., Penedo, F. J., & Schneiderman, N. (2005). A stress and coping model of medication adherence and viral load in HIV-positive men and women on highly active antiretroviral therapy (HAART). *Health Psychology*, *24*(4), 385–392.

Webber, M. P., Schoenbaum, E. E., Gourevitch, M. N., Buono, D., & Klein, R. S. (1999). A prospective study of HIV disease progression in female and male drug users. *AIDS*, *13*, 257–262.

34 HIV and African American Women in the U.S. South[1]

A Social Determinants Approach to Population-Level HIV Prevention and Intervention Efforts

Vickie M. Mays, Regan M. Maas,
Joni Ricks, and Susan D. Cochran
University of California, Los Angeles

The year 2011 marks the 30th anniversary of the discovery of the HIV/AIDS virus (Centers for Disease Control and Prevention [CDC], 1981; Gottlieb, 1981; Gottlieb, Schanker, Fan, Saxon, & Weisman, 1981). Although the United States has invested substantial efforts in reducing and eliminating HIV infections and AIDS-related morbidity and mortality, these efforts have had less than optimal success among subpopulations of some racial/ethnic minorities (Dean & Fenton, 2010; Mays, Cochran, & Zamudio, 2004; Sutton et al., 2009). Indeed, CDC surveillance data paint an alarming picture of increasing disparities in HIV/AIDS cases both in terms of such individual characteristics as race and ethnicity and by geographic region. Sadly, for some subpopulations, such as African American women, the incidence and prevalence of HIV infections is worse now than in the early years of the HIV epidemic (Mays & Cochran, 1987, 1988, 1993). In recent data examining new infections from just 2005 to 2008, African American women accounted for 64% of new infections. This trend of increasing proportions of new cases of HIV occurring in African American women cries out for changes in the way the state, county, and federal agencies approach HIV prevention and intervention (CDC, 2010).

Throughout the history of the HIV epidemic in the United States, different subpopulations of Black women have experienced a level of vulnerability unmatched by women of other ethnic and racial groups. In the early years of the epidemic, the enormous impact of the disease among men who have sex with men (MSMs) and the rapidly emerging epidemic among injection drug users were readily apparent. This drew research dollars as the public health system mounted a multipronged attack on the new population health threat. Black women, initially small in number in the HIV statistics, were sometimes an afterthought as scientific attention concentrated elsewhere. Some Black women were infected by sexual partners who were injection drug users or MSMs, behaviors in their partners that the women may or may not have been aware of fully. Some Black women were at risk from their own unsafe injection practices, often without full knowledge of or control over methods to effectively reduce their risks. And some were part of the sex work industry, fueled by the pernicious crack epidemic raging coincidentally in poor urban communities (Cochran & Mays,

---

[1] 1 A version of this work was presented as an APA Master Lecture by the senior author (Mays, V. M. [2007, August]. *The next twenty five years of the HIV epidemic: African American women in the deep south*. Invited Master Lecturer, 115th Annual Convention of the American Psychological Association, San Francisco, CA).

1989; Cochran, Mays, & Roberts, 1988; Mays & Cochran, 1988, 1993; Mays, Cochran, & Bellinger, 1989; Mays, Cochran, & Roberts, 1988a, 1988b).

Eventually, knowledge of how to reduce risk of transmission and effective interventions to do so were developed in the course of the public health response. With maturation of the epidemic, interventions in the intravenous drug use (IDU) community became more effective, especially in urban areas. Hence, for the last two decades, the greatest risk for African American women has increasingly been associated with known heterosexual transmission. However, African American women continue to have the highest number of cases attributed to unknown causes (CDC, 2004; Millett, Malebranche, Mason, & Spikes, 2005). The latter route creates special problems for developing efficacious individual-level public health interventions as it is particularly difficult to counsel women on how to reduce their personal risk when the source of that risk is to them unknown and not necessarily personal. Even more challenging is the complex picture emerging that the cause of these infections is not just male sex partners on the "down low," as previously assumed, but also that there is a greater risk profile in general of heterosexual Black men (Millett, Malebranche, Mason, & Spikes, 2005) with an overall lower rate of condom usage (CDC, 1990; Cornelius, Okundaye, & Manning, 2000; Grinstead, Peterson, Faigeles, & Catania, 1997; Peterson, Catania, Dolcini, & Faigeles, 1993), higher rate of sex partners compared with other racial and ethnic groups (Dolcini, Coates, Catania, Kegeles, & Hauck, 1995; Leigh, Temple, & Trocki, 1993; Peterson et al., 1993), greater participation in concurrent and nonmonogamous sexual relationships (Adimora & Schoenbach, 2002; Norris & Ford, 1999), trading of sex for drugs or money (Lewis & Watters, 1991), active sexually transmitted infections (STIs), and even participation in anal sex (Adimora & Schoenbach, 2002; Jaffe, Seehaus, Wagner, & Leadbeater, 1988). In the face of these dynamics, compared to other racial/ethnic groups' heterosexual women, African American women have the highest numbers of cases. Figure 34.1 shows that of new HIV

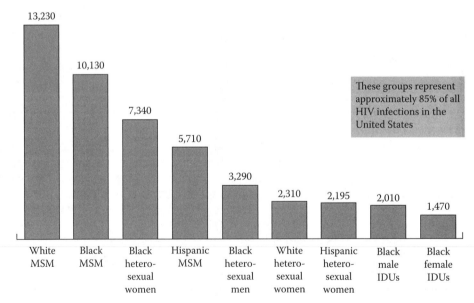

FIGURE 34.1 Numbers of annual HIV infections by high-risk groups (2006). MSM, men who have sex with men (gay and bisexual men); IDU, injection drug user. Sources: *Morbidity and Mortality Weekly Report*, October 3, 2008 and June 5, 2009, with the addition of incidence data from Puerto Rico based on an analysis by Holgrave, D., Johns Hopkins Bloomberg School of Public Health. For this analysis, all Puerto Rico cases were classified as Hispanic. Chart based upon Centers for Disease Control, *HIV Prevention in the United States at a Critical Crossroads*, 2009. (From Office of National AIDS Policy, National HIV/AIDS Strategy for the United States, *The White House Office of National AIDS Policy*, http://www.whitehouse.gov/sites/default/files/uploads/NHAS.pdf, 2011.)

infections in 2006, the pattern is that of all women, African American women have the highest number of cases, a pattern that is continuing in the epidemic. These numbers argue against HIV prevention efforts for African American women continuing to rely heavily on individual responsibility for condom use. To change the circumstances that serve to fuel the infection rate in African American women, we need population-based strategies to address the population vulnerabilities that exist within African Americans communities (El-Bassel, Caldeira, Ruglass, & Gilbert, 2009; Mays, Cochran, & Barnes, 2007; Mays, Cochran, & Zamudio, 2004). It is from within the boundaries of the African American population that most African American women draw their sexual partners, their confidants for social support who serve as their sources of health information, and their social community-based norms.

Despite the tremendous gains in the public health fight again the HIV/AIDS epidemic in the United States, Black women remain a vulnerable population for HIV infection. In this chapter, we focus on two major issues in understanding the HIV epidemic among African American women. The first is context: Over the last three decades, many excellent papers have been published highlighting the importance of individual and social factors in the HIV/AIDS epidemic (Adimora & Schoenbach, 2002; Lightfoot & Milburn, 2009), including as it affects Black women in particular (Bhatta, Vermund, & Hoesley, 2010). Here, we add to the mix the intersection of place—in this instance, the American South—to highlight how social and individual determinants are also shaped by their physical location in America (Qian, Taylor, Fawal, & Vermund, 2006; Whetten & Reif, 2006). We argue that the concentration of overlapping sources of disadvantage and pathways to HIV infection in the South have created an environmental threat to the health of Black women living there. Our second focus is on the ways in which a social determinants approach at a population level can be employed by various branches of the federal government, which must be enlisted to break the cycle of HIV transmission in the South, where the context of HIV risks requires interventions beyond the individual level. The branches of government are oft-overlooked as potential partners in HIV prevention that could, under the leadership of the Department of Health and Human Services, move beyond the traditional focus on individual-level health interventions. Given our focus here, we hope to highlight a potential pathway to improving HIV prevention for the future that can meet and exceed the goals of the President's National Strategy for the Elimination of HIV Infection. (Office of National AIDS Policy [ONAP], 2010).

In this chapter, we propose eliminating and reducing HIV/AIDS disparities in African American women in the South through efforts made at the population level. Often the focus for reducing and eliminating health disparities for African American women is individual, dyadic, or familial, even involving circles of influence of family, friends, and community groups. We have chosen to employ a social determinants approach emphasizing how the confluence of issues cluster together to create a "risk environment" (Blankenship, Bray, & Merson, 2000; Diez-Roux, 1998; Farley, 2006; Rhodes, 2002; Rhodes, Stimson, & Ball, 2001). This notion of thinking about risk environment in the reduction of HIV infection has been employed in developing countries, where we realize that women who have no economic means of sustaining themselves need jobs in order to protect themselves against HIV infection. In developing contexts, we realize the importance of women going to school and becoming educated, the importance of clean water and viable methods of transportation to sell goods, and so on, as necessary structural interventions for reducing women's risk of getting infected. We have also seen an emphasis on HIV prevention at a multivariate structural level that emphasizes risk environment as a framework for reducing drug-related harm (Rhodes, 2002). Whereas we recognize these approaches as sensible to use in developing countries, we fail to understand that they also apply here, in the United States. There are many conditions in the U.S. South, for example, that come together for women in a unique and compelling way that creates an almost inescapable set of risks for HIV infection that require structural interventions at a policy level.

To contextualize the risk of African American women in the South, we have included two mediational models. First, Farley's (2006) clustering risk helps to illustrate that it is not each risk factor that by itself puts African American women in such great jeopardy for HIV infection but, rather, the circumstances of how the factors cluster together to create an almost inescapable vulnerability. Although these individual risk factors are such regardless of gender, socioeconomic status, and so on, it is the intersectionality of the statuses that African American women bring to the table that makes their vulnerability not only different from but also unique relative to other racial and ethnic groups and relative to other women. It is the intersectionality of Black women's statuses of their race, their gender, and their history in U.S. society, particularly in the Deep South, that has left a legacy of vulnerabilities ranging from legal policies that still fail to protect Black women equally even to Black men, to structural forces within the African American community of "color caste" systems, sex ratio imbalances, and overall intimate injustices that are outgrowths of racism and social injustices uniquely experienced by African American women (Rose, 1998, 2004). Then second, Hammonds (1994) helps us to understand the uniqueness of the experience of Black women's sexuality, especially in the Deep South, with its history of Black women's bodies as colonized. Although it is beyond the scope of this chapter to consider in depth, we must note that Hammond (1994) traces themes around Black women's sexuality that in the face of clustering facilitate risk unlike that of any other group. First is the theme of Black women's silence about their sexuality, that is, their inability to give historical voice to their experiences, such that even when abused and raped they found silence far safer than sharing information or seeking justice for these sexual injustices. This tendency of silence about sexualty continues even today in that historical narratives of Black women's sexuality are often alive and well as their sexuality is pathologized, eroticized, and labeled dark when compared to other women, particularly White women. So, in the service of avoiding stereotypes and the negative consequence of being "other," there is a resistance to admitting sexuality as an attempt to portray proper behavior in search of respect. This contested nature of Black women's sexuality, particular in the South, with its set of rules of engagement, reinforces a silence around sexuality that is detrimental to individualized risk reduction.

RACE, PLACE, AND HIV INFECTION

Social determinant models of health (Brunner & Marmot, 1999; Gehlert et al., 2008; Kaplan, Everson, & Lynch, 2000) emphasize that social and individual factors influence both the likelihood that an individual will develop a particular disease or will, having experienced illness or its precursors, receive optimal care from health care settings. Influential social characteristics include such constructs as poverty, family support, cultural values, and availability of health care resources. Influential individual characteristics include a laundry list of demographic characteristics that have been linked repeatedly to health, as, for example, age, race and ethnicity, immigration status, and gender. As well, intrapsychic factors, including attitudes and beliefs, and individual behaviors, such as engaging in HIV risk behaviors, play important roles in the prevention of HIV infection.

In recent years, "place," the focus on *where* people live, has evolved as an additional key contextual factor that is a determinant of health (Acevedo-Garcia, Lochner, Osypuk, & Subramanian, 2003; Acevedo-Garcia & Osypuk, 2008a, 2008b; Acevedo-Garcia, Osypuk, McArdle, & Williams, 2008; Acevedo-Garcia et al., 2004). Place is an organizing structure that reflects the social, cultural, and economic capital locally available to individuals, as well as the contextual forces that help shape their options and experiences of health. Critical to this perspective is that some persons, located in particular geographic spaces, are impacted more than others by policies, procedures, or deficits in social, economic, and legal resources, which hinder them from obtaining optimal benefit of their individual choices. Or in terms of the HIV epidemic, some locations, such as the Deep South, are more efficient incubators than others of the conditions that encourage and facilitate the spread of HIV infection. Further, we assert that this condition is especially relevant for African American women.

The South occupies a particularly important place in African American life. In 1870, in the first U.S. census following the American Civil War, 90% of Blacks lived in the South (Gibson & Jung, 2002). Thus, the majority of today's Black population can trace its historical roots to the South. Further, in the 1860 census just prior to the Civil War, 89% of Blacks lived in slavery, including 94% of those slaves residing in the South. The legacy of slavery, too, is thus intimately woven into the Black experience and can be seen in the multiple social, political, and economic race-based disadvantages that persist even today. Although in the eyes of many individuals, and perhaps true for them, slavery is an experience relegated to the past, the legacy of slavery in policies, procedures, attitudes, and resources remains, unfortunately, alive and well.

An example of how past practices influence current economic resources is evident in the states that have adopted or are in the process of developing slavery-era disclosure laws in recognition of how particular businesses built their wealth on commerce related to slavery. The most famous cases of such businesses are insurance companies whose early success and profit came from insuring slaves (Quinn, 2000), thereby allowing the companies to amass wealth. However, modern analyses of the benefits of employment and education exemplify that despite current acquisition of equal salaries or education, Black Americans derive far less benefit in society from their education or salaries compared to Whites (Shapiro & Oliver, 2006). As Shapiro and Oliver (2006) so eloquently illustrate, the foundations of early benefits as well as current policies and procedures continue to disadvantage African Americans such that they derive less benefit per dollar earned or per year of education. The South has a history of enacting policies that range from devaluing African Americans' ability to be free, amass property, and pass those benefits forward to heirs, to maintaining equity policies in education, health care, and other vital support services that are today, by default, both separate and unequal to those who have benefited from early race discrimination. The result is a South, particularly a Deep South, in which African Americans bear a tremendous cumulative disadvantage resulting in higher levels of negative health outcomes.

As Farley's (2006) model of risk clustering (see Figure 34.2) illustrates, several factors associated with the transmission of sexually transmitted infections (STIs) are clustered among African American populations in the southeastern states. These factors include a number of socioeconomic

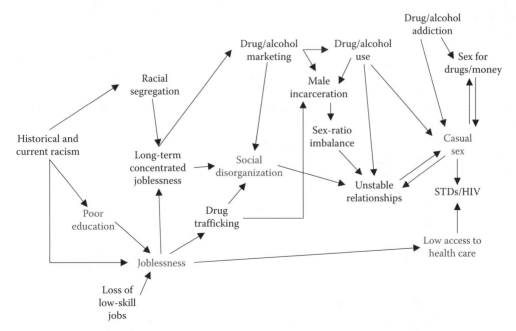

FIGURE 34.2 Risk clustering of social-contextual issues in HIV infection in African American women in the U.S. South. (Adapted from Farley, T., *Sexually Transmitted Diseases*, 33, 7, S58–S64, 2006.)

disadvantages as well as a co-occurring drug network. The intersection of these factors, within the context of social and political neglect born of centuries of racism, provides a ready breeding ground for HIV transmission. In looking at the risk clustering, we also see emerging the intersectionality of different domains of responsibilities that come together to create environments of risk. If the goal were to disrupt or break up connections in this model of risk clustering, doing so would require a multiagency approach to reduce the risk of acquiring HIV infection. Yet we focus more of our efforts on asking individuals alone or in their dyadic relationships to break these connections. Clearly, in the South, this latter approach may be insufficient to stem the tide of STI and HIV in African American women because of the extent to which their social status puts them at the crux of vulnerability in this multisectorial clustering of potential sources of risk. To break or reduce their risk clearly cannot be accomplished only through efforts tailored to those responsible for their own health. Broadening efforts to include prevention strategies spanning multiple levels to simultaneously reduce and eliminate as many of the risk factors in the cluster as possible, as well as by evaluating success as a long-term goal, could increase the country's capacity to reduce the number of new infections in the African American population.

HIV/AIDS IN THE AMERICAN SOUTH

Of the HIV/AIDS epidemic, it has been said that it "moves along the fault lines of our society and becomes a metaphor for understanding that society" (Bateson & Goldsby, 1988, p. 16). Had we heeded that warning more than two decades ago, we would have predicted that the U.S. Southern states, particularly the Deep South, with its unique history and social position of African Americans, would be the harbinger of the conditions that facilitate and complicate the prevention of HIV infection for African Americans (Adimora & Schoenbach, 2002; Adimora, Schoenbach, & Martinson, 2006; Aral, O'Leary, & Baker, 2006; Dean & Fenton, 2010; Doherty, Leone, & Aral, 2007; Hightow et al., 2005; McKinney, 2002; Morris & Monroe, 2009; Reif, Geonnotti, & Whetten, 2006; Reif, Whetten, Ostermann, & Raper, 2006).

Today, 9 of the 16 Southern states are represented among the 15 states with the highest prevalence of HIV cases; 16 of the 20 metropolitan areas, with the highest number of AIDS cases; and for women, 6 of the 10 states with the highest AIDS case rate (Hall & McKenna, 2005; Magnus et al., 2009; Southern AIDS Coalition, 2008). Nationally, although new HIV infections have been occurring at a relatively stable rate since the year 2000, with approximately 56,000 per year (CDC, 2008; Hall et al., 2008), the rate of new infections among Black women is nearly 15 times as great as that of White women and approximately four times that of Latina women (CDC, 2010). It is within this context that one out of every 30 Black women will be HIV infected in the United States, with this likelihood being even higher for those Black women who live in the South (Fleming, Lansky, Lee, & Nakashima, 2006), where the case rate of new infections is increasing.

On another front, the South is home to approximately 68% of all AIDS cases among rural populations but represents only 35% of that population (Phillips & Forti, 2004). The case rate is three times greater in this region than in any other rural area in the United States (Bowen, Gambrell, & DeCarlo, 2006; DeCarlo, 1998).

From the initial years of the HIV epidemic, there were warning signs that the South was an HIV incubator. Data since the mid-1980s consistently showed a growing number of cases of STIs and HIV/AIDS in the South (Rural Center for HIV/AIDS Prevention, 2002). Data from the early 1990s demonstrated as well an increase in cases among rural communities in the South. Yet despite these data, the case numbers continued to grow to become an epidemic for Black women in the South.

So, what is it about the South, particularly the Deep South, that makes control of the HIV/AIDS epidemic among African American women so difficult? We argue here that it is the intersection of several distinct social conditions and accumulated disadvantages that sets the stage for this occurrence (Diallo et al., 2010; Doherty et al., 2007; Whetten & Reif, 2006). When considered in the context of clustering, theses factors, presented in Figure 34.2, create a unique, place-specific risk context.

THE SOUTH AS AN INCUBATOR OF THE HIV EPIDEMIC

As Farley (2006) has argued, multiple factors contribute synergistically to creating HIV risk in the South. Table 34.1 presents some of the most compelling social determinants identified by community agencies and drawn from research studies conducted in the South. Although each of these social determinants is a problem individually, in its own domain, it is how they cluster together in the South as a function of history, policies, regional attitudes, quality or lack of resources, and even the legacy of the relationships of the South in general with its African American residents that creates the biggest HIV risk. These social determinants are addressed in the next sections.

Low Educational Attainment

Even before the appearance of the HIV epidemic, levels of educational attainment among African Americans in the South were persistently low. About half of the African American population of the United States lived in the South, and nearly all (91%) African Americans who reside in rural areas are in the Deep South—623 counties in 11 Old South states: Alabama, Arkansas, Florida, Georgia, Louisiana, Mississippi, North Carolina, South Carolina, Tennessee, Texas, and Virginia (Kismo, 1999). Over half (54%) of all rural African Americans aged 25 or older living in those regions as of the 1990s, when HIV was taking a foothold, did not have high school diplomas (Kuismo, 1999; Wimberley & Morris, 1996). The dreams of liberal America, whose advocates fought so hard in the Southern civil rights movement in the 1960s and early 1970s, were that all Americans, but in particular rural Southern African Americans, would benefit from increased educational opportunity as a result of the *Brown v. Board of Education* (1954) decision. This result was not the case. Rural African Americans aged 25 to 34 had the least educational attainment in both 1980 and 1990 when compared with urban Blacks and both urban and rural Whites (Kuismo, 1999). This group also had the lowest proportion of college graduates (6.1%, down nearly two percentage points from 1980), and the highest proportion of young adults who had not completed high school (29.4%; Butler, 1997; Kuismo, 1999). When HIV was blazing through the U.S. South, African Americans lacked the ben-

---

TABLE 34.1
Unique Factors in the HIV/AIDS Epidemic in the U.S. South

- Migration of African American men
- Low levels of economic opportunities
- Sex ratio imbalances/unequal relationship opportunities/racial preferences
- Rural and periurban areas
- High rates of other STDs
- Low educational attainment
- Lack of cultural competency in HIV prevention, education, and interventions
- Prison complexes
- Drug trade corridors
- HIV/AIDS stigma
- Inadequate health infrastructure

Source: Adapted from State AIDS/STD Directors Work Group, Southern States Manifesto, 1, http://www.southernaidscoalition.org/policy/SouthernStatesManifesto_2003.pdf, 2003; Hall, H., Li, J., & McKenna, M. *Journal of Rural Health*, 21, 3, 2005.

---

efits of health maintenance that are associated with education (Egerter, Braverman, Sadegh-Nobari, Grossman-Kahn, & Dekker, 2009) to help stave off HIV infection.

This lack of educational attainment reflected a long-standing political disenfranchisement that resulted in race-segregated and inferior schools for African American children. Eventually, the 1954 Supreme Court decision in *Brown v. Board of Education* outlawed discriminatory practices, thereby leading to the desegregation of public schools. In delivering the unanimous opinion of the Court, Chief Justice Earl Warren noted that the aim of ending segregation was not just to eliminate the disparities in resources and educational quality that characterized White and Black schools. It was also to affect the "intangible" qualities that make segregation particularly pernicious. Chief Justice Warren argued, "To separate [children] from others of similar age and qualifications solely because of their race generates a feeling of inferiority as to their status in the community that may affect their hearts and minds in a way unlikely ever to be undone" (*Brown v. Board of Education*, 1954, p. 6).

Although the intervention successfully ended state-sanctioned segregation, school enrollment bifurcated into private versus public settings that retained the effects of segregation. Fifty years later, the South has some of the lowest expenditures per public school student in K–12 grades and the highest drop-out rates in the country (Greenwald, Hedges, & Laine, 1994; Hedges, Laine, & Greenwald, 1994; Morris & Monroe, 2009; Southern Education Foundation, 2007). Indeed, as of 2005, children in the South made up over 40% of all school dropouts in the nation. The legacy of inadequate educational venues for African Americans, restricted by Whites for many years to the teaching of vocational careers and currently receiving low levels of public financing, continues to limit the educational opportunities for African American children (Morris & Monroe, 2009).

Low levels of educational attainment are associated with poorer outcomes for a multitude of health conditions (Currie & Enrico, 2003; Kubzansky, Berkman, Glass, & Seeman, 1998; Mirowsky & Ross, 2003; Reynolds & Ross, 1998; Ross & Mirowsky, 1999; Ross & Wu, 1995, 1996). It is estimated that even a small one-year increase in education for a mother, for example, is associated with a 7%–9% reduction in mortality for children less than 5 years of age (Cleland & Van Ginneken, 1988; Gakidou, Cowling, Lozano, & Murray, 2010; Ross & Van Willigen, 1997). Of particular significance for African American women at risk for HIV is that educational attainment is also associated with a delay in pregnancy. Each year of delay in becoming pregnant at a young age means that more young women are able to obtain the necessary skills and resources to be more capable mothers.

A lack educational attainment also results in a lack of preparation and competitiveness for the workforce that is also associated with difficulties in employment, especially in obtaining and keeping jobs paying a living wage and being covered by health insurance (Wyn & Peckman, 2010). For women, this burden can lead to economic dependence on a man for financial support (Adimora & Schoenbach, 2002; Adimora, Schoenbach, & Doherty, 2006; Adimora et al., 2001; Farley, 2006). This economic dependence may, in turn, have direct consequences for the choices that women make surrounding sexual behaviors with sexual partners, behaviors that may put them at risk for STIs and HIV (Annang, Walsemann, Maitra, & Kerr, 2010).

The critical role that educational attainment plays in overall health is illustrated in Figure 34.2, which is drawn from the Robert Wood Johnson Commission on Social Determinants Brief on Education and Health (Egerter, Braverman, Sadegh-Nobari, Grossman-Kahn, & Dekker, 2009). Drawing on results from a series of studies, the commission compiled Figure 34.3 to show three possible models of how educational attainment may be linked with health through three interrelated pathways: (1) Model 1: health knowledge and behavior; (2) Model 2: employment and income; and (3) Model 3: social and psychological factors. Each model has a clear implication for ways to think about how education is related to reducing HIV infection. In Model 1, the assumption is that knowledge increases healthy behaviors. Although knowledge is not by itself sufficient for behavior change, it is nonetheless a necessary component of behavior change. In Model 2, employment and resources act in a protective manner for women by reducing their likelihood of being in positions of

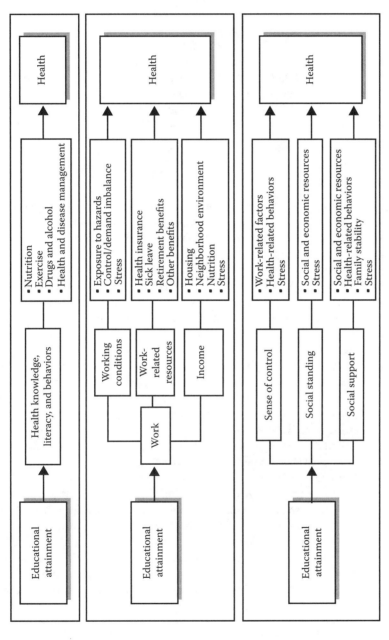

FIGURE 34.3 Models of how education possibly affects health. (From Egerter, S., Braverman, P., Sadegh-Nobari, T., Grossman-Kahn, R., & Dekker, M., *Education matters for health* [Issue Brief No. 6]. Princeton, NJ: Robert Wood Johnson Foundation, 2009.)

vulnerability. As discussed earlier, poverty and a lack of resources place women in risk-prone situations. The third model is one that addresses the socioemotional contributions to risk avoidance and risk engagement. The use of drugs, participation in sexual behaviors, and relationship dynamics are related to a lack of social support, social standing, and sense of personal control.

Educational attainment is a key factor for addressing many of the social determinants that increase the vulnerability of African American women to HIV infection. If school systems are failing African American women, the loss in this country is not just a group of people who fall short on educational standards but also women at greater risk for negative health outcomes.

The importance of education for HIV can be seen in a 2005 study by Peterman, Lindsey, and Selik that compared social factors among counties with the smallest increase in AIDS incidence and those with largest increase in AIDS incidence between the periods 1981–1990 and 1995–1999. The researchers observed that counties with higher incidence included a larger proportion of African Americans, a greater percentage of individuals in the lowest literacy levels, and a higher proportion of individuals reporting less than a ninth-grade education. The education statistics show at least a twofold difference.

FEWER ECONOMIC OPPORTUNITIES

As the United States continues to outsource employment, there are fewer jobs for those individuals without higher levels of education. African American women compared to women of other races are more likely to exceed the national average for living in poverty. Approximately one in four African American women currently live in poverty, including 32% of women aged 18 and older residing in the South (U.S. Census Bureau, 2009). African Americans residing in rural areas in the South have lower incomes than do Whites of similar educational backgrounds (Beaulieu, Barfield, & Stone, 2001; Probst et al., 2002).

Poverty is a known correlate of increasing the likelihood that women and adolescent girls will engage in transactional and nonconsensual sex, use condoms less frequently, and begin sexual activity at an earlier age (Hallman, 2005). As well as being a measure of income, poverty is also a proxy for many things that are related to vulnerability to HIV/AIDS (Smith, 2002). For example, living in poverty decreases resources for the purchase of condoms and for transportation to access condoms. It is also often a sign of lack of employment and the need to rely on others for financial subsidies. Poverty is the underlying basis for many of the factors appearing in Farley's risk clusters, which are the proxies for poverty. In the South, particularly in rural areas, poverty characterizes not only individuals but also large segments of communities, making it difficult for individuals to improve their economic status short of moving out of the area (Probst et al., 2002). A study by the U.S. Department of Agriculture notes that individuals in rural and nonmetropolitan areas are more likely to receive greater funds from the government in the areas of income subsidies (e.g., medical benefits, social security, and public assistance) than are individuals living in metropolitan areas. In contrast, metropolitan centers are more likely than rural areas to receive business assistance and funds for community and regional development. This pattern makes it much more difficult for people in rural areas to change their life circumstances (Probst et al., 2002) and thereby reduce their risk for HIV infection. The characteristics associated with poverty and limited resources are more likely to be associated with HIV infection in African American women in the rural South than with others.

Living in Rural and Peri-Urban Areas

Because in comparison to other regions the South has the greatest proportion of its population living in rural areas, there are unique challenges for HIV-prevention activities (Agee et al., 2006; Crosby, Yarber, DiClemente, Wingood, & Meyerson, 2002; Krawczyk, Funkhouser, Kilby, & Vermund, 2006). These activities include geographic isolation and limited access to health care and social services (Bowen et al., 2006; Decarlo, 1998; Rural Center of HIV/AIDS Prevention, 2002). Social isolation puts young girls, particularly when they are less socially connected, at greater risk of sexual coercion (Hallman & Diers, 2004) and is characteristic of some rural areas. Some of the issues facing rural areas, such as a lack of economic opportunities, high rates of STIs, and low rates of safe-sex practices, have been discussed at length in the literature (Doherty et al., 2007; Napravnik & et al., 2006; Phillips & Forti, 2004; Rural Center of HIV/AIDS Prevention, 2002; Thomas, 2006; Thomas et al., 1999; Thomas & Sampson, 2005; Thomas & Thomas, 1999). These issues apply especially to African Americans; for although only 12% of African Americans live in rural areas nationally, 90% of that 12% reside in the South (Cromartie & Beale, 1996; Morris & Monroe, 2009). This demographic has implications as well for HIV prevention methods. The great majority of culturally appropriate interventions developed for African Americans are based on urban models. For example, the notion of using condoms is often predicated on the assumption that drugstores and places of condom purchase or distribution are within short distances and therefore condoms are easy to obtain. However, in rural areas getting to a drugstore or a neighborhood store to buy condoms can be difficult and require preplanning. Rural bus service is limited. Many young people have no or restricted access to cars for transportation. Further, the store clerk might be a friend or acquaintance of the family, making if difficult for married males or young adults to purchase condoms without raising suspicions.

Other issues arise with peri-urban areas, which are often transition or interaction zones, where urban and rural activities mix. Peri-urban areas have landscape features that are subject to rapid modifications because as cities develop, much of their growth is located in such areas. Transportation systems are often minimal, restricting the radius of social interactions and access to such simple prevention resources as condoms purchasable from drug stores. In very recent times, the place variable of peri-urban areas has become a focus in health research as studies examine walkability, physical inactivity, and obesity (World Health Organization [WHO], 2001). It may also be to our advantage to consider how accessibility in peri-urban areas affects social networks and access to resources, as well as the role of this space in the development of effective prevention strategies. Studies of peri-urban and rural areas in the South indicate a different picture than that we are accustomed to seeing in urban areas. For example, in the South, rural patients infected with HIV/AIDS were more likely be female, heterosexual, young, and African American or Latino (Cohn, Klein, Mohr, Van de Horst, & Weber, 1994; Elmore, 2006). Peri-urban spaces may facilitate finding potential sexual partners as a function of restricted access in the neighborhood; but because of their suburban rural nature, such peri-urban spaces do not necessarily facilitate HIV prevention services and educational outreach activities.

HIV/AIDS STIGMA

Several studies have indicated that fear of HIV/AIDS-related stigma plays a significant role in controlling the HIV epidemic (Herek, 2007; Herek, Capitanio, & Widaman, 2002; Mahajan et al., 2008). This type of control happens at multiple levels, including reducing willingness to be tested for HIV infection status and fear that disclosure of one's HIV status will lead to discrimination (Mahajan et al., 2008). However, we have yet to fully investigate experiences with HIV/AIDS stigma in the rural or peri-rural environment (Whetten, Reif, Whetten, & Murphy-Miller, 2008). A qualitative study of persons living with HIV/AIDS (PWH/A) in the Southern town of Wilmington, North Carolina, found that when individuals perceived the community to be nonsupportive, few were willing to reveal their HIV status because they feared being stigmatized for having HIV/AIDS (Elmore, 2006). Some individuals were even reluctant to share their HIV status with family and close friends for fear that they would then share the information with others. This fear is realistic because in small towns anonymity is likely to be lower than it is in urban settings.

Deficits in economic and job opportunities and low population densities may constrain individuals' opportunities for both privacy and disclosure. Further, it is not entirely clear that providing resources within an HIV/AIDS-specialized context, as is typically done in urban settings, is the best approach in rural and peri-urban areas, where blending prevention, care, and treatment into general public services may work better. There are pros and cons to offering stand-alone HIV education and prevention services, rather than making them a part of other health services or health promotion and outreach community groups, as a method for addressing stigma. Again, much of the research literature that has identified best practices for dealing with concerns around stigma has been developed in urban or international rural settings.

Southern Black culture, too, has a complex but functional set of social rules that operate to offer support as well as sanction behaviors, including homosexuality and sexual infidelities (Glick & Golden, 2010; Herek, Widaman, & Capitanio, 2005). One of the particular pressures on individuals is the push not to bring shame or embarrassment to the race as a group (Gilbert, Harvey, & Belgrave, 2009; Pitt, 2010). Whereas such large urban areas in the Deep South as Atlanta might reflect a mixture of cultures and enhanced tolerance of "stigmatized" sexual behaviors, this situation is not true for much of the Bible Belt. Black conservative church congregations, where traditionally sex outside of marriage and homosexuality are frowned on, abound in the Deep South (Lemelle & Battle, 2004; Pitt, 2010; Wilson & Moore, 2009). Further, sex education is relegated to the purview of parents, and sexual abstinence until marriage might be the preferred method of school-based and parental education for reducing HIV risk behaviors (Haberland & Rogow, 2007; Kirby et al., 1994). These social conditions can make it difficult to address HIV prevention in a forthright manner and can make HIV-infected individuals reluctant to acknowledge their status publicly (Akers et al., 2010).

CONTEXTUAL ISSUES IN INTIMATE RELATIONSHIPS

Among African American women in general, the risk for HIV infection through sexual contact is influenced by the prevalence of the infectious agent in their social networks, their choice of sexual partners, and the intraracial and intrapersonal relationship dynamics that influence both their own choice of behaviors and the normative behaviors of their sexual network (Adimora & Schoenbach, 2002; Adimora, Schoenbach, & Doherty, 2006; Adimora, Schoenbach, Martinson, et al., 2006; Adimor et al., 2001; Adimora et al. 2003, 2004; Aiello, Simanek, & Galea, 2010; Diallo et al., 2010; Mays & Cochran, 1988). Estimates are that approximately 1 in 30 Black women in the United States will become HIV infected, most often through heterosexual sex and often with a partner of unknown HIV status (CDC, 2010). Hence, encouraging these women to take precautions to reduce their risk through behavior change is critical.

But there are a number obstacles African American women face in pursuing this path. Apart from the well-known difficulties in creating individual behavior change, recent efforts to target dyadic change (Karney et al., 2010) are likely to prove especially difficult for African American women. The new focus on dyadic approaches is an attempt to recognize that one of the primary prevention tools for reducing contact with such infectious agents as HIV relies on condom use, which is not under the control of women. Developing dyadic HIV interventions in which protective behavior changes are achieved is best accomplished for African Americans, it has been argued, if these interventions are couched in Afrocentric approaches (Gilbert et al., 2009; Taylor, Harvery, & Belgrave, 2009). Significant support exists for using culturally specific or culturally relevant Afrocentric approaches based in values and beliefs drawn from the religion and philosophy of ancient African traditions—useful mechanisms by which to achieve prosocial and healthy behaviors in African Americans (for a fuller discussion, see the works of Myers, 1988; Nobles, 1980).

However, the efficacy of these Afrocentric dyadic approaches is dependent, to some extent, on whether relationships are long term and monogamous as opposed to short term and serial. Census data analyzed by the Joint Center for Political and Economic Studies (2001) suggest that this limitation is more likely to impact African American women. Black women's marriage rates between 1950 and 2000 dropped from 62% to 36.1%. Although White women experienced a decline as well (66% to 57.4%), the decline was not as severe. Between 1950 and 2000, the prevalence of never-married Black women doubled, from 20.7% to 42.4%. Thus, the experience for many Black women is that they will never marry but will instead experience a number of serial partnerships over the course of their lifespan. African American women also are least likely, when compared to women in other racial and ethnic groups, to marry or date outside of their race (Adimora et al., 2004; Cornwell & Cunningham, 2006; Mays & Cochran, 1988). Over 93% of African Americans marry within their race, however (Joint Center for Political and Economic Studies, 2001). Finally, even married African Americans are more likely (21%) than similar Whites (16%) to report having had sex outside the marriage at some point (ARDA, 2008). The effect of these factors (i.e., serial relationships and lower rates of marriage, lower rates of monogamous marriage, and same-race partner choices) and the greater prevalence of HIV infection among Blacks (Millett et al., 2005) increases Black women's HIV risk because they are more likely than women from other racial and ethnic groups to be exposed to an HIV-infected partner.

Indeed, one of the ways to quantify the pressures on African American women's choices in intimate relationships is the sex-ratio imbalance. (Cornwell & Cunningham, 2008). The sex ratio is the ratio of partnership-eligible women to partnership-eligible men. As can be seen in Figure 34.4, throughout much of the South, African American women face an intensely competitive market for relationship partners. Findings from one study (Adimora, Schoenbach, & Doherty, 2006) in North Carolina underscore that the sexual networks of African Americans in the South are more likely than among other racial and ethnic groups to be dissassortive relative to STIs, mixing low and high risk for individuals. As well, nearly a quarter of women in the study reported being in concurrent relationships in the previous year. In Figure 34.4 we also see the overlay of the limited market and the prevalence of AIDS, indicating a potential linkage between the two. Place, race, and social determinants of health are clearly at work in the increasing new cases of HIV infection in African American women.

A TRADITION OF INADEQUATE HEALTH CARE SERVICES

The South has long suffered from a lack of major medical centers and from academic programs that turn out large numbers of African American health care providers (Probst et al., 2002). In rural areas in the South, 84% of the counties where African Americans are the majority are health professions shortage areas (Probst et al., 2002). One out of eight African Americans lives in an area without a hospital in comparison to 1 out 10 White Americans in the rural South (Probst et al., 2002). One of the ironies is that a large number of historically Black colleges and medical schools are located in the South. However, they are persistently in need of greater levels of infrastructure assistance in order to expand and increase adequate health care services to African Americans in this geographic region. In the United States, top-ranked hospitals are typically affiliated with major academic institutions, few of which call the Deep South their home.

In parallel with the relative deficiency in health care infrastructure, over the years major investments by the Centers for Disease Control and the National Institutes of Health in HIV prevention efforts typically bifurcated along two lines of attack that bypassed many African Americans in the South. One major focus was predominantly urban MSMs; a second was predominantly urban intravenous drug users. Neither focus was likely to optimally target the needs of many Southern Blacks. The issue is not just delivery of services, such as extra resources for testing and counseling that come with research investments, but also a potential lack of full development of culturally efficacious approaches. What works in New York City among predominantly young, African American MSMs may not have the same effect in a rural or peri-urban African American setting. Even some of the earliest efforts to develop appropriately targeted rural interventions (Heckman et al., 1998; Williams, Bowen, & Horvath, 2005) were often focused on young, White MSMs.

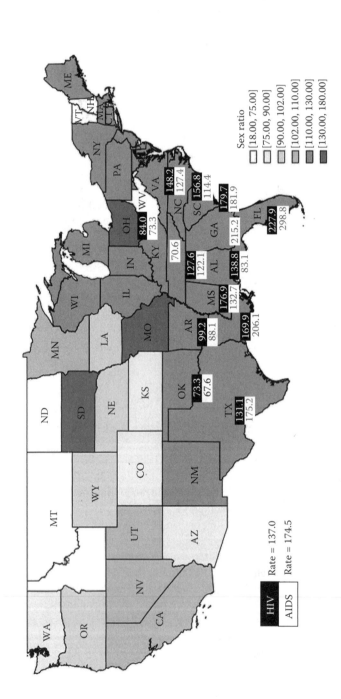

FIGURE 34.4   African American sex ratios (18–24 year olds). (From Cornwell, C., & Cunningham, S. A., *Sex ratios and risky sexual behavior* [Working paper], Department of Economics, University of Georgia, 2006.)

HIGH RATES OF OTHER STIs

The HIV epidemic in the South co-occurred with other outbreaks of STIs, including gonorrhea and syphilis (Aral, 1996; Newman & Berman, 2008; Thomas, Kulik, & Schoenbach, 1995; Thomas & Thomas, 1999). As noted earlier, several factors in partner selection and opportunities serve to accelerate sexually transmitted disease epidemics among African Americans in the South (Aral, Adimora, & Fenton, 2008; Aral et al., 2006; Crepaz et al., 2009). Sexual mixing across class, age, educational, and risk-behavior status boundaries is fueled by limited partner choices (Blanchard & Aral, 2010; Kraut-Becher & Aral, 2006; Nelson et al., 2007). Further, early detection and treatment is hampered by deficiencies in the health care structure. Indeed, in 2005, approximately 68% of gonorrhea cases and 42% of all primary and secondary syphilis infections in the United States reported to the Centers for Disease Control occurred among African Americans (Newman & Berman, 2008). African American women were nearly 15 times as likely as White women to experience a syphilis infection. To some extent, these statistics reflect reporting bias associated with public clinic use (Newman & Berman, 2008), but other population-based surveys also indicate rates of some STIs 2.6 to 21 times greater in African Americans compared to other racial and ethnic groups. More than a third of these infections occur in the South, where most of the high African American density counties (defined as 15% or greater of residents) exist. In more than 95% of these high African American density counties, rates of reported gonorrhea infections are greater than 100 per 100,000 persons. In contrast, among high White density counties (defined as 80% or greater of residents) in the United States, only 0.5% experience this great a gonorrhea case reporting prevalence. Newman and Berman (2008) note that the effect of this enormous difference in the widespread prevalence of gonorrhea may function to reduce pressure on public health agencies to intervene.

MIGRATION OF PERSONS, DRUGS, AND RISKS

Migration of persons in and out of the South has always been a significant factor in the history of African Americans in the United States (Frey, 2004; Grossman, 2001). Large-scale migrations in the early 20th century to cities in the North, Midwest, and West followed economic and social opportunities that offered better lives. In the end of the 20th century, the migration pattern reversed as Blacks sought economic and social opportunities in the new South. This pattern can be seen in the 2000 census, where compared to all other regions of the United States, the South had the largest net growth in its Black population (Morris & Monroe, 2009; U.S. Census Bureau, 2003). Gang abatement efforts in the Northeast and such other urban areas as Chicago and Los Angeles pushed African American and Latino males with histories of gang affiliation and/or incarceration to live with family members in the South. Migration, too, from high-HIV-prevalence areas like the Northeast brought greater numbers of HIV-infected persons into high Black density communities. Data from 1994 show that even then a large proportion of HIV-infected individuals in the rural South reported that they were infected elsewhere (Cohn et al., 1994).

Not only do people move through the South, but drugs, drug trafficking, and drug cultures do as well. Drug trafficking brings with it increased drug use by persons in the community, transitional sex for drugs or money, increased rates of STIs in general and HIV in particular, and increased rates of incarceration.

In the South, a major drug-trade corridor follows I-95, an interstate highway that runs from New York to Miami (Cook, Royce, Thomas, & Hanusa, 1999). To demonstrate the effects of this drug corridor on syphilis rates, Cook and colleagues (1999) divided counties in North Carolina into one of three mutually exclusive groups: (1) counties transversed by or within 5 miles of I-95; (2) counties not transversed by or close to I-95; and (3) counties containing urban settings, that is, cities of populations greater then >100,000. Counties classified as I-95 counties were the only counties that had syphilis rates above the state average. This finding was so even though many other counties also contained interstate highways. In addition, their yearly average syphilis rates were considerably higher than those rates found in non-I-95 counties. Thus, this major migration and drug corridor, like truck routes in Africa (Bwayo et al., 1994; Gouws, 2002), concentrates probabilities of infection among a highly mobile population.

Evidence for this mobility of higher risk persons comes as well from a study by McCoy, Correa, and Fritz (1996). In this investigation, the researchers interviewed intravenous drug users and their sexual partners in cities with low, moderate, and high HIV prevalence. Individuals were asked about any travel in the last two years as well as high-risk activities they had engaged in while traveling. McCoy and colleagues observed that two regions evidenced the highest rates of visitation by respondents: the Middle Atlantic (including New York, Pennsylvania, and New Jersey) and the West South-Central (including Texas, Oklahoma, Louisiana, and Arkansas). Both regions reported relatively elevated cases of HIV infection at the time of the study. Many of their respondents also reported engaging in high-risk activities during their travels. A little over one half reported never using condoms, a third reported engaging in sex for money, about a fourth engaged in sex to obtain drugs, and most concerning, two thirds shared needles. These rates were significantly higher than the rates reported by nontravelers.

CONCENTRATION OF CORRECTIONAL AND PRISON COMPLEXES AND HIGH RATES OF INCARCERATION

The last 20 years have seen an exponential increase in the number people in prison in the United States, with an incarceration rate of 497 per 100,000 persons (Sabol, Minton, & Harrison, 2007). The impact has been greatest in the South, which has a rate of incarceration of 540 per 100,000 persons (Sabol, Contrere, & Harrison, 2007). Further, this increase has had the most impact on the African American population (Hogg, Druyts, Burris, Drucker, & Strathdee, 2008; Rosen et al., 2009). In state and federal facilities, even when stratified by type of facility, the rates are highest among African Americans; Black men are especially affected. In correctional facilities, African American men outnumber White men by a factor of 7; African American women outnumber White women by a factor of 3.5 (Beck, 2000; Beck & Karberg, 2001; Beck, Karberg, & Harrison, 2002; Harrison & Beck, 2006).

Approximately one quarter of HIV positive people in this country have been incarcerated in some type of correctional facility. In addition, HIV seroprevalence in U.S. prisons parallels the uneven geographic distribution found in may regions of the United States (Kantor, 2006). Even though many inmates are infected prior to entry into a correctional system, inmates are still at risk of exposure during incarceration through injection drug use, tattooing, body piercing, or sexual activity. These behaviors, risky on the outside, are even more risky in the incarceration environment because of the much higher numbers of people living with HIV/AIDS in these crowded facilities than in the general U.S. population. Between 1991 and 1997, the prevalence of HIV infection among women who were incarcerated rose 88%, whereas the rate among men rose only 28% (Degroot, Jackson, & Stubblefield, 2000; Gilliard, 1999). During this same period, the South had the second-highest HIV prevalence among inmates, second only to the Northeast. By 2004, Black women made up the largest percentage of female inmates testing positive for HIV in both state (3.4%) and federal facilities (2.6%) nationwide (Maruschak, 2005). The relatively high prevalence of HIV infection in correctional facilities among women is not surprising, given that the majority of women are incarcerated for drug use, prostitution, or both (Hammett, Harmon, & Rhodes, 2002; Maruschak, 2005).

For African American women, the high rate of incarceration of Black men reflects another correlate of HIV risk. Studies have shown that there is a positive relationship between incarceration rates of Black men and HIV/AIDS infection among Black women (Freudenberg, 2002; Johnson & Raphael, 2006). Other work has demonstrated that policies enacting early prisoner release because of prison overcrowding were followed 5 to 10 years later by increases in cases of HIV/AIDS infection among women and African Americans in general (Johnson & Raphael, 2006). A second study investigating the connection between sexually transmitted infections and rates of incarceration reported that counties with high rates of incarceration also tended to report high rates of gonorrhea, chlamydia, and AIDS (Thomas & Sampson, 2005). A second way in which incarceration has harmful effects on African American women is that it changes the sex ratio. When African American men in large numbers are incarcerated, their removal as eligible mates increases the sex-ratio imbalance, and the very relationship dynamics that leads to risk taking by the women who compete for the relatively few Black men not incarcerated increases the women's risk of HIV infection (Mays & Cochran, 1988; Pouget, Kershaw, Niccolai, Ickovics, & Blankenship, 2010).

The building of prisons, jails, and other correctional facilities is, on the one hand, made necessary by increasing densities of population and local rates of crime and punishment. Further, these facilities are also sources of economic support for the communities in which they are housed. As can be seen in Figure 34.5, the South has become home for numerous incarceration facilities providing well-paying jobs in communities where lost manufacturing, agricultural, and blue-collar jobs have contributed to economic stagnation (Beck, 2000; Beck & Karberg, 2001; Beck et al., 2002; Harrison & Beck, 2006). In addition, incarceration close to home allows inmates better access to family support while incarcerated. Thus, some aspects of the high density of incarceration facilities have positive benefits on local communities. Still, these facilities can also function inadvertently to intensify the effect of the HIV epidemic for African American women. This result can occur in three ways. First, incarceration of Black males contributes to the sex-ratio imbalance described earlier. Stability of relationships can be disrupted by incarceration as well (Harawa & Adimora, 2008). Second, housing men in higher risk HIV environments may lead to avoidable HIV infections and STIs. Also, to the extent that pre-release programs do not target HIV-prevention efforts, a teachable moment in the controlling the epidemic is lost. Third, release of both men and women into communities with few employment or educational opportunities or access to prevention and health care services increases the likelihood of recidivism, including a return to intravenous drug use, prostitution, and HIV-related risk taking (Adkins, 1978). Prison, correctional facilities, and jail can enhance HIV prevention efforts, both in incarcerated setting and in preparing individuals for managing HIV risk postincarceration.

SUMMARY

In 2008, 87% of new HIV infections in African American women likely arose from heterosexual transmission and 69% women with presumptive heterosexual transmission were African American (CDC, 2008). Many of the individual factors that shape African American women's risk that we describe in the foregoing sections are not limited to the South. But what is unique about the South is the concentration of contextual issues that are linked to risk for HIV within a relatively confined geographic place. Individuals are often resilient in the face of one social disadvantage, or even two or three social disadvantages. As the layers of disadvantage deepen, however, threats to health become endemic and targeting one risk or another in isolation can rapidly lose effectiveness. For the past 30 years, much of the investment in the control of the HIV epidemic has done just that, focusing on control and change of individual risk behaviors, particularly within known high-risk populations (Dean & Fenton, 2010). But for African American women, a reliance on changing individual exposures, individual lifestyles, and individual risk is unlikely to be optimally effective. Many women are concerned about the sexual histories of their partners (Adimora, Schoenbach, & Doherty, 2006). African Americans, in general, are more concerned than other ethnic and racial groups in the HIV epidemic. However, since the 1990s, personal concern about getting an HIV infection has declined among Blacks (Kaiser Family Foundation, 2007). This response does not portend well for HIV control efforts in the future that continue to rely on individual or even dyadic interventions to reduce HIV risk. We offer next several recommendations to better help reduce Black women's risk for HIV infection by targeting contextual risk factors. Our suggestions focus on the additional opportunities available in institutional structures targeting interventions at the population level.

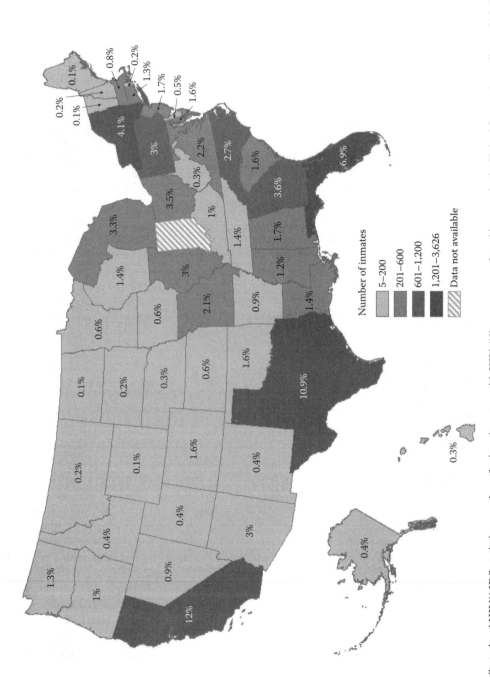

FIGURE 34.5 State-level HIV/AIDS statistics: number of prison inmates with HIV. #%, percentage of total inmates in the United States. According to U.S. Department of Justice, Bureau of Statistics data, 2,292,133 inmates were incarcerated in U.S. prisons and jails at the end of 2009 (Glaze, 2010; International Centre for Prison Studies, 2011; U.S. Bureau of Justice Statistics, 2011).

FEDERAL LEADERSHIP OPPORTUNITIES TO REDUCE SOUTHERN BLACK WOMEN'S RISK FOR HIV INFECTIONS

African American's women's societal inequities often place them in dependent relationships with governmental institutions and systems (e.g., prisons, health care facilities, and federal assistance program), where policies and procedures can either enhance or reduce their risk for HIV infection (Albarracin, Tannenbaum, Glasman, & Rothman, 2010; Aral et al., 2008; Auerbach, 2009; Dean & Fenton, 2010; Diallo et al., 2010; Gupta, Parkhurst, Ogden, Aggleton, & Mahal, 2008; Hillemeier, Lynch, Harper, & Casper, 2003; Latkin, Weeks, Glasman, Galletty, & Albarracin, 2010; Mays & Cochran, 1987, 1988). The Personal Responsibility and Work Opportunity Reconciliation Act of 1996 (an ineffective program that resulted in the loss of support and subsidies for women and their families), National Drug Control Strategies (the so-called war on drugs and the criminalization of drug use without access to treatment), Three Strikes Sentencing (which increased incarceration of men of color), state laws criminalizing HIV/AIDS transmission (thus pregnant women are convicted of exposing their babies, jailed during pregnancy, and in danger of losing their children)—all are examples of policies that make women more vulnerable in society to some of the social determinants that can increase risk of contracting HIV infection.

Many of the issues examined in this chapter are not about the individual-level determinants of sexual risk taking or unsafe injection use, practices that from an infectious-agent disease model are the principal drivers of the HIV/AIDS epidemic. We instead focused our attention on the social, structural, and psychological determinants that serve to increase the vulnerability of African American women in the South to HIV/AIDS. However, focusing on a social determinants perspective for the prevention and reduction of HIV/AIDS means taking a culturally relevant approach in examining social determinants in which we understand how factors associated with the South are related to HIV vulnerability for African American women. Taking this perspective is about realizing that confining our efforts to the parameters of a biomedical model with leadership predominantly from only the U.S. Department of Health and Human Services (DHHS) will serve only to continue the disproportionate cases of new HIV infections in African Americans. Why? Because DHHS does not have responsibility for many of the contextual factors discussed earlier. In a commentary on socially determinant health and HIV/AIDS, former surgeon general David Satcher (2010) advocated that social determinants of health be integrated into all policies, not just health policies. He called for public health to create and establish better working partnerships with nontraditional partners among governmental entities, in the private sector, and in industry (Satcher, 2010). Government entities have previously crossed into partnerships in both industry and business, but only with modest success (Satcher, 2010). This success is often modest because the U.S. government, which should be the natural leader in the fight against HIV/AIDS for vulnerable populations, has yet to effectively institute Satcher's (2010) call for a social determinants health perspective in all policies that require cross-agency partnerships. In order to successfully engage a social determinants health perspective in HIV/AIDS for women for whom social determinants often leave them more vulnerable to structural and social factors, leadership is needed across federal departments previously ignored in HIV/AIDS efforts. In the White House's Office of National AIDS Policy (ONAP) HIV/AIDS Strategy Federal Implementation Plan of July 2010, there is a clear and compelling call for federal agencies to develop not only cross-agency partnerships but also a culture where working relationships are geared toward policy and functional operations that can best change the rate of new HIV infections and facilitate efficacious care and treatment. Numerous federal agencies were targeted for efforts in 2010 and 2011: Agency for Healthcare Research and Quality (AHRQ), Bureau of Prisons, Centers for Disease Control (CDC), Centers for Medicare and Medicaid Services (CMS), Department of Justice (DOJ), Department of Labor (DOL), Equal Employment Opportunity Commission (EEOC), Health and Human Services (HHS) and HHS Office of the Secretary, Health Resources and Services Administration (HRSA), Department of Housing and Human Development (HUD), National Institutes of Health (NIH), Office of the Global AIDS Coordinator, Office of

Management and Budget (OMB), President's Advisory Council on HIV/AIDS, Substance Abuse and Mental Health Services (SAMSHA), Social Security Administration, and the Department of Veterans Affairs (VA).

This demand for cross-agency partnerships has emerged as a central recommendation in the response of several women's organizations to DHHS's request for comments on the July 2010 National HIV/AIDS Strategy Federal Implementation Plan (henceforth, the National HIV/AIDS Strategy; ONAP, 2010; Office of Women's Health [OWH], 2010). Thirteen women's organizations came together to issue the report card on the National HIV/AIDS Strategy, "A Gender Monitoring Tool for the U.S. National HIV/AIDS Strategy" (Positive Womens Network, 2010). Similarly, the Office of Women's Health brought a national group of women together to provide feedback. The National HIV/AIDS Strategy and the women's groups identified DOL, DOJ, CDC, and HRSA as critical partnership agencies. However, when we come back to the issues of place, race, and HIV infection, even though the requested partnerships are with the same agency specified in the National HIV/AIDS Strategy, in some instances what is needed from that agency to reduce new HIV infections and increase efficacious care and treatment for African American women in the South would differ. Conspicuously absent from suggested partnerships is the U.S. Department of Education. Although educational attainment alone is not a magic bullet in the prevention of HIV/AIDS in women, particularly African American women in the South, it is probably an important and necessary factor for resource-poor women.

Schools are often a site for HIV education and sexuality as a part of health curriculum. One study across developed and undeveloped countries found approximately two thirds of HIV- and sex-education programs reduced risk associated with sexual behaviors (Kirby, Laris, & Rolleri, 2006). Sex-education programs can be the vehicle for teaching about gender awareness, gender norms, and gender equality, all of which have a positive effect on men's condom use and men's more egalitarian behaviors in their interpersonal relationships with women (Haberland & Rogow, 2007; Karim, Magani, Morgan, & Bond, 2003; Pulerwitz, Barker, Segundo, & Nascimento, 2006; Pulerwitz et al., 2010). Partnerships with the U.S. Department of Education promoting policies for evidenced-based sex-education programs in early grades would benefit African American women in efforts to reduce HIV infection.

How partnerships with agencies other than DHHS can help in reducing HIV infections in African Americans is best thought about by matching agency responsibilities to the social determinants that result in Black women's greater vulnerability to HIV infection. We have, thus far in our chapter, attempted to illustrate some of the social determinants that put African American women in the South at greater risk for HIV infection (see Figure 34.4). We now illustrate actions that could, if taken by federal agencies, address some of these social determinants. For example, although the National HIV/AIDS Strategy did not mention the U.S. Department of Agriculture as a potential partner in the South, it might consider doing so, particularly because rural-area food insecurity is a serious problem experienced by all. The DHHS could encourage the U.S. Department of Agriculture to examine how its policies and procedures intersect with race, place, and HIV infection in areas where women are having sex to feed themselves and their families. Through the Office of Rural Development, the U.S. Department of Agriculture is responsible for developing programs to improve the economy and quality of life in rural America. Thus, in partnership with this department, DHHS could launch programs that decrease the very conditions that create negative social determinants of HIV infection for Black women in rural areas. A number of federal as well as foundation efforts specifically designed to determine the social determinants that can create healthy communities in order to reduce the incidents of particular health crises could be tried in rural areas in the South where we see growing numbers of cases of new infections and AIDS death (Lantz & Pritchard, 2010; Mokdad & Remington, 2010; Parrish, 2010).

Another sector of the U.S. Department of Agriculture, the Rural Housing Program, could also aid in intervention efforts through cross-agency collaboration at the population level. The Rural Housing Program, which is responsible for encouraging homeownership options and housing rehabilitation, as well as helping developers of multifamily housing projects, overseeing assisted housing for the elderly and disabled or apartment buildings and such community facilities as libraries, child care centers, or schools, could be engaged much like HUD, with allocations for the provision of housing for African American women who are uninfected but highly vulnerable to HIV infection. In the early days of examining women's vulnerability to HIV infection, discussion centered on whether providing resources specific to HIV/AIDS was creating exceptionalism. The concern was that women who were poor, minority, and without many social options in taking care of themselves and their families were intentionally becoming infected to access the resources associated with HIV (Mays, 1993). However, creating profiles for African American women in rural areas of risk for HIV infection and the likely benefit and success of interventions—that is, marrying education and information to housing and such other benefits as education, vocational training, and health literacy, for example, much along the lines of the healthy cities efforts—could reduce new infections.

Not mentioned in the National HIV/AIDS Strategy but, as already noted, one of the key partnerships that could contribute to reducing HIV infections in African American women in the South is with the U.S. Department of Education. The department could, as a partner in the battle against new HIV infections, be engaged to develop policies that specify best practices for the teaching of health and sexual-health literacy. The Office of Women's Health consultation to the National HIV/AIDS Strategy recommended specific activities for the U.S. Department of Education (OWH, 2010). These activities included a request for comprehensive sex education for all school-aged children, with sex education mandated in juvenile detention centers and foster care facilities. They recommended that mandated comprehensive health and sex education be included in the reauthorization of the Elementary and Secondary Education Act (ESEA). These health and sex-education programs, which should be age and gender appropriate and culturally relevant, could become part of the yearly assessment that students must pass to be promoted. The U. S. Department of Education could examine ways to enrich schools in states with low pupil expenditure either through encouraging partnerships with foundations or identifying community efforts that can raise the proportion of Black women who complete some level of college education in fields where there are highly employable careers.

The U.S. Department of Justice could work with DHHS to ensure case management as HIV-infected individuals move from the correctional system back into society. All too often HIV-infected individuals who were treated in the correctional setting may find that upon release, they are provided with a limited supply of medication and expected to find their own way into treatment. Linkage to care as these individuals transition out of correctional custody to general society could help prevent new infections. When this is lacking, opportunities for the management of treatment and care and the reduction in the spread of new infections are lost. The DHHS is working with the U.S. Department of Justice and the Bureau of Prisons to fund the development and evaluation of family reunification programs (which prerelease inmates, whether or not they have tested positive) in which HIV testing, counseling, and education about safer sex and sexual health are part of the curriculum.

Another department, the U.S. Department of Labor, could focus on skill development and job training to move women along a path of a livable wage with benefits and could develop programs for women engaged in high-risk activities driven by economic needs. Training programs developed with not only DHHS but also the U.S. Department of Education to provide completion of GED, if needed, along with entrance into college associate-degree programs, could provide training for career paths with livable wages. Further, the U.S. Department of Transportation, with its Research and Innovative Technology Administration, could be charged with employment impact assessments in Southern rural areas where HIV infections are high. The department could monitor whether public transportation meets individuals' needs to travel to where jobs are developing and could address gaps that affect the chronically unemployed, especially in rural areas, where people may have no way to reach suburban growth areas that are often the site of new jobs.

Although many people tout the improved quality of life outside inner urban cities, sometimes these areas are unreachable because of the lack of public transportation. This situation might be remedied by engaging the U.S. Department of Housing and Urban Development, which already works with DHHS through the Housing Opportunities for Persons with AIDS (PWAs) Program, to use its power to reengineer inner urban neighborhoods with high indicators of crime, violence against women, and broken windows and other indicators of neglect. This area of development is ripe for partnership with the foundations currently engaged in developing healthy communities. Also, we should not forget to call upon the U.S. Department of Commerce to enact small-business microloan systems, especially in rural areas and tribal communities, where economic stimulation and infrastructure building are critical interventions to reducing vulnerability to the risk of HIV infection.

The U.S. Department of Commerce also includes among its offices the National Telecommunications and Information Administration, which advises the president on telecommunication policies. An area where we have seen the benefits of technology for young adults has been SEXTECH (http://sextech.org) run by ISIS, which develops the technology and messages for HIV prevention virtually, such as texting to find answers to questions about health and sexuality. Technology should be more in the forefront of bringing to women and girls information to keep them safe, help them make decisions about how to reduce their STI risk, and tell them where they can go for testing, counseling, and support. One can imagine a free service that allows accessing HIV information by anyone who owns a phone, rather than envisioning only a bricks-and-mortar center where women must go to ask for resources. Why has the U.S. Department of Defense, which is home to some of the most cutting-edge national laboratories in the world, not lead efforts to model the HIV epidemic and thereby develop projections that can identify the spread and risk of the disease so other departments can intervene in the structural ways necessary to slow down the rate of the epidemic? Our suggestion requires unprecedented leadership by the federal government, which appears not to be up the challenge. Our suggestion is, in short, about realizing that the strategies employed to help women in underdeveloped countries—that is, approaches that seek to reduce women's vulnerability through skill attainment, employment, and ability to earn income, all hampered by their poverty and lack of infrastructure—would actually work in some U.S. communities, particularly in the rural South.

CONCLUSION

Race and geographic place also form a critical nexus for the conditions of HIV infection because, as so eloquently pointed out by Dean and Fenton (2010), the conditions that increase the likelihood of the risk of infection occur because of the nature of people's lives, such as where they live and work, as well as where and with whom they carry on their social relationships (Mays, Cochran, & Barnes, 2007). Equally true is that the likelihood of HIV infection or, conversely, the ability to protect against it is connected to societal resources in place for assistance, education, and health care, resources that are shaped by social, political, legal, racialized, and economic dynamics (Dean & Fenton, 2010; Gupta et al., 2008; Morris & Monroe, 2009).

If we are to accomplish the White House vision of the National HIV/AIDS Strategy (2010)—namely that "the United States will become a place where new HIV infections are rare and when they do occur, every person, regardless of age, gender, race/ethnicity, sexual orientation, gender identity or socio-economic circumstance, will have unfettered access to high quality, life-extending care, free from stigma and discrimination" (p. 4)—we must employ a social determinants approach to strategies that are multisectoral and population based.

ACKNOWLEDGMENTS

This work was funded by the National Institute of Drug Abuse (DA 15539, DA 20826) and the National Center for Minority Health and Health Disparities (MD 00508) at the National Institutes of Health. We would like to thank Francisco Robles for his assistance with the graphics and content and Justin Kwok for his help.

REFERENCES

Acevedo-Garcia, D., Lochner, K. A., Osypuk, T. L., & Subramanian, S. V. (2003). Future directions in residential segregation and health research: A multilevel approach. *American Journal of Public Health, 93*(2), 215–221.

Acevedo-Garcia, D., & Osypuk, T. L. (2008a). Impacts of housing and neighborhoods on health: Pathways, racial/ethnic disparities, and policy directions. In J. H. Carr & N. K. Kutty (Eds.), *Segregation: The rising costs for America* (pp. 197–235). New York, NY: Routledge.

Acevedo-Garcia, D., & Osypuk, T. L. (2008b). Invited commentary: Residential segregation and health: The complexity of modeling separate social contexts. *American Journal of Epidemiology, 168*(11), 1255–1258.

Acevedo-Garcia, D., Osypuk, T. L., McArdle, N., & Williams, D. (2008). Toward a policy-relevant analysis of geographic and racial/ethnic disparities in child health, *Health Affairs, 27*(2), 321–333.

Acevedo-Garcia, D., Osypuk, T. L., Werbel, R. E., Meara, E. R., Cutler, D. M., & Berkman, L. F. (2004). Does housing mobility policy improve health? *Housing Policy Debate, 15*(1), 49–98.

Adimora, A. A., & Schoenbach, V. J. (2002). Contextual factors and the Black–White disparity in heterosexual HIV transmission. *Epidemiology, 13*(6), 707–712.

Adimora, A. A., Schoenbach, V. J., & Doherty, I. A. (2006). HIV and African Americans in the southern United States: Sexual networks and social context. *Sexually Transmitted Diseases, 33*(7), S39–S45.

Adimora, A. A., Schoenbach, V. J., Martinson, F. E., Coyne-Beasley, T., Doherty, I., Stancil, T. R., & Fulilove, R. E. (2006). Heterosexually transmitted HIV infection among African Americans in North Carolina. *Journal of Acquired Immune Deficiency Syndromes, 41*(5), 616–623.

Adimora, A. A., Schoenbach, V. J., Martinson, F., Donaldson, K., Fullilove, R., & Aral, S. (2001). Social context of sexual relationships among rural African Americans. *Sexually Transmitted Diseases, 28*(2), 69–76.

Adimora, A. A., Schoenbach, V. J., Martinson, F., Donaldson, K., Stancil, T., & Fullilove, R. (2003). Concurrent partnerships among rural African Americans with recently reported heterosexually transmitted HIV infection. *Journal of Acquired Immune Deficiency Syndromes, 34*(4), 423–429.

Adimora, A. A., Schoenbach, V. J., Martinson, F., Donaldson, K., Stancil, T. R., & Fullilove, R. E. (2004). Concurrent sexual partnerships among African Americans in the rural South. *Annual Epidemiology, 14*(3), 155–160.

Adkins, G. (1978). Prisons: What's going on behind the walls? *Illinois Periodical Online, 4*(3), 7–12. Retrieved from http://www.lib.niu.edu/1978/ii780307.html

Agee, B. S., Funkhouser, E., Roseman, J. M., Fawal, H., Holmberg, S. D., & Vermund, S. H. (2006). Migration patterns following HIV diagnosis among adults residing in the nonurban Deep South. *AIDS Care, 18*(Suppl. 1), 51–58.

Aiello, A. E., Simanek, A., & Galea, S. (2010). Population levels of psychological stress, herpes virus reactivation and HIV. *AIDS and Behavior, 14*(2), 308–317.

Akers, A. Y., Youmans, S., Lloyd, S. W., Smith, D. M., Banks, B., Blumenthal, C., … Adimora, A. A. (2010). Views of young, rural African Americans of the role of community social institutions in HIV prevention. *Journal of Health Care for the Poor and Underserved, 21*(2 Suppl.), 1–12.

Albarracin, D., Tannenbaum, M. B., Glasman, L. R., & Rothman, A. J. (2010). Modeling structural, dyadic, and individual factors: The inclusion and exclusion model of HIV related behavior. *AIDS and Behavior, 14*, 239–249.

Annang, L., Walsemann, K. M., Maitra, D., & Kerr, J. C. (2010). Does education matter? Examining racial differences in the association between education and STI diagnosis among Black and White young adult females in the US. *Public Health Reports, 125*, 110–121.

Aral, S. O. (1996). The social context of syphilis persistence in the southeastern United States. *Sexually Transmitted Diseases, 23*(1), 9–15.

Aral, S. O., Adimora, A. A., & Fenton, K. A. (2008). Understanding and responding to disparities in HIV and other sexually transmitted infections in African Americans. *Lancet, 372*(9635), 337–340.

Aral, S., O'Leary, A., & Baker, C. (2006). Sexually transmitted infections and HIV in the southern United States: An overview. *Sexually Transmitted Diseases, 33*(7), S1–S5.

Association of Religious Data Archives. (2008). *Sex before marriage.* Retrieved from http://www.thearda.com/quickstats/qs_120.asp

Auerbach, J. (2009). Transforming social structures and environments to help in HIV prevention. *Health Affairs, 28*(6), 1655–1665.

Bateson, M. C., & Goldsby, R. (1988). *Thinking AIDS: The social response to the biological threat.* Reading, MA: Addison-Wesley.

Beaulieu, L. J., Barfield, M. A., & Stone, K. L. (2001). Educated workforce, quality jobs: Still elusive goals in the rural South. *Rural America, 15*(4), 28–35.

Beck, A. J. (2000). *Prison and jail inmates at midyear 1999* (NCJ Publication No. 181643). *Prison and Jail Inmates at Midyear Series.* Washington, DC: U.S. Department of Justice.

Beck, A. J., & Karberg, J. C. (2001). *Prison and jail inmates at midyear 2000* (NCJ Publication No. 185989). *Prison and Jail Inmates at Midyear Series.* Washington, DC: U.S. Department of Justice.

Beck, A. J., Karberg, J. C., & Harrison, P. M. (2002). *Prison and jail inmates at midyear 2001* (NCJ Publication No. 191702). *Prison and Jail Inmates at Midyear Series.* Washington, DC: U.S. Department of Justice.

Bhatta, M. P., Vermund, S. H., & Hoesley, C. J. (2010). Human immunodeficiency virus in Alabama women: Sociodemographic, behavioral, and reproductive health characteristics associated with the lakc of human immodefiency virus-1 viral control. *American Journal of Medicine, 338*(2), 133–140.

Blanchard, J. F., & Aral, S. O. (2010). Emergent properties and structural patterns in sexually transmitted infection and HIV research. *Sexually Transmitted Infections, 86*(Suppl. 3), 4–9.

Blankenship, K. M., Bray, S., & Merson, M. H. (2000). Structural interventions in public health. *AIDS, 14*(Suppl. A), S11–S21.

Bowen, A., Gambrell, A., & DeCarlo, P. (2006). What are rural HIV prevention needs? *Center for AIDS Research Studies.* Retrieved November 21, 2010, from http://www.caps.ucsf.edu/pubs/FS/pdf/revruralFS.pdf

Brown et al. v. Board of Education of Topeka et al. (1954). 347 U.S. 483.

Bruce, J. (2007). *Transitions to adulthood: Child marriage in the context of the HIV epidemic.* Retrieved from http://www.popcouncil.org/pdfs/TABriefs/PGY_Brief11_ChildMarriageHIV.pdf

Brunner, E. J., & Marmot, M. G. (1999). Social organisation, stress and health. In M. Marmot & R. Wilkinson (Eds.), *Social determinants of health* (pp. 17–43). Oxford: Oxford University Press.

Butler, M. (1997). Education and the economic status of Blacks. In L. Swanson (Ed.), *Racial/ethnic minorities in rural areas: Progress and stagnation, 1980–90* (Agricultural Economic Report No. 731, pp. 77–86). Washington, DC: U.S. Department of Agriculture.

Bwayo, J., Plummer, F., Omari, M., Mutere, A., Moses, S., Ndinya-Achola, J., … Kreiss, J. (1994). Human immunodeficiency virus infection in long-distance truck drivers in east Africa. *Archives of Internal Medicine, 154*(12), 1391–1396.

Centers for Disease Control and Prevention (CDC). (1981). Kaposi"s sarcoma and Pneumocystis pneumonia among homosexual men: New City and California. *Morbidity and Mortality Weekly Report, 30*, 305–308.

Centers for Disease Control and Prevention (CDC). (1990). Current trends: Heterosexual behaviors and factors that influence condom use among patients attending a sexually transmitted disease clinic—San Francisco. *Morbidity and Mortality Weekly Report, 39*, 685–689.

Centers for Disease Control and Prevention. (2004). *HIV/AIDS Surveillance Report, 2003*, Vol. 15. U.S. Department of Health and Human Services. Retrieved from http://www.cdc.gov/hiv/stats/hasrlink.htm.

Centers for Disease Control and Prevention (CDC). (2008). *Diagnoses of HIV infection, by race/ethnicity and selected characteristics, 2008—37 states with confidential name-based HIV infection reporting.* Retrieved from http://www.cdc.gov/hiv/surveillance/resources/reports/2008report/table3a.htm

Centers for Disease Control and Prevention (CDC). (2010). *HIV among African-Americans.* Retrieved from http://www.cdc.gov/hiv/topics/aa/pdf/aa.pdf

Cleland, J. G., & Van Ginneken, J. K. (1988). Maternal education and child survival in developing countries: The search for pathways of influence. *Social Science and Medicine, 27*(12), 1357–1368.

Cochran, S. D., & Mays, V. M. (1989). Women and AIDS-related concerns: Roles for psychologists in helping the worried well. *American Psychologist, 44*(12), 529–535.

Cochran, S. D., Mays, V. M., & Roberts, V. (1988). Ethnic minorities and AIDS. In A. Lewis (Ed.), *Nursing care of the patient with AIDS/ARC* (pp. 17–24). Rockville, MD: Aspen.

Cohn, S., Berk, M., Bozzette, S., Berry, S., Duan, N., Frankel, M., & Bozzette, S. A. (2001). The care of HIV-infected adults in rural areas of the United States. *Journal of Acquired Immune Deficiency Syndromes, 28*(4), 385–392.

Cohn, S. E., Klein, J. D., Mohr, J. E., Van der Horst, C. M., & Weber, D. J. (1994). The geography of AIDS: Patterns of urban and rural migration. *Southern Medical Journal, 87*(6), 599–606.

Cook, R., Royce, R., Thomas, J., & Hanusa, B. (1999). What's driving an epidemic? The spread of syphilis along an interstate highway in rural North Carolina. *American Journal of Public Health, 89*(3), 369–373.

Cornelius, L. J., Okundaye, J. N., & Manning, M. C. (2000). HIV related risk behavior among African American females and the changing face of HIV/AIDS in the third decade of the pandemic. *Journal of the National Medical Association, 92*(4), 183–195.

Cornwell, C., & Cunningham, S. A. (2006). *Sex ratios and risky sexual behavior* [Working paper]. Athens, GA: University of Georgia.

Crepaz, N., Marshall, K. J., Aupont, L. W., Jacobs, E. D., Mizuno, Y., Kay, L. S., … O'Leary A. (2009). The efficacy of HIV/STI behavioral interventions for African American females in the United States: A meta-analysis. *American Journal of Public Health, 99*(11), 2069–2078.

Cromartie, J. B., & Beale, C. L.(1996). Increasing black-white separation in the plantation south. In L. Swanson (Ed.), *Racial/ethnic minorities in rural areas: Progress and stagnation, 1980–90.* (Economic Research Service, Agricultural Economic Report No. 73, pp. 54–64). Washington, DC: U.S. Department of Agriculture.

Crosby, R. A., Yarber, W. L., DiClemente, R. J., Wingood, G. M., & Meyerson, B. (2002). HIV-associated histories, perceptions, and practices among low-income African American women: Does rural residence matter? *American Journal of Public Health, 92*(4), 655–659.

Currie, J., & Enrico M. (2003) Mother's education and the intergenerational transmission of capital: Evidence from college openings. *Quarterly Journal of Economics, 118*(4), 1495–1532.

Dean, H. D., & Fenton, K. A. (2010). Addressing social determinants of health in the prevention and control of HIV/AIDS, viral hepatitis, sexually transmitted infections, and tuberculosis. *Public Health Reports, 125*(Suppl. 4), 1–5.

DeCarlo, P. (1998, February). What are rural HIV prevention needs? *World*, No. 82, 7.

DeGroot, A. S., Jackson, E. H., & Stubblefield, E. (2000). Clinical trials in correctional settings: Proceedings of a conference held in Providence, Rhode Island, October 13–15, 1999. *Medical Health Rhode Island, 83*(12), 376–379.

Diallo, D. D., Moore, T. W., Ngalame, P. M., White, L. D., Herbst, J. H., & Painter, T. M. (2010). Efficacy of a single-session HIV prevention intervention for Black women: A group randomized controlled trial. *AIDS and Behavior, 14*(3), 518–529.

Diez-Roux, A. V. (1998). Bringing context back into epidemiology: Variables and fallacies in multilevel analysis. *American Journal of Public Health, 88*, 216–222.

Doherty, I. A., Leone, P. A., & Aral, S. O. (2007). Social determinants of HIV infection in the Deep South. *American Journal of Public Health, 97*(3), 391–392.

Dolcini, M. M., Coates, T. J., Catania, J. A., Kegeles, S. M., & Hauck, W. W. (1995). Multiple sexual partners and their psychosocial correlates: The population-based AIDS in Multiethnic Neighborhoods (AMEN) Study. *Health Psychology, 14*(1), 22–31.

Egerter, S., Braverman, P., Sadegh-Nobari, T., Grossman-Kahn, R., & Dekker, M. (2009). *Education matters for health* (Issue Brief No. 6). Princeton, NJ: Robert Wood Johnson Foundation.

El-Bassel, N., Caldeira, N. A., Ruglass, L. M., & Gilbert, L. (2009). Addressing the unique needs of African American women in HIV prevention. *American Journal of Public Health, 99*(6), 996–1001.

Elmore, K. (2006). The migratory experiences of people with HIV/AIDS (PWHA) in Wilmington, North Carolina. *Health and Place, 12*(4), 570–579.

Farley, T. (2006). Sexually transmitted diseases in the southeastern United States: Location, race, and social context. *Sexually Transmitted Diseases, 33*(Suppl. 7), S58–S64.

Fleming, P. L., Lansky, A., Lee, L. M., & Nakashima, A. K. (2006). The epidemiology of HIV/AIDS in women in the southern United States. *Sex Transmitted Diseases, 33*(7 Suppl.), S32–S38.

Freudenberg, N. (2002). Adverse effects of US jail and prison policies on the health and well-being of color. *American Journal of Public Health, 92*(12), 1895–1899.

Frey, W. H. (with the Brookings Institution). (2004). *The new great migration: Black Americans' return to the South, 1965–2000. Living Cities Census Series.* Washington, DC: Center on Urban and Metropolitan Policy, Brookings Institution.

Gakidou, E., Cowling, K., Lozano, R., & Murray, C. (2010). Increased educational attainment and its effect on child mortality in 175 countries between 1970 and 2009: A systematic analysis. *The Lancet, 376*(9745), 959–974.

Gehlert, S., Sohmer, D., Sacks, T., Mininger, C., McClintock, M., & Olopade, O. (2008). Targeting health disparities: A model linking upstream determinants to downstream interventions. *Health Affairs (Millwood), 27*(2), 339–349.

Gibson, C., & Jung, K. (2002). *Historical census statistics on population totals by race, 1790 to 1990, and by Hispanic origin, 1970 to 1990, for the United States, regions, divisions, and states.* Retrieved October 25, 2010, from http://www.census.gov/population/www/documentation/twps0056/twps0056.html

Gilbert, D. J., Harvey, A. R., & Belgrave, F. Z. (2009). Advancing the Africentric paradigm shift discourse: Building toward evidence-based Africentric interventions in social work practice with African Americans. *National Association of Social Workers, 54*(3), 243–252.

Gilliard, D. K. (1999). *Prison and jail inmates at midyear 1998* (NCJ Publication No. 173414). *Prison and Jail Inmates at Midyear Series.*

Glaze, L. (2010). *Total correctional population in the United States, 2009.* U.S. Bureau of Justice Statistics. Retrieved from http://bjs.ojp.usdoj.gov/index.cfm?ty=tp&tid=11

Glick, S. N., & Golden, M. R. (2010). Persistence of racial differences in attitudes toward homosexuality in the United States. *Journal of Acquired Immune Deficiency Syndrome, 55*(4), 516–523.

Gottlieb, M. S. (1981). Pneumocystis carini pneumonia and muscosal candidiasis in previously healthy homosexual men: Evidence of a new acquired cellular immunodeficiency. *New England Journal of Medicine, 305*, 1425–1431.

Gottlieb, M. S., Schanker, H. M., Fan, P. T., Saxon, A., & Weisman, D. O. (1981) Pneumocystis pneumonia. *Morbidity and Mortality Weekly Report, 45*(34), 729–731,

Gouws, R. G. (2002). Prevalence of HIV among truck drivers visiting sex workers in KwaZulu-Natal, South Africa. *Sex Transmitted Diseases, 29*(1), 44–49.

Greenwald, R., Hedges, L. V., & Laine, R. D. (1994) When reinventing the wheel is not necessary: A case study in the use of meta-analysis in education finance. *Journal of Education Finance, 20*(1), 1–20.

Grinstead, O. A., Peterson, J. L., Faigeles, B., & Catania, J. A. (1997). Antibody testing and condom use among heterosexual African Americans at risk for HIV infection. *American Journal of Public Health, 87*(5), 857–859.

Grossman, J. R. (2001). *Land of hope: Chicago, Black Southerners, and the Great Migration.* Chicago, Il: University of Chicago Press.

Gupta, G. R., Parkhurst, J. O., Ogden, J. A., Aggleton, P., & Mahal, A. (2008). Structural approaches to HIV prevention. *Lancet, 372*(9640), 764–765.

Haberland, N., & Rogow, D. (2007). *Sexuality and education: Time for a paradigm shift.* Retrieved from http://www.popcouncil.org/pdfs/TABriefs/PGY_Brief22_SexEducation.pdf

Hall, H., Li, J., & McKenna, M. (2005). HIV in predominantly rural areas of the United States. *Journal of Rural Health, 21*(3), 245–253.

Hall, H., Song, R., Rhodes, P., Prejean, J., An, Q., Lee, L. M., ... Janssen, R. S. (2008). Estimation of HIV incidence in the United States. *JAMA, 300*(5), 520–529.

Hallman, K. (2005). Gendered socioeconomic conditions and HIV risk behaviors among young people in South Africa. *African Journal of AIDS Research, 4*(1), 37–50.

Hallman, K., & Diers, J. (2004). *Social isolation and economic vulnerability: Adolescent HIV and pregnancy risk factors in South Africa.* Presentation at the annual meeting of the Population Association of America, Boston, MA.

Hammett, T. M., Harmon, P., & Rhodes, W. (2002). The burden of infectious disease among inmates of and releasees from US correctional facilities, 1997. *American Journal of Public Health, 92*(11), 1789–1794.

Hammonds, E. (1994). Black (w)holes and the geometry of Black female sexuality. *Differences: A Journal of Feminist Cultural Studies, 6*(2–3), 126–147.

Harawa, N., & Adimora, A. (2008). Incarceration, African Americans and HIV: Advancing a research agenda. *Journal of the National Medical Association, 100*(1), 57–62.

Harrison, P. M., & Beck, A. J. (2005). *Prison and jail inmates at midyear 2004* (NCJ Publication No. 208801). *Prison and Jail Inmates at Midyear Series.* Retrieved from http://bjs.ojp.usdoj.gov/content/pub/pdf/pjim04.pdf

Harrison, P. M., & Beck, A. J. (2006). *Prison and jail inmates at midyear 2005* (NCJ Publication No. 213133). *Prison and Jail Inmates at Midyear Series.* Retrieved from http://bjs.ojp.usdoj.gov/content/pub/pdf/pjim05.pdf

Harrison, P. M., & Karberg, J. C. (2003). *Prison and jail inmates at midyear 2002* (NCJ Publication No. 198877). *Prison and Jail Inmates at Midyear Series.* Retrieved from http://bjs.ojp.usdoj.gov/index.cfm?ty=pbdetail&iid=865

Heckman T. G., Somlai, A. M., Peters, J., Walker, J., Otto-Salaj, L., Galdabini, C. A., & Kelly, J. A. (1998). Barriers to care among persons living with HIV/AIDS in urban and rural areas. *AIDS Care, 10*(3), 365–375.

Hedges, L. V., Laine, R. D., & Greenwald, R. (1994). Does money matter? A meta-analysis of studies of the effects of differential school inputs on student outcomes. *Educational Researcher, 23*(3), 5–14.

Herek, G. M. (2007). Confronting sexual stigma and prejudice: Theory and practice. *Journal of Social Issues, 63*(4), 905–925.

Herek, G. M., Capitanio, J. P., & Widaman, K. F. (2002). HIV-related stigma and knowledge in the United States: Prevalence and trends, 1991–1999. *American Journal of Public Health*, *92*(3), 371–377.

Herek, G. M., Widaman, K. F., & Capitanio, J. P. (2005). When sex equals AIDS: Symbolic stigma and heterosexual adults' inaccurate beliefs about sexual transmission of AIDS. *Social Problems*, *52*(1), 15–37.

Hightow, L., MacDonald, P., Pilcher, C., Kaplan, A., Foust, E., Nguyen, T., & Leone, P. A. (2005). The unexpected movement of the HIV epidemic in the southeastern United States: Transmission among college students. *Journal of Acquired Immune Deficiency Syndromes*, *38*(5), 531–537.

Hillemeier, M. M., Lynch, J., Harper, S., & Casper, M. (2003). Measuring contextual characteristics for community health. *Health Services Research*, *38*(6, Pt 2), 1645–1717.

Hogg, R. S., Druyts, E. F., Burris, S., Drucker, E., & Strathdee, S. A. (2008). Years of life lost to prison: Racial and gender gradients in the United States of America. *Harm Reduction Journal*, *1*(5), 4.

International Centre for Prison Studies. (2011). *Prison brief for United States of America*. School of Law, King's College London. Retrieved from http://www.kcl.ac.uk/depsta/law/research/icps/worldbrief/wpb_country.php?country=190

Jaffe, L. R., Seehaus, M., Wagner, C., & Leadbeater, B. J. (1988). Anal intercourse and knowledge of acquired immunodeficiency syndrome among minority group female adolescents. *Journal of Pediatrics*, *112*(6), 1005–1007.

Johnson, R. C., & Raphael, S. (2006). *The effects of male incarceration dynamics on AIDS infection rates among African-American women and men*. National Poverty Center Working Paper #06-22, University of Michigan, Ann Arbor.

Joint Center for Political and Economic Studies. (2001). *Marriage and African Americans*. Retrieved from http://www.jointcenter.org/DB/factsheet/marital.htm

Kaiser Family Foundation. (2007). *HIV/AIDS policy fact sheet*. Retrieved from http://www.kff.org/hivaids/upload/6089-04.pdf

Kantor, E. (2006). *HIV transmission and prevention in prisons* [HIV in-site knowledge base chapter 2006]. Retrieved from http://hivinsite.ucsf.edu/InSite?page=kb-07-04-13#

Kaplan, G., Everson, S. A., & Lynch, J. W. (2000). The contribution of social and behavioral research to an understanding of the distribution of disease: A multilevel approach. In B. D. Smedley & S. L. Syme (Eds.), *Promoting health: Intervention strategies* (pp. 37–80). Washington, DC: National Academies Press.

Karim, A. M., Magani, R., Morgan, G., & Bond, K. (2003). Reproductive health and protective factors among unmarried youth in Ghana. *International Family Planning Perspectives*, *29*(1), 14–24.

Karney, B. R., Hops, H., Redding, C. A., Reis, H. T., Rothman, A. J., & Simpson, J. A. (2010). A framework for incorporating dyads in models of HIV-prevention. *AIDS and Behavior*, *14*(Suppl. 2), 189–203.

Kirby, D., Laris, B. A., & Rolleri, L. (2006). *Impact of sex and HIV education programs on sexual behaviors of youth in developing and developed countries*. FHI Youth Research Working Paper # 2, Family Health International (Youth Net Program), Research Triangle Park, North Carolina.

Kirby, D., Short, L., Collins, J., Rugg, D., Kolbe, L., Howard, M., … Zabin, L. S. (1994). School-based programs to reduce sexual risk behaviors: A review of effectiveness. *Public Health Reports*, *109*(3), 339–360.

Kraut-Becher, J. R., & Aral, S. O. (2006). Patterns of age mixing and sexually transmitted infections. *International Journal of STD & AIDS*, *17*(6), 378–383.

Krawczyk, C., Funkhouser, E., Kilby, J., & Vermund, S. (2006). Delayed access to HIV diagnosis and care: Special concerns for the southern United States. *AIDS Care*, *18*(1), S35–S44.

Kubzansky, L. D., Berkman, L. F., Glass, A., & Seeman, T. E. (1998). Is educational attainment associated with shared determinants of health in the elderly? Findings from the MacArthur Studies of Successful Aging. *Psychosomatic Medicine*, *60*(5), 578–585.

Kuisimo, P. S. (1999). *Rural African Americans and education: The legacy of the Brown decision*. Charleston, WV: ERIC Clearinghouse on Rural Education and Small Schools.

Lantz, P. M., & Pritchard, A. (2010). Socioeconomic indicators that matter for public health. *Preventing Chronic Disease*, *7*(4), A74. Retrieved from http://www.cdc.gov/pcd/issues/2010/jul/09_0246.html

Latkin, C., Weeks, M. R., Glasman, L., Galletty, C., & Albarracin, D. (2010). A dynamic systems model for considering structural factors in HIV prevention and detection. *AIDS Behavior*, *14*(2), 222–238.

Leigh, B. C., Temple, M. T., & Trocki, K. F. (1993). The sexual behavior of U.S. adults: Results from a national survey. *American Journal of Public Health*, *83*(10), 1400–1408.

Lemelle, A. J., & Battle, J. (2004). Black masculinity matters in attitudes toward gay males. *Journal of Homosexuality*, *47*(1), 39–51.

Lewis, D. K., & Watters, D. K. (1991). Sexual risk behavior among heterosexual intravenous drug users: Ethnic and gender variations. *AIDS*, *5*(1), 77–83.

Lightfoot, M. A., & Milburn, N. G. (2009). HIV prevention and African American youth: Examination of individual-level behavior is not the only answer. *Culture, Health & Sexuality, 11*(7), 731–742.

Magnus, M., Kuo, I., Shelley, K., Rawls, A., Peterson, J., Montanez, L., ... Greenberg, A. E. (2009). Risk factors driving the emergence of a generalized heterosexual HIV epidemic in Washington, District of Columbia networks at risk. *AIDS, 23*(10), 1277–1284.

Mahajan, A. P., Sayles, J. N., Patel, V. A., Remien, R. H., Ortiz, D., Szekeres, G., & Coates, T. J. (2008). Stigma in the HIV/AIDS epidemic: A review of the literature and recommendations for the way forward. *AIDS, 22*(Suppl. 2), S67–S69.

Maruschak, L. M. (2005). HIV in prisons, 2003. *Bureau of Justice Statistics Bulletin* (NCJ Publication No. 210344). Retrieved from http://bjs.ojp.usdoj.gov/content/pub/pdf/hivp03.pdf

Maruschak, L. M. (2006). HIV in prisons, 2004. *Bureau of Justice Statistics Bulletin* (NCJ Publication No. 213897). Retreived from http://bjs.ojp.usdoj.gov/content/pub/pdf/hivp04.pdf

Maruschak, L. M., & Beaver, R. (2009). HIV in prisons, 2007–2008. *Bureau of Justice Statistics Bulletin* (NCJ Publication No. 228307). Retrieved from http://bjs.ojp.usdoj.gov/content/pub/pdf/hivp08.pdf

Mays, V. M. (1993). Women and HIV: Policy and AIDS exceptionalism. Paper presented at the 121st annual meeting of the American Public Health Association, San Francisco, CA.

Mays, V. M., & Cochran, S. D. (1987). Acquired immunodeficiency syndrome and Black Americans: Special psychosocial issues. *Public Health Reports, 102*(2), 224–231.

Mays, V. M., & Cochran, S. D. (1988). Issues in the perception of AIDS risk and risk reduction by Black and Hispanic/Latina women. *American Psychologist, 43*(11), 949–957.

Mays, V. M., & Cochran, S. D. (1993). Issues in the perception of AIDS risk and risk reduction by Black and Hispanic/Latina women. In M. Berer (Ed.), *Women and HIV/AIDS: An international resource book* (pp. 215–244). London, England: Pandora Press.

Mays, V. M., Cochran, S. D., & Bellinger, G. (1989). Factors influencing AIDS risk perception of Black gay men. *Proceedings of the Fifth International Conference on AIDS* (p. 802; abstract no. D.644). Montreal, Canada.

Mays, V. M., Cochran, S. D., & Roberts, V. (1988). Heterosexuals and AIDS. In A. Lewis (Ed.), *Nursing care of the patient with AIDS/ARC* (pp. 31–37). Rockville, MD: Aspen Publications.

Mays, V. M., Cochran, S. D., & Zamudio, A. (2004). HIV prevention research: Are we meeting the needs of African American men who have sex with men? *Journal of Black Psychology, 30*(1), 78–105.

McCoy, H. V., Correa, R., & Fritz, E. (1996). HIV diffusion patterns and mobility: Gender differences among drug users. *Population Research and Policy Review, 15*(3), 249–264.

McKinney, M. M. (2002). Variations in AIDS epidemiology and service models in the United States. *Journal of Rural Health, 18*(3), 455–466.

Millett, G., Malebranche, D., Mason, B., & Spikes, P. (2005). Focusing "low down": Bisexual Black men, HIV risk and heterosexual transmission. *Journal National Medical Association, 97*(7), S52–S59.

Mirowsky, J., & Ross, C. (2003). *Education, social status, and health*. New York, NY: Walter de Gruyter.

Mokdad, A., & Remington, P. L. (2010) Measuring health behaviors in populations. *Preventing Chronic Disease, 7*(4), A75. Retrieved from http://www.cdc.gov/pcd/issues/2010/jul/10_0010.htm

Morris, J. E., & Monroe, C. R. (2009). Why study the U.S. South? The nexus of race and place in investigating Black student achievement. *Educational Researcher, 38*(1), 21–36.

Myers, L. J. (1988). *Understanding an Afrocentric worldview: Introduction to an optimal psychology*. Dubuque, IA: Kendall/Hunt.

Napravnik, S., Eron, J. J., McKaig, R., Heine, A., Menezes, P., & Quinlivan, E. (2006). Factors associated with fewer visits for HIV primary care at a tertiary care center in the southeastern U.S. *AIDS Care, 18*(Suppl. 1), S45–S50.

Nelson, S. J., Manhart, L. E., Gorbach, P. M., Martin, D. H., Stoner, B. P., Aral, S. O., & Holmes, K. K. (2007). Measuring sex partner concurrency: It's what's missing that counts. *Sexually Transmitted Diseases, 34*(10), 801–807.

Newman, L. M., & Berman, S. M. (2008). Epidemiology of STD disparities in African American communities. *Sexually Transmitted Diseases, 35*(12 Suppl.), S4–S12.

Nobles, W. (1980). African philosophy: Foundations for Black psychology. In R. Jones (Ed.), *Black psychology* (2nd ed., pp. 23–26). New York, NY: Harper & Row.

Norris, A. E., & Ford, K. (1999). Sexual experiences and condom use of heterosexual, low-income African-American and Hispanic youth practicing relative monogamy, serial monogamy and monogamy. *Sexually Transmitted Diseases, 26*(1),17–25.

Office of National AIDS Policy (ONAP). (2010). *National HIV/AIDS Strategy for the United States*. Washington, DC: White House Office of National AIDS Policy. Retrieved from http://www.whitehouse.gov/sites/default/files/uploads/NHAS.pdf

Office of Women's Health (OWH). (2010). *Recommendations for the White House: National HIV/AIDS strategy implementation.* Unpublished document available from the U.S. Department of Health and Human Services, Office of Women's Health, Washington, DC.

Parrish, R. G. (2010) Measuring population health outcomes. *Preventing Chronic Disease, 7*(4), A71. Retrieved from http://www.cdc.gov/pcd/issues/2010/jul/10_0005.htm

Peterman, T., Lindsey, C., & Selik, R. (2005). This place is killing me: A comparison of counties where the incidence rates of AIDS increased the most and the least. *Journal of Infectious Diseases, 191*(Suppl. 1), S123–S126.

Peterson, J. L., Catania, J. A., Dolcini, M. M., & Faigeles, B. (1993). Multiple sexual partners among Blacks in high-risk cities. *Family Planning Perspective, 25*(6), 263–267.

Phillips, D. M., & Forti, E. (2004). *HIV/AIDS in rural America disproportionate impact on minority and multicultural populations.* Washington, DC: National Rural Health Association. Retrieved from http://www.ruralhealthweb.org/go/left/programs-and-events/programs-and-events-overview/rural-hiv/aids-resource-center/rural-hiv/aids-resource-center

Pitt, R. N. (2010). Still looking for my Jonathan: Gay Black men's management of religious and sexual identity conflicts. *Journal of Homosexuality, 57*(1), 39–53.

Positive Womens Network. (2010). *A gender monitoring tool for the U.S. national HIV/AIDS strategy.* Retrieved from http://www.pwn-usa.org/wp-content/uploads/2011/02/Gender-Monitoring-Tool-June-2010.pdf

Pouget, E. R., Kershaw, T. S., Niccolai, L. M., Ickovics, J. R., & Blankenship, K. M. (2010). Associations of sex ratios and male incarceration rates with multiple opposite-sex partners: Potential social determinants of HIV/STI transmission. *Public Health Reports, 125*(Suppl. 4), 70–80.

Probst, J. C., Samuels, M., Jepersen, K. P., Willert, K., Swann, R. S., & McDuffie, J. A. (2002). *Minorities in rural America: An overview of population characteristics.* Columbia, SC: South Carolina Rural Health Research Center.

Pulerwitz, J., Barker, G., Segundo, M., & Nascimento, M. (2006). Promoting more gender-equitable norms and behaviors among young men as an HIV/AIDS prevention strategy. Horizons Final Report. Washington DC: Population Council.

Pulerwitz, J., Michaelis, A., & Weiss, E. (with the International Center for Research on Women). (2010). *Promoting gender equity to fight HIV.* New York, NY: The Population Council.

Qian, H., Taylor, R. D., Fawal, H. J., & Vermund, S. H. (2006). Increasing AIDS case reports in the South: U.S. trends from 1981–2004. *AIDS Care, 18*(Suppl. 1), S6–S9.

Quinn, M. S. (2000). Slavery & insurance examining slave insurance in a world 150 years removed, *Insurance Journal.* Retrieved from http://www.insurancejournal.com/magazines/southcentral/legalbeat/2000/05/15/21120.htm

Reif, S., Geonnotti, K. L., & Whetten, K. (2006). HIV infection and AIDS in the Deep South. *American Journal of Public Health, 96*(6), 970–973.

Reif, S., Whetten, K., Ostermann, J., & Raper, J. L. (2006). Characteristics of HIV-infected adults in the Deep South and their utilization of mental health services: A rural vs. urban comparison. *AIDS Care, 18*(Suppl. 1), S10–S17.

Reynolds, J., & Ross, C. (1998) Social stratification and health: Education's benefits beyond economic status and social origins. *Social Problems, 45*(2), 221–248.

Rhodes, T. (2002). The "risk environment": A framework for understanding and reducing drug-related harm. *International Journal of Drug Policy, 13*, 85–94.

Rhodes, T., Stimson, G. V., & Ball, A. (2001). From risk behaviour to risk environment: Assessing the social determinants of HIV associated with drug injecting. In *Global Networks on HIV prevention in drug-using populations.* Rockville, MD: National Institute of Drug Abuse.

Rose, T. (1998). Race, class and the pleasure/danger dialectic: Rewriting black female teenage sexuality in the popular imagination. In Elizabeth Long (Ed.), *Sociology of culture* (pp. 185–202). Malden, MA: Blackwell Press.

Rose, T. (2004). *Longing to tell: Black women talk about sexuality and intimacy.* New York, NY: MacMillan Press.

Ross, C. E., & Mirowsky, J. (1998). Refining the association between education and health: The effects of quantity, credential, and selectivity. *Demography, 36*(4), 445–460.

Ross. C. E,, & Wu, C. (1995). The links between education and health [Review]. *American Journal of Sociology, 60*(5), 719–745.

Ross, C. E., & Wu, C. (1996). Education, age, and the cumulative advantage in health. *Journal of Sociological Behavior, 37*(1), 104–120.

Rural Center of HIV/AIDS Prevention. (2002). *AIDS and sexually transmitted diseases in the rural South* (Fact Sheet No. 14). Retrieved from http://www.indiana.edu/~aids/factsheets/042228_fact%20sheet.pdf

Sabol, W. J., Couture, H., & Harrison, P. M. (2007). *Prisoners in 2006* (NCJ Publication No. 219416). Bureau of Justice Statistics Report. Retrieved from http://74.53.234.131/attachments/ex-offender-corrections-industry-reference-publications/620d1227735238-prisoners-united-states-2006-bureau-justice-statistics-report-prisoners.2006.pdf

Sabol, W. J., Minton, T. D., & Harrison, P. M. (2007). *Prison and jail inmates at midyear 2006* (NCJ Publication No. 217675). *Prison and Jail Inmates at Midyear Series.* Retrieved from http://bjs.ojp.usdoj.gov/content/pub/pdf/pjim06.pdf

Satcher, D. (2010). Include a social determinants of health approach to reduce health inequities. *Public Health Reports, 125*(4), 6–7.

Shapiro, T. M., & Oliver, M. L. (2006). *Black wealth, White wealth: A new perspective on racial inequality.* New York, NY: Routledge.

Smith, M. K. (2002) Gender, poverty, and intergenerational vulnerability to HIV/AIDS. *Gender and Development, 10*(3), 63–70.

Southern AIDS Coalition. (2008). *Southern states manifesto: Update 2008 HIV/AIDS and sexually transmitted diseases in the South.* Birmingham, AL: Southern AIDS Coalition.

Southern Education Foundation. (2007). *The new majority: Low income students in the South's public schools.* Retrieved from http://www.southerneducation.org/pdf/A%20New%20Majority%20Report-Final.pdf

State AIDS/STD Directors Work Group. (2003). HIV/AIDS and STDs in the South: A call to action. *Southern States Manifesto, 1.* Retrieved from http://www.southernaidscoalition.org/policy/SouthernStatesManifesto_2003.pdf

Sutton, M. Y., Jones, R. L., Woltski, R. J., Cleveland, J. C., Dean, H. D., & Fenton, K. A. (2009). A review of the Center for Disease Control and Prevention's response to the HIV/AIDS crisis among Blacks in the United States, 1981–2009. *American Journal of Public Health, 99*(Suppl. 2), S351–S359.

Thomas, J. C. (2006). From slavery to incarceration: Social forces affecting the epidemiology of sexually transmitted diseases in the rural South. *Sexually Transmitted Diseases, 33*(7), S6–S10.

Thomas, J. C., Clark, M., Robinson, J., Monnett, M., Kilmarx, P., & Peterman, T. (1999). The social ecology of syphilis. *Social Science & Medicine, 48*(8), 1081–1094.

Thomas, J. C., Kulik, A. L., & Schoenbach, V. J. (1995). Syphilis in the South: Rural rates surpass urban rates in North Carolina. *American Journal of Public Health, 85*(8, Pt. 1), 1119–1122.

Thomas, J. C., & Sampson, L. C. (2005). High rates of incarceration as a social force associated with community rates of sexually transmitted infection. *Journal of Infectious Diseases, 191*(Suppl. 1), S55–S60.

Thomas, J., & Thomas, K. (1999). Things ain't what they ought to be: Social forces underlying racial disparities in rates of sexually transmitted diseases in a rural North Carolina county. *Social Science & Medicine, 49*(8), 1075–1084.

U.S. Bureau of Justice Statistics. (2011). *Correctional populations trend charts.* Retrieved from http://bjs.ojp.usdoj.gov/content/glance/tables/corr2tab.cfm

U.S. Census Bureau. (2003). *Migration by race and hispanic origin: 1995 to 2000.* Retrieved from http://www.census.gov/prod/2003pubs/censr-13.pdf

U.S. Census Bureau. (2009). *2009 American community survey.* Retrieved from http://factfinder.census.gov/servlet/DatasetMainPageServlet?_program=ACS&_submenuId=&_lang=en&_ds_name=ACS_2009_1YR_G00_&ts=

U.S. Census Bureau. (n.d.). *Access data: Data tables: Data profiles, 2003* [U.S. Census Bureau home page]. Retrieved from http://www.census.gov/acs/www/Products/Profiles/Single/2003/ACS/

Whetten, K., & Reif, S. (2006). Overview: HIV/AIDS in the Deep South region of the United States. *AIDS Care, 18*(Suppl. 1), S1–S5.

Whetten, K., Reif, S., Whetten, R. A., & Murphy-Miller, L. K. (2008). Trauma, mental health, distrust, and stigma among HIV-positive persons: Implications for effective care. *Psychosomatic Medicine, 70,* 531–538.

Williams, M. L., Bowen, A. M., & Horvath, K. J. (2005). The social/sexual environment of gay men residing in a rural frontier state: implications for the development of HIV prevention programs. *Journal of Rural Health, 21*(1), 48–55.

Wilson, P. A., & Moore, T. E. (2009). Public health responses to the HIV epidemic among Black men who have sex with men: A qualitative study of US health departments and communities. *American Journal of Public Health, 99*(6), 1013–1022.

Wimberley, R., & Morris, L. (1996). *The reference book on regional well-being: U.S. regions, the Black Belt, and Appalachia.* Washington, DC: Southern Rural Development Center.

World Health Organization (WHO). (2001). *Urban and peri-urban food and nutrition action plan: Elements for community action to promote social cohesion and reduce inequalities through local production for local consumption.* Retrieved from http://www.euro.who.int/__data/assets/pdf_file/0016/101626/E72949.pdf

Wyn, R., & Peckman, E. (2010). *Nearly 2.5 million nonelderly California women uninsured at some time during 2007.* Los Angeles, CA: UCLA Center for Health Policy Research.

Author Index

Subject Index